ETHNICITY AND FAMILY THERAPY

Ethnicity & Family Therapy

THIRD EDITION

edited by
Monica McGoldrick
Joe Giordano
Nydia Garcia-Preto

THE GUILFORD PRESS
New York   London

© 2005 Monica McGoldrick, Joe Giordano, and Nydia Garcia-Preto
Published by The Guilford Press
A Division of Guilford Publications, Inc.
72 Spring Street, New York, NY 10012
www.guilford.com

Printed in the United States of America

This book is printed on acid-free paper.

Last digit is print number: 9 8 7 6 5 4 3

Library of Congress Cataloging-in-Publication Data

Ethnicity and family therapy / edited by Monica McGoldrick, Joe Giordano, Nydia Garcia-Preto.—3rd ed.
    p. cm.
  Includes bibliographical references and index.
  ISBN 1-59385-020-4 (hardcover)
  1. Minorities—Mental health services—United States. 2. Family psychotherapy—United States. 3. Minorities—United States—Family relationships. I. McGoldrick, Monica.
II. Giordano, Joseph. III. Garcia-Preto, Nydia.
  RC451.5.A2E83 2005
  362.2′089′00973—dc22

                                  2004029338

To the memory of Evelyn Lee, EdD, LCSW (1944–2003)

Friend, colleague, author, trainer,
community worker, researcher

An inspiration to so many of us
in doing work to build cultural bridges

About the Editors

Monica McGoldrick, LCSW, PhD (h.c.), Director of the Multicultural Family Institute in Highland Park, New Jersey, is also Associate Professor of Clinical Psychiatry at the University of Medicine and Dentistry of New Jersey–Robert Wood Johnson Medical School. She served as Visiting Professor at Fordham University School of Social Service for 12 years. Ms. McGoldrick received her MSW in 1969 from Smith College School for Social Work, which later granted her one of the few honorary doctorates awarded by the school in its 60-year history. She has also received many other awards, including the American Family Therapy Academy's award for Distinguished Contribution to Family Therapy Theory and Practice. Known internationally for her many books, she has spoken widely on a variety of topics, including culture, class, gender, the family life cycle, loss, genograms, remarried families, and sibling relationships.

Joe Giordano, MSW, is a family therapist in private practice in Bronxville, New York. He was formerly Director of the American Jewish Committee's Center on Ethnicity, Behavior, and Communications, where he conducted pioneering studies on the psychological nature of ethnic identity and group behavior. Widely published, his articles on ethnicity, family, and the media have appeared in national magazines and newspapers. Mr. Giordano also served as host of *Proud to Be Me*, a PBS television program for adolescents on race and ethnic identity, and as producer of the audio series *Growing Up in America*.

Nydia Garcia-Preto, LCSW, is cofounder and Clinical Director of the Multicultural Family Institute, where she serves on the faculty and has a private practice. She has served as Visiting Professor at the Rutgers Graduate School of Social Work and as Director of the Adolescent Day Hospital at the University of Medicine and Dentistry of New Jersey. A noted family therapist, author, teacher, and lecturer, Ms. Garcia-Preto has published in textbooks and journals and has presented nationally on Puerto Rican and Latino families, Latinas, ethnic intermarriage, and families with adolescents. She is a highly respected trainer in the areas of cultural competence and organizational team building.

Contributors

Nuha Abudabbeh, PhD, NAIM Foundation, Washington, DC

Anna M. Agathangelou, PhD, Department of Political Science, York University, Toronto, Ontario, Canada

Rhea Almeida, PhD, LCSW, Institute for Family Services, Somerset, New Jersey; Multicultural Family Institute, Highland Park, New Jersey

Zarita Araújo-Lane, MSW, LCSW, Cross Cultural Communication Systems, Inc., Winchester, Massachusetts

Guillermo Bernal, PhD, University Center for Psychological Services and Research and Department of Psychology, University of Puerto Rico, Rio Piedras, Puerto Rico

Lascelles Black, MSW, private practice, New Rochelle, New York, and New York, New York

James K. Boehnlein, MD, Department of Psychiatry, Oregon Health and Science University, Portland, Oregon

Nancy Boyd-Franklin, PhD, Graduate School of Psychology, Rutgers, The State University of New Jersey, Piscataway, New Jersey

Janet R. Brice-Baker, PhD, Department of Psychology, Yeshiva University, Bronx, New York

Mary Anne Broken Nose, BA, COPSA Institute for Alzheimer's Disease and Related Disorders, University of Medicine and Dentistry of New Jersey–University Behavioral HealthCare, Piscataway, New Jersey

Steve Dagirmanjian, PhD, Catskill Family Institute, Kingston, New York

Sean D. Davis, PhD, Marriage and Family Therapy Program, Department of Family Studies, University of Kentucky, Lexington, Kentucky

Conrad De Master, LCSW, private practice, Waldwick, New Jersey

Ann Del Vecchio, PhD, Alpha Assessment Associates, Albuquerque, New Mexico

Jenny Duncan-Rojano, MS, LCSW, School-Based Centers, Hartford Public Schools, Hartford, Connecticut

Beth M. Erickson, PhD, Erickson Consulting, Edina, Minnesota, and Ramsey, Minnesota

Celia Jaes Falicov, PhD, Department of Psychiatry, University of California, San Diego, San Diego, California

John Folwarski, LCSW, Raritan Bay Mental Health Center, Perth Amboy, New Jersey

Nydia Garcia-Preto, LCSW, Multicultural Family Institute, Highland Park, New Jersey

Rita Mae Gazarik, LCSW, private practice, New York, New York; Columbia University School of Social Work, New York, New York; Hunter College School of Social Work, City University of New York, New York, New York

Joe Giordano, MSW, private practice, Bronxville, New York

MaryAnn Dros Giordano, MSW, private practice, Bronxville, New York

Karen L. Haboush, PsyD, Graduate School of Applied and Professional Psychology, Rutgers, The State University of New Jersey, Piscataway, New Jersey; private practice, Highland Park, New Jersey

Miguel Hernandez, LCSW, Roberto Clemente Center, Sylvia Del Villard Program, Gouverneur Healthcare Service, New York, New York; Ackerman Institute for the Family, New York, New York

Paulette Moore Hines, PhD, Center for Healthy Schools, Families, and Communities and Office of Prevention Services and Research, University of Medicine and Dentistry of New Jersey–University Behavioral HealthCare, Piscataway, New Jersey; Multicultural Family Institute, Highland Park, New Jersey

Vanessa Jackson, LCSW, private practice, Atlanta, Georgia

Behnaz Jalali, MD, Department of Psychiary, University of California, Los Angeles, Los Angeles, California

Hugo Kamya, PhD, Graduate School of Social Work, Boston College, Boston, Massachusetts

Valli Kalei Kanuha, PhD, School of Social Work, University of Hawaii, Honolulu, Hawaii

Kyle D. Killian, PhD, Department of Family Therapy and Psychology, University of Houston–Clear Lake, Houston, Texas

Bok-Lim C. Kim, MSW, private practice, San Diego, California

Joanne Guarino Klages, LCSW, Multicultural Family Institute, Highland Park, New Jersey; private practice, Highland Park, New Jersey, and Staten Island, New York

Eliana Catão de Korin, DiplPsic, Department of Family and Social Medicine, Montefiore Medical Center, Albert Einstein College of Medicine, Bronx, New York

Jo-Ann Krestan, MA, private practice, Center for Creative Change, Ellsworth, Maine

Daniel Kusnir, MD, New College of California School of Graduate Psychology, San Francisco, California; La Familia Counseling Service, Hayward, California; Survivors International, San Francisco, California

Pamela Langelier, PhD, Department of Family Medicine, College of Medicine, University of New England, Biddeford, Maine; private practice, Saco, Maine

Régis Langelier, PhD, private practice, Saco, Maine

Tracey A. Laszloffy, PhD, Marriage and Family Therapy Program, Seton Hill University, Greenberg, Pennsylvania

Evelyn Lee, EdD (deceased), Richmond Area Multi Services, Inc., San Francisco, California

Paul K. Leung, MD, Department of Psychiatry, Oregon Health and Science University, Portland, Oregon

Catherine D. M. Limansubroto, MS, private practice, Tangerang, Indonesia

Vanessa McAdams-Mahmoud, MSW, private practice and Director of Counseling, Spelman College, Atlanta, Georgia

David W. McGill, PsyD, Couples and Family Center, Cambridge Hospital, Cambridge, Massachusetts; Department of Psychiatry, Harvard Medical School, Cambridge, Massachusetts

Monica McGoldrick, LCSW, PhD (h.c.), Multicultural Family Institute, Highland Park, New Jersey; Department of Psychiatry, University of Medicine and Dentistry of New Jersey–Robert Wood Johnson Medical School, Piscataway, New Jersey

Lorna McKenzie-Pollock, MSW, MA, School of Social Work, Boston University, Boston, Massachusetts; private practice, Brookline, Massachusetts

Josiane Menos, PsyD, Staten Island Office of Children and Family Services, Staten Island, New York; New York City Department of Education, New York, New York; Multicultural Family Institute, Highland Park, New Jersey

Marsha Pravder Mirkin, PhD, Women's Studies Research Center, Brandeis University, Waltham, Massachusetts; Lasell College, Newton, Massachusetts

Matthew R. Mock, PhD, Family, Youth, Children's and Multicultural Services, Berkeley, California; Graduate School of Professional Psychology, John F. Kennedy University, Orinda, California; private practice, Berkeley, California

Shivani Nath, MS, Department of Professional Psychology and Family Therapy, College of Education and Human Services, Seton Hall University, South Orange, New Jersey; Asian American Federation of New York, New York

Leonid Newhouse, LCSW, private practice, Boston, Massachusetts

Barbara F. Okun, PhD, Department of Counseling and Applied Psychology, Northeastern University, Boston, Massachusetts

John K. Pearce, MD, Psychiatric Group of the North Shore, Lynn, Massachusetts; Island Counseling, Martha's Vineyard, Massachusetts

Sueli S. de Carvalho Petry, PhD, Department of Psychology and Family Therapy, College of Education and Human Services, Seton Hall University, South Orange, New Jersey; Multicultural Family Institute, Highland Park, New Jersey

Fred P. Piercy, PhD, Department of Human Development, Virginia Polytechnic Institute and State University, Blacksburg, Virginia

Vimala Pillari, DSW, LCSW, Graduate School of Social Work, Dominican University, River Forest, Illinois

Ramón Rojano, MD, City of Hartford, Hartford, Connecticut; University of Connecticut School of Community Medicine, Storrs, Connecticut; Marriage and Family Therapy Program, Central Connecticut State University, New Britain, Connecticut; Institute for the Hispanic Family, Hartford, Connecticut

Maria P. P. Root, PhD, private practice, Seattle, Washington

Elliott J. Rosen, EdD, private practice, Scarsdale, New York

Eunjung Ryu, LCSW, Department of Couples and Family Therapy, College of Nursing and Health Professions, Drexel University, Philadelphia, Pennsylvania; private practice, Highland Park, New Jersey

Ester Shapiro, PhD, Department of Psychology, University of Massachusetts, Boston, Massachusetts

Tazuko Shibusawa, PhD, Columbia University School of Social Work, New York, New York

Joseph Smolinski, Jr., MSW, Psychotherapy and Spirituality Institute, New York, New York

Adriana Soekandar, MS, Mandiri School and private practice, Jakarta, Indonesia

CharlesEtta T. Sutton, MSW, LCSW, Multicultural Family Institute, Highland Park, New Jersey; private practice, Plainfield, New Jersey; Turtle Island Project, Phoenix, Arizona

Nadine Tafoya, MSW, private practice, Espagnola, New Mexico

Morris Taggart, PhD, retired, Houston, Texas

Carmen Inoa Vazquez, PhD, private practice and Department of Psychiatry, New York University School of Medicine, New York, New York

Susan F. Weltman, LCSW, private practice, Metuchen, New Jersey

Norbert A. Wetzel, ThD, Center for Family, Community, and Social Justice, Princeton, New Jersey

Hinda Winawer, MSW, LCSW, LMFT, Center for Family, Community, and Social Justice, Princeton, New Jersey; Ackerman Institute for the Family, New York, New York

Anat Ziv, MSc, private practice, Ra'anana, Israel

Acknowledgments

Many people have supported us in our efforts to produce this third edition of *Ethnicity and Family Therapy*, particularly Senior Editor Jim Nageotte and the staff at The Guilford Press. Fran Snyder and Irene Umbel, at the Multicultural Family Institute, provided assistance both direct and indirect to make this book come to fruition.

I (M. M.) thank my husband, Sophocles Orfanidis, for the ongoing emotional and physical support he has given me over more than 35 years, which have made my endeavors, including this major life effort, possible. And I thank my Greek-Irish son, John, for growing into such a wonderful man.

I (J. G.) want to thank my wife, MaryAnn, who generously has given her love, support, and clinical insights in all my professional and creative endeavors. I also want to thank Irving Levine, my dearest friend and colleague for the past 35 years, for his continued counsel, and David Szonyi, whose help in editing this book was invaluable. And finally, I am grateful to the Maurice Falk Medical Fund and the American Jewish Committee, whose financial and organizational support contributed to the success of this book.

I (N. G.-P.) want to thank my children, Sara and David, for challenging my ideas about culture, gender, and class, and my parents, who taught me to love and to be proud of my Puerto Rican roots. I would also like to thank all the Latin American families who have given me the opportunity to learn about the struggles and strengths of Latino immigrants in this country.

We are also deeply indebted to Mary Anne Broken Nose, who has for many years been our major research consultant on materials for our work. We don't know how this edition would have come to fruition without her. Her positive energy, intelligence, and skill in finding relevant materials were indispensable.

David McGill, a wonderful friend, came through as he always has, offering counsel and specific suggestions regarding the book. His behind-the-scenes support was a major factor in making this third edition possible.

And we thank the authors for all their efforts in providing so much creativity and wisdom in their cultural descriptions. Some of them had to put up with our calls and critiques over and over again and we thank them for persevering. We owe a special debt to those authors who helped out in a pinch by delivering a chapter in the nick of time when we were at our wits' end about filling in the gap for missing material. We also thank the network of therapists and trainers who have participated in the Multicultural Family Institute's Annual Culture Conferences over the years, for the underlying support they have given that is the subtext of all our work. They have given us roots and wings and we would not be publishing this without their loyalty and ongoing challenges to our thinking.

We are very proud of the work of so many colleagues and hope the readers will appreciate the efforts made by so many people to speak clearly and practically on a subject that is so very complex.

Contents

1. Overview: Ethnicity and Family Therapy   1
   Monica McGoldrick, Joe Giordano, and Nydia Garcia-Preto

I.
AMERICAN INDIAN AND PACIFIC ISLANDER FAMILIES

2. American Indian Families: An Overview   43
   CharlesEtta T. Sutton and Mary Anne Broken Nose

3. Back to the Future: An Examination of the Native American   55
   Holocaust Experience
   Nadine Tafoya and Ann Del Vecchio

4. *Nā 'Ohana*: Native Hawaiian Families   64
   Valli Kalei Kanuha

II.
FAMILIES OF AFRICAN ORIGIN

5. Families of African Origin: An Overview   77
   Lascelles Black and Vanessa Jackson

6. African American Families   87
   Paulette Moore Hines and Nancy Boyd-Franklin

7. African Immigrant Families   101
   Hugo Kamya

8. British West Indian Families   117
   Janet R. Brice-Baker

  9. Haitian Families   127
     Josiane Menos

 10. African American Muslim Families   138
     Vanessa McAdams-Mahmoud

III.
LATINO FAMILIES

 11. Latino Families: An Overview   153
     Nydia Garcia-Preto

 12. Brazilian Families   166
     Eliana Catão de Korin and Sueli S. de Carvalho Petry

 13. Central American Families   178
     Miguel Hernandez

 14. Colombian Families   192
     Ramón Rojano and Jenny Duncan-Rojano

 15. Cuban Families   202
     Guillermo Bernal and Ester Shapiro

 16. Dominican Families   216
     Carmen Inoa Vazquez

 17. Mexican Families   229
     Celia Jaes Falicov

 18. Puerto Rican Families   242
     Nydia Garcia-Preto

 19. Salvadoran Families   256
     Daniel Kusnir

IV.
ASIAN FAMILIES

 20. Asian Families: An Overview   269
     Evelyn Lee and Matthew R. Mock

 21. Cambodian Families   290
     Lorna McKenzie-Pollock

22. Chinese Families   302
    Evelyn Lee and Matthew R. Mock

23. Filipino Families   319
    Maria P. P. Root

24. Indonesian Families   332
    Fred P. Piercy, Adriana Soekandar, Catherine D. M. Limansubroto,
    and Sean D. Davis

25. Japanese Families   339
    Tazuko Shibusawa

26. Korean Families   349
    Bok-Lim C. Kim and Eunjung Ryu

27. Vietnamese Families   363
    Paul K. Leung and James K. Boehnlein

V.
ASIAN INDIAN AND PAKISTANI FAMILIES

28. Asian Indian Families: An Overview   377
    Rhea Almeida

29. Indian Hindu Families   395
    Vimala Pillari

30. Pakistani Families   407
    Shivani Nath

VI.
MIDDLE EASTERN FAMILIES

31. Arab Families: An Overview   423
    Nuha Abudabbeh

32. Armenian Families   437
    Steve Dagirmanjian

33. Iranian Families   451
    Behnaz Jalali

34. Lebanese and Syrian Families   468
    Karen L. Haboush

35. Palestinian Families   487
    Nuha Abudabbeh

VII.
FAMILIES OF EUROPEAN ORIGIN

36. Families of European Origin: An Overview   501
    Joe Giordano and Monica McGoldrick

37. American Families with English Ancestors from the Colonial Era: 520
    Anglo Americans
    David W. McGill and John K. Pearce

38. Dutch Families   534
    Conrad De Master and MaryAnn Dros Giordano

39. French Canadian Families   545
    Régis Langelier and Pamela Langelier

40. German Families   555
    Hinda Winawer and Norbert A. Wetzel

41. Greek Families   573
    Kyle D. Killian and Anna M. Agathangelou

42. Hungarian Families   586
    Tracey A. Laszloffy

43. Irish Families   595
    Monica McGoldrick

44. Italian Families   616
    Joe Giordano, Monica McGoldrick, and Joanne Guarino Klages

45. Portuguese Families   629
    Zarita Araújo-Lane

46. Scandinavian Families: Plain and Simple   641
    Beth M. Erickson

47. Scots-Irish Families   654
    Morris Taggart

VIII.
JEWISH FAMILIES

48. Jewish Families: An Overview   667
Elliott J. Rosen and Susan F. Weltman

49. Israeli Families   680
Anat Ziv

50. Orthodox Jewish Families   689
Marsha Pravder Mirkin and Barbara F. Okun

51. Russian Jewish Families   701
Leonid Newhouse

IX.
SLAVIC FAMILIES

52. Slavic Families: An Overview   711
Leonid Newhouse

53. Czech and Slovak Families   724
Jo-Ann Krestan and Rita Mae Gazarik

54. Polish Families   741
John Folwarski and Joseph Smolinski Jr.

APPENDIX. CULTURAL ASSESSMENT   757

AUTHOR INDEX   765

SUBJECT INDEX   776

CHAPTER I

Overview
Ethnicity and Family Therapy

Monica McGoldrick
Joe Giordano
Nydia Garcia-Preto

The future of our earth may depend on the ability of all [of us] to identify and develop
new . . . patterns of relating across difference.
—LORDE (1992, p. 502)

What would it be like to have not only color vision but culture vision, the ability to see
the multiple worlds of others?
—BATESON (1995, p. 53)

Cultural identity has a profound impact on our sense of well-being within our society
and on our mental and physical health. Our cultural background refers to our ethnicity,
but it is also profoundly influenced by social class, religion, migration, geography, gender
oppression, racism, and sexual orientation, as well as by family dynamics. All these factors influence people's social location in our society—their access to resources, their
inclusion in dominant definitions of "belonging," and the extent to which they will be
privileged or oppressed within the larger society. These factors also influence how family
members relate to their cultural heritage, to others of their cultural group, and to preserving cultural traditions. Furthermore, we live in a society in which our high rates of cultural intermarriage mean that citizens of the United States increasingly reflect multiple
cultural backgrounds. Nevertheless, because of our society's political, economic, and
racial dynamics, our country is still highly segregated; we tend to live in communities segregated communities by race, culture, and class, which also have a profound influence on
our sense of ethnic identity.

It is now more than two decades since the first edition of *Ethnicity and Family Therapy* was published; in these decades our awareness of cultural diversity in our society and

I

world has changed profoundly. We have witnessed amazing attempts at transforming ethnic group relationships in South Africa, Northern Ireland, the Middle East, and the former Soviet Union, as well as tragic ethnic devastation in the Sudan, Rwanda, Kosovo, Russia, the Middle East, and Latin America. Meanwhile, the United States is being transformed by rapidly changing demographics and has played a most ethnocentric role in going to war in Iraq. This is a role it has unfortunately played in many other regions at other times, most especially in Central and South America, in some of the Caribbean island nations, the Phillipines, and Vietnam (see Chapters 11–19, 23, and 27).

THE MEANING OF ETHNICITY

Why have we as a people been able to continue to exist? Because we know where we come from. By having roots, you can see the direction in which you want to go.
—JOENIA BATISTE DE CARVAHLO, first Indian woman lawyer in Brazil,
 who is fighting for the rights of her people.
 (*New York Times*, November 13, 2004, p. 7)

Having a sense of belonging, of historical continuity, and of identity with one's own people is a basic psychological need. Ethnicity, the concept of a group's "peoplehood," refers to a group's commonality of ancestry and history, through which people have evolved shared values and customs over the centuries. Based on a combination of race, religion, and cultural history, ethnicity is retained, whether or not members realize their commonalities with one another. Its values are transmitted over generations by the family and reinforced by the surrounding community. It is a powerful influence in determining identity. It patterns our thinking, feeling, and behavior in both obvious and subtle ways, although generally we are not aware of it. It plays a major role in determining how we eat, work, celebrate, make love, and die.

The subject of ethnicity tends to evoke deep feelings, and discussion frequently becomes polarized or judgmental. As Greeley (1969) has described it, using presumed common origin to define "we" and "they" seems to touch on something basic and primordial in the human psyche. Irving Levine (personal communication, February 15, 1981) observed: "Ethnicity can be equated along with sex and death as a subject that touches off deep unconscious feelings in most people." When there has been discussion of ethnicity, it has tended to focus on nondominant groups' "otherness," emphasizing their deficits, rather than their adaptive strengths or their place in the larger society, and how so-called "minorities" differ from the "dominant" societal definitions of "normality."

Our approach is to emphasize instead that ethnicity pertains to everyone, and influences everyone's values, not only those who are at the margins of this society. From this perspective cultural understanding requires examining everyone's ethnic assumptions. No one stands outside the category of ethnicity, because everyone has a cultural background that influences his or her values and behavior.

Those born White, who conform to the dominant societal norms, probably grew up believing that "ethnicity" referred to others who were different from them. Whites were the definition of "regular." As Tataki (1993, 2002) has pointed out, we have always tended to view Americans as European in ancestry. We will not be culturally competent until we let go of that myth. Many in our country are left with a sense of cultural homelessness because their heritage is not acknowledged within our society.

Our very definitions of human development are ethnoculturally based. Eastern cultures tend to define the person as a social being and categorize development by growth in the human capacity for empathy and connection. Many Western cultures, in contrast, begin by positing the individual as a psychological being and define development as growth in the capacity for autonomous functioning. Even the definitions "Eastern" and "Western," as well as our world maps (Kaiser, 2001), reflect an ethnocentric view of the universe with Britain and the United States as the center.

African Americans (see Chapter 6; Boyd-Franklin, 2003; Carter, 1995; Franklin, 2004) have a very different foundation for their sense of identity, expressed as a communal sense of "We are, therefore I am," contrasting starkly with the individualistic European ideal: "I think, therefore I am." In the United States, the dominant cultural assumptions have generally been derived from a few European cultures, primarily German (Chapter 40), Dutch (Chapter 38), and, above all, British (Chapter 37), which are taken to be the universal standard. The values of these few European groups have tended to be viewed as "normal," and values derived from other cultures have tended to be viewed as "ethnic." These other values have tended to be marginalized, even though they reflect the traditional values of the majority of the population.

Although human behavior results from intrapsychic, interpersonal, familial, socio-economic, and cultural forces, the mental health field has paid greatest attention to the first of these—the personality factors that shape life experiences and behavior. DSM-IV, although for the first time considering culture in assessing and treating patients, allows one to conduct the entire course of diagnosis and therapy with no thought of the patient's culture at all. Much of the authors' work on culture was omitted from the published manual, and the "culture-bound" syndromes they did mention tended to "exoticize the role of culture" (Lopez & Guarnaccia, 2000). Indeed, the authors decided to exclude disorders seen as primarily North American disorders (anorexia nervosa and chronic fatigue syndrome) from the glossary of culture-bound syndromes because they wanted to restrict the term to problems of "ethnic minorities" (Lopez & Guarnaccia, 2000)!

As things stand now, most mental health record-keeping systems do not even record patients' ethnic backgrounds, settling for minimal reference to race as the only background marker. No other reference is generally made to immigration or heritage. In the broader mental health field, there was a great increase in attention paid to ethnicity in the 1980s. However, since then there has been a distinct retreat from attention to culture as managed care, pharmaceutical, and insurance companies took control of most mental health services and intentionally minimized attention to family, context, and even service for those who cannot afford to pay. Since the early 1990s, the mental health professions in general pay only lip service to the importance of cultural competence. The study of cultural influences on human emotional functioning has been left primarily to the cultural anthropologists. Yet they have preferred to explore remote cultural enclaves, rather than examining culture within our own diverse society.

Even mental health professionals who have considered culture have often been more interested in examining international, cross-cultural comparisons than in studying the ethnic groups within our own society. Our therapeutic models are generally presented as having universal applicability. Only recently have we begun to consider the underlying cultural assumptions of our therapeutic models and of ourselves as therapists. And even now, reference to "cultural competence" varies from complete acceptance to outright derision (Betancourt, 2004).

We must incorporate cultural acknowledgment into our theories and into our therapies, so that clients not of the dominant culture will not have to feel lost, displaced, or mystified. Working toward multicultural frameworks in our theories, research, and clinical practice requires that we challenge our society's dominant universalist assumptions, as we must challenge our other societal institutions as well in order for democracy to survive (Dilworth-Anderson, Burton, & Johnson, 1993; Hitchcock, 2003; Pinderhughes, 1989).

It is unfortunate that society's rules have made it difficult for us to focus our vision on ourselves in this way, but it is essential if we are to become culturally effective clinicians. As Bernard Lewis (2002) has put it:

> When things go wrong in our society, our response is usually to place the blame on external or domestic scapegoats—foreigners abroad or minorities at home. We might ask a different question: What did we do wrong? (pp. 22–23)

This question, which leads us to look in every situation to see what we contribute to misunderstandings, is essential to expanding our cultural awareness. We must understand where we have been and the cultural assumptions and blinders our own history has given us before we can begin to understand those who are culturally different from us.

This book presents a kind of "road map" for understanding families in relation to their ethnic heritage. The paradigms here are not presented as "truth," but rather as maps to some aspects of the terrain, intended as a guide for the explorer seeking a path. They draw on historical traits, residues of which linger in the psyche of families many generations after immigration, long after its members have become outwardly "Americanized" and cease to identify with their ethnic backgrounds. Although families are changing very rapidly in today's world, our focus here is on the continuities, the ways in which families retain the cultural characteristics of their heritage, often without even noticing these patterns. Of course, the clinical suggestions offered by the authors of this book will not be relevant in every case, but they will, it is hoped, expand the readers' ways of thinking about their own clinical assumptions and the thinking of the families with whom they work. Space limitations have made it necessary for us to emphasize characteristics that may be problematic. Thus, we do not always present families in their best light. We are well aware that this can lead to misunderstandings and feed negative stereotypes. We trust the reader to take the information in the spirit in which it is meant—not to limit our thinking, but to expand it.

There has been a growing realization since this book's first edition that a positive sense of ethnic and racial identity is essential for developing a healthy personal and group identity, and for effective clinical practice. So far, more in the field of health care than in mental health, the concept of "cultural competence" has begun to become an accepted value. In recognition of the overwhelming evidence of racial and ethnic disparities in health care, there is a beginning acknowledgment that with every illness and on virtually every measure of functioning, the cultural disparities in health care are staggering and it is time to rethink our cultural attitudes and to address these realities. A new field of "cultural competence" in health care has been emerging, a field that defines the "culturally competent health care system" as one that acknowledges the importance of culture throughout the system and is vigilant in dealing with the dynamics that result from cultural differences, the expansion of cultural knowledge, and the adaptation of services to meet culturally unique needs (Betancourt, Green, Carrillo, & Ananeh-Firempong, 2003).

This field of culturally competent health care seeks to identify sociocultural barriers to health care and to address them at every level of the system, including the cultural congruity of the interventions provided and the degree to which the leadership and workforce reflect the diversity of the general population (Betancourt et al., 2003).

Within the mental health field, recognition of the importance of culture has been much slower. Family therapy, which was rocked to its foundations by the feminist critique (Luepnitz, 1992; McGoldrick, Anderson, & Walsh, 1989; Wheeler, Avis, Miller, & Chaney, 1985), has been moving toward an awareness of the essential dimension of culture as well as gender. Unfortunately, most of the institutions in the field, such as the major training programs, the publications, and the professional organizations, still view ethnicity as an "add-on" to family therapy, a "special topic," rather than as basic to all discussion. Reactions to the upsurge in "diversity" presentations at the annual Family Therapy Academy meetings have included a frequently articulated request by members to "get back to basics." In our view there is no such thing as moving "back" to basics. Rather, we must re-envision the "basics" from more inclusive perspectives, so that the cultural underpinnings of all therapeutic endeavors will inform our work, allowing us to deal theoretically and clinically with all our clients (see the Appendix on cultural clinical assessment).

For many, the earlier editions of *Ethnicity and Family Therapy* provided an "ah ha!"—a recognition of their own cultural background or that of spouses, friends, or clients. Still, when it was first written, we were all fairly naive about the meaning of culture in our complex world. Some feared that our book reinforced cultural stereotypes, but we believed then, and believe now, that exploring cultural patterns and hypotheses is essential to all our clinical work.

We also recognize that ethnicity is not the only dimension of culture. In this book we illustrate how gender, socioeconomic status, geography, race, religion, and politics have influenced cultural groups in adapting to American life. Knowing that no single book could possibly provide clinicians with all they need to know to work with those who are culturally different, we gave the authors of the chapters the following instructions:

We have become increasingly convinced that we learn about culture primarily not by learning the "facts" of another's culture, but rather by changing our attitude. Our underlying openness to those who are culturally different is the key to expanding our cultural understanding. Thus, cultural paradigms are useful to the extent that they help us recognize patterns we may have only vaguely sensed before. They can challenge our long-held beliefs about "the way things are." Thus, we ask you to write your chapter with the following aims in mind:

1. Describe the particular characteristics and values of the group with some context of history, geography, politics, and economics as they are pertinent to understanding the patterns of the group.
2. Emphasize especially values and patterns that are relevant for therapy—those an uninformed therapist might be most likely to misunderstand (e.g, related to problems, help seeking, and what is seen as the "cure" when people are in trouble).
3. Describe patterns that relate to clinical situations, especially couple relationships; parent–child issues, sibling relationships, three-generational relationships; how families deal with loss, conflict, affection, homosexuality, and intermarriage.
4. Include relevant information on the impact of race, class and class change, religion, gender roles, sexual orientation, and migration experiences.
5. Offer guidelines for intervention to facilitate client well-being, demonstrating respect for both the historical circumstances and the current adaptive needs of families in the United States at the beginning of the 21st century.

Clinicians should never feel that, armed with a small chapter about another cultural group, they are adequately informed to do effective therapy. The chapters that follow are not intended as recipes for relating to other ethnic groups, which is far more influenced by respect, curiosity, and especially humility, than by "information." It has been said that some individuals are blessed with a certain magic that enables them to break down the natural reserve we all feel toward those of another language, another culture, another economic stratum. This is the blessing we wish to impart to our readers.

THE COMPLEXITY OF ETHNICITY

If we look carefully enough, each of us is a "hodgepodge." Developing cultural competence requires us to question the dominant values and explore the complexities of cultural identity. All of us are migrants, moving between our ancestors' traditions, the worlds we inhabit, and the world we will leave to those who come after us. The consciousness of ethnic identity varies greatly within groups and from one group to another. Many people in the United States grow up not even knowing their ethnicity or being descended from many different ethnic backgrounds. Our clinical work of healing may entail helping clients to locate themselves culturally so that they can overcome the sense of mystification, invalidation, or alienation that comes from not being able to feel culturally at home in our society. But everyone has a culture. As family therapists, we work to help clients clarify the multiple facets of their identity to increase their flexibility to adapt to America's multicultural society. We help them appreciate and value the complex web of connections within which their identities are formed and which cushion them as they move through life. Our clients' personal contexts are largely shaped by the ethnic cultures from which they have descended.

For most of us, finding out who we are means putting together a unique internal combination of cultural identities. Ethnicity is a continuous evolution. We are all always in a process of changing ethnic identity, incorporating ancestral influences while forging new and emerging group identities, in a complex interplay of members' relationships with each other and with outsiders. Every family's background is multicultural, and all marriages are, to a degree at least, cultural intermarriages. No two families share exactly the same cultural roots. Each of us belongs to many groups. We need to find a balance that allows us to validate the differences between us, while appreciating the common forces that bind us together, because the sense of belonging is vital to our identity. At the same time, the profound cultural differences between us must also be acknowledged. It is when the exclusion of others becomes primary to group identity that group identity becomes negative and dysfunctional, based on exclusion of others through moral superiority, such as White supremacy groups, or on elite social status, such as secret societies. The multiple parts of our cultural heritage often do not fit easily into the description of any one group. In addition, to define oneself as belonging to a single ethnic group, such as "Irish," "Anglo," "African American," is to greatly oversimplify matters, inasmuch as the process of cultural evolution never stands still. We are always evolving ethnically. We offer ourselves as illustrations:

Monica: My Irish ancestors had roots in Celtic tribes, who probably came from what is now Switzerland, and Viking communities in what is now Norway. My husband emigrated from Greece at age 19, his family having lived in Turkey for generations until the

1920s. Our son speaks some Greek, but no Gaelic, and has had to struggle to put together the differences between Greek patriarchy and Irish matriarchal values.

Joe: My grandparents came from Italy—grandpa from Naples and grandma from Genoa. (Some would say that was a mixed marriage!) I married a Puerto Rican-Italian woman; my second wife's mother was Scots Irish, and her father was born in Holland of a Jewish mother and a Protestant father. I also have three grandchildren whose mother is African American with roots in the Baptist South.

Nydia: My ancestors were Spanish colonizers, African slaves, Corsicans, and Taino Indians who met in Borinquen, the island known today as Puerto Rico. I came with my interracial parents and brother to Columbus, Georgia, in 1956, for my father was in the U.S. Army. I married a second-generation Italian, and my two children identify themselves mainly as Puerto Rican. My grandson's mother is African American.

Each generational cohort also has a different "culture," shaped by the historical forces that defined it (the Depression, World War II, Vietnam, etc.), as do people of different geographic regions, urban and rural areas, socioeconomic contexts, and religious affiliations. Upper-middle-class Jewish families in Northeast cities, middle-class German and Scandinavian families on Midwestern farms, African Americans and Anglo families in small Southern towns, poor Mexican migrant farm workers in rural Texas, and Asian Indian and Iranian professionals in California suburbs all have had very different experiences. In addition, we are all being influenced by the "culture" of the Internet and television, which is replacing family and community relationships to an ever increasing extent.

So when we ask people to identify themselves ethnically, we are really asking them to oversimplify, to highlight a part of their identity in order to make certain themes of cultural continuity more apparent. We believe that ethnically respectful clinical work helps people to evolve a sense of whom they belong to. Thus, therapy involves helping people clarify their self-identities in relation to family, community, and their ancestors, while also adapting to changing circumstances as they move forward in time.

We need to go beyond many of our cultural labels and develop a more flexible language that allows people to define themselves in ways that more accurately reflect their heritage and cultural practices. Such labels as "minorities," "Blacks," and "Americans," and one of the more recent additions to our lexicon, "non-Hispanic Whites," reflect the biases embedded in our society's dominant beliefs. The term "minority" marginalizes groups whose heritage is not European. The term "Black" obliterates the ancestral roots of Americans of African heritage altogether and defines them only by their color. And the use of the term "American" to describe people of the United States makes invisible Canadians, Mexicans, and all other people of the Western Hemisphere. We might use the term "United Statesan," but we have instead claimed only for ourselves the descriptor for people of all the Americas. The term "non-Hispanic White" for people of European origin forces them to define themselves always in relation to "Hispanics." Hispanics are defined as a cultural group, although they thought of themselves as a racial group in the 2000 census, but were forced to define themselves by races that included Filipino and Guamanian but not Hispanic or Latino.

Ethnicity is, indeed, a complex concept. Jewish ethnicity, for example, is a meaningful term to millions of people (Chapter 48). Yet it refers to people who have no single country of origin, no single language of origin, no single set of religious practices. Jews in the United States may come from Argentina, Russia, Greece, or Japan and have Ashkenazic roots. Or they may be Sephardic Jews from North Africa or Spain, who have very different cultural traditions and migration patterns within the United States. There are similar difficulties with definitions of Arabs (Chapter 31), who may be Eastern Orthodox Syrians, Roman Catholic Lebanese (Chapter 34), or Turkish, Jordanian, Egyptian, or Palestinian Muslims (Chapter 35). There is, however, some sense of cultural connection between these groups. Moreover, the shared ethnic history of families of these backgrounds is not irrelevant to their adaptation in the United States.

We may feel negative toward, or proud and appreciative of, our cultural heritage, or we may be unaware of which cultural groups we even belong to. But our relationship to our cultural heritage will influence our well-being, as will our sense of our relationship to the dominant culture. People's sense of their ethnicity is affected by their relationship (unaware, negative, proud, appreciative) to the groups they come from, and their relationship (a sense of belonging, feeling like an outsider, or feeling inferior) to the dominant culture. Are we members of it? Are we "passing" as members? Do we feel like marginalized outsiders? Or are we outsiders who have so absorbed the dominant culture's norms and values that we do not even recognize that our internalized values reflect its members' prejudices and attempts to suppress cultural difference? Individuals should not have to suppress parts of themselves in order to "pass" for normal according to someone else's standards. Being "at home" means people having a sense of being at peace with who they really are, not being assigned to rigidly defined group identities, which strains people's basic loyalties. Maria Root (2003) has developed a "Bill of Rights" for racially mixed people, which includes the right

- to identify myself differently than strangers expect
- to identify myself differently than my parents identify me
- to identify myself differently than my brothers and sisters identify me
- to identify myself differently in different situations
- to create a vocabulary to communicate about being multiracial
- to change my identity over my lifetime and more than once
- to have loyalties and identify with more than one group of people

As family therapists, we believe in helping clients understand their ethnicity as a fluid, ever-changing aspect of who they are. Louise Erdrich (Erdrich & Dorris, 1991), has described the complexity this entails through one of her characters:

> I belong to the lost tribe of mixed bloods, that hodgepodge amalgam of hue and cry that defies easy placement. When the DNA of my various ancestors—Irish and Coeur d'Alene and Spanish and Navajo and God knows what else—combined to form me, the result was not some genteel indecipherable puree that comes from a Cuisinart. You know what they say on the side of the Bisquick box, under instructions for pancakes? Mix with fork. Leave lumps. That was me. There are advantages to not being this or that. You have a million stories, one for every occasion, and in a way they're all lies and in another way they're all true. When Indians say to me, "What are you?" I know exactly what they're asking and answer Coeur D'Alene. I don't add, "Between a quarter and a half," because that's information they don't require, first off— though it may come later if I screw up and they're looking for reasons why. If one of my Dartmouth colleagues wonders, "Where did you study?" I pick the best place, the hardest one to get into, in order to establish that I belong. If a stranger on the street questions where [my daughter] gets her light brown hair and dark skin, I say the Olde Sodde and let them figure it out. There are times when I control who I'll be, and times when I let other people decide. I'm

not all anything, but I'm a little bit of a lot. My roots spread in every direction, and if I water one set of them more often than others, it's because they need it more. . . . I've read anthropological papers written about people like me. We're called marginal, as if we exist anywhere but on the center of the page. We're parked on the bleachers looking into the arena, never the main players, but there are bonuses to peripheral vision. Out beyond the normal bounds, you at least know where you're not. You escape the claustrophobia of belonging, and what you lack in security you gain by realizing—as those insiders never do—that security is an illusion. . . . "Caught between two worlds," is the way we're often characterized, but I'd put it differently. We are the catch. (pp. 166–167)

This brilliant expression of a multifaceted cultural identity, composed of complex heritages, illustrates the impact of one's social location on the need to highlight one or another aspect of one's cultural background in a given context, in response to others' projections. The illustration also points out what those who belong have to learn from those who are marginalized.

Most of us are somewhat ambivalent about our ethnic identification. But even those who appear indifferent to their ethnic background would be proud to be identified with their group in some situations and embarrassed or defensive in others. Those most exposed to prejudice and discrimination are most likely to internalize negative feelings about their ethnic identity. Often ethnicity becomes such a toxic issue that people do not even want to mention it, for fear of sounding prejudiced, even in situations where it is primary. Some families will hold onto their ethnic identification, becoming clannish or prejudiced in response to a perceived threat to their integrity. Others use ethnic identification to push for family loyalty. They might say: "If you do that, you're betraying the Jews." For other groups, for example, Scots, Irish, or French Canadians, such an emotional demand for ethnic loyalty would probably not hold much weight.

Awareness of ethnicity within a United States context is always associated with loss. In the case of the indigenous peoples of the Americas, their cultures were destroyed by the European immigrants or by the illnesses they brought, or they were uprooted and great efforts were made to destroy them, so the preservation of their ethnicities has been a profound struggle (Tataki, 2002; Zinn, 2003). Those who came from elsewhere came because of political or religious oppression in their original culture, economic need, or, as in the case of African Americans, enslavement. For many, the memories and associations with their own cultural group or homeland are fraught with pain for their ancestors or relatives left behind or for the plight of their group, which may lead them to distance themselves from this history and perhaps even hide it from their children and grandchildren.

Stuart Hall (1987) has said that every immigrant must face two classic questions: "Why are you here?" and "When are you going back home?"

No migrant ever knows the answer to the second question until asked. Only then does she or he know that really, in the deep sense [he or she is] never going back. Migration is a one-way trip. There is no "home" to go back to. There never was. (p. 44)

What Hall is referring to is that those who come, especially from poor, war torn, or oppressive situations can never really go back, because the circumstances in the culture of origin remain devastating, but also because they will never again have the same relationship to the culture of origin they left; so the connection with their heritage necessarily involves pain, and their homeland is a place where that pain often continues. Thus, connecting to one's ethnic roots has a different meaning, depending on the situation in the culture of origin. The Irish who are now 150 years away from the poverty and desperation that led to their migration may look to their ethnic roots with nostalgia and find in them a source of strength for their ancestors' courage, while feeling supported by our society's social institutions when they need assistance (Chapter 43). Immigrants of Latino origin rarely feel that their cultural values are supported by the community institutions on which they become dependent when in need. Their experience is often of ineffective, inadequate, and at times blatantly hostile, antifamily social service bureaucracies (Ortiz, Simmons, & Hinton, 1999; Chapter 11).

Given the harsh circumstances many immigrants face, and the painful, traumatic history they have left behind, it is not surprising that many people ignore or deny their ethnicity by changing their names and rejecting their families and social backgrounds, but they do so to the detriment of their sense of themselves. Those who have experienced the stigma of prejudice and racism may attempt to "pass" as members of the more highly valued majority culture. Groups that have experienced prejudice and discrimination, such as Jews, Latinos, Asians, and African Americans, may absorb the larger society's prejudice and become conflicted about their own identities, internalizing racial or ethnic hatred.

Family members may even turn against each other, with some trying to "pass" and others resenting them for doing so. Those who are close enough in appearance to the dominant group's characteristics may experience a sense of choice about what group to identify with, whereas others have no choice, because of their skin color or other physical characteristics. Examples of ethnic conflict include some group members' attempts to change their appearance through plastic surgery or other means to obtain "valued" characteristics. Families that are not of the dominant culture are always under pressure to give up their values and conform to the norms of the more powerful group. Intrafamily conflicts over the level of accommodation should be viewed not just as family conflicts, but also as reflecting explicit or implicit pressure from the dominant culture.

A few years ago Ann Fadiman wrote a book about the experience of a Hmong family in Merced, California, with the health care system, which may serve as a primary guide to cultural competence for family therapists and other health care professions. Fadiman (1997) shows how an understanding of culture challenges all our assumptions, beginning with our decisions on how far back in history we go to assess the presenting problem:

> If I were Hmong, I might feel that what happened when Lia Lee and her family encountered the American medical system could be understood fully only by beginning with the first beginning of the world. But since I am not Hmong, I will go back only a few hundred generations to the time when the Hmong were living in the river plains of north-central China. (p. 13)

Here, in two simple sentences, Fadiman expresses a most profound understanding of "cultural competence" as she refers to the astounding difference in worldview between the dominant culture's managed care values, whereby an impersonal health care professional is expected to do an assessment in 15 to 30 minutes, focusing almost exclusively on current symptoms, whereas the Hmong patient's framework includes a history going back a thousand years:

For as long as it has been recorded, the history of the Hmong has been a marathon series of bloody scrimmages, punctuated by occasional periods of peace, though hardly any of plenty. Over and over again, the Hmong have responded to persecution and to pressures to assimilate by either fighting or migrating—a pattern that has been repeated so many times, in so many different eras and places, that it begins to seem almost a genetic trait, as inevitable in its recurrence as their straight hair or their short, sturdy stature. The Chinese viewed the Hmong as fearless, uncouth, and recalcitrant. . . . The Hmong never had any interest in ruling over the Chinese or anyone else; they wanted merely to be left alone, which, as their later history was also to illustrate, may be the most difficult request any minority can make of a majority culture. (p. 14)

Here too is a profound insight into cross-cultural understanding, demonstrating the main problem: how to see past our assumptions in order to understand the experience of others. The Lee family experienced repeated violations by well-meaning but ethnocentric health care personnel who saw this loving family as uncaring, abusive, negligent, and ignorant, only because the yardstick they used to measure the family's values and relationships was that of the dominant U.S. psychological theories. The health care system's unwitting imposition of its own values on this family shows us how limited our perspectives are, unless we add a cultural lens to our psychological assessments.

Sukey Waller, one of the few clinicians who managed to connect with the Lee family, demonstrated an amazing natural creativity as a culture broker:

Psychological problems do not exist for the Hmong, because they do not distinguish between mental and physical illness. Everything is a spiritual problem. I've made a million errors. When I came here everyone said you can't touch people on the head, you can't talk to a man, you can't do this, you can't do that, and I finally said, this is crazy! I can't be restricted like that! So I just threw it all out. Now I have only one rule. Before I do anything I ask, Is it okay? Because I'm an American woman and they don't expect me to act like a Hmong anyway, they usually give me plenty of leeway. (quoted in Fadiman, 1997, p. 95)

Waller's guidelines urge openness to others and reflect the certain knowledge that we will make mistakes. But the dominant culture makes it hard to open oneself to the possibility of mistakes, our only hope for increasing our learning about groups that are different.

In the 1990s, Robert McNamara, defense secretary during the Vietnam War, met with his Vietnamese counterpart of 30 years earlier. He reports that it was in that conversation that he for the first time understood the cultural misunderstanding between the United States and the Vietnamese. The United States viewed the Vietnamese as pawns of the Chinese communists in the Cold War. The Vietnamese leader said to McNamara:

Haven't you ever read a history book? Don't you know we've been fighting the Chinese for 1,000 years? We saw you as coming to dominate us as everyone else always had and were willing to fight to the death. (Morris, 2002)

Here was a lesson in cultural humility that corresponds completely with the message of this book for family therapists: We must work to see the limitations of our own view so we can open our minds to the experience of others.

Cultural meanings may persist many generations after migration and after people have ceased to be aware of their heritage. Indeed, the suppression of their cultural history may lead to cultural patterns they themselves fail to appreciate. They may perceive their behavior as resulting purely from intrapsychic or familial factors, when, in fact, it derives from hidden cultural history. Tom Hayden, co-founder of the Students for a Democratic Society in the early 1960s, a fourth-generation Irish American, who became a committed spokesperson for the power of the hidden cultural identity, discussed the experience of so many in our country who have had to live with their deepest cultural history denied:

> What price do we pay when those who pull the curtains of history allow us to know our history only dimly or with shame. [Ours is a] . . . story . . . of identity forever blurred by the winds of silence and the sands of amnesia. It is also a universal story of being rooted in uprootedness. . . . Themes of personal identity being threatened first with destruction and later by assimilation appear throughout our literature. . . . Themes that reverberate in each story are those of near destruction and survival, shame and guilt, the long fuse of unresolved anger, the recovery of pride and identity. (1998, pp. 8–9)

Hayden himself grew up experiencing himself as Catholic, but not Irish, thinking that he was "post-ethnic in an ethnic world," only to realize years later that he carried his suppressed ethnicity within:

> I had no historic rationale for why I was rebelling against my parents' achievement of respectability and middle-class comfort. There was no one teaching the Irish dimension of my radical discontent, in contrast to Jews and blacks who were instilled with values of their ancestors. . . . The Irish tradition . . . seemed more past than present, more sentimental than serious, more Catholic than political. (2001, pp. 68–69)

It was years until Hayden realized that his family had sought "respectability" as a way to "pass" for the dominant group. It had required his family, and indeed his whole cultural group, to appear to assimilate into the melting pot, but it had cost them their sense of who they were. Feeling himself an outsider in young adulthood, he joined the civil rights movement. His first task was to bring food to Black sharecroppers who had been evicted from their lands in Tennessee.

> Was it only coincidental that I responded to a crisis reminiscent of my evicted, starving Irish ancestors? So effective was the assimilation process that my parents couldn't comprehend why I would risk a career to prevent hunger, eviction and prejudice. I was Irish on the inside, though I couldn't name it at the time. (2001, p. 68)

Hayden grew up mystified about his identity. His father too was mystified about what made Tom do what he did, saying, "I don't know what influenced him when he went away, but it's not the way he was raised." Hayden's example illustrates the mystifying effect that attempts to deny or ignore cultural history have on people's sense of their own identity. Cultural competence requires not a cookbook approach to cultural differences, but an appreciation for the often hidden cultural aspects of our psychological, spiritual, and social selves, a profound respect for the limitations of our own cultural perspective, and an ability to deal respectfully with those whose values differ from our own.

Maya Angelou (1986), who, as a young African American, not surprisingly found it hard to feel culturally at home in the United States, went to live in Africa, hoping in some way to find home. What she found there was that who she was could not be encompassed by that important part of her heritage:

If the heart of Africa still remained elusive, my search for it had brought me closer to understanding myself and other human beings. The ache for home lives in all of us, the safe place
where we can go as we are and not be questioned. It impels mighty ambitions and dangerous
capers. . . . We shout in Baptist churches, wear yarmulkes and wigs and argue even the tiniest
points in the Torah, or worship the sun and refuse to kill cows for the starving. Hoping that
by doing these things, home will find us acceptable or that barring that, we will forget our
awful yearning for it. (p. 196)

Those who try to assimilate at the price of forgetting their connections to their heritage are likely to have more problems than those who maintain their heritage. Simpson
(1987) has said that:

The United States, which has been called the home of the persecuted and the dispossessed, has
been since its founding an asylum for emotional orphans. . . . Many who have assimilated by
changing their names and forgoing their roots, have no way of estimating their spiritual loss.
(pp. 221, 225)

We often see people in therapy who have become disconnected from their history and
don't even know it, because belonging to your context is not a value in the dominant culture. When people are secure in their own identity, they tend to act with greater flexibility
and openness to those of other cultural backgrounds. However, if people receive negative
or distorted images of their ethnic group, they often develop a sense of inferiority, even
self-hate, that can lead to aggressive behavior and discrimination toward outsiders.

STEREOTYPING

Although generalizing about groups has often been used to reinforce prejudices, one cannot discuss ethnic cultures without generalizing. The only alternative is to ignore this
level of analysis of group patterns, which mystifies and disqualifies the experience of
groups at the margins, perpetuating covert negative stereotyping, as does the failure to
address culture explicitly in our everyday work. Yet many have eschewed the value of discussing ethnicity per se, considering socioeconomic, political, and religious influences
more important. Others avoid discussion of group characteristics altogether, in favor of
individual family patterns, maintaining, "I prefer to think of each family as unique" or "I
prefer to think of family members as human beings rather than pigeonholing them in categories." Of course, we all prefer to be treated as unique human beings. But such assumptions prevent us from acknowledging the influence of cultural and group history on every
person's experience. Some have the privilege to belong, with access to society's resources
and the ability to trust that society's institutions will work for them. Others are disqualified by society at every turn, because they are judged not as human beings, but by particular group characteristics such as culture or race.

The values, beliefs, status, and privileges of families in our society are profoundly
influenced by their socioeconomic and cultural location, making these issues essential to
our clinical assessment and intervention. Discussing cultural generalizations or stereotypes is as important as discussing any other norms of behavior. Without some concept of
norms, which are always cultural norms, we would have no compass for our clinical
work at all.

OUR EVOLVING CONCEPT OF ETHNICITY

We live in the most ethnically diverse society that has ever existed on the planet and have struggled since its beginning over issues of ethnicity. It has not been only since September 11, 2001, and the massive reactivity against people from Middle Eastern and Asian Indian cultures that ethnicity has been a source of great conflict. Our nation was founded by people seeking change from their ancestors' cultures. But it was also built on conflict, prejudice, and attempts to oppress and destroy ethnic groups that were perceived as "other," even as we attempted to set up the most culturally tolerant society that had ever been imagined. Tataki (1993) states:

> Indians were already here, while blacks were forcibly transported to America, and Mexicans were initially enclosed by America's expanding border. The other groups came here as immigrants: for them, America represented liminality—a new world where they could pursue extravagant urges to do things they had thought beyond their capabilities. Like the land itself, they found themselves "betwixt and between all fixed points of classification." No longer fastened as fiercely to their old countries, they felt a stirring to become new people in a society still being defined and formed. (p. 6)

Conflicts between different groups in the United States have been built into our nation from the beginning. The Naturalization Law of 1790 restricted citizenship to Whites (Tataki, 1993). We attempted to destroy Native American cultures (see Chapters 2, 3, and 11), and we built into the interior of our governmental institutions, the dehumanization and disqualification of many cultural groups that had been brought here from Africa as slaves (see especially Chapters 5 and 6). When, only a few years after our own revolution, the slaves in Haiti fought for their freedom in a revolt very similar to our own, we saw them as dangerous and did everything we could to hinder it (see Chapter 9). The idea of "liberty and justice for all" was never more than an idea that we found impossible to truly believe. Benjamin Franklin, like so many of the founders of our democracy, owned slaves and advertised slave sales in his newspaper, though he later became president of the first abolition society. His ethnic prejudice extended also to Europeans. Dismayed by the mass immigration of Germans, he expressed fear that "this will in a few years become a German colony: Instead of their learning our language, we must learn theirs, or live as in a foreign country" (cited in Morgan, 2002, p. 77).

> Why should Pennsylvania, founded by the English, become a colony of Aliens, who will shortly be so numerous as to Germanize us instead of our Anglifying them, and will never adopt our language or customs, any more than they can acquire our complexion? Which leads me to add one remark: That the number of purely white people in the world is proportionably very small. All Africa is black or tawny. Asia chiefly tawny. America (exclusive of the new comers) wholly so. And in Europe, the Spaniards, Italians, French, Russians and Swedes are generally of what we call a swarthy complexion; as are the Germans also, the Saxons only excepted, who with the English make the principal body of white people on the face of the earth. I could wish their numbers were increased. And while we are, as I may call it, scouring our planet, by clearing America of woods, and so making this side of our globe reflect a brighter light to the eyes of inhabitants on Mars or Venus, why should we in the sight of superior beings, darken its people? Why increase the sons of Africa, by planting them in America, where we have so fair an opportunity, by excluding all blacks and tawnys, of increasing the

lovely white and red? But perhaps I am partial to the complexion of my Country, for such kind of partiality is natural to Mankind. (1918, cited and discussed in Malcomson, 2000, p. 177)

Franklin's attitudes help us understand the pervasive yet unacknowledged way racism and prejudice have been embedded in our nation. Alexis de Tocqueville, the great 19th-century observer of American ethnic traits, found it striking how Whites were able to deprive Indians of their rights and exterminate them "with singular felicity, tranquility, legally, philanthropically, without shedding blood, and without violating a single great principle of morality in the eyes of the world." Tocqueville wryly remarked that no other people could destroy men with "more respect for the laws of humanity" (Tocqueville, 1835, reprinted 1945, pp. 352–353, cited in Tataki, 1993, p. 92).

Over the centuries we have greatly expanded the category of "White" cultures to include Europeans previously considered "ethnic," such as Poles, Italians, Irish, and Jews. People of mixed heritage are often pressed to identify with a single cultural group, rather than being free to claim the true complexity of their cultural heritage (Chapter 31; Root, 1992, 1996).

The majority group has often asserted its power through an assimilationist "melting pot" ideology, and we have remained ambivalent about the value of ethnic pluralism, as indicated also in recent attempts to roll back affirmative action, which have decreased the diversity of the college population even as the nation is becoming more diverse. Yet ethnicity remains a major form of group identification and a major determinant of our family patterns and belief systems. The American premise of equality required us to give primary allegiance to our national identity, fostering the myth of the melting pot—the notion that group distinctions between people should ultimately disappear. The idea that we were all equal led to pressure to see ourselves as all the same. But we have not "melted." Some have said that ethnicity, especially among European Americans, the only ones always free to become "American," is more symbolic than real (Alba, 1990). Indeed, some research on ethnicity lumps all European Americans together into one group. This book asserts a different view, that it will be a long while before ethnicity disappears as a factor relevant to understanding European Americans as well as other groups (Chapter 36).

The way our census counts people has always been a volatile issue in the United States. The reason is, said former bureau chief Kenneth Prewitt, that "throughout American history, starting with the 1790 Census, a classification of racial groups has been used to regulate relations among the races and to support discriminatory policies designed to protect the numerical and political supremacy of white Americans of European Ancestry" (Roberts, 2004, p. 143). In the 2000 census people were asked to identify themselves ethnically/racially and to list up to two ancestries. Some 7.6 million people nationwide answered simply "American" or "USA," and millions more left the question blank (Roberts, 2004). In our definition, however, everyone is ethnic, whether they choose to identify with their background or not. Not acknowledging our ethnic background is like not acknowledging our grandparents; it is a fact of identity over which we have no choice.

The 2000 census was the first to allow people to acknowledge mixed heritage at all, though it was done in a completely inadequate way. Many have feared that the reason was only that the United States is in need of further expansion of the category of "White," which will otherwise soon become a minority of the population. The census, which has enormous power to determine the dominant cultural definitions of race and ethnicity, has severe limitations in its cultural categorizations. A glaring illustration is its definition of "White," which includes all those who have origins in Europe, the Middle East, and North Africa. The term "Asian" is used to include a wide spectrum of groups, ranging from Hmong to Pakistani. Cultural groups from Middle Eastern countries such as Afghanistan or Iraq are classed as White, although they are much more closely related to cultural groups in Pakistan that we have labeled "Asian," making one wonder whose interests it serves to use the categorization "White" at all. The only ethnicity explored at all by the latest census was "Hispanic." This is a very problematic category (Chapter 11), which many consider racist, since it emphasizes the connection to Spain. It is so general that it is about as relevant as using "American" to describe people of so many heritages. Second, the census forced "Hispanics" to define themselves racially using categories that did not include Hispanic, Latino, or Native American. Their only choices were Black, White, American Indian, Asian, or Other, the last of which they generally saw as their only option. Furthermore, this categorization by the U.S. Census Bureau forced Brazilians (Chapter 12) to label themselves "White" rather than "Hispanic," even though the cultural history of Puerto Ricans (Chapter 18), Cubans (Chapter 15), Dominicans (Chapter 16), Colombians (Chapter 14), and other groups in Latin America (Chapter 13) undoubtedly have much more in common with Brazilian cultures than with "White" cultures.

The census has been a conservative force within our society for 200 years, putting people in categories that oversimplify their heritage and cultural connections to each other and to their ancestors. People have been pressed into racial categories that have no basis whatsoever except to stratify people by the meaningless difference of skin color. These categorizations have been developed to promote White supremacy in our society (Malcomson, 2000). Racial categorization was first articulated in Germany by Johann Blumenbach (Frederickson, 2002), an anatomist who divided the world into four racial categories by geography (Gould, 1994):

- The Caucasian variety for the light-skinned people of Europe and the adjacent parts of Asia and Africa.
- The Mongolian variety for the other inhabitants of Asia, including China and Japan.
- The Ethiopian variety for the dark-skinned people of Africa.
- The American variety for most native populations of the "New World."

In his second edition he added a fifth Malay category for the Polynesians and Melanesians of the Pacific and the aborigines of Australia. This clarified a hierarchy with White at the apex and the American variety on the way to the Mongolian extreme on one side, and, quite illogically, labeled the Malay as in the direction of the other extreme, the Ethiopian. Blumenbach's categories had no basis whatsoever in science. They were based on his judgment of the beauty of the people of the Caucasus! He said:

> I have taken the name of this variety from Mount Caucasus, both because its neighborhood, and especially its southern slope, produces the most beautiful race of men, I mean the Georgian, and because . . . in that region, if anywhere, it seems, we ought with greatest probability to place the aotochthones (original forms) of mankind. (cited in Gould, 1994, p. 1)

During the 18th century, Europeans and Americans were in serious need of a categorization of races that would provide justification for Whites to treat people of color as not human. This was especially important at a time when, with the Enlightenment, there was a focus on the "inalienable" rights of human beings. Having a hierarchy of races helped rationalize slavery. This insidious categorization persists to this day and continues to promote White power because unlike the definition of ethnicity, U.S. official definitions of race have no scientific or historically cultural basis. Maria Root (1992, 1996, 2001), one of the prime researchers on ethnicity and multuculturalism, has defined a special bill of rights for people of mixed race, asserting their right to define themselves for themselves and not be limited by society's racial and ethnic stereotypes and caricatures.

THE CHANGING FACE OF ETHNICITY IN
THE UNITED STATES AT THE START OF THE 21st CENTURY

The late 20th century saw the greatest rise in immigration in 100 years. More than one million legal and undocumented immigrants came annually, most from Asia and Latin America. And although there has been a great upturn in negativity toward immigrants since September 11, 2001 (Gallup Organization, 2004), the 2000 census counted about 28 million first-generation immigrants in the United States, equaling 10% of the population—not the highest percentage of foreign born in the overall population, which occurred in 1907, when the percentage was 14% (Martinez, 2004). With streams of new immigrants imparting their unique cultures, American society has become characterized by unparalleled diversity. Asians, Latin Americans, and other newcomers have become "the new face of America."

Respect for ethnic diversity has flourished during certain periods in American history and has been stifled at others. The backlash against multiculturalism has also waxed and waned, depending on the economics and politics of the moment. Anti-Arab and Anti-Muslim feelings escalated to an extreme degree in the wake of September 11, 2001, and various governmental initiatives related to Homeland Security and the Patriot Act increased fear and negative feelings about certain nondominant groups in our society. White extremist skinheads and neo-Nazi groups periodically escalate their fostering of racial and ethnic hatred, and we experience periodic increases of anti-immigrant reactions, depending on the labor needs of the country.

The impact of ethnicity varies geographically. In the Pacific region, for example, one fifth of Americans are foreign born, whereas in the Midwestern farm belt, this is true of only one person in 50. In Los Angeles, 4 in 10 residents are foreign born; in New York, 3 in 10. Before the end of this century, White Americans will be a minority. In 1900, outside of the South, all states but Arizona had a population that was more than 90% White. Roberts (2004) reports that, by 2000, only 10 states had that ratio and 5 states beyond the South had a population that was less than 70% White. African Americans have increased to 12.3% of the population, with record-high proportions in the Northeast, Midwest, and West, and record lows in the South (Roberts, 2004). Latinos have increased dramatically to become 13.4%, in contrast to 9% in 1990, whereas Asians have increased to 3.6% of the population, one third of whom live in California. Only about 69% of Americans are "non-Hispanic Whites," a decrease of more than 6% in a decade, although fully one in 4 Americans believe they were descended from the Pilgrims!

However, this includes almost 50% of Hispanics who, as stated earlier, had no way to identify themselves in the 2000 census except as White, Black or "Other race." They could not identify themselves racially as "Hispanic." Of the 31 million foreign-born Americans, only 15% are European, 26% are Asian, and 51% are Latino. Thirty-three ancestry groups reported populations of over 1 million in 2000. The Arab population rose by 41% in the 1980s and by 38% in the 1990s, but still accounts for only 0.5% of the general population.

Concomitantly, there has been a rapid rise of multicultural consciousness in the United States. When Queens, New York, the most diverse county in the nation, launched its new telephone information line, it boasted providing service in 170 different languages (Roberts, 2004).

The changing ethnic demographics are having a significant impact on all aspects of our society. Of new workers entering the workforce, 80% are women, minorities, or new immigrants. In other words, our workforce is becoming culturally diverse in ways we never imagined. This reality in the context of a growing global economy and the presence of many international corporations helps explain the upsurge in business literature on managing a culturally diverse workforce (Jamieson & O'Mara, 1991, Thiederman, 1991; Thomas, 1991). Twenty percent of the nation's children have at least one foreign-born parent! The foreign-born population has increased to more than 31 million, making the United States now the least "American," by conventional definitions, or the most American it has ever been when we consider Latinos as Americans (Roberts, 2004). Twenty percent of schoolchildren speak a language other than English at home, mostly Spanish, although more than 150 languages are represented in America's schools (Roberts, 2004). Multicultural education, although controversial, is increasingly being included in school curricula (Banks, 1991).

FACTORS INFLUENCING ETHNICITY

Essential to understanding culture is learning about the interaction between ethnicity, gender, sexual orientation, class, race, religion, geography, migration, and politics and how they have together influenced families in adapting to life in the United States. All these components are also influenced by the length of time since migration, a group's specific historical experience, and the degree of discrimination its members have experienced in this society. Generally, people move closer to the dominant value system the longer they remain in the United States and the more they rise in social class. Families that remain within an ethnic neighborhood, that work and socialize with members of their groups, and those whose religion reinforces ethnic values, will probably maintain their ethnicity longer than those who live in heterogeneous settings. When family members move from an ethnic enclave, even several generations after immigration, the stresses of adaptation are likely to be severe. The therapist should learn about the community's ethnic network and, where appropriate, encourage the rebuilding of social and informal connections through family visits, letters, or creating new networks.

Those who are systematically excluded from the dominant group, or from the groups to which they belong because of racism, anti-Semitism, sexism, homophobia, or other institutionalized bias, will continue to show the effects of this exclusion in their psychological and social makeup.

MIGRATION

No one leaves his or her world without having been transfixed by its roots, or with a vacuum for a soul. We carry with us the memory of many fabrics, a self soaked in our history, our culture; a memory, sometimes scattered, sometimes sharp and clear, of the streets of our childhood.

—FREIRE (1994, p. 32)

All Americans have experienced the complex stresses of migration. And the hidden effects of this history, especially when it goes unacknowledged, may linger for many generations. Families' migration experiences have a major influence on their cultural values. Why did the family migrate? What were they seeking (e.g., survival, adventure, wealth)? What were they leaving behind (e.g., religious or political persecution, or poverty)? An immigrating family's dreams and fears become part of its heritage. Parents' attitudes toward what came before and what lies ahead will have a profound impact on the expressed or tacit messages they transmit to their children. Families that have migrated before tend to adapt more easily, such as the Jews who migrated first to South America and later to the United States. Their previous migration probably taught them something about flexibility. Those who come as refugees, fleeing political persecution or the trauma of war and who have no possibility of returning to their homeland, may have very different adaptations to American life than those who come seeking economic advancement with the idea of returning to their homeland to retire. The political history surrounding migration may intensify cultural traits for a particular group, strengthening their tendency to hold onto cultural traits if they experienced the threat of cultural annihilation, as happened for Cubans, African Americans, Poles, Native Americans, and Jews, for example.

Adaptation is also affected by whether one family member has migrated alone or whether a large portion of the family, community, or nation has come together. Frequently, educated immigrants who come for professional opportunities move to places where there is no one with whom they can speak their native language or share family customs and rituals. Families that migrate alone usually have a greater need to adapt to the new situation, and their losses are often more hidden. On the other hand, when a number of families migrate together, as happened with the Scandinavians who settled in the Midwest (Chapter 46), they are often able to preserve much of their traditional heritage.

When members of a large part of a population or nation come together, as happened in the waves of Irish (Chapter 43), Polish (Chapter 54), Italian (Chapter 44), and Jewish migration (Chapter 48), discrimination against the group may be especially intense. The newest immigrants always pose a threat to those who came just before, who fear losing their tenuous economic security. Sometimes more recent immigrants of the same background have conflicts with their older compatriots because of class differences, as has been true for Cubans, Iranians, Poles, and other groups. Some groups have a back-and-forth pattern of migration, like Puerto Ricans and Mexicans, and are more transnational, meaning that they are always incorporating two cultures rather than only adjusting to the new one.

The East and West coasts, the entry points for most immigrants, are likely to have greater ethnic diversity and defined ethnic neighborhoods, and people in these areas are more often aware of ethnic differences. The ethnic neighborhood provides a temporary cushion against the stresses of migration, which are likely to surface in the second generation. Those immigrant families that moved to an area where the population was relatively stable, for example, the South, generally had more trouble adjusting or were forced to assimilate very rapidly.

RACE AND RACISM

> Racial bars build a wall not only around . . . [people of color] but around white people as well, cramping their spirits and causing them to grow in distorted shapes.
> —BRADEN (1999, p. 24)

> Prejudice is a burden which confuses the past, threatens the future, and renders the present inaccessible.
> —ANGELOU (1986, p. 155)

> Race, reality and relationships are often complexly entangled in ways that are difficult to discern. The volatility of race as a phenomenon, the acute silence that often accompanies racial interactions, and the general lack of attention devoted to the intricacies of relationship development and maintenance all contribute to the difficulty of deconstructing this enganglement, which is a powerful and pervasive force in our personal lives and in our clinical practices.
> —HARDY (2004, p. 87)

Race, unlike culture, is not an internal issue, but rather a political issue, operating to privilege certain people at the expense of others. It is a bogus construct, created and kept in place by White people, and it creates walls that lock us all in. Ann Braden (1999), one of the White sheroes of the antiracism movement, puts it this way: Racism "is the assumption that everything should be run by white people for the benefit of white people" (p. 340). Unlike culture, which operates from the inside out, influencing us because it represents values that have been passed down to us through generations of our ancestors, race is a construct which imposes judgment on us from the outside in, based on nothing more than our color or physical features. Many who come to the United States are deeply troubled when they experience racism here for the first time. Over time reactions to our society's racism, which stratifies people by skin color, tends to be internalized. As Hardy (2004) puts it, "although seldom explicitly acknowledged, race is often one of the factors that determines who participates in certain interactions, and how" (p. 87). Expectations of privilege and entitlement or invalidation tend to become internalized assumptions in response to this social force. For people of color, race becomes "like the invisible fences that pet owners use to keep their dogs contained within a given circumscribed space. After a very short while, dogs learn where the boundaries are that should not be crossed unless they are willing to be shocked" (Hardy, 2004, p. 88). Race is an issue of political oppression, not a cultural or genetic issue. Ignatiev (1995) has said, "No biologist has ever been able to provide a satisfactory definition of 'race'—that is, a definition that includes all members of a given race and excludes all others." Categorizing people by race serves, rather, to justify reducing all members of one group to an undifferentiated social status, beneath that of all members of another group. Racism operates like sexism, a similar system of privilege and oppression, justified within the dominant society as a biological or cultural phenomenon, which functions systematically to advantage White members of society at the expense of members of color (Chapter 36; Hardy & Laszloffy, 1992; Hitchcock, 2003; Katz, 1978; Mahmoud, 1998).

Although racism may be more subtle and covert today, the politics of race continue to be complex and divisive, and, unfortunately, Whites remain generally unaware of the problems our society creates for people of color. Just as patriarchy, classism, and heterosexism have been invisible structural definers of all European groups' ethnicity, race and racism have also been invisible definers of European groups' cultural values. The invisible knapsack of privilege (McIntosh, 1998) granted to all White Americans, just by the color of their skin, is something that most White ethnics do not acknowledge (Chapter 36).

Although there is a rapidly increasing rate of intermarriage among European groups and of Whites with people of color, the percentages are still small. And the level of segregation in the United States between European Americans and people of color, especially African Americans, remains profound, a problem that most Whites do not notice. Racism and poverty have always dominated the lives of ethnic minorities in the United States. Race has always been a major cultural definer and divider in our society, inasmuch as those whose skin color marked them as different always suffered more discrimination than others. They could not "pass," as other immigrants might, leaving them with an "obligatory" ethnic and racial identification.

Racial bigotry and discrimination continue to be terrible facts of American life, from college campuses to corporate boardrooms. Although Blacks are no longer forbidden to drink from the same water fountains as Whites or to attend integrated schools, we still live in a highly segregated society. The racial divide continues to be a painful chasm, creating profoundly different consciousness for people of color than for Whites (Tatum, 2003). People find it even more difficult to talk to each other about racism than about ethnicity. Each new racial incident ignites feelings and expressions of anger and rage, helplessness and frustration. Exploring our own ethnicity is vital to overcoming our prejudices and expanding our understanding of ourselves in context, but in our pursuit of multicultural understanding, we must also take care not to diminish our efforts to overcome racism (Hitchcock, 2003; Katz, 1978; Kivel, 2002).

RELIGION

The United States is a very religious country. Normally, such an advanced society would over time become more secular, but this has not been the case. About 95% of Americans profess a belief in God, most of them belong to a church or synagogue, and most say that they pray on a daily basis (Gallup & Lindsay, 1999). According to the 2001 American Religious Identity Survey (Kosmin & Lackman, 2001), 76.5% of Americans, or 159 million people, identify themselves as Christians; 13.2%, or 27.5 million, identify themselves as nonreligious or secular. In order, the major Christian denominations are Catholic, Baptist, Methodist, Lutheran, Presbyterian, Pentecostal (charismatic or evangelical), Episcopalian, Mormon, Church of Christ, and Congregationalist. Other major religious groups include Jews, 2.8 million; Muslims, 1 million; Buddhists, 1 million; Hindus, 766,000; and Unitarian Universalists, 629,000. There are also an estimated 991,000 agnostics and 902,000 atheists. There are indications that public interest in spirituality is increasing (Miller & Thoreson, 2003). Religion, for many groups, roots its participants in the family and community, and thus in their own histories and cultural traditions (Aponte, 1994; Boyd-Franklin & Lockwood, 1999; Walsh, 1999; Walsh & Pryce, 2002).

For many ethnic groups, their religion has been a major force for transmitting their cultural heritage, even where, as with African Americans (Jones, 1993), Haitians (Chapter 9), Cubans (Chapter 15), Puerto Ricans (Chapter 18), and others, they had to hide their ancestral beliefs in a new religion. Many Latino groups, for example, maintained their earlier gods hidden in the guise of Catholic saints. Religion and cultural tradition have been largely intertwined, although there are cultural groups, such as Koreans (Chapter 26), that may practice very different religions (Buddhism, Methodism, Catholicism) even within the same family. Walsh (Walsh & Pryce, 2002) notes:

> Spirituality . . . like culture and ethnicity, involves streams of experience that flow through all aspects of life, from family heritage to personal belief systems, rituals and practices, and shared faith communities. Spiritual beliefs influence ways of dealing with adversity, the experience of pain and suffering and the meaning of symptoms. (p. 337)

Most Europeans share the dominant American Judeo-Christian belief in one God, and in the separation of church and state. Today, however, with the flood of new immigrants coming to the United States, other religions are making an impact on established religious institutions. Islam, the third great monotheistic faith, while expanding through immigration and African American conversions, will soon supplant Judaism as this country's third largest faith, including people of widely different ethnic backgrounds: African Americans with roots in the southern United States and Africa (Chapter 10), Pakistanis (Chapter 30), Asian Indian families (Chapters 28 and 29), Arab families from many different countries (Chapters 31 and 32), Albania, Turkey, and Indonesia, the world's largest Muslim nation (Chapter 24).

The Catholic Church, which has absorbed floods of immigrants, is particularly feeling the impact of the new immigration. Today mass is heard in 30 languages in New York City. Millions of Latinos with a fervent approach to worship are challenging the church hierarchy. The Catholic Church also has contingents of African immigrant families and African Americans, Filipinos, Latinos and others. These groups are also increasingly being attracted to the Pentecostal and Baptist faiths, creating new competition for the Catholic Church. Likewise, Koreans are changing the nature of both Protestant and Catholic church communities, with their evangelical zeal and religious traditionalism. And many Jews and former Catholics of European heritage are embracing Buddhism and altering the practice of this and other religious communities of Asian origin. Thus, the interaction between religion and ethnicity is profound, and it is essential to understand the interplay as one explores families' cultural contexts.

People use religion as a means of coping with stress or powerlessness, as well as for spiritual fulfillment and emotional support. Institutionalized religion also meets social needs. Unfortunately, clinicians often fail to utilize appropriate religious tenets and support systems that give comfort and meaning to the family (Hodge, 2001; Miller & Thoresen, 2003; Walsh, 1999). Given Americans' strong spiritual beliefs and their religious institutions' social service networks, it is surprising that many family therapists treat faith as a private affair that has little or no impact on treatment; we hope that this book will help clinicians appreciate that spiritual values are fundamental to healing for most of the cultural groups in the United States.

SOCIAL CLASS AND SOCIOECONOMIC STATUS

Social class and socioeconomic status increasingly organize the United States in very insidious ways, including structuring the relationships between ethnic groups, often pitting less powerful groups against each other, or members of a less powerful group against one another. The distance between the very rich and everyone else has been increasing dramatically in the last two decades. It has been estimated that the richest 20% of American households now own more than 80% of our country's wealth (Vermeulen, 1995). With this trend continuing, poor as well as middle-class families will find themselves in more vulnerable and precarious situations. These class differences will have a serious impact on family relations. The top one million people in the United States make as much money as the next 100 million put together. And the share of wealth of the top 1% of the population (40% of the nation's wealth) has doubled since 1970 (Thurow, 1995). Twenty years ago, the typical CEO made 40 times the amount of the typical American worker. That ratio has swelled to 190 times as much (Hacker, 1995). Inequalities in earnings between the top 20% of wage earners and the bottom 20% doubled in the last two decades (Thurow, 1995). Derrick Bell (1993) has suggested that intergroup conflicts, especially racial conflicts, are promoted by those at the top to keep everyone not at the top from realizing their commonalties and shared interests, because, if they did, it would create a revolution. It is much safer for the dominant group to promulgate the myth that it is the Black man we really have to fear, rather than the power structure that holds our dominant class in place.

Class intersects powerfully with ethnicity and must always be considered when one is trying to understand a family's problems. The influence of class on the cultural position of groups in the United States is extreme. Of the 1,000 people who have ever appeared on *Forbes* magazine's list of the 400 richest people in America, only 5 have been Black (Hacker, 1995). Some have maintained that class, more than ethnicity, determines people's values and behavior. Class is important, but not all differences can be ascribed to class alone. Boyd-Franklin (2002) makes extremely clear the powerful interaction between race and class in the case of African Americans. Ethnic distinctions generally play a less powerful role among the most educated and upwardly mobile segments of a given group, who are more likely to dissociate themselves from their ethnic roots. This may create hidden problems in a family, pitting one generation against another, or one segment of a group against another. It is also more difficult to rise into the upper classes if your skin is dark, because of the institutionalized racism in this country.

Upward mobility is part of the "American dream." Although you cannot change your ethnicity, changing class is even an expectation in our society. You may deny your gender or culture, you may not conform to stereotypic patterns of your gender or cultural group, but you cannot change who you are on these dimensions. Yet changes in class, which are among the most profound we experience, are generally not talked about, even among people within the same family. Silence about class transitions can become very painful. Parents and children or siblings from the same family often end up in different socioeconomic groups when the children are either highly successful or disabled and dysfunctional.

Groups also differ in the extent to which they value education or "getting ahead." Family members may feel compelled to make a choice between moving ahead and loyalty to their group, which can be a major source of identity or intrafamilial conflict. For important historical reasons, certain groups, such as Irish, Italians, Poles, and African Americans, may have a distinct ambivalence or discomfort about moving up in class, whereas others embrace it wholeheartedly.

CULTURAL DIFFERENCES IN WORLDVIEW AND BASIC VALUES

It is almost impossible to understand the meaning of behavior unless one knows something of the cultural values of a family. Even the definition of "family" differs greatly from group to group. The dominant American (Anglo) definition focuses on the intact nuclear family, whereas for Italians there is no such thing as the "nuclear" family. To them, family means a strong, tightly knit three- or four-generational family, which also includes godparents and old friends. African American families focus on an even wider network of kin and community. And Asian families include all ancestors, going all the way back to the beginning of time, and all descendants, or at least male ancestors and descendents, reflecting a sense of time that is almost inconceivable to most other Americans.

Ethnic groups' distinctive problems are often the result of cultural traits that are conspicuous strengths in other contexts. For example, British American optimism leads to confidence and flexibility in taking initiative. But the same preference for an upbeat outlook may also lead to the inability to cope with tragedy or to engage in mourning. Historically, the British have perhaps had much reason to feel fortunate as a people. But optimism becomes a vulnerability when they must contend with major losses. They have few philosophical or expressive ways to deal with situations in which optimism, rationality, and belief in the efficacy of individuality are insufficient. Thus, they may feel lost when dependence on the group is the only way to ensure survival.

Families from different ethnic groups may experience diverse kinds of intergenerational struggles. British American families are likely to feel that they have failed if their children *do not* move away from the family and become independent, whereas Italians generally believe they have failed if their children *do* move away. Jewish families often foster a relatively democratic atmosphere in which children are free to challenge parents and discuss their feelings openly. Greek and Chinese families, in contrast, do not generally expect or desire open communication between generations and would disapprove of a therapist's getting everyone together to discuss and "resolve" their conflicts. Children are expected to respect parental authority, which is reinforced by the distance parents maintain from their children.

Cultural groups vary greatly in the emphasis they place on various life transitions (Carter & McGoldrick, 2005; Dilworth-Anderson et al., 1996). Irish and African Americans have always considered death the most important life cycle transition (McGoldrick et al., 2004). Italians, Asian Indians, and Poles tend to emphasize weddings, whereas Jews often pay particular attention to the bar or bat mitzvah, and Puerto Ricans to the *Quinceanero*, the 15th birthday, celebrating transitions from childhood, which other groups hardly mark at all. Families' ways of celebrating these events differ as well. The Irish tend to celebrate weddings (and every other occasion) by drinking, the Poles by dancing, the Italians by eating, and the Jews by eating and talking. Mexican Americans (Chapter 17) may see early and middle childhood as extending longer than the dominant American pattern, while adolescence is shorter and leads more quickly into adulthood than in the dominant American structure, in which courtship is generally longer and middle age extends into what Americans generally think of as older age. Any life cycle transition can spark conflicts in regard to ethnic identity, because it puts a person in touch with his or her family traditions (Carter & McGoldrick, 2005). A divorce, marriage, childbirth, illness, job loss, death, or retirement can exacerbate ethnic identity conflicts, causing people to lose a sense of who they are. A therapist who tries to help a family to preserve cultural continuities will assist its members in maintaining and building upon their ethnic identity (Cushing & McGoldrick, 2004).

MIGRATION AT DIFFERENT PHASES OF THE LIFE CYCLE

Migration is so disruptive that it seems to add an entire extra stage to the life cycle for those who must negotiate it (Hernandez & McGoldrick, 2005). Adjusting to a new culture is not a single event, but rather a prolonged developmental process (Falicov, 2002) that affects family members differently, depending on their life cycle phase when they are going through the process.

Young Adult Phase

When individuals immigrate during the young adult phase, they have the greatest potential for adapting to a new culture in terms of career and marital choice, but they may also be most vulnerable to cutting off their heritage.

Families with Young Children

Families that migrate with young children are often strengthened by having each other, but they are vulnerable to the reversal of hierarchies. Parents may acculturate more slowly than their children, creating a problematic power inversion. When children interpret the new culture for their parents, parental leadership may be threatened, as children are left without effective adult authority to support them and without a positive ethnic identity to ease their adaptation to life in the new culture. If the parents are supported in their cultural adjustment, through their workplaces or extended family and friends, their children's adjustment will go more easily, since young people generally adapt well to new situations even when doing so involves learning a new language. But in adolescence, when the children are drawn toward their peer culture, problems may surface. Coaching the younger generation to show respect for their elders' values is usually the first step in negotiating such conflicts.

Families with Adolescents

Families migrating with adolescents may have more difficulty, because they will have less time together as a unit before the children move out on their own. A family can struggle with multiple transitions and generational conflicts at once. Families' distance from the grandparents in their home country may be particular distressing as the grandparents become ill, dependent, or die, and their children may experience guilt or other stresses in not being able to fulfill their filial obligations. At times adolescents develop symptoms in reaction to their parents' distress.

Launching Phase

Families with young adult children are less likely to migrate seeking a better way of life. More often, if families migrate at this phase, it is because circumstances in the country of origin make remaining there impossible. Migration at this phase may be especially hard, because it is much more difficult for the parents to adapt to a new language, job situation, relationships, and customs. Again, if their aging parents are left behind, the stresses of migration will be intensified. This phase may be more complex if children date or marry individuals from other backgrounds. This is naturally perceived as a threat by many, if not most, parents, because it means a loss of the cultural heritage in the next generation. One cannot underestimate the stress parents experience in their children's intermarriage when they themselves have lost the culture in which they grew up.

Later Life

Migration in later life can be especially difficult because at this point families are leaving a great deal of their life experience and sociocultural resources behind. Even those who might migrate at a young age have a strong need to reclaim their ethnic roots at this phase, particularly because they are losing other supports. For those who have not mastered English, it can be extremely isolating to be dependent on strangers for health care services when they cannot communicate easily. When older immigrants live in an ethnic neighborhood, acculturation conflicts may be postponed. Members of the next generation, particularly during adolescence, are likely to reject their parents' "ethnic" values and strive to become "Americanized." Intergenerational conflicts often reflect the families' struggles over values in adapting to the United States. The third and fourth generations are usually freer to reclaim aspects of their identities that were sacrificed in previous generations because of the need to assimilate.

CULTURAL AND RACIAL INTERMARRIAGE

The degree of ethnic intermarriage in the family also plays a role in the evolution of cultural patterns (Crohn, 1995; Kennedy, 2003; McGoldrick & Garcia-Preto, 1984; Petsonk & Remsen, 1988; Root, 2001). Although, as a nation, we have a long history of intercultural relationships, until 1967 our society explicitly forbade racial intermarriage, and discouraged cultural intermarriage as well, because it challenged White supremacy. But traditional ethnic and racial categories are now increasingly being challenged by the cultural and racial mixing that has been a long submerged part of our history. Intimate relationships between people of different ethnic, religious, and racial backgrounds offer convincing evidence that Americans' tolerance of cultural differences may be much higher than most people think (Alibhai-Brown & Montague, 1992; Crohn, 1995; McGoldrick & Garcia-Preto, 1984; Petsonk & Remson, 1988; Schneider, 1989). Intermarriage is occurring at triple the rate of the early 1970s. More than 50% of Americans are marrying out of their ethnic groups; 33 million American adults live in households where at least one other adult has a different religious identity. Intermarriage greatly complicates those issues that partners from a single ethnic group face.

Generally, the greater the cultural difference between spouses, the more trouble they will have in adjusting to marriage.

Knowledge about ethnic/cultural differences can be helpful to spouses who take each other's behavior too personally. Typically, we tolerate differences when we are not under stress; in fact, we may find them appealing. However, when stress occurs, tolerance for differences diminishes. Not to be understood in ways that conform with our wishes and expectations frustrates us. For example, when upset, Anglos tend to move toward stoical isolation to mobilize their powers of reason. In contrast, Jewish spouses seek to analyze their experience together. Italians may seek solace in food or in emotionally and dramatically expressing their feelings, and Asians may become very silent, fearing loss of face. Members of these groups sometimes perceive each other's reactions as offensive or insensitive, although, within each group's ethnic norms, such reactions make perfect sense. Much of therapy involves helping family members recognize each other's behavior as largely a reaction from a different frame of reference.

Many cultural and religious groups have prohibitions against intermarriage, which is seen as a threat to group survival. Until 1967, when such laws were declared unconstitutional, 19 states prohibited racial intermarriage. Until 1970, the Catholic Church did not recognize out-marriages, unless the non-Catholic partner promised to raise the couple's children in the Catholic faith. Members of many Jewish groups have also feared that intermarriage would threaten the group's survival. In earlier generations the intermarriage rate in Jewish families was very low, though it has increased dramatically for the current generation. According to the 1990 National Jewish Population Studies, 52% of new marriages were to non-Jews. The likelihood of ethnic intermarriage increases with the length of time individuals have lived in this country, as well as with higher educational and occupational status.

Couples who choose to "marry out" are usually seeking to rebalance their own ethnic characteristics, moving away from some values as well as toward others. During courtship, a person may be attracted precisely to the loved one's differentness, but when he or she is in a marital relationship the same qualities can seem grating.

Consider an Anglo Italian couple in which the Anglo husband takes literally the dramatic expressiveness of the Italian wife, whereas she finds his emotional distancing intolerable. The husband may label the Italian "hysterical" or "crazy" and in return be labeled "cold" or "catatonic." Knowledge about differences in cultural belief systems can help spouses who take each other's behavior too personally. Couples may experience great relief when they can come to see the spouse's behavior fitting into a larger ethnic context rather than as a personal attack. Yet cultural traits may also be used as an excuse for not taking responsibility in a relationship: "I'm Italian. I can't help it" (i.e., the yelling, abusive language, impulsiveness), or "I'm a WASP. It is just the way I am" (lack of emotional response, rationalization, and workaholism), or "I can't help being late. We Puerto Ricans have a different conception of time."

CLINICAL INTERVENTION FROM A CULTURAL PERSPECTIVE

Appreciation of cultural variability leads to a radically new conceptual model of clinical intervention. Helping a person achieve a stronger sense of self may require resolving internalized negative cultural attitudes or cultural conflicts within the family, between the family and the community, or in the wider context in which the family is embedded. A part of this process involves identifying and consciously selecting ethnic values we wish to retain and carry on. Families may need coaching to distinguish deeply held convictions from values asserted for dysfunctional emotional reasons.

What is adaptive in a given situation? Answering this requires an appreciation of the total context in which a behavior occurs. For example, Puerto Ricans may see returning to the island as a solution to their problems. A child who misbehaves may be sent back to live with an extended family member. This solution may be viewed as dysfunctional if the therapist considers only that the child will be isolated from the immediate family, or that the relative in Puerto Rico may have fewer resources to meet the child's developmental needs. Rather than counter the parents' plan, the therapist may encourage them to strengthen their connectedness with family members in Puerto Rico with whom their child will be staying, for they will be using a culturally sanctioned network for support. The therapist's role in such situations may be that of a culture broker, helping family members to recognize their own ethnic values and to resolve the conflicts that evolve out of different perceptions and experiences.

There are many examples of such misunderstood behavior. Puerto Rican women are taught to lower their eyes and avoid eye contact, which American therapists are often taught to read as indicating an inability to relate interpersonally. Jewish patients may consider it essential to inquire about the therapist's credentials; many other groups would perceive this as an affront, but for these patients it is a needed reassurance. Iranian and Greek patients may ask for medication, give every indication of taking it, but then go home and not take it as prescribed. Irish families may not praise or show overt affection to their children for fear of giving them "swelled heads," which therapists may misread as lack of caring. Physical punishment, routinely used to keep children in line by many groups, including, until recently, the dominant groups in the United States, may be perceived as idiosyncratic pathological behavior, rather than as culturally accepted behavior, albeit a violation of human rights. This is not to justify child beatings, which have been widely accepted by many cultures. Rather, we must consider the cultural context in which a behavior evolves, even as we try to shape it, when it does not reflect humanitarian or equitable values. The point is that therapists, especially those of dominant groups, who tend to take their own values as the norm, must be extremely cautious in judging the meaning of behavior they observe and in imposing their own methods and time table for change.

Almost all of us have multiple belief systems to which we turn when we need help. Besides medical or psychotherapeutic systems, we turn to religion, self-help groups, alcohol, yoga, chiropractors, crystals, special foods, and remedies our mothers taught us or those suggested by our friends. Various factors influence our choice of solutions that we will rely on at any given time. Many studies have shown that people differ in the following:

1. Their experience of pain.
2. What they label as a symptom.
3. How they communicate about their pain or symptoms.
4. Their beliefs about its cause.
5. Their attitudes toward helpers (doctors and therapists).
6. The treatment they desire or expect.

Yet a group whose characteristic response to illness is different from that of the dominant culture is likely to be labeled "abnormal." For example, one researcher found that doctors frequently labeled Italian patients as having psychiatric problems, although no evidence existed that such disorders occurred more frequently among them (Zola, 1966). Another classic study (Zborowski, 1969) found that Italian and Jewish patients complained much more than Irish or Anglo patients, who considered complaining to be "bad form."

CULTURAL ATTITUDES TOWARD "TALK" AND THERAPY

Another obvious and essential variable is the family's attitude toward therapy. The dominant assumption is that talk is good and can heal a person. Therapy has even been referred to as "the talking cure." Talking to the therapist or to other family members is seen as the path to healing. A high level of verbal interaction is expected in Jewish, Italian, and Greek families, whereas Anglo, Irish, and Scandinavian families have much less intense interaction and are more likely to deal with problems by distancing. Therapists need to take these potential differences into account in making an assessment, considering carefully their own biases and their clients' values. Clients may not talk openly in therapy for many different reasons related to their cultural background or values. Consider various cultures and the value they assign to talk:

• African American clients may be uncommunicative, not because they cannot deal with their feelings, but because the context involves a representative of a traditional "White" institution that they never had reason to trust (Chapter 6).

• In Jewish culture, analyzing and discussing one's experience may be as important as the experience itself for important historical reasons. Jews have long valued cognitive clarity. Analyzing and sharing ideas and perceptions help them find meaning in life. Given the anti-Semitic societies in which Jews have lived over the centuries, with their rights and experiences often invalidated, one can understand that they came to place great importance on analyzing, understanding, and acknowledgment of what has happened (Chapter 48).

• In families of English descent, words tend to be used primarily to accomplish one's goals (Chapter 37). They are valued mainly as utilitarian tools. As the son says about his brother's death in the movie *Ordinary People*: "What's the point of talking about it? It doesn't change anything."

• In Chinese culture, families may tend to avoid the dominant American idea of "laying your cards on the table" verbally. They have many other symbolic ways of communicating, such as with food, rather than with words, so the talking cure, as we have known it, would be a very foreign concept (Chapter 22).

• Italians often use words primarily for drama, to convey the emotional intensity of an experience. They may be mystified when others, who may take verbal expression at face value, hold them to their words, because for them it is the interaction and the emotional relationship, not the words, that have the deepest meaning (Chapter 44).

• An Irish client's failure to talk may have to do with embarrassment about admitting his or her feelings to anyone, most especially to other family members. The Irish were forced by the British, who ruled them for centuries, to give up their language, which they found a cruel punishment. They are perhaps the world's greatest poets, using words to buffer experience—poetry and humor somehow make reality more tolerable. They have tended to use words not particularly to tell the truth, but often, rather, to cover it up or embellish it. The Irish have raised poetry, mystification, double meanings, humorous indirection, and ambiguity to an art form, in part, perhaps, because their history of oppression led them to realize that telling the truth could be dangerous (Chapter 43).

• Norwegians may withhold verbal expression out of respect and politeness, which for them involves not openly stating negative feelings they have about other family members. Such a custom may have nothing to do with guilt about "unacceptable" feelings or awkwardness in a therapy context, as it might for the Irish (Chapter 46).

• In Sioux Indian culture, talking is actually proscribed in certain family relationships. A wife does not talk directly to her father-in-law, for example, yet she may experience deep intimacy with him, a relationship that is almost inconceivable in our pragmatic world. The reduced emphasis on verbal expression seems to free Native American families for other kinds of experiences of each other, of nature, and of the spiritual realm (Chapters 2 and 3).

CULTURAL DIFFERENCES IN WHAT IS VIEWED AS A PROBLEM

Concomitantly, groups vary in what they view as problematic behavior. Anglos may be uncomfortable with dependency or emotionality; the Irish are distressed by a family member "making a scene"; Italians, about disloyalty to the family; Greeks, about any insult to their pride or *filotimo*; Jews, about their children not being "successful"; Puerto Ricans, about their children not showing respect; Arabs, about their daughters' virginity. For Chinese families harmony is a key dimension, and for African Americans bearing witness and testifying about their suffering is a central concept.

Of course, cultural groups also vary in how they respond to problems. Anglos see work, reason, and stoicism as the best responses, whereas Jews often consult doctors and therapists to gain understanding and insight. Until recently, the Irish responded to problems by going to the priest for confession, "offering up" their suffering in prayers, or, especially for men, seeking solace through drink. Italians may prefer to rely on family support, eating, and expressing themselves. West Indians may see hard work, thrift, or consulting with their elders as the solution, and Norwegians may prefer fresh air or exercise. Asian Indians may focus on sacrifice or purity, and the Chinese, on food or prayer to their ancestors.

Groups differ as well in attitudes toward seeking help. In general, Italians rely primarily on the family and turn to an outsider only as a last resort. African Americans have long mistrusted the help they can receive from traditional institutions, except the church, the only institution that was "theirs." Puerto Ricans and Chinese may somatize when under stress and seek medical rather than mental health services. Norwegians, too, often convert emotional tensions into physical symptoms, which they consider more acceptable; thus their preference for doctors over psychotherapists. Likewise, Iranians may view medication and vitamins as a necessary part of treating symptoms. And some groups tend to see their problems as the result of their own sin, action, or inadequacy (Irish, African Americans, Norwegians) or someone else's (Greeks, Iranians, Puerto Ricans).

CULTURAL DIFFERENCES IN SOCIAL ORGANIZATION AND GROUP BOUNDARIES

Cultures differ also in their attitudes about group boundaries. Many Puerto Ricans, Italians, and Greeks have similar rural, peasant backgrounds, yet there are important ethnic differences among these groups. Puerto Ricans tend to have flexible boundaries between the family and the surrounding community, so that informal adoption is a common and accepted practice. Italians have much clearer boundaries within the family and draw rigid lines between insiders and outsiders. Greeks have very definite family boundaries, are disinclined to adopt children, and have deep feelings about the "bloodline." They are also strongly nationalistic, a value that relates to a nostalgic vision of ancient Greece and to the country they lost after hundreds of years under Ottoman oppression. In contrast, Italians in the "old country" defined themselves first by family ties, second, by their village, and, third, if at all, by the region of Italy from which they came. It was only within a U.S. context that defining themselves by their ethnicity became relevant as they experienced discrimination by others. Puerto Ricans' group identity has coalesced only within the past century, primarily in reaction to the United States' oppression. Each group's way of relating to therapy will reflect its differing attitudes toward family, group identity, and outsiders, although certain family characteristics, such as male dominance and role complementarity, are similar for all three of these groups.

Groups differ in other patterns of social organization as well. African Americans and Jewish families tend to be more democratic, with greater role flexibility, whereas Greeks (Chapter 41) and Asian cultures (Chapter 20) tend to be structured in a much more hierarchical fashion. Such differences will significantly influence how a person may respond to meetings of the whole family together versus individual coaching or meeting with same-sex subgroups of family members. Therapists need to be aware of how their methods of intervention fit for clients of different backgrounds.

NOT ROMANTICIZING CULTURE

Just because a culture espouses certain values or beliefs does not make them sacrosanct. All cultural practices are not ethical. Mistreatment of women or children, or gays or lesbians, through disrespect, as well as physical or sexual abuse, is a human rights issue, no matter in what cultural context it occurs. Every intervention we make is value laden. We must not use notions of neutrality or "deconstruction" to shy away from committing ourselves to the values we believe in. We must have the courage of our convictions, even while realizing that we can never be completely certain that our perspective is the "correct" one. It means we must learn to tolerate ambiguities and continue to question our stance in relation to the positions and values of our clients. And we must be especially careful about the power differential if we are part of the dominant group, since the voices of those who are marginalized are harder to hear. The disenfranchised need more support to have their position heard than do those who feel they are entitled because theirs are the dominant values.

In addressing racism, we must also deal with the oppression of women of color and of homosexual, bisexual, and transgender people. This cannot be blamed solely on White society, for patriarchy and heterosexism are deeply embedded in African, Asian, and

Latin American cultures. We must work for the right of every person to a voice and a sense of safety and belonging. We must challenge those who argue that cultural groups should be allowed to "speak for themselves." This ignores the issue of who speaks for a group, which is usually determined largely by patriarchal and class factors. Helping families define what is normal, in the sense of healthy, may require supporting marginalized voices within the cultural group that express liberating possibilities for family adaptation. This requires making a careful cultural assessment (see the Appendix).

ETHNICITY TRAINING

Although there has been a burgeoning literature on ethnicity since the first edition of this book was published in 1982, integration of material on ethnicity in mental health professional training remains a "special issue," ignored for the most part in research, taught at the periphery of psychotherapy training, and rarely written about or recognized as crucial by or for therapists of European origin (Chambless et al., 1996; Murry, Smith, & Hill, 2001). For this perspective to become truly integrated into our work will require a transformation of our field, which has barely begun (Green, 1998a, 1998b).

In our view, the most important part of ethnicity training involves the therapist coming to understand his or her own ethnic identity (Hardy & Laszloffy, 1992, 1995a; Laszloffy & Hardy, 2000). Just as clinicians must sort out the relationships in their own families of origin, developing cultural competence requires coming to terms with one's own ethnic identity. Ideally, therapists would no longer be "triggered" by ethnic characteristics they may have regarded negatively, or caught in the ethnocentric view that their own cultural values are more "right" or "true" than those of others. Ethnically self-aware therapists achieve a multiethnic perspective, which opens them to understanding values that differ from their own, so that they neither need to convert others to their view, nor give up their own values. Our underlying openness to those who are culturally different is the key to expanding our cultural understanding. We learn about culture primarily not by learning the "facts" of another's culture, but rather by changing our own attitudes about cultural difference. Indeed, David McGill (Chapter 37) has suggested that the best training for family therapists might be to live in another culture and learn a foreign language. That experience might best help the clinician achieve the humility necessary for respectful cultural interactions that are based on more than a one-way hierarchy of normality, truth, and wisdom. The best cultural training for family therapists may be to experience what it is like to not be part of the dominant culture.

Cultural paradigms are useful to the extent that they help us challenge our long-held beliefs about "the way things are." But we cannot learn about culture cookbook fashion, through memorizing recipes for relating to other ethnic groups. Information we learn about cultural differences will, we hope, expand our respect, curiosity, and humility regarding cultural differences.

Our experience has taught us repeatedly that theoretical discussions about the importance of ethnicity are practically useless in training clinicians (McGoldrick, 1998). We come to appreciate the relativity of values best through specifics that connect with our lived experience of group differences. Thus, in our training we try to fit any illustration of a cultural trait into the context of historical and cultural experiences in which that value or behavior evolved. We ask trainees to think about how their own groups, and perhaps those of their spouses or close friends, differ in responding to pain, in their attitudes about doctors, and in their beliefs about suffering. Do they prefer a formal or informal style in dealing with strangers? Do they tend to feel positive about their bodies, about work, about physical, sexual, psychological, or spiritual intimacy, or about children expressing their feelings? Then we try to help them broaden this understanding to other groups through readings, films, and conversations that illustrate other ways of viewing the same phenomena.

When beginning cultural training, it is extremely important to set up a safe context, which allows for generalizing about cultural differences. Of course, all generalizations represent only partial truths. We begin by personal sharing, conveying that everyone has grown up influenced by culture, class, race, gender, and sexual orientation. We discuss the problem of stereotyping (e.g., becoming stuck in an overgeneralization) and the problem of not generalizing (e.g., that it prevents culture from being discussed at all).

As the training evolves, we discuss the implications of people's social location, which becomes a core part of our assessment of each case, both for ourselves and the client. A power analysis of cultural, racial, class and gender politics becomes a core part of all training, so that clinicians can see how power affects all clinical interactions (Hardy & Laszloffy, 1992, 1995b; Laszloffy & Hardy, 2000).

The training usually proceeds from the personal, to the theoretical, to the clinical implications. We frequently use an exercise in which trainees discuss their own social location and how it has shifted over the course of their own and their family's cultural journey in the United States since immigration. We do this by actually spreading index cards on the floor showing a hierarchical listing of social locations by class (from the upper class—those who live on inherited wealth, to the poor—who may grow up without even the hope of employment), with subhierarchies for gender, race, and sexual orientation. Trainees take turns moving along this hierarchy on the floor as they describe their personal and family evolution. As they do this, they explore the influence of ethnicity and religion on the hierarchies of class, race, gender, and sexual orientation. They also show how education, migration, employment, finances, health, and marital status have influenced their positions. This exercise helps trainees understand that cultural dimensions are not individual issues, but are socially structured within the sociopolitical context.

We have found that to organize training only around "minority" ethnicities, as has so often been done, is not helpful. Such training perpetuates the marginalization of groups that are already at the periphery, because they continue the myth that Western theories (developed by Europeans and White Americans) are the norm from which all other cultures deviate. Instead, training entails considerable deconstruction of "Western" ways of thought to challenge the dominant psychological structures as an essential part of freeing people to become more culturally competent.

We have found a number of common pitfalls in discussions of diversity:

1. The discussion may become polarized, particularly in regard to the Black experience of White racism, leaving other people of color feeling invisible or excluded. People get lost in arguments over which oppression is the worst or most important, This typically leads to the withdrawal of those who feel that their own issues of oppression are marginalized in such a dialogue.

2. People tend to think much more easily about their oppression than about their privilege, and are thus likely to move quickly from acknowledgment of racism and White

supremacy to talk about the impact of sexual abuse, sexual orientation, poverty, or some other disadvantage. This has the effect of short-circuiting the discussion of racism. As other differences are discussed, racism becomes submerged and sidelined.

3. We believe that staying at the table is everything, and we make great efforts to explain that if we are to succeed in moving conversations about race and other oppression forward, staying in the conversation is the primary requirement. We try to emphasize that the conversations may get sticky, uncomfortable, or intense and that we will all make mistakes as we go along. But persevering with the conversation is everything—not letting the issues get resubmerged, which, as Ken Hardy puts it, always leads to cutoff, war, destruction, and, ultimately, death (Hardy & Laszloffy, 2000).

We consider it essential to keep a multidimensional perspective that highlights the overwhelming reality of institutionalized racism while also including other forms of oppression. At the same time we have found that it helps to let the group know about the dynamics of power, privilege, and oppression early in the conversation and to say that in terms of social location, all of us have privilege on certain dimensions and experience oppression on others. We then share guidelines that may help trainees notice how these power dynamics work and how people can monitor themselves. They can notice their own inclination to shift a discussion from a dimension on which they have privilege to one on which they are oppressed. The following are some of the guidelines we lay out in training to help participants monitor their own reactions and increase their sensitivity to others:

The impact of privilege on our vision

- The more privilege we have, the harder it is to think about how our own actions have affected others with less privilege.
- We take our privilege for granted—our right to safety, acknowledgment, being heard, being treated fairly, being taken care of; our right to take up the available time, space, and resources, etc.
- The more power and privilege we have, the harder it is to think about the meaning of the rage of the powerless.

How Whites often respond to attempts to discuss racism

- They distinguish themselves from those with power and privilege by emphasizing their other oppressions: They refer to their great-grandfather, who was Cherokee, their own history of oppression as Irish, Jewish, gay, poor, disabled, or being from an abusive or mentally ill family. We experience oppression ourselves, they say, why focus only on racism?
- They shift the discussion to the internalized racism of people of color against themselves or of one group against another: the issue of skin color within African American families, conflicts between Latinos or Koreans and African Americans, etc.).
- They resist group categories, saying, "We're just human beings." "We do not think of people by color, culture, or class, but as unique human beings." "You're creating the problem by forcing us into categories. It's stereotyping." "I don't identify as White. It's not fair to force me into this categorization. It's reverse racism."

"How can you blame a whole race for a few individuals? My ancestors weren't even here during slavery. It's not fair for you to blame me for these problems."

- They say they feel "unsafe" in an atmosphere of "political correctness," that it makes them feel they are walking on egg shells, which focuses the discussion on their discomfort, implicitly blaming those who are attempting to discuss oppression for making them uncomfortable. Such assertions make it impossible to have a discussion about their privilege.
- They accept criticism, but then assume a talking position, refocusing the discussion on their feelings of shame. By doing so, they are implicitly asking others to listen or to take care of their pain about their racist behavior, and thus keep the focus on themselves.
- They disqualify the issue or the one who raises it, by saying things like:

  "Why do people always have to bring up the past? Slavery ended 140 years ago."

  "People of color get so angry when they talk about these issues that it's impossible to talk with them. I don't want to talk until they can deal with these issues in a more appropriate way."

  "They never point out the clinical implications of these issues."

- They feel confused, thinking, "I'm certainly not a racist. I can't think of anything to say on this topic."

African American responses to a discussion of racism

- "It's too painful and overwhelming. I feel so weary always having to lead Whites in these discussions, and they never get it anyway."
- "Even when they claim to acknowledge racism, they always go back to individual thinking when they assess the behavior of a person of color. They don't get excited about Rodney King or Amadou Diallo, but are apalled about O. J. Simpson."
- "Racism makes me feel so much rage. I hate to get into it. I have to choose my battles. Why should I go into it here?"
- "When I was a child we could not even eat next to a White person or use the Whites' drinking fountain, and they still don't get it."
- "I wish I knew how to protect my children from racism. I worry about how I will handle it the first time my child comes home having experienced a racist insult."

What White people need to do in response to people of color discussing their experiences of racism (Hardy, 2004)

- Resist the temptation to equalize the experience with a description of their own suffering.
- Resist refocusing the conversation on their good intentions.
- Listen and believe. Resist any response that could negate the experience that is being described. The only reasonable position for people of privilege to take is to "listen and believe."

Guidelines for accountability in training

- Racist patterns are most likely to be replicated when there is only one member of a traditionally oppressed group present. Whites are more likely to learn about oppression and privilege in a group where the majority are people of color, a context that rarely occurs for White people.

- The most culturally competent structure has people of color at every level of the hierarchy.
- If that is not possible, consultation to the upper levels of the hierarchy from an outside group with experience in dealing with racism, and partnerships at other levels with consultants of color, can help the organization move in this direction as well.
- It helps to have at least three perspectives present in any discussion to minimize polarization.

In our experience presentations on a single group are rarely successful, because participants tend to focus on the exceptions to the "rule." We find that presenting two groups is also problematic, because it leads to polarizing so-called opposites. Discussion becomes more meaningful when three or more groups are discussed together, at least until there is a general acceptance by the trainees of the importance of culture in clinical discussions. This is especially important because of our society's tendency to polarize: Black/White, male/female, gay/straight, rich/poor. It is always valuable to create a context in which overlapping and ambiguous differences cannot easily be resolved, because that fits better with the complexities of human experience. Presenting several groups also tends to help students see the pattern, rather than the exception. Thus, although not all Dominicans may be alike, they may have certain similarities when compared with Haitians, Russians, or Greeks.

In training groups we often ask participants to (1) describe themselves ethnically, (2) describe who in their families influenced their sense of ethnic identity, (3) discuss which groups other than their own they think they understand best, (4) discuss the characteristics of their ethnic group they like most, and which they like least, and (5) discuss how they think their own families would react to having to go to family therapy and what kind of approach they would prefer.

CONCLUSION

The following guidelines, based on our years of clinical experience, suggest the kind of inclusive thinking necessary for judging family problems and normal adaptation in a cultural context (Giordano & Giordano, 1995; McGoldrick, 1998):

- Assume that the family's cultural, class, religious, and political background influences how its members view their problems until you have evidence to the contrary.
- Assume that having a positive awareness of one's cultural heritage, just like a positive connection to one's family of origin, contributes to one's sense of mental health and well-being.
- Assume that a negative feeling or lack of awareness of one's cultural heritage is probably reflective of cutoffs, oppression, or traumatic experiences that have led to suppression of the person's history.
- Assume that no one can ever fully understand another's culture, but that curiosity,

humility, and awareness of one's own cultural values and history will contribute to sensitive interviewing.

- Assume that clients from marginalized cultures have probably internalized society's prejudices about them and that those from dominant cultural groups have probably internalized assumptions about their own superiority and right to be privileged within our society.

Respectful clinical work involves helping people clarify their cultural identity and self-identity in relation to family, community, and their history, while also adapting to changing circumstances as they move through life.

REFERENCES

Alba, R. D. (1990). *Ethnic identity: The transformation of white America*. New Haven, CT: Yale University Press.

Alibhai-Brown, Y., & Montague, A. (1992). *The colour of love: Mixed race relationships*. London: Virago Press.

Angelou, M. (1986). *All God's children need traveling shoes*. New York: Vintage.

Aponte, H. (1994). *Bread and spirit*. New York: Norton.

Banks, J. A. (1991). *Teaching strategies for ethnic studies* (5th ed.). Boston: Allyn & Bacon.

Bateson, M. C. (1995). *Peripheral vision: Learning along the way*. New York: Perennial.

Bell, D. (1993). *Faces at the bottom of the well: The permanence of racism*. New York: Basic Books.

Betancourt, J. R. (2004). Cultural competence: Marginal or mainstream movement? *New England Journal of Medicine, 351*(10), 953–954.

Betancourt, J. R, Green, A. R., Carrillo, J. E., & Ananeh-Firempong, O. (2003). Defining cultural competence: A practical framework for addressing racial/ethnic disparities in health and healthcare. *Public Health Reports, 118*(4), 293–302.

Boyd-Franklin, N. (2002). Race, class and poverty. In F. Walsh (Ed.), *Normal family processes: Growing diversity and complexity* (3rd ed., pp. 260–279). New York: Guilford Press.

Boyd-Franklin, N. (2003). *Black families in therapy: Understanding the African American experience* (2nd ed.). New York: Guilford Press.

Boyd-Franklin, N., & Lockwood, T. W. (1999). Spirituality and religion: Implications for psychotherapy with African American clients and families. In F. Walsh (Ed.), *Spiritual resources in family therapy* (pp. 90–103). New York: Guilford Press.

Braden, A. (1999). *The wall between*. Knoxville: University of Tennessee Press.

Carter, B., & McGoldrick, M. (Eds.). (2005). *The expanded family life cycle: Individual, family and social perspectives* (Classic ed.). Boston: Allyn & Bacon.

Carter, R. T. (1995). *The influence of race and racial identity in psychotherapy*. New York: Wiley.

Chambless, D. L., Crits-Cristoph, P., Baker, M., Johnson, B., Woody, S. R., Sue, S., et al. (1996). An update on empirically validated therapies. *Clinical Psychologist, 49*, 5–18.

Crohn, J. (1995). *Mixed matches: How to create successful interracial, interethnic, and interfaith relationships*. New York: Fawcett Columbine.

Cushing, B., & McGoldrick, M. (2004). The differentiation of self and faith in young adulthood. In F. B. Kelcourse (Ed.), *Human development and faith*. St. Louis, MO: Chalice.

Dilworth-Anderson, P., & Burton, L. M. (1996). Rethinking family development: Critical conceptual issues in the study of diverse groups. *Journal of Social and Personal Relationships, 13*(3), 325–334.

Dilworth-Anderson, P., Burton, L., & Johnson, L. (1993). Reframing theories for understanding race, ethnicity and families. In P. G. Boss, W. J. Doherty, R. LaRossa, W. R. Schumm, & S. K. Steinmetz (Eds.), *Sourcebook of family theories and methods: A contextual approach*. New York: Plenum Press.

Erdrich, L., & Dorris, M. (1991). *The crown of Columbus*. New York: Harper.

Fadiman, A. (1997). *The spirit catches you and you fall down*. New York: Farrar, Straus & Giroux.

Falicov, C. J. (2002). Immigrant family processes. In F. Walsh (Ed.), *Normal family processes: Growing diversity and complexity* (3rd ed., pp. 280–300). New York: Guilford Press.

Franklin, A. J. (2004). *From brotherhood to manhood: How Black men resuce their relationships and dreams from the invisibility syndrome*. Hoboken, NJ: Wiley.

Frederickson, G. M. (2002). *Racism: A short history*. Princeton, NJ: Princeton University Press.

Freire, P. (1994). *The pedagogy of hope*. New York: Continuum.

Gallup, G., Jr., & Lindsay, D. M. (1999). *Surveying the religious landscape: Trends in U. S. beliefs*. Harrisburg, PA: Morehouse.

Gallup Organization. (2004, July 22). *Americans divided on immigration*. Princeton: Gallup Poll News Service.

Giordano, J., & Giordano, M. A. (1995). Ethnic dimensions in family therapy. In R. Mikesell, D. Lusterman, & S. McDaniel (Eds.), *Integrating family therapy*. Washington, DC: American Psychological Association.

Goldner, V. (1988). Generation and gender: Normative and covert hierarchies. In M. McGoldrick, C. Anderson, & F. Walsh (Eds.), *Women in families*. New York: Norton.

Gould, S. J. (1994, November). The geometer or race. *Discover*, p. 1.

Greeley, A. (1969). *Why can't they be like us?* New York: American Jewish Committee.

Green, R.-J. (1998a). Race and the field of family therapy. In M. McGoldrick (Ed.), *Re-visioning family therapy: Race, culture, and gender in clinical practice* (pp. 93–110). New York: Guilford Press.

Green, R.-J. (1998b). Training program: Guidelines for multicultural transformation. In M. McGoldrick (Ed.), *Re-visioning family therapy: Race, culture, and gender in clinical practice* (pp. 111–117). New York: Guilford Press.

Hacker, Andrew (1995, November 19). Who they are. *New York Times Magazine*, pp. 70–71.

Hall, S. (1987). Minimal selves. In H. K. Bhabe et al. (Eds.), *Identity: The real me: Post-modernism and the question of identity* (ICA Documents, No. 6, pp. 44–46). London: Institute of Contemporary Arts.

Hardy, K. V. (2004). Race, reality, and relationships: Implications for family therapists. In S. Madigan (Ed.), *Therapeutic conversations 5: Therapy from the outside in* (pp. 87–98). Vancouver, BC, Canada: Yaletown Family Therapy.

Hardy, K. V., & Laszloffy, T. A. (1992). Training racially sensitive family therapists: Context, content and contact. *Families in Society, 73*(6), 363–370.

Hardy, K. V., & Laszloffy, T. A. (1995). The cultural genogram: Key to training culturally competent family therapists. *Journal of Marital and Family Therapy, 21*(3), 227–237.

Hardy, K. V., & Laszloffy, T. A. (1995). Deconstructing race in family therapy. *Journal of Feminist Family Therapy, 5*(3–4), 5–33.

Hayden, T. (Ed.). (1998). *Irish hunger*. Boulder, CO: Roberts Reinhart.

Hayden, T. (2001). *Irish on the inside: In search of the soul of Irish America*. New York: Verso.

Hernandez, M., & McGoldrick, M. (2005). Migration and the family life cycle. In B. Carter & M. McGoldrick (Eds.), *The expanded family life cycle*. Boston: Allyn & Bacon.

Hitchcock, J. (2003). *Lifting the white veil: An exploration of white American culture in a multiracial context*. Roselle, NJ: Crandall Dostie & Douglass Books.

Hodge, D. R. (2001). Spiritual genograms: A genenerational approach to assessing spirituality. *Families in Society: The Journal of Contemporary Human Services*, pp. 35–48.

Ignatiev, N. (1995). *How the Irish became white*. New York: Routledge.

Jamieson, D., & O'Mara, J. (1991). *Managing workforce 2000*. San Francisco: Jossey-Bass.

Jones, A. C. (1993). *Wade in the water: The wisdom of the spirituals*. Maryknoll, NY: Orbis.

Kaiser, W. L. (2001). *A new view of the world: Handbook to the Peters projection world map*. New York: Friendship Press.

Katz, J. H. (1978). *White awareness: Handbook for anti-racism training.* Norman: University of Oklahoma Press.

Kennedy, R. (2003). *Interracial intimacies: Sex, marriage, identity, and adoption.* New York: Pantheon.

Kivel, P. (2002). *Uprooting racism: How White people can work for racial justice.* New York: New Society.

Kosmin, B., & Lachman, S. (2001). *American Religious Identity Survey (ARIS).* New York: Graduate School of the City University of New York. www.gc.cuny.edu/studies/aris_index.htm

Laszloffy, T. A., & Hardy, K. V. (2000). Uncommon strategies for a common problem: Addressing racism in family therapy. *Family Process, 39*(1), 35–50.

Lewis, B. (2002). *What went wrong: Western impact and Middle Eastern response.* New York: Oxford University Press.

Lopez, S. R., & Guarnaccia, P. (2000). Cultural psychopathology: Uncovering the social world of mental illness. *American Review of Psychology, 51,* 571–598.

Lorde, A. (1992). Age, race, class, and sex: Women redefining difference. In M. Anderson & P. H. Collins (Eds.), *Race, class, and gender: An anthology* (pp. 495–502). Belmont, CA: Wadsworth.

Luepnitz, D. (1992). *The family interpreted.* New York: Basic Books.

Mahmoud, V. M. (1998). The double binds of wisdom. In M. McGoldrick (Ed.), *Re-visioning family therapy: Race, culture, gender, and clinical practice* (pp. 255–267). New York: Guilford Press.

Malcomson, S. (2000). *One drop of blood. The American misadventure of race.* New York: Farrar, Straus & Giroux.

Martinez, R. (2004). *The new Americans.* New York: The New Press.

McGoldrick, M. (Ed.). (1998). *Re-visioning family therapy: Race, culture, and gender in clinical practice.* New York: Guilford Press.

McGoldrick, M. (2002). Culture: A challenge to concepts of normality. In F. Walsh (Ed.), *Normal family processes: Growing diversity and complexity* (3rd ed., pp. 235–259). New York: Guilford Press.

McGoldrick, M., Anderson, C., & Walsh, F. (Eds.). (1989). *Women in families.* New York: Norton.

McGoldrick, M., & Garcia-Preto, N. (1984). Ethnic intermarriage. *Family Process, 23*(3), 347–362.

McGoldrick, M., Gerson, R., & Schellenberger, S. (1999). *Genograms: Assessment and intervention.* New York: Norton.

McGoldrick, M., Marsh Schlesinger, J., Hines, P., Lee, E., Chan, J., Almeida, R., et al. (2004). Mourning in different cultures: English, Irish, African American, Chinese, Asian Indian, Jewish, Latino, and Brazilian. In F. Walsh & M. McGoldrick (Eds.), *Living beyond loss* (2nd ed.). New York: Norton.

McGoldrick, M., & Rohrbaugh, M. (1987). Researching ethnic family stereotypes. *Family Process, 26,* 89–98.

McIntosh, P. (1998). White privilege: Unpacking the invisible knapsack. In M. McGoldrick (Ed.), *Re-visioning family therapy: Race, culture, and gender in clinical practice* (pp. 147–152). New York: Guilford Press.

Miller, W. R., & Thoresen, C. E. (2003). Spirituality, religion and health. *American Psychologist, 58*(1), 24–35.

Morgan, E. S. (2002). *Benjamin Franklin.* New Haven, CT: Yale University Press.

Morris, E. (Producer & Director). (2003). *The fog of war* [Film]. Available from Sony Pictures.

Murry, V. M., Smith, E. P., & Hill, N. E. (2001). Race, ethnicity and culture in studies of families in context. *Journal of Marriage and the Family, 63*(4), 911–914.

Ortiz, A., Simmons, J., & Hinton, W. L. (1999). Locations of remorse and homelands of resilience: Notes on grief and sense of loss of place of Latino and Irish-American caregivers of demented elders. *Culture, Medicine and Psychiatry, 23,* 477–500.

Petsonk, J., & Remsen, J. (1988). *The intermarriage handbook: A guide for Jews and Christians.* New York: William Morrow.

Pinderhughes, E. (1989). *Understanding race, ethnicity and power*. New York: Free Press.

Roberts, S. (2004). *Who we are now: The changing face of America in the 21st century*. New York: Times Books.

Root, M. P. P. (Ed.). (1992). *Racially mixed people in America*. Thousand Oaks, CA: Sage.

Root, M. P. P. (Ed) (1996). *The multiracial experience: Racial borders as the new frontier*. Thousand Oaks, CA: Sage.

Root, M. P. P. (2001). *Love's revolution: Interracial marriage*. Philadelphia: Temple University Press.

Root, M. P. P. (2003). Bill of rights for racially mixed people. In M. P. P. Root & M. Kelley (Eds.), *Multiracial child resource book*. Seattle, WA: Mavin.

Schneider, S. W. (1989). *Intermarriage: The challenge of living with differences*. New York: Free Press.

Simpson, E. (1987). *Orphans: Real and imaginary*. New York: New American Library.

Tatum, B. D. (2003). *"Why are all the Black kids sitting together in the cafeteria?": And other conversations about race* (rev. ed.). New York: Basic Books.

Tataki, R. (1993). *A different mirror: A history of multicultural America*. Boston: Little, Brown.

Tataki. R. (2002). *Debating diversity: Clashing perspectives on race and ethnicity in America* (3rd ed.). New York: Oxford.

Thiederman, S. (1991). *Profiting in America's multicultural marketplace: How to do business across cultural lines*. New York: Lexington.

Thomas, R. (1991). *Beyond race and gender*. New York: American Management Association.

Thurow, L. (1995, November 19). Why their world might crumble. *New York Times Magazine*.

Vermuelen, M. (1995, June 18). What people earn. *Parade Magazine*, pp. 4–6.

Walsh, F. (Ed.). (1999). *Spiritual resources in family therapy*. New York: Guilford Press.

Walsh, F., & Pryce, J. (2002). The spiritual dimension of family life. In F. Walsh (Ed.), *Normal family processes: Growing diversity and complexity* (3rd ed., pp. 337–372). New York: Guilford Press.

Wheeler, D., Avis, J., Miller, L., & Chaney, S. (1985). Rethinking family therapy training and supervision: A feminist model. *Journal of Psychotherapy and the Family*, 1, 53–71.

Zborowski, M. (1969). *People in pain*. San Francisco: Jossey-Bass.

Zinn, H. (2003). *A people's history of the United States* (rev. ed.). New York: Harper.

Zola, I. K. (1966). Culture and symptoms: An analysis of patients' presenting complaints. *American Sociological Review*, 5, 615–630.

PART I

AMERICAN INDIAN AND PACIFIC ISLANDER FAMILIES

CHAPTER 2

American Indian Families

An Overview

CharlesEtta T. Sutton

Mary Anne Broken Nose

An objective of the Decade is the promotion and protection of the rights of indigenous people and their empowerment to make choices which enable them to retain their cultural identity while participating in political, economic and social life, with full respect for their cultural values, languages, traditions and forms of social organization.

—General Assembly Resolution 50/157 (December 21, 1995)

You were born here, she was born here, and so was I. We are all Native Americans. My relatives were here when Columbus and other explorers discovered the Americas. I like to be called an Indigenous person belonging to an Indigenous Nation, the Poncas, in North America.

—Parrish Williams, Ponca Elder, personal communication (December 3, 2002)

Since the time of Columbus, inaccurate and conflicting images have characterized the dominant culture's concept of American Indians. Europeans thought of Indians as either, innocent savages living in a primitive paradise or as heathens and bloodthirsty fiends. Explorers, settlers, missionaries, and political leaders all exploited these images for their own purposes. When viewed through the lens of European beliefs and customs, Europeans saw Indian culture generally as barbaric. Even the design of "humanistic" policies of Indian advocates, such as those of 18th-century reformers, was to "educate the Indian out of the Indian." In retrospect, their impact was almost as devastating as the U.S. army's genocidal policies (Berkhoffer, 1978).

Early Spanish explorers first gave one name, "Indios," to all the indigenous peoples living in America, rather than seeing them as diverse ethnic groups. When the Europeans first sailed to this land, at least "two thousand cultures and more societies practiced a multiplicity of customs and life styles, held an enormous variety of values and beliefs, spoke numerous languages mutually unintelligible to the many speakers, and did not conceive of themselves as a single people—if they knew about each other at all" (Berkhoffer, 1978, p. 3).

Europeans' concern was that the new people they encountered were neither Christian nor culturally familiar. By labeling these aboriginal people as "uncivilized," they were able to make decisions concerning them more easily, as well as to justify the atrocities they committed. This blurring of distinctions between tribal groups continues today.

The entertainment industry has offered a distortion of American Indian customs and culture. The images created by the early dime novelists and, later, by movies had little to do with reality. They sometimes placed tribes in the wrong parts of the country or had a character who was supposed to be Cherokee speak Lakota and practice Mohawk ceremonies. What they often portrayed was not an Arapaho, Cheyenne, or Ute, but a generic "Indian." Unfortunately, most Americans having very little day-to-day contact with American Indians and often obtain their main and largely inaccurate impressions through the media.

Indians are changing this view by using the very institutions that have done so much to malign them to portray a more accurate picture of their history and society. Many school systems are developing curricula featuring Indian history. Documentaries produced by American Indians tell the stories of their individual nations. There are now Indian-owned and operated radio stations, TV networks, newspapers, and publishing companies. A new respect for Indians' positive influences on the dominant culture is replacing old concepts and stereotypes (Adams, 2002).

Environmental groups applaud Indians' respect for nature. Theologians, as well as New Age spiritualists, embrace Indian ceremonial life. Feminists and sociologists study many of the first nations' democratic social structures. Educational and behavioral health care settings are incorporating Native American teachings and rituals, such as sweat lodge ceremonies and talking circles, into their practices. More dominant culture and mixed-race people are searching their family histories for Indian roots.

NATIVE AMERICANS IN HISTORICAL AND CULTURAL CONTEXT

Demographics

The terms "Native American" and "American Indian" are labels that encompass a diversity of languages, lifestyles, religions kinship systems, and community structures (Polacca, 1995). Many tribes are sovereign nations, both in law and through treaties.

There are many ways of defining "Indian": by genetic definition—having a certain percentage of Indian blood as established by the Federal Register of the United States; by community recognition—being recognized as Indian by other Indians is paramount, because federal and state governments do not recognize all tribes; by enrollment in a recognized tribe; and by self-declaration, the method used by the Census Bureau.

According to the 2000 Census, 2.5 million people identified themselves being American Indian, with another 1.6 million reporting they were Indian and of another race. (U.S. Bureau of the Census, 2000). There are 562 federally recognized tribes (U.S. Department of the Interior, 2004). Many tribal members live in urban areas, and those on the reservations may spend time away looking for work, education, and other opportunities. Most major cities have a substantial Indian population, with New York and Los Angeles having the largest.

There is a wide range of cultural identification among Indians. Some consider themselves American Indian because they have a great-grandparent who was Indian. Others are born on reservations and enter school speaking a mixture of their native language and English. Still others grow up in the city and have no knowledge of tribal language or customs. A large group, however, move in and out of both worlds, trying to maintain a precarious balance between their Indian and American identities.

Family Structure and Obligations

Family represents the cornerstone for the social and emotional well-being of individuals and communities.

—RED HORSE (1981, p. 1)

The ultimate aim of Dakota life, stripped of accessories, was quite simple: One must obey kinship rules; one must be a good relative. No Dakota who has participated in that life will dispute that. In the last analysis every other consideration was secondary—property, personal ambition, glory, good times, life itself. Without that aim and the constant struggle to attain it, the people would no longer be Dakota in truth. They would no longer even be human. To be a good Dakota, then, was to be humanized, civilized. And to be civilized was to keep the rules imposed by kinship for achieving civility, good manners and a sense of responsibility toward every individual dealt with. Thus only was it possible to live communally with success, that is to say, a minimum of friction and a maximum of good will.

—DELORIA (1944, cited in Gunn, 1989, p. 11)

Although the extended family is typical of American Indians, its core is quite different from that of the dominant culture. Family therapist Terry Tafoya (1989) explains: "In many Native American languages, cousins are all referred to as brother and sister. The primary relationship is not the parents, but rather that of grandparents" (p. 32). This reflects the grandparents' role as caregiver and provider of training and discipline.

The grandparent role is not limited to what is called a "grandparent" in English, but is opened up to include other relations such as a "grand aunt," and could be extended to include . . . a "Godparent." Parent roles include not only the biological parents, but also those who have a sibling relation to the biological parents. The biological parents of the central siblings would then have specific responsibility over their nieces and nephews. . . . (pp. 32–33)

Many Indian cultures do not have a term for in-law; rather, a daughter-in-law is a daughter; a sister-in-law, a sister. Families make no distinctions between natural and inducted by marriage family members once one marries into an Indian family. This concept is foreign to White Anglo-Saxon, Protestant family norms. Thus, families blend, not join, through marriage. Medicine people[1] and non-blood relatives are sometimes made part of the family. This is similar to what happens in African American and Latino families, where the relationship, not blood, determines the family role.

A therapist working with a Lakota Sioux couple obtained an initial family history. When Joseph, the father, learned that one of his grandfathers had died, the therapist pulled out the genogram and did not find his name listed as a grandfather. For the non-Indian therapist, the deceased was the client's paternal great-uncle. The client explained that all his grandfather's brothers were his grandfathers. "So, you call your great-uncles 'grandfather'?" inquired the therapist. "No," replied Joseph, "I don't call them that; that is what they are, my grandfathers." At this moment, the therapist understood that the client's emotional relationship and sense of respect was to a grandfather, not a great-uncle.

The individual tribe determines roles and family obligations. For example, in Hopi society, an uncle is a family leader who provides guidance, nurturance, and support to other family members. A person unable to meet these role obligations can experience a great deal of anxiety and guilt. Two-Spirit is the contemporary name for lesbian, gay, bisexual, and transgender Native Americans. This contemporary term, adopted in 1990 from the Northern Algonquin word *niizh manitoag*, proposes to signify the embodiment of both feminine and masculine spirits within one person (Anguksuar, 1997). Traditionally, many Indian cultures respect lesbian, gay, bisexual, and transgender (LGBT) persons and believe these persons hold sacred and ceremonial roles. Healer is often one of such roles. Many scholars believe the suppression of these traditional indigenous values of acceptance and honor is another result of compulsory Christianity and colonization. According to Walters (1997), most LBGT Native Americans face homophobic oppression from both mainstream U.S. society and their own tribes and communities, especially those who live off their reservations and in urban areas. Adopting the label Two-Spirit for many LGBT Native Americans is an act of decolonization and reclamation of tradition for future generations.

A non-Indian therapist may have difficulty recognizing these different roles. It helps to take a good family history, a nonthreatening activity with which an American Indian client usually feels comfortable and which demonstrates the therapist's concern for the extended family. Traditionally, when strangers meet, they often identify themselves through their relatives: "I am a Navaho. My name is Tiana Bighorn. My hometown is Tuba City, Arizona. I belong to the Deer Springs Clan, born for the Rocky Gap Clan" (Benet & Maloney, 1994, p. 9). As therapy proceeds, the professional who is sensitive and willing to listen intently will gradually learn more about the family structure and dynamics. Therapist–client rapport, does not happen in one session but gradually develops over time. The therapist might begin by modeling the process. It is very important to say who you are and where you come from in an accessible, nonthreatening way. Napoli (1999) and Warner (2003) stress the importance of the clinician's self-disclosure in establishing a working alliance and trust with the family.

The Spiritual Relationship of Man and Nature

Mitakuye Oyasin, Lakota for "To all my relations," is a salutation and a saying one commonly hears at the end of prayer. It acknowledges the spiritual bond between the speaker and all people present. It affirms the importance of the relationship of the speaker to his or her blood relatives, the forbears' tribe, the family of man, and Mother Nature. It bespeaks a life-affirming philosophy that all life forces are valuable and interdependent. Western civilization's orientation is toward control over nature, whereas traditional Indian culture sees harmony with natural forces as a way of life. A belief is that only a few human beings have control over nature's forces, those gifted with a special bond to and an unusual understanding of nature. The acceptance of overwhelming, uncontrollable natural events is an integral part of life.

For the American Indian, sacred beings may include animals, plants, mountains, and bodies of water, which are part of the universal family and, as such, involved in a reciprocal system; we care for Mother Earth and she nurtures us. Just as a person strives to be in harmony with his or her human relatives, so should that person try to be in harmony with his or her spiritual and natural relatives: "My mother told me, every part of this earth is sacred to our people. Every pine needle. Every sandy shore. Every mist in the dark woods. Every meadow and humming insect. The Earth is our mother" (Jeffers, 1991, p. 3).

Genocide

Contact with Europeans was devastating for North America's indigenous peoples. Millions died through disease and genocidal warfare that destroyed entire communities and tribes. They subjected survivors to an insidious plan of coerced assimilation and cultural genocide, with many tribes forced to live on reservations distant from their native lands. They tore thousands of Indian children from their families and placed them in boarding schools. White authorities denigrated Indian languages, customs, and religions and forbade their practice. These policies led to a profound cultural trauma, because American Indian cultures are rooted in family ties, a unique attachment and respect for their natural surroundings, and a distinct spirituality (La Due, 1994).

Efforts at forced assimilation did not end in the 1800s. During the 1950s and 1960s the federal government developed a termination and relocation plan, taking many Indians from their homes and families and relocating them to urban centers (Tafoya & Del Vecchio, 1966). Alcoholism rates soared. One scholar concluded: "This was another significant loss heaped upon the already present losses of language, elders, family and culture. Suicide, violence, and homicide all increased to epidemic proportions. School dropout rates, teen pregnancies and high rates of unemployment all became markers of a legacy of trauma experienced throughout this country by Indian people" (La Due, 1994, p. 99). The implications of this "soul wound" are far-reaching, passed down through each generation (Duran, Duran, Brave Heart, & Yellow Horse-Davis, 1998).

Today, Indian cultures continue to survive in a hostile environment, as evident in the controversy over court cases that adjudicate treaty rights, the unapologetic use of Indian mascots for sports teams, and the need for civil rights investigations in areas that border reservations. Contrary to the typical pattern of violence in which most acts are committed between members of one ethnic group, the members of another group, primarily Whites, victimize American Indians (Greenfield & Smith, 1999). The therapist should be aware of such phenomena as suicide, depression, and alcoholism within the context of ongoing oppression combined with a genocidal history. Labeling and naming are powerful methods of creating subjectivity and "life worlds," which may "be contributing to the invalidation of the pain and suffering that is directly connected to generations of genocide" (Duran et al., 1998, p. 346).

Tribal Identity

Although many may think of Indians as a homogenous group, Indians identify themselves as belonging to a particular tribe, band, or clan. Each tribe's customs and values are critical to individual identity and affect family dynamics (Red Horse, 1981). This tradition of thinking in terms of "we" instead of "I" is a great strength of Indian culture.

All tribes, even those in the same geographic area, have distinctive worldviews and practices. For example, the Hopi, Dine'h (Navaho), Havasupai, Pima, Yaqui, and Apache all share the desert of the Southwest, but differ in terms of religious practices, customs, and family structures. When a Hopi or Dine'h man marries, he usually moves in with his wife's family. However, the opposite is true of the Havasupai; the woman lives with her husband's relatives. The particular American Indian worldview has major implications for therapy. The Dine'h have a legend indicating that epileptic seizures result from a brother and sister being involved in incest. Recent studies comparing attitudes of Apaches, Dine'h, and Hopis toward epilepsy reveal that Dine'h Indians with epilepsy feel more stigmatized, are more ashamed of their illness, and are less likely to seek treatment (Levy, 1987). The Mvskoke Creek believe that animals cause all illnesses and diseases (P. Coser, personal communication, February 26, 2004).

American Indian tribes' diversity sometimes leads to conflict. For example, the Sioux and the Ponca are both Plains Indian Nations that may seem similar to outsiders, but they are traditional enemies. Each nation has legends about its own warriors, heroes, medicine men, and medicine women. Each has its own horror stories about encounters with Whites and tales of military, moral, or spiritual triumph. Through tribal traditions, Indian people are offered a radically different view of themselves than that created by the dominant culture. This view helps sustain them in their encounters with White society.

> Families succeeding best in this migration (into the White culture) have two characteristics. Not surprisingly, one is openness to learning and to using the social and technical skills of the White culture. A second, more startling characteristic is the interest that these families show in keeping alive the language, folkways, crafts, and values associated with their tribal identities. (Attneave, 1982, p. 82)

Some Indians struggle to maintain their cultural identity in a foreign environment, and others may try to recapture nearly extinct languages and customs. Because a therapist cannot be familiar with all the nuances of a particular Indian culture, when on unfamiliar ground he or she might ask the client such questions, "What particular cultural traits do you value most and wish to maintain: language, spirituality, family ties?" The therapist might explore such practical resources as a language class, participation in local ceremonies and traditional events such as Pow Wow, Sun Dance, and Sweat Lodge, or involvement with Indian organizations and centers. The therapist would do well to acknowledge the depth of a client's loss of his or her culture, even for those who have assimilated and are yearning for what they never had.

Communal Sharing

"When I was little, I learned very early that what's yours is mine and what's mine is everybody's" (Ivern Takes the Shield, traditional Oglala Lakota, personal communication, June 1989). Traditionally, Indians accord great respect to those who give the most to other individuals and families, and then to the band, tribe, or community. "Giveaways," an ancient custom whereby many gifts are presented to others for their help or achievements, persist in many tribes. They are a way of marking climactic events in the life cycle such as birth, naming, marriage, and death. On a day-to-day basis, Indians share material goods. Each traveler and visitor is always fed, housed, and even clothed and transported (Attneave, 1982, p. 69).

This value of sharing contrasts sharply with the dominant culture's capitalist emphasis on acquisition and can make it difficult for Indians on reservations to operate businesses. For example, a cafe started by a Dine'h (Navaho) couple should have been very successful, given the lack of competition and the availability of patrons. Nevertheless, the owners felt an obligation to provide food gratis for family members. Because "family" often includes in-laws and their families, it was difficult to find paying customers. People who are either part Indian or nontraditionalists, however, run many successful businesses on reservations.

Similar issues often arise when the head(s) of an urban Indian family finds steady work or a student receives a stipend or fellowship. Whereas White culture focuses on carefully managing cash flow and savings, American Indians are prone to share liquid assets. "Unemployed parents may move in; siblings consume food, wear out clothing, and take up time needed for study. Students realize they can hardly pay tuition or study in this kind of environment. However, they feel that they cannot be Indian, yet be selfish about helping others whose needs are greater" (Attneave, 1982, p. 69).

THERAPY ISSUES

Many family therapy models are akin to the "Indian way," which consists of extended families and often entire tribal groups working together to resolve problems. Family therapy, with its emphasis on relationships, is particularly effective in working with Indians, whose life cycle orientation blends well with the life cycle approach of family therapy. We suggest that the therapist use culturally sensitive, nondirective approaches. It is helpful to incorporate the use of storytelling, metaphor, and paradoxical interventions. Networking and the use of ritual and ceremony are favored over strategic interventions and brief therapy models.

Studies show that Indians come to treatment hoping that the therapist is an expert who can give them concrete, practical advice about their problems and be sensitive to their cultural beliefs and differences (Attneave, 1982; DuBray, 1993; La Fromboise, Trimble, & Mohatt, 1990; Polacca, 1995; Tafoya, 1989). Historically, racism has marred the relationship between American Indians and the helping professions. Missionaries, teachers, and social workers usually try to "help" Indians by changing their value systems, thus alienating them from the strength and support of their own people and traditions (La Fromboise et al., 1990). This has understandably led many to feel wary of therapists and therapy.

Professionals with impeccable credentials have victimized American Indians, who sometimes judge therapists by who, not what, they are. When Indian clients enter a clinician's office, they will more likely look for behavioral indications of who the therapist is rather than for a particular diploma on the wall. Personal authenticity, genuine respect, and concern for the client are essential.

There are three important elements for successful therapy with American Indians. The first is to be aware of the impact of genocide. The second is to understand the differences between the dominant culture and that of American Indian clients. The third is to consider each individual client and family's level of assimilation.

Who Comes to Therapy and Why?

American Indians come to therapy for the same reasons other Americans do, including marital problems, chemical dependency issues, and depression. An American Indian family's underlying racial and cultural characteristics may resemble those of an immigrant family that has acculturated for several generations. Nevertheless, the Indian client may still be very close to his or her reservation roots (Attneave, 1982). Yet, as in Oklahoma, many Native families of mixed-blood ancestry have no connection to their communities (P. Coser, personal communication, February 26, 2004).

The stress of intermarriage often brings couples to therapy. Working out the details of everyday life can result in the collision of Indian and dissonant cultural values.

Ruben, a Cheyenne, and his wife Angie, a Hungarian, were at an impasse. Living on the East Coast and childless, with financial problems, they came to therapy when Ruben was offered an apprentice job with a large manufacturer, a position arranged by a member of Angie's family. Angie worked as a secretary, while Ruben held a series of temporary jobs. Instead of being happy about the new position, Ruben was depressed and even was thinking of turning it down. Furious, Angie was threatening to leave him.

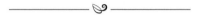

In this case, the therapist and clients explored how problems were resolved in their families of origin. Angie came from a family in which women typically made decisions about work and finances and thus helped to direct the family's mobility (socioeconomic and/or upward mobility). For her, financial stability was critical.

In Ruben's family, asking for guidance and direction through healing rituals was a way to begin to find answers to problems. Before he and Angie married, Ruben had made a commitment to Sun Dance, a religious purification and peace ceremony of his tribe, which sometimes requires a year or more of preparation. The sun dancer fasts, prays, and dances in the hot sun under the guidance of a medicine man. Sun Dance grounds are usually located on reservations. As in most Indian ceremonies, the sun dancer's family and community participate and provide emotional and spiritual support. The time, travel, and expense involved in keeping this kind of commitment often conflict with the demands of employment or education in the non-Indian world.

Ruben wished to sun dance to provide blessings for his family and as a way of promising himself that although he was moving into the dominant culture, he would not abandon his ceremonial ways. He felt that if he did not keep this commitment, something bad might happen to someone he loved or he might lose the marriage he valued so highly. He thus found himself caught in a difficult conflict.

Here is a classic example of the counterpoint between the American Indian value of spirituality expressed through ceremonial life versus financial security, as well as the Indian way of thinking in terms of "we" instead of "I." Ruben fears that not fulfilling his commitment will hurt someone he loves. If Ruben does not perform the Sun Dance and his father subsequently dies, he may well feel responsible. However, if he tells his non-Indian therapist this, the therapist is likely to think that Ruben is overreacting and will try to diffuse his guilt. That will not work, for Ruben has a culturally defined problem that requires a culturally acceptable solution. The therapist's primary task is to allow him to talk about his feelings and explore acceptable ways for him to resolve the situation. The therapist may also encourage Ruben to seek support from family and friends who may want to pray with him. Angie also needs support in learning about the sacredness of the Sun Dance and its significance for Ruben. Understanding this ritual may make her feel more comfortable about discussing possible alternatives with her family.

Living in the dominant society can make following culturally prescribed solutions difficult. The therapist can help by supporting such values and rituals and assisting the client in determining ways of using them to become "unstuck." "Until traditional indigenous therapies are implemented and considered legitimate, there will be a struggle" (Duran et al., 1998, p. 341).

Communicative Style

My grandmother always told me that the white man never listens to anyone, but expects everyone to listen to him. So, we listen! My father always told me that an Eskimo is a listener. We have survived here because we know how to listen. The white people in the lower forty-eight talk. They are like the wind, they sweep over everything.
—COLES (1978, cited in Nabokov, 1991, p. 431)

Native cultures value listening. Long periods of silence during a session can be confusing for the therapist. Yet silence may connote respect, that the client is forming thoughts, or that the client is waiting for a sign that it is the right time to speak. Indians can be very indirect. Some native cultures consider it disrespectful for one relative to mention the name of another. A Lakota woman may refer to her father-in-law as "he" rather than speak his name.

The non-Indian therapist may treat silence, embellished metaphors, and indirectness as signs of resistance, when in fact they often represent important forms of communication (Attneave, 1982). The professional needs to monitor his or her feelings about these differences and resist the urge to interrupt. Otherwise, Indians may experience the therapist as disrespectful, insensitive, and opinionated. The therapist can counter this perception by joining with the client and following his or her directive and by being willing to admit to confusion and misunderstanding.

Professionals also need to be especially aware of nonverbal communication, particularly when "nothing is taking place." For an Indian client, everything one does, no matter how subtle, communicates something (Sutton & Mills, 2001). How the therapist enters a room, what is in that room, and how the therapist responds to silence reveals something about him or her to the client. Everything influences the therapy. In addition, having coffee and food available for clients can make an office seem more welcoming and comfortable.

Treatment: Native and Western

Until the passage of the American Indian Freedom of Religion Act (1978), Indians who practiced their own religion through Sun Dance ceremonies, Native American Church practices, Sweat Lodge rituals, and the like, risked, and sometimes suffered, imprisonment. Despite such hardships, Indian religion endured and is thriving today. Some traditional American Indians seek the guidance of medicine people in times of crisis or major decision making, or when seeking spiritual growth. Others may not even know what a medicine person is, much less have contact with one (Polacca, 1995). Often we assume that a family follows traditional cultural practices. However cultural orientation can vary on a continuum ranging from the traditional to the contemporary (Weibel-Orlando, 1987).

"Indian medicine refers to a traditional and specific cultural approach to health and life for a person, rather than a treatment for a disease or illness" (DuBray, 1985). Generally, a medicine person's approach is holistic, involving healing the body and the troubled soul. Therapists should be alert to any contact that their clients may have with medicine people and should usually consider it beneficial.

In 1980, the American Medical Association revised its code of ethics, giving physicians permission to consult, and to take referrals from and make referrals to, nonphysician healers, including American Indian medicine people (Polacca, 1995). Even practicing Christians may have an ongoing relationship with medicine people, which may positively or negatively affect a therapist's work with a family, as the following case reveals:

The Shields are a Navajo family who relocated to a large city from a rural reservation on a mesa; they are practicing Catholics, with three children: Tony, 16; Kensil, 12; and Shell, 9. The children attend a parochial school system with a large Indian population. The school's guidance counselor referred them because Tony clearly had a substance abuse problem affecting his school performance. After initially feeling that things were going well, the therapist began to sense that the family had become resistant, particularly after placing Tony in a juvenile detention facility because of a drinking episode. The therapist instructed the family to keep Tony in the detention center, as an intervention designed to allow him to experience the consequences of his actions. Without notifying the therapist, the family withdrew Tony from the detention facility and took him to the reservation to stay with an aunt and uncle. When the therapist contacted the family about this action, they scheduled an appointment, but did not show up. When Tony returned to school, the family resumed therapy, only to have the same pattern repeat itself.

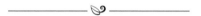

In this case, the Shields brought their son home to be with an uncle, a person who traditionally plays an important role in a son's upbringing. They also utilized the services of a medicine man and were involved in the Native American Church. The Native American Church is a recognized religion that uses peyote as a sacrament instead of wine or juice and wafers or bread. The Shields were reluctant to discuss these involvements with the therapist, feeling that she would not understand their decision and would reject their ceremonial approach. Rather than having to explain why they had not followed her instructions, the family tried to avoid her. The therapist began to explore the reasons behind the missed appointments instead of assuming the family was rejecting treatment. Upon discovery of the family's reason, she began to integrate some of their healing methods into therapy.

Many Indians utilize traditional and Western practices, viewing both as vital to the healing process. Using the clients' own language, the therapist can strongly support such approaches as prayer meetings and the use of herbal medicines, as well as encourage American Indian healing rituals. With regard to the Shields, the therapist might say something like, "The ceremonies you are performing to get rid of these bad spirits, while Tony is in treatment, are helpful. It is good that you are helping him in this way."

Family therapists must also examine their own personal values. How do their religious beliefs affect those of their clients? Therapists need to respect and value cultural differences and help clients to use their own traditions for personal or familial healing.

Today, American Indians are developing their own approaches to treatment and to preventing alcohol, drug abuse, and suicide. They are also incorporating recovery techniques used in the broader society. The Native American Church, for example, described as "the most important pan-Indian movement in this country, is political, cultural and spiritual, a source of pride, power, and psychological health" (Hammerschlag, 1988, p. 60). The Native American Church has many members throughout the country.

CONCLUSION

Therapists wishing to work effectively with American Indian clients not only need to discard the stereotypes perpetuated by our Eurocentric historical legacy and by the media, but must also be willing to suspend their assumptions regarding family roles, relationships, and what is considered as an appropriate style of communication. Therapists must fully understand and respect each native client's degree of identification with his or her own tribe. Therapists should listen carefully, ask questions, and assume nothing when gathering information about American Indian clients, all of which will provide them with important information. In addition, this helps to foster the trust of American Indian clients, who often are wary of non-Indian therapists. To become more effective in understanding and determining the best course of treatment, we encourage therapists to read the literature about individual tribes, about historical trauma, about rituals and ceremonies, and about the religion, beliefs, and customs of the client family. When invited, the therapist should take the opportunity to participate and attend the ceremonies, rituals, and other events important to a family.

ACKNOWLEDGMENTS

We both would like to express our gratitude to Mona Polacca, Hopi-Havasupai; Pete G. Coser, Mvskoke Creek; Parrish Williams, Ponca; and Helen Rende, Kahnewke-Mohawk, for their reviews and suggestions regarding this chapter.

NOTE

1. *Medicine people* refers to men or women who practice indigenous healing that focuses on physical or spiritual health or both. Practitioners may also be members of the mainstream medical community.

REFERENCES

Adams, J. (2002). Coast Indian film festival highlights banner year. *Indian Country Today*. Retrieved March 4, 2002, from www.indiancountry.com/?1038415793

Anguksuar, L. R. (1997). A postcolonial perspective on Western [mis]conceptions of the cosmos and the restoration of indigenous taxonomies. In S. E. Jacobs, W. Thomas, & S. Lang (Eds.), *Two-spirit people: Native American gender identity, sexuality, and spirituality* (pp. 217–222). Chicago: University of Illinois Press.

Attneave, C. (1982). American Indians and Alaska Native families: Emigrants in their own homeland. In M. McGoldrick, J. K. Pearce, & J. Giordano (Eds.), *Ethnicity and family therapy* (pp. 55–83). New York: Guilford Press.

Benet, N., & Maloney, S. (1994). Keeper of the culture. *Intertribal America*. Collectors Edition.

Berkhoffer, R. (1978). *The White man's Indian: Images of the American Indian from Columbus to the present*. New York: Vintage Press.

DuBray, W. (1985). American Indian values: Critical factors in casework. *Social Casework: The Journal of Contemporary Social Work*, 66(1), 30–38.

DuBray, W. (1993). *American Indian values: Mental health interventions with people of color*. St. Paul, MN: West.

Duran, E., Duran, B., Brave Heart, M., & Yellow Horse-Davis, S. (1998). Healing the American Indian soul wound. In Y. Danieli (Ed.), *International handbook of multigenerational legacies of trauma* (pp. 341–354). New York: Plenum Press.

Gunn, P. A. (Ed.). (1989). *Spider Woman's granddaughters: Traditional tales and contemporary writing by Native American women*. New York: Fawcett Columbine.

Hammerschlag, C. (1988). *The dancing healers: A doctor's journey of healing with Native Americans*. New York: HarperCollins.

Jeffers, S. (1991). *Brother Eagle, Sister Sky: A message from Chief Seattle*. New York: Dial Books.

La Due, R. (1994). Coyote returns: Twenty sweats does not an Indian expert make, bringing ethics alive. *Feminist Ethics in Psychotherapy Practice*, 15(1), 93–111.

La Fromboise, T., Trimble, J., & Mohatt, G. (1990). Counseling intervention and American Indian tradition: An integrative approach. *Counseling Psychologist*, 18(4), 628–654.

Levy, J. (1987). Psychological and social problems of epileptic children in four Southwestern Indian tribes. *Journal of Community Psychology*, 15(3), 307–315.

Nabokov, P. (Ed.). (1991). *Native American testimony: A chronicle of Indian–White relations from prophecy to the present*. New York: Penguin.

Napoli, M. (1999). The non-Indian therapist working with American Indian clients: Transference–counter transference implications. *Psychoanalytic Social Work*, 6(1), 25–47.

Polacca, M. (1995). *Cross cultural variation in mental health treatment of aging Native Americans*. Unpublished manuscript, School of Social Work, Arizona State University.

Red Horse, J. (1981, April). *American Indian families*. Paper presented at the conference on American Indian Family Strengths and Stress, Tempe, AZ.

Sutton, C., & Mills, J. (2001) *Take hart (healing and recovery after trauma): An emergency response to terrorist the United States—A training manual*. Piscataway, NJ: University of Medicine and Dentistry of New Jersey.

Tafoya, N., & Del Vecchio, A. (1996). Back to the future: An examination of the Native American holocaust. In M. McGoldrick, J. Giordiano, & J. K. Pearce (Eds.), *Ethnicity and family therapy* (2nd ed., pp. 45–54). New York: Guilford Press.

Tafoya, T. (1989). Coyote's eyes: Native cognition styles. *Journal of American Indian Education* [Special issue], pp. 29–40.

U.S. Bureau of the Census. (2000, February). *The American Indian and Alaska Native population: 2000*. Washington, DC: U.S. Department of Commerce, Economics and Statistics Administration.

U.S. Department of the Interior. (2004). Bureau of Indian Affairs. Retrieved March 2, 2004, from www.doi.gov/bureau-indian-affairs.html

Walters, K. L. (1997). Urban lesbian and gay American Indian identity: Implications for mental health service delivery. *Journal of Gay and Lesbian Social Services*, 6(2), 43–65.

Warner, J. C. (2003). Group therapy with Native Americans: Understanding essential differences. *Group*, 27(4), 191–202.

Weibel-Orlando, J. (1987). Culture-specific treatment modalities: Assessing client-to-treatment fit in alcoholism programs. In W. M. Cox (Ed.), *Treatment and prevention of alcohol problems: A resource manual* (pp. 261–283). Orlando, FL: Academic Press.

CHAPTER 3

Back to the Future

An Examination
of the Native American Holocaust Experience

Nadine Tafoya
Ann Del Vecchio

NATIVE AMERICANS TODAY: ROSE P.'S STORY

What is it like to be an Indian in today's society? I live in shame and feel oppressed. I know that the stress and strain of oppression takes its toll on my psyche, on my sense of self, and on my ability to live a good life.

"When I was thinking about this question, I remembered a time when my son was about 4 years old. He was angry at me. He wasn't ready to come in from playing outside. He was very angry and crying in his rage. I sternly told him to go to his room until he could calm down. As he headed for his room, he narrowed his eyes at me and whispered something under his breath. He stood before his bedroom door and raised his little fist in the air and shook it wildly at me. I will always picture that raised fist clearly in my mind.

"That raised fist is what comes to mind first when I think about being a Native American in America today. I have been scorned and squashed down because my culture, my traditions, and my identity are different from mainstream America's. My son raised his fist to me. To whom do I shake my fist in rage at the daily frustration of being humiliated for simply being Native American? My boss? My husband? My teacher? My tribal leaders?

"I learned very young that I was different. In school, I learned not to try to answer the teacher's questions. The teacher only called on the blond children. When she looked at me, I saw disgust, or worse, pity. I felt dirty and stupid. If I had tried once in the past to raise my hand and offer my answers, I learned to stop trying. I hid my pride, my pain, and my tears. I didn't talk to the other Native kids about it. We all kept quiet.

"As an adult, I don't try much. I don't shake my fist but the pain is still there. I see the teacher's look of disgust on my boss's face. I drink alcohol. I gamble. One of my cousins killed herself. I think about how easy it would be to kill myself too. The pain would be gone then.

"For 500 years my people have been told in so many ways, 'You're no good. You're a savage. You're ways are not Christian.' My parents met in boarding school and relocated from their reservations (they came from different tribes) to Los Angeles after they were married. The government promised them training and jobs, housing, and education. These promises, like the federal treaties made years before, never materialized and my father began to drink, beat my mother and us kids. We grew up away from our tribal reservation, languages, and culture. We never spoke the language of my mother or father, we never spent enough time with our grandparents to learn the old ways. This bitter legacy is mine to pass on to my own children and grandchildren today.

"We have found systematic oppression and racism. We have found depression and anxiety. We have lost ourselves again in alcohol, drugs, and suicide. We are survivors of multigenerational loss and only through acknowledging our losses will we ever be able to heal."

DOCUMENTING OUR HISTORICAL LOSS AND THE DYNAMICS OF UNRESOLVED GRIEF

> Memories are all we have. And when the memories are dreadful—when they hold images of the pain we have suffered or, perhaps even worse, inflicted—they are what we try to escape.
>
> —CORLISS (1993, p. 110)

In a review of the movie *Schindler's List* in the popular press, Corliss makes the point that the movie is essentially a plea to remember, and that to remember is to speed the healing. This is the case for Native Americans in the United States today. We are at a crossroads, and actively remembering our past and the historic trauma that is our legacy is one way we can recover a happy, healthy, and productive existence as a separate and distinct ethnic/cultural group.

As a result of the genocidal U.S. policies toward native peoples, unresolved grief is a day-to-day dynamic that affects the lives of Native Americans. Historical trauma involves the impact and social transmission of one generation's trauma to subsequent generations. As a result of federal boarding school policies, this trauma included the destruction of native language and culture.

The dynamics of unresolved grief include symptoms and manifestations that affect every aspect of an individual's life, including:

- Somatic symptoms such as migraines, stomachaches, joint pain, dizziness, and chronic fatigue
- Physical stress and vulnerability to chronic health problems, such as Type II diabetes
- Depression
- Substance abuse
- Preoccupation with death
- Suicidal ideation and gestures
- Chronic, delayed, or impaired grief process, including searching and pining behaviors

Trauma response, as documented in survivors of the Nazi Holocaust, among Vietnam veterans, and the survivors of war, involves both psychological and physical responses (DeBruyn & Brave Heart, in press). Duran and colleagues (2004) identified the prevalence and correlates of mental health disorders among Native American women in primary care, and although they did not find a direct link between boarding school experiences and mental health disorders, they did posit that the high prevalence of anxiety disorders in this group may be effected by a complex interaction of individual and community-level variables. The following list of trauma response behaviors was derived from the literature:

- Psychic numbing
- Hypervigilance
- Disassociation
- Intense fear, free-floating anxiety
- Survivor guilt
- Fixation on the trauma
- Victim identity, death identity, and identification with the dead
- Low self-esteem
- Anger
- Self-destructive behavior
- Weakened immune system and chronic disease processes
- Depression
- Substance abuse

These processes, signs, and symptoms of both unresolved grief and the trauma response are endemic on reservations and among urban Indian populations in the United States. No family is untouched by these problems, and the manifestations are evident community-wide. A lack of public infrastructure on reservations compounds the problem with a lack of critical behavioral health services and providers to address this multigenerational holocaust.

It has been only within the last two decades that historians have begun to detail the legacy of oppressive and racist federal policies that were aimed at forcibly and nonnegotiably assimilating and/or annihilating the indigenous peoples of the North American continent. Ethnohistorical methods of inquiry have helped to paint a picture of the historical trauma visited upon Native Americans without further victimization. "Ethnohistory enables scholars to move beyond traditional methods in providing a balanced assessment of cultures meeting in the arena of contact" (Axtell, 1981, p. 5). Ethnohistory has allowed a more balanced and complete rendering of the historic trauma to enter mainstream America through video, audio, and other forms of commercial mass media (television and movies), as well as through history and social studies textbooks and the popular press.

LIFE BEFORE CONTACT BETWEEN NATIVE AMERICAN AND EUROPEAN CULTURES

Prior to any contact with Europeans, the tribes of North America existed with an intact community self-awareness and purpose that included a complete educational system for raising their children. Each tribal group lived in relative isolation from the other native peoples, and most tribes had a name for themselves in their own languages that, translated loosely, meant "the people" or "the true people." Some groups—for example, members of the Tewa-speaking San Juan Pueblo—had ritual precautions and purification ceremonies that were used when they returned from hunting or foraging expeditions that put them in contact with "other people" (Szasz, 1988). These other native groups were not always recognized as people; rather, they were identified as a source of contamination or sometimes as a source of trade goods, slaves, different foods, and other ways of life. Some tribes were more receptive to the cultural ways and innovations of other people.

Although each tribal group used distinct linguistic and cultural methods to educate their children, all tribes required that certain skills be mastered before a youth was accepted as an adult member of the tribe. These knowledge requirements and skills can be loosely categorized in three areas: (1) knowledge of cultural heritage, (2) spiritual/religious practices, and (3) economic survival skills (Szasz, 1988). This tripartite emphasis provided an effective educational system for child rearing and the transmission of indigenous languages and cultures. The child's special skills, temperament, or proclivities might shape his or her role in the community. However, each child was expected to be knowledgeable and competent in all three areas. A child who was an exceptionally good hunter might spend more time hunting and supplying meat to the community, but that child was also expected to know the tribe's ethics, values, and religion and to practice them accordingly.

These competencies were interwoven. Religious rituals were performed to ensure abundant harvests and hunts. Storytelling during cold winter months entertained the adults and youth confined because of the weather, simultaneously passing on the traditions and beliefs of the tribe. Cultural ideals, mundane lessons, and moral instruction were passed on through a rich oral tradition (Szasz, 1988). Cultural continuity was ensured by the accumulation of stories told each winter as a child grew up. Economic/survival skills were passed on through stories and through direct, hands-on instruction with supervised practice throughout the year. When the European explorers first encountered Native Americans, they were exposed to these traditions, beliefs, and skills, but most viewed indigenous ways of life as primitive, and only a few explorers were able to experience and understand the Native American ways of life as complete, elaborate, practical cultures that were intact and not in need of "civilization."

LIFE AFTER CONTACT BETWEEN NATIVE AMERICANS AND EUROPEANS

Traditional history books are full of details about the conquest of the New World by European immigrants. However, the French, Spanish, English, and other European settlers who arrived in the New World were rarely referred to as immigrants in the history books. To the indigenous cultural groups who lived in the New World, these settlers were immigrants to begin with, and later, interlopers and usurpers.

Ethnohistory documents the persistent pressure from the European immigrants on the Native Americans to give up their land. Once the homelands were usurped by the Europeans, pressure was exerted on Native Americans to conform to the immigrants' European customs. With a loss of traditional lands as the foundation of Native American economic survival, and with associated policies and pressure to assume European ways and means of economic survival, Native Americans were caught in a vise that crushed the traditional tripartite educational systems for the transmission of tribal cultures and ways of life.

By the 1800s, the press of European immigrants had become massive in scale and was reaching the Great Plains west of the Mississippi River. Pushed into the domains of neighboring tribes, which resulted in bloody conflict between tribes, attacked by Old World diseases such as smallpox, exposed to the insidious corruption of alcohol abuse, ravaged by starvation and malnutrition, the Native American population of the New World was decimated; Native Americans numbered some 600,000 in the 1840s, and the population dropped again to about 250,000 by 1850. European "civilization" resulted directly in more Native American deaths than the actual warfare between the immigrants and the North American tribes (New, 1964).

THE MISSIONARY SYSTEM OF ASSIMILATION

A concomitant of the European immigrants' greed for the tribes' lands was the need to Christianize the heathens. The underlying assumption was that Native Americans would fit better with the immigrants' schemes for the New World if they practiced a "real" religion and gave up their savage religious customs. The U.S. government approached the Indian pragmatically by encouraging missions.

Missionaries cost the government little beyond minimal military support to suppress any hostility on the part of the indigenous population, and the missionary system of education bought the government a ready means of annihilating the rest of the tripartite tribal system of educating children. Through missionary schools, Indian children lost their languages, their tribal customs and beliefs, and came home strangers to their parents, clans, and tribal communities. Szasz (1988) provides an excellent ethnohistorical description of the missionary system of schooling Indians from 1607 to 1783. Beyond 1783 missionary schools continued to educate Native American children and can be found today on reservations throughout the United States. However, the missionary schools proved to be insufficient as a means of assimilation and annihilation of the tenacious Native American cultures.

THE BOARDING SCHOOL PHENOMENON

It was 1915, during the harvest season. I was a little girl. I remember it was in October and we had a pile of red chile and we were tying chile into fours. And then my grandfather was putting them onto a longer string. We were doing that when they came to get me. Then right away my grandmother and mother started to cry, "Her? She's just a little girl! She's just a little girl, you can't take her" . . . I was 5 years old.
　　　　　　　　　　　　　　　　　　　　　　—HYER (1990, pp. 5–6)

The boarding school method of removing the Indian from the child was implemented toward the end of the 1800s. Tribal leaders were informed that all Indian children were required to be formally educated, and that this would be accomplished through boarding schools. The Carlisle School in Carlisle, Pennsylvania, was established in 1879. By 1902 a total of 25 Indian boarding schools had been established in 15 states. The schools were often located in old army forts and commonly staffed by ex-military personnel (old army types).

Native American children, parents, and tribes were not given a choice or a voice in the matter of the education of Indian children. The aim of this system was twofold: (1) to remove all traces of Indian from the child and (2) to immerse the child totally in Western culture, thought, and tradition. Thus, the Indian problem would be solved by raising the children in a Western, civilized manner and away from their wanton, savage ways. The boarding school system was one of the most ruthless and inhumane methods of assimilation available to the U.S. government. All-out warfare, with associated atrocities, was a much more humane method of dealing with Native Americans. McLaughlin (1994) included this description from a 40-year-old Navajo parent who was left at boarding school at 7 years of age. At the time, she spoke only Navajo, no English.

> It was the first time I've seen a brick building that was not a trading post. The ceilings were so high and the rooms so big an empty. There was no warmth. Not as far as "brrrr, I'm cold," but in a sense of emotional cold. Kind of an emptiness, when you're hanging on to your mom's skirt and trying hard not to cry. Then when you get up to your turn, she thumbprints the paper and she leaves and you watch her go out the big metal doors . . . you see her get into the truck and the truck starts moving and all the home smell goes with it. . . . Then them women takes you by the hand and takes you inside and the first thing they do is take down your bun. The first thing they do is cut off your hair and you been told your whole life that you never cut your hair recklessly because that is your life. . . . And you see that long, black hair drop, and it's like they take out your heart and they give you this cold thing that beats inside. And now you're gonna to be just like them. You're gonna be cold. You're never gonna be happy or have that warm feeling and attitude towards life anymore. That's what it feels like, like taking your heart out and putting in a cold river pebble. When you go into the shower, you leave your squaw skirt and blouse right there at the shower door. When you come out, it's gone. . . . They cut your hair, now they take your squaw skirt. They take from the beginning. When you first walk in there, they take everything that you're about. They jerk it away from you. They don't ask how you feel about it. They never tell you anything. They barely speak to you. They take everything away from you. . . . (pp. 47–48)

The trauma described in this passage was typical of the boarding school experience. The boarding school system was inhumane by virtue of the fact that children as young as 5 years of age were separated from their parents and transported far from home. As most Native American families lived on poverty-level incomes, traveling to these schools to visit was impossible. A multifaceted process of assimilation commenced as soon as the children reached their destination. The process involved the following features:

- English language immersion with punishment for speaking tribal languages.
- Destruction of traditional garments and replacement with alien, Western clothing.
- Braids and traditional hairstyles shaved and replaced with Western-style haircuts.
- Buildings, dormitories, campuses, and furnishings of Western design.
- Forced physical labor in the kitchens, stables, gardens, and shops, necessary to run the schools.
- Corporal punishment for the infraction of rules or for not following the work and school schedules.

- Immersion in a Western educational curriculum with associated alien goals and philosophy.
- Regimented, time-bound schedules.

This list is not exhaustive. Szasz (1977) described the boarding school experience as one in which the physical conditions were almost always inadequate. Food was scarce, children were overcrowded, and the improper treatment of sick children led to frequent epidemics. Preadolescent children worked long hours to care for the facilities and produce food, because congressional appropriations were woefully inadequate. Staff were usually not prepared with any understanding of the children, their languages, and traditions. In addition, boarding school staff members and teachers lacked coping strategies and skills for working with confused and sometimes defiant children. At times, the staff disciplined the children brutally.

As a result of the boarding school system, several generations of Native Americans were raised without family ties. Nurturing, the most essential element of healthy development for young children, was nonexistent and was replaced with forced assimilation, hard physical labor, harsh discipline, and physical, sexual, and emotional abuse. A variety of negative coping strategies have been adopted by Native Americans as a result of the historical trauma and internalized oppression. These survival skills include some of the same behaviors itemized earlier as features of unresolved grief and trauma response. Substance abuse, depression, and suicide are endemic on our reservations are resorted to in order to cope.

The boarding school generations of Native Americans survived, but at the cost of thousands of lives lived in the misery and doubt of damaged self-esteem and linguistic and cultural annihilation. This is the legacy of Native American communities today.

It is the fallout from the historical trauma of the boarding school system with which we, as mental health professionals, must contend. Our awareness of this trauma and our ability to assist Native American clients to become aware of it must be used as a foundation to *speed the healing*.

IMPLICATIONS FOR TREATMENT

Middelton-Moz (1986) describes some of the emotional and psychological scarring produced by forced assimilation. She states that children who were sent to boarding school institutions became strangers to their parents. The children gave up their traditional cultural values and ways and assumed the values of the majority culture. The children found themselves ill prepared to cope with either culture and often felt confused and alienated from both the Western and the Indian ways of life. Middelton-Moz found that adults in the therapeutic setting who had been educated through the boarding school system suffered from a pervasive sense of low self-worth, powerlessness, depression, and alienation from the power and strength of cultural values. Indian adults in therapy were confused about their family roots and traditions and felt abandoned. The young adults who had not been raised by their own parents felt increased confusion when faced with the need to parent their own children.

DeBryun and Braveheart (in press) have extended work in the area of historical trauma to encompass four principal elements for dealing with the trauma response and for addressing the symptoms of unresolved grief and historical trauma. These authors suggest that, as mental health professionals, we can assist Native American individuals and communities to develop positive methods and models, using the following framework.

1. Treatment must provide for cathartic release of affect during the initial process. Some discussion of the history of genocide against Native Americans and the boarding school experience may be necessary to orient clients to the effect that trauma has had on the families and communities. Repression and racism should be identified as concomitant to the trauma process, and the impact of racist behavior on daily life should be investigated.

2. Treatment must provide an emotional container so that the client feels safe and competent to handle the feelings that emerge. Therapists must acknowledge the impact historical trauma has had on Native people and must act as educators and resources when necessary. Therapists must guard against judgmental statements and affect and should cultivate nonjudgmental acceptance.

3. Timing is critical to ensuring that the client can cope with the feelings and knowledge associated with multigenerational trauma. Sessions should end with a debriefing time, and during this time the clinician can impart hope and confidence that the client is capable of handling the negative feelings that arise in the process. It is important to reflect on the accomplishments of the client, who may need to be reminded of what he or she has achieved.

4. Traditional ceremonies and healing processes provide a grounding for clients linked to their culture and history. The client should be encouraged to access the cultural ways that will facilitate healing and to become involved in traditions that provide anchoring and emotional support. The traditional ways and ceremonies help to facilitate the cathartic release of unresolved grief and feelings as well.

This framework is a simple beginning to use with Native American clients who seek professional mental health care for problems or for growth and wellness. However, on a larger scale, it is important to apply the framework's principles to the larger context of whole communities, reservations, and pueblos. As our tribal governments, social service workers, religious leaders, and other community members have all been through the historical trauma and the fallout from oppressive racist policies to one degree or another, healing must occur at the level of the whole community. Remembering and acknowledging the impact of our past is the first step on our road back to the future.

REFERENCES

Axtell, J. (1981). *The European and the Indian: Essays in the ethnohistory of colonial America*. New York: Oxford University Press.

Corliss, R. (1993, March 14). Schindler comes home. *Time*, p. 110.

DeBruyn, L. M., & Brave Heart, M. Y. H. (in press). Suicide as a manifestation of historical trauma. In M. Y. H. Brave Heart, B. Segal, L. M. DeBruyn, J. Taylor, & R. Daw (Eds.), *Historical trauma within the American experience: Roots, effects, and healing*. New York: Haworth Press.

Duran B., Sanders, M., Skipper, B., Waitzkin, H., Halinka Malcoe, L., Paine, S., & Yager, J. (2004). Prevalence and correlates of mental disorders among Native American women in primary care. *American Journal of Public Health*, 94(1), 71–77.

Hyer, S. (1990). *One house, one voice, one heart: Native American education at the Santa Fe Indian School*. Albuquerque: University of New Mexico Press.

McLaughlin, D. (1994). Critical literacy for Navajo and other American Indian learners. *Journal of American Indian Education*, 33(3), 47–59.

Middelton-Moz, J. (1986). Wisdom of the elders. In R. J. Ackerman (Ed.), *Growing up in the shadow: Children of alcoholics* (pp. 57–70). Deerfield Beach, FL: Health Communications.

Szasz, C. M. (1977). *Education and the American Indian: The road to self-determination since 1928* (2nd ed.) Albuquerque: University of New Mexico Press.

Szasz, C. M. (1988). *Indian education in the American colonies, 1607–1783*. Albuquerque: University of New Mexico Press.

༄

CHAPTER 4

Nā ʻOhana:
Native Hawaiian Families

Valli Kalei Kanuha

Ola nā iwi.
The bones live.
(Said of a respected oldster who is well cared for by his family.)
—PUKUI (1983)

The 2000 U.S. Census marked the first time national population data were collected about Native Hawaiians, who are the indigenous people of Hawaiʻi (Greico, 2001). The Hawaiʻi Revised Statutes define "Hawaiian" as "any descendant of the aboriginal peoples inhabiting the Hawaiian Islands which exercised sovereignty and subsisted in the Hawaiian Islands in 1778, and which peoples thereafter have continued to reside in Hawaiʻi" (Office of Hawaiian Affairs, 2002). The terms "native Hawaiian," "Hawaiian," Kanaka Māoli (first or original people) (Blaisdell & Mokuau, 1990), and Nā ʻŌiwi or Kanaka ʻŌiwi, literally, "the bones" or ancestors, are used interchangeably.

According to the U.S. Census Bureau, 874,000 or 0.3% of Americans claim Native Hawaiian or Pacific Islander (NH/PI) as their primary racial/ethnic category (United States Census Bureau, 2003). The largest subcategory chose Native Hawaiian as their only ethnicity (141,000 or 16%), with an additional 261,000 (30%) who identified themselves as Native Hawaiian and other Pacific Islander (Greico, 2001). Fifty-eight percent of NH/PIs live in Hawaiʻi or California, with the majority residing in Hawaiʻi (283,000; 23%). Native Hawaiians also live in major U.S. cities such as Seattle, New York, Salt Lake City, and Chicago. The majority of NH/PIs have at least a high school diploma (79%), but only 17% have baccalaureate degrees. Although almost 50% of NH/PIs own their own homes, 18% lived below the poverty line in 1999. It is important to note, however, that most U.S. Census-based statistics on the NH/PI population are aggregated and therefore do not accurately describe Native Hawaiians as a separate ethnic group from the broader Pacific Island category.

As with many indigenous peoples, 79% of Hawaiians and Pacific Islanders live in families (U.S. Census Bureau, 2003). Families, or *nā 'ohana*, are fundamental to Native Hawaiians because, as many Hawaiians learn from an early age, "*'ohana* is the center of all things Hawaiian" (Santos, 2002). This chapter on Kanaka Māoli families begins with a brief historical overview of pre- and post-Western contact Hawai'i, describes central values, beliefs, and customs associated with traditional Native Hawaiian society, and presents key issues of practice for clinicians working with Native Hawaiians today.

A HISTORY OF NATIVE HAWAIIANS

The area known as the Polynesian Triangle, "the largest nation on Earth" (Polynesian Voyaging Society, 2004) covers 10 million square miles of the eastern Pacific Ocean. The triangle is composed of three island points, with Hawai'i at the northernmost apex, New Zealand to the west, and Easter Island, or Rapa Nui, in the east. The peopling of the Hawaiian Islands is attributed to forbears from the Marquesas, one of the largest island groups of French Polynesia, located about 500 miles south of the equator almost midway between Rapa Nui and Hawai'i, and 3,000 miles from California. Around 500 A.D., skilled navigators from this island group sailed double-hulled canoes almost 2,000 miles to the north for Hawai'i, guided only by the stars, tides, and their highly advanced knowledge of "wayfaring" passed on orally by their ancestors (Finney, 1994; Kyselka, 1987). The first Europeans who traveled to Hawai'i in the late 1700s described the native people as

> radiantly healthy and of near physical perfection. They were genial, affectionate and generous. A highly developed agricultural system and skillful and intensive fishing methods provided the food needed for a relatively large population. (Mitchell, 1992, p. 250)

Ancient Hawaiian social life centered on a complex cosmology linking human beings, animal and plants, the skies, sea, and land, as well as ancestral spirits, in a holistic existence ruled by gods (*akua*) and spiritual powers/forces (*mana*). Various estimates put the population of precontact Hawai'i at 400,000 to almost one million (Nordyke, 1977; Smith, 1978; Stannard, 1988). However, after the first foreign arrival to Hawai'i by English explorer Captain James Cook in 1778, exposure to contagious diseases to which the people had no natural immunities reduced the Kanaka Māoli population to 40,000 in just 100 years.

Following this decimation of the Native Hawaiian race, Caucasian industrialists designed a land-registration policy known as the Great Mahele of 1848, a single act that many Kanaka Māoli historians believe marked the end of Hawaiian self-rule (Kame'eleihiwa, 1986). Hawaiians who had resided for generations on land tracts with deeply spiritual origins not only lost their homesteads because they did not understand the concept of land ownership, but were subsequently forbidden from fishing, gathering, planting, or engaging in other cultural practices. These prohibitions, coupled with the influx of Protestant missionary doctrines in the mid-1800s, resulted in the condemnation and subsequent deterioration of the Kanaka Māoli belief systems and traditions so integral to the social stability of Hawaiian life. Over a brief century untold numbers of

Native Hawaiian practices and sacred sites were lost through Western colonization, however many values and beliefs still prevail today.

STRUCTURE, VALUES, AND TRADITIONS OF HAWAIIAN FAMILIES

The literal translation of the Hawaiian word for "family," *'ohana*, has its origins in the taro plant, the staple of ancient Kanaka Māoli. An indigenous plant of Hawai'i, taro (*kalo*) is one of the few edible sources from which the emerging shoots, or *'oha*, sprout from the mature corm, or *makua*, which is also the Hawaiian word for "parent." When joined with *nā* to form the plural "many," *nā 'ohana* attests to the symbolic meaning of the family as a collective that gives life, nourishment, and support for the growth and prosperity of blood relatives as well as extended family, those joined in marriage, adopted children or adults, and ancestors living and deceased (Pukui, Haertig, & Lee, 1972, 1979).

Young (1980) suggests that the emphasis on the family is inherently linked to the necessity for and significance of the connection between people, not only to those who are biologically related, but to the community of Native Hawaiians as a people. The foundation of *nā 'ohana* is its children and their relationship to elders (*kūpuna*), their ancestors, and their physical, spiritual, and material surroundings. Core values that maintain the necessary balance between family members and their natural environment include *aloha* (love and affinity), *mālama* (care), *kokua* (help, aid), *lōkahi* (unity, connection), *lokomaika' i* (generosity), *ha'aha'a* (humility), *ho'omana* (spirituality), and *pono* (righteousness or "right") (Blaisdell & Mokuau, 1990; Pukui et al., 1972, 1979; Rezentes, 1999).

Traditional Hawaiian families functioned within a well-defined structure based on "generation, genealogical superiority, and sex" (Handy & Pukui, 1998 p. 43). Therefore, older Hawaiians were viewed as more deserving of respect than the younger generations, Hawaiians of royal lineage were accorded higher status than commoners, and males and females were assigned distinct roles and tasks in family and social life. *Kūpuna* (elders or grandparents) were so revered that the first-born child in a family was often given to grandparents to be raised with indigenous Hawaiian beliefs and traditions (Kamakau, 1991).

As in other Pacific Islander cultures, in early adolescence males and females were relegated to sex-designated residences to learn expected sex and gender roles. Hawaiian men fished or dived from reefs far out in the ocean, and women and children gathered mollusks and seaweed near the shore. Both men and women cultivated plants and animals for eating; however, foods were prepared and consumed according to clearly delineated sex/gender customs. For example, only males could eat pork, bananas, coconuts, and turtle, because these foods were thought to represent male gods and characteristics. Food preparation was solely the domain of Hawaiian men, a function carried out separately for males and females, who were not permitted to eat together until 1820, when one of the most powerful Hawaiian queens, Ka'ahumanu, abolished the practice along with many other then-sacred rules of behavior, or *kapu* (Kamakau, 1992; Kame'eleihiwa, 1999b).

Ancient Hawaiians espoused a joyous and open attitude toward sexuality. Historian Kame'elihiwa states: "Sexual possession was rare in Hawai'i, where marriage did not exist, where men and women did not 'own' one another because they were lovers" (1999b, p. 5). Sex and mating with blood kin was not only allowed but preferred among members of the royal class—"for how could a high chief be sure of passing on equally high *mana* (supernatural powers) unless he conceived a child with his own kin?" (Pukui et al., 1979, p. 86). Couples could have more than one sexual and intimate partner as long as all parties agreed to the arrangement. Among Hawaiian royalty same-sex relationships were well known; however, there are conflicting accounts about whether such relationships were socially accepted across different social strata, such as among commoners (Handy & Pukui, 1998; Kame'eleihiwa, 1999a; Pukui et al., 1979).

Caring for family members over the lifespan was a key value and practice for the Kanaka Māoli. The ancients believed, as do many modern-day Hawaiians, that because humans are related to all elements in nature, we are required to care for the land, plants, and oceans as we would our own families. When ill health befell a family member, the ailment might be attributed to possession by spirits, failure to abide by social rules of conduct (*kapu*), or the harboring of negative thoughts such as jealousy or anger toward others (Pukui et al., 1979).

To facilitate healing, Hawaiians used herbs, physical treatments such as massage (*lomilomi*), and prayer to ancestors and gods. They also employed *ho'oponopono* (Ii, 1959; Kamakau, 1991; Mitchell, 1992; Rezentes, 1999), an indigenous family conflict-mediation strategy, which is described in more detail later in this chapter.

CRITICAL ISSUES IN INTERVENTION WITH KANAKA MAOLI FAMILIES

There are two basic requirements in any clinical intervention with Native Hawaiian individuals, couples, or families. The first is to have a working knowledge of the key events in the history of the Kanaka Māoli and the islands of Hawai'i as unique cultural and geographic entities. Clinicians must also acknowledge the importance of Hawaiian values and traditions to which most Kanaka Māoli have access, whether or not they actively believe in or practice them. Whether having lived for many generations in the islands or having been raised exclusively elsewhere, most Hawaiians maintain some bond to their cultural roots. There are Hawaiian social clubs, community associations, and cultural activities (traditional Hawaiian dance or *hula* schools; annual *lū'au* or parties) in almost every major U.S. city. These gatherings of primarily expatriate Native Hawaiians, their families, and friends are crucial to maintaining Hawaiian values and traditions for those who live away from the islands (Dudoit, 1997; Halualani, 2002).

Cultural Conflict between Traditional and Contemporary Belief Systems

For Hawaiians, the notion of family, or *'ohana*, has always been central to their worldview. However, the rapid evolution of American life due to expanding technologies and the impact of globalization has resulted in some daunting challenges for Native Hawaiians, as for all families. Long-established customs regarding child–parent relations, sex/gender roles, and even how family life was prioritized within other social relationships (such as work) have transformed traditional Hawaiian families into modern-day Hawaiian families.

Peter is a 16-year-old Native Hawaiian–Japanese American youth, born and raised in Hawai'i. Two years ago Peter's father, Clyde, a Hawai'i-born Japanese American and career Marine, transferred his family from Hawai'i to North Carolina. Peter was always described as "a sensitive boy" who was very close to both of his parents. In the past 6 months, Peter has begun wearing makeup on weekend outings to clubs, laughing it off to his parents as "something all the kids are doing these days."

Peter's Hawaiian mother, Pua, has long thought that Peter might be *māhū*, Hawaiian for transgendered. Pua grew up in a predominantly Native Hawaiian community, where *māhū* were well accepted by most families. Her husband, Clyde, grew up in a more traditional Japanese American household in a rural area of Hawai'i where sexuality was not discussed.

Peter has begun to have arguments with his father about his makeup and "girly" mannerisms, much of the conflict focused on Clyde's embarrassment about Peter being seen around the base. Tensions are rising between Clyde and Pua about Pua's support for Peter's gender development versus the impact Peter's behavior might have on Clyde's status with his Marine peers and supervisors.

Peter has finally begun talking to his mother about his emerging sexual and gender identity and asking Pua to tell him more about her *māhū* relatives. He is afraid of being "different" and is already being taunted in school. He is also worried about the discord with his father and between his parents. Over the past few weeks Peter has started to distance himself from his parents and has been staying out late with his friends. More recently Peter has asked to move back to Hawai'i to live with Pua's extended Hawaiian family.

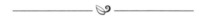

A key developmental issue for adolescents coming of age focuses on individual emancipation and the simultaneous reconfiguring of family roles and expectations. Sexual and gender identity development is a critical issue for teens, and particularly for Native Hawaiians who traditionally were much more tolerant of sex and gender variability than those of many other cultures. Clinicians working with Hawaiian families in which homosexuality, transgender, and/or other sexual issues are present must be knowledgeable about how Hawaiian families once and still do understand sex and gender. Many contemporary Hawaiians accept *māhū* in their families, partly because of being socialized to the belief that the special nature of *aloha*, or love, is unconditional, particularly in regard to *'ohana* (Anbe & Xian, 2001; Matzner, 2001). Hawaiian families are taught to value the enduring connection of family members with each other, no matter what conflicts, disagreements, or hurts transpire between them.

Over the past two decades there have been many changes in societal norms and attitudes in response to the long-standing bigotry and discrimination against gay men, lesbians, and transgendered persons. However, homophobia, sexism, and oppression of anyone with an alternative sexual or gender identity are still rampant in Hawai'i and throughout the United States. Even in the relatively tolerant environment of Hawai'i, in which vestiges of Hawaiian open-mindedness about sexuality still exist, a recent constitutional amendment to allow same-sex marriage was roundly defeated (Goldberg-Hiller, 2002). The "don't ask, don't tell" policy of the U.S. military is especially relevant in Peter's case, as it foreshadows the challenges ahead for Peter and his Marine father.

In this case study, conflicting belief systems about sex/gender are highlighted against the Hawaiian cultural background of Peter and his mother's family, the deeply entrenched nature of homophobia in today's Hawaiian and American societies, and the already existing challenge of launching adolescents in the family life cycle (Carter & McGoldrick, 1999). Practitioners working with Hawaiian families such as Peter's should not only acknowledge the historical culturally positive view toward *māhū*, particularly with an already supportive Hawaiian parent, but should also encourage the mobilization of Hawaiian values such as *aloha* and *lōkahi* from Hawaiian family traditions to mediate those tensions resulting from "culture clashes" in today's Kanaka Māoli families.

Cultural Conflict Related to Multiethnic/Multicultural Identity

Alika is a 20-year-old college student in Wisconsin who has never lived in Hawai'i. His Native Hawaiian father and Caucasian mother left the islands in the mid-1970s but maintain family ties in Hawai'i, where they both grew up. Alika has always felt out of place in the Midwest, particularly because of mispronunciations of his name and questions about his racial/ethnic background. Alika recently sought counseling at the student health center for anxiety, resentment, and anger after taking a sociology course on minority ethnic identity. As the only Native Hawaiian in the class, Alika was subject to many questions about Hawaiians and Pacific Islanders and was also expected to be a "spokesperson" about contemporary topics such as Hawaiian sovereignty and the movement for Native Hawaiian political and economic self-rule, about which other students knew more than he did.

During the early stage of therapy, Alika reported ambivalence about his Hawaiian identity, in part because his father had always been reluctant to share much about his own family history. His father was sometimes disparaging of Hawaiians, saying, "We left Hawai'i for a new life so we wouldn't have to be poor and on welfare like other Hawaiians at home." In addition, Alika described conflicting feelings about being Hawaiian and Caucasian, particularly given the negative history of White colonization in Hawai'i. The sometimes racist situations he experienced as a part-Hawaiian male growing up in the Midwest only exacerbated his social and emotional detachment from his Native Hawaiian heritage. However, although he did not often admit it to others, he also yearned to know more about his Native Hawaiian roots and culture.

Like many indigenous and First Nations peoples in the United States, Hawaiians are overrepresented in negative indices of health, education, and crime (Office of Hawaiian Affairs, 2002). According to the Office of Hawaiian Affairs:

- Native Hawaiian students in 8th to 12th grade use more tobacco, alcohol, and other drugs than any other ethnic group in Hawai'i.
- Only half of Kanaka Māoli who reside in the state complete high school, and of those who attend college, only 15% graduate.
- Native Hawaiians are among those with the highest rates of obesity, diabetes, hypertension, and cancer-related deaths in the United States.
- Hawaiians make up 39% of the inmate population in Hawai'i correctional facilities, more than any other ethnic group in the state.

The long-standing stigma associated with being Native Hawaiian is evidenced among Kanaka Māoli in Hawai'i, who report anxiety about seeking help because of the shame associated with being "another Hawaiian" with problems (Bell et al., 2001;

Crabbe, 1998; Mokuau, 1996; Nahulu et al., 1995). Hawaiians who are multiracial, particularly those who are part Caucasian, also struggle, as all mixed-race peoples do, with having to "choose identities" and never feeling a sense of belonging to any of their racial/ ethnic communities (Root, 1995). In addition, some Native Hawaiians who are raised away from Hawai'i and who lack knowledge of or, especially, direct experience with their own indigenous cultural practices sometimes reject or distance themselves from their Hawaiian heritage (Ahlo, 1996; Dudoit, 1997).

This psychosocial dynamic of denying the cultural norms or practices associated with one's stigmatized or oppressed identity group is often referred to as internalized oppression. Internalized oppression has been conceptualized as a mechanism wherein those of an oppressed class assume and enact the negative characteristics and stereotypes of their class as defined by those classes with more social power (Lipsky, 2004; Pheterson, 1990). In the preceding case study, Alika's father, as a Hawaiian himself, has expressed disdain for other Hawaiians, resulting in Alika's confusion about his own Hawaiian identity. Particularly in this post–civil rights era of racial pride, it is not uncommon for people of color to condemn those who reject their own minority racial/ethnic heritage.

I suggest, however, that internalized oppression is a survival mechanism resulting solely from living in oppressive conditions reinforced by societal institutions and norms (Kanuha, 1999). In Alika's case, rather than attribute his ambivalence and shame about his Hawaiian identity to his negative self-concept, our focus should be on the courage and resiliency required for any subjugated person to keep his or her spirit alive in the face of oppression. Internalized oppression is an indictment of societal racism, sexism, classism, and all systems of oppression that force persons such as Alika to assume a persona and belief system that daily results in self-hatred and rejection of others similar to oneself. As clinicians, we need to be cautious about not revictimizing survivors of racism by accusing them of consorting with the beliefs and behavior of their oppressors when they, like many of us, must sometimes choose to act against their true selves under circumstances of subjugation and fear of retaliation.

Family therapists working with Hawaiians must understand the historical milieu in which coping mechanisms such as distancing from one's ethnic heritage emerge. That is, when deluged with abysmal social, health, and economic data about Native Hawaiians, as reported here, it should not be surprising that some Kanaka Māoli might reject their own cultural values, beliefs, and traditions. In a therapeutic situation, Hawaiians, like all minority groups, require culturally skilled practitioners to help them utilize the resiliency and strengths of their values and traditions to overcome the health and mental health consequences of centuries-old colonization.

Cultural Conflict
between Traditional and Contemporary Helping Approaches

A challenging aspect of working with Kanaka Māoli families is the balancing of traditional Hawaiian understandings and strategies with modern-day therapeutic approaches. For example, because of the disconnect between many Native Hawaiians and their lands, language, and cultural practices, they may lack familiarity with values and traditions that are sometimes more accessible to a well-informed family therapist (Hawaiian or not) than to the Native Hawaiian client him- or herself.

As introduced earlier, an ancient Native Hawaiian approach to family conflict is *ho'oponopono*, which is translated as "to make right" (Meyer & Davis, 1994; Mokuau,

1990; Omuro-Yamamoto, 2001; Pukui et al., 1972; Shook, 1992). This unique Hawaiian family intervention includes a fundamental spiritual overlay, clearly delineated process stages, and well-defined roles and functions for all participants, which are performed in the context of Hawaiian values such as *aloha* (love and affinity), *mālama* (care), *lōkahi* (unity, connection), *lokomaika'i* (generosity), and *pono* (righteousness or "right"). The goal of *ho'oponopono* is to address pain and hurt among family members through a structured process in which those who have offended make amends to others, and aggrieved family members accept those acts of contrition through forgiveness.

In traditional *ho'oponopono* sessions, all interactions are grounded in spirituality. Guidance is sought from a Christian deity and/or Hawaiian ancestral gods throughout each session. There is a pivotal role played by the facilitator, or *haku*, who was traditionally a respected family *kupuna* (elder) but who now may be a community member or social worker trained in the process and chosen by consensus of all family members. Although similar in function to a Western family therapist, in *ho'oponopono* the *haku* assumes a more directive and prescribed role during sessions. For example, all interaction and dialogue are mediated through the *haku*; that is, at no time do participants speak directly to each other. *Ho'oponopono* may be employed deftly by a parent to quickly resolve disagreements between children or may involve sessions that extend for hours over a period of months. Sharing a meal upon completion of a session is a tradition that continues to be fundamental to the process.

The ideal outcome of *ho'oponopono* is healing and reconciliation among family members, but occasionally an impasse that cannot be resolved can result in banishment, or *mō ka piko*—literally, the severing of the umbilical cord. According to renowned scholar Mary Kawena Pukui (1979) this most extreme consequence "was not pronounced lightly" (p. 221) because "the ultimate heartbreak came with the total severance of family ties" (p. 220).

Until recently, this approach was not promoted in clinical settings. The present-day availability and use of *ho'oponopono* may sometimes produce anxiety among some Native Hawaiian clients who are not only unfamiliar with the practice, but are more comfortable with "talking therapy" led by Western-trained family therapists. With the growing acceptance of indigenous approaches to address many types of health and social issues, practitioners must be cognizant of the variety of traditional Native Hawaiian clinical approaches now available, as well as how, when, where, and with what types of social problems those strategies might complement or supplant Western models of healing.

CONCLUSION

Native Hawaiian families today only vaguely resemble Kanaka Māoli of ancient times. Whereas the lives of most Native Hawaiians were traditionally defined by bloodline, many Hawaiians today have no knowledge of nor interest in their genealogy. It is inconceivable that Hawaiian women were once not allowed to eat with men and that certain foods were *kapu* (forbidden) to them. Men slept with men without fear of homophobic retribution. And, most important, elders and grandparents were once integral to family life, not cast off to nursing homes or regarded as long-forgotten memories.

As the case examples illustrate, Native Hawaiian families today not only have culturally specific traditions that distinguish them from other ethnic groups, but are equally diverse within Hawaiians as a subgroup. Software developers of Hawaiian ancestry living in Seattle may still listen to Hawaiian music and dance the *hula*. Multiethnic offspring of African American and Hawaiian parents who've lived most of their lives in Chicago may wish one day to return to Hawai'i or may be disinterested in Hawaiian culture. A Native Hawaiian youth living in Honolulu may know a few Hawaiian words, or as a graduate of a Hawaiian language immersion school be equally adept in English and Hawaiian.

Clinicians working with Native Hawaiians are not necessarily required to be "competent" in their knowledge of *nā mea Hawai'i* (Hawaiian things), but should think and practice with understanding, sensitivity, and openness to Hawaiian culture. All Native Hawaiians, whether they reside in Hawai'i or elsewhere, have some connection to their Hawaiian cultural roots. For some, a deep understanding of their Hawaiian ancestry may be elusive because of the stigma attached to Native Hawaiians and Hawaiian culture in a colonial context. For others, who have the opportunity and/or support to retain and, most important, practice their Hawaiian heritage, "Hawaiian pride" may be the predominant aspect of their lives. Clinicians who work with Native Hawaiians today must acknowledge the historical losses associated with colonization of the Hawaiian Islands, as well as the challenges that contemporary Hawaiians face in realizing what it means to reclaim and live those belief systems and traditions of old.

As this chapter is being written, Kanaka Māoli are poised at a critical juncture in U.S. history. Today, Native Hawaiian sovereignty and the legal relationship of the Hawaiian people to the American government are being hotly and passionately debated in the U.S. Congress and, especially, among Native Hawaiians everywhere (Kelly, 2003; Office of Hawaiian Affairs, 2004; Sai, 2004). Shall Native Hawaiians establish legal status with the United States similar to other First Nations people? What type of self-governance should Hawaiians, now Americans, expect when until 1893 Hawai'i was an independent nation with distinct diplomatic ties to other countries?

Sovereignty as an issue of self-determination for the Native Hawaiian people is also reflected at the individual and family levels. Native Hawaiians must determine for themselves how they will nurture their relationships with each other, with non-Hawaiians, and with their global brothers and sisters in the broadest sense of *'ohana*. They must learn how to preserve and practice such values as *lokomaika'i* (generosity), *ha'aha'a* (humility), and *pono* (righteousness or "moral right") in their families and communities just as they did in ancient times. Self-determination means that, as a people, they must grapple with the conundrums of determining how to balance the "old ways" with the new.

The role of family therapists and clinicians is to support, empower, and facilitate healing for Native Hawaiian individuals and *nā 'ohana* through acknowledgement and affirmation of indigenous cultural values and beliefs, coupled with present-day "best practices."

REFERENCES

Ahlo, M. N. (1996). *Aloha spirit past and present: Two generations of Native Hawaiians discuss the issue of aloha in the context of cultural crisis.* Unpublished master's thesis, University of Hawaii, Honolulu.

Anbe, B., & Xian, K. (2001). *Ke kulana he māhū* (Film). Honolulu, HI: Zang Pictures.

Bell, C. K., Goebert, D., Miyamoto, R. H., Hishinuma, E. S., Andrade, N. N., Johnson, R. C., &

McDermott, J. F. J. (2001). Sociocultural and community factors influencing the use of Native Hawaiian healers and healing practices among adolescents in Hawaii. *Pacific Health Dialog, 8*(2), 249–259.

Blaisdell, K., & Mokuau, N. (1990). Kanaka Māoli: Indigenous Hawaiians. In N. Mokuau (Ed.), *Handbook of social services for Asian and Pacific Islanders*. Westport, CT: Greenwood Press.

Carter, B., & McGoldrick, M. (1999). *The expanded family life cycle: Individual, family and social perspectives* (3rd ed.). Needham Heights, MA: Allyn & Bacon.

Crabbe, K. M. (1998). Etiology of depression in Native Hawaiians. *Pacific Health Dialog, 5*(2), 341–345.

Dudoit, M. R. (1997). *Cultural identity and cultural practices of Hawaiians and part-Hawaiians in Southern California and Hawai'i*. Unpublished master's thesis, California State University, Long Beach.

Finney, B. R. (1994). *Voyage of discovery: A cultural odyssey through Polynesia*. Berkeley: University of California Press.

Goldberg-Hiller, J. (2002). *The limits to union: Same-sex marriage and the politics of civil rights*. Ann Arbor: University of Michigan Press.

Greico, E. M. (2001). *The Native Hawaiian and other Pacific Islander population: Census 2000 Brief*. Washington, DC: U.S. Department of Commerce, Economics and Statistics Administration, U.S. Census Bureau. Retrieved March 2, 2004, from www.census.gov/prod/2001pubs/c2kbr01-14.pdf

Halualani, R. T. (2002). *In the name of Hawaiians: Native identities and cultural politics*. Minneapolis: University of Minnesota Press.

Handy, E. S. C., & Pukui, M. K. (1998). *The Polynesian family system in Ka'u Hawai'i*. Honolulu, HI: Mutual.

Ii, J. P. (1959). *Fragments of Hawaiian history* (M. K. Pukui, Trans.). Honolulu, HI: Bishop Museum Press.

Kamakau, S. M. (1991). *Ka po'e Kahiko: The people of old* (M. K. Pukui, Trans.). Honolulu, HI: Bishop Museum Press.

Kamakau, S. M. (1992). *Ruling chiefs of Hawai'i* (rev. ed.). Honolulu, HI: Kamehameha Schools Press.

Kame'eleihiwa, L. (1986). *Land and the promise of capitalism: A dilemma for the Hawaiian chiefs of the 1848 Mahele*. Honolulu, HI: University of Hawaii Press.

Kame'eleihiwa, L. (1999a, September 20–22). *Le'ale'a o na kupuna (The pleasures of our ancestors)*. Paper presented at the *Lei Ānuenue*: Community Building with Groups at Risk for HIV conference, Honolulu, HI.

Kame'eleihiwa, L. (1999b). *Nā wahine kapu: Divine Hawaiian women*. Honolulu, HI: 'Ai Pohaku Press.

Kanuha, V. K. (1999). The social process of "passing" as a stigma management strategy: Acts of internalized oppression or acts of resistance? *Journal of Sociology and Social Welfare, 26*(4), 27–46.

Kelly, A. K. (2003). From Native Hawaiian to Native American? *Hawai'i Island Journal*. Retrieved September 24, 2004, from www.hawaiiislandjournal.com/stories/8a03a.html

Kyselka, W. (1987). *An ocean in mind*. Honolulu: University of Hawaii Press.

Lipsky, S. (2004). Internalized racism: A major breakthrough has been achieved. *FUSE*. Retrieved September 24, 2004, from focusonfreedom.org/resources/consciousness/breakthrough.html

Matzner, A. (2001). *'O au no kēia: Voices from Hawai'i's māhū and transgender communities*. Philadelphia: Xlibris.

Meyer, M., & Davis, A. (1994, Fall). Talking story: Mediation, peacemaking and culture. *American Bar Association Dispute Resolution Magazine*, pp. 5–9.

Mitchell, D. D. K. (1992). *Resource units in Hawaiian culture* (rev. ed.). Honolulu, HI: Kamehameha Schools Press.

Mokuau, N. (1990). Family-centered approach in native Hawaiian culture. *Families in Society: Journal of Contemporary Human Services, 71*(10), 607–613.

Mokuau, N. (1996). Health and well-being for Pacific Islanders: Status, barriers, and resolutions. *Asian American and Pacific Islander Journal of Health, 4*(1–3), 55–67.

Nahulu, L. B., Andrade, N. N., Makini, G. K. J., Yuen, N. Y. C., McDermott, J. F. J., Johnson, R. C., &

Waldron, J. A. (1995). Psychosocial risk and protective influences in Hawaiian adolescent psychopathology. *Cultural Diversity and Mental Health*, 2(2), 107–114.

Nordyke, E. C. (1977). *The peopling of Hawaii*. Honolulu: University of Hawaii Press.

Office of Hawaiian Affairs. (2002, June). *Native Hawaiian data book*. Honolulu: Author.

Office of Hawaiian Affairs. (2004). *The Hawaiian federal recognition bill*. Honolulu: Author. Retrieved May 20, 2004, from www.nativehawaiians.com/fedrecindex.html.

Omuro-Yamamoto, L. K. (2001). *Ho'oponopono: A phenomenological investigation of a Native Hawaiian harmony restoration process for families*. Unpublished doctoral dissertation, University of Wisconsin, Madison.

Pheterson, G. (1990). Alliances between women: Overcoming internalized oppression and internalized domination. In L. Albrecht & R. Brewer (Eds.), *Bridges of power: Women's multicultural alliances*. Philadelphia: New Society.

Polynesian Voyaging Society. (2004). *History of the Polynesian Voyaging Society: 1973–1998*. Retrieved September 21, 2004, from www.pvs-hawaii.com/about_pvshistory.htm

Pukui, M. K., Haertig, E. W., & Lee, C. A. (1972). *Nānā i ke kumu (Look to the source)* (Vol. 1). Honolulu, HI: Queen Lili'uokalani Children's Center.

Pukui, M. K., Haertig, E. W., & Lee, C. A. (1979). *Nānā i ke kumu (Look to the source)* (Vol. 2). Honolulu, HI: Queen Lili'uokalani Children's Center.

Rezentes, W. C. (1999). *Ka lama kukui (Hawaiian psychology): An introduction*. Honolulu, HI: 'A'ali'i Books.

Root, M. P. P. (Ed.). (1995). *The multiracial experience*. Thousand Oaks: Sage.

Sai, D. K. (2004). *The Hawaiian kingdom*. Retrieved September 25, 2004, from hawaiiankingdom.org

Santos, B. (2002). *'Ohana: Hawaiian proverbs and inspirational quotes celebrating family in Hawai'i*. Honolulu, HI: Mutual.

Shook, V. E. (1992). *Ho'oponopono*. Honolulu: University of Hawaii Press.

Smith, R. C. (1978). *Historical statistics of Hawaii*. Honolulu: University of Hawaii Press.

Stannard, D. E. (1988). *Before the horror: The population of Hawai'i on the eve of Western contact*. Honolulu: University of Hawaii Press.

U.S. Census Bureau. (2003). *Minority links: Facts on the Native Hawaiian and other Pacific Islander population*. Retrieved March 20, 2003, from www.census.gov

Young, B. B. C. (1980). The Hawaiians. In J. F. McDermott, W.-S. Tseng, & T. W. Maretzki (Eds.), *People and cultures of Hawaii: A psychosocial profile*. Honolulu: John A. Burns School of Medicine and University of Hawaii Press.

PART II

❧

FAMILIES OF AFRICAN ORIGIN

CHAPTER 5

Families of African Origin
An Overview

Lascelles Black
Vanessa Jackson

Unlike other immigrants, the ancestors of most people of African descent came to the Americas in a migration not of choice, but of capture. The slave trade that flourished from the 15th to the 19th centuries brought African captives to the Caribbean and the Americas and scattered them throughout the hemisphere. Efforts were made to break the spirits of those captured by erasing their history (Bennett, 2003; Van Sertima, 1976) and denying the validity of their culture.

Zinn (2003, p. 26) writes that African civilization was as advanced in its own way as that of Europe in the 16th and early 17th centuries. It contained 100 million people, some in large cities. Before the slave trade, the kingdoms of Timbuktu, Mali, and Benin were stable, well organized, and prosperous at a time when European states were just beginning to develop into modern nations. These and other African nations were sought out for trade by European nations (Bennett, 2003).

Early European settlers in the Americas were mostly unskilled in agriculture and "were so little inclined to work the land that in Virginia John Smith had to declare martial law . . . and force them into the fields for survival" (Zinn, 2003, p. 25). Yet this proved insufficient, and there were too few indentured White servants to make the plantations profitable. After attempts to enslave the native population proved futile, plantation owners saw African slaves as the solution. By 1619 a million enslaved Africans had already been transported to South America and the Caribbean.

AFRICAN AMERICANS
IN HISTORICAL AND CULTURAL CONTEXT

In his essay "Before Color Prejudice," Frank M. Snowden Jr. (1983) notes that, in early Christian sources, skin color contrasts were viewed as part of the natural order. However, in England, sometime before the 15th century, often sinister qualities were attributed to the color black, whereas the color white became symbolic of goodness, beauty, and purity. Everything "white," symbolizing European and Christian, was perceived to be good and superior, and everything "black," symbolizing African and non-Christian, was perceived as bad and inferior. Prejudice against skin color became the justification for brutality and hatred, and racism became important in building the nations of the Americas (Zinn, 2003).

It is estimated that Africa lost about 50 million of her people to death and slavery during the 16th through the 19th centuries; they usually lived in horrible conditions at the hands of slave traders and plantation owners (Zinn, 2003, p. 29). Estimates of the mortality rate during the journey from Africa to the Americas, called the Middle Passage, ranged from 20% (Lovejoy, 1989) to 33.3% (Zinn, 2003, p. 29). Despite the loss of life, investors saw huge profits, sometimes double their investments.

After the Declaration of Independence in 1776, six states banned the importation of Africans. In 1808 the federal government did so as well, but permitted the institution of slavery in those states that maintained it and allowed slavery to spread unrestricted south of the Ohio River.

In 1860 the population of the slave-owning states and the District of Columbia was 12.3 million, of whom 8.1 million were Whites, 4 million were slaves, and 250,000 were "free colored." In the South slave ownership was practiced by just 25% of Whites, but the majority of Whites defended slavery because they believed that their prosperity depended on it. Slavery also provided even the poorest of Whites with a sense of superiority over the African population, a false superiority based on skin color.

There were many uprisings over the years in all countries that practiced slavery. In 1605, Africans in northern Brazil freed themselves and founded the kingdom of Palmares, which was independent until 1694, when its people were defeated by the Portuguese and enslaved again. Between 1712 and 1801, slave uprisings took place in New York City, South Carolina, Virginia, and elsewhere. In 1791, François-Dominique Toussaint-Louverture led a successful slave rebellion and founded the island nation of Haiti. The Maroons of Jamaica, a group of escaped slaves who fought the British for more than a century, won the recognition of their right to live in their own communities as free and independent citizens, paying no taxes.

An important avenue to freedom in this country was the Underground Railroad, a secret network that helped escaped slaves to make their way to the free states and Canada. Between 1810 and 1860 as many as 100,000 enslaved African Americans were guided to freedom by the workers of the network, such as Harriet Tubman, William Wells Brown, and Josiah Henson (Koslow, 1999).

The Emancipation Proclamation of 1863 and the passage of the Thirteenth Amendment in 1865 ended the institution of slavery in the United States. The Civil Rights Act of 1866 and the Fourteenth Amendment in 1868 decreed all African Americans to be citizens with full civil and voting rights. Although these rights existed in law, they were not honored in practice in many parts of the country for decades. Throughout the South, Jim Crow laws denied African Americans their rights and severely limited their access to basic services. The struggle for recognized freedom and equality continued into the 20th century. The passage of the 1964 Civil Rights Act and the Voting Rights Act of 1965 focused attention on the de facto segregation and racism prevalent in the entire country. The modern civil rights movement under leaders such as Dr. Martin Luther King Jr., Malcolm X, Rev. Jesse Jackson, and others, starting in the 1960s, revitalized the struggle for justice and equality.

Demographics

Many older African Americans, especially those who are products of the rural South, often orient themselves to a new acquaintance by asking, "Who are your people?" This is a layered question that moves beyond family name and geography; it highlights the importance of looking at individuals and communities within a context of their connections.

The 2000 U.S. Census reports that 34.7 million people, or 12.3% of the U.S. population, identify themselves as Black. This number is projected to double in the next 50 years (U.S. Census Bureau, 1998). People of African origin include individuals from Africa, South and Central America, the Caribbean, and elsewhere.

Immigration statistics can augment this snapshot data of the census. For example, between 1972 and 1996, approximately 1.1 million persons of African origin migrated to the United States from Jamaica, Haiti, Guyana, Trinidad and Tobago, and Nigeria. (Schomburg Center, 1999). A colleague of Jamaican descent, raised to adulthood in Canada and currently living in the United States, described a sense of "invisibility" that she experiences when listed in the category "African American." This woman did not reject her African past or distance herself from a stigmatized racial identity; rather, she felt loyalty to and pride in her heritage.

Brice-Baker (Chapter 8, this volume) highlights the complexity of relationships between African Americans (especially individuals with a family history of enslavement in America) and immigrants of African origin from Africa, the Caribbean, and Latin America. Although sharing an experience with enslavement and/or colonization, these communities have very different historical, political, and economic experiences that shape their relationship with racism. In addition, perceptions of economic competition in America and the limited or distorted information about the history and experiences of different African descendent groups contribute to intergroup tensions. One university counseling center established a support group for African, African American, and Caribbean women to provide an opportunity for dialogue and healing between these communities (P. Freeman, personal communication, January 25, 2004).

Biracial and multiracial categories were included for the first time in the 2000 U.S. Census. An additional 1.8 million people identified themselves as multiracial (Black and at least one other race). As noted by Root (2004), the inclusion of a multiracial category challenges a race system wedded to notions of racial purity and acknowledges the fluidity of racial identity in America.

Approximately 2% of psychiatrists and psychologists and 4% of social workers identify themselves as African American (Holzer et al., 1998, in U.S. Department of

Health and Human Services, 2001). The dearth of mental health providers of African origin creates a significant barrier for members of those communities who prefer to work with a therapist of similar racial, ethnic, and cultural origin.

Migration to the United States

Throughout the 19th and 20th centuries, and continuing in this century, immigration from Africa and the countries of the African diaspora in the Americas has increased. Some came as political refugees; most were seeking a better standard of living. In 1998, 5% of Black people in this country were foreign born (Pollard & O'Hare, 1999). It is critical in therapy to understand the meaning migration has for individuals and for the family system as a whole, both in the United States and in their country of origin. Migration for educational or economic opportunities can create contexts for grief and a deep sense of emotional dislocation. It is important to understand that government polices have also shaped the entry of people of African origin into the United States beyond the forced distribution of Africans through the slave trade.

From 1924 to 1965, the U.S. immigration policies severely restricted the entry of people of color and those of the less desirable European populations. The significant immigration of Africans and people of African descent from the Caribbean coincides with the movement of African American communities due to the softening of residential segregation in this country. Increased housing and job opportunities have led to the intensification of urban renewal and the resulting dislocation of more than 1,600 African American communities (Fullilove, 2004).

Those who left family members behind in the South endeavored to sustain the familial bonds. A tremendous emotional toll is exacted when people leave family members behind in their country of origin. Often, women must separate from their children for many years until they get their residency and citizenship. These children, deprived of an ongoing parent–child bond, have been known to grow up with a sense of abandonment and resentment for the years they were separated from their mothers and fathers. The immigrant parents struggle to maintain the family connections through financial support and gifts, as well as phone calls and letters. The children are usually raised by caring members of the extended family or by trusted friends. But parents are still worried because of the uncertainty of how their children are being raised, and they miss sharing the love and experiencing the growth of their children (Larmer & Moses, 1996).

Themes frequently dealt with when working with these immigrants are the sense of loss of the actual family bond and the family fragmentation; social dislocation; economic advancement that has come at a very high emotional cost; the difficulties of assimilation; and anger that grows from the frustration of coping with all of these issues. But above all such concerns looms the issue of legitimacy; that is, do they have documented status, the green card? Without this legitimacy there is always the fear of discovery and deportation.

An invitation to share their immigration story is not only important in engaging the families, it is also an opportunity for them to listen to each other tell their experiences, because sometimes these stories are not shared in the home. Often the joy of reuniting the family pushes aside the tales of the difficulties each person suffered during the separation (Black, 2000, 2003).

To facilitate this sharing, the following questions may be asked:

- What were the circumstances of your migration? How was the decision made, and who was involved in the process?
- What have been the benefits of migration?
- What was lost to acquire these benefits?
- How has your sense of yourself as a Black person been affected by your migration?
- How connected are you to other immigrants from your country of origin?

It is important for both the children and the parents to tell their stories, to express their ways of grieving the separation from their original home, and to realize that celebrating their new home is not being disloyal. They need to know that the relationships left behind can be honored and sustained through frequent communication.

Spirituality

Spirituality has historically been an important factor in the lives of Africans. The myth that Africans were godless heathens before exposure to missionaries and coming to the Americas was concocted to ease the consciences of slavery's perpetrators. The form of Christianity introduced by the missionaries became a tool of oppression. However, Judaism, Islam, and Christianity were already well established in Africa alongside other indigenous religions. In this country three of every four African Americans say that religion is significant in their lives (Billingsley, 1992). Most are Christians, even if many do not identify themselves as members of a specific religious denomination (Moore Hines, 1998). The Black church was the first institution that belonged exclusively to people of African descent, and it provided not only spiritual refuge and counseling, but also a place from which to organize their community (Boyd-Franklin, 1989). Islam is also a significant religious influence in the lives of a growing number of African Americans (Daneshpour, 2003), and there are more than 110,000 Black Jews.

A family's strong spiritual values may influence the meaning it assigns to a crisis and the options for resolution it considers. Clinicians' understanding of these spiritual values is essential, both in terms of how a problem may challenge or threaten spiritual beliefs, and how spiritual values can be drawn on to resolve problems.

THERAPY ISSUES

Gender

Gender relations in communities of African origin are colored by the subjugation of males and females during enslavement and colonization and the constant impingement of European values on African descendent communities. As in most cultures of the world, patriarchal values shaped male–female relationships in many African nations prior to European contact and imposed significant limitations on social, economic, and political opportunities for women. However, there are also numerous examples of more fluid gender roles related to the importance of women's labor in the economic life of many African communities (Patterson, 1998). The misinterpretation of gender role flexibility within families of African origin and racist barriers to employment for males fed the stereotype of Black families as a "tangle of pathology." Willie and Reddick (2003) note that one of the greatest gifts of Blacks to the culture of the nation has been the egalitarian family model in which neither the husband nor the wife is always in charge.

Jones and Shorter-Gooden (2003) offer insights into Black women in America as they negotiate gender and race. The term "shifting" refers to the practice of dissimulation historically utilized by Africans in situations of oppression as a key survival strategy. However, over time this strategy can serve to separate the shifted from his or her essential self; he or she becomes self-alienated to accommodate others' needs.

McAdams-Mahmoud (Chapter 10, this volume) notes that social separation among African American Muslim families serves as a tool for providing support and reinforcing intimacy, and offers insights into practices that are frequently written off as sexist and oppressive. An African American man she interviewed described a ritual he attended with a group of African American Muslim men, who had had no previous connection, in which there was an amazingly high level of self-disclosure as they shared perspectives on marriage and men's roles.

Despite fairly egalitarian values related to gender and work, families of African origin continue to struggle with issues of patriarchal control. Male violence against women is a frequent presenting problem in family therapy. Families of African origin may be inhibited from seeking services related to emotional or physical abuse because of concerns about exposing men to a racist criminal justice system or confronting negative attitudes about their domineering behavior toward Black women. Assisting families in exploring gender role expectations and understanding the impact of institutionalized racism may be a crucial role for clinicians who are working with families of African origin. Head (2004) described the challenges faced by Black men and the contribution of racism to their experiences with clinical depression.

In *Standing the Test of Time* (2001), Julie Rainbow offers loving and honest portrayals of long-term African American couples. Her work serves as a guide for eliciting stories of commitment, resilience, and love from couples and families seeking new ways to relate to each other.

A genogram, which can be a useful tool in exploring intergenerational family stories related to gender roles, marital ties, and power, should include non-nuclear family members, because they contribute to a family's strength and emotional life (Watts-Jones, 1997).

Class

America is a class-saturated, class-silent, and consumption-focused society. Census data consistently point to the asset accumulation gap between Blacks and Whites in America. Immigration to this country often brings with it changes in class status. Individuals holding professional positions in their countries of birth, but whose credentials have not been accepted here, may be required to accept low-wage jobs. The quest for economic security and advancement may be the impetus for migration to, and within, the United States, resulting in family separations and isolation. What does it mean for a family to have to start over and rebuild an economic and social base? Brice-Baker (Chapter 8, this volume) offers insights into the unique class issues of families that immigrated to the United States.

Prior to residential desegregation, African American communities were economically diverse. Integration opened up a wider range of residential choices, resulting in a significant level of "green flight" (i.e., when businesses, and therefore money, leave a community) and the abandonment of traditionally Black neighborhoods by members with means to move to previously all-White settings. Clinicians might explore with a family the rationale for migration out of predominately Black neighborhoods, and its impact on the family. In addition, in most extended family networks, there are some who have done well and others who may continue to struggle economically.

Education and socioeconomic advancement continue to be highly valued among people of African origin, although some individuals entrenched in multigenerational poverty may have more negative attitudes regarding education and upward mobility.

Sexual Orientation/Heterosexism

Within communities of African origin, lesbian, gay, bisexual, and transgendered (LGBT) individuals continue to fight for visibility as marginalized members within their families, communities, and the wider society. Black gays and lesbians have made substantial contributions to their communities but rarely are acknowledged for them. Cohen (1999) states that gay and lesbian acceptance of this conditional status in Black communities is critical because of the racism that they face on the outside.

Homosexuality is considered taboo in many communities of African origin, resulting in its often being kept hidden. Clinicians must balance respect for the cultural and spiritual values of people of African origin with the needs of LGBT members for support in dealing with heterosexism. Clinical issues related to sexual orientation include coming out, gay and lesbian parenting, depression and anxiety, and posttraumatic stress disorder related to physical and emotional abuse based on sexual orientation.

One of the few studies of Black LGBT experiences (Battle, Cohen, Warren, Fergerson, & Audam, 2002) reported that 40 percent of women and 18 percent of men interviewed reported having at least one child. Although she does not specifically address the issue of race and ethnicity, Bernstein (2000) advocates a "cultural literacy" model for heterosexual clinicians working with LGBT clients. To engage in progressive and potentially healing interactions with clients, clinicians should challenge their heterosexist assumptions and develop an understanding of the economic, social, political, and emotional impact of homophobia.

Response to Treatment

Jackson (2002) provides a historic overview of mental health services for Africans in America that was characterized by brutality, segregation, overreliance on institutionalization, and racist application of psychiatric diagnoses. In 1851, Samuel Cartwright, a fierce proponent of slavery, coined the term *Drapetomania*, the "mental disease" causing slaves to run away (Cartwright, 2001). People of African origin have a long history of being labeled pathological because of their efforts to resist racial and economic oppression or their attempts to adapt to such conditions. In addition, people of African origin are vulnerable to the same emotional and family problems that affect non-African-descendent populations.

Family conflicts are primary presenting problems for many families of African origin. It is especially critical for clients who have been mandated to family counseling to share their unique stories about their families, including their encounters with the social welfare and mental health systems. In the engagement process, they should be encouraged to state what they value about their families, and what needs to change to increase a sense of connection and healing (Black, 2003).

Social/Political/Economic Impact

Families of African origin frequently have experiences with social, economic, and political oppression that affect their emotional health. Their giving voice to feelings of fear and outrage at the injustices they experience may result in their being told that they are acting as "victims" or "playing the race card." Some individuals, who have internalized these messages, may need assistance in linking current emotional difficulties to broader social, economic, and political realities. Akinyela (2002) emphasizes the need to place the experiences of people of African origin seeking clinical consultation within a historical and political context. Specifically, he calls for a creation of therapeutic space free from the interpretations and judgments of the dominant Eurocentric culture.

Grief/Rage/Loss

Therapists should acknowledge the resilience of people of African origin, which is reflected in loving familial bonds, economic survival, professional success, and deeply held spiritual values. However, there are deep, unacknowledged pools of grief, rage, and loss that color the experiences of many people of African descent. Enslavement, colonization, migration, and the emotional and physical separation from their homeland, whether by force or by choice, create a need for reflecting on losses even while accomplishments should be celebrated.

Some people of African origin experience internalized rage that can be the result of a lifetime accumulation of micro-aggressions, real and perceived slights and insults, subtle acts of dismissal, and implied suggestions to "stay in your place." Therapists need to provide a safety zone for speaking about these experiences, which often lie beneath conflicts, confusion and disillusionment, depression, and substance abuse. A. J. Franklin outlines strategies and interventions for helping men of African descent to cope and support each other with these complex issues (Franklin, 2004).

Pemina Yellow Bird of the Three Affiliated Tribes (Mandan, Hidatsa, and Arikara) offers three questions that emerged from the healing tradition of the indigenous peoples of America. Makungu Akinyela, an African American activist/therapist suggests an additional question that emerged from testimonial rituals within the Black church:

- What happened to you (your people)?
- How does what happen to you (your people) affect you now?
- In spite of what happened, how were you (your people) able to triumph?
- What do you need to heal?

These questions create a framework for the creation of individual, family, and community narratives. Most people of African origin have had limited opportunity to have their experiences of trauma, struggle, or triumph witnessed to and validated. The therapeutic encounter should serve as an opportunity for families of African origin to share their stories, construct meaning, and identify internal and external change strategies. The clinician should evaluate his or her role in facilitating or inhibiting these therapeutic processes.

CONCLUSION

Therapists must delve into the complex historical, cultural, and linguistic realities of clients of African descent, including the invisibility syndrome that often haunts them, in order to provide culturally competent interventions. The depth of their presenting problems may not be recognized by a therapist who is unaware that a slight to a White person can be an emotional wound to a Black person because of the weight of history and a lifetime of subtle and sharp injuries (Franklin, 2004). Culturally competent therapists can serve a crucial role in helping families of African descent to reconnect with their unique histories and values.

REFERENCES

Akinyela, M. (2002). Decolonizing our lives: Divining a post-colonial therapy. *International Journal of Narrative Therapy and Community Work, 2,* 32.

Battle, J., Cohen, C., Warren, D., Fergerson, G., & Audam, S. (2002). *Say it loud: I'm Black and I'm proud: Black Pride Survey 2000.* New York: Policy Institute of the National Gay and Lesbian Task Force.

Bennett, L., Jr. (2003). *Before the Mayflower: A history of Black America.* Chicago: Johnson.

Bernstein, A. C. (2000). Straight therapist working with lesbians and gays in family therapy. *Journal of Marital and Family Therapy, 25*(4), 443.

Billingsley, A. (1992). *Climbing Jacob's ladder: The enduring legacy of African-American families.* New York: Simon & Schuster.

Black, L. W. (2000). Therapy with African American couples. In P. Papp (Ed.), *Couples on the fault line* (pp. 205–221). New York: Guilford Press.

Black, L. W. (2003). Rituals for bicultural couples and families. In E. Imber-Black, J. Roberts, & R. Whiting (Eds.), *Rituals in families and family therapy.* New York: Norton.

Boyd-Franklin, N. (1989). *Black families in therapy; A multisystems approach.* New York: Guilford Press.

Cohen, C. J. (1999). *The boundaries of Blackness: AIDS and the breakdown of Black politics.* Chicago: University of Chicago Press.

Daneshpour, M. (2003). Lives together, worlds apart? The lives of multicultural Muslim couples. In V. Thomas, T. Karis, & J. Wetchler (Eds.), *Clinical issues with interracial couples: Theories and research.* New York: Haworth Press.

Franklin, A. J. (2004). *From brotherhood to manhood.* Hoboken, NJ: Wiley.

Fullilove, M. T. (2004). *Root shock: How tearing up city neighborhoods hurts American and what we can do about it.* New York: One World/Ballantine.

Gaines, S. O. (1995). Prejudice: From Allport to DuBois. *American Psychologist, 5*(2), 96–103.

Head, J. (2004). *Standing in the shadows: Understanding and overcoming depression in Black men.* New York: Broadway Books.

Jackson, V. (2002). In our own voice: African American stories of oppression, survival and recovery in mental health systems. *International Journal of Narrative Therapy and Community Work, 2,* 11–31.

Jones, C., & Shorter-Gooden, K.(2003). *Shifting: The double lives of Black women in America.* New York: HarperCollins.

Koslow, P. (1999). *The African American desk reference.* New York: Wiley.

Larmer, B., & Moses, K. (1996, February 19). The barrel children. *Newsweek,* p. 45.

Lovejoy, P. E. (1989). The impact of the Atlantic slave trade on Africa: A review from the literature. *Journal of African History,* p. 30.

Moore Hines, P. (1998). Climbing up the rough side of the mountain: Hope, culture, and therapy. In M. McGoldrick (Ed.), *Re-visioning family therapy: Race, culture, and gender in clinical practice* (pp. 78–90). New York: Guilford Press.

Patterson, O. (1998). *Rituals of blood: Consequences of slavery in two American centuries.* Washington, DC: Civitas/Counterpoint.

Rainbow, J. (2001). *Standing the test of time.* Cleveland, OH: Pilgrim Press.

Root, M. P. P. (2004). Multiracial families and children: Implications for educational research and practice. In J. A. Banks (Ed.), *Handbook of research on multicultural education* (2nd ed., pp. 574–597). San Francisco: Jossey-Bass.

Schomburg Center for Research on Black Culture. (1999). *The African American desk reference.* New York: Wiley.

Snowden, F. M., Jr. (1983). *Before color prejudice: The ancient view of Blacks.* Cambridge, MA: Harvard University Press.

U.S. Census Bureau. (1998). *Statistical abstract of the United States.* Washington, DC: Author.

Van Sertina, I. (1976). *They came before Columbus: The African presence in ancient America.* New York: Random House.

Watts-Jones, D. (1997). Towards an African American genogram. *Family Process, 36*(4), 375–383.

Willie, C. V., & Reddick, R. J. (2003). *A new look at Black families* (5th ed.). Walnut Creek, CA: Altimira Press.

Zinn, H. (2003). *A people's history of the United States.* New York: HarperCollins.

CHAPTER 6

African American Families

Paulette Moore Hines
Nancy Boyd-Franklin

Families of African heritage come to the United States from many different countries and are therefore very diverse in terms of geographic origin, acculturation, religious background, skin color, socioeconomic status, and in the implementation of strategies employed to cope with racism and discrimination. The largest group, and our focus here, are descendants of African slaves.

Many early studies of African American families reflected a pejorative view that characterized them as "disorganized, deprived, disadvantaged" (Deutsch & Brown, 1964; Frazier, 1966; Moynihan, 1965). In recent years, African American researchers and scholars have reexamined this deficit view and have presented a more balanced perspective that includes the strengths inherent in these families (Billingsley, 1968, 1992; Boyd-Franklin, 2003; Hill, 1972, 1999; Hines, 1999; Hines & Boyd-Franklin, 1996; Hines, Garcia-Preto, McGoldrick, Almeida, & Weltman, 1992; Jones, 2004; McAdoo, 1996, 2002; Staples, 1994; White, 2004). A number of researchers have also explored the stages of racial identity development among African Americans (Carter, 1995; Cross, 1991; Cross, Parham, & Helms, 1998; Helms & Cook, 1999; Jones, 1998; Parham, 1992).

Afrocentric scholars (Akbar, 1984, 1985; Ani, 1994; Asante, 1988, 1990; Kambon, 1998; Karenga, 1997; Mbiti, 1970; Nobles, 1985, 2004) have concluded that the recognition of ancient African culture and history is paramount to fully comprehending African Americans. This emerging scholarly movement believes that the family and the spiritual dimension of life are essential for the individual's existence (Nobles, 2004).

FAMILY AND CULTURAL CONTEXT OF AFRICAN AMERICANS IN THE 21st CENTURY

African Americans make up about 13.3% of Americans (U.S. Bureau of the Census, 2004). Between 1940 and 1970, more than 1.5 million African Americans migrated from the South, most frequently to the North and sometimes to the West, in pursuit of greater economic opportunities. Currently, more than half (55%) live in the South and a majority live in the central city of a metropolitan area (McKinnon, 2003).

The result of this migration was the emergence of a substantial number of African Americans moving into the middle class. According to the 2000 census, 33% of all Black families were considered middle-income families (earning $50,000–$99,999 annually), as compared with 11.4% in 1970. Blacks also made major advances in education, employment, home ownership, and voter participation (Billingsley, 1992; Staples, 1994). In addition, between 1990 and 2000, the percentage of African Americans living below the poverty level decreased from 27.0 to 22.7% (McKinnon, 2003; U.S. Bureau of the Census, 2000, 2001).

Still, institutional racism exerts a significant impact on the lives and well-being of African Americans. For example, in 2000, African Americans averaged just 66% of the income of Whites ($30,439 vs. $ 45,904). Twenty-three percent of all African American families lived below the poverty level in 2001, as compared with 8% of non-Hispanic Whites, and the unemployment rate for African Americans, aged 16 and over, was almost twice that for their White counterparts (11% vs. 5%) (McKinnon, 2003). Disparities based on race continue to exist on a host of key quality of life indicators, including home and business ownership, physical health, children living at or below the poverty level, number employed in professional and managerial specialty occupations, and others (McKinnon, 2003).

The average life expectancy of African Americans remains substantially lower than that of Whites, and the rate of death among African Americans due to AIDS and homicide exceeds that of any other group (Arias, 2002; Rockeymoore, 2002).The disillusionment and frustration generated by persistent poverty and oppression have resulted in a high rate of drug and alcohol abuse among African Americans, a dependence that makes for what we view as "psychological slavery." Yet, as Billingsley (1968) noted, African Americans generally are noteworthy for their "amazing ability to survive in the face of impossible conditions." Hill (1999), a researcher who focuses on the adaptive strengths in African American families, attributed the group's survival to strong kinship bonds, flexibility of family roles, and the high value placed on religion, education, and work.

KINSHIP BONDS

Strong African American kinship bonds are traceable to Africa, where various tribes shared "commonalities" (e.g., worldview) that were broader than bloodlines (Akbar, 1985; Nobles, 2004). In contrast to the European premise "I think, therefore I am," the prevailing African philosophy is "We are, therefore I am." In effect, individuals owed their existence to the tribe (Nobles, 2004).

Torn from their homelands and tribal connections by slavery, men, women, and children had to abandon their native languages, names, occupations, mates, religions, foods, and customs. Mortality rates were high and life expectancies were low. Families were frequently dissolved by the sale of members to slaveholders on different plantations. Afrocentric scholars (Ani, 1994; Kambon, 1998) have referred to slavery as the *Maafa*, a Kiswahili word meaning "great disaster." The *Maafa* was the African holocaust, with a catastrophic loss of life estimated at 25 to 100 million (Ani, 1994; Boyd-Franklin, 2003; Kambon, 1998).

With male and female slaves prohibited from marrying, frequent changes of partner became the rule. Black men were used as breeders to increase the labor supply, and their owners sexually exploited Black women. Despite these extreme hardships, slaves sought to form new family units to compensate for losses due to death and slavery. Even after emancipation, many former slaves remained on plantations, hoping that lost family members might return.

Access to and use of their kinship network, which is much broader than traditional "bloodlines," has always been a critical resource for African Americans, given the persistent need to cope with the pressures of an oppressive society (Billingsley, 1992; Boyd-Franklin, 2003; Staples, 1994). White (2004) has noted the number of "uncles, aunts, big mamas, boyfriends, older brothers and sisters, deacons, preachers, and others who operate in and out of the African American home."

Therapists working with African Americans must be willing to take into account, and sometimes work with, an extended kinship system. Because of characteristic extended family orientation and the role flexibility, emotional ties are not predictable solely on the basis of biological relationship. Relatives often live in close proximity and rely on one another in times of need (McAdoo, 2002). The therapist should ask who is in the family, who lives in the home, and what family members and significant others live elsewhere. Often the question, "Whom can you depend on for help when needed?" will uncover key individuals in the family's support system.

A genogram can aid the therapist in gathering information about relationships and the roles of different family members (Boyd-Franklin, 2003; McGoldrick & Gerson, 1999). However, information generally should be gathered only after the therapist senses that a bond of trust has been established with the family (Boyd-Franklin, 2003; Hines, 1999). The therapist should look for natural openings to obtain information, rather than force data gathering, for many African Americans are suspicious about the motivation underlying what they perceive as "prying." Illegitimate births, parents' marital status, the incarceration of family members, or deaths due to AIDS, violence, or substance abuse, may be "secrets" unknown to all family members or information that members are hesitant to discuss with an outsider.

Within the African American family system, it is fairly common for a child to be informally adopted by a grandparent or other extended family member, who may be better able than the child's parents to provide nurture and/or a wholesome environment (Billingsley, 1992; Boyd-Franklin, 2003). Young adults frequently rely on the extended-kin network's support to achieve a college education. This support may also facilitate the transition into adulthood and the work world.

Such role flexibility is often mobilized in times of crisis, such as separation, illness, hospitalization, or the death of a family member. However, for far too many African Americans, there is a growing gap between the cultural ideology that encourages extending help and their ability to be responsive to family members' needs. African American families, particularly those who are poor or of the working class, are disproportionately affected by high unemployment and health crises (e.g., mothers unable to care for their children because of drug addiction and/or AIDS) that financially and emotionally overtax their networks. Sometimes, even when family members can provide assistance, bureaucratic or legal obstacles in school or health and human services policies can impede the involvement of family members (Hill, 1999).

Family therapists must explore and select carefully the core and extended family members to include in family therapy. Often, key family members may be unwilling or unable to keep appointments on a regular basis. The therapist might therefore schedule a family session in the home, provided key family members consent.

Too frequently, outsiders assume that certain family structures are inherently dysfunctional (e.g., multigenerational, single-parent). Therapists need to recognize that what matters most is not the structure but the functioning of a family. Sometimes, however, family boundaries and authority lines become quite blurred. Role confusion occurs most frequently in families that include a parental child and three generations, as described in the following sections.

GENDER ROLES AND COUPLE RELATIONSHIPS

Despite stereotypes that characterize African American men negatively, there is considerable variability among African American men, as there is in all ethnic groups. Some live in the home and are very active in child rearing; some live in the home but are peripheral to their children's lives; some are involved but live outside the home.

It is safe to say that the high rate of unemployment among African American men has greatly influenced the willingness of African American women and men to marry (Testa & Krogh, 1995; Tucker & Mitchell-Kernan, 1995) and to assume a central role in the lives of their children. This reality can easily give rise to perceptions of Black men as non-family-oriented or uncaring. Franklin (1993, 2004) coined the term "invisibility syndrome" in his discussion of the marginalization of African American men. White Americans have often been taught to fear Black males in particular and to treat them as if they were "invisible," thus marginalizing them in the larger societal context.

African American women, who are often more actively religious than their mates, are frequently regarded as the "strength of the family." More easily employed than their male counterparts, Black women historically have worked outside the home, sometimes as the sole wage earners, particularly in times of high unemployment (Boyd-Franklin, 2003; Hines, 1999). Still, these relationships are affected by the male–female power differential that characterizes our patriarchal society. Shelton and John (1993) found that, in contrast to European American and Hispanic males, the more time married African American males spent in paid labor, the more time they spent in household labor as well.

Because African American men have a much lower life expectancy than African American women or Whites of either sex (Arias, 2002), the gender ratio among African American adults is quite skewed. The availability of African American men to participate in relationships is affected by incarceration, mental and physical disabilities, drug and alcohol abuse, and deaths on jobs involving a high degree of danger or health hazards (e.g., military service, blue-collar work in hazardous waste, chemical production, or mining), as well as violence of many kinds.

Professional African American women are often left with the choice of marrying less educated, lower-status men or remaining single. Even if a woman is willing to marry, the gender ratio is so skewed that she may not be successful in finding a partner, maintaining a relationship, or remarrying. In addition, African American couples often experience relationship stress because of the added burden of racism and their own internalization of negative projections about each other (Boyd-Franklin, 2003; Hines, 1999; Pinderhughes, 1982).

Children and, hence, the role of mothers are highly valued within African American culture (Hines, 1990). Across income groups, a growing number of women are choosing to become single parents rather than remain childless. In 2002, 48% of Black children were living with a single mother, as compared with 16% of non-Hispanic White children (Fields, 2003).

The identity of African American fathers, regardless of income, is linked to their ability to fulfill traditional gender functions and to provide for their families. Success in being a provider, however, continues to be influenced by systematic discrimination. They are constantly challenged with negative stereotypes, including the notion that they are absent or, at best, peripheral in their children's lives.

Therapists are particularly likely to overlook noncustodial fathers, as well as other males in the extended family system, particularly a noncustodial father's kinship network. Therapists should involve male partners, fathers, and other significant adult males in family assessment and treatment. However, many African American men are reluctant to enter therapy, because they associate it with distrusted mainstream organizations.

Therapists should explore signs of ambivalence and respond with creativity, sensitivity, and flexibility. A father who is regarded as "unavailable" may more easily be persuaded to attend if a therapy session is scheduled to accommodate his work schedule, perhaps in the evening, or if the request is that he attend a single, problem-focused session (Hines, Richman, Maxim, & Hays, 1989). Recognizing a father's role can decrease sabotaging of the therapeutic process; even limited involvement may facilitate positive individual or family structural changes.

Usually, when relationship issues between adult heterosexual partners are the central concern, African American women initiate the therapy process. It may both surprise and frustrate therapists when women express considerable dissatisfaction, yet exhibit ambivalence toward, if not an outright rejection of, ending unsatisfactory and even dysfunctional relationships. Two contributing factors may be an absence of hope that they can find more rewarding relationships, and anxiety about surviving financially on their own. In some cases, women may be concerned about joining society in "beating their men further down" (Boyd-Franklin, 2003; McGoldrick, Garcia-Preto, Hines, & Lee, 1989). Their discontent is often coupled with an awareness of the pervasive effects that generations of racism have had for both African American men and women.

One task for therapists, in such an instance, is to help the woman to differentiate between empathy for her partner's frustration and sense of powerlessness, and encouraging or enabling the continuation of self- and relationship-defeating behaviors.

PARENT–CHILD SYSTEMS

Sometimes a child is "parentified," particularly when parents work or when there are many children in the home. Parents may consciously decide to have a child assume or assist with parental responsibilities, or the child may take on this responsibility without the adults' direct encouragement. The parental child structure can enhance the parental child's sense of responsibility, competence, and autonomy. However, if there is no explicit delegation of authority, the child may lack power to carry out the responsibilities he or she attempts to assume. Alternatively, if parents abdicate their responsibilities, the child may be forced to become the main source of guidance, control, and decision making, even if developmentally unprepared to do so (Minuchin, 1974). Such children often "act out" in school during late adolescence through delinquency, sexual impulsiveness, or inappropriate intervention with younger siblings when household demands conflict with their own developmental needs.

In such a situations, the goal of therapy should not be to eliminate a child's parental role, which may be essential to a family's survival, but rather to redistribute the child's burdens by helping the family to better use other resources. Parents must also strive to ensure that the responsibilities assumed by the parental child do not interfere with the fulfillment of the child's developmental needs.

THE THREE-GENERATION SYSTEM

The role of the grandmother is often central in African American families. The three-generation system, as well as other forms of the extended family system, can clearly be a source of strength and support (Jones, 2004; Logan, 2001; White, 2004). As the following case reveals, these three-generation systems may also present sensitive boundary issues.

The Gallop Family

The family consisted of Ms. LaVerne Frazier; her two children, Charlie (age 11) and Mary (age 5); her mother, Mrs. Sarah Gallop; and her aunt, Frances Pierre. In addition, Charlie had contact with his father, Jeffrey Frazier, who had major input in decision making concerning him. Ms. Frazier reported that Charlie was "out of control" at home and frequently truant from school; moreover, he never listened to her and was involved in many fights.

Charlie's grandmother had functioned as his mother during his earlier years, but could not do so in the last year because she had been forced to switch from a day shift to an evening shift at her job. However, it became clear during the family session that Mrs. Gallop believed that her daughter was incapable of parenting Charlie. It was also obvious that both Charlie and his mother responded to Mrs. Gallop as the real power in the home.

At the second session, the therapist learned that in Mrs. Gallop's absence, Mr. Frazier and Ms. Pierre often undermined Ms. Frazier's discipline. For example, Mr. Frazier took Charlie on outings even when he knew Charlie was being punished and didn't have his mother's permission to leave the house. Ms. Pierre, a warm, nurturing person who had cared for Charlie when his grandmother was ill, would allow Charlie to stay at her home when he became angry with his mother and often supported his refusal to obey her.

With Ms. Frazier's and Mrs. Gallop's permission, a session was scheduled with Charlie's father and Ms. Pierre. The therapist became instantly aware of the animosity between Ms. Frazier and Mr. Frazier, and that no family member, including Charlie, responded to Ms. Frazier as Charlie's parent.

When the adults were asked to discuss Charlie's most serious problem, they eventually agreed that it was truancy. Mrs. Gallop and Ms. Frazier were asked to confer on and establish rules for Charlie. Charlie's father agreed that he would take Charlie to the movies and bowling only if he had a positive report from the boy's mother. Ms. Pierre was helped to see how she had contributed to Charlie's acting out; she agreed to return Charlie if he ran away to her home.

Mrs. Gallop offered to help her daughter learn how to parent effectively. Ms. Frazier was asked to discuss the plan with Charlie and to gain his agreement to try it, without other adults intervening. When Charlie became angry at his mother at one point, and both his grandmother and his aunt attempted to intervene, the therapist blocked their intervention and encouraged Ms. Frazier to complete her discussion and to obtain Charlie's consent.

During treatment, various family members were seen in different subgroups to reinforce the new structure that had been established. For example, Mr. and Ms. Frazier were seen together for two sessions to help them stop triangulating Charlie in their conflicts.

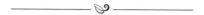

This case illustrates the importance of working with subsystems in African American extended families. Mrs. Gallop's role as a grandmother, as opposed to functional mother, had only recently evolved, and Charlie's mother had functioned more as a sibling, so that a clear parental structure needed to be introduced, with well-defined roles for Charlie's father and other close relatives involved in helping to raise Charlie.

RELIGION AND SPIRITUALITY

A strong spiritual orientation was a major aspect of life for Blacks in Africa and in the United States during the slavery era. Highly emotional religious services were of great importance in dealing with oppression during the years of slavery. Often, signals as to the time and place of an escape were transmitted through sermons and music. Spirituals contained hidden messages (e.g., about times and places of escape) and a language of resistance (e.g., "Wade in the Water" and "Steal Away"). The ecstatic celebration of Christ's gift of salvation provided African slaves with an outlet for expressing feelings of pain, humiliation, and anger.

Churches continue to serve numerous functions for members of the African American community in modern times. African Americans today belong to many different religious groups, including Baptists, Roman Catholics, Seventh-Day Adventists, Pentecostal churches, and numerous Islamic sects (Billingsley, 1992; Boyd-Franklin, 2003).

The largest religious affiliation is Baptist. In a Baptist church, an African American family finds a complete support system, including the minister, deacons, deaconesses, and other church members. Many churches also include social activities for the entire family. There are often special groups for youth, young adults, single parents, men, women, and couples, along with opportunities for participation in choirs, Sunday school, Bible study, and varied ministries (e.g., working with homeless people, foster children). Congregates also organize health promotion classes, day-care centers, health fairs, economic development initiatives, tutoring programs, and support groups (e.g., for unemployment, alcohol and drug abuse, grief). Even the smallest church provides a network of people who are available to a family in times of crisis.

Mental health professionals are increasingly aware that a strong spiritual base can enhance personal resilience. Bergin (1991) notes that the values promoted by mental health professionals are very consistent with spiritual values, including sensitivity to others' feelings, responsibility for one's actions, personal fulfillment and satisfaction, self-discipline, forgiveness of others, healthy sexual fulfillment, and striving for a sense of purpose.

Yet therapists may encounter instances when clients espouse interpretations of religious doctrine that have deleterious effects on their personal and family functioning. Their spiritual orientation may be a source of, as well as a haven from, stress. Larsen (1976), for example, notes that some clients may "spiritualize" problems by defining difficulties as "God's will," passively trusting that the problems will somehow be resolved. Wimberly (1997) suggests that therapists work within the confines of a family's belief system, rather than attempt to modify their beliefs.

Larsen (1976) notes that some clients may "spiritualize" problems by defining difficulties as "God's will," passively trusting that the problems will somehow be resolved. Even when individuals are not actively involved in organized religion, their core beliefs may be intricately intertwined with religious doctrine. Therapists should also be aware that when individuals convert from one denomination or religious group to another, conflicts with family members who have different beliefs and practices can become a treatment issue.

In their book *Soul Theology* (1986), Mitchell and Lewter provide clinical examples for therapists interested in learning more about the extent to which biblical narratives provide a frame of reference that can serve as a source of affirmation, hope, freedom, and positive behavioral change. Hines (1998) underscores the paramount importance of hope for clients and therapists alike. She also delineates strategies (e.g., the use of music, images, proverbs, biblical scriptures, and stories) to assist clients in tapping into their personal, familial, and cultural reservoirs to discover and foster hope.

WORK AND EDUCATION

A number of writers emphasize that African Americans have traditionally viewed hard work and education as critical to success (Billingsley, 1992; Boyd-Franklin, 2003; Hill, 1999; Staples, 1994). Yet many Americans believe that most African Americans survive only because of welfare, despite the fact that the overwhelming majority work, often having more than one job. Unfortunately, they often secure less desirable jobs, receive less pay for the same work, are the last hired, and are more likely to be underemployed and/or stuck under "glass or cement ceilings" than their White counterparts. Most African Americans no longer believe that the American dream is intended to include them.

African American parents generally expect their children to pursue careers offering security and to surpass them in achieving the comforts of life. Those who succeed are held in high regard. Yet because African Americans place great value on character and generally believe in the basic worth of every individual, children who earn an honest living and are self-supporting may win as much parental approval as those who are professionals.

As a result of this value, then, concern about the consequences of poor school adjustment often leads African American families to treatment. Low-income African American youth may act out in school as they face an oppressive society and the expectations of parents who have limited resources to assist them (Hines, 1999). Middle-class African American youth may encounter conflicts with peers and family members related to differences in socioeconomic status, Afrocentricity, how racism has been experienced, and the style of coping with it (Boyd-Franklin, 2003).

Their parents, who often enter the middle class without sufficient financial assets, and struggle to retain even a tenuous hold on their status, are likely to demand high achievement from their children. Parents' concerns for their children's futures and an awareness of their limited capacity to protect their children may heighten parents' sense of powerlessness and rage about racism. Some may respond in ways that are detrimental (e.g., overprotection, constant lecturing) to their relationships with their children, resulting in self-defeating behaviors (Boyd-Franklin, Franklin, & Toussaint, 2001).

Therapists can assist parents in managing their own stress and anger, in distinguishing between their own and their children's issues and goals, and in engaging their children in joint dialogue about the positive strategies that helped the parents and their ancestors to transcend difficult circumstances.

Believing that "to whom much is given, much is expected," African Americans often feel that they have a responsibility to "give back," especially to less economically advantaged family members. Their sense of responsibility is linked to the belief that individual well-being is tied to the collective welfare. For African Americans, personal accomplishments often are attributed to the sacrifices of others, as well as to individual effort. Some individuals may experience difficulty because their efforts to help extended family members leave them feeling depleted emotionally, physically, and/or financially. In such instances, culturally congruent therapists will support their clients' capacity to develop or maintain a balance between extending help and taking care of themselves, rather than encouraging emotional cutoffs and attention only to individual needs.

A MULTISYSTEM APPROACH TO THE TREATMENT OF AFRICAN AMERICAN FAMILIES

In working with African American families, therapists must be particularly willing to expand the context of therapy to include the impact of social, political, socioeconomic, and other environmental conditions. Aponte (1994) described this broader treatment approach as "ecostructural." Boyd-Franklin (2003) used the term "multisystems," given that poor inner-city African American families are likely to be involved with numerous external systems. Both ask therapists always to consider a family's environment and community in diagnosis and treatment.

Inner-city African American families are often faced with overwhelming socioeconomic problems, such as eviction or termination of public assistance. When these survival issues take precedence over family conflicts, clinicians should not assume responsibility, but rather should act as guides to help families learn how to negotiate complex bureaucratic systems. This sometimes requires the therapists to engage in outreach and often involves substantial amounts of time and energy.

Middle-class African Americans, like their lower-income peers, contend with circumstances that are shaped by racism, even if of a more subtle kind. They are likely to have few or no role models as they enter "unchartered territories' in their workplaces and/or neighborhoods. For some, the stress of having to discern and respond to subtle and overt prejudice may result in social and psychological isolation. Others derive from their experience exceptional strength, flexibility, and tolerance for diversity.

OTHER CONSIDERATIONS FOR FAMILY THERAPISTS

Given the aforementioned cultural and ecological considerations, African Americans' reliance on individuals within their natural support systems can probably better mitigate feelings of guilt, defeat, humiliation, and powerlessness than the use of mental health services.

Many African Americans view therapy as being for "crazy people." Some assume that clinicians will operate in the same way as do professionals in other agencies (e.g., welfare system, schools), who have been intrusive in telling families what they can or cannot do and own (e.g., telephone or television). Others may view serious emotional difficulties as "the wages of sin"; the person who manifests psychiatric symptoms may be seen as "mean" or "possessed by the devil" (particularly if he or she engages in antisocial behavior). For some, seeking help from a mental health professional rather than through prayer may signify a lack of trust in God. For still others, turning to family therapy is perceived as turning to "the system" that has negatively influenced African American well-being.

African Americans may also fear misdiagnosis, the prescribing of medication for behavioral and population control, and governmental abuse. These concerns arise out of oral stories about abuse in psychiatric facilities and from incidents such as the "Tuskegee Study" in which, for four decades, black men infected with syphilis were monitored, but not treated, in a program that involved the complicity of doctors and government officials (Jackson, 2000).

Still, African Americans have been utilizing mental health services in greater numbers than ever before in history. Their most frequent major presenting problems include poor school adjustment, acting-out behavior, depression, "nervous breakdowns" or psychotic behaviors, drug addiction, and alcoholism. Among low-income and working-class families, the identified patient is frequently a child who has been referred by a school, welfare department, court, or the police. Because some families feel that they have been forced into therapy, and as a result are very ambivalent about treatment, therapists should discuss families' feelings, expectations, and priorities.

African American families often need to be oriented to mental health services; myths must be discussed and dispelled. They are likely to be most responsive to time-limited, problem-solving therapy approaches with an active, directive therapist. Aponte (1978, 1994) emphasizes the need to help a family experience therapy as a process that can help produce immediate change(s) in their lives.

A therapist who requests total family involvement may heighten a family's feelings of responsibility and guilt, so the therapist should be flexible when families resist. Otherwise, those who are participating in therapy may decide that it is not worth trying to coerce unwilling family members to join them. Clinicians should clarify their rationales for requesting family involvement and invite questions about the entire process. African American families are quite aware of larger systems influences, and therapists who do not acknowledge their context are likely to lose credibility.

Communicating respect is critical to successfully engaging families. Therapists should openly acknowledge family strengths, avoid professional jargon, relate in a directive but supportive manner, and avoid addressing adults by their first names, especially in their children's presence, without their consent. The refusal to acknowledge African American adults with the titles routinely used with their White counterparts was a standard way for Whites, during and after slavery, to communicate that they regarded African Americans as inferior beings.

A non-African American therapist may wish to acknowledge his or her different racial/ethnic background and to discuss the family's feelings about it early in therapy. When the therapist senses discomfort on the part of one or more family members, he or she probably should move in this direction. The risk of raising the race issue and finding it to be irrelevant is not likely to have a devastating effect if the therapist conveys respect and genuineness and can handle suspiciousness and challenges to his or her authority in a nondefensive manner.

In addition, a well-meaning therapist may unwittingly undermine much-needed parental authority because of concern about parents' "harsh" handling of their children. Many African American parents believe that our society allows African American youth a very narrow "window for error." The principle "Spare the rod, spoil the child" is a common rule of thumb, and physical punishment is often an accepted mode of discipline. Rather than argue for the elimination of physical punishment, the therapist is urged to convey an appreciation for parents' concerns about their child's misbehavior, to frame physical punishment as a residual of slavery, and to emphasize the benefits of positive discipline approaches.

A family's concerns about investing time and money in the therapeutic process may stem from negative experiences with "helping" professionals or a desire to avoid an additional expense whose value hasn't been proven. Moreover, some families may not recognize the importance of being punctual for an appointment or may not call to cancel or reschedule without being informed of the importance of doing so.

Low-income families, in particular, are likely to approach mental health services using a medical clinic as their frame of reference, where they are used to waiting long hours for service. "Resistance" also may well be grounded in the difficulties of balancing parenting, household tasks, and one or more jobs.

Therapists frequently characterize African Americans as nonverbal and incapable of dealing with feelings. Sometimes, African Americans who appear almost mute in the therapy room may talk endlessly on their home turf (White, 2004). Furthermore, a lack of trust may limit family members' willingness to "open up." Grier and Cobbs (1968) coined the term "healthy cultural paranoia" to refer to the suspiciousness that, in fact, has facilitated the survival of African Americans' survival over time, given the extent to which they face constant threats to their well-being.

Minuchin, Montalvo, Guerney, Rosman, and Schumer (1967) have noted that for many low-income families, "affect is communicated mostly through paraverbal channels in the pitch, tempo, and intensity of the verbal messages and the accompanying kinesthetic modifiers" (p. 206), a description that applies to many African American families. Tracking relationships, messages, and joining a family can be a difficult and complex process. When the larger family group's messages are so vague, complex, or incomplete that the family, as well as the therapist, becomes overwhelmed, the therapist might consider working with family subgroups.

The therapist might also consider having family members observe each other behind the one-way mirror or using videotape playback to promote improved communication. Because of African American families' suspiciousness about therapy, therapists should clarify how audiotapes and videotapes will be used.

Therapists may well "burn out" when working with families who live under oppressive life circumstances if they do not exercise caution to avoid this outcome. Although managed care introduces many billing constraints, a team treatment model with these families can have many advantages (Hines et al., 1989). When this approach is not possible, even experienced therapists will benefit from peer supervision and the opportunity to confer with a consulting team.

CONCLUSION

Disparities in treatment access (e.g., choice of provider) and outcomes (e.g., diagnostic accuracy) for African Americans are well documented and should compel practitioners to move beyond the complacency that promotes ethnocentric mental health practices (U.S. Department of Health and Human Services, 1999). As noted, African Americans have maintained a sense of peoplehood, as well as a distinctive set of core values, traditions, and sociopolitical realities that are still affected by institutional racism. They have accomplished much in the face of centuries of institutionalized oppression.

Therapists should be sensitive to the diversity within the African American culture. We have attempted to sensitize clinicians about African Americans' experience and to introduce a strengths-based framework for assessing and intervening with these clients. Key to effective engagement, assessment, and intervention with African Americans is to convey genuine respect, to move beyond generalizations, to communicate interest in learning about clients' specific realities, and to help them reclaim and retain a sense of hope while moving toward the changes that will enhance their well-being.

REFERENCES

Akbar, N. (1984). *Chains and images of psychological slavery.* Chicago: Third World Press.
Akbar, N. (1985). Nile Valley origins of the science of the mind. In I. Van Sertima (Ed.), *Nile Valley civilizations.* New York: Journal of African Civilization.
Ani, M. (1994). *Yurugu: An African-centered critique of European cultural thought and behavior.* Trenton, NJ: Africa World Press.
Aponte, H. (1978). Diagnosis in family therapy. In C. B. Germain (Ed.), *Social work practice: People and environments.* New York: Columbia University Press.
Aponte, H. (1994). *Bread and spirit: Therapy with the new poor.* New York: Morton Press.
Arias, E. (2002). United States life tables: 2000. *National Vital Statistics Reports, 52*(3). Hyattsville, MD: National Center for Health Statistics.
Asante, M. (1988). *Afrocentricity.* Trenton, NJ: Africa World Press.
Asante, M. (1990). *Kemet, Afrocentricity, and knowledge.* Trenton, NJ: Africa World Press.
Bergin, A. (1991). Values and religious issues in psychotherapy and mental health. *American Psychologist, 46*(4), 394–403.
Billingsley, A. (1968). *Black families in White America.* Englewood Cliffs, NJ: Prentice-Hall.
Billingsley, A. (1992). *Climbing Jacob's ladder: The enduring legacy of African-American families.* New York: Simon & Schuster.
Boyd-Franklin, N. (2003). *Black families in therapy: Understanding the African American experience* (2nd ed.). New York: Guilford Press.
Boyd-Franklin, N., Franklin, A. J., & Toussaint, P. (2001). *Boys into men: Raising our African American teenage sons.* New York: Plume.

Carter, R. T. (1995). *The influence of race and racial identity in psychotherapy: Toward a racially inclusive model*. New York: Wiley.

Cross, W. E. (1991). *Shades of black*. Philadelphia: Temple University Press.

Cross, W. E., Parham, T. A., & Helms, J. E. (1998). Nigrescence revisited: Theory and research. In R. Jones (Ed.), *African American identity development*. Hampton, VA: Cobb & Henry.

Deutsch, M., & Brown, B. (1964). Social influences in Negro–White intellectual differences. *Social Issues*, 20(2), 24–36.

Fields, J. (2003). *Children's living arrangements and characteristics: March 2002*. Current Population Reports, Series P20-547. Washington, DC: U.s. Bureau of the Census.

Franklin, A. J. (1993, July/August). The invisibility syndrome. *Family Therapy Network*, 17(4), 33–39.

Franklin, A. J. (2004). *From brotherhood to manhood: How Black men rescue their dreams and relationships from the invisibility syndrome*. Hoboken, NJ: Wiley.

Frazier, E. F. (1966). *The Negro family in the United States*. Chicago: University of Chicago Press.

Grier, W., & Cobbs, P. (1968). *Black rage*. New York: Basic Books.

Helms, J. E., & Cook, D. A. (1999). *Using race and culture in counseling and psychotherapy: Theory and process*. Boston: Allyn & Bacon.

Hill, R. (1972). *The strengths of African American families*. New York: Emerson-Hall.

Hill, R. (1999). *The strengths of African American families: Twenty-five years later*. Lanham, MD: University Press of America.

Hines, P. (1990). African-American mothers. *Journal of Feminist Family Therapy*, 2(2), 23–32.

Hines, P. (1999). The family life cycle of African American families living in poverty. In B. Carter & M. McGoldrick (Eds.), *The expanded family life cycle: Individual, family, and social perspectives* (3rd ed., pp. 327–345). Boston: Allyn & Bacon.

Hines, P., Garcia-Preto, N., McGoldrick, M., Almeida, R., & Weltman, S. (1992). Intergenerational relationships across cultures. *Families in Society*, 73(6), 323–338.

Hines, P., Richman, P., Maxim, K., & Hays, H. (1989). Multi-impact family therapy: An approach to working with multi-problem families. *Journal of Psychotherapy and the Family*, 6, 161–175.

Hines, P. M. (1998). Climbing up the rough side of the mountain: Hope, culture and therapy. In M. McGoldrick (Ed.), *Re-visioning family therapy: Race, culture, class and gender* (pp. 78–90). New York: Guilford Press.

Hines, P. M., & Boyd-Franklin, N. (1996). African American families. In M. McGoldrick, J. Giordano, & J. K. Pearce (Eds.), *Ethnicity and family therapy* (2nd ed., pp. 66–84). New York: Guilford Press.

Jackson, V. (2000). *Separate and unequal: The legacy of racially segregated psychiatric hospitals*. Unpublished manuscript. Available at www.healingcircles.org

Jones, R. (1998). *African American identity development*. Hampton, VA: Cobb & Henry Press.

Jones, R. (2004). *Black psychology* (4th ed.). Hampton, VA: Cobb & Henry Press.

Kambon, K. K. (1998). *African/Black psychology in the American context: An African-centered approach*. Tallahassee, FL: Nubian Nation Publications.

Karenga, M. (1997). *Kwanzaa: A celebration of family, community, and culture*. Philadelphia: University of Sankore Press.

Larsen, J. (1976, October). *Dysfunction in the evangelical family: Treatment considerations*. Paper presented at the annual meeting of the American Association of Marriage and Family Counselors, Philadelphia.

Logan, S. L. (Ed.). (2001). *The Black family: Strength, self-help, and positive change* (2nd ed.). Boulder, CO: Westview Press.

Mbiti, J. S. (1970). *African religions and philosophies*. Garden City, NY: Anchor Books/Doubleday.

McAdoo, H. P. (Ed.). (1996). *Black families* (3rd ed.). Thousand Oaks, CA: Sage.

Mc Adoo, H. P. (Ed.). (2002). *Black children: Social, educational, and parental environments* (2nd ed.). Thousand Oaks, CA: Sage.

McGoldrick, M., Garcia-Preto, N., Hines, P., & Lee, E. (1989). Ethnicity and women. In M. McGoldrick, C. Anderson, & F. Walsh (Eds.), *Women in families*. New York: Norton.

McGoldrick, M., & Gerson, R. (1999). *Genograms: Assessment and intervention* (2nd ed.). New York: Norton.

McKinnon, J. (2003). *The Black population in the United States: March 2002.* Current Population Reports, Series P20-541. Washington, DC: U.S. Bureau of the Census.

Minuchin, S. (1974). *Families and family therapy.* Cambridge, MA: Harvard University Press.

Minchin, S., Montalvo, B., Guerney, B. G., Jr., Rosman, B. L., & Schumer, F. (1967). *Families of the slums.* New York: Basic Books.

Mitchell, H., & Lewter, N. (1986). *Soul theology: The heart of American Black culture.* San Fransico: Harper & Row.

Moynihan, D. P. (1965). *The Negro family: The case for national action.* Washington, DC: U.S. Department of Labor.

Nobles, W. (1985). *Africanicity and the Black family: The development of a theoretical model.* Oakland, CA: Black Family Institute.

Nobles, W. (2004). African philosophy: Foundations for Black psychology. In R. Jones (Ed.), *Black psychology* (4th ed.). New York: Harper & Row.

Parham, T. A. (1992). Cycles of psychological nigrescence. *Counseling Psychologist, 17*(2), 187–226.

Pinderhughes, E. (1982). Afro American families and the victim system. In M. McGoldrick, J. K. Pearce, & J. Giordano (Eds.), *Ethnicity and family therapy* (pp. 108–122). New York: Guilford Press. ·

Rockeymoore, M. (2002). African Americans confront a pandemic: Assessing community impact, organization, and advocacy in the second decade of AIDS. In L. A. Daniels (Ed.), *The state of Black America.* New York: National Urban League.

Shelton, B. A., & John, D. (1993). Ethnicity, race, and difference: A comparison of White, Black, and Hispanic men's household labor time. In J. Hood (Ed.), *Men, work, and family.* Newbury Park, CA: Sage.

Staples, R. (1994). *Black family: Essays and studies* (5th ed.). New York: Van Nostrand Reinhold.

Testa, M., & Krogh, M. (1995). The effect of employment on marriage among Black males in inner-city Chicago. In M. B. Tucker & C. Mitchell-Kernan (Eds.), *The decline in marriage among African Americans.* New York: Russell Sage Foundation.

Tucker, M. B., & Mitchell-Kernan, C. (Eds.). (1995). *The decline in marriage among African Americans* (pp. 59–95). New York: Russell Sage Foundation.

U.S. Bureau of Census. (2000). *The Black population in the United States. Current population reports* (Series P20-530). Washington, DC: U.S. Government Printing Office.

U.S. Bureau of Census. (2001). *Minority-owned business enterprises. Economic census: 1997.* Washington, DC: U.S. Government Printing Office.

U.S. Bureau of Census. (2004). African American history month: February 2003. Press Release. Washington, DC: U.S. Government Printing Office.

U.S. Department of Health and Human Services, Office of the Surgeon General. (1999). *Mental health: A report of the Surgeon General.* Washington, DC: U.S. Government Printing Office.

White, J. (2004). Towards a Black psychology. In R. Jones (Ed.), *Black psychology* (4th ed.). Hampton, VA: Cobb & Henry Press.

Wimberly, E. P. (1997). *Counseling African American marriages and families.* Louisville, Ky: Westminster John Knox Press.

CHAPTER 7

African Immigrant Families

Hugo Kamya

One evening, a group of armed men stormed into our family's house while we were having dinner. A small light illumined our little dinner room. The intruders, who wore military uniforms and carried guns, which they waved at us, were very loud. They demanded to see the man of the house; they were looking for my father. Scared, we ran to hide in the corners of the tiny room.

My father ran into the bedroom; the men followed him. The next thing I heard was a gunshot in the bedroom. After what seemed to be a long time, the men walked out, stepping all over the plates (we had been eating on the floor) and telling us that they would be back. We sat motionless, praying for courage. Then, quietly, one by one, we walked into the bedroom. There was a crack in the window and a streak of blood on the floor. There was no sign of our father.

The traumatic story of my family from Uganda, a country in eastern Africa with more than 24 million people and more than 15 ethnic/tribal groups, is common among African immigrants. Fear, loss, grief, anger, militarism, and colonialism are pervasive. The immigrants relate other, untold stories of illness, death, and oppression. There are also stories of privilege, and political affiliation based on patriarchy, the domination of one religion over others, and the hardships of a particular social class or ethnicity. They also capture the destruction and changing structure of families, as well as the large-scale wars, mass migrations, displacement, hunger, and poverty, which are the lingering effects of racist colonialism and slavery.

Other important, but less noticed stories are those of hope, opportunity, and possibility. Musake's story is not unlike mine. Musake is a 45-year-old native of Rwanda, a country devastated by war and ethnic conflicts between the Hutu and Tutsi peoples. Musake, whose father was killed by military soldiers at a roadblock, wept bitterly as he described his inability to mourn because his brother had died of AIDS shortly thereafter. He reported with great frustration how much he wished he had "more life" in him. He struggles to go to school at night as he works two jobs to make ends meet. "I have lost everything, my father was killed and I lost a brother. I have to make my father's dreams come true. Going to school is one way of doing what my family would have liked me to do."

Other stories, such as Muzibu's, combine despair, courage, and resilience. He belongs to the Batoro, a pastoral tribe in western Uganda, and arrived in the United States after being tortured by the military government of Idi Amin in the late 1970s. He had also witnessed three of his children being tortured. Soldiers had raped his wife in front him as they pressed him to disclose information he did not have.

Muzibu himself was forced to sit in cold water for days and was beaten repeatedly to make him give information about the rebels. He was also taken to execution sites to intimidate him. His home was ransacked. When the government received no confession, soldiers went after his extended family and associates. Today, Muzibu has trouble sleeping, lives with constant nightmares, and has great difficulty in developing intimate relationships and trusting care providers or anyone else. His wife left him and returned to her parents, referring to the "terrible shame" that had happened to her. New situations and people around him frighten him. Sometimes he says, "I am so afraid of who I am."

Muzibu's situation resembles that of many African refugees in the United States. His trauma has had a pervasive effect on him, undermining his sense of safety, trust, control, and intimacy. His sense of meaning and purpose, his spiritual well-being, has been disrupted.

COLONIALISM

My family's story, like those of Musake and Muzibu, reflects some factors that are key to understanding Africa and its immigrants. Africans carry with them the lingering effects of racist colonialism from many years of European rule. Britain, France, Italy, Germany, Belgium, and other countries divided Africa into mainly small nations, devised to suit European trading interests, and otherwise ruled the continent heavy-handedly. Colonialism ultimately destroyed the social contracts that were made with African nations, and after independence European nations did little to help them rebuild (Nwidor, Nwidor, & Wiwa-Lawani, 2004).

Postcolonial African rulers modeled their regimes on those of their colonial masters and thus, for the most part, had very little respect for life. Corruption abounded. The supposed superiority of European conquerors had deleterious effects on Africans (McCulloch, 1995). Despite European efforts to destroy the African spirit, many Africans held, and still hold, a strong spirit of collectivism and communalism, as well as a will to live no matter what the odds.

Over the years, Africans have struggled to maintain their culture and traditional communal structure as they transitioned from tribal and colonial to national governments. These struggles also characterize African immigrants in the United States. The effects of the HIV/AIDS epidemic, alcohol abuse, sex trafficking, hunger, poverty, war, human rights violations, and other personal trauma compound the mental health issues affecting African immigrants. Such oppression also has affected African immigrants' family structures, child-rearing practices, gender roles, and social class.

AFRICANS IN THE UNITED STATES

There are about 800,000 African immigrant families in the United States, which come from 52 countries, a population that has increased over the past two decades (Djamba, 1999). Since 1946, more than 80,000 Africans who were persecuted by their governments or ethnic groups other than their own have sought asylum or refuge in the United States (www.uscis.gov). The largest numbers have come from Nigeria, Egypt, Ethiopia, South Africa, and Ghana (Takyi, 2002), though many Africans are from such war-devastated regions as Rwanda, Liberia, and Somalia. They often arrive in the United States traumatized, without resources, and with compromised immune systems, because many African countries have endured wars and other highly destabilizing conditions.

Although some Africans have come to the United States for economic and educational reasons, more have had to flee their homelands, often against their will and under horrific conditions. When they arrive, they may find that the professional status that assured them economic stability in their home countries is not valued here. Moreover, immigration laws and economic difficulties often prevent family members from joining their relatives in the United States.

Families may have to shoulder the burden of bringing others to this country, who, without appropriate immigration papers, fear deportation. Parents' long work hours may leave them little time or energy to pass on the cultural traditions, values, and rituals that traditionally have sustained African families in their homelands.

ACCULTURATION

African immigrants encounter many stressors as they begin to adapt to American life. A recent immigrant from Nigeria, one of the largest and richest African countries, with more than 100 million people, reported, "I feel so helpless," describing how drastically his life had changed. He felt that because his skills did not matter in America, he did not belong. Another Nigerian man, a member of the Yoruba (one of the largest Nigerian tribes, which also has members elsewhere in West Africa), has been in the United States for more than 10 years. Recently, he was joined by his wife and three children. In one session with a therapist, the parents expressed their frustration with their children, who constantly remind them that they are hard to understand; other children had said their parents "speak funny." The children were learning at an early age that something is "wrong" with their parents, who, in turn, felt inadequate.

Africans, like other immigrants, experience a deep sense of loss of their culture, which is partly associated with loss of a common language with their children. Parents lament their inability to communicate with their sons and daughters, as they could in their home countries, and are pained when their Americanized children fail to learn their language.

A family from Kenya spent several sessions discussing difficulties in providing opportunities for their children to use their native language because "life is so hectic between our four jobs that we cannot afford time together." The prolonged separation of family members also can create gaps in the shared family history and can make family members strangers to each other, which leads to major strains. Most frightening of all for those who have arrived illegally is the fear of deportation.

The relocation involved in immigration typically produces depression and insecurity along with excitement and hope (Baker, 1999; Luthke & Cropley, 1990; Magwaza & Bhana, 1991; Ritsner, Ponizovsky, Chemelevsky, & Zetser, 1996). Immigrants must adjust both attitudinally and behaviorally to a new culture and environment (Kim, 1978; Padilla, 1980). They often have difficulty in locating housing and jobs, and poverty and unfamiliarity with American society sometimes leaves them vulnerable to crime.

Posttraumatic stress associated with their premigration experience adds to the difficulty of adapting to the American environment. Maria, a Ugandan woman, described witnessing the rape and abduction of her sister, whom a warlord later used as a sex slave:

> "She was only a little girl, but I recall soldiers attacking our school and pulling aside all the girls. They took us into a room where they raped all the girls except those who had acne. I had acne so they did not rape me. I can recall seeing my sister being taken away into the camp. I never saw her again."

Some parents who have experienced trauma displace their anguish onto their children in ways they may not realize. One Ugandan who suffered torture under Idi Amin's dictatorial regime often screamed at his children for both big and little offenses. He realized this only when he finally spoke about the humiliation he had suffered.

THE RELATIONSHIP BETWEEN THE HOME COUNTRY AND THE UNITED STATES

Therapists need to understand African immigrants' sense of obligation to relatives in their country of origin. Family members in Africa may expect relatives in America to support them and so put financial pressure on immigrants. This pressure may be expressed in terms of an appeal to a person's cultural, family, and community values. These loyalties are often the issues for which families seek therapeutic help. Kliman (2005) describes such a struggle between a Yoruba man from Cameroon, whose relatives kept arriving at his doorstep to stay for extended periods, and his Scottish American wife, who saw them as intruders rather than welcome family guests.

For many African immigrants, the politics of their home countries often have a negative effect on how they are perceived in America. A man from Sierra Leone reported how his neighbors in a small New England town identified him with the fighting and warring tribes in his native country. He commented, "I cannot go anywhere without becoming a spokesperson for my country. I am asked about all the atrocities that are going on in my country. Some I know about. Some I do not and do not care to. They remind me of a lot of painful things."

Many African immigrants struggle with the tension between taking on a new identity in America, and at the same time maintaining the identity of their African roots. A married couple from Kenya, Mwangi and Wanjiko, both 32, fled their land because of their opposition to the government and have had three children since arriving in the United States. As their children entered school, the couple were happy that their children would live a better life than their parents did. At the same time, they experienced shame because they could no longer see themselves as fully Kenyan. At times, they have contemplated returning to Kenya to reclaim their full ethnic identity.

RACE, RACE RELATIONS, AND RACISM

Because of Africa's colonialist legacy, Africans' attitudes toward Whites often depend on their class, as well as the particular politics of their home countries. For example, Njoroge, a 32-year-old Kenyan man whose father fought and was killed in his country's war for independence, says, "It is hard for me to trust any White man. They lied to us." He speaks with great sadness as he describes his grandfather telling him that Whites told him to close his eyes, and when he opened them, his land was gone. He said, "I have nothing I can call my own."

There is a different story for most Ugandans. Their experience can only be understood in the context of a different history. They were not a colonized group. As a British protectorate, Uganda was allowed a degree of self-rule, enjoying limited self-governance. In contrast, Kenya, as a British colony, was denied any measure of political sovereignty.

Africans' sense of political powerlessness comes in part from the wounds of colonialism in their countries of origin, which is often reflected in feelings of inferiority, anger, and mistrust. For many African immigrants, experiencing racism in the United States recreates the earlier feelings of lack of power, privilege, and political oppression.

Most African immigrants, like Black Americans, suffer racial discrimination; for example, their professional credentials may be viewed with suspicion. On several occasions, I, a PhD and tenured professor, have sat through academic meetings where I made points that were dismissed until they were echoed by a White colleague. When I co-teach with White colleagues, I often see course participants responding to questions I have posed while looking at my White colleague, as if he or she had asked the questions. Yet my colleagues do not seem to consider—or even to notice—the impact of this form of oppression on me or on our relationship.

Still, some social distance usually exists between Africans and American Blacks, in part because Africans experience some Blacks as uninformed about Africa. In addition, some Africans perceive American Blacks as resentful because Whites seem to treat Africans more favorably than they treat them, thus driving a wedge between the two groups. At the same time, some Africans report being marginalized as compared with West Indian immigrants.

Most Africans see American Blacks as more culturally similar to Europeans than to Africans. They see American Blacks as sharing in the lifestyle they associate with affluent Europeans in Africa. Moreover, the forces leading Africans to immigrate here in recent decades differ profoundly from the forcible removal and enslavement of Blacks' African ancestors, as do the respective social and psychological consequences.

Sometimes there are misunderstandings between American Blacks and African immigrants about cultural and religious issues, as the following case illustrates:

Natasha, an African American woman, and her husband, Kwaku, who is from Sierra Leone, a country plagued by civil war, came to therapy because they were having difficulties managing their 5-year-old son. It became clear that Natasha was angry at Kwaku for refusing to attend her church. He reported that Natasha's church "did not do it for me," but could not explain what the "it" was. This made her even angrier, inasmuch as she knew that Kwaku read the Bible and often quoted from scriptures.

Kwaku did not want to hurt Natasha by telling her what really irked him about her church. But he finally blurted out that he disliked the congregation's responses of "Halleluiah!" following every utterance in the church service, which contrasted sharply with his experience of worship in Sierra Leone. She was relieved that what troubled her husband was "no reflection on me or on my relationship with Kwaku." Once Kwaku had explained his discomfort, the couple were able to discuss their different relationships to their respective forms of church worship, spirituality, and the scriptures. Natasha was able to explain to Kwaku her own spiritual background, and he could own his relationship to the scriptures.

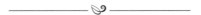

Exploring such cultural similarities and differences contributes greatly to achieving harmony in a relationship (Black, 1996). Helping Kwaku and Natasha see what they did, and did not, share, and exploring Christian practices in Africa, helped Natasha to respect the ways in which Kwaku's experience of Christian worship in Africa differed from her own. Kwaku was soon able to honor Natasha's American ways of worship.

African Americans' forms of worship in the United States reflect their people's experience of coming to Christianity while enslaved and are thus necessarily different from the Christianity that emerged in Africa. Indeed, the Exodus theme of redemption from slavery permeated slaves' Christianity, gave them hope for freedom, and even provided a code to communicate their escape plans. Those "Halleluiahs" were not only spiritual communion, but also a call to freedom.

AFRICANS IN THE UNITED STATES: A DIFFERENT SOCIAL CONTEXT

Having to renegotiate their ethnic culture in the United States can leave Africans highly vulnerable to emotional distress. Worrying about how they will fare in a foreign land, they often manifest social anxiety and mistrust of others. Such suspiciousness may have begun in their countries of origin, where their sense of safety was first violated. Having to continually explain themselves in the United States also feeds mistrust. A woman from Nigeria reported frequently hearing inquisitive comments about her unfamiliar dress, accent, and speech. She told how people responded with dismay and disbelief when she talked about each detail on her dress, and then asked her more questions, which suggested there was something more they should learn.

Downward job mobility is a major frustration for many African immigrants. Even those with excellent credentials often cannot find employment commensurate with their training or education and so must work in low-status jobs to support their families here and back at home. Undocumented immigrants must also worry about being discovered by the Immigration and Naturalization Service (especially since September 11, 2001). Such circumstances can create intense feelings of resentment.

Because American society links health insurance to employment, many immigrants have only limited access to medical and mental health services. It can take enormous energy just to keep up one's self-esteem at work. Many Africans work several jobs, for example, as nannies, janitors, or security guards, to make ends meet while also pursuing educational opportunities to earn new credentials. Class, gender role, and life cycle expectations further compound these issues (Kliman & Madsen, 1999). One Ugandan immigrant woman spends several hours a day working as a nanny and many evening hours cleaning houses. She sometimes weeps as she cares for other people's children while her own children hardly ever get to see her.

Because of financial pressures or long work hours, some parents send their children back to their countries of origin for extended periods. This practice reconnects the children to members of their extended family, who often play a major role in raising them. However, children may suffer many losses as a result of such family separations. Some inadequately bond with parents if the separation takes place too early in life. Family therapists should carefully explore children's attachments, disruption in parental relationships, including feelings of loss and grief by both generations.

VALUES

Most African families believe that values are mainly learned in the context of family, where they are passed on from one generation to the next. Proverbs and stories, which are told on many occasions, help transmit these values. From a very young age, children learn the meaning of these sayings, which are sometimes communicated playfully, sometimes seriously. Besides parents, community members contribute to this process via such occasions as coming-of-age ceremonies, holiday gatherings, and worship cerebrations.

SPIRITUALITY AND SPIRITUAL BELIEFS

In the first couple therapy session with his White American girlfriend, Mboa, a 30-year-old man from the Central African Republic, described at great length how much he missed his late mother's cooking: "No one, not even my girlfriend, could ever cook as well as my mother did for me. However, I know she [his mother] is up there in heaven watching over me. I pray to her. It is so much easier to talk to her than even this White God I see everywhere in their [White American] churches. She smiles to me and I smile back. She is my strength and my hope. When I have children someday I will tell them about my mother's cooking. I will cook for them. I will give them something of her. "

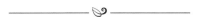

Traditional religious beliefs, which permeate all areas of life, comfort many Africans facing life's hardships. Africans believe in the power of both the natural and the spiritual worlds. Africa has about a thousand tribes, each with its own religious system (Mbiti, 1970). Worshipers invoke and pray to various spiritual powers—the supreme God, other divinities, the spirits, and ancestors; sometimes libations are poured to honor them.

One must then understand these religious systems in the context of Africa's history, including the effects of colonialism, Islam, and Christianity. Traditional religions tended to be tribal or national, but with the migration and intermarriage of peoples, tribal groups often have embraced the religious ideas of other groups.

African religions can be described as animistic, meaning soul- or spirit-derived, from *animus*, the Latin word for "breath" (Mbiti, 1970, p. 9). Because Africans believed in the existence of several spirits residing in mountains, rivers, lakes, trees, rocks, and other objects, the monotheistic West has placed the continent's religions on the low end of religious evolution toward monotheism, below the three monotheistic faiths. Colonialists often dismissed African traditions and rituals as "pagan" or uncouth. This perception of European and American religious superiority created tension between African spiritual beliefs and the major monotheistic religions.

For Africans, religion is expressed through mystical power, magic, witchcraft, and sorcery, which many in the Western world would consider outside the boundaries of religion. African peoples are intimately aware of the mystical powers in the universe.

Some Africans' belief in divine or spiritual beings translates into a commitment to worship in its varied forms, whether in churches or mosques, or in smaller groups that sustain a sense of connection, purpose, and meaning. Many Africans attend worship services and celebrate their relationship to the divine, which they also understand as their relationship to nature and community. Holding spiritual beliefs is often done more for commitment to one's entire community than for the sake of individual meaning.

The spiritual world of Africans is populated with spiritual beings, spirits, and the living-dead (Mbiti, 1970), all of which play a major role in African culture. Many Africans find their sense of purpose and meaning in the relationships of the community with the spiritual beings and spirits, which are seen as guides to a well-lived life.

Some Africans consider major objects in nature, like the sun or the moon, as spiritual beings. Indeed, many Africans revere these objects of nature. They name children for such objects out of respect for them and to seek their protection. Most Africans believe that spiritual beings are powerful, transcendent forces and view them with reverence. Spirits guide the family throughout the life cycle, which includes assisting with child-rearing practices. For example, when parents lose control of their children, they invoke spirits to provide guidance and give solutions to the problem.

Among the Baganda of Uganda, the living-dead, who are believed to dwell around homesteads, are considered to be benevolent spirits. Some Africans live out their spirituality through elaborate dances that invoke these spirits. Other people enter into trances or other meditative states believed to connect them to spiritual beings. Spirituality and spiritual beings are also intimately connected to the notion of community. African immigrants in the United States hold onto at least some of these African beliefs, even while embracing one of the major faith traditions.

COMMUNITY IDENTITY AS A SPIRITUAL IDENTITY

For Africans, their community is at the core of their spiritual identity. Africans believe in a communal identity that involves both the living and the dead. Mbiti (1970) noted that African personal identity is found in the context of their community's identity. An African proverb found in many languages states: "I am because we are." Africans try to integrate the sacred and the secular into one harmonious, cooperative, and communal whole, without formal distinction between the religious and the nonreligious, or the spiritual and the material, areas of life (Mbiti, 1970).

In the United States, African immigrants frequently engage relatives and friends from their native country in planning celebrations around births, marriages, and funerals and mourning rituals, as well as family reunions. Invited guests will travel long distances to attend these key moments. Elaborate meals and meetings mark family get-togethers with the serving of traditional ethnic foods. Recently, some ethnic groups like the Baganda of

Uganda and the Yoruba of Nigeria have dedicated time to teaching children about their respective cultures, histories, and traditions. At marriages or funerals, the meanings of rituals are explained to children, often through the use of plays and other artistic productions.

FAMILY LIFE

The survival of the family is almost a mystery, given the harsh colonial oppression of Africans. Africans place great importance on the family, which includes kin relationships that extend beyond ties of blood or marriage to include other individuals, especially members of the tribe or clan.

Tribes often speak distinct languages, with members having a shared history and social or political organizations. One is born in a tribe and remains part of it. In the past, tribes occupied distinct geographical regions, but because of widespread migration, they are no longer confined to geographical areas. Some tribes were herders; others were farmers. Europeans' rule over Africa led to an artificial division of tribal groups as the colonialists created arbitrary borders within them.

The clan is a subdivision of the tribe; it is composed of several families that may be united by a shared lineal heritage, which can be either patriarchal or matriarchal. Certain animals, plants, or rocks serve as totemic identification symbols of the clan's strengths, hopes, and dreams.

Many Africans believe that the propagation of life is key to their long-term survival. Because European colonial domination of Africa has divided families and groups, nearly extinguishing some, many Africans see having large families as an obligation.

Unfortunately, the number of African immigrants to the United States has been limited, because the narrow American definition of "family" has not allowed many already settled here to bring fellow clan or tribe members into the United States.

Bot, a 17-year-old refugee from Sudan, was a member of a group that included five other children who escaped from the war in Sudan. Bot, who saw himself as a member of a tribe and clan, suspected that everyone wanted him to forget his roots because he had come to a "land of opportunity." He was clearly angry whenever his host foster family asked him about his "biological" family. "The war wiped away my family, but I do have it [a larger family]," he would say. "They are everywhere. I wish they could have come with me like these brothers" (pointing to the rest of the group). His host family's obsession with such a restrictive understanding of family made Bot long for connection with clan and tribe, whom he often telephoned to in Sudan and elsewhere to ask for guidance about many things, especially about how to survive in the United States.

Hospitality as a Community Spiritual Calling

Hospitality is a powerful aspect of family and community life in Africa. An African proverb states: "Home is no highway stop. To stop is to arrive." This proverb underscores the importance of welcoming with open arms every person who comes to one's home. This tradition recognizes others' vulnerability and acknowledges each person's humanity. African hospitality also reflects the idea that people are valued for who they are rather than for what they have or own. Underlying this belief is the value of stewardship, which is lived out as service and hospitality to all human beings. Children are taught very early to be responsible and hospitable to peers, to adults, and, most important, to strangers. Given this tradition, it is no wonder that many Africans struggle with the expectations of their extended families.

Any experiences that challenge these cultural expressions of meaning, belief, spiritual practices, or values are primary sources of stress and psychological distress. A story is told of an African man who traveled a great distance to visit his long-lost son. Upon his arrival, his daughter-in-law, who did not remember him, treated him with disdain. When it became clear that a family elder had been mistreated, a curse descended upon the family, which suffered many mishaps, including the loss of livestock. Until a spiritual cleansing was done for the entire family, misfortune after misfortune plagued it.

GENDER ROLES, HIERARCHY, AND COMMUNICATION

Most Africans have clearly defined gender roles. Men, the clear heads of families and clans, adjudicate and settle disputes and officiate at most major life cycle events. Fathers often designate an oldest son as the rightful heir.

Women tend to dominate at birth rituals and are caregivers and nurturers to children and elderly people. They also do most household chores with the help of children. In some societies, women tend to be the chief breadwinners as well as homemakers. In some cases, especially in rural areas, the hard physical labor is left to women.

Females may prefer to talk away from the males in their lives, either because of fear of the males or as a sign of respect. Public displays of affection are uncommon among African couples; instead, humor is often used to communicate such emotions. In general, happiness or excitement is often tempered with humility, and the expression of anger or rage is frowned upon.

Although African women are often confined to the home in their countries of origin, in the United States they may be forced to take jobs to support their families. Employment augments family income; it also dramatically changes the dynamics of male–female relationships. Child care is often left to recently arrived family members or to paid caregivers.

African women in the United States generally tend to have more legal rights, and better financial, educational, and social opportunities, than in their home countries. These new possibilities can excite them, but they often frighten their husbands. In such cases, both the husband and wife need to formulate new understandings of themselves.

With African families always evolving, men and women sometimes share responsibilities, although marked differences remain in their prescribed roles. Because women have invested wisely in more income-generating activities, such as small businesses, their economic position is sometimes stronger than that of men. This encourages them to state their needs and feelings to men and helps them to achieve greater decision-making power about family matters.

African women in the United States are also making important choices about life partners. Some choose to partner with other women, defying traditional heterosexual conventions. However, Africans rarely discuss sexual orientation and some people are oblivious to homosexuality in their community. Other women choose to be single parents rather than remain childless.

New powers and possibilities have created a sense of liberation for most African women. However, the level of domestic abuse, especially in heterosexual relationships, has increased greatly. Family therapists must examine the larger social, economic, political, and cultural environments in which the battering takes place (Almeida, 1998; Bograd, 1984), so as to provide men and women alike opportunities to deconstruct issues of power, control, and hierarchy.

Today, men in heterosexual relationships often feel less effective and struggle to adjust to new roles. Therapists might engage them in identifying new responsibilities that both work for them and are fair to their partners. Storytelling, which is important to most Africans, can be used to explore cultural ideas about gender roles.

Family structures have traditionally been divided along generational as well as gender lines, going beyond the nuclear family. Grandparents command great respect because they are seen as wiser than others, more knowledgeable, and closer to God. Their perspective and experience is often sought by children, other family members, and village folk.

In the wake of war and the AIDS epidemic, grandparent- and even child-headed households are becoming more common as increasing numbers of children are orphaned. Wars throughout the continent have killed many adults and children and exacerbated the oppression and suppression of girls and women.

Wars also have created militarized societies in which soldiers, as a means of intimidation, abduct and rape girls and women. Females have been targeted and forced into sexual slavery. When a woman is raped, she is often ostracized from society. Because rape stigmatizes women, shaming them and denying them status in society, raped women and their families rarely report the rapes for fear of reprisals. Such women may not be able to marry. Instead, their trauma continues, stigmatizing them and their communities.

Some African groups practice female genital cutting or mutilation. Although this practice is outlawed in many African countries, it continues to affect numerous women, who may have little or no say in its being carried out. This procedure is often performed in unsanitary conditions that present serious dangers to women's health. Cultural sanctions prohibit both women and men from talking about these practices. Thus, therapists must be clinically skillful in opening discussions on this issue. A stance that offers respectful invitation to all conversations is necessary. Such a stance embraces a "both–and" thinking and emphasizes interactional processes at both the micro/interpersonal level and the macro/sociocultural level (Hardy & Laszloffy, 2002).

Boys have been used to perform dangerous tasks in wars they may not even understand, such as being spies, weapon carriers, and mine detectors. Premature deaths among African men and women has affected traditional culture and contributed to serious mental health issues for Africans.

THE FAMILY LIFE CYCLE, MARRIAGE PRACTICES, AND TRADITIONS

In African cultures, elaborate rituals often mark major life transitions. The naming ceremony for a newborn brings together extended family members and village folk. Men, women, and children dance to drums and other music to welcome the infant to the community.

The birth of twins in a family is considered an extraordinary event and a celebration that takes on greater meaning. It is believed that twins possess certain unique powers. Families can be struck with calamities if the twins are mistreated or if the rituals at different life cycles are not appropriately performed for them. Twins are also given different last names, which thus affects the names given to children born after them.

In most families, the newborn's name reflects events surrounding its birth. Rituals from native and major world religions are often combined. Among the Baganda of Uganda, boys are named "Musisi" and girls are named "Namusisi" when they are born soon after an earthquake occurs.

Most families also hold a second naming ceremony as children reach adolescence, initiating them into manhood or womanhood. The children spend days or weeks under instruction by tribal elders, who teach them about sex, tribal folklore, and religious traditions. The second naming ritual affirms the parents' dreams and expectations for their children.

Marriage is a complex affair involving the two families' economic situation, social status, and religion (Mbiti, 1970) For many Africans, marriage ensures economic and social survival for families via the children the couple produces.

Most African immigrants marry later than those in their native countries. Marriage in Africa is almost always between individuals from different clans; it is taboo for people from the same clan to marry each other. Intertribal marriage has come to be accepted throughout the continent, ensuring that no closely related persons marry each other. In the United States such marriages help to solidify kinship bonds between families. Yet there are many African immigrants who are marrying non-Africans, challenging parents and children to negotiate new multiracial/cultural contexts.

Many African groups practice polygamy. Polygamy tends to be polygynous, meaning that a man has more than one woman. Polyandry, in which a woman marries more than one man, is considerably less common. These practices serve several purposes, including the assurance that such families will be blessed with many children. Polygamy is also seen as helping women, who in traditional families do almost all the domestic labor, to share these tasks.

But polygamous families can engage in bitter quarrels that often separate them and create enmity among feuding family subunits. The resources of such families are stretched further than those of nonpolygamous families when they migrate. Moreover, women in polygamous families have less power than their husbands. There are also hierarchical differences, in terms of love and support from the husband, among the wives and among their children. Most African immigrant families are monogamous, but family therapists should inquire about possible polygamous situations in their families of origin.

African families living in the United States usually do not engage in the practice of offering a dowry or paying a bride price. In this traditional practice, donations are made to secure a woman in marriage, usually in the form of cash, cattle, land, or material goods. The gradual disappearance of this practice has diluted some family bonds, but has also alleviated families' monetary burdens.

Africans celebrate various rituals, including birth, naming, marriage, and death. Death rituals require specific gender roles and spiritual and community practices. Death was common during the history of colonialism in Africa, during which many people perished at the hands of colonists. Today, war, hunger, poverty, and disease have intensified Africans' encounters with death. Many Africans have relatives and friends who have died prematurely and fear they too will die at a young age. Pain and loss have surrounded most Africans as they have fled wartorn countries, as my own story and the stories of Musake and Muzibu attest.

Family therapists need to listen very carefully to the ways in which trauma is expressed among African immigrants. Many are plagued by sequelae of traumatic events, as in the case of Musake and Muzibu. It is clear that they carry both their own personal trauma and that of their extended families and entire community (Kamya & Trimble, 2002; Weingarten, 2003).

I know that the day intruders invaded our home has left an indelible mark on my life. The events of that day created both chaos and opportunity. The crack in the window shattered my hopes of ever seeing my father again. But it also ultimately provided me a sense of hope and determination to live on. Family therapists must understand and work with African families grieving over losses and trauma and carefully explore their pain and their possibilities for the future.

CLINICAL IMPLICATIONS

In general, Africans live through the stories they tell. Many need assistance in learning how to relate to others and to new institutions through the development of narratives that empower them to value their life. The therapist must learn to listen deeply to and understand their stories of social isolation, adjusting to their new locations, and dealing with financial difficulties and job barriers.

Therapists should develop a "listening-and-learning" stance as they enter into the African family's narratives of life and culture in the homeland and the stories of their migration. To do this, they must be prepared to explore and understand the family's frame of reference. African families engage well when they experience the therapeutic encounter as a mutual learning process, one in which they are encouraged to ask questions just as the therapist does. Therapy must be, in part, an invitation to clients to make meaning of their experiences through telling their stories and to understand the significance of people's context and nature of their existence (Hardy & Laszloffy, 2002).

Africans love to talk about their names and the meanings associated with them, and therapists should explore this as well. Their names often capture their ancestry, their clan, or the circumstances and events surrounding their birth. Such interaction is often nonthreatening and opens the way for therapeutic trust and relationship building.

Understanding the cultural legacies and loyalties of Africans as they endured colonialism is important for therapists (Hardy & Laszloffy, 2002). A therapeutic goal is to honor the clients' history, culture, and traditions. Doing so may afford clients emotional reparation for the internalized disrespect that many African families have experienced. The therapist should listen carefully to the family's values regarding the importance of such issues as kinship, gender, generational roles, class, politics, spirituality, work, and leisure time.

The oppression that many African families have experienced in their home countries has led them to be suspicious of anyone who seems to have power over them. Conversely, as a reaction to colonialism, African clients may try hard to please the therapist in their early work.

The therapist might do well to articulate the possible awkwardness or "foreignness" of therapy for the family. Most Africans have informal ways of addressing stress and other major issues in their lives without undertaking formal treatment with a stranger such as a therapist.

A clinician's knowledge of some African sayings may break the ice in developing a therapeutic relationship. The proverbs vary from group to group. Many African ethnic groups, however, share sayings that suggest caution as one enters a relationship. Through exploring these proverbs with clients, therapists can ask clients about their reservations in entering treatment.

It is important for therapists to be aware of the complicated immigration status of many African families, which often prohibits them from fully disclosing their situations in the United States. Family members may talk selectively about their lives until they come to trust the therapist. The clinician may need to assure African clients that he or she will not report information to the Immigration and Naturalization Service, and to empathize in regard to immigration issues or lingering feelings of mistrust.

The clinician also should determine who in the family feels emotional stress with respect to immigration or other issues, and who in the family is not "in the know" about these matters. Parents may choose to keep certain stressors secret to protect their children. Similarly, some African couples may not want in-laws to know of any difficulties they are having. Thus, therapists ought to ask about relatives beyond the immediate family, yet must also be careful in determining who should attend sessions.

Therapists might ask about reasons for migration, although some Africans may not want to discuss them, especially if they involve trauma. Thus, therapists should be very careful not to retraumatize clients by asking too many questions. In general, they might ask, "What would be helpful for me to know to work with you?" to open up conversation on these issues.

Dealing with loss on a variety of levels is important. Therapists should offer families opportunities to talk about the loss of relationships, possessions, and status, among other things, during and after the migration process. Because many African families have not been able to return to their countries of origin, such narratives offer ways to put the past in perspective, to cope in the present, and to create a hopeful vision of the future that preserves the integrity of the client family and culture.

Therapists should be open to discussions of race and racism and the "invisible wounds of oppression" (Hardy & Laszloffy, 2002) as they affect African clients. Recent African immigrants may encounter racism quite differently from both earlier immigrants and African Americans whose ancestors were brought here as slaves.

One way to enter the discussion of race and racism is to link it to tribalism in African cultures. Many tribes have disdain for other tribes, based on stereotypes such as perceived lack of education or etiquette. As in the case of racism, many tribes internalize these perceptions about themselves, creating suspicions about each other. Still others are constantly walking a fine line between acceptance and seeking a sense of belonging.

Akot, a 25-year-old woman from Kenya's western tribe of the Luo, has a very dark-skinned father and a White American mother. She, on the other hand, is very light-skinned. Akot tells the story of never fitting in either with her African peers or with her American ones, and she finds that the age-old animosity between some tribes in Kenya persists in the United States. She also straddles two or more worlds as she negotiates a sense of loyalty to both her roots in Kenya and her new-found place in the United States.

Many African families are reluctant to initiate family therapy. They may be referred to a therapist because of issues with children at school or work-related matters. The clinician should address these concerns before tackling couple issues. Once trust has been established, many African couples are more willing to explore the issues affecting them. Moreover, to establish and maintain trust, couples and families need to be repeatedly assured that their anonymity will be preserved.

Work and education are important values for many African families. They often look to therapists for help in developing concrete solutions to such issues as obtaining gainful employment or education to better the family's circumstances. Because they may be averse to therapy to begin with, some families terminate therapy as soon as they feel they are on the road to their desired goals.

CONCLUSION

African families, like other immigrant families, embark on a difficult journey when they enter American culture. Therapists working with them must examine and recognize their own and the dominant culture's value biases. Clinicians must learn to respond to differences as valuable and necessary learning opportunities. Most important, therapists must seek to engage Africans through collaboration in understanding their experiences (Anderson, 1997), attend to the particular language a client uses, allow opportunities for rich story and spiritual development (White, 1995), and respect their perceptions of themselves not only as individuals, but also as members of a larger community.

REFERENCES

Almeida, R. V. (Ed.). (1998). Transformations of gender and race: Family and developmental perspectives [Special issue]. *Journal of Feminist Family Therapy, 10*(1).

Anderson, H. (1997). *Conversation, language, and possibilities: A postmodern approach to therapy.* New York: Basic Books.

Baker, K. (1999). Acculturation and re-acculturation influence: Multilayer contexts in therapy. *Clinical Psychology Review, 19,* 951–967.

Black, L. (1996). Families of African origin: An overview. In M. McGoldrick, J. Giordano, & J. K. Pearce (Eds.), *Ethnicity and family therapy* (pp. 57–65). New York: Guilford Press.

Bograd, M. (1984). Family systems approaches to wife battering: A feminist critique. *American Journal of Orthopsychiatry, 54*(4), 558–568.

Djamba, Y. (1999). African immigrants in the United States: A socio-demographic profile in comparison to native Blacks. *Journal of Asian and African Studies, 34,* 210–216.

Hardy, K. V., & Laszloffy, T. A. (2002). Couple therapy using a multicultural perspective. In A. S. Gurman & N. S. Jacobson (Eds.), *Clinical handbook of couple therapy* (3rd ed., pp. 569–593). New York: Guilford Press.

Kamya, H., & Trimble, D. (2002). Response to injury: Toward ethical construction of the other. *Journal of Systemic Therapies, 21,* 19–29.

Kim, Y. (1978). A communication approach to the acculturation process: A study of Korean immigrants in Chicago. *International Journal of Intercultural Relations, 2,* 197–223.

Kliman, J. (2005). Many differences, many voices: Toward social justice in family therapy. In M. P. Mirkin, K. L. Suyemoto, & B. F. Okun (Eds.), *Psychotherapy with women: Exploring diverse contexts and identities* (pp. 42–63). New York: Guilford Press.

Kliman, J., & Madsen, W. (1999). Social class and the family life cycle. In B. Carter & M. McGoldrick (Eds.), *The expanded family life cycle: Individual, family, and social perspectives* (pp. 88–105). Boston: Allyn & Bacon.

Luthke, M., & Cropley, A. (1990). Decision-making and adjustment difficulties: A counseling strategy for working with migrants. *Australian Psychologist, 25,* 147–164.

Magwaza, A., & Bhana, K. (1991). Stress, loss of control, and psychological status in Black South African migrants. *Journal of Social Psychology, 131,* 157–164

Mbiti, J. S. (1970). *African religions and philosophy.* New York: Doubleday.

McCulloch, J. (1995). *Colonial psychiatry and the African mind.* Cambridge, UK: Cambridge University Press.

McGoldrick, M., & Giordano, J. (1996). Overview: Ethnicity and family therapy. In M. McGoldrick, J. Giordano, & J. K. Pearce (Eds.), *Ethnicity and family therapy* (pp. 1–30). New York: Guilford Press.

Migration Policy Institute. Migration information source. Available online at www.migrationinformation.org

Nwidor, I., Nwidor, N., & Wiwa-Lawani, B. (2004). Nigeria to Chicago. In R. Martinez (Ed.), *The new Americans.* New York: The New Press.

Padilla, A. (1980). *Acculturation: Theory, models and some new findings.* Boulder, CO: Westview Press.

Ritsner, M., Ponizovsky, A., Chemelevsky, M., & Zetser, F. (1996). *37,* 17–22.

Takyi, B. (2002). The making of the second diaspora: On the recent African American immigrant community in the United States of America. *Western Journal of Black Studies, 26,* 32–44.

U.S. Citizenship and Immigration Services. Available online at www.uscis.gov

Weingarten, K. (2003). *Common shock: Witnessing violence every day.* New York: Dutton.

White, M. (1995). *Reauthoring lives: Interviews and essays.* Adelaide, Australia: Duluth.

CHAPTER 8

British West Indian Families

Janet R. Brice-Baker

We can only hypothesize on the paucity of new material related to Jamaicans living in America. One possible factor is their invisibility. As Black people who speak English, they probably do not stand out as a group different enough to warrant investigation. (Non-English-speaking Black people from the Caribbean or elsewhere appear more culturally disparate.) In addition, like many other groups, Jamaicans are disinclined to disclose their problems to others.

HISTORY AND SOCIOLOGY

Jamaica is the third largest island in the West Indies, and the largest island in the British West Indies (GoPaul-McNicol, 1993). Originally settled by the Arawak and subsequently colonized by Spain and then by Great Britain, Jamaica achieved independence in 1962 (Galens, Sheets, & Young, 1995).

The diseases brought by the colonizing Europeans, along with hard labor and abuse, killed off the original inhabitants of the island, the Indians. As the numbers of Indians diminished, Africans were brought to Jamaica as slaves. They probably originated in the Ashanti, Fanti, Zbo, and Yoruba tribes. The minority communities on the island include the Chinese, East Indians, French, German, Irish, Sephardic Jews, and some Ashkenazi Jews. Many of these groups were brought to Jamaica as indentured laborers, particularly after the emancipation of the African slaves after the Civil War.

Jamaica's current population is more than 2.5 million. According to Galens and colleagues (1995), "As many as 90% of all Jamaicans can lay claim to African ancestry. About 26% of the population is mixed" (p. 783). The people speak English and a patois combining English and various African dialects, which are often spoken in intimate situations or when one does not want to be understood by non-Jamaicans. Jamaicans fre-

117

quently say that they are from a particular region of Jamaica or claim to be British or from the West Indies. They assert these identities to distinguish themselves from other Blacks in America and from Whites.

Jamaicans also place great value on all things English. An English person represents dignity, grace under fire, an exceptional education, and a class second to none. Jamaicans most often view non-English Whites and Blacks as being crude and lacking refinement.

MIGRATION

Historically, Jamaicans have migrated to Great Britain, Canada, and the United States. The initial reasons were related to the destruction of Jamaica's economy by colonialism and slavery. The first knowledge of Jamaicans in the "New World" occurred in 1619. Since then there have been three major periods of migration: between 1900 and 1920, in the 1930s, and from 1965 until the present (Galens et al., 1995) According to Levinson and Ember (1997):

> In Jamaica, there have been too many people with too few opportunities to earn a decent living. Unequal land distribution patterns, for example, mean that small farmers do not have enough land. When Jamaicans look to other, or additional, ways to make a living (and increasing numbers of young people are leaving rural parishes for Kingston), they are often disappointed. The big growth industries of the past World War II decades in the nonagricultural sector—bauxite, manufacturing, and tourism—have not created many new jobs. In the 1980s and the 1990s economic conditions worsened with, among other things, a fall in prices for exports and increasing foreign debt. (pp. 491–492)

Migration to the United States during the 1930s declined sharply because of restrictive U.S. immigration laws.

From 1981 to 1991, approximately 250,000 Jamaicans emigrated to the United States. In 1991, their median age was 28 and the proportion of men to women was fairly even. Jamaican immigration was characterized by long family separations, feelings of dislocation, adjustment to urban settings, and encounters with much colder weather. Therapists in large metropolitan areas are now likely to encounter Jamaicans as clients.

Often, a family member would travel to America, sometimes with other relatives, and become established. Other family members were sent for later. It was fairly common for several Jamaican families to share an apartment or house, with each family occupying a bedroom. However, when a family moved out, the remaining families did not necessarily move into the other rooms; rather, in an effort to save money, they might rent out the extra bedroom.

Earlier periods of migration were often characterized by feelings of isolation and disconnection. The new immigrants spent long hours working, and fellow Jamaicans were not necessarily nearby. Many returned to the island. More recently, large Jamaican communities of legal and illegal immigrants have arisen in many American cities, particularly in the North and South. These communities are providing access to Jamaican food stores, social groups, and houses of worship. The proximity of so many Jamaicans to each other has also helped their economic survival (Galens et al., 1995).

The rotating credit association, a West African institution that survived in vigorous form among British West Indians, played an important role in the development of West Indian business enterprises in the United States. In this informal savings system, known by Jamaicans as "partners" and by other West Indians as *"susu,"* a dozen or so trusted members pooled individual contributions to form a mutual fund which was then "rotated" by lottery at regular intervals among members to finance business activities. (Ueda, 1980)

Today, too, many urban communities of Jamaican Americans have large religious and business associations. The ever-increasing poverty on the island has reconciled many immigrants to the idea that they are not returning home. As a result, there is a greater investment in the United States as "home." Some become involved in local and state politics to try to make a difference for themselves, their families, and their community.

JAMAICAN AND AMERICAN BLACKS: ISSUES OF IDENTITY

The relationship between Jamaican and American Blacks is often ambivalent. On one hand, persistent racism in the United States has made it not only useful but also necessary for Jamaican immigrants and Blacks to present a united front to defend their interests. On the other hand, the two groups are divided over certain matters. Perhaps most important, White society has frequently put Jamaicans on pedestals as examples of "the good and industrious Black," while American-born Blacks have been stereotyped as lazy, criminal, and willing to live on public assistance.

Another issue concerns basic racial definitions. Jamaicans and American Blacks alike are very sensitive to skin hue and tend to make at least three broad distinctions, Black, Colored, and White, representing a continuum from African skin color to European skin color. The lighter-skinned a person is, the closer he or she is perceived to be at the European end of the continuum and the higher that individual's status is in Caribbean society (Garvey, 1973). But in the United States such color shadings, and the meanings assigned to them, are ignored, at least publicly, and people are more generally classified as Black or White.

A light-skinned Jamaican who comes to the United States experiences a dilemma. On the island, he or she probably had a certain amount of status, at least more than a dark-skinned Black person. In the United States, however, Whites might reject the Jamaican as "another Black"; while at the same time Blacks might reject or look down on the Jamaican because of what seems to be his or her refusal to identify with other Blacks.

Jamaicans, who are sensitive to potential exploitation by a powerful nation (Dominquez, 1975), share with Blacks ambivalent feelings about the United States. Unlike American Blacks, who were brought to this country in slave ships and have endured a long history of oppression, Jamaicans have come here voluntarily, looking for educational and occupational advancement. Like American Blacks, they are cut off from their African roots, but in contrast, Jamaicans retain an ethnic identity associated with Jamaica and view themselves as immigrants (Best, 1975).

Recent studies have found that Jamaicans are more likely to maintain the identity of their home country. They identify themselves by the island from which they came (Thompson & Bauer, 2003; Wallen, 2001). A study that looked at the relationships between Black identity, Afrocentric values, and self-esteem found some gender differences. "Results indicated that Afro-centric values, black identity and self-esteem were correlated for female adolescents but not for male adolescents. Unexpectedly, self-esteem accounted for more variability in black female identity, thus serving as a better predictor than Afro-centric values"(Akbar, Chambers, & Thompson, 2001).

The two groups differ considerably in their attitudes toward the possibility of social mobility. Although both have a strong desire to advance, they disagree on the extent to which they can control their own destinies in a country with a White majority. Many American Blacks believe that no matter how hard Black people work, their color will prevent them from being justly rewarded. For some, the frustration has resulted in "learned helplessness," so that they view efforts to break the cycle of poverty as futile.

Jamaicans, however, have a sense of empowerment derived from their successful efforts at casting off the mantle of colonialism. The Maroons, a tribe of enslaved Africans who were discharged from ships in Jamaica, are a particularly vivid example of this outlook. They did not accept bondage easily and fought ardently to escape their captors. Although many died in the process, substantial numbers lived and carved out an existence for themselves in the hills. The Maroons have come to symbolize ethnic pride and strong survival skills. More important, they provided a legacy of Jamaicans who were never enslaved, which has had a tremendous impact on the self-esteem of Blacks from the island.

Having lived in a predominantly Black society, Jamaicans in general have had different experiences than American Blacks. Even if Jamaicans are not well educated, they have come to hope, and sometimes expect, that their children and grandchildren will achieve more than they did. Thus, Jamaicans and other West Indians "have been disproportionately over-represented among black professionals" (Sowell, 1981). And the U.S. ethos of working hard, which was learned primarily from the British, is believed in and practiced by Jamaicans.

It is generally those Jamaicans who are most acculturated and familiar with European culture who "make it" in the Caribbean or in the United States (Glantz, 1978). Consequently, Jamaican immigrants to the United States are not only more apt to be enterprising than either the native American Black or the island Jamaican, but are also more likely to believe that hard work and self-denial can lead to prominence as a professional, local leader, small property owner, small business person, or landlord (Bryce-LaPorte, 1972). And because Jamaicans are oriented toward the future and advancement, they have been very thrifty, and they make sacrifices today in order to have resources for tomorrow.

FAMILY RELATIONSHIPS

Jamaican family relationships can be understood only if one is familiar with their family and social class structure, which is based on an English model. During the long British colonial period, the elite class was composed of planters and attorneys who saw to the administration of each estate. The absence of "quality White women," who might become the wives of these men, led to sexual liaisons with female slaves (Smith, 1998); other such unions occurred because White men were simply attracted to Black women.

The progeny of these unions created a mixed-colored (Creole) middle class, which, 70 years after the emancipation of slaves, enjoyed the benefits of better education and opportunities to go into the professions. Blacks who were laborers and who could not trace their family origins to White ancestors, however, filled the lower classes (Smith, 1998).

In Jamaica, upward mobility could be achieved in one of two ways: education and/or intermarriage with members of the elite class. Before educational opportunities became more widespread, a key factor in the identification of elites, or members of Creole society, was a white or near-white complexion. Jamaican Blacks wishing to improve their social status strove to "lighten" the family gene pool. Thus, intermarriage of Black Jamaicans with White or Asian Jamaicans is often looked upon favorably in the Black community.

GoPaul-McNicol (1993) writes about another type of intermarriage, that between individuals from different islands. She points out that the existence of problems in a couple's relationship may be influenced by the spouses' islands of origin. GoPaul-McNicol also points out that marriage between Jamaican Blacks and American Blacks is considered intercultural. Studies show that unions between Black American men and West Indian women are generally more successful than those between Black American women and West Indian men.

Jamaica is a society of gender role paradoxes. On the surface, sex roles are very traditional, varying little by class, race, or age (Smith, 1998). Girls are taught obedience and discouraged from being too assertive. Their domestic training is emphasized in the belief that confining a young girl to the house and garden will keep her out of trouble (Henry & Wilson, 1975; Schlesinger, 1968).

Girls are expected to be pretty, but never sexually alluring, and are usually denied sex education. They often date boys whom their parents know very well. If the community does not provide opportunities for a girl to meet appropriate young men, she is not permitted to go out.

Yet despite the emphasis on propriety, there are many unplanned, out-of-wedlock pregnancies and extramarital affairs. For a man, having a mistress is an indication of his level of success. His ability to clothe, feed, and house his mistress and the children they might have together reflects his status and wealth.

Two other hypotheses have been offered to explain the prevalence of extramarital relationships. One suggests that because of the practical considerations in the selection of a spouse, upper-class men resort to affairs to find true love, as well as sexual satisfaction. In contrast, women's happiness and satisfaction with their mates are not taken into consideration. The other theory holds that many Jamaican men believe that normative sexual acts are appropriately performed with one's wife. The assumption is that a "good" woman neither desires nor cares much for sex to begin with. Mistresses, who are usually drawn from the lower class, are considered suitable partners with whom to explore the full range of the male's sexual appetite (Henriques, 1957).

Upper-class wives are often mysterious about how they feel about their husbands' arrangements. Therapists need to tread carefully here. For example, making an issue of an affair during a session could be a mistake if the couple has an agreement that the husband is permitted to have such a liaison, provided he is discreet, that is, that he does everything possible to keep the affair a secret from his wife, her friends, and everyone in their social circle. If the therapist has any suspicions about an affair, or concerning the couple's agreement, he or she might have a separate discussion with each spouse.

Another glaring inconsistency is the stated Jamaican attitude toward fidelity. On one hand, fidelity is seen as important, and adultery is grounds for dissolving a marriage. On the other hand, there is a double standard for men and women; a woman's extramarital affair is viewed significantly more negatively than a man's extramarital affair (Voyandoff & Rodman, 1978).

The Jamaican woman often enters marriage totally ignorant about sex and is far more concerned with being a good mother than being a good sexual partner to her husband (Henry & Wilson, 1975). In the minds of most Jamaicans, womanhood and femininity are connected with motherhood. A married woman's duties revolve around child rearing, and a wife without children is often viewed as deviant.

The job of child rearing includes discipline. Among Jamaicans, spankings are the primary form of punishment and are often accompanied by a scolding or "tongue lashing." These punishments are not viewed by Jamaicans as abusive. In fact, a prevailing sentiment among parents is that spankings are a necessary means of teaching children to distinguish right from wrong and to learn respect for their elders and other authority figures (Go-Paul-McNicol, 1993, pp. 109–110).

GoPaul-McNicol (1993) cites Payne's (1989) study, which lists the following types of corporal punishment: lashing with a belt, slapping the hand, spanking with shoes, and hitting the knuckles or palm of the hand with a ruler. Although the study was done in Barbados, not in Jamaica, it still yields some interesting information. First, the subjects were teachers and child care workers, as opposed to parents. The majority endorsed flogging with a belt or strap as an approved disciplinary method, with the buttocks most frequently identified as part of the anatomy to which it should be administered (p. 109). This suggests that parents and teachers on the island are similarly disposed in their attitudes toward disciplining children.

A study that appeared in 1999 examined attitudes toward physical discipline among Jamaican American and African American college-age students. The results suggested that there were "no significant differences between the two groups on measures of the severity of physical discipline and the occurrence of physical abuse" (Cicone, 1999). However, Jamaicans were less likely than Americans to rate physical discipline, no matter how harsh, as abuse (Cicone, 1999; Wallen, 2001).

In the United States, many Jamaican immigrants sometimes find themselves at odds with teachers, child care workers, and health professionals. If abuse is defined as any and all forms of corporal punishment, therapists may be inclined to condemn parents for these behaviors without giving them closer scrutiny. Jamaican parents may find themselves in the embarrassing position of having to explain themselves to authorities outside the family sphere.

Children are expected to show great respect for their elders. It is considered impolite for them to talk back to or disagree with an older person, because adults are certain that their life experience guarantees that they know what is best for children. Boys are socialized to be responsible. Educational achievement is valued as a means to an end, not as a goal in and of itself. Boys are encouraged to seek respectable, stable professions and to choose fields of study that offer opportunities for advancement and upward mobility.

There is often a strong bond between mothers and sons, and a boy is sometimes doted on regardless of his sibling position. If her husband is absent, the mother may rely on her male children. A son's closeness to his mother continues even as he becomes older, and he is expected to take care of her when she ages.

British West Indian children usually have warm and loving relationships with their fathers, though unfortunately this close relationship is frequently disrupted by lengthy separations. The family's economic situation determines the likelihood of separation; the poorer the family, the likelier it is that the father will have to search for work away from the community.

"Child lending," whereby school-aged children are sent to live with extended family members, is a fairly common occurrence in the Islands. In some families this is done because the mother may be forced to work or has died at a young age. In other situations, a child may be sent to live with a relative in order to have easier access to education. Sometimes the arrangement may be made for the relative's benefit. For example, a child may be sent to be a companion to a childless woman or a woman whose children are grown (Sanford, 1974).

HELP-SEEKING BEHAVIOR

Jamaicans often do not recognize mental, psychological, or psychiatric problems. Usually, a significant change in an individual's functioning, particularly in aspects of daily living, serves as a sign that something is wrong. The family may cease to refer to this individual. Relatives and certain outsiders eventually learn not to inquire about this person.

Mavis, the oldest of three children in a middle-class Kingston family, had always talked about becoming a physician and had the grades, deportment, and motivation to achieve her goal. Her parents were very proud of her and mentioned her aspirations at every opportunity.

At the end of her second year of college, something changed. She was not able to get up on time for classes, spoke very little, had few friends, stopped studying, and no longer performed her extracurricular pre-med activities. Mavis's hygiene deteriorated; she kept to herself and eventually stopped going to classes altogether. Her family did not understand.

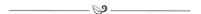

In this case, many mental health professionals would have tried to rule out some type of depressive disorder. However, a common explanation is that Jamaican families tend to "blame the victim." Mavis might have been viewed as losing her motivation. She would have been cared for by her family, but she would not have been "showcased" like her achieving brothers, sisters, or cousins.

What the American mental health field labels as a "psychological problem" Jamaicans may view as either a medical or a spiritual disturbance. (GoPaul-McNicol, 1993). This dichotomous system of classification makes it important for the therapist to understand the role of religion in Jamaican's lives.

On the island, the members of the middle and elite classes are predominantly Protestant, mostly Presbyterian, Baptist, Methodist, and Anglican (Lowenthal, 1972). A minority are Roman Catholic. Members of the lower classes are strongly influenced by folk beliefs of African origin.

One African rite that survived throughout slavery to the present day is witchcraft or *obeah*. (Practitioners are referred to as *obeahmen*, *obeahwomen*, or witch doctors.) They are consulted for a variety of reasons: to cure illness, predict the future, interpret dreams, allay fears, exact revenge, or grant a favor. Many of these goals are similar to the reasons for which individuals seek psychotherapy—to instill hope in their lives and increase feel-ings of self-efficacy (Brice-Baker, 1994).

The people who consult the witch doctor come from all segments of society. *Obeah* is widespread throughout the island, as well as throughout the Jamaican American popu-lation, though its exact prevalence has never been studied.

During slavery it was necessary for *obeah* practitioners to hide their activities from the White plantation owners, and slaves on the plantation had a hand in protecting their identity. A strong inducement against betrayal was the individual slave's fear of retribu-tion by the *obeah* practitioner. To this day Jamaicans continue to be reluctant to discuss *obeah* (Henriques, 1957). Middle-class Jamaicans often distance themselves from what the White majority society would consider "heathen superstition" (Lowenthal, 1972).

Neki and colleagues (1986) note that *obeah* can be used by clients to explain an unfavorable plight over which they feel they have no control. It can also come up in ther-apy when individuals want to relinquish responsibility for bad and overwhelming feelings they harbor against another person. Clients can claim that these feelings are coming from the witch doctor and can thus claim innocence of any wrongdoing.

Jamaicans also often use witchcraft and spiritual possession to explain aberrant behavior and illnesses for which no organic cause can be found. They sometimes view mental illness as a form of possession by evil spirits. It is fairly uncommon for Jamaican clients to consult a spiritist at the same time they are in psychotherapy:

> For people who endorse the "spiritual unrest" view, the duration can range from one day to several years. The major point is that West Indians believe a spiritist can remove the evil spirit and free the individual from this "evil force." (GoPaul-McNicol, 1993, p. 100)

Although the Jamaican family may find it difficult to admit that there is a problem it cannot handle, a family often goes to a mental health professional for a child's problem. Such a problem may surface at the child's school, as the result of a medical complaint, or at the suggestion of a physician unable to find a physiological basis for the client's symp-toms.

The immigration process is often a significant source of stress. Of course, not all families in which parents and children have been separated for a period of time are dys-functional. But the therapist needs to consider several factors that may have contributed to emotional problems: the length of the separation, the reason for it, how old the child was at its beginning, how the separation was explained, who was responsible for the child's physical care, and whether the parents continued to make major decisions about the child. Also important are the nature and frequency of contact during a separation and whether the child had a sense of when the family would be reunified.

Today government agencies in the United States have forced Jamaicans to deal with what they may think of as unacceptable interference by nonfamily members. of an indi-vidual with a mental illness becomes dangerous and someone reports this, then a state agency is likely to get involved.

Once a family is referred, the therapist should have little trouble getting members to come in, because Jamaicans take seriously the advice of professionals (e.g., teachers and doctors). However, the therapist must choose an appointment time that will not require the father or mother to miss work. Jamaicans take the adage "time is money" very seri-ously.

It is difficult to determine the impact of the therapist's race on the outcome of family therapy, largely because of the paucity of research on the subject. (The research that has been done has focused primarily on individual treatment as opposed to family therapy [Davis & Proctor, 1989].) The consensus is that racial similarity between client and therapist is an important, but perhaps not the most important, factor. What is perhaps more critical to the Jamaican client is the similarity of culture and values of the therapist and client. As for the effect of the therapist's gender on treatment, little is known.

SUMMARY

Therapists who treat Jamaicans should be sensitive to their unique heritage, their history of enslavement, the colonization of their land by Europeans, migratory labor, and migration to the United States, all of which have had profound effects on their family system and their behavior.

The strength of Jamaican families lies in their being so closely knit, something that can work to a therapist's advantage. Throughout history, extended family members have been an important resource for Jamaican families. What therapists of the dominant culture often refer to as "enmeshment" usually has been, and still is, adaptive, because it has provided individuals with emotional and practical support in times of stress. Therapists treating these families will find their work rewarding, inasmuch as individuals are often truly motivated to help one another.

Another strength of Jamaican American families is their resiliency. Perhaps this is in large part due to their "transnationality," or citizenship in multiple countries, the fact that they often have close relatives in more than one land, and their frequent movement from one nation to another. The three major countries in which Jamaican immigrants reside are England, Canada, and the United States.

In this day and age "transnationality" changes the meaning of migratory stress. Family separations do not necessarily become emotional baggage for the family members. People who are transnational are more flexible and adapt more readily to change. They are also more readily able to determine and prioritize what must be done to have their needs met.

REFERENCES

Akbar, M., Chambers, J., & Thompson, V. (2001). Racial identity, Africentric values, and self-esteem in Jamaican children. *Journal of Black Psychology, 27*(3), 341–358.

Best, T. (1975). West Indians and Afro-Americans: A partnership. *Crisis, 82,* 389.

Brice-Baker, J. R. (1994). West Indian women: The Jamaican woman. In L. Comas Diaz & B. Greene (Eds.), *Women of color: Integrating ethnic and gender identities in psychotherapy* (pp. 72–113). New York: Guilford Press.

Bryce-LaPorte, R. S. (1972). Black immigrants: The experience of invisibility and inequality. *Journal of Black Studies, 3,* 29–56.

Cicone, J. (1999). Self-reported differences in physical discipline between Jamaican American and African American college students. *Dissertation Abstracts International: Section B: The Sciences and Engineering, 59*(8-B), 44–57.

Dominquez, V. (1975). *From neighbor to strangers.* New Haven, CT: Yale University, Antilles Research Program.

Galens, J., Sheets, A., & Young, R. (Eds.). (1995). *Gale encyclopedia of multicultural America* (Vol. 2, pp. 783–797). New York: Gale Research.

Garvey, M. (1973). The race question in Jamaica. In D. Lowenthal & L. Comitas (Eds.), *The consequences of class and color.* New York: Anchor Books.

Glantz, O. (1978). Native sons and immigrants: Some beliefs and values of American-born and West Indian Blacks at Brooklyn College. *Ethnicity, 5,* 189–202.

GoPaul-McNicol, S.-A. (1993). *Working with West Indian families.* New York: Guilford Press.

Henriques, F. (1957). *Jamaica: Land of wood and water.* London: MacGibbon & Kee.

Henry, F., & Wilson, P. (1975). Status of women in Caribbean societies: An overview of their social, economic, and sexual roles. *Social and Economic Studies, 24,* 165–198.

Levinson, D., & Ember, M. (1997). *American immigrant cultures: Builders of a nation.* New York: Simon & Schuster.

Lowenthal, D. (1972). *West Indian societies.* New York: Oxford University Press.

Sanford, M. (1974). A socialization in ambiguity: Child lending in a British West Indian society. *Ethnology, 13*(4), 393–400.

Schlesinger, B. (1968). Family patterns in the English-speaking Caribbean. *Journal of Marriage and the Family, 30,* 149–154.

Smith, R. (1988). *Kinship and class in the West Indies.* New York: Cambridge University Press.

Sowell, T.(1981). *Ethnic America.* New York: Basic Books.

Ueda, R. (1980). West Indians. In S. Thernstrom, A. Orlov, & O. Handlin (Eds.), *Harvard encyclopedia of American ethnic groups* (p. 4). Cambridge, MA: Harvard University Press.

Voyandoff, P., & Rodman, H. (1978). Marital careers in Trinidad. *Journal of Marriage and the Family, 40,* 157.

Wallen, V. (2001). Ethnic identity, self-esteem and academic factors in second generation post-1970 Jamaican immigrants. *Dissertation Abstracts International, 62*(4-A), 1586.

CHAPTER 9

Haitian Families

Josiane Menos

Haitians were the first, and remain the only enslaved people in human history to have overthrown slavery and established an independent polity ruled by former slaves in place of the one controlled by their masters.

—SIDBURY (quoted in Wills, 2003, p. 45)

In the 18th century, Saint Dominique, known to the natives as Haiti and to Columbus as Hispaniola, was the richest colony in the Caribbean, supplying half the world's sugar and coffee and having the densest slave population in the Western Hemisphere. By the beginning of the 19th century, it had created a unique revolution, one of the most thorough examples of dramatic change in a country's social, political, intellectual, and economic life in modern history (Knight, 2000).

To its shame, the United States, which just two decades before had been created through a revolution, which espoused the rights of liberty, chose to do everything in its power to undermine Haiti's revolution (Wills, 2003). In fact, European powers and America had exploited and undermined Haiti from Columbus's time. Thus, Haiti today is the poorest country in the Americas, torn by strife and struggling to survive. The United States still does not acknowledge or accept this reality, which contributes to the plight of Haitian immigrants.

The chapter focuses primarily on low-income Haitian families, who generally do not voluntarily seek mental health services. Rather, they are often referred by child protective services and schools as a result of domestic violence and child abuse, issues seldom talked about in patriarchal Haitian society. Based on extensive interaction with Haitians, clinical work with Haitian families in New York City, and personal experience, I present my observations of Haitian history and culture and their implications for therapy. To work effectively with the great diversity of Haitian families, the therapist must pay attention to the joint effects of history, politics, economics, class, time of immigration, the immigration experience, and ties to Haiti. These elements add to each family's unique story.

HISTORICAL BACKGROUND

Haiti has been besieged with 400 years of struggle. When Columbus landed in Haiti in 1492, the island was populated by the Taino Indians, who also lived in parts of Cuba and Puerto Rico, and who, in Haiti, had developed an advanced civilization. During the 50 years that Spain controlled Haiti, most of the Tainos died from diseases brought by the Europeans and from the atrocities of slavery. A Spanish priest, Bartolomew Las Casas, appalled by the treatment of the Tainos, promoted the end of Native American slavery by, paradoxically, supporting the importation of Black slaves from Spain.

In 1503, the first Blacks landed on the island. Later, in the early and mid-17th century, most Spanish settlers left Haiti, now renamed Hispaniola, in search of gold mines in South America. In 1697, after losing a war with France, Spain surrendered the western part of the island (known to the natives as Haiti, or mountainous land) to that country. (The French had been involved in island affairs since the early 17th century and had imported large numbers of African slaves.)

To sustain this industry involved in the exportation of sugar and coffee, the small island had 500,000 slaves (Wills, 2003), as compared with 700,000 in the entire United States. Slaveholders probably used harsh measures of control, since the ratio of slaves to masters in Haiti was higher than anywhere else in the world.

In 1791, the slaves revolted against their French plantation owners. Yet although the United States had just gone through its own rebellion for freedom, it gave its support to the slave owners. Even the English, then at war with France, sent an army and supplies to the slaveholders. Both nations feared that a successful slave uprising would endanger their own slaveholdings.

In August 1791, Boukman, a rebel slave, priest, and political leader, organized a secret meeting and religious ceremony, which impelled many Haitian slaves to revolt against the slave owners. They ultimately gained their freedom, and Haiti its independence from France, making it the first Black nation, on January 1, 1804. Many Haitians attributed the victory to their faith in their African gods. Their victory also resulted in a surge of pride in native Haitian culture. To honor the memory of the original Taino population, which had been destroyed, the island took back its original name, Haiti.

The Haitian army, composed of slaves, mulattos, and free Blacks, had battled against one of the most powerful armies of the time and won. Yet, President Jefferson refused to recognize this achievement and directed Congress to suspend trade with Haiti (Wills, 2003), and to deny diplomatic recognition. The United States finally acknowledged Haiti's independence in 1862.

This long period of isolation from commerce and a 150 million franc debt owed to France in return for its official recognition of Haiti as an independent country, began Haiti's turbulent journey toward a failed economy, political instability, and its sad distinction as the poorest country in the Western Hemisphere. Had it been granted recognition by the world powers at the time, rather than enduring 68 years of postindependence isolation and a huge debt, Haiti could have evaded two centuries of turmoil and been less vulnerable to the American occupation. Had this been the case, Haiti could have thrived.

After its independence the country's population was composed of two classes: the mulatto bourgeoisie and wealthy elite, who were mostly the offspring of slave women and French colonists, and the primarily dark-skinned peasants. The mulattoes were often provided with educational opportunities by their French fathers, sent to France for higher education, and often were left their fathers' wealth. Their influence resonates in Haitian culture to this day. Composed of several thousand families, the Haitian bourgeoisie, which is predominantly mulatto, yet also includes some Blacks, makes up less than 1% of the Haitian population but controls nearly 50% of the country's wealth.

Haiti went through 22 heads of state and 14 revolutions between 1843 and 1915, when American forces occupied the country, largely in response to what was seen as the threat of German economic interest in the country. The occupation lasted almost two decades, until 1934 (Cosgray, 1999). After the United States left Haiti there was more political turmoil until 1957, the beginning of François "Papa Doc" Duvallier's brutal dictatorship.

Duvallier, who declared himself president for life in 1964, established a military police force known as the *tonton macoutes*, which brought terror to the Haitian people through random acts of cruelty. In 1971, his 19-year-old son, Jean Claude "Baby Doc" Duvallier, became president following his father's death.

In 1986, the U.S. withdrawal of support of the Duvallier regime and peasant revolts led to its end. Four years later, a Catholic priest, Jean Bertrand Aristide, was elected president (Heinl & Heinl, 1996). From that time until now, the country remained in dire straits, economically and politically. The latest episode of upheaval was the 2004 bloody uprising of armed rebels determined to unseat President Aristide, who, facing pressure from the United States and France, finally left Haiti.

LANGUAGE

In 1987, Creole, the language of the people, became Haiti's official language (Stepick, 1998). Its origins are unclear. One theory claims that Creole was developed by slaves and is a blend of African dialects and French (Pierce & Elisme, 1997). Creole is also believed to have African, Spanish, Portuguese, English, and French origins.

Only a small percentage of Haitians are fluent in French, although the language is highly esteemed by all Haitians and is a sign of social class.

Even some individuals who speak only Creole have been resistant to public schools teaching the language, viewing it as the language of the poor and believing that the ability to speak French could help to raise their child's social standing. The Haitian Creole language is replete with proverbs, metaphors, and colorful images that lend it a melodic rhythm.

HAITIAN PROVERBS

Creole proverbs in particular provide critical insights into Haitian history, culture, and spiritual beliefs. A fatalistic (or, for some, optimistic) view is indicated in the phrase "*Bondye bon*" ("God is good"), often said when something dreadful happens. It expresses the idea that whatever happens is God's choice and is for the best, which reflects Haitians' deep faith that, because of divine providence, things will always work out in the end.

Another proverb states, "*Nan tan grangou patat pa gen po*" ("During times of hunger, sweet potatoes have no skin"). It means that when one is starving, one will eat anything, including the skin of a potato, and is also said during very difficult times. This proverb too conveys the Haitian's strong will to survive even in the face of insurmountable troubles. For if poorly armed slaves could triumph over the once powerful French army, then no problem is so great that it cannot be resolved.

REASONS FOR IMMIGRATION

Political and economic instability in Haiti resulted in waves of Haitian immigration into the United States. Between 1915 and 1934 the first group of Haitians immigrants came to this country; they were primarily individuals escaping the terror imposed during the American occupation of Haiti. Many settled in Harlem, where they integrated into the African American community (Pierce & Elisme, 1997).

Hurbon (1994) reports that in his book, *The White King of La Gonave*, Lt. Faustin Wirkus, a Marine, gave an account of the damage he inflicted during the American occupation to "save" the Haitian people from cannibalism. The book sold 10 million copies in the United States, Europe, and Japan. Reportedly, the U.S. Marines prided themselves on pillaging religious temples and destroying the "idols" of the African ancestors.

The next wave of immigration, between 1957 and 1964, resulted from the oppression and turmoil brought about by François Duvallier's dictatorship. The majority were upper-class opponents of his rule, whose mass departure resulted in Haiti's loss of a many well-educated people (Stepick, 1998).

During the late 1960s, another wave of Haitian immigrants arrived, due to the increased horror of Duvallier's terrorist regime, the relative ease with which they could enter the United States (thanks to the 1965 immigration law), and the need for skilled workers as a result of the Vietnam War. These individuals were mostly from the middle and poorer classes (Colin & Paperwalla, 1996).

The educated mulatto elite and middle-class Haitians who came during the 1960s did not view themselves as having a common heritage with other Haitians. Rather, the elite valued the social privileges they had had in Haiti. To safeguard their social status and power, they avoided socializing with Haitians who were not of their class.

Divisions between Haitian social classes have continued in the United States. During the late 1970s and the 1980s—in fact, until Aristide's election in 1990—the immigrant population fleeing Haiti was composed of rural peasants and urban dwellers escaping the violence of Baby Doc's reign. This population, which reached the American shores in small, flimsy boats, came to be known as the "boat people" (Colin & Paperwalla, 1996).

In October 1980, the United States instituted a policy stating that Haitians who arrived here were economic refugees and subject to deportation. In 1991, President George H. W. Bush continued the policy to turn away Haitian immigrants from American shores by ordering the Coast Guard to return all Haitian boats without screening their passengers. President Bush's order preceded a Supreme Court ruling that deportation was legal and that Haitians who entered the country illegally could be sent back (Cosgray, 1999).

Between 1991 and 1994 more than 65,000 Haitians were intercepted at sea by the Coast Guard (Pain, 2004). Most had sacrificed everything to come to the United States, risking their lives in leaky boats and sailing on treacherous waters to escape further political terror. They had the added hope of reunification with family members who were already living in the United States. Edwidge Danticat, a Haitian author who was 12 years old when she moved to the United States to be reunited with her parents, wrote:

> There was a swell of people coming by boat from Haiti to Florida to escape the dictatorship, the first large exodus of the 1980s. Every night on the six o'clock news, you could see dead, bloated bodies washing up on Miami beaches. This was often followed by some type of report on AIDS, still a fresh news topic then too. Both items would keep all the members of my family anxious. The boat people, because coming from a poor Haitian family, any of those faces could have been one of our relatives. So we watched the television screen with great interest as the Coast Guard's white sheets were thrown over the dark, dead faces, already half buried in the Florida sand. And we watched with great interest those who had survived the boat journey to America and were able to walk away, only to be processed into detention centers in New York and Miami. We leaned in to observe their gait, their height, their body type, and we searched for traces of ourselves in them. (Excerpted from a lecture presented at the Inter-American Development Bank's Cultural Center in Washington, D.C., on December 7, 1995)

When working with Haitian families, a therapist should remember that most recent immigrants are escaping political persecution and economic devastation, as well as such traumas as rape, assault, and death threats, and have been witness to horrifying crimes (Desrosiers & St. Fleurose, 2002). The immense difficulties that some Haitians have experienced in acquiring legal status have had harsh consequences for them and their families. Children may be separated from parents, and spouses from each other, for more than a decade. Reunification is often discordant because of the lengthy separation and the acculturation of family members already living in the United States. Still, Haitians have kept coming to these shores, and today there are more than one million Haitians living in the United States, with the largest number in Illinois.

STIGMA

In 1982, the U.S. Centers for Disease Control (CDC) erroneously classified Haitians as a high-risk group for AIDS, partly because earlier studies incorrectly suggested that the disease originated in Haiti. The removal of Haitians from the CDC's risk list in 1985 did not receive the same publicity as their placement on it; in fact, very few people, including Haitians, know that the CDC has issued a retraction. As late as the early 1990s, Haitians continued to be labeled as an AIDS risk group.

In the United States, some Haitian patients admitted to hospitals were immediately placed in isolation, regardless of their presenting symptoms. Blood donors were specifically asked if they were Haitian, for Haitians were not permitted to donate blood. Some Haitian women were turned away from beauty parlors. Non-Haitian parents did not want their children to play with Haitian children. Farmer and Kim (1991) reported that some families of color apparently were evicted from their homes, and others were fired from their jobs. To avoid rejection and stigmatization by the dominant culture, many Haitians were reluctant to mention their ethnic background. The stigma of being associated with AIDS has had an enormous impact on the emotional development of Haitian Americans.

MARRIAGE

The man is viewed as the head of the family. When Haitian families immigrate to the United States, a husband can feel threatened by his wife's acculturation to American life, particularly if she becomes established financially. The therapist can help the couple to recognize and adjust to a new dynamic of power, while stressing the benefits of joint planning and decision making.

When a woman appears to be satisfied with her role as a wife, the therapist should be cautious about inserting his or her own values, but should draw his or her cues from the clients themselves. In cases where the man is abusive, the woman can be empowered to stop the abuse.

ECONOMIC SUPPORT

Many Haitians in the United States share a moral obligation to financially support relatives living in on the island who may have no resources of their own because of unemployment. Schiller and Fouron (2001) stress that Haitians living in the United States can affirm their humanity by fulfilling "kinship responsibilities." Those who ignore the needs of family members still in Haiti, who live in very difficult circumstances, are seen as manifesting a callous indifference. Thus, not only a love of family propels distribution of funds by Haitians living in the United States, but also a "morality of obligation."

Those who provide economic support are given respect and status, whereas those unable to do so must sometimes cut ties with family living in Haiti (Schiller & Fouron, 2001). And those helping to sustain more than one family often require other sources of income in addition to full-time employment, which, as the following case study shows, can limit their family and leisure time.

Jean, whose parents came to a New York City clinic for an intake, was an eighth-grade Haitian American boy who was referred by his school for fighting, being disruptive in class, and not completing his schoolwork. His behavior led to a suspension from the school's basketball team. Jean's father, Claude, explained that he and his wife worked long hours to support themselves and their three children. They also regularly sent money to relatives who lived in Haiti, who depended on this money to survive.

According to school records and the parents' report, Jean's behavior started to deteriorate at the beginning of seventh grade. His father labeled him an "ingrate" because his behavior showed that he did not appreciate the efforts his parents had made for him. Jean recognized that his parents worked hard, yet expressed disappointment that his father had never attended his basketball games and that his parents were never around, or complained of being too tired when they were home.

Recognizing the parents' commitment to hard work, the therapist validated their feeling that their time was stretched thin. She also applauded the parents' remarkable skill at structuring their financial resources so well and conveyed respect for the family's strong work ethic, in which Jean took increasing pride. Gradually, through the therapist's gentle coaching, Jean was able to convey to his parents his sense of being neglected by them and his desire for his father to see him play basketball. The therapist helped Jean and his parents to find small, yet impor-

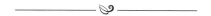

tant, ways to increase family time together, which in turn resulted in Jean's improved behavior in school.

DISCIPLINE AND EDUCATION OF CHILDREN

Children are valued in Haitian culture, and the entire family participates in raising a child. It is common for certain parents in the United States to send their children to live with relatives on the island if they feel that the children would have a better life there. It is equally common for individuals from the island to host a child whose parents live in Haiti.

Older family members are respected for their wisdom, and their guidance is often sought. Haitians view their entire extended family as a source of support and miss it when the family is split. The "togetherness" of extended families is sometimes viewed as "enmeshment" by a non-Haitian therapist.

In general, parents, who have near absolute power in Haiti, raise children with an understanding that they must be obedient and sometimes administer physical discipline with a belt or switch when they misbehave, which may on occasion be viewed as abuse in this country. When child protective services intervene, parents can be stunned. If this happens, the therapist must become a change agent and teacher. To do so, the therapist might teach parents American laws regarding the treatment of children. Haitian parents living in the United States benefit from information on alternatives to corporal punishment. However, it should be noted that many Haitian families do not practice harsh discipline with their children.

Haitian adolescents, in particular, acculturate easily through their exposure to school and the larger society and often rebel against their parents' ways. The therapist's role is to help to ease intergenerational conflicts between children and parents. To do so, advises Garcia-Preto (1996), in addition to promoting open lines of communication between the generations, the therapist helps the parents to maintain a balance that respects parents' responsibility to protect adolescents yet acknowledge adolescents' need for independence. Asking families to identify the cultural values that create the greatest conflict at home can lead them to think about a compromise (Garcia-Preto, 1996).

Haitians place a great value on education. Haitian families may work long hours at multiple jobs to pay their children's tuition at parochial or other private schools. They also view academic advancement with pride, seeing it as a source of social mobility. However, many families, struggling to meet day-to-day needs, cannot afford to obtain the advanced training for themselves required to achieve professional advancement (Schiller & Fouron, 2001).

RELIGION AND MENTAL HEALTH

Most Haitians are Roman Catholic, though others have converted to Protestantism as a result of the efforts of missionaries. Much of the population also practices voodoo, whose roots are in West Africa and which Haitians believe can coexist with Christian beliefs.

Voodoo includes a belief in one God, similar to the God of Christianity. It also recognizes three types of spirits: the *loa* or *lwa*, (protective spirits of ancestors); the twins, who are the descendants of God and represent the poles of good and evil, and the spirits of deceased family members. Voodoo believers ask the *loa* for protection and good fortune. Each *loa* functions independently and has the power to control the forces of nature. During religious ceremonies the *loa* send messages through their devotees and are given food and drink offerings, as well as other gifts, in return for their protection.

The *loa*, an intermediary between God and mortals, is seen as being present in all spheres of nature—trees, streams, mountains, air, water, and fire—and controlling human affairs and the agricultural cycle. One's fate is believed to be predetermined by the *loa*, and only by paying homage to them through religious ceremonies can one influence one's own destiny. Individual families have their own *loa*, who protect the them from malevolent spirits. Bad fortune may occur if one does not honor one's *loa* (Laguerre, 1981). The twins (good and evil) are believed to have more power than the *loa* because of the union they symbolize. They are believed to be endowed with extraordinary powers, such as making the rain fall and providing remedies to the sick. All of the religious rituals include them. They are extremely finicky about the services they require, and the slightest inattention shown by their living relatives brings retribution. They regularly require offerings of specific meals served in special dishes. When the twins have been satisfied, they provide recipes for medicines made from plants or herbs (Hurbon, 1994). It is critical for family members to remember the souls of their departed ancestors, for they too may exert a malevolent influence if ignored. In return, the family honors its *loa* with a yearly ceremonial feast that includes drums, singing, dancing, food, and drink (Laguerre, 1984). Ritual objects as well as ritualistic chants, dances, and foods are necessary for the spiritual intervention to occur. Deren (1953) stresses, for example, that it is the rhythm of the drums themselves, which are the sacred voice of address to the *loa*. Any individual ancestor or being of power may ultimately become a *loa* (Miller, 2000). Catholic Haitians often associate *loa* with saints. For instance, Dumballah, the snake *loa* is represented by St. Patrick, and Erzulie, the earth mother *loa*, is represented by the Virgin Mary (Stepick, 1998).

For certain Haitians, it is their cultural legacy that is the foundation of their life force, it is their history that arms them for their activities, and it is from their ancestral *loa* that they draw the psychic energy and wisdom they rely on to empower and instruct them in their daily lives. To ask a Haitian if he or she believes in voodoo is a pointless question. The person answers, "I serve the *loa*." Followers respect the degree of knowledge of the *houngan* (priest) and the *mambo* (priestess) who help to summon and to control the *loa* (Deren, 1953).

The realm of a religious person is directed by moral reason. The voodoo believer does not believe that well-being will result from a certain ritual, but that well-being will be a reward for the performance of it. Service to the *loa* strengthens a believer's relationship with his or her ancestors, history, and community, leading to a revitalized sense of the believer's union to spiritual, social, and personal elements. The rituals, which the believer understands as supernatural intervention, actually do work, very often, and the main effect of the ritual is on the doer. "The miracle is, in a sense, interior. It is the doer who is changed by the ritual, and for him, therefore, the world changes accordingly" (Deren, 1953).

The most sensational aspect of voodoo is the creation of zombies, a practice that is highly exaggerated in the media and a racial stereotype characterizing African ways as savage. In fact, Haitians usually do not discuss the notion of zombies, and only a very small percentage of *hougans* practice magic and sorcery (Hurbon, 1994).

DEPRESSION AND SOMATIC DISORDERS

Haitians tend to view depression as a state of general fatigue and discouragement caused by anemia or constant anxiety about problems. As previously noted, the work ethic is important to most Haitians, who place great value on fulfilling their familial obligations both at home and on the island. To respond to their feelings, somatization is the most common representation of a mood disorder. Primary care providers are consulted about headaches and other pains. Reports of an "empty head" or "my head is not there," fatigue, insomnia, and poor appetite are common.

Inconclusive test results may lead to a mental health referral. The client often needs to be given information about the impact of stress on physical and mental health and the great effect that the repressed past has on the present (Desrosiers & St. Fleurose, 2002). Haitian clients can be helped to acknowledge the stress of migration, racism, and the continued need to financially support relatives in Haiti. Discussion of these issues can help to normalize their feelings.

THE NEED FOR CONCRETE SERVICES

The initial visit with a therapist should deal with the referral question. Unaccustomed to counseling and therapy, Haitian families need to feel that practical services have been provided to them before there is any possibility of engagement in therapy, as shown in the following case study.

Lucie, a 39-year-old single parent, was referred by the New Jersey Division of Youth and Family Services for child neglect. She had been living in the United States for 10 years and had three children, Daniel, 9; Serge, 7; and Jacinthe, 5. A neighbor reported her for leaving the children home alone after school.

Lucie explained that she could not afford after-school services for her children and noted that Daniel was highly responsible and could take care of his younger siblings until she returned home. The therapist arranged a meeting between Lucie and the school's social worker, who offered information on community agencies that provided sliding-scale after-school care and homework help. Helping Lucie to find a solution to her immediate stress enabled her to realize that a continuation of therapy could benefit her family.

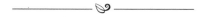

CONCLUSION

Haitian families are often separated by long distances. Although most family members may still be in Haiti or otherwise not in proximity to the client family, it is important to involve the extended family through a genogram. Most Haitian families know their family history, yet make few connections to intergenerational patterns. Developing a genogram offers them a nonthreatening context that enables them to tell their stories.

Haitians Americans have experienced much trauma, racial prejudice, and cultural bias, both in Haiti and in the United States. To a large extent, these injustices have caused many Haitian Americans to feel a sense of shame, leading some to keep their ethnic identity a secret as a means of protecting themselves. Some Haitians may need a voice to help them articulate why they should be proud, particularly in the face of their many struggles.

Many Haitians believe in the power of God to alleviate problems. They may also need help in creating religious and psychological rituals to deal with their problems. An example of a ritual that might help Haitian clients cope with distress is: Write down your problem, then throw it in the river and watch it float away, or put it in a bottle and freeze it.

Therapists working with Haitians should avoid making assumptions. Because of the many class, religious, and other subcultures in Haitian society, therapists should be open to asking many questions about emotional dynamics, religious beliefs, and other aspects of family life.

Questions will also help the therapist to uncover incidents of trauma, which clients do not always associate with their symptoms. Haiti's long history of political problems makes it important to ask detailed questions to uncover possible human rights violations experienced or witnessed in Haiti. The therapist's intervention can make the association between past trauma and present problems and help to normalize the client's feelings.

Haitians are not usually avid consumers of psychotherapy, partly as a result of their belief that families should solve problems on their own. The family therapist working with Haitian families needs to recognize that therapy alone is not the answer. Haitian families referred by outside agencies require practical resources to help them deal with the issues they present.

REFERENCES

Colin, J. M., & Paperwalla, G. (1996). Haitians. In J. G. Lipson, S. L. Dibble, & P. A. Minarik (Eds.), *Culture and nursing care: A pocket guide* (pp. 139–154). San Francisco: UCSF Nursing Press.

Colin, J. M., & Paperwalla, G. (2003). People of Haitian heritage. In L. D. Purnell & B. J. Paulanka (Eds.), *Transcultural health care: A culturally competent approach* (pp. 70–84). Philadelphia: F. A. Davis.

Cosgray, R. E. (1999). Haitian Americans. In J. N. Giger & R. E. Davidhizar (Eds.), *Transcultural nursing: Assessment and intervention* (3rd ed., pp. 482–507). St. Louis, MO: Mosby.

Deren, M. (1953). *Divine horsemen: The living gods of Haiti*. New York: McPherson.

Desrosiers, A., & St. Fleurose, S. (2002). Treating Haitian patients: Key cultural aspects. *American Journal of Psychotherapy*, 56(4), 508–522.

Farmer, P., & Kim, J. Y. (1991). Anthropology, accountability, and the prevention of AIDS. *Journal of Sex Research*, 28(2), 203–221.

Garcia-Preto, N. (1996). Transformation of the family system during adolescence. In B. Carter & M. McGoldrick (Eds.), *The expanded family life cycle* (3rd ed., pp. 274–286). Needham Heights, MA: Allyn & Bacon.

Heinl, R. D., Jr., & Heinl, N. G. (1996). *Written in blood: The story of the Haitian people, 1492–1995* (Revised and expanded by M. Heinl). Lanham, MD: University Press of America.

Hurbon, L. (1994). *Voodoo—search for the spirit*. New York: Abrams.

Knight, F. W. (2000, February). The Haitian revolution. *American Historical Review*, pp. 103, 105.

Laguerre, M. S. (1981). Haitian Americans. In A. Harwood (Ed.), *Ethnicity and medical care* (pp. 172–210). Cambridge, MA: Harvard University Press.

Laguerre, M. S. (1984). *American odyssey: Haitians in New York City.* Ithaca, NY: Cornell University Press.

Miller, N. L. (2000). Haitian ethnomedical systems and biomedical practitioners: Directions for clinicians. *Journal of Transcultural Nursing, 11*(3), 204–211.

Pain, J. (2004, February 27). US Haitian immigration policy condemned. *Associated Press.*

Pierce, W. J., & Elisme, E. (1997). Understanding and working with Haitian immigrant families. *Journal of Family Social Work, 2*(1), 49–65.

Schiller, N. G., & Fouron, G. E. (2001). *Georges woke up laughing: Long distance nationalism and the search for home.* Durham, NC: Duke University Press.

Stepick, A. (1998). *Pride against prejudice: Haitians in the United States.* Needham Heights, MA: Allyn & Bacon.

Wills, G. (2003). *Negro president: Jefferson and the slave power.* Boston: Houghton Miflin.

CHAPTER 10

African American Muslim Families

Vanessa McAdams-Mahmoud

Many African Americans have found themselves influenced by Islam and Islamic values in their search for identity and self-determination. Much of what African Americans are taught about Islam has come through organizations or individuals who have attempted to blend the culture of African Americans with the practice of Islam. This reconciliation of culture and religion is not unusual in the Islamic world. Although the tenets of the religion do not change from culture to culture, there is usually a distinct cultural stamp placed on the everyday habits and practices of the religion. The Chinese Islamic community will vary in cultural practices from the Pakistani, and the Sudanese from the Egyptian, but all are Muslim, perform the same *salat*, or prayer, and read from the same book, the Holy Qur'an.

Islam first arrived in America with the enslaved Africans Yorro Mahmoud, Ayub Ibn Sulayman Diallo, and Abdul Rahman (Nyang, 1985, cited in Rashad, 1991). There were numerous others, whose practice of Islam was often done in secret and passed down to others surreptitiously in oral history or through family members imitating behaviors, without indicating its origins. Often, when I have done genogram work with African Americans, a story might surface of a distant relative, who refused to eat pork, always prayed facing east, named his or her children "funny" names, or refused to allow them to be baptized.

This behavior was often remembered because it caused some dissension in the family, which was usually seeking to acculturate and conform to dominant community norms. Other family members had no way of placing such behavior in context, because the practice of traditional African religions, as well as the speaking and writing of Arabic, were all generally suppressed and punished by slave owners. There is some evidence, however, that a very few slave owners valued the habits of Muslim slaves, except when they sought their freedom (Rashad, 1991).

Some African American families preserved some fragments of Islamic practices. The most famous example of such an occurrence is told in Alex Haley's *Roots*. Haley's ancestor, Kunta Kinte, fiercely fought to maintain his identity and his Islamic faith. He also passed down the practice of maintaining one's lineage in one's memory as did the *griots* (recorders of history) of his people, the Muslims of Gambia. Thanks to his tenacious practice, one of his descendants was able to journey back to Gambia and be reunited with his relatives.

In addition to the anecdotal and behavioral remnants of Islam that persist within African American family life and culture, there have been a number of attempts to reestablish Islam among African Americans. Although Muslims of other nationalities settled in the United States (e.g., Arabs, Albanians, Indian Muslims, etc.), there was no recorded effort by those communities to establish Islam among African Americans until 1928, when Sheikh Dau'wd was granted a charter by Sheikh Khalid of Jordan and King Saud of Saudi Arabia to establish an Islamic mission in the Western Hemisphere (Rashad, 1991).

The most powerful combination of cultural necessity and Islamic principles came about in the pairing of Black nationalism and Islam. Noble Drew Ali founded the Moorish American Science Temples in 1913. He was influenced heavily by Marcus Garvey's movement, the United Negro Improvement Association.

Elijah Muhammad was taught by a man named Wallace Fard and built his organization based on the principles of both Garvey and Ali. All three sought to:

- Reverse the effects of enslavement by introducing an alternative set of values about oneself (adopting new names, alternative explanations of history, self-pride, nationalism and loyalty) for a people long alienated and denied access to full citizenship.
- Introduce an alternative social milieu in which to practice these values and set goals that expanded the people's aspirations.
- Develop a family life and models of ideal male and female behavior.
- Establish bases of economic independence from the dominant culture.
- Protest and fight against the oppression of African American people.
- Educate children and indoctrinate them with these values, so that they would base their lives on these principles.
- Establish a secure homeland that could be controlled by African Americans.

Elijah Muhammad promised his followers "money, good homes and friendship in all walks of life" if they adhered to his program and to Islamic principles. Malcolm X, or Al-Hajj Malik al-Shabazz, the son of a Garveyite, was murdered for his principles. His break with Elijah Muhammad later in his life was mirrored the experience of many Muslims who were first attracted to the combination of Black nationalism and Al-Islam. Many of his followers later began to study and to practice orthodox Islam.

The son of the Honorable Elijah Muhammad, Warith Deen Muhammad, led a massive number of his father's followers into the orthodox practice of Islam in the late 1970s. Minister Louis Farrakhan, a protégé of the Elijah Muhammad, continued in his tradition and maintained the blend of Black nationalism and Islam among his followers.

The growth of orthodox Islam has been rapid in the last 30 years. Today, in every major American city and large town, there are African American Muslims who identify themselves as *Sunni*, or orthodox, or those who follow the example of the prophet

Muhammad. Other schools of thought, such as the Ahmadiyya and the Hanafi, as well as members of esoteric Sufi circles, are flourishing in establishing religious academies, *masajid* (places of worship and congregation), and other aspects of communal life..

A family therapist who works with a Muslim African American should know to which community the family belongs and how they feel about their particular religious community. African American Muslims are grouped in very broad categories:

1. *Cultural nationalists* stress Black nationalism and Islam, as well as separation and independence from the dominant community.
2. *Sunni or orthodox Muslims (African American–centered leadership)* adhere to the traditional practice of Islam, stressing self-determination and pride, and are defined by their faith. Their communities are usually led by an African American.
3. *Sunni or orthodox Muslims (African- or Arab-centered leadership)* practice and adhere to the traditional practice of Islam, but stress the religion's universality and are most comfortable in an international, multicultural Islamic community.

Conscious adoption of African and Islamic practices, customs, habits, dress, and symbolism is on the increase in many African American Muslim families.

IMPACT ON FAMILY LIFE

The adoption of the *adab* (Islamic behavior, manners, and customs) by African American families can sometimes alter family life. In a cultural nationalist family, there are changes in diet (no pork or pork products, emphasis on "eating to live," one meal per day, fasting for religious and health reasons), dress (conservative suits, uniforms for men; long dresses, head coverings, uniforms for women), and relationships with non-Muslim family members (sometimes encouraging socialization only with Muslims, nonparticipation in Christian religious holidays that might be celebrated by other family members).

A strong personal commitment to the group's goals is expected. Chivalry, marriage, and traditional gender and parent–child roles are emphasized. Scholarship is prized when it encompasses a strong knowledge of African/African American history and Afrocentric views. Cultural nationalists also stress the development of small businesses, salesmanship, economic self-sufficiency, and an appreciation of African American cultural identity.

Sunni Muslims base their family life on the five principles of Islam (Al-Qaradawi, 1960):

1. *Shahadah:* The declaration of faith that there is no god but Allah, and Muhammad is the Messenger of God.
2. *Salah:* The five daily prayers.
3. *Zakah:* The giving of charity (about 2% of annual income) to the needy.
4. *Sawm:* Fasting during the month of Ramadan, the time when the Holy Qur'an was revealed).
5. *Hajj:* The performance of the pilgrimage to Mecca once in a person's lifetime.

Commitment to these traditional tenets means that each family must reconcile the demands made upon them by everyday life, with the requirements placed upon them as

Muslims and as African Americans. Of course, the ability to fulfill these demands varies with each family and each individual.

The stress of living as a African American Muslim on the individual should not be minimized. Traditional Islam also includes dietary restrictions (prohibition of pork or pork by-products, meat with any trace of blood, or food that is intended for sacrifice.), ritual cleanliness (for prayer, after sexual contact, and sleep), and prohibitions against alcohol and gambling. Also important are modest dress and behavior for both men and women (head covering for women, so that only the face and hands are seen, as well as modest dress that covers the body; *kufi* [hats] for men; and prohibitions against wearing silk and the colors red and gold). Believers must be familiar with Muslim greetings and common phrases, such as *Al hamdu lillah* (All praise is due to God), *Allah U Akbar* (God is great), and *As salaam uAlaikum* (Peace be unto you).

Shoes are not worn in a Muslim home, but are left at the door. The home decoration should be free of human images of people. Still other cultural and religious rules in the lives and homes of Muslims are based on the *hadith* and *sunna* (sayings, practices, and example) of Prophet Muhammad.

The ability to adapt and synthesize these aspects of their faith varies from family to family, individual to individual. The decision to wear *hijab* (full ritual covering) for women, in a society that sees such covering as oppressive, is quite stressful for some women, but for others it is not. Finding a place to pray is difficult when the individual works in certain settings or is in school all day.

African American Muslims must endure the stereotypes and distorted images projected upon them as Muslims, as well as those they endure as African Americans. It is very difficult when these views are held by other African Muslims, particularly by relatives who are not Muslim. However, there is also genuine respect for their moral standards and practices, as well as for their staunch pride and their belief in standing firm against oppression.

Cultural Nationalist Muslim Family

A young couple had come for their initial visit with me after being referred by a friend. They sought me out because I was African American and Muslim. Samuel, 23, was dressed in a suit and wore a bow tie. Mary, 21, was dressed in a long skirt and a blouse that covered her hips. They had been having marital troubles, after having been married for only a year. Samuel had converted to Islam 3 years earlier, and she had done so a year earlier.

When asked what had been disturbing them, Samuel, a jewelry vendor who also sold his organization's newspapers, stated that his wife, Mary, did not support his work. She wanted him to get a more regular job and to sell his jewelry part-time. She stated that she wanted to be supportive and would help him part of the time, but that she also wanted more security.

Samuel accused Mary of not having faith and being materialistic. He also stated that he was the provider and that she had married him knowing how important his business was to him. She admitted that she was sometimes ashamed of not living in a better place and of her family's giving her a hard time because she had "married one of those Muslims." She had been close to her family before her conversion, but had recently had an argument with her mother, who had put pork in her food without telling her. Mary's father often muttered about her going to hell and said ugly things about her husband.

She stated that she was so proud of her husband for what he was trying to do for their community, but did not like feeling that she had to choose between her husband and family. Samuel felt that she should just leave her family alone, associate more with Muslims, and cultivate Muslim friends, but Mary felt that other Muslims could not take the place of her family.

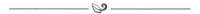

In this couple, the stresses of adopting a new set of values were straining their relationship. They had changed their last name to an Islamic one, changed their diet, stopped drinking and smoking, avoided nightclubs, changed some of the music they listened to, and attended their mosque regularly. The hostility of Mary's family to these changes in her life was a great source of pain for her. I explored with Samuel and Mary their experiences to determine if the conversion had been a well-thought-out action and decision, an attempt to rebel, or an effort to achieve some boundary or cutoff from the family of origin. We explored the kind of mother each had and also looked at the influences of their fathers on their relationship.

We were able to talk about their concept of the "ideal Muslim couple" and consider how closely their relationship resembled that ideal, as well as the difficulties of living up to that ideal. With Samuel, I looked at what kind of provider his father was and the contrast between that and the type of provider he wished to be.

We also talked about the meaning of their conversion to Islam and the spiritual aspects of their relationship. Mary was able to reveal that her family was afraid that she would be dominated by her husband and made a prisoner in her home. She also thought that members of her family were offended because she would not eat certain foods anymore, for one of her mother's primary ways of expressing affection was to prepare elaborate meals. She was aware that she was still seeking her parents' approval in many ways and still felt in need of her mother's guidance. Samuel was concerned about being a good influence on his own family, for he was the oldest of four sons. His mother was a widow and his father had been ill with cancer for a long time before he died. He felt that the model of manhood he found in his community was one he could emulate and teach to his brothers, who looked to him for leadership. His family was enthusiastic about his involvement and very supportive. He was also able to reveal how much he admired Mary's father, who owned a scrap metal business. We decided to have Samuel approach Mary's father formally, discuss his plans for providing for her, and ask for his advice in getting started with a stable business. Mary decided to go back to nursing school to further her own needs for autonomy and economic stability. They agreed to postpone having children until Samuel was better established financially, and that she would stay home with any children they had.

We talked about the importance of internalizing the ideal roles of Muslim husband and wife, but stressed the fact that they were human beings and therefore fallible and still learning.

Both seemed relieved to have a safe place where they felt understood, accepted, and not judged. They felt that it was helpful to express their beliefs without censure and judgment from other people. We met for only four sessions, but the tension was relieved greatly as we strategized about how Samuel could assist Mary in bridging the gap with her parents. The couple decided to continue demonstrating their positive regard for them, inviting them into their home and lifestyle, and reassuring them that Mary was happy but still needed them.

African American Sunni Muslim Family

A family was referred for therapy by a local *imam* (religious teacher), who was also the head of a local *masjid* (place of worship and congregation). The husband, Na'im, his wife of past years, Amira, and his new wife, Salima, came to the first session. All had been Muslims for more than 15 years, performed daily *salat*, and attended *masjid* regularly. Both women wore *hijab* (traditional Islamic dress that allows the uncovering of only the face and hands), and Na'im wore a *kufi*.

Salima, a widow, had approached Amira and asked if she would consider her as a co-wife. Salima had two sons, and her husband had been friends with Na'im. Amira liked Salima, and after consultation with the *imam*, agreed to the marriage. Na'im also expressed his attraction for Salima, and soon they had a lovely wedding ceremony, which Amira helped to plan.

However, 8 months into the marriage, Amira began to have second thoughts. The women maintained separate households, and Na'im struggled to provide for both families. He and Amira had four children of their own. Because Salima was younger, Amira began to feel more like her mother than her co-wife. Salima was extremely dependent and somewhat lazy with housework.

Over five or six sessions, it became clear that Na'im was getting increasingly irritated with Salima. However, when he argued with her, she would regress and begin to talk in a baby-like voice. At one point, he found her in a closet, curled up in a fetal position. It was clear that she had severe emotional problems that had been exacerbated by her husband's death. Na'im did not feel it would be right to divorce her at this point, but things becamse increasingly worse between them.

Salima had also discovered that she was pregnant, and an Islamic divorce would be impossible while she was pregnant anyway. The couple thought that they should seek counseling because both households were in turmoil.

In this family, it was clear that another value system and even another legal code than that of the dominant culture were operative. Islamic law recognizes marriages with as many as four wives. Although such marriages are not recognized by secular legal institutions, they are formally accepted by the Islamic community. Most African American Muslims have only one wife, for the practice of polygamy is viewed with hostility and/or mistrust by many African American Muslim women. However, other African American Muslim women believe that polygamy is justified in their communities because of the shortage of eligible African American Muslim men.

In Islamic countries, the *Shariah*, or code of Islamic law, carries more weight, and custom supports the practice. In therapy, it is important to know how each individual feels about the marriage and whether the customary limits of fairness to all wives are being observed.

The way this polygamous marriage was contracted was proper in the eyes of all parties, their *imam*, and their religious community. The main problem was the co-wife's emotional impairment and the additional strain this put on the extended family finances and family harmony.

Because of Salima's dysfunction, Amira had to care for her children. Amira felt overwhelmed, resentful, and guilty about agreeing to a situation with which she could not live. She wanted to help Salima, but also desired to regain the peace that she and Na'im had developed over the past 13 years, prior to her addition to the family. Na'im felt as if he were trapped, but also felt obligated to live up to his duties. He began to feel alienated from both women because he could find little peace with either.

I worked on setting priorities in the family and arranged to have Salima evaluated by a psychiatrist and tested by a psychologist. She was severely depressed and was experiencing dissociative episodes. Salima disclosed that she had been sexually abused as a child and that her first husband had rescued her from a very dysfunctional family. While he was alive, she was able to function well and put her past behind her. After he died, Salima felt as if she could no longer function. She was still grieving his loss.

She began attending individual therapy, which continued throughout her pregnancy, and was hospitalized once during this time. Amira arranged for the children to go to a preschool during the day so that she could have some time for herself. She also started a small business, sewing garments for other Muslim women and children. Salima's mother came to live with her after the baby was born, which gave her the support that she needed, and she began a course of antidepressants. Na'im remained married to both women, but he and Amira recognized that theirs was the primary relationship and realized that they had not lost each other by bringing Salima into their lives. They maintained a boundary between their relationship and Salima, by refusing to discuss their relationship with her, and also took some trips together.

Na'im and Salima settled into a nonsexual relationship. He maintained his financial support of her and her children, but both realized that neither wanted to be intimate anymore. Salima continued to work on her survivor issues in therapy and gradually became more capable as a woman and a mother.

Salima and Amira are cordial but formal with another. They occasionally do things with the children as an extended family during Ramadan and at other times, but not on a daily basis. At this point, the family is no longer in therapy.

Being a co-wife is honorable in Islam, because it allows women to live their lives not deprived of the company and support of, and sexual relations with, men or to become only girlfriends to whom men have no social or moral responsibility. Sex outside of marriage is considered *haram*, forbidden, in Islam.

Therapists should not impose their values on these arrangements that are consistent with this belief system, unless they are being used as a cover for abusive behavior. I have witnessed occasions in which that is the case. Of course, it is un-Islamic for women to suffer oppression at the hands of men who use polygamy as a cover to have more than one woman in their lives.

The *shariah*, or Islamic codes of law, are extensive and based on the Holy Qur'an and the *hadith* (collections of observations of the life and sayings of Prophet Muhammad) by authors such as Al-Bukhari and Sahih Muslim. The following practices are based on these sacred writings:

1. Contraception is allowed for Muslims, but abortion is forbidden after the fetus is fully formed.
2. The best male believers are good to their wives.
3. Among all lawful things, divorce is most hated by Allah (God).
4. A representative from the husband's family and one from the wife's family are often appointed to settle marital disputes that the couple cannot solve themselves.
5. Fathers retain custody of their children after divorce, unless otherwise arranged by the couple.

6. Muslims are not allowed to change the birth name of adopted children, for the children should always know their lineage.
7. Anything that intoxicates, including alcohol and other mood-altering drugs, is forbidden (*haram*).
8. It is considered modest for a man or a woman who is not married to look down and away when speaking directly to a member of the opposite sex.

There are many other traditions and customs derived from this belief system, and within many Islamic communities there are scholars who are experts on them. Violations of these traditions sometimes constitute a source of guilt in Muslims who struggle to be devout.

PARENT–CHILD ISSUES

Raising children in an Islamic family, but not in an Islamic society, is a difficult task. Some African American Muslims send their children to public or private secular schools; others may do home schooling or educate their children in private Islamic schools. In Islamic schools classes are separated by sex and, along with their regular curricula, Arabic and Qur'anic studies are taught. In general, Muslim families emphasize education, and studious, well-behaved children are prized.

As in any religion, parents who are too strict or shaming in their parenting often raise rebellious children who may be attracted to all the things their parents forbid. Children are also subject to all of the pressures that maturation brings and may have to struggle to define their identity and the place Islam has in their lives.

Because of restriction on dress, girls often struggle with wearing *hijab* in their adolescence, unless they are in a community where this practice is supported. Muslim girls who go to secular high schools sometimes wear *hijab*, but others choose not to do so because of the negative stereotypes attached to covering one's hair.

Observing *salat* five times a day is also difficult for children who attend a secular school. Cafeteria lunches that contain pork may cause a child to go hungry, and the schools are not always supportive of special religious diets.

Pressures to date, which is not allowed in Islam unless there is intent to marry, are also difficult issues for both sexes. Parents must work very hard to ensure that their children have a large enough peer group with which to relate.

Muslim girls are not supposed to marry non-Muslims, but Muslim men can marry non-Muslims if they are believers in monotheism (Christians and Jews). Because the man is supposed to be the spiritual leader of the home, a girl is thought vulnerable to oppression for her beliefs if she marries a non-Muslim.

As the following case demonstrates, parents must be sensitive to the issues, pressures, and emotions of young people who are struggling to synthesize their sense of personal and cultural identity with their religious and spiritual beliefs.

Identity Issues in Adolescence

A 14-year-old boy, Mustafa, who had attended an Islamic elementary school and had to transfer to a public high school, was brought to therapy by his parents. They complained that he had been skipping school and lying about it. Sullen and angry since the school transfer, he began to pay attention in the session when we started to talk about all of the changes he was going through and how difficult they must be for him.

Mustafa slowly began to admit hating his new school. He talked about how rude and profane some of his classmates were, about how he had been teased because of his dark skin color and because of the way his mother and sister dressed. Mustafa was also upset because of the things his teacher had said about Islam and the way people at school mispronounced his name, Mustafa ibn Abdul Rahman. In addition, he was shamed by news reports that always portrayed Muslims as evil terrorists, especially when he had to do a report on them for his class. His parents were shocked that his feelings were so intense, because he had always been a relatively happy, obedient son.

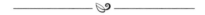

His mother and father resolved to advocate for Mustafa with his teachers and the principal. His mother and sister volunteered to go with him to school when he did his report so that they could explain the significance of their dress and answer questions about the myths surrounding Muslim men and women.

Mustafa was surprised at the support he received, for he had felt that he had to handle the situation and stand up for Islam on his own, although he was ashamed to admit that he was scared to do so. His father was able to share with him his experiences at work and how he dealt with prejudice, and gave Mustafa some suggestions. Both parents reassured him that they were a team and that they had to help him stand up for who he was. This, they taught him, was the truest meaning of *jihad* (holy war).

BIRTH AND DEATH

In *Sunni* Muslim families, the first words a child hears after birth should be the *adhan*, or the call to prayer, and, often, Al-Fatiha, the first *sura* (chapter) in the Holy Qur'an. Both are usually said by the father. Boys are circumcised.

Seven days after birth, the *aqeeqah*, or naming ceremony, is celebrated by the ritual sacrifice of a lamb and the distribution of the meat to the community in a feast provided by the father or grandfathers. The names given the child are usually Arabic and chosen for values the parents hope their child will embody For example, *Abdul* means "servant of," and when followed by *Rahman* (the beneficent), the name means "servant of the most Beneficent."

The highest title for a Muslim is to be considered a faithful servant of Allah; therefore, many Muslims have taken on one of the 99 names of Allah's attributes.

Muslims bury the dead as quickly as possible, preferably before sundown on the day of death. The corpse should be cleansed by persons of the same sex as the deceased and given a ritual ablution, as if preparing for prayer.

COURTSHIP, ENGAGEMENT, AND MARRIAGE

In Islam, marriage is considered a religious duty, engaged in via contract, and seen as a social necessity, fulfilling half of the personal religious obligations of a Muslim. Muslims generally do not regard celibacy as a desirable state.

Given that Muslims do not date, how do they select a mate? Often, friends and family will recommend someone to a person who is seeking a wife or husband. At other times, the individual may actively seek out someone he or she has noticed in the religious community. Marriages may be arranged, but the partners must see each other.

An unmarried woman is expected to have a *wali*, or guardian, usually her father, who helps her investigate the prospective partner's suitability and negotiate the written marriage contract. In this contract, the couple specify the amount agreed upon for *mahr*, or the dowry, that the prospective husband gives his fiancée as proof of the seriousness of his intent and as insurance against any future economic need she may have.

African American Muslims are adopting and adapting some traditional Muslim wedding ceremonies, including the henna party prior to the wedding night. During this party, the bride is adorned with intricate henna designs all over the body as a surprise for her new husband.

Both parties must consent to the marriage, a dowry must be paid, at least two witnesses should be present during the ceremony, and the marriage must be public. A *waleemah*, or wedding feast, is held after the wedding and, in more traditional families, after consummation of the marriage.

After marriage, the husband becomes responsible for the wife's maintenance according to his means. The wife may work outside the home if the couple agrees; however, any money she earns is considered hers. If she contributes money to the household, it is considered a gift to her husband.

Social Separation of the Sexes

On most social and religious occasions, separation of the sexes is observed. At a party, women will be in one room and men in the another. This seems to reinforce intimacy within the sexes and gives each emotional support and security. Muslims do not view such gender segregation as oppressive, but rather as natural and modest. In the homes of Muslims who are cultural nationalists, however, separation is observed publicly but may not be practiced at social events within the home.

In general, gender roles are clear in all types of Muslim homes, groups, and strong identification with one's role is encouraged—the husband as protector and provider, and the wife as nurturer. For women who work outside the home, this traditional split is maintained as well.

Conflict can result from the inability of a husband and wife to manage their individual interpretations of what constitutes a balance of gender-role expectations with career aspirations. Within the extended families of African American Muslims, there are expectations according to social class and blood relationship that can conflict with the individual's interpretation of his or her obligations as a Muslim. For example, parents may wish a college-educated daughter to pursue a career rather than stay home and raise a family, whereas other members of the extended family may oppose this choice.

HOMOSEXUALITY

Islam forbids homosexuality and considers it abominable; thus, Muslim communities in no way acknowledge practicing homosexuals. It is difficult, therefore, if not impossible, for a person who has homosexual feelings to reconcile them with Islamic law. A homosexual orientation without actual homosexual practice, however, is considered a matter between the individual and Allah. Some parents and siblings accept adult children who are homosexual and who wish to be accepted; others do not.

BARRIERS TO TREATMENT

Within African American Muslim communities, both cultural nationalist and *Sunni*, there is much suspicion of Euro-American therapists. Rarely do members go outside their community for advice or guidance. I believe this suspiciousness has grown out of the acute awareness of the oppression African Americans have experienced, the association of Islam in this country with cultural nationalism, and individual experiences with racism, which may have contributed to their conversion. In addition, prejudicial articles and books, as well as media attention, foster fear and dislike of Muslims and do little to educate the public about the religion as it is practiced by different groups.

The relationship between African American Muslims and other ethnic Muslims is generally polite and cordial. There are sometimes tensions between African American Muslims and American Jews because of the former's identification with the Palestinians; in addition, some African Americans have felt exploited by some Jewish and other individuals who have taken money out of their communities and really don't care about their development. Muslims usually resent economic dependence in any form and view it as a form of oppression.

Distrust of the therapist, skepticism about his or her attitude toward Muslims and African Americans, and sensitivity to being misperceived are common among Muslim clients. Knowing even a little about Islam and about African American culture may take the therapist a long way in forming a positive relationship with this population.

A therapist should explore the belief system of a Muslim client by asking such questions as:

- How did you first hear about Islam?
- How long have you been a Muslim?
- What difference has being Muslim made in your life?
- What members of your family are Muslim?
- What are your experiences and perceptions of how Muslims are viewed by others?

CONCLUSION

Family therapy with African American Muslims is greatly facilitated by the therapist's collaboratively developing genograms and gathering extensive family histories with the client. Particular attention should be paid to the client's subcultural style, dialect and Arabic phrases, style of dress, sensitivity to nonverbal cues, double-consciousness, and sensitivity to race and power issues within the therapeutic relationship and setting.

As in any therapeutic relationship, the therapist should be aware of prejudice or other countertransference issues related to the client, particularly to one whose belief system is distasteful to the therapist. But a therapist who sincerely wishes to help the client, and who is interested in and open to his or her presenting issues, can perform appropriate and helpful interventions.

If Muslims remain wary of non-Muslim therapists, that may be because of the two sets of negative stereotypes—about African Americans and about Muslims—with which the dominant culture characterizes them and which may interfere with accurate assessment and intervention. Both groups experience frequent scapegoating by the dominant society, which informs the self-perceptions of some White and Black Americans, serves as a source of gratification, defines social meaning, absorbs aggression, and facilitates a sense of virtue, as observed by Kovel (1970; cited in Pinderhughes, 1989). Bowen's (1982) theory of the societal projection process is also operative in the dynamics of the dominant society's perception of both of these groups.

Muslims are often the targets of self-appointed patriots when negative reports appear about Islamic political activity. In addition, African Americans are frequently subjected to police harassment and suspicion by the general public whenever crime increases. The therapist's willingness to listen and affirm the experiences of the client subjected to racism and cultural oppression is essential to a good therapeutic alliance. If Islamic customs and behaviors are exhibited that the therapist does not understand, his or her respectful request for explanation will usually be answered.

Of course, some people use religion as a way to run away from certain difficulties in their lives or as a defense against personal growth. In such cases, the therapist should explore the extent to which adherence to religious tenets masks other problems.

Respect for the patriarchal nature of Islamic family life is important. Most African American Muslim women are familiar with feminist concepts, but have consciously chosen the Muslim lifestyle as more meaningful for them. In fact, they often view themselves as more fortunate than women who have chosen less traditional lifestyles. Feminist therapists should have respect for their different model of womanhood and femininity. If clients are uncomfortable with the way their relationships are constructed, therapists need to pay attention to what they feel is painful to them and reserve judgment for clinical sessions.

Prayer, fasting, and rituals are important in the lives of Muslims. Worship is often communal, with the entire family praying together. Increasing occasions for prayers sometimes increases contact between family members. Suggesting that participants pray, especially for their relationships, is often an appropriate intervention.

Female therapists should pay particular attention to their dress during family therapy sessions. Low necklines, short skirts, and bare arms will lessen clients' respect for them. Male therapists should pay particular attention to acknowledging the husband's place in the family by asking him if he has any objection to the therapist's addressing questions to his wife or daughters. Doing so does not imply support for male dominance, but rather is viewed as respecting what Muslims consider good manners.

In the Holy Qur'an, the first *sura* includes the phrase "Guide us along the straight path." The idea of "the straight path" is dear to Muslims and speaks to their belief in the duty of unswerving devotion and conviction in the path to Allah's grace and blessings. Encouraging Muslims to continue on that straight path in ways that support healthy family life, communication, personal growth, and wisdom is consistent with the goals of family therapists interested in family preservation, even though the constellation of that family life may be vastly different from the therapist's own.

African Americans who practice traditional Islam usually became attracted to the faith as an outgrowth of their study of African and/or African American history. Interest in and conversion to Islam is growing rapidly in the United States, and therapists in urban areas are increasingly likely to have an opportunity to work with this population. Many

African Americans identify positively with the values of Muslims and have relatives who are Muslim. Elijah Muhammad, referring to the millions of slaves brought to this country who were Muslim, called them as the "lost–found" Nation of Islam, giving his organization, now headed by Louis Farrakhan, that name.

Muslims emphasize community, or *ummat*, among all followers of the faith. Obligations to the group sometimes compete with obligations to the family. Family therapists should explore how the family relates to the greater *ummat* in order to fully assess its functioning.

It is my hope that this chapter will contribute, in some small way, to better understanding of this growing and interesting group of Americans.

REFERENCES

Al-Qaradawi, Y. (1960). *The lawful and prohibited in Islam*. Indianapolis, IN: American Trust Publications.

Bowen, M. (1982). *Family therapy in clinical practice*. New York: Aronson.

Pinderhughes, E. (1989). *Race, ethnicity and power*. New York: Free Press.

Rashad, A. (1991). *The history of Islam and Black nationalism in the Americas*. Beltsville, MD: Writers Inc.

Rouse, C. M. (2004). *Engaged surrender: African American women and Islam*. Berkeley: University of California Press.

PART III

LATINO FAMILIES

CHAPTER 11

Latino Families

An Overview

Nydia Garcia-Preto

During the past decade the Latino population in the United States has grown at an incredible rate of 3% a year, or about 400,000 new immigrants a year. According to the U.S. Census Bureau there were 39.9 million Hispanics as of July 1, 2003, making people of Hispanic origin, as the government labels them, the nation's largest race or ethnic minority (U.S. Bureau of the Census, 2003). These numbers, however, do not reflect the undocumented and illegal migrants who come into this country daily and cannot be adequately counted. When this rapid growth in population is combined with the fact that one third of all Hispanics are below the age of 18 (U.S. Bureau of the Census, 2004), we can see why Latinos are the fastest growing ethnic group in the United States and why they have recently been compared to the baby boomer generation (Grow, 2004).

Although the majority of Latinos in this country continue to have little access to political and economic power, their vote has begun to have a much greater impact on national elections. In 1996 their vote astounded political experts with both its explosive growth and its unpredictability (Gonzalez, 2000). Since the late 1990s there has been a steady rise in the number of Latinos who have become citizens, and in their voter participation. This trend has been in response to various factors, among which is the increased social oppression that many have faced resulting from the effects of laws such as Proposition 187—former California governor Wilson's 1994 initiative denying public educational, medical, and social services to undocumented immigrants. In 1998, Judge Marianne Pfaelzer overturned some of its major provisions, but the effects continued, inasmuch as President Clinton, in 1996, had signed the Personal Responsibility and Work Opportunity Reconciliation Act, imposing restrictions on immigration rights that duplicated many of the provisions of Proposition 187 (Ono & Sloop, 2002). English-only laws intending to limit or prohibit schools and government agencies from using Spanish have been passed in some 18 states. Most of these efforts have been ineffective, but are likely to continue as the Latino population increases (Grow, 2004).

According to the U.S. census, Mexicans, Puerto Ricans, and Cubans continue to be the three largest Latino groups in this country, but the increase in the number of Dominicans, Central Americans, and some South American groups, such as Colombians and Brazilians, raises questions about the numbers. Considering these changes, we have expanded the section on Latino families in this third edition of *Ethnicity and Family Therapy* to include chapters on Colombians, Dominicans, and Salvadorans. Colombians are a growing group who have established vibrant communities that are flourishing economically in Queens, New York City, and in various other cities. Chapter 14, which discusses this group, gives attention to the controversial relationship between Colombia and the United States, and to the meaning of violence in that culture that has caused fear and dislocations in the lives of the immigrant population here.

Chapter 16, on Dominicans, acquaints us with that country's sociopolitical history and the effect that its conflictual relationship with Haiti has had on the Dominicans' experience of racism. The chapter focuses on clinical interventions with an immigrant group that may soon outnumber Cubans in this country. Chapter 19, on Salvadorans, discusses the specific problems of a group of people who came here mostly to escape the devastating effects of war and natural disasters in their country, but of whom only 2.3% have been granted the status of "refugee." In contrast, 77% of Cuban immigrants admitted from 1981 to 1998 were granted refugee status, allowing them to gain permanent residency and welfare benefits (Chapter 15). The largest Central American group here, Salvadorans are one of the top five foreign-born populations in the United States, and the majority have settled in California.

The chapters on Brazilians (Chapter 12), Central Americans (Chapter 13), Cubans (Chapter 15), Mexicans (Chapter 17), and Puerto Ricans (Chapter 18) have also been revised to reflect changes in society that have affected family organization and functioning. This overview provides some perspective on the migration, socioeconomic, and political history of Latinos in this country, and on cultural factors that may influence the treatment of their families.

LATINO FAMILIES IN HISTORICAL AND CULTURAL CONTEXT

Hispanic or Latino?: A Sociopolitical Perspective

Hispanic and *Latino* are adjectives used to describe people who come from different countries with different cultures and sociopolitical histories, and who in their countries of origin would never describe themselves that way. They are Cubans, Chicanos, Mexicans, Puerto Ricans, Argentinians, Colombians, Dominicans, Brazilians, Guatemalans, Costa Ricans, Nicaraguans, Salvadorans, and the people of all the other nationalities who make up South America, Central America, and the Caribbean. Proclaiming their nationality is very important to Latinos; it provides a sense of pride and identity that is reflected in the stories they tell, their music, and their poetry. Longing for their homeland is more pronounced when they are unable to return to their homes either because they are here as political exiles, or illegally, or because they are unable to afford the cost of travel. In therapy, asking the question, "What is your country of origin?" and listening to the client's stories of immigration helps to engage the family and gives the therapist an opportunity to learn about the country the client left behind, the culture, and the reasons for leaving.

Although Latinos may hold onto their national heritage with pride, when they arrive in this country, what is most apparent to others are their similarities. They speak Spanish, except for Brazilians, who speak Portuguese, and do not think of themselves as Latinos, but as people of a separate country. In this society the fact that they come from a country in South America makes them Latinos and political allies. Most are Roman Catholic and have in common values and beliefs rooted in a history of conquest and colonization. To outsiders Latinos look alike because their physical features, such as skin color, facial structure, and hair texture are often similar as a result of the mixing of races that has occurred in most of these countries. Once they arrive in the United States, they are officially categorized as "Hispanic." This label, established in the 1970s by the U.S. Department of Education, has been used by the U.S. Census Bureau to track population growth, as well as trends in education and socioeconomic levels. *Hispanic* refers to the influence of the Spanish culture and language on a group of people who suffered years of colonization. The term doesn't take into account indigenous cultures, therefore prioritizing the dominant European cultures (Quinones-Rosado, 2000).

In contrast, *Latino/Latina* does not refer to Spain, but rather to Spain's former colonies in Latin America, indicating people who come from South America, Central America, and Mexico, including territories in the United States that were taken from Mexico, and some of the Caribbean islands. It takes into account the influences of indigenous cultures and African ancestry on people who share a history of colonization by Spain, and of economic and political oppression by the United States. Brazilians are the exception because they were colonized by the Portuguese. However, upon entering the United States they are often seen as Latinos because of their Latin American background. They resent the lack of recognition by U.S. citizens of their unique heritage and often resist this classification because the "Latino" label is mostly associated with Spanish speakers and ignores their particular history and cultural background. However, when confronted with racial and social oppression in this society, many accept the label as a way of locating themselves within a sociopolitical context (Chapter 12). It is a term that is chosen by some of us living in the United States that implies an awareness of our shared struggle against oppression, and recognition of the effects of racism on our lives. It is a political term reflecting defiance against White supremacy (Quinones-Rosado, 2002).

For many of us, the label, whether Latino/Latina or Hispanic, takes away our nationality and symbolizes a loss of identity. However, the benefit is that it provides a way for the Latinos of various nationalities in this country to have some unity in order to gain political power, especially because, as a group, they are significantly oppressed socially.

The history of Latinos in the United States, as well as in the Caribbean, Central America, and South America, has followed a cycle of conquest, oppression, defeat, and struggle for liberation. Social oppression has been deeply rooted in Latin American history. Latinos are the descendants of the oppressors and the oppressed, and for generations they have struggled for liberation. The destruction of the culture and religion of native inhabitants was rampant as the Spaniards and Portuguese took the land, raped the women, and killed the men. In the Caribbean, especially, the Tainos, Arawaks, and Caribes were enslaved, killed, and disappeared within 50 years after the conquest; African slaves were then brought to do the work. Slaves were also brought to Central and South America, mostly along the coastline, and in large numbers to Brazil (Chasteen & Tulchin, 1994). As in the United States, the power was held by White European immigrants who owned the land. Wanting control of their own government, the landowners led revolutions against Spain, fighting and winning wars for independence. The liberation movement swept across Latin America, giving the promise of hope and independence to a population of mostly impoverished and uneducated peasants who owned no land and had no power. The power remained in the hands of the wealthy White Europeans, who, in turn, oppressed the indigenous population, the slaves, and the racially mixed people known as *mestizos*. Socioeconomic and political oppression persists in many Latin American countries, and as the poor struggle for survival, many look to emigration to the United States as a possible solution.

U.S. Immigration and Social Oppression

For many Latinos, the United States has represented a place in the sun, a place to be free, yet upon arrival they are dismayed by the attitude of non-Hispanics toward them. Their color, language, and culture, essentials to their being, become cause for oppression. A majority see themselves as victims of discrimination and at the bottom of the social ladder, below Blacks. They often view the American people as cold and the American way of life as hostile to what they describe as their tradition of family unity, personal warmth, respect for their elders, and for their own and other people's dignity. For most, especially those with darker complexions and less money and education, feeling respected for who they are outside their families, out there in the street among the gringos, is a daily struggle. It is not surprising that in an attempt to protect their self-respect, many are unwilling to call themselves American or to let their language, traditions, or way of life disappear. Actually, Latinos are less likely to assimilate than to acculturate, or to become "transnational," because they maintain multiple relations (familial, economic, religious, organizational, and political) that span countries. Transmigrants take actions, make decisions, and feel concerns within a social field that links their country of origin and their country of settlement (Chapter 17). It is also significant that 97% of Mexican children whose parents are immigrants, and 76% of other Hispanic immigrant children, know Spanish, even as nearly 90% also speak English very well, according to a decade-long study by University of California (Irvine) sociologist Ruben G. Rumbaut (Grow, 2004).

The history of Latinos in the United States dates back to the 1500s, when the Spaniards settled Santa Fe, conquering and oppressing the indigenous population of what is today New Mexico, Texas, and California. Spain lost the territory to Mexico in the 1800s during the Mexican War for independence, and in the same century the Mexicans lost it to the United States. By the time the Mexicans lost the war with the United States, their possession of land had expanded to include New Mexico, California, Texas, Nevada, Utah, parts of Arizona, Colorado, Kansas, Oklahoma, and Wyoming (Calvert & Calvert, 1993). Although the Treaty of Guadalupe Hidalgo promised citizenship, freedom of religion and language, and maintenance of their lands, the Mexicans who lived in these territories became subject to discrimination and social injustice soon after the war. They became strangers, or immigrants, in their own land, losing their rights and private property (Falicov, 1982).

Although there are Spaniards and Mexicans who have lived in the United States since before the *Mayflower* landed (Shorris, 1992), the major waves of Latino immigrants came after World War II. Mexicans, Puerto Ricans, Cubans, Dominicans, Colombians, Brazilians, Argentinians, other South Americans, and more recently, growing numbers from Central America, have made the journey north. The greatest migration usually follows economic depression or political revolution. Those who come are usually the poor, the wealthy who are able to flee with their money, and the intellectuals who are persecuted for the expression of their religious or political ideas. The majority, however, are the very poor.

Once they are in the United States, poverty is a way of life for the majority of Latinos who live in this society, and their inability to access resources keeps them locked in a cycle that is oppressive and demoralizing. Jobs are scarce, even when they are willing to work for peanuts; housing is substandard and unaffordable; they have no health benefits; and difficulties with understanding and speaking English often keep them on the periphery. Inability to speak English lowers their potential to earn higher wages and to attain higher-paying jobs (Bean & Tienda, 1987; Grow, 2004; Reimers, 1985). Without English, they are relegated to low-skill-level jobs. According to the 2000 U.S. Census, Latinos as a group continue to be more than likely unemployed, and one quarter of their children under 18 live in poverty. Those who work are trapped in low-wage service jobs with little chance for advancement. There has been a hopeful gain of 12% since 1980 in the number of Latino students who graduate from high school, but 57%, as compared with 88% for non-Hispanic White and 80% for African Americans is still a significant difference (U.S. Bureau of the Census, 2000).

Latinos come looking for a place in the sun, but are burned by the scalding rays of oppression. Somehow the institutions that provide help are not sheltering; instead, they tend to reinforce the feelings of shame and failure that Latinos feel when their dreams about improving their lives are truncated. Extended family members, when present, are usually caught in the cycle themselves, unable to provide the emotional and financial support that has traditionally been an expectation in Latino cultures. Resentments between family members about lack of support cause cutoffs and exacerbate Latinos' feelings of isolation. Those who are White or educated and have financial resources are in a better position to live out their dreams, especially if they understand and speak English. And, depending on how much emotional support they have at home from their families and friends, they may experience less isolation and a greater connection to the community in which they live.

Differences between Groups

Although Latinos, once they are in the United States, may experience similar injustices, there is often competition between the different groups. The conflict is sometimes related to a history of war between the countries of origin due to struggles over natural resources such as land or access to waterways, or because of opposing political ideologies. Distinct sociopolitical histories and different historical ties to the United States have affected Latinos' entrance and acceptance in this country, leading to resentment and distrust among the groups. Racism and classism influence relationships within and among the groups and contribute to a pecking order marked by prejudice and stereotypes. One group may be afraid that another will take over jobs, businesses, and control of neighborhoods, receive more help from the government, or attain a higher education. Often the prejudice is subtle and the groups coexist peacefully; however, resentments can quickly surface. Intermarriage between groups is one of those triggers that can make prejudice between groups salient.

The prospect of defining unique cultural characteristics that describe different Latino groups is intriguing and can raise painfully controversial issues. Differences can be subtle and complex, making it difficult to tease out specific and categorical statements about each group. It would be an injustice and clinically detrimental to make a chart assigning values, patterns, and attitudes to certain groups without being careful to analyze, compare, and define the sociopolitical context in which the cultures have evolved. It would be ludicrous to assume that this type of summary could do justice to such rich heritage. However, in the following sections I offer a brief introduction to the history and pattern of migration of some of the major groups we may encounter in treatment. The next few chapters offer more specific information about several groups.

Mexicans

Mexicans have been in this country since the 1600s and 1700s, when with the Spaniards they established missions and communities that later became important cities in the United States (Chapter 17). However, they first came to this country in large numbers in the early 1900s, attempting to escape the economic depression that Mexico was experiencing and the violence of the Mexican Revolution of 1910 (Chapter 17; Shorris, 1992). The wealthy, as well as the poor, settled mostly in Texas, California, New Mexico, and Arizona. They constitute the largest group of Latinos in this country and have been here the longest. According to the latest U.S. Bureau of the Census report (2000), 66.9% of Latinos in the United States are of Mexican birth or ancestry. Mexican Americans, or Chicanos, are mostly *mestizos*, that is, of mixed Native American (Mayan, Aztec, Hopi) and White European descent (Novas, 1994). The major concentration of Mexican Americans remains in California and the Southwest. The latest official count shows that 54% of Mexican Americans live in the West and 34.3% live in the South (U.S. Bureau of the Census, 2000). It is difficult to accurately ascertain how many Mexican Americans live in this country, inasmuch as many of them are here illegally or have become assimilated and may not identify themselves as Latino.

Although some Mexican Americans have been able to move up socioeconomically, the majority of the population remains below the poverty line. After World War II, Mexican Americans made more efforts to gain political power in towns where they were in the majority, and to assert their rights, especially after their men had fought so valiantly in the war. There was a reawakening to the historical cruelty and unfairness by which they had lost their land, language, and culture after the Mexican War. The descendants of those early residents who lost all they had are often among the poorest today. In the 1960s, the Chicano movement emerged, progressive and radical, but it did not become a unifying force for Mexican Americans because many could not identify with its politics (Shorris, 1992). There continues to be a constant movement north, across the Mexican border and into this country, even though deterrence at the gates has become stronger and opportunities for finding jobs here have lessened (Massey, 1993). In recent years, apprehensions at the border have multiplied as new immigrants have been lured by unclear government statements that promise legalization to temporary workers (Chapter 17; Gonzalez, 2000).

Puerto Ricans

Puerto Ricans, the second largest Latino group, began to arrive in great numbers after the depression and the war, in the late 1940s and early 1950s. According to the 2000 U.S. Census, there are about 3.2 million Puerto Ricans in the United States, which amounts to

8.6% of the Latino population. Most are settled in the Northeast, especially in New York City. Puerto Rican communities, however, are also found in other states such as Texas, Florida, and Illinois. Puerto Ricans say, "We are like white rice; you can find us anywhere you go." Many are racially mixed, representing the native Tainos, African slaves, and the White Europeans, mostly Spaniards, who settled the island. Unlike other Latinos, they do not need special papers to come into the United States. U.S. citizenship was granted to them in 1917, when the island, a possession of the United States since 1898, gained more participation in its own government and obtained a bill of rights. Their pattern of immigration has been characterized by a back-and-forth movement, different from that of other groups who must establish residency in this country before they can move about freely. For Puerto Ricans, going back to the island often represents a solution to the problems they face here, an oasis from the prejudice, discrimination, and isolation that plague their lives.

Although they have citizenship, they are not acknowledged as citizens. Instead, most are relegated to an existence of marginality and hold the status of being the poorest among the Latino groups (U.S. Bureau of the Census, 2000). One-third of all Puerto Ricans living on the mainland live in poverty, and of great concern is that their unemployment rate is the highest among Latinos in the United States (U.S. Bureau of the Census, 2000). Another compounding problem is that of all the Latino men in jail in New York, the majority are Puerto Rican (Novas, 1994). Drug addiction, alcoholism, and AIDS have also plagued Puerto Ricans both at home and on the mainland. It is interesting that those Puerto Ricans who migrate to regions in the United States other than New York seem to fare better economically than other Latinos in those areas. In Texas, for instance, Puerto Ricans graduate from college at a higher rate than Mexicans and have a higher income per capita. In Lorain, Ohio, and in San Francisco, they also have done well economically (Novas, 1994). Perhaps the high rate of unemployment and crime in New York City, as well as the history of discrimination they have experienced there, has led those with some potential to seek advancement elsewhere.

Cubans

Cubans are the third largest group of Latinos in the United States. According to the 2000 U.S. Census, Cubans make up 3.7% of the U.S. population residing in this country, and their population is concentrated in Florida, New York, and New Jersey. They began to arrive in large numbers in the 1960s, after Fidel Castro led a successful revolution in 1959 and established a socialist government. The United States, fearing the threat of communism so close to its shores and having to face its loss of economic control of the island, opened its doors to Cubans fleeing the new government (Chapter 15).

Those who first arrived were mainly White, from the upper socioeconomic classes, with educational resources, business know-how, and financial backing (Chapter 12.) Most settled in Miami, in what became known as "Little Havana," and saw themselves as exiles waiting to return when the revolution was over. In the meantime, they used their skills, knowledge, and desire for enterprise to adjust and prosper. Unlike any other immigrant or exile group in the history of the United States, they also had the benefit of favorable legislation—the Cuban Adjustment Act of 1966, which helped legalize their status here, and the Cuban Refugee Program (Shorris, 1992). In fact, the $2.1 billion in aid for Cubans was greater than the entire budget for the Alliance for Progress, designed to finance what President Kennedy called "a true revolution for progress and freedom" throughout the whole of Latin America (Allman, 1987).

The common belief among Latinos that all Cubans are rich is, however, a fallacy. Despite the fact that Cubans are more affluent and have the highest rate of incorporation into the labor force of any Latino group, their average family income still falls below the national average (Novas, 1994). This is especially true when one considers the second wave of Cuban immigrants who came in 1980, known as *Marielitos*, a pejorative label given to them after the name of the port in Cuba from which they departed. They differed from the first wave of Cuban immigrants in that the majority came from a lower socio-economic background and were more racially mixed. In the 1990s, after the disintegration of the Soviet Union and the end of its aid to Cuba, with the situation compounded by the U. S. economic blockade, thousands of Cubans took the risk of reaching this country via makeshift rafts. Many were captured by the United States before reaching land and returned to Guantanamo Bay. Although the political situation between the two countries continues to be polarized, there seems to be more communication between the two Cuban communities and a move toward new transnational alliances (Chapter 15).

Dominicans

The number of Dominicans arriving in the United States has steadily increased in recent years as the economic situation in Santo Domingo worsens. In 2000 an estimated 1, 000, 000 lived primarily in Washington Heights in New York City (U. S. Bureau of the Census, 2000; Chapter 16). The Dominican Republic occupies two-thirds of the island of Hispaniola, whereas Haiti occupies one third on the western side. Columbus landed there in 1492, and it became the first colony settled by Spaniards in the New World. However, it soon became neglected after Mexico and Cuba were discovered, which made it easier for the French to settle the western part of the island. They brought massive numbers of slaves to work the land. Eventually, the slaves rebelled against their owners and proclaimed Haiti's independence. In 1822, the Haitians took over the eastern part of the island but lost it in 1844, when the Spanish-speaking people rebelled against them and proclaimed their independence as the Dominican Republic.

A source of conflict for many Dominicans has been that even though about 80% of the population is mulatto, a mixture of Black and White races, the government has held an unofficial policy against negritude, or descendants of African slaves, and an official policy in favor of the island's Spanish roots (Novas, 1994). This may be partly in reaction to the 1822 invasion by Haiti, a nation built by African slaves. Unlike the governments of other Caribbean islands, the Dominican government seems to have a pro-Columbus attitude and almost a denial of the cruelty and devastation that the indigenous population and slaves suffered under the Spaniards.

To escape poverty and economic devastation, Dominicans often take the risk of crossing the ocean to Puerto Rico. If they are not caught by the patrols on the coast or killed in the treacherous waters, travel to the United States is almost guaranteed, because they can easily pass for Puerto Rican. Like Puerto Ricans, they tend to be more racially mixed than Cubans, who have traditionally maintained a greater separation between the races. Also similar to Puerto Ricans, those who migrate tend to be of lower socioeconomic status. Among other Latinos, they are known to be industrious and, like Cubans, are perceived to be aggressive. Most Dominican immigrants have continued to settle in New York and New Jersey.

Central Americans

There are seven countries that constitute Central America: Belize, Costa Rica, El Salvador, Guatemala, Honduras, Nicaragua, and Panama. As of 2000, Central and South Americans represented 14.3% of the total Latino population in the United States (U.S Bureau of the Census, 2000). During the 1990s many Central Americans left their countries in desperation and arrived as refugees, settling in cities where they found sanctuary. Most did not receive the status of refugee and are here illegally. The aid and welcoming that the government offers to these groups is a far cry from that which Cubans received when they first came in the 1960s. The movie *El Norte* portrays with much accuracy and sensitivity the struggle of many Central Americans as they make the journey north. The character Rosa conveys the hopelessness that many experienced, as she sadly tells her brother prior to her death, "We couldn't stay in our village because they wanted to kill us, and we couldn't stay in Mexico because of the extreme poverty, and here we can't find a home because they don't accept us. Perhaps the only place where we will be able to find a home is when we die."

Foreign intervention and nationalism fueled the war in Nicaragua, and ideology, class tension, and poverty did the same in El Salvador, where, as in Guatemala, racial wars between the Mayan Indians and the White Ladinos (the Guatemalan term for all non-Indians, including Whites and mestizos) devastated the Mayans (Krauss, 1991). Thousands of Nicaraguans have settled in Florida (Shorris, 1992), whereas the largest concentration of Salvadorans is in Los Angeles. Some studies indicate that they number almost one million, but their numbers, like those of many other Latino groups, cannot be documented because of their illegal status (Montes Mozo & Garcia Vasquez, 1988; Chapter 16). In California, some of the agencies dealing with Central Americans, such as the Central American Refugee Committee and the Central American Refugee Center, are confronted daily with the traumatic effects of war on many of the refugees (Shorris, 1992; Chapter 19). In therapy, their experiences with torture and terror are frequently major themes for treatment.

South Americans

South Americans represent a complexity of cultures that are markedly affected by geography and climate, as well as by the different races and groups of people who settled in the specific countries. "Differences in land, climate, and resources in pre-Columbian societies, and in degrees of a cultural influence by European colonial administrations led to major political and economic variations in South America" (Hopkins, 1987, p. 39). Colombians, for example, especially those on the Caribbean coast, seem to have more in common with Costa Ricans than with Argentinians, or Uruguayans, probably due in part to their location on the Caribbean and the effect of slavery on their cultures. The foods they eat and some of the linguistic colloquialisms they use are similar. Ecuador, Bolivia, and Peru have large indigenous populations that have significantly influenced the culture of these groups, yet they have also been at war with each other. Argentina, Chile, and Uruguay tend to be more European in character, and their culture reflects the separation of immigrant groups and races (Calvert & Calvert, 1993). Brazil (Chapter 12) is the only country in South America that was colonized by Portugal, and the Portuguese influence can still be seen in the music, food, and language. As in the Caribbean nations, the indigenous population was killed by hard labor and punishment, and African slaves were brought to do the work. The mixture of races is reflected in the population, and there are also very strong indications of indigenous and African cultures in the beliefs, values, and religious practices in Brazil (Chapter 12). There are also South American Jews here whose families had initially emigrated from Europe around the turn of the century or later. Although members of this group identify themselves as Latino, their experiences in those countries often kept them marginalized.

These differences are acknowledged among Latinos, but once they are in this country, they become identified as one group by the rest of society. Becoming citizens, or legal residents, does not necessarily stop others from perceiving them as "aliens" who are not as good as other citizens. In response to their experience of prejudice and discrimination, many change their names and try passing for White or Black "Americans," depending on their skin color and ability to speak English well. Others react by holding on very tightly to their native language and traditions as protection against the unwelcoming outside world. The majority, however, become acculturated or transcultural, as many of the authors in this section indicate (Chapters, 12, 13, 14, and 17). Regardless of differences, living in a country that is racist and unwelcoming, and that does not acknowledge their history, is a common experience.

TREATMENT IMPLICATIONS

Although it is crucial to differentiate the ethnic identity of Latino families in therapy, there are certain commonalities that can inform therapeutic interventions. Spanish is a common language, except for Brazilians who speak Portuguese, and most belong to the Roman Catholic Church. Although religion is valued and has greatly influenced gender roles, family values, and rules of behavior, most Latinos tend to emphasize spirituality and to express a willingness to sacrifice material satisfactions for spiritual goals. Another value Latinos seem to have in common is personalism, a form of individualism that values those inner qualities in people that make them unique and give them a sense of self-worth. In contrast, American individualism values achievement. Dignity of the individual and respect for authority are closely linked to personalism. Most Latinos also agree that *machismo* and *marianismo* are constructs that tend to organize gender roles in their culture.

Perhaps the most significant value they share is the importance given to family unity, welfare, and honor. The emphasis is on the group rather than on the individual. There is a deep sense of family commitment, obligation, and responsibility. The family guarantees protection and caretaking for life as long as a person stays in the system. It also offers individuals a measure of control for aggression and violence. The expectation is that when a person is having problems, others will help, especially those in stable positions. The family is usually an extended system that encompasses not only those related by blood and marriage, but also *compadres* (godparents) and *hijos de crianza* (adopted children, whose adoption is not necessarily legal). *Compadrazco* (godparenthood) is a system of ritual kinship with binding mutual obligations for economic assistance, encouragement, and even personal correction. *Hijos de crianza* refers to the practice of transferring children from one nuclear family to another within the extended system in times of crisis. The relatives assume responsibility, as if children were their own, and do not view the practice as neglectful.

Often their respect for authority, a value that many of these groups have in common, keeps them from speaking up and asserting their rights. Especially for those who are here illegally, this becomes more problematic because they live in constant fear of being caught and sent back to situations that may be extremely dangerous and oppressive, both socially and politically. With the passing of laws such as the aforementioned Proposition 187 in California, the Personal Responsibility and Work Opportunity Reconciliation Act of 1966, and the recent Patriot Act (Chapter 13) this fear has escalated, causing increased stress for families already feeling displaced.

For people in these situations, coming to therapy, or seeking social services or health care, becomes a threat; moreover, for most Latinos, going outside the family for help is done only as a last resort. In general, Latinos are more likely to have a holistic view of health, not necessarily separating body, mind, and spirit. They may prefer to go to a physician or a spiritual healer for help than to a mental health professional when they feel anxious, depressed, or have emotional problems that are affecting family relationships.

Like members of any other group, the most important concern they bring to therapy is a wish to improve their lives. Research by Santisteban, Muir-Malcom, Mitrani, and Szapocznik (2002) suggests that there is a constellation of immigration- and acculturation-related life experiences and stressors that tend to disproportionately affect Hispanic families. Living in communities that are infested with crime, drugs, rape, and AIDS, most are frightened, especially for their children. Many are experiencing intense feelings of loss, missing the family left behind, or even fearing that they may never be able to see them again because of politics or immigration laws. There is also a feeling of loss for the social status and connections in their country of origin, for the smells and sounds of their former surroundings, and for their friends and neighbors. For a significant number, as in the case of Salvadorans and other Central Americans, the effects of postwar trauma continue to be part of their experience (Chapters 13 and 19). Feeling isolated and pressured to change, in ways that are not always understood, often causes disruption and conflict in their lives. Adjustment to this culture depends on the reasons for coming to the United States, plans for staying or returning, the support received from family and friends, and their ability to assimilate new values without giving up the strengths of the old culture.

In therapy, eliciting, listening, and validating stories about how their lives are affected by living in this country will help families to view themselves and their problems in relation to a larger context, to see themselves beyond their problems, not circumscribed by them (Chapter 15). Some may experience living here as being caught between two worlds, without a secure foundation in either (Chapter 14). Helping them to understand the cultural journey they have embarked upon is essential, because many, even after living here for decades, are still struggling with cultural shock (Chapter 13) and feel encumbered by unresolved resentments and hurt by separations. This is especially true when parents and adolescents reunite after years of separation and have to reestablish relationships (Mitrani, Santisteban, & Muir, 2004; Suarez-Orozco, Todorova, & Louie,

2002; Chapter 17). Problems also tend to arise in Latino families when female adolescents who have spent their childhood here and are more acculturated expect freedoms that their parents oppose because of their more traditional cultural expectations.

Couples, too, often find themselves struggling with conflicting cultural values. Engaging them in discussions that force them to reflect on cultural contrasts, and on what they see as positive and negative about each culture, may lead them to ways of relating that take from the old and the new. The idea that to make it in this country both men and women have to struggle, and must struggle together, is generally accepted by Latinos and can be used to join the couple in a more egalitarian relationship. The metaphor of building bridges to connect the world they come from to the world they live in now helps them to take what is needed from both (Garcia-Preto, 1994). Validating the positives in their culture is essential in helping Latinos rid themselves of shame, regain their dignity, make connections, and have a sense of community.

Another reason that may bring Latinos to family therapy has to do with the cultural problems engendered in ethnic intermarriage. Although the similarities among Latinos can be a source of strength to the couple, differences in sociopolitical histories, social class, race, religion, and legal status in this country can generate conflicts. These problems become more complicated when Latinos marry non-Latinos. Only 12% of Latino immigrants marry non-Latinos, but the number grows to more than 50% by the third generation (Roberts, 2004.) Helping them to identify some of these differences, and ways in which they may be affecting their relationship, can be effective.

CONCLUSION

Assuming that the number of Latinos continues to grow as has been predicted, by the year 2100 they will compose about half the population of the United States (Gonzalez, 2000; Roberts, 2004). It is also estimated that as their numbers increase, so will their influence on the social and political structure of this society. This country's welfare will greatly depend on their contributions, and for those contributions to be positive, a shift in the present social position of marginalization and oppression that the majority of Latinos experience is necessary. Engaging Latinos in a process of change that will help them use their spiritual power to access internal and external resources can be beneficial and may lead to their feeling more connected to their history, family, and community. For Latinos to embrace this nation and work toward its betterment, they must feel embraced.

REFERENCES

Allman, T. D. (1987). *Miami*. New York: Atlantic Monthly Press.

Bean, F. D., & Tienda, M. (1987). *The Hispanic population of the United States*. New York: Russell Sage.

Calvert, S., & Calvert, P. (1993). *Latin America in the 20th century*. New York: St. Martin's Press.

Chasteen, J. C., & Tulchin, J. S. (1994). *Problems in modern Latin America*. Washington, DC: Scholarly Resources.

Falicov, C. (1982). Mexican families. In M. McGoldrick, J. K. Pearce, & J. Giordano (Eds.), *Ethnicity and family therapy* (pp. 134–163). New York: Guilford Press.

Garcia-Preto, N. (1994). On the bridge. *Family Therapy Networker, 18*(4), 35–37.

Gonzalez, J. (2000). A History of Latinos in America: Harvest of empire. New York: Viking.

Grow, B. (2004, March 15). Is America ready? *Business Week*, pp. 59–70.

Hopkins, J. W. (1987). *Latin America: Perspectives on a region*. New York: Holmes & Meier.

Krauss, C. (1991). *Inside Central America*. New York: Summit Books.

Massey, D. S. (1993). Latinos, poverty and the underclass: A new agenda for research. *Hispanic Journal of Behavioral Sciences*, *15*(4), 449–475.

Mitrani, V. B., Santisteban, D. A., & Muir, J. S. (2004). Addressing immigration-related separations in Hispanic families with a behavior problem adolescent. *American Journal of Orthopsychiatry*, *74*(3), 219–229.

Montes Mozo, S., & Garcia Vasquez, J. (1988). *Salvadoran migration to the U.S.: An exploratory study*. Washington, DC: Center for Immigration Policy and Refugee Assistance.

Novas, H. (1994). *Everything you need to know about Latino history*. New York: Plume/Penguin Books.

Ono, K. A., & Sloop, J. M. (2002, January). Shifting borders: Rhetoric, immigration and California. *American Journal of Sociology*. Available at: www.temple.edu/tempress

Quinones-Rosado, R. (2002). *Empowerment, Latino identity, and the process of transformation: Writing for people in the struggle against racism*. Caguas, PR: Institute for Latino Empowerement.

Reimers, C. W. (1985). A comparative analysis of the wages of Hispanics, Blacks, and non-Hispanic Whites. In G. J. Borjas & M. Tienda (Eds.), *Hispanics in the U.S. economy* (pp. 27–76). Orlando, FL: Academic Press.

Roberts, S. (2004). *Who are we now: The changing face of America in the twenty-first century*. New York: Times Books.

Santisteban, D. A., Muir-Malcom, J. S., Mitrani, V. B., & Szapocnik, J. (2002). Integrating the study of ethnic culture and family psychology intervention science. In H. Liddle, R. Levant, D. A. Santisteban, & J. Bray (Eds.), *Family psychology intervention science* (pp. 331–351). Washington, DC: American Psychological Association.

Shorris, E. (1992). *Latinos*. New York: Norton.

Suarez-Orozco, C., Todorova, I. L. G., & Louie, J. (2002). Making up for lost time: The experience of separation and reunification among immigrant families. *Family Process*, *41*, 625–643.

U.S. Bureau of the Census. (2000). Public Information Office. Washington, DC: Government Printing Office.

U.S. Bureau of the Census. (2003). The Hispanic Population, Public Information Office. Washington, DC: Government Printing Office.

U.S. Bureau of the Census. (2004, September 8). *Hispanic heritage month 2004: Sept. 15–Oct. 15*. Public Information Office. Washington, DC: Government Printing Office.

CHAPTER 12

Brazilian Families

Eliana Catão de Korin
Sueli S. de Carvalho Petry

Over the last two decades an increasing number of Brazilians have migrated to the United States, making this population one of the fastest-growing immigrant groups in many U.S. cities. Brazilians have migrated to this country before, but since the mid-1980s their immigration rate has risen considerably as new economic policies emerged in Brazil, threatening the middle class and making its standard of living difficult to maintain (Goza, 1999; Margolis, 1994; Martes, 1999).

Often confused with Hispanics and Portuguese, it is only recently that Brazilians have started to be noticed as a distinct group in the diverse cultural mosaic of this country. Brazilians, of course, do not speak Spanish, and their culture is quite different from those of other Portuguese-speaking people. In spite of their culture or language affinity with these two groups, Brazilians resent the lack of recognition by U.S. citizens of their unique heritage. Upon entering the United States, Brazilians are often seen as Latinos because of their Latin American background. However, they often resist this classification because the Latino label is mostly associated with Spanish speakers and ignores their particular history and cultural background. Furthermore, for some Brazilian immigrants successful Americanization means not becoming part of a disenfranchised immigrant group—in this case Latinos—often associated with low socioeconomic status. A recent study found that second-generation Brazilians are most likely to say they are Brazilian American, and White or Black, rather than Latino, in order to become more "American" (Marrow, 2003). However, when confronted with the limitations of the U.S. racial/ethnic schema, some Brazilian immigrants may opt to accept the Latino label in response to a need to affirm themselves within a sociopolitical context in this country.

This immigrant group is relatively small—estimated to be between 600,000 and 1,000,000[1]—but its impact is becoming quite noticeable in some communities because of its concentration and visibility in particular areas, where Brazilian restaurants, small businesses, and news publications have proliferated. The largest concentrations of Brazilians are in the New York City metropolitan area and Massachusetts, with significant numbers found in Connecticut; Newark, New Jersey, and surrounding communities; Miami and other cities in South Florida; and California, particularly the San Francisco Bay Area and Los Angeles (Margolis, 1994, 1998; Martes, 1999, 2001; Sacks, 1993).

Initially mostly male, this group now includes an increasing number of women and families. Most recent arrivals are from urban, middle-class, relatively educated backgrounds. Most enter legally as tourists and become "visa overstayers." Brazilians migrating to larger cities are mostly from the middle or lower-middle class, are more racially mixed, and come mostly from large urban centers. Those from the interior prefer to settle in small towns in the United States, where larger numbers of lower- and working-class Brazilians are concentrated. The majority of Brazilian immigrants have at least a high school education, and others have had some years of college and have held professional or semiprofessional positions back home. In contrast, recent immigrants, most often lacking proper documentation and English language skills, are confined to menial and dead-end jobs, positions considered undesirable by U.S. workers (Margolis, 1994; Messias, 2001; Vaughan, 2003). They work hard, usually at two or three jobs, so they are able to make enough money to pay debts related to their immigration expenses and to help their families in Brazil. They see themselves at least initially as "sojourners" rather than "settlers" (Cwerner, 2001; Margolis, 1994; Martes, 1999, 2001), planning to return when they have saved enough money to buy a home or start a business back home. Many wealthy Brazilians have also emigrated to escape economic uncertainty and a surge of violence (such as recurrent kidnappings for ransom) threatening the stability of their lives. A number of upper-middle-class and professional people have also come with plans to continue their professional careers or to invest in businesses.

Class, regional, and educational background, conditions of migration, and immigrant status are all determining factors regarding the needs and adaptation of this group to the new culture. The recency of their immigration, fear of the authorities, and linguistic barriers are factors restricting most Brazilians' access to and contact with mental health and human services.

This chapter describes the Brazilian immigrant population in the United States, presents an overview of the Brazilian culture, and discusses its implication for clinical work.

BRAZIL: A SOCIOPOLITICAL PERSPECTIVE

Brazil is a large and populous country, almost the size of the United States. Its population of almost 178 million[2] is mostly concentrated in large urban areas close to the Atlantic. Brazil is comprised of distinct subcultures, sharing the Portuguese language as a common denominator.

Although colonized by the Portuguese in the 1500s, Brazilians are descendants of a mixture of people. Portuguese colonizers mixed with the indigenous population and African slaves, mostly of Yoruba and Quimbundu (West African) origin, from whom they borrowed many customs and words. Brief Dutch and French colonization in the northeast, and the 19th-century waves of German, Italian, Polish, Ukrainian, Lebanese, Japanese, and other immigrants added new elements to this mixture. Brazilian culture is therefore a composite of rich ethnic traditions that have blended differently in various regions. The African influence is most visible in Bahia (a northeastern state), in contrast to the European south. The southeast reflects a confluence of all cultures and races, with a Portuguese African predominance. Brazilian culture, in general, while predominantly of Portuguese origin, maintains strong African influences. Whites, along with Brazilians of color, share this Portuguese African culture, seeing the African elements as an integral part of the national culture (Telles, 1993).

Though the majority of Brazilians are Catholic, their religious practices are influenced by spiritualist religions of African origin. Candomblé and Umbanda, Afro-Brazilian faiths, have a powerful presence in Brazilian spiritual and cultural life. Brazilians do not necessarily follow all church dogmas. For example, contraceptive practices are widely accepted and sexuality is openly expressed. Moreover, Catholicism in Brazil has been largely influenced by the ideology of Liberation Theology, a movement led by priests working in Latin America to address the needs of the poor.[3] During times of extreme political and cultural repression the Brazilian church, led by liberal theologians, was the only voice defending the rights of the oppressed groups. In spite of the predominance of Catholicism in Brazil, other faiths are also present, such as Protestant, Jewish, and *Espiritismo*.[4] In addition, the Evangelical Christian movement has gained an increasing number of adherents among Brazilians both in the United States and in Brazil.

Initially an agrarian society, Brazil has evolved since World War II into a mostly industrialized society, becoming the largest economy in Latin America. Nowadays it is a well-developed and modern country with a relatively advanced infrastructure, modern educational institutions, and well-equipped health facilities, where large cosmopolitan urban centers flourish and many Brazilians enjoy a high standard of living. But there is also another Brazil: a country where enormous wealth coexists with visible poverty, where an internationally competitive industry is shadowed by a huge external debt, and where social opportunities are limited for many because of well-defined class and racial hierarchies.

The social fabric of the country is maintained by a system of privileges according to class status and racial background. Higher-status Brazilians (most likely White or light-skinned) always expect special treatment, and social inferiors (Brown, Black, or poor White) easily yield to elites. In Brazil, authority and hierarchy rule, as contrasted with the United States, where a pervasive, although idealized, egalitarian ethos prevails (Da Matta, 1991). A system of patronage and favors becomes an acceptable way to get on in life. This system, in which some are privileged (rich and mostly White) and many are excluded (poor White, many Brown, Black, and indigenous Brazilians), becomes the social norm. A Brazilian's social identity and power are mostly determined by family/social connections, which are inevitably related to class and racial background.

As compared with other countries, Brazil has often been recognized for its harmonious race relations. The Portuguese colonizers' acceptance of intermarriage, the absence of outright segregation, the national consensus against public discrimination, and a racial classification system that distinguishes between shades of color[5] are factors that have contributed to racial integration in Brazil. However, racism and racial inequality still remain unquestionable realities (Telles, 1993). Although the society recognizes and values the African contribution to its culture, especially in food, religion, music, dance, and arts in general, few Blacks are in positions of power and privilege. Brazilians are also confronted with the fact that the average non-White person in Brazil is poorer and less educated than the average White person. Nonetheless, most Brazilians (Whites, Browns, and most Blacks) would deny or disregard the presence of racism in Brazil, which is often obscured by high levels of racial interaction. Some Afro-Brazilian scholars have recently begun to examine this racial inequality, noting that racism, internalized racism, and racial ambiguity serve as mechanisms to preserve the status quo (Hanchard, 1999; Marx, 1998; Telles, 1999, 2002).

Race relations in Brazil are far more ambiguous than in the United States. Because of miscegenation, the interplay of shades of blackness and the complex perceptions of social standing, race is defined differently in Brazil. Brazilians understand race as a continuous color variable rather than as a categorical variable, as it is in the United States (Nobles, 2000; Telles, 1993). Moreover, racial identification is somewhat flexible and may reflect a tendency toward "whitening." Persons near the boundaries of color are likely to identify with the lighter category. For instance, middle-class darker Brazilians may be classified as Black—and eventually discriminated against—for the first time in their lives on coming to the United States, in contrast with their experiences in Brazil, where they may be seen and identify themselves as White or mulatto. Discrimination is not simply racially determined in Brazil; it also requires class considerations. Afro-Brazilians are more likely to choose class over racial identity (Telles, 1993, 2002). Brazilians of all shades often say, "He is a Black of good position," meaning that he can be accepted by an elite group in spite of his color. Race and class are two intertwined realities in Brazil; they both determine racial identity and social status.

Paradoxically, in Brazil's highly hierarchical society, money and social power are not absolute values. For instance, music, dance, and play are equally important elements, acting as social regulators of power between different social groups. This is a culture full of contradictions, where opposing values maintain each other, and where special rituals (such as Carnival) provide outlets that question and reaffirm a hierarchical social order. Public social spaces such as the beaches, soccer games, and "the schools of samba" are also places where hierarchies are ignored and people of all colors and classes congregate, becoming part of the same world. As the Brazilian anthropologist Roberto Da Matta (1991) noted, "[Brazilians] unlike the people of the U.S., never say 'separate but equal'; instead we say 'different but united,' which is the golden rule of a hierarchical and relational universe such as ours" (p. 4).

CULTURAL VALUES

The descriptions that follow refer primarily to middle-class Brazilians, mostly from the southeast region, from which the majority of U.S. Brazilian immigrants come. Ethnic distinctions are not highlighted because in Brazil, unlike the situation in the United States, there is a tendency toward cultural integration and/or biculturality. For instance, German, Jewish, Italian, and Japanese immigrants, in spite of their higher levels of ethnic identity, tend to acculturate upon contact with the mainstream culture. Intermarriage (usually to native Whites) among second-generation immigrants is common.

The importance and value of the family is probably the most central element of Brazilian culture. Indeed, the family constitutes the most important source of support throughout a person's life. Brazilians maintain a close relationship with their families, even when distant geographically. This close-knit unit includes nuclear and extended family members, as well as non-blood kin. Personal needs and issues are dealt with in the context of the family. Social life commonly involves weekly family meals and celebrations of special occasions, when stories are shared, games are played, and problems are addressed and solved. Concepts of loyalty and obligation or accountability toward the family influence personal choices and often compromise individual aspirations. Generational or marital conflicts often involve mediation by other relatives or family friends. Children receive a lot of attention, nurturance, and protection. Traditionally, family life has been based on a patriarchal structure, thereby reinforcing hierarchical relations within the family. Nevertheless, sex roles among Brazilian men and women have been changing. Younger couples tend to adopt a more egalitarian view of marriage, abandoning the idea that a woman should always accede to her husband's demands (Miller, 1979). Although many Brazilian women hold public positions of power, most agree with prevailing attitudes, commonly accepting the burden of most responsibilities for family caretaking functions. Certainly, the balance of power in any marriage is largely dependent on the wife's level of education and employment. Among middle-class urban groups, marriage tends to be postponed until after education and employment are secured by both women and men. Parenthood is highly valued, but the marital relationship also involves mutual fulfillment through a sense of intimacy and sexual love.

Brazilians are extremely gregarious people; they enjoy being together, sharing tasks, and helping others at times of need. Solidarity, empathy, and hospitality are important values in this culture. They are also known for a basically positive outlook on life. For every problem there is a solution, or a way out (*um jeitinho*—"a clever dodge,"[6] as Brazilians often say). If there is no solution, problems are accepted as an inevitable part of life, and life goes on (*fatalismo*). Avoidance of conflict and denial of problems can be a result of this sense of optimism. When sufferings, frustrations, and losses occur, the norm is not to dwell on suffering or negative feelings.

Brazilians differ from Americans regarding notions of privacy. They are not usually very concerned about "having their own space." They prefer physical closeness, touching often when talking, standing close to strangers, and hugging and kissing when greeting friends or expressing affection. Boundaries are also defined differently at an emotional level. People are expected to acknowledge others' problems and needs—to "be considerate"—even when they are not expressed verbally. As in other Latin cultures, social interactions between Brazilians are guided by the concept of *personalismo* (Garcia-Preto, 1996), which means that relationships are more important than accomplishments. Whereas in the United States identity emerges from *what one does*, social identities in Brazil are based on *what one is*. American anthropologist Conrad Kottak (1990) has said that the contrast is one of "doing" (United States) versus "being" (Brazil). Good social standing is established by gaining *respeito* (respect) from others through recognition of personal values such as honor and dignity, and not necessarily through achievement. However, to "be somebody in life" (*ser alguém na vida*), meaning to succeed through work and education, is a value reinforced especially by the middle and lower-middle classes.

Sexuality is more openly expressed in Brazil: Nudity and graphic scenes in the theater, in movies, and on TV are usually acceptable (Kottak, 1990), and sexual language is commonly used in lyrics and plays. Both men and women tend to be very expressive with their bodies, especially those who come from urban areas. Despite the patriarchal nature of the society, women are not necessarily assigned passive roles. Virginity before marriage is usually expected for young women, but adolescents are not as closely supervised as in other cultures. On the surface, homosexuality is accepted, and gay communities have become more visible recently in some cities (Parker, 1999). However, homosexuality is not legitimized. Within the family, it is dealt with as a secret that everybody knows. In general, Brazilian culture allows for greater fluidity of sexual roles than other cultures, in spite of its patriarchal norms.

BRAZILIANS IN THE UNITED STATES

Most Brazilians' lives in the United States are shaped by the typical challenges faced by first-generation, middle-class immigrants arriving in this country, such as poor English language skills, issues related to immigration and occupational status, and economic difficulties. Isolation, fear of deportation, and loss of social status are specific stresses that affect many Brazilians here. Brazilian immigrants often succeed, counting on their disposition to hard work, their sense of determination, and their capacity to improvise when faced with unexpected problems. However, they are often unaware of some of the challenges awaiting them in this country. Coming from a culture where emotional closeness, fun, and reciprocity are important values, loneliness, absence of social life, and lack of nurturance and support by loved ones can be major blows to their sense of well-being. A common dilemma constantly voiced by Brazilians who come searching for the American dream, independent of class, occupational status, or, to a certain extent, their success in the new country, is "Is it better to live poor and happy in Brazil or rich and unhappy in the United States?"

Juvenal, a man in his mid-30s, who immigrated to the United States 3 years ago, leaving behind his wife and children, shared his dilemma of "here or there." "Here I am making more money than I was in Brazil. I work hard but I make enough money to send to the kids and survive here. But this is not life! Here is just work, work and money. No respect and consideration for you at work. Nobody cares for anybody."

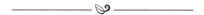

The opportunities offered in the United States are offset for Brazilians by the loss of a nurturing and stimulating culture, which they have had to leave behind and for which they continue to yearn. The dream of return is always present among most Brazilians, even when they are well adjusted to this society.

The patterned and programmed style of American culture is also difficult for many Brazilians, who are accustomed to a more spontaneous social life. Loneliness is particularly acute for those many individuals who immigrated alone, leaving behind their spouses and/or children (Sacks, 1993). The immigrant's adjustment to a new culture depends a great deal on whether one family member migrated alone or whether a large portion of the family, community, or a nation came together (Chapter 1).

Juvenal, in his report, was also referring to his frustration with the lack of support among Brazilians here and his experiences of discrimination at work. Unfortunately, lack of solidarity among members of their community here is definitely a source of major stress for Brazilian immigrants (Sacks, 1993). Negative experiences with compatriots, which often involve loss of money or abuses of some sort, are not infrequent among Brazilian immigrants. Lack of support in a highly competitive environment may promote these maladaptive behaviors. Typically, Brazilian communities are not as well organized and supportive as other ethnic communities that were able to develop an economic enclave in the United States (Margolis, 1994, 1998). Churches, in general, are the major source of support to Brazilian immigrants (Martes, 2001). Increased religiosity and, at the other extreme, alcohol intake are coping mechanisms used to deal with loneliness and lack of support.

When families come to this country together, both parents often work extensive shifts and children may be neglected or overwhelmed by the responsibility of taking care of siblings. A sense of mutual nurturance and connection is often eroded in this new life situation. Marital distress may result, especially when one member of the couple is not awarded the same opportunity as the other or if there were previous disagreements about the very idea of migration. However, most couples overcome initial stresses, renegotiating relationships to adjust to the new reality. This is especially the case in achieving, goal-oriented families.

Stresses are obviously worse for families for whom the American dream is not accessible. Without a job or income, these families feel trapped, unable to earn enough money to pay for migration debts at home and survive and, at the same time, unable to return home because of a lack of resources.

CLINICAL IMPLICATIONS

Most Brazilians come to treatment when an acute emotional crisis occurs and support is not available in their immediate network. Nonetheless, psychotherapy or counseling for emotional and family problems is not an alien concept for most middle-class Brazilians, especially the younger generation. As compared with other ethnic groups, Brazilians in the United States seem to be more receptive to the idea of psychotherapy if a personal connection is provided with a particular therapist, someone who can relate to them culturally and linguistically. However, linguistic barriers, time and financial constraints (Sacks, 1993), lack of information about resources, and the scarcity of culturally sensitive professionals keep Brazilians away from clinical settings. Although sometimes grouped together in clinical settings (McIntyre & Augusto, 1999), Brazilians are culturally very different from Portuguese (European) immigrants.

Brazilians are a proud and self-reliant immigrant group; they avoid being viewed as a problem and do not want to be dependent on social services. Brazilians respond better to a friendly, personal manner than to a business-like one, expecting the therapist to be personally interested in their problems and to take an active role in their lives. Curiosity about Brazilian culture, reinforced by empathic statements regarding the cultural differences between the therapist—as well as the dominant society—and the family can be instrumental in facilitating the therapeutic relationship. Most Brazilians tend to be initially deferential with authorities but will exhibit a casual and spontaneous style once a relationship is established. People from the interior of the country are more formal: personable and cordial, but reserved and less verbal. Those from the coastal areas are more expansive and demonstrative. They are likely to be very open and trusting about sharing their vulnerabilities and personal problems. This spontaneous and easy dialogue may change in family sessions, however, where fear of conflict and a need of mutual protection may interfere with the communication flow. These mechanisms are intensified in the first years after migration. Together with an acknowledgement of family strengths, indirect techniques such as the use of circular questions are useful to address conflicts without direct confrontations, which do not work well with this group. Reflecting Brazilian immigrant patterns, adults represent the largest number of clients coming for treatment in the United States. Common reasons for seeking therapy include depression, family problems, anxiety, somatization, grief, and issues related to sexual dysfunction and sexual identity. Referrals for family treatment are increasing as families are formed here, and as more families migrate together. Many Brazilians come to treatment for problems related to marital conflicts. Couples who migrate together may experience increased closeness in the period just after migration, each becoming a major source of support for the other, but as new life opportunities emerge in the new culture, they are challenged to revise previous modes of partnership and to renegotiate their relationship. Some are successful; however, separation and divorce occur in many families. Among recent immigrants, marriage is sought as a buffer for loneliness and other stresses. Many Brazilian women marry non-Brazilian men, thus facing additional difficulties related to cultural differences between partners (Sacks, 1993).

School referrals are often generated by conflicted and depressed adolescents who have difficulties adjusting here and want to return to Brazil. Antisocial behaviors are not usual among first-generation adolescent immigrants, which most Brazilian adolescents here are. Adolescents may also immigrate alone, joining a parent who has constituted a new family here. These reunions tend to be very distressing for the adolescent, who faces losses, has to accept a new family, and whose idealized dream of coming to the United States contrasts with the reality of the daily lives of families here.

The current wave of immigrants is younger than previous waves; therefore, more young adults are coming for therapy. Depression, usually related to loneliness and separation from their families of origin, is the most common presenting complaint. Coming from a culture with a different model of individuation, in which a young adult could live many years with his or her parents, this sudden separation, with many miles in between, can be a disorienting experience for many Brazilians and can cause unanticipated distress.

As with other immigrants, in assessing the emotional problems presented by Brazilian immigrants and their families, it is crucial that the therapist examine the interface of family, life cycle, and cultural transitional issues. Furthermore, situational stresses need to be distinguished from dysfunctional patterns already existent before migration, in order to determine the type and level of intervention required.

Life cycle issues are usually amplified by the stress of migration. For instance, an adolescent with problems of school adjustment might be challenging his parents in dealing with their own developmental dilemmas in the context of cultural transition: "Did we make the right choice by immigrating? How can we cope with these feelings of loss and uncertainty?" The therapy has to include a consideration of both the impact of cultural and developmental stresses affecting the individual and of the family at a particular stage.

Fortunately, many crises are situational, requiring only brief counseling. There are, however, cases in which the cultural conflict involves complex, unresolved past issues.

In a family whose depressed and suicidal adolescent daughter insisted to her parents that she wanted to return to Brazil, a focus on the parents' adolescence uncovered an important secret (unknown to the daughter): When her mother was about her age, her grandfather had abandoned the family and was never seen again. The mother avoided any family and marital con-

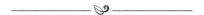

flict for fear of a new abandonment. Typically, as with other less functional families, these parents blamed the new culture for their child's problems.

In these situations, the therapist's initial "acceptance" and validation of the cultural conflicts are crucial for building a therapeutic alliance. An inquiry focused on pre- and postmigratory stresses is most relevant to facilitate an understanding of the migration in the context of the unfolding life script.

Often the very idea of the migration comes about as a way to deal with a particular conflict. Fortunately, though, migration may also provide a successful "solution" for individual and family impasses. For example, a gay man who immigrated as an attempt to legitimize his sexual identity, thus escaping constant criticisms by his father, was able to achieve success and change his image in his family of origin after coming to the United States.

Class, gender, and skin-color dynamics, as well as stages of migration and immigration status, are important factors to be considered in formulating problems and designing therapeutic interventions with Brazilians. The following case illustrates how the therapist's attention to these issues elicited crucial information for the understanding of the conflicts faced by this family.

Fernando is a White 38-year-old man with a technical degree, who arrived in the United States 8 years ago with his wife, a specialized nurse, and two children. Well adjusted to this country and speaking English fluently, he has been able to provide for his family with a modest but stable income, working as a carpenter for a small contractor. Very depressed and facing escalating marital fights, he came for therapy, referred by his employer. In therapy, Fernando shared his pain of seeing his marriage fail and his disillusionment with his limited financial accomplishments. "I should never have left," he said, an untimely statement for an immigrant who would soon receive permanent resident status in this country.

At this migration stage, earlier immigrants are reexamining their initial goals and considering new life directions. When dreams are not fulfilled, unresolved family conflicts and the fantasy of return may emerge.

When asked about the fights with his wife, Fernando described her as the instigator, easily upset with his family and sensitive about being excluded from family social events. She was portrayed as prone to emotional outbursts whenever "she does not get her way." He blamed her for alienating his family and others with her angry outbursts. Initially, migration brought them back together, but the fights had escalated during the last 2 years as she started to become more independent.

In eliciting his story, we learned that Fernando met his wife in São Paulo after migrating from a small conservative town in the interior of Brazil. He, a serious and quiet man, was attracted (and still seemed to be) to her vivacious and engaging manner. In response to the therapist's questions about her background, he reported that he had chosen a type of woman his "proper" family did not consider to be a good enough match for him: She was an illegitimate child raised by a poor, Black, adoptive, single mother. Her qualifications as a specialized nurse and main provider had been dismissed by both Fernando and his family.

This case shows how Brazilians' concerns with family status and social class affect personal and family dynamics, requiring the therapist's understanding of the peculiarities of gender, class, and skin-color dynamics in Brazil. Marly, the wife, considered a *mulata* (born to White and Black parents, often regarded as a symbol of beauty in Brazil), was discriminated against mostly for her poor and illegitimate background and less for her skin color, which, in the Brazilian context, gave her some social power.

In describing her drama, Marly, a woman of high aspirations, but who has been unable to advance professionally here, revealed that all along what had mattered most to her was to be treated "as a wife should be." Her personal history (illegitimacy) and racial background (dark in a country where to be White is best) made her more vulnerable to being dependent for legitimacy and affirmation on the acceptance of her husband and others of higher social status.

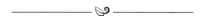

Therapy with this couple involved a process of life review to examine their individual behaviors in relation to their specific family and cultural legacies and to power differences dictated by gender and skin color. A narrative model integrating Paulo Freire's problem-posing method (Korin, 1994) is most valuable in the treatment of Brazilians, as it provides a framework to relate their personal conflicts to a larger sociocultural context. This approach involves therapist and client in a process of reflection and mutual learning about the client's personal and social realities. The client and family's migration story is validated and reexamined within a historical and sociocultural context to promote empowerment. Therapy with Brazilians will always require a family orientation. Family-of-origin work, with a focus on losses related to cultural transition, social status, and changes of racial identity, is a necessary approach in doing therapy with this immigrant group.

CONCLUSION

The formulations outlined in this chapter are presented as an initial map for orienting therapists' work with Brazilian clients and their families. Clients themselves are always the best source of information about their culture (Korin, 1994).

Therapists need to examine and recognize the impact of their own value orientation, and that of the dominant society, in assessing their clients' problems; they should avoid ethnic stereotyping and be aware of pathologizing normal processes. The individualist orientation predominant in middle-class U.S. culture is not a universal value; in many cultures, attachment to one's family of origin continues throughout life, in spite of the inevitable changes of relationships that occur over time. Brazilian clients in treatment with U.S. therapists often find that their attachment to their family of origin is misunderstood and pathologized. Discussing differences in communication style, many Brazilian women have expressed their dissatisfaction with the ways in which their more demonstrative and body-oriented communication style has often been misunderstood by therapists and supervisors. This style has been interpreted as sexualized/seductive behavior, contributing to stereotyping and discomfort in therapeutic and professional relationships.

It is our belief that a culture-sensitive practice requires therapists' self-reflection and knowledge about their own cultural values as much as their knowledge about their clients' culture. A final reminder: It is important to bear in mind that the therapeutic encounter is an interactive process that always involves the interface of three cultures: the client/family's, the therapist's, and the dominant culture (Sluzki, 1979).

NOTES

1. There are no reliable data regarding the total number of Brazilians living in the United States. In the categories offered by the 2000 census, Brazilians are not precisely classified; in addition, many Brazilians are undocumented and are therefore not included in official reports.
2. Based on the 2000 census, the 2004 population has been projected at 178,269,286 (Instituto Brasileiro de Estatística e Geografia, Censo Demográfico).
3. This movement gave rise to many leading voices in Brazil, such as those of Bishop Helder Camara and educator Paulo Freire, who became known around the world for their work with disenfranchised populations.
4. A spiritual practice founded by Allan Kardec in the 19th century in France that combined with the Catholic and African religions in Brazil, Cuba, and Puerto Rico.
5. The Brazilian census includes five racial categories: White (53.8%), Brown (39.1%), Black (6.2%), Yellow (0.5%), and Indigenous (0.4%). Afro-Brazilians, almost half of the national population, are usually considered the Brown and Black categories taken together. The Brown category includes primarily mixed-raced people. Whites are often not purely White, as in the U.S. definition, but relatively White (Telles, 2002).
6. This famous expression, *dar um jeitinho*, may be translated as "find a way out," "clever dodge," or "bypass," and may also imply the use of playful "chicanery" (*malandragem*).

REFERENCES

Cwerner, S. B. (2001). The times of migration. *Journal of Ethnic and Migration Studies*, 27(1), 7–36.

Da Matta, R. (1991). *Carnival, rogues and heroes: An interpretation of the Brazilian dilemma*. Notre Dame, IN: University of Notre Dame Press.

Garcia-Preto, N. (1996). Puerto Rican families. In M. McGoldrick, J. K. Pearce, & J. Giordano (Eds.), *Ethnicity and family therapy* (2nd ed., pp. 183–199). New York: Guilford Press.

Goza, F. (1999). Brazilian immigration to Ontario. *International Migration*, 37(4), 765–789.

Hanchard, M. (1999). Introduction. In M. Hanchard (Ed.), *Racial politics in contemporary Brazil* (pp. 1–29). Durham, NC: Duke University Press.

Korin, E. C. (1994). Social inequalities and therapeutic relationship: Applying Freire's ideas in clinical practice. In R. Almeida (Ed.), *Expansions of feminist family therapy through diversity* (pp. 75–88). New York: Haworth Press. (Published simultaneously in *Journal of Feminist Family Therapy*, 3/4, 75–88).

Kottak, C. P. (1990). *Prime society: An anthropological analysis of television and culture*. Belmont, CA: Wadsworth.

Margolis, M. (1994). *Little Brazil: An ethnography of Brazilian immigrants in New York City*. Princeton, NJ: Princeton University Press.

Margolis, M. (1998). *An invisible minority: Brazilian immigrants in New York City*. Boston: Allyn & Bacon.

Marrow, H. (2003). To be or not to be (Hispanic or Latino): Brazilian racial and ethnic identity in the United State. *Ethnicities*, 3(4), 427–464.

Martes, A. C. B. (1999). *Brasileiros nos Estados Unidos: Um estudo sobre imigrantes em Massachussets* [Brazilians in the United States: A study of immigrants in Massachusetts]. São Paulo, Brazil: Editora Paz e Terra.

Martes, A. C. B. (2001). Migration and religion a safe place for sociability: Brazilian immigrants and church affiliation in Massachusetts. *Migration World*, 29(5), 28–39.

Marx, A. W. (1998). *Making race and nation: A comparison of South Africa, the United States, and Brazil*. Cambridge, UK: Cambridge University Press.

McIntyre, T. M., & Augusto, F. (1999). The martyr adaptation syndrome: Psychological sequelae in the adaptation of Portuguese-speaking immigrant women. *Cultural Diversity and Ethnic Minority Psychology, 5*(4), 387–402.

Messias, D. K. H. (2001). Transnational perspectives on women's domestic work: Experiences of Brazilian immigrants in the United States. *Women and Health, 33*(1/2), 1–20.

Miller, C. (1979). The function of middle-class extended family networks in Brazilian urban society. In M. Margolis & W. Carter (Eds.), *Brazil: Anthropological perspectives* (pp. 305–316). New York: Columbia University Press.

Nobles, M. (2000). History counts: A comparative analysis of racial/color categorizations in US and Brazilian censuses. *American Journal of Public Health, 90*(11), 1738–1745.

Parker, R. (1999). *Beneath the equator: Cultures of desire, male homosexuality, and emerging gay communities in Brazil.* New York: Routledge.

Sacks, D. (1993). *Recent Brazilian immigrants to the United States: Human service needs and help-seeking behaviors.* Unpublished doctoral dissertation, Rutgers University, Piscataway, NJ.

Sluzki, C. E. (1979). Migration and family conflict. *Family Process, 18*(4), 379–390.

Telles, E. E. (1993). *Afro-Brazilian identity and segregation.* Paper presented at the Conference on Racial Politics in Brazil, Austin, TX.

Telles, E. E. (1999). Ethnic boundaries and political mobilization among African Brazilians: Comparisons with the U.S. case. In M. Hanchard (Ed.), *Racial politics in contemporary Brazil* (pp. 83–97). Durham, NC: Duke University Press.

Telles, E. E. (2002). Racial ambiguity among the Brazilian population. *Ethnic and Racial Studies, 25*(3), 415–441.

Vaughan, J. (2003). Shortcuts to immigration: The "temporary" visa program is broken. *Backgrounder.* Washington, DC: Center for Immigration Studies.

CHAPTER 13

Central American Families

Miguel Hernandez

According to the U.S. Bureau of the Census in the year 2000, there are more than two million Central Americans living in the United States. Yet it is impossible to have an accurate number because so many Central American families live in the United States without legal documentation and do not want to be counted (Suarez-Orozco & Suarez-Orozco, 2001). Central Americans have been a mobile population, dating back to the Spanish conquest and to centuries of political and socioeconomic upheaval. In an earlier era, many Central Americans, especially the professional, educated, and skilled-worker classes, followed the path northward on the heels of economic recession and political repression, seeking socioeconomic advancement in the United States. Furthermore, the Immigration Act of 1965, which eliminated the preference for immigrants of European extraction (mostly White) and changed the system to one of equal quotas for all nationalities, facilitated the possibilities for many Central Americans to obtain visas and become legal residents in the United States. However, the situation changed during the 1970s when revolution and war erupted in several Central American countries and the United States developed new restrictive migration policies denying political asylum to Central American refugees. According to Booth and Walker (1993), U.S. foreign policy toward Central America changed as a result of the Soviet Union's support of the revolutions and fear of the spread of communism in the developing countries of the region. These restrictions resulted in the increase of undocumented migration of people from countries such as Nicaragua, Honduras, El Salvador, and Guatemala, fleeing from war and political oppression.

From 1998 to 2000, the U.S. Immigration and Naturalization Service (INS) reported apprehending more than 1.5 million undocumented immigrants each year at the southwestern border. Many were Central American refugees escaping from complex sociopolitical situations, severe poverty, and lack of basic resources. Close to half of the undocumented Central Americans arrested at the border were from Honduras, El Salvador, Nicaragua, and Guatemala (Valch, 2003). Those seeking political asylum tended to be mainly Salvadoran and Guatemalan (INS Border Apprehensions, n.d.). In 1990, the INS detained 8,500 children at the southwestern U.S. border, 70% of whom were unaccompanied and were from Central America (Therrien & Ramirez, 2001).

Today Central Americans are a minority (about 5%) of the total Latino population in the United States. They are somewhat more scattered geographically than other Latino groups. Regions of highest Central American concentration are the South (34.6%), the Northeast (32.3%), and the West (28.2%) (U.S. Bureau of the Census, 2001). The increased diaspora of indigenous Maya throughout Central America, as well as the United States, has been a contemporary phenomenon of note (Loucky, Moors, & Moors, 2000). Although they share similar cultural aspects and migration and adaptation experiences with other Latino groups in the United States, Central American families have in common two important distinctions that are usually overlooked by clinicians. One is the legacy of a violent war and, consequently, a very unstable sociopolitical and economic situation. Another is the psychosocial impact of a traumatic migration experience and the stresses of their undocumented status (Valch, 2003).

This chapter focuses on the unique challenges Central American refugee families experience in adapting to and integrating into United States society. I explore here the complex historical events that triggered their migration to the United States, the impact of their exposure to war, the difficulties emanating from their political status in the United States, and the effects of migration on individual and family life. The suggestions made in this chapter are intended to be a general clinical framework from which to approach Central American refugee families living in the United States.

HISTORICAL BACKGROUND

Central America, the region that links North and South America, includes seven countries: Belize, Guatemala, El Salvador, Honduras, Nicaragua, Costa Rica, and Panama. Belize and Panama, although geographically part of Central America, have fairly distinct histories from those of the other countries in the region. Belize is an English-speaking republic that became independent from Great Britain in 1981 and does not figure significantly in what has been called the "Central American problem." Panama, although often lumped with the other countries of the region, is not technically Central American; its pre-Columbian indigenous cultures were South American and, until 1903, it was part of Colombia (Booth & Walker, 1993).

Nicaragua, Honduras, El Salvador, and Guatemala were conquered two decades after the first Spanish penetration in 1522. Costa Rica was not settled until the 1560s because, unlike other areas, it offered no easily exploitable gold or Indian slaves. Its geographical isolation from the rest of the isthmus probably contributed to the total extermination of its native inhabitants. The Indian population had been oppressed and marginalized by the Spaniards who took its people's land and agricultural resources. Through the crimes of colonization, the Spanish devalued their cultural traditions and imposed a Western European culture. This led to a distinctive political, economic, and social history in Costa Rica, where a dominant Iberian society developed without a racially distinct or exploited underclass (Booth & Walker, 1993).

Elsewhere in Central America, Spaniards were able to impose their domination without destroying the entire native population. By the end of the conquest, however, fighting, diseases, and enslavement caused a drastic reduction of the Indian population. Only in

Guatemala did a large number of Indians survive. This, perhaps, was due to the greater difficulty Spaniards had in subjugating completely the relatively more advanced society they encountered in the region, which resisted colonization by defending and claiming their lands and culture in a more politically organized system that addressed issues of human rights (Booth & Walker, 1993). Today, Guatemala continues to have a large native Indian population, which has kept its culture and language alive and has made others feel its presence in the political history of the country.

During the colonial period, Spain ruled Guatemala, Nicaragua, El Salvador, Honduras, and Costa Rica. The region was controlled by a Spanish-born elite class, and everyone else belonged to a downtrodden lower class. Biological unions between Spaniards and Indians produced *mestizos* (of Spanish Indian blood), who were never considered equals to Spaniards, but were nonetheless of higher social status than pure Indians. This class configuration changed drastically as new groups were added to the population: African slaves and, later, the mulatto offspring of White–Black unions. Today there are still clear racial divisions whereby non-White people are socially, politically, and racially discriminated against and the sociopolitical hierarchy of power continues to be dominated by race, giving social, economic, and political privilege to those who are White and belong to an elite that is defined by their historical connection to the colonizers.

The White elite controlled the human and natural resources. The economy became focused on exportation of products that were not essential for supporting the lower-class population. For instance, it concentrated on cultivating coffee, sugar, and other products that had greater value for exportation to European countries but were not relevant to the diet of the Indian population. After the region's independence from Spain in the 1820s, those who had inherited economic power and social standing perpetuated an unregulated agro-export economy for their own benefit. Out of this pattern, complex social, political, and economic conflicts later developed (Booth & Walker, 1993).

The 19th century was characterized by American and British efforts to expand their political influence in the region. Laissez-faire liberals, who advocated unregulated free enterprise, dominated Central American nations during the late 19th century and part of the 20th, introduced new export products such as coffee and bananas, and advocated modernization, development of governmental institutions, and the infrastructure that could facilitate their economic plan. By the century's end, their coffee business had produced a large class of wealthy landowners who tolerated military and civilian dictatorships and the oppressive sociopolitical system that contributed to important revolutions in the 20th century (Skidmore & Smith, 1992).

In Costa Rica, political reforms, begun in the late 19th century, culminated in 1948 with the abolition of the army and the development of local democratic reforms. The rest of the region, however, made limited progress toward democracy in the 1950s, only to witness a renewal of military rule in the 1960s (Skidmore & Smith, 1992).

During the mid-20th century, changes in the export crops took land away from the rural poor, provoking an exodus to the cities. Landownership and agricultural production became even more concentrated. To varying degrees in each nation, the surge in domestic and foreign investment was concentrated in the production of consumer goods. The number of factory and middle-class jobs grew as the region became more industrialized during the 1970s, but rural and urban unemployment rose because of urban migrations by unemployable peasants (Booth & Walker, 1993).

Nicaragua, Guatemala, and El Salvador entered the 1970s with numerous common problems, including even greater concentration of wealth, increased rural and urban lower-class unemployment, and decreased agricultural self-sufficiency among large segments of the rural poor. The rapid accumulation of wealth by the bourgeoisie in these three countries increased the growth of the upper and middle classes and improved their standard of living, causing a dramatic rise in socioeconomic inequality that stimulated class conflict and widespread protests throughout the region (Booth & Walker, 1993).

Supported by the United States, the governments in these countries responded to the massive rebellions by sharply escalating military force and violence. Subjected to repression and the governments' refusal to carry out political and economic reforms, the aggrieved began to organize, mobilize economic resources from poor and wealthy opposition leaders, and engage in armed resistance (Booth & Walker, 1993). The escalating conflicts resulted in two decades (1970–1990) of civil wars within the three countries.

During the wars, many human rights crimes were committed. Physical and psychological torture, intimidation, massive killings, and other persecution of individuals, families, and communities left many with profound psychological and physical wounds (Booth & Walker, 1993; Garcia & Rodriguez, 1989). With the wars, poor socioeconomic conditions and human terror increased, and record numbers of refugees escaped to the United States. From the early 1970s throughout the late 1980s, more than one million Salvadorans, Nicaraguans, and Guatemalans entered the United States (Arredondo, Orjuela, & Moore, 1989). Yet the U.S. government did not recognize these people as political refugees, but as illegal aliens who came to the United States for economic gain. Thus, they did not have the benefit of the Refugee Act, which provides political asylum to individuals who flee their homeland because of well-founded fear of social or political persecution (Drachman, 1995). Consequently, many Central Americans have been forced to remain hidden without proper legal documentation (Conover, 1993).

During the last decade serious sociopolitical and economic changes have affected the region. Severe poverty, an increase in the drug subculture, crime, and the impact of devastating hurricanes and other disasters have been related to a constant pattern of undocumented migration from Central America. Although it has never been easy to live undocumented in the United States, the situation has become worse since September 11, 2001, with the passing of the Patriot Act, which has declared a war against immigrants. U.S. immigration policies have become stricter, and the number of deportations of undocumented immigrants has increased dramatically. The new U.S. national paranoia in regard to immigrants has affected Central Americans in many ways. They have experienced increased hostility at the southern U.S. border and by mistreatment of detainees at the border detention camps. Approval of civilians for patrolling the border has especially resulted in the murdering of many immigrants who were crossing the border through private U.S. property. Generally, the greater intolerance for groups that are racially different has affected Central American immigrants. These families live now in fear and are victims of ethnic prejudice and socioeconomic oppression by the increasing intolerance of the U.S. policies in regard to welcoming immigrants, especially racially different newcomers (Ferrari, 2004).

TREATMENT CONSIDERATIONS

Assessment and therapy with Central American families in the United States require an understanding of their status as political refugees (Arredondo et al., 1989; Valch, 2003). Therapists should be alert to the complex psychosocial stresses that many Central American families have experienced before, during, and after migration.

Whether or not an immigrant family fled illegally, its members may have witnessed the terror and violence that have recently dominated the region. Families generally have experienced the loss of family members or friends and the horrors of torture and other crimes. Profound political and socioeconomic repression have left deep emotional and relational wounds among those who came to the United States (Garcia & Rodriguez, 1989; Valch, 2003). In addition to the trauma of war, losses, and disruptions, refugees suffer from survivor's guilt, self-recrimination, unresolved grief, dissociation, and severe stress, which are transmitted multigenerationally (Hernandez, 1996).

When the way we understand ourselves, others, and the world is disrupted, and when we feel fear, horror, or terror, intense stress can produce a traumatic response. This is a normal response to abnormal events and experiences (Weingarten, 2003). Common reactions to trauma are sadness, shame, helplessness, negative reactivity, and aggression. The unspoken impact of trauma affects each family member who unconsciously keeps silent about the trauma, and family members develop different ways of acting out the impact of the trauma.

Therapists commonly observe alliances and coalitions among family members concerning "untold stories" about the family's experience or history with political and socioeconomic repression. Like some Holocaust survivors and other victims of common shock, many Central American refugee families come to therapy with an impenetrable silence that can perpetuate the trauma and create a culture of fear, secrecy, numbness, memory effects, sadness, helplessness, shame, and even inexplicable aggression among family members. They may develop rigid family boundaries, which results in social isolation and the development of a convoluted language that revisits emotional and physical symptoms. These can be startlingly specific metaphors for the unspoken truths and the multigenerational legacy of psychological trauma (Hernandez, 1996; Lang, 1995; Weingarten, 2003).

Families that were victims of direct persecution often remain anchored in a state of permanent collective remembrance and mourning, engaged in a constant conversation about the circumstances from which they escaped while others did not. Survivor's guilt can produce two mayor impacts on refugee families. For those who witnessed the loss of family members, friends, and loved ones, there usually is an unspoken emotional search for the meaning of their survival. The sense of guilt often stops them from living and leaves them with feelings of anger, sadness, and an existential need to find some meaning as to why they survived while those whom they loved died. Usually the legacy of their trauma is to have high expectations of their children, as if they should pay back spiritually and emotionally for their ancestors' death. Parents often expect their children to make amends for their (the parents') losses and to honor their good luck to be alive. The following vignette is an example:

Olga, a 34-year-old Salvadoran client, had lost her parents, her two brothers, and their wives to the guerillas. After escaping El Salvador as an illegal refugee, she was trying very hard to reestablish her life in New York City. Her husband, Juan, abandoned her a few months after their arrival. Her only daughter, Raquel, was 16 years old when referred to treatment. Olga worked two shifts in a local bodega. Undocumented and with limited resources, her main life project was her daughter's education and future. She was planning for her daughter to achieve "the American Dream." Her unspoken expectation was that achieving the "dream" would give some meaning to their tragedy and offer reparation for their luck of being alive. However, these unspoken reasons that justified her mother's obsession with success and reparation made

Raquel rebellious, a school truant, and defiant. She felt that it was not her responsibility to pay back an unspoken debt of which she had not been aware. In therapy, once the mother was able to share her story, her guilt and her expectations for reparation by changing the family's story through her daughter' success, helped Raquel understand her mother's context better. Helping the mother to share her guilt about losing her family due to their political commitment to resist the U.S. intervention in controlling their country's future, and exploring why Raquel remained so aloof to that political reality because of her young age, facilitated Raquel's understanding about the source of her mother's distress and her need to repair the trauma by achieving the American Dream.

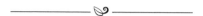

Although a fixation on the trauma can sometimes be detrimental to a family, talking about it in therapy can provide context of the source of its members' relational conflicts and therefore provide some healing in regard to their misunderstandings. It is important for the therapist to acknowledge and provide empathy about the impact the trauma has had on their clients' lives. It is also helpful to explore the effect and emotional meaning of keeping secrets about unresolved legacies and how this affects the rules and expectations families develop for their children. It is important to discuss why the legacies of these children are usually different from those of other Latino children living in the United States whose families have not experienced the trauma of war. Otherwise, the children will not understand how certain family rules and beliefs systems have become central to their story and meaning of success in their host country. As Almeida, Woods, Messineo, and Font (1998) have demonstrated in their work, if we help our clients to become involved and to participate in political and social activism by speaking out and sharing their personal testimony with other survivors, the healing becomes more communal. Helping the victims of trauma share their personal stories with their families, and then in some type of public forum where their experience of survival is validated, facilitates their moving from feeling like victims to feeling empowered. Their personal experiences are thus framed within a sociopolitical context that helps them to retell their stories from a different perspective and reclaim power over their lives. Sharing their personal trauma in this way can free families from the power of secrets and helps them integrate their pride and resiliency into the family story. This process can also normalize their anxiety and fears about whom to blame for the trauma and/or whom to make accountable for their lives.

Lack of legal status adds another level of stress to the psychosocial strain experienced during the postmigration period. Unlike most other refugees, Central American families usually lack access to federally funded medical, educational, or food programs, which has a direct impact on their adaptation and integration into U.S. society (Garcia & Rodriguez, 1989; Valch, 2003). U.S. immigration policy makes it easy for employers to exploit immigrant workers. They are denied adequate health care and/or access to higher education for young people, which further separates and impoverishes families. These conditions tend to make women and children vulnerable to sexual abuse and to exclude immigrants' voices from decisions that affect their lives. Undocumented immigrants are particularly vulnerable to discrimination based on their illegal status, which is particularly true for Central Americans because of their race, ethnicity, and class (Ferrari, 2004). The Immigration Reform and Control Act of 1986, which penalizes employers who hire illegal immigrants, forces many Central American refugees to work illegally in low-paying jobs where exploitation and abuse are common. The fear of being captured and deported forces them to hide, live in silence about their past, violate various laws, and tolerate abusive conditions. In addition, as mentioned earlier, the new Patriot Act allows detention and deportation without judicial review, and immigrants with minor criminal records face deportation, resulting in the breakup of intact families when they lose the main breadwinner (American Family Therapy Academy, 2004). During the last 3 years many immigrant men have been deported from the United States because of minor criminal records, leaving their families without the financial resources needed to survive (Ferrari, 2004).

José, age 40, a union organizer who had been actively involved in the Nicaraguan revolution, escaped his country after surviving incarceration, torture, and various other forms of persecution. To protect his wife and two children, José left his family and remained hidden while preparing for his long journey. His goal was to secure a job and housing and obtain some legal status in order to bring the rest of the family to the United States legally.

Three months after leaving Nicaragua, José arrived in the United States and presented a well-documented case for political asylum, but his petition was denied. Motivated by his fear of being deported, he moved to a different state. In order to find work and housing, and to save money to pay for his family's trip, José obtained a false Social Security card, thereby committing fraud. He also obtained a driver's license and lied to his landlord when he assumed a new identity as a Puerto Rican. His efforts to remain inconspicuous and silent about his past and his true identity had a profound psychological impact. In addition, the pressure to make money, the difficulty in keeping in contact with his family, and the long hours at two demanding jobs finally triggered an emotional collapse.

José fell into a severe depression and began to have nightmares, anxiety attacks, and flashbacks about his traumatic experiences in Nicaragua. Overwhelmed by the intensity of his memories, he dealt with his symptoms by drinking heavily every night. Fifteen years after immigration, José had become a different person. Later he would tell his therapist that he came to the United States to escape death from persecution, only to die in a more painful way. He was bitter and felt cheated by the U.S. government, which he accused of invalidating his experiences and forcing him to live in a constant lie. Today José still fears being deported because he continues to be illegal, and since September 11, 2001, he worries even more about becoming the target of racism and being deported.

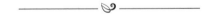

THE MIGRATION EXPERIENCE

The events preceding migration are often just as distressful as the act of migrating. Many Central American refugee families have to depart suddenly, with no time for farewells. Their fear of not ever returning, the uncertain future of those left behind, and expectations of freedom increase their anxiety and make their experience of being uprooted and expatriated more difficult. These experiences are usually unspoken and repressed for the sake of adaptation and survival. Repressed feelings of loss, however, affect their ability to adapt to their new context. Repressing their losses and focusing on adaptation evoke meaningful family conflicts. In my work with Central American families, I have found that the main reason for their uprooteness is never discussed. Very often the children and the parents collude by explaining their migration as a way of finding a better life. When family members become aware that life is more difficult in the United States than they had expected and that language, cultural beliefs, lifestyles, and even personal goals are different, family conflicts develop. This often causes negative coalitions between parents and children (Hernandez, 1996).

Because most Central American refugees cannot enter the United States legally, they have to resort to the services of "coyotes," guides who offer to take them via risky alternative routes. During the trip, which sometimes lasts weeks or months, the travelers are frequently mistreated, robbed, and raped by their guides. The final part of the trip, the border crossing, is usually undertaken under inhuman conditions (Garcia & Rodriguez, 1989). Many refugees are captured by officers of the U.S. Immigration and Naturalization Service and are either imprisoned or deported to their country of origin (Conover, 1993).

This mode of migration has a direct impact on the refugee family's structure and development. Often, a few members of the family emigrate first. Those who stay behind are forced to assume new roles and responsibilities for keeping the family functioning. Women often become the sole breadwinners and assume responsibility for the family's financial and emotional support. The oldest child may take a parental role, and the family's dependence on the extended networks increases.

If the family is eventually reunited, it will need to reorganize as a new structure and to negotiate new roles and functions in order to include the newly arrived members. It is important to remember that family members almost certainly will go through readjustment conflicts as they struggle with the new cultural environment (Garcia & Rodriguez, 1989).

Luisa, a 44-year-old Nicaraguan woman who had survived the Sandinista revolution and the U.S.-supported Contra war, decided to leave her country in the year 2000 in order to look for a better life for her children. Having survived the "situation," which euphemistically refers to the personal experiences of arrest, torture, threatened conscription, seeing dead bodies, rape, and economic exploitation, she was a woman of extraordinary resilience. With six children, no husband, and very limited financial resources to support her family, she first fled to Costa Rica alone, illegally and with false documentation, to work and save money to pay for her illegal entrance to the United States. While in Costa Rica, Luisa worked as a maid in a large resort that catered fancy services for North American tourists. For 2 years she was able to save enough money to pay her coyote to bring her to the United States through the Arizona dessert. She had learned some basic English, had a decent amount of cash money to resettle in the United States, and was determined that the difficulties ahead would be worthwhile if they led to her children's well-being and their reunification in the land of liberty and opportunity. However, as her coyote had told her, the trip was difficult and dangerous. The long walks under the dessert sun, the heat, and the hiding from U.S. Border Patrol delayed what was supposed to have been a week's journey, which then took 15 days after their departure before she was able to make a successful crossing. During her journey Luisa witnessed the death of four illegal immigrants, who, like her, were full of hopes for a better future. A very traumatic experience for Luisa was witnessing the killing of a man, one of the last group members who survived the journey, by a civilian; while trying to cross the border, he had invaded a private ranch in Arizona.

Two weeks after Luisa arrived at her friend's house in New York, she was numb, suffered intense nightmares, could not eat, and refused to leave the house. She became depressed and overwhelmed by the memories of her journey to a point where she needed psychiatric hospitalization. When Luisa recounted her traumatic experiences, she was diagnosed as having psychotic delusions. Later, after being discharged to a partial hospitalization program, diagnosed with major depression with psychotic features, with the help of a caring clinician she began to contextualize her traumatic experience of migration and its impact on her emotional health. Through validation, empathy, care, and support, she was able to understand how her personal experience was connected to her decision to escape a sociopolitical reality of oppression and imperialism that affected the well-being of her family. Expanding her personal experience to include how political realities have a direct impact on people's personal stories helped Luisa to reframe her sense of feeling mentally disabled, disorganized, and a victim and moved her to understand and redefine her struggles from a more positive perspective. Focusing on her strengths, her resilience, and her ability to overcome trauma, and validing her experiences as a way to rescue her family, gave her a sense of empowerment and moved her from a reactive stance to a more reflective mode of understanding and reorganizing her story. Today we still struggle in helping Luisa to achieve legal status in the United States. However, we have helped her reconnect with her family through letters that strengthen her efforts to reunite the family. A shared hope by Luisa and her children has made them closer, allowing an open communication that includes detailed descriptions of their different realities.

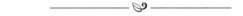

SETTLEMENT AND ACCULTURATION

Once a refugee family enters the United States, a complex psychological process begins. Not having time to process the traumatic experiences accumulated during their migration, the family is now confronted with the stresses of survival, adaptation, and integration into a new environment. During this time many refugees feel cheated, as the "Land of Liberty" is not as welcoming as they were told (Garcia & Rodriguez, 1989; Hernandez, 1996; Hernandez & McGoldrick, 1999). Central American refugees often end up in marginal positions within the U.S. social structure because they lack legal documentation, support networks, or access to social and economic resources.

Perhaps the greatest difficulties result from trying to adapt to the new culture. Acculturation is a complex, multigenerational process in which constant negotiation between the culture of origin and the new culture forces the family to reshape values, behaviors, belief systems, relational patterns, and attitudes (Hernandez, 1996; Hernandez & McGoldrick, 1999; Rogler, 1994). The process usually triggers relational and emotional conflicts as family roles, rules, and values that were culturally congruent and effective in Central America become less functional in the United States (Hernandez, 1996; Hernandez & McGoldrick, 1999).

Although the Central American family's cultural context largely varies with each country, along with the family's social class (pre- and postmigration) and the historical factors surrounding migration, the legacy of Latino cultural values remains strong. There are probably more similarities than differences between Central Americans, Mexicans, and South Americans in language, religion, spiritual beliefs that incorporate indigenous rituals with Catholic rituals, family values, sex roles, and life philosophy. In this sense, clinicians need to be attuned to central organizing cultural values such as familism, *machismo* and *marianismo*; the importance of extended family and other social networks; the values of respect, dignity, and honor; and the impact of patriarchal and agrarian ideologies on the distribution of power between men and women. These values are discussed in depth elsewhere (Bernal, 1982; Falicov, 1998; Garcia-Preto, 1996; Hernandez, 1996; Valch, 2003).

An important factor to consider is that, as in the Andes and in southern Mexico, there is a strong Indian heritage in Central America. In countries such as Guatemala, the Indian population continues to be sufficiently concentrated to preserve its traditional cultural and social identity. Thus, many of the cultural values discussed in this chapter are not necessarily relevant when the families have a Mayan, rather than a Latino, cultural heritage (Hernandez, 1996; Valch, 2003).

Another important difference is the unique political and economic history of Central America and its impact on family values. For instance, during the revolutions in Nicaragua, El Salvador, and Guatemala, the concept of acceptable social behavior for women greatly broadened. Many women, who had been confined to the private sphere, joined the guerrillas and became important participants in the region's political transformation. Some became heads of household after their husbands were killed or disappeared during the wars. The impact of this shift in gender roles on Central American society is uncertain. But it is clear that with the crushing of the revolutions, women have been redirected toward more traditional roles (Hernandez, 1996).

ACCULTURATION AND FAMILY CONFLICT

Central American refugees are often forced to assume unaccustomed roles in U.S. society. Women are often the first to obtain jobs, because they are more open to performing menial tasks, or because the available jobs are seen as more appropriate for females. Through their work, they usually develop an outside network that allows a more rapid learning of the new culture. Even when they are not part of the workforce, women are quicker to develop social relationships through traditional duties such as shopping and involvement with their children's school (Garcia & Rodriguez, 1989; Hernandez, 1996). This exposure and newly developed strategies to negotiate their traditional gender roles are felt in the family when women begin to demand more participation of their children and husbands in home care.

As expected, new behaviors unbalance the family, particularly the marital dyad's traditional power structure. For example, traditional husbands, who are used to being considered the main providers and protectors of the family, resent the changes and challenge the newly acquired independence of their wives by reclaiming old role patterns. Women are often accused of abandoning their culture and family. In my experience, out of guilt and confusion, many women try to resume old roles, isolate themselves from friends, and work extra hard to please their husbands. Their resulting discontent is usually manifested in somatization, depressive symptoms, or relational conflicts.

Traditional Central American masculine gender roles are also challenged by the new cultural environment. Without the public recognition given to the cultural norms of *machismo* or to the strong patriarchal ideology to which they are accustomed, many Central American men feel they have lost their power. Their new ethnic-minority status and social invisibility invalidate their domain in the public sphere. Losing power in the public sphere because of racism, ethnic prejudice, and, paradoxically, societal changes toward gender equity, has a direct impact on the men's family life. Their new context does not support the rigid ideology of male-dominant power as it was in the machismo culture in their country of origin. Laws protecting against domestic violence and child abuse, and governing financial support for children, make men accountable for their misuse of gender power. Confusion, anxiety and depression, substance abuse, and overall psychosocial underfunctioning are common manifestations of the effects of loosing status and power.

Central American families also experience change in their traditional hierarchical structure when they acculturate. Through formal education, children generally become proficient in English before their parents do and often become their culture brokers; parents become dependent on their children to negotiate with the outside world.

As they acculturate, children demand to be heard in the home and begin to challenge their parents' traditional values and cultural beliefs (Garcia & Rodriguez, 1989; Hernandez, 1996). Parents frequently feel that they have lost their credibility as authority figures when children move toward a more "American" way, becoming increasingly "lost" to the new culture. These conflicts usually generate family tension and disorganization. A breakdown in family cohesion leaves members without support and at risk of developing emotional, psychological, and relational symptoms.

An important issue to be considered for Central American families is that although we are grouping countries that are somewhat similar, we must keep in mind that there are very significant differences, according to whether a family is from Guatemala, El Salvador, Panama, Nicaragua, or Belize, because of their specific cultures and histories. What is common, however, is that they all share fragmented identities as a result of mixed racial and class backgrounds, which affected their values and their cultural and historical contexts. There are four main ethnic groups to be found throughout the Central American region. There are the descendants of the indigenous Maya, predominating in the highland regions and who speak some 23 different and distinctive languages; the Afro-Caribbean populations of mixed Black and indigenous heritage; the descendents of European immigrants (mainly Spanish); and the *mestizos*, or the racially mixed population of European and indigenous people (Valch, 2003). These mixed identities become even more complex as they are exposed to new alternatives through the acculturation process.

Usually the problem is that, like many other Latinos, Central American families are exposed to new and different role models that may help them fit into their new cultural context, but can also create conflicts. For example, women are forced to become more liberal and independent, and men have to learn to share their patriarchal power. Children and adolescents also have to choose from contradictory influences that include alternative lifestyles such as the Latino hip-hop culture, the stereotyped macho or Latin sex symbol, the cool gang fighter, or the very often not available successful professional, which is usually rejected as a possibility because it is associated with selling out and becoming "a White dressing brown traitor" (Inclan & Quiñones, 2003). Deciding which role models to choose as a way to fit into the new cultural context can create personal and intrafamilial conflicts as individuals try adapting in their own ways to their particular situations. The choices they make may cause conflict when they are dissonant with the family's culture or when they put into question its identity as a Central American family.

Carlina, a 15-year-old Guatemalan adolescent with skin too dark and features too indigenous to be a Christina Aguilera lookalike, tried to be White and look like her role model but could not fit the prototype. She was not White, and her body had a different shape. Even when she tried diets and body sculpting classes at her local YMCA, she could not achieve the slim, sexy image of her idol. Then she began to hear how other Latina pop singers were closer to her physical reality and tried to transform herself in the image of Selena and Jennifer Lopez. When she began to sexualize her image by wearing revealing outfits and becoming the stereotyped Latina bombshell, her parents and brother reacted negatively to her new identity. Her parents complained that she was too sexualized, rebellious, and disrespectful of her cultural traditions. Her brother, who had overidentified with the Afro-American rap culture, accused her of becoming a caricature of the stereotypical Latina easy girl. Carlina felt misunderstood, because in school and among her friends she was a "hot girl." In her family's view, however, she was violating cultural codes and adopting an identity that was shameful to her family.

After Carlina met with a Latina therapist, she began to expand on the role models she had been given by her sociocultural reality and learn new alternatives for adaptation, which included a working woman, an educated professional, and a new vision of a wife and a mother that, although respectful to her cultural traditions, had a pro-feminist view. Working with a successful Latina therapist provided Carlina with a new role model and possibilities to adapt in a different way to her new reality.

A THERAPEUTIC ALTERNATIVE

Consistent with my work with other immigrants and with the ideas I developed with Jaime Inclan, I believe that the Culture and Migration Dialogue Technique is a most efficient and clinically relevant method for working with Central American families. This approach emphasizes a psychohistorical account of the family's migration experience. Beginning with an exploration of the family members' lives before migration and the circumstances surrounding their decision to leave their country, they recount their migration experience. They talk about the social and economic changes they have experienced through the process of adaptation and acculturation, and about losses, especially their loss of a social network (Hernandez & McGoldrick, 1999). As they retell their story, the therapist must pay attention to the affect and emotional impact of the events. I have found that retelling the story is very important to process the unresolved feelings that have become unconscious for the sake of adaptation. Processing such repressed feelings provides an opportunity for the family members to transform their feelings of failure into a sense of survival,

In doing this work we found (Hernandez & McGoldrick, 1999; Inclan, 2001) that an emphasis on empathy at two different levels elicits the healing. We first emphasize human empathy. At that level we validate, support, and provide some corrective emotional experience for the individuals' collective experience of trauma and distress. At another level we provide "social empathy." Social empathy goes beyond understanding and supporting the client's individual feelings. It refers to the ability of a therapist to learn and understand the emotional impact of the historical context on the family experience. This includes learning about how the family's original context, as well as the new context, affects the lives of its members. It includes learning what it is like for a family to leave everything behind for the sake of a better future, a dream that is usually unrealistic, and to understand the impact it has on individuals and families (Inclan, 2001). Social empathy is not achieved by just collecting information from family members; the therapist has to be willing to learn about their realities, their history, values, and cultural beliefs, and their struggles in adapting to a new country. It really means that the therapist has to read and learn about the group with whom he or she is working, and then check with the clients to determine whether the information he or she has about them is correct and not stereotyped (Inclan, 2001).

Another important clinical strategy in working with Central Americans is to help them contextualize their personal and family experiences by expanding the view to explore and understand the impact of sociopolitical contexts in shaping and defining their personal experiences. This provides a liberating experience, as well as an opportunity to help clients move from self-blame to sociopolitical accountability. In doing this, individuals and families who have been traumatized can first contextualize their experiences within a sociopolitical context and then define the impact of the trauma. The validation they feel by talking about it often helps them move toward working on forgiveness and reparation. Forgiveness is an important value for many Latino groups, and consistent with their religious and spiritual beliefs. Forgiveness provides spiritual permission for a person to let go and move on with his or her life. It can also free clients to hold their oppressors accountable for what happened before and after migration. Redirecting their anger and reactivity to the source of their oppression facilitates the process of empowerment.

Regaining a sense of mastery by being able to contextualize their individual and family misfortune stories within the larger sociopolitical forces that have affected their lives can provide clients an opportunity to repair their present stories. Once that goal is achieved, the family, or at least one of its members, is usually ready to commit in some way to social and political activism. As therapists, if we are committed to principles of social justice, we can hope that by using this process we can start changing our present oppressive reality, especially for undocumented immigrants and families that are victims of oppression.

REFERENCES

Almeida, R., Woods, R., Messineo, T., & Font, R. (1998). The cultural context model: An overview. In M. McGoldrick (Ed.), *Re-visioning family therapy: Race, culture, and gender in clinical practice* (pp. 414–432). New York: Guilford Press.

American Family Therapy Academy. (2004). *Position statement supporting the rights of immigrants.* Paper presented at the Joint Human Rights and Family Policy Forum at the AFTA 2004 annual meeting, San Francisco.

Arredondo, P., Orjuela, E., & Moore, L. (1989). Family therapy with Central American refugee families. *Journal of Strategic and Systemic Therapies, 8*(2), 28–35.

Bernal, G. (1982). Cuban families. In M. McGoldrick, J. K. Pearce, & J. Giordano (Eds.), *Ethnicity and family therapy* (pp. 187–206). New York: Guilford Press.

Booth, J., & Walker, T. (1993). *Understanding Central America* (2nd ed.). Boulder, CO: Westview Press.

Conover, T. (1993, September 19). The United States of asylum. *New York Times Magazine,* pp. 56–58, 74–78.

Drachman, D. (1995). Immigration statuses and their influence on service provision, access and use. *Social Work, 40*(2), 188–197.

Falicov, C. (1998). *Latino families in therapy: A guide to multicultural practice.* New York: Guilford Press

Ferrari, S. (2004). La esperanza sigue estando abajo: 25 anos despues de la revolucion Centro Americana. *Claridad, 2683,* 22–25.

Garcia, M., & Rodriguez, P. (1989). Psychological effects of political repression in Argentina and El Salvador. In D. R. Koslow & E. P. Slett (Ed.), *Crossing culture and mental health* (pp. 64–83). Washington, DC: International Society for Education, Training, and Research.

Garcia-Preto, N. (1996). Puerto Rican families. In M. McGoldrick, J. Giordano, & J. K. Pearce (Eds.), *Ethnicity and family therapy* (2nd ed., pp. 183–199). New York: Guilford Press.

Hernandez, M. (1996). Central American families. In M. McGoldrick, J. Giordano, & J. K. Pearce (Eds.), *Ethnicity and family therapy* (2nd ed., pp. 214–224). New York: Guilford Press.

Hernandez, M., & McGoldrick, M. (1999). Migration and the life cycle. In B. Carter & M. McGoldrick (Eds.), *The expanded family life cycle: Individual, family and social perspectives* (3rd ed., pp. 169–184). Boston: Allyn & Bacon.

Inclan, J. (2001). Steps toward a culture and migration dialogue for therapy with immigrant families. In S. H. McDaniel, D-D. Lusterman, & C. I. Philpot (Eds.), *Casebook for integrating family therapy: An ecosystemic approach* (pp. 229–245). Washington, DC: American Psychological Association.

Inclan, J., & Hernandez, M. (1992). Cross-cultural perspectives and codependence: The case of poor Hispanics. *American Journal of Orthopsychiatry, 16*(2), 245–255.

Inclan, J., & Quinones, M. (2003). Puerto Rican children and adolescents. In J. T. Gibbs, L. N. Huang, & Associates (Eds.), *Children of color: Psychological interventions with culturally diverse youth* (2nd ed., pp. 382–408). San Francisco: Jossey-Bass.

INS Border Apprehensions. (n.d.). Available online from United States Immigration and Naturalization Service at www.ins.gov

Lang, M. (1995, September–October). The shadow of evil. *Family Therapy Networker*, pp. 55–65.

Loucky, J., Moors, J., & Moors, M. (Eds.) (2000). *The Mayan diaspora: Guatemalan roots/new American lives*. Philadelphia: Temple University Press.

Rogler, L. (1994). International migrations: A framework for directing research. *American Psychologist, 49*(8), 701–708.

Skidmore, T., & Smith, P. (1992). *Modern Latin America* (3rd ed.). New York: Oxford University Press.

Suarez-Orozco, C., & Suarez-Orozco, M. (2001). *Children of immigration*. Cambridge, MA: Harvard University Press.

Therrien, M., & Ramirez, R. R. (2001). *The Hispanic population in the United States: March 2000 current population reports*. Washington, DC: U.S. Bureau of the Census. Available online at www.census .gov/prod/2001 pubs/p 20-535.pdf

U.S. Bureau of the Census 2000. (2001). *Summary file*. Washington, DC: U.S. Goverment Printing Office, 2001.

Valch, N. (2003). Central American children and adolescents. In J. T. Gibbs, L. N. Huand, & Associates (Eds.), *Children of color: Psychological interventions with culturally diverse youth* (2nd ed., pp. 301–343). San Francisco: Jossey-Bass.

Weingarten, K. (2003). *Common shock: Witnessing violence every day, wow we are harmed, how we can heal*. New York: Dutton.

CHAPTER 14

Colombian Families

Ramón Rojano
Jenny Duncan-Rojano

During the last three decades the population of Colombians residing in United States experienced a dramatic growth. By 2004, combining the numbers of permanent residents, U.S.-born and naturalized citizens, refugees, students, temporary workers, quasipermanent visitors, and undocumented residents, the Colombian U.S. population might have already surpassed the 1.5 million figure. This extraordinary demographic boom has elevated the visibility of Colombians in local communities across the country and has underscored the need to learn more about this particular population group.

HISTORY AND SOCIOCULTURAL CONTEXT
Basic Facts about Colombia

Located in the northwest corner of South America, Colombia is a beautiful and geographically diverse country with coasts on both the Atlantic and Pacific oceans. It borders five countries: Panama, Venezuela, Ecuador, Peru, and Brazil. The country's area of 440,381 square miles equals the combined areas of Spain, Portugal, and France. Colombia lies above the equator, and the climate varies significantly from one region to another, given the complexity and richness of its land and the presence of different levels of altitude (World Book, 2001).

Colombia has a rich and fascinating history. Precolonial Colombia was the home of powerful Indian cultures, which included among others the Chibchas, Calimas, Pijaos, and Aruacos. The first Spanish settlements were established in 1509, and the viceroyalty of Nueva Granada was established. A new ethnicity—the *criollos* or *mestizos*—was born out of the mix of Indians, Europeans, and Africans. Led by Simon Bolívar, the national independence movement was successful and the Spaniards were defeated. In 1819 the independent republic of "La Gran Colombia" (the Great Colombia) was declared, including Colombia, Ecuador, Panama, and Venezuela. In 1830, Venezuela and Ecuador

192

became separate nations, and in 1903, Panama also became independent. Since its inception, Colombia has been almost uninterruptedly a democratic country that elects a president every four years (Williams & Guerrieri, 1999).

In 2001, with an estimated population of 42,321,386 inhabitants, Colombia became the second most highly populated Spanish-speaking country of the world, after Mexico. Colombia is a country rich in natural resources, but a very poor one for many of its people. It is a nation of contrasts with major social class differences. Although some are very wealthy, the majority of the people struggle to survive and a middle class is almost nonexistent. Roman Catholicism continues to be the most common religion, with a reported affiliation of about 90% of the population (Rojano, 2001).

As a social phenomenum, *La violencia* has been constant in the background of Colombia's history for more than a half century. Its history dates back to fighting between Liberals and Conservatives, the two major political parties in the country. In 1903, the violence escalated after Panama gained its independence with the help of the United States, which had gained the rights to build the Panama Canal. The fighting between these groups increased further when, in 1948, Jorge Eliézer Gaitán, the Liberal Party's leader and a leftist, was assassinated. Starting in the late 1940s, there was also large-scale guerilla activity by rebels. Political violence turned into pure criminality, especially in the rural areas. A military junta in 1957, backed by both parties, took control after a military coup had overtaken the government and imposed repressive measures. Inflation continued to be a problem, leading to much social unrest, increased guerrilla fighting, and the growth of the drug cartels and their amassing of money, weapons, and influence. In 1998, Pastrana, a Conservative, became president and tried to negotiate a treaty with the Revolutionary Armed Forces of Colombia, the main guerrilla group. However, the fighting has continued until the present, along with the production of cocaine. Pastrana has gone ahead with his "Plan Colombia," a $7 billion social and antidrug program that included $1.3 billion largely in military aid from the United States. These chronic forms of violence have been a perturbing and distressing reality that has altered the lives of many communities. During the last decade, approximately 2 million Colombians were displaced from their homes because of the intensification of the war. It has been estimated that at least 500,000 moved to other countries, including the United States (Grupo Temático de Desplazamiento, 2000).

Colombians have also been battered by the war on drugs. According to the U.S. Drug Enforcement Administration (DEA), "organized crime groups operating in Colombia control the worldwide supply of cocaine. These organizations use a sophisticated infrastructure to move cocaine into the United States" (DEA, 2001). Both the Colombian government and the population at large have traditionally been against the drug cartels, and the war on drugs has resulted in the deaths of thousands of government officials, politicians, law enforcement agencies, journalists, and many other members of Colombian society. It is believed that the affiliation between armed groups and drug traffickers has had a lot to do with the widespread increase in violence during the last decade.

Diverse Populations

The present Colombian population resulted from mixes of the native aborigines, the conquering Europeans, and the Africans who were brought as slaves. Colombian demographers have classified the various types of mixes as follows: *mestizos* (Indians and Whites), *mulatos* (Whites and Blacks), and *zambos* (Indians and Blacks). The population has been estimated to split as follows: *mestizos*, 58%; Whites, 20%; *mulatos*, 14%; Blacks, 4%; *zambos*, 3%; and Indians, 1% (CIDEIBER, 1998). In Colombia there are 81 Indian tribes, which some believe have a total population of more than one million people.

Even though Colombia's 1991 constitution recognized the "multiethnic and pluricultural character of the nation and created mandates for the protection and development of the diverse populations, the socioeconomic conditions and quality of life of both the indigenous and Afrocolombian communities continue to be inferior to the one for whites and Mestizos" (Fundacion Hemera, 2004). An estimated 80% of Afro-Colombians live in conditions of extreme poverty, and nationwide less than 59% of the total population lives below the poverty line (U.S. Office on Colombia, 2003).

The 1991 constitution also provided for equal protection of the right to "personal and family intimacy" and the right to "the free development of one's personality." Colombia also has had openly gay politicians and an active Gay and Lesbian Information Network. However, traditional Colombian society continues to be opposed to homosexual, bisexual, and transgender lifestyles, and over the past few years, prejudice toward homosexuals has hardened (GAYTIMES, 2003).

COLOMBIANS IN THE UNITED STATES

In the 2000 U.S. census, 470,684 individuals identified themselves as Colombians. However, there was a major flaw in the process, and a large proportion of Latinos (6,211,800, or 17.6 %) listed themselves in the newly introduced category "Other Latino Group." This resulted in a potentially massive undercount of Colombians and people of other nationalities. Subsequently, in 2002, the U.S. Bureau of the Census estimated that the number of just Colombian-born individuals in the United States was 510,158. Colombians are concentrated primarily in four states: Florida, 29%; New York, 22%; New Jersey, 13%; and California, 7%.

The average size of Colombian families in the United States was reported to be 3.21 persons, which is larger than the average size of American families (2.59). The majority (54.2%) are female. The median household income of Colombians in the United States is 38,514, which is 91.7% of the average for U.S. citizens ($41,994). The poorest Colombians seem to be those living in Miami, with an income of $23,483. The majority, or 61.6%, are adults and young adults between 20 and 55 years of age. Children below 18 years of age make up only 22.1% of the population. Colombians' high interest in education is underscored by the following statistics: 74.5% of the U.S. Colombian population have at least a high school diploma, and 23.7% a bachelor's or higher degree. In comparison, the average education attainments for the Latino U.S. population are 52.4% and 10.4%, respectively (U.S. Bureau of the Census, 2000).

Reasons for Migration

A survey of Colombian immigrants showed the following reasons for migration: seeking a better job or higher education, escaping from violence or difficult family situations, and looking for an international experience (Rojano, 1993). Recently, exposure to higher levels of violence, experiences related to kidnappings, death threats, and the intensification of the political conflict have contributed to a massive migration out of Colombia (Forero, 2001; Velez et al., 1997).

Legal Status

The majority of Colombians live legally in the United States. In 1991, the new Colombian constitution allowing for dual citizenship was adopted (Gaviria, 1991). As a consequence, a surge in naturalizations occurred and the level of political participation increased in the United States. Simultaneously, the number of American-born Colombians has continued to grow. Others live here as legal residents or with temporary visitor, worker, or student status. Just in 2002, more than 400,000 Colombians entered this country with temporary visas (Office of Immigration Statistics, 2003.) In regard to the undocumented population, the U.S. Immigration and Naturalization Service (2003) has estimated that approximately 141,000 Colombians stayed in this country without having appropriate documentation in the year 2000. Practitioners should be aware that many Colombian families have a "fluid" status. With temporary visitor's visas, many have a quasi-permanent residence in the United States and go to Colombia once or twice a year. Yearly, an unspecified number of temporary visitors or undocumented migrants change their status to students, refugees, or permanent residents. Along with many other countries, Colombia has almost uninterruptedly enjoyed strong support from Washington. Political and economic agreements that have been negotiated between the two countries provide for the annual admittance of a good number of migrants into the United States.

CULTURAL PATTERNS

The country's diversity in history, geography, ethnicity, and socioeconomic conditions poses a challenge to the notion of a unique profile for Colombians. Nevertheless, various attempts have been made to study the Colombian culture, and descriptions of socioeconomic characteristics and cultural patterns of specific regional groups are available (Gutiérrez de Pineda, 1975). These patterns show a separation of male–female roles, with behaviors previously described as *machismo* and *marianismo* (Rojano, 1985a; Rojas de Gonzáles, 1985). However, these traditional patterns are changing rapidly, with women now playing a more active role in the labor market and in society in general (Rojano, 1985b).

The following sections describe cultural patterns, values, and behaviors that are observable with some frequency in Colombian families.

Adventurous and Entrepreneurial Spirit

Always enduring high unemployment rates, Colombians are trained early to be creative and entrepreneurial. Additional sources of income are generated through home-based business or other creative ventures. *Rebuscarse* (to reseek for something) is a fundamental way of surviving and coping. Historically, geographic circumstances required people to work in places distant from their homes such as mines, farms, and rivers. With this background, Colombians find the United States a fertile ground for the development of many projects. This attitude is a primary cultural asset that can be used positively in the implementation of any family development plan. Yet a negative aspect is that the search for creative ways of succeeding may hinder the potential to follow traditional paths to success and may also cause family instability. Marital discord usually stems from the relocating-versus-staying dilemma.

Endurance and Sacrifice

From the traditional Catholic teachings, Colombians derived a major tendency to sacrifice and usually show high levels of endurance to painful situations or the troubles of life. They don't accept defeat easily and tend to be persistent and relentless. Many engage in "lost causes" and have difficulty in giving them up and moving forward.

Leadership and Altruism

Colombians tend to be dynamic, passionate, courageous, and generous. Leadership is spontaneously displayed in cases of natural disasters and is manifested at a micro-level in response to personal or family crises. Colombians are also very idealistic and patriotic and tend to feel responsible for helping other family members and friends.

Festive Spirit

Colombians are typically high spirited and enjoy life as much as they can. Their joyful and enthusiastic spirit can even be contagious. Colombian music, particularly the *Cumbia*, is played and danced around the world. Colombians, always ready to celebrate, frequently organize weekend family parties that help boost their spirits. These parties may also serve as distractions that prevent them from dealing directly with family conflicts.

High Interest in Education and Language

Being one of the major viceroyalties of the continent, the Great Colombia became the intellectual epicenter of this "new world," and Santa Fé de Bogotá was known as the "Athens of South America." From this period, Colombians inherited great pride in intellectual achievement and superior language skills. Working and sacrificing to help children attain college graduation is culturally conceived as both a family responsibility and a legacy. Colombians also tend to make a great efforts to speak almost perfectly. The high expectation for children's performance is a natural source of conflicts, and the expected perfection in their own language sometimes prevents them from trying to practice English as a new language.

Diplomacy

Although some other cultural groups value the ability to be sincere and frank, many Colombians, especially those coming from the interior of the country, try to be diplomatic and avoid open disagreement with other people. This diplomatic tendency helps to perpetuate family secrets and hide disagreements with family members, friends, neighbors, or coworkers. The result can be a low level of assertiveness and failure to openly address personal needs.

Social Status

Upon the inception of the "Nueva Granada," the Spaniards organized a society of various social classes. Those belonging or related to royalty were considered "high class" and enjoyed special privileges. Once Colombia achieved its independence, the *Criollo* leaders (children of Spaniards) reproduced the same structure, and a privileged elite seized domain over most of the land. The development of the oligarchy is the main reason for the uprising of armed groups that 50 years ago organized the peasants and rebelled against the landowners. Because in 1819 Blacks were declared independent along with the mainstream population, racism was never formally institutionalized. However, the Black population remains segregated in various regions of the country, and a correlation between lighter skin color and better social status is easily observable.

Regionalism

Regional differences are marked by geography, climate, race, and ethnicity and also depend on the regional origin of the Spaniards who settled in specific Colombian areas. For example, in the Andean mountains social behaviors tend to resemble those of other Andean countries, such as Peru or Chile. Mediterranean and African influences are felt on the Caribbean coast, where people exhibit cultural patterns similar to those of other Caribbean countries such as Cuba, Puerto Rico, or the Dominican Republic (Gutiérrez de Pineda, 1975; López, Rojano, Hoyos, & Colorado, 1982). Regional differences are also related to ethnic backgrounds. For example, mestizos vastly predominate in the interior, whereas a good proportion of mulatos and zambos live on the Atlantic and Pacific coasts, respectively. Colombians in the United States tend to socialize and organize according to these regional differences, and there is still some animosity between the various groups. Conflicts are related to different levels of access to power and resources and to long-lasting interregional stereotypes.

Attitude toward Stereotypes

The increase in drug trafficking and violence has affected the way in which Colombians are viewed. They frequently have to endure rumors and jokes and must deal with the negative stereotype that associates them with drugs, as well as worry about being wrongfully targeted for investigations and searches. This reality now shapes many behavioral patterns of Colombians in the United States.

The Impact of Violence

More recently, a substantial number of Colombians in therapy relate symptoms in response to existing violence. Many have been directly affected by the experiences of kidnapping, life threats, assaults, and loss of loved ones. Others live in constant fear for the safety and lives of close relatives and friends who remain in Colombia.

Commonalities

The following characteristics of Latino families in general are also observed in Colombians: strong family orientation, spirituality, humor, friendliness, warmth, and passion for sports. They also tend to present adaptation problems, nostalgia, machismo, over-involvement with children, shame, and guilt.

TREATMENT IMPLICATIONS

Reasons for Seeking Help

Colombian families may seek help for marital conflicts, difficulties with teenage children, and posttraumatic stress symptoms. Other frequent problems include alcohol abuse, passive–aggressiveness, shame, guilt, family violence, depression, and somatization. Alcoholism tends to be common in males, and depression occurs frequently in women (León, 1993). Colombians may show somatization resulting from postmigration stress. Higher somatization indices among Colombian patients with major depression, as compared with North American patients, have been reported (Escobar, 1987; Escobar, Gomez, & Tuason, 1983). Lack of insurance coverage, limited knowledge, prejudice against mental illness, and shame are factors that prevent Colombians from seeking mental health therapy. Initially, they try to resolve issues within the extended family and/or with friends, and, if necessary, they tend to consult with their doctors.

Mauricio Correa was a 17-year-old teenager who lived in New York with his parents, a 10-year-old sister, and a 7-year-old brother. He was referred to counseling by a schoolteacher whom he had approached, seeking information about legal ways of becoming emancipated from his parents. Sensing a major family conflict, the teacher referred him for family counseling. The entire family had come to this country 5 years earlier as legal residents under the auspices of Mrs. Correa's sister, who was an American citizen. His parents, both in their late 40s, were still struggling with acculturation issues, finding it quite difficult to learn English. Their hope was to work very hard, buy a house, and put their children through college. Mr. Correa worked during the day in a factory and in the evenings cleaned buildings with his wife. Mrs. Correa baby-sat a friend's child, and on Saturdays both worked cleaning family homes. Previously, in Colombia, Mr. Correa had obtained a college degree and worked in his own furniture store. Mrs. Correa had worked as a day-care teacher.

    Mauricio was a low-performing high school senior who seemed more interested in music than anything else. Based on tradition, both parents were already saving money to buy a house and to finance Mauricio's education. They expected him to be a successful professional, who in return would help them pay for his siblings' college tuitions. Everything was working fairly well until the father's brother was kidnapped and murdered in Colombia, leaving a wife and three children. Mr. Correa thought it was his responsibility to take care of this family and developed the idea of moving to Miami to start a furniture business with a friend who lived in south Florida. He would bring his relatives to this country and use the business to provide employment opportunities for the entire family. For this venture, he planned to use existing family savings. This plan created a major distress for the entire family. Mauricio and his siblings opposed the plan. Mrs. Correa was also in disagreement, but she did not dare talk against it. She did not want her husband or the relatives in Colombia to think she was being inconsiderate of their feelings and needs. Mauricio seemed to be the only one capable of expressing disagreement, and arguments with his father were frequent. The conflict escalated even further when Mauricio announced that soon after completing high school he planned to find a job and move with a friend. His parents joined in disagreement with this plan. At that moment, two major issues were at stake. First, middle-class Colombian families traditionally have a major interest in sending their children to college. Second, launching a child is expected to be smooth and fully approved by parents. Unless children move to another city, they are not expected to leave their parents' house until graduating from college or after getting married. Having a teenager go to work and move out of the home without any clear college plans is culturally unacceptable and is considered as a major family crisis.

During the first session, the therapist learned that this was a middle-class family from the interior of Colombia, experiencing problems in two areas: (1) They were experiencing acculturation problems (limited English skills, limited professional development, lack of social networks, and their adolescent's search for independent living), and (2) right here in the United States, they were also directly suffering the impact of the Colombian violence. The therapist invited the family to conjointly explore ways to deal effectively with both situations. He devoted one session to helping the father talk about his humiliation and shame about his current jobs. Seeing his father cry helped Mauricio to understand his father better and to reconcile with him. In a subsequent session the family was able to let Mr. Correa know why they did not want to leave. He was able to understand that his entire family was more deeply rooted in New York City than he could ever have believed.

Both parents agreed to use part of the savings to bring the relatives to this country and hire a lawyer to file a petition for political asylum. They also decided to seek other types of jobs and take some English classes that were available. This general plan worked well. One year later, the relatives had established legal residency in New York and had their own apartment. Mrs. Correa completed specialized courses and had started a licensed home-based day-care business. Mr. Correa was working as a driver for a large furniture store, had joined a Colombian club, and was making progress in English. Mauricio was still living at home while enrolled in a city college, worked part time, and was paying for his own new car. He was also planning to spend his last 2 years of study at the college campus.

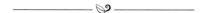

This case had a successful outcome because of the following factors:

1. The therapist identified and focused on two primary issues.
2. The acculturation issue was worked out well. A middle ground was negotiated between the traditional, rigid family values and the need for the client's independence.
3. The harmonious and respectful planning approach matched the culture of this family.
4. The intervention provided for skill development and careful financial planning.
5. The therapist validated various Colombian family values, such as loyalty to their relatives in trouble and the quest for educational achievement.

CONCLUSION

To work effectively with Colombians, it is necessary to depart from traditional treatment modalities and use comprehensive and creative approaches that deal with particular issues, simultaneously working on increasing the level of functioning and acculturation within the American society. For example, we have successfully tried the tridimensional Community Family Therapy (CFT) method with Colombian families. This approach assesses three basic areas: psychological clearance and drive, support systems, and skills and strengths. CFT focuses on three treatment goals: (1) constructing an autobiography that focuses on strengths and a life plan that invites positive action and family development, (2) developing a functional and effective network of supportive resources, and (3) providing for leadership development and civic engagement (Rojano, 2004).

Any other approach that covers the aforementioned areas can be also helpful. However, regardless of the approach used, it is important always to check the following four categories: regional origin, social class, legal status, and reason for migration. Interventions must also assess and treat previous traumatic experiences. Colombian identity must be reinforced while simultaneously building bridges with the mainstream community.

REFERENCES

CIDEIBER. (Centro de Información y Documentación Empresarial sobre Iberoamérica). (1998). *Colombia, perfil demografico y social.* Available at www.cideiber.com/infopaises/Colombia/Colombia-02-01.html

Drug Enforcement Administration (DEA). (2001). *Drug trafficking in the United States.* Available at www.usdoj.gov/dea/pubs/intel/01020/#c1

Escobar, J. (1987, February). Cross-cultural aspects of the somatization trait. *Hospital and Community Psychiatry, 38*(2), 174–180.

Escobar, J. I., Gomez, J., & Tuason, V. B. (1983). Depressive phenomenology in North and South American patients. *American Journal of Psychiatry, 40,* 47–51.

Forero, J. (2001, April 10). Prosperous Colombians flee. Many to U.S. to escape war. *New York Times,* p. A1.

Fundacion Hemera. (2004). *Etnias de Colombia: Afrocolombianos.* Available at www.etniasdecolombia.org/grupos_afro_poblacion.asp

Gaviria, C. (1991). *Constitución Política de Colombia.* Santa Fe de Bogota, Colombia: Ediciones J. Bernal.

GAYTIMES. (2003). *Lesbian and Gay Colombia.* Available at www.gaytimes.co.uk/gt/default.asp?topic=country&country=284

Grupo Temático de Desplazamiento. (2000). *Datos sobre desplazamiento en Colombia.* Available at www.col.ops-oms.org/desplazados/cifras/default.htm

Gutiérrez de Pineda, V. (1975). *Familia y Cultura en Colombia: Tipologías, funciones y Dinámica de las Familia* (Vol. 2). Bogota, Colombia: Instituto Colombiano de Cultura.

León, C. A. (1993). The clinical profile of disthymia in a group of Latin American women: Worldwide therapeutic strategies in atypical depressive syndromes. *European Psychiatry, 8*(5), 257–255.

López, O., Rojano, R., Hoyos, D., & Colorado, G. (1983). *Algunas características socioeconómicas y culturales de las familias del área urbana del municipio de Medellín.* Medellín, Colombia: Universidad de Antioquia. Facultad de Medicina.

Office of Immigration Statistics. (2003). *Yearbook of immigration statistics.* Available at www.uscis.gov/graphics/shared/aboutus/statistics/TEMP02yrbk/TEMPExcel/Table25.xls

Rojano, R. (1985a). El conflicto conyugal a través del ciclo vital en Colombia. *Revista Colombiana de Psiquiatría, 14*(4), 453–462.

Rojano, R. (1985b). Problemas socioculturales de la familia y tres alternativas de la terapia de familia en Colombia. *Revista Colombiana de Psiquiatría, 14*(1) 143–169.

Rojano, R. (1993). *Migration and acculturation patterns of Colombian families in the United States.* Paper presented at the 32nd annual meeting of the Colombian Psychiatric Association. Medellín, Colombia.

Rojano, R. (2001). Colombians. In A Lopez & E. Carrasquillo (Eds.), *The Hispanic patient.* Washington, DC: American Psychiatric Association.

Rojano, R. (2004). The practice of community family therapy. *Family Process, 43*(1), 59–75.

Rojas de González, N. (1985). *Conflictos de pareja y familia.* Bogota, Colombia: U. Publicaciones.

U.S. Bureau of the Census. (1999a). *Statistical abstract of the United States, 1998.* Washington, DC: U.S. Bureau of the Census.

U.S. Bureau of the Census. (1999b). Statistical abstract of the United States. Washington, DC. In T. B. Heaton, B. A. Chadwick, & C. K. Jacobson (2000). *Statistical handbook on racial groups in the United States.* Phoenix, AZ: Oryx Press.

U.S. Bureau of the Census. (1999c). *World population profile: 1998.* Report WP/98. Washington, DC: U.S. Government Printing Office.

U.S. Bureau of the Census. (2000). *DP-1. Profile of the general demographic characteristics: 2000. Census 2000 Summary File 2 (SF2) 100 Percent Data. And DP-2. Profile of selected social characteristics: 2000. Census 2000 Summary File 4 (SF 4)—Sample data. Geographic Area: United States. Racial or ethnic grouping: Colombian.* Available at www.factfinder.census.gov

U.S. Immigration and Naturalization Service, Office of Policy and Planning. (2003). *Estimates of the unauthorized immigrant population residing in the United States: 1990 to 2000.* Available at www.uscis.gov/graphics/shared/aboutus/statistics/Ill_Report_1211.pdf

U.S. Office on Colombia. (2003). *Afro-Colombians.* Available at usofficeoncolombia.org/afro-colombianos.htm

Velez, L., McAllister, A., & Hu, S. (1997, August). Measuring attitudes toward violence in Colombia. *Journal of Social Psychology, 137*(4), 533–534.

Williams, R. L., & Guerrieri, K. G. (1999). *Culture and customs of Colombia.* Wesport, CT: Greenwood Press.

World Book 2001. (2001). *Colombia* (Vol. 4). Chicago: World Book.

CHAPTER 15

Cuban Families

Guillermo Bernal
Ester Shapiro

Family development occurs at the crossroads of politics and history, yet the Cuban American family experience has been uniquely shaped by the highly polarized political struggle between the United States and Fidel Castro's socialist government. Starting with the triumph of the Cuban revolution in 1959, Cuban immigration to the United States has been described as a "cold war faucet . . . abruptly turned off and on at the will of those in power in Havana and Washington in response to political considerations" (Perez, 2001, p. 92). A recent iconic example of this struggle and its tragic consequences was evident in the custody battle over Elian Gonzalez, a 5-year-old Cuban child who washed up in Miami on Thanksgiving Day in 1999. Elian was the sole survivor of an attempt to flee Cuba by raft in which his mother, stepfather, and 10 others drowned. Elian's mother, encouraged by the U.S. government's "dry feet/wet feet" policy, whereby Cubans landing on U.S. soil are awarded legal residency after a year, had taken her son and left Cuba on a flimsy, overcrowded boat without notifying the boy's father or his paternal grandparents. When Elian landed on the Miami shore, a divisive, highly politicized, and emotionally explosive custody battle began between Elian's father (supported by Castro, who wanted to bring the deeply traumatized boy home to his family) and Elian's great-uncle and other family members in Miami (supported by the anti-Castro Cuban American exile community, who insisted that Elian's mother had died for freedom and only her son's freedom would honor her sacrifice). The agonizing, fascinating, media-fueled global spectacle included the sanctification of Elian's rescue by magical dolphins, the demonization of Cuban Communism as represented by Fidel Castro, and the crass manipulation of a deeply traumatized boy with a shower of consumer products, as if total strangers could replace the family, friends, and landscape he knew and loved. The ordeal finally ended with Elian's return to Cuba, but only because the U.S. attorney general's office ordered that the child be forcibly seized in an armed raid on the Gonzalez home, which was being guarded by members of Alpha 66, a Cuban exile terrorist organization.

For many in the Cuban American "one-and-a-half generation," that is, Cubans born on the island who had come to the United States as children (including us, the authors of this chapter), the battle over Elian's future undermined an emerging reconciliation in our embattled communities and magnified the intense hatreds, longings, and distortions of reality that characterize our transnational family feud. Perhaps the most painful distress at how Elian Gonzalez's losses were compounded by political intransigence on both sides was experienced by the 14,000 Cuban Americans who had been sent to the United States alone as children during the 1960–1962 Operation Pedro Pan (Peter Pan) (Torres, 2003b). Most of them, now adults in their 40s and 50s with children of their own, relived the anguish of their own traumatic separation from their parents and in many cases empathized with Elian's father as he fought to avoid losing custody of his child for political reasons. After a March 2000 panel on Cuban identity, which was held during the height of the controversy at the Latin American Studies Association meeting in Miami, an organizer of the South Florida Pedro Pan Association shared a moving experience. Two weeks after Elian's arrival and shortly after his 6th birthday, she had been invited to visit him at his relatives' home in Miami. When she tried to explain to him how her own story of exile as an unaccompanied minor connected to his plight, she realized that he had no idea of who Peter Pan was, and she explained that he was a boy who never grew up and knew how to fly. Elian ran excitedly around the room, flapping his "wings," declaring that he too would learn how to fly so he could fly home to his family. As she left, he followed her and sat in the back seat of her car, believing she could get him home. Still shaken by this poignant memory, she remarked that in subsequent television footage, Elian was filmed outside in the fenced yard, flapping his arms and practicing his flying.

The story of the Cuban American family experience must be told as an intergenerational narrative of love, loyalty, and longing, within which memory is a highly contested political territory. Socioeconomic, political, cultural, and historical events spanning centuries, though accelerating in the last 45 years, have directly impacted intimate family relationships and their expression in the developmental pathways of all its members. Intergenerational tensions within Cuban families have been documented not only within the family therapy field, but also by Cuban American writers, many of whom evocatively describe their struggles to preserve family loyalty while defining their own relationship to both Cuban and American identities. Carlos Eire began writing his award-winning memoir, *Waiting for Snow in Havana* (2003), when Elian Gonzalez's plight coincided with his children's reaching the age he was when he had left Cuba with Operation Pedro Pan, opening a floodgate of vivid memories about his many family losses. Growing up in Cuba, a privileged son in a wealthy, eccentric, deeply Catholic family, Eire's exile ended his childhood and scattered his family, and Fidel Castro remains portrayed as the demonic force at the heart of this violent betrayal. Others, like the women who contributed to Maria de los Angeles Torres's *By Heart/De Memoria* (2003a), represent a more complicated reckoning with the thwarted dreams and desires of Cubans on both sides of the ideological divide. Performance artist Alina Troyano, who created the outrageous theatrical persona Carmelita Tropicana, documents in her autobiographical *Milk of Amnesia/Leche de Amnesia* (1995) her own problematic attempts at Americanization and the return of her repressed *cubanidad*. Cuban American critic and performance artist Coco Fusco (1994, 1995) displays a photograph of her mother carrying her as an infant as they descend from the plane after leaving Cuba. Like Ester Rebeca Shapiro Rok's photo (Shapiro, 1994a) of her family's last Purim in a Havana synagogue, Fusco's photograph marks a moment of migration frozen in time; a moment to which the family returns, again and again, in its process of building and rebuilding the dislocated intergenerational relationships that make up Cuban American family life. This chapter draws from literary sources such as *testimonios* and memoirs, as well as social science and family therapy sources, to describe the Cuban American family experience and to suggest effective therapeutic responses that understand our families within a socioeconomic, political, cultural, and historical context. Because we believe that an understanding of the broader social context is an inseparable aspect of working with Cuban families, we begin with a brief description of the context.

Cuba is the largest island in the Caribbean, with a total area of 44,218 square miles (approximately the size of Pennsylvania). Because of its unique geographical position between the Florida and Yucatan peninsulas, some historians have suggested that Cuba's historical significance is out of proportion to its size (Foner, 1962). To the Spanish, Cuba was quite literally the "key" to the Americas, inasmuch as traffic bound to and from Mexico, Peru, and other points in South America was generally routed through Havana. Indeed, at different moments in history, access to the Americas was possible only through Cuba.

To the newly emerging nation of the United States, only 90 miles away from Cuba, it was becoming quite evident in the mid-1800s that the island held great strategic economic, political, and military significance for Spain. In 1898, Cuba's War of Independence from Spain attracted a major U.S. intervention. During the course of the Spanish-American War, the United States invaded Cuba, as well as Puerto Rico, the Philippines, and Guam. These islands became U.S. colonies, but Cuba was able to achieve independence. However, independence came at the price of a military base (Guantánamo Bay) and an amendment to the Cuban Constitution that granted the United States the right to intervene in internal Cuban affairs (repealed in 1933).

Cuba remained bound to U.S. interests until the revolution in 1959. An analysis of the historical developments that preceded the revolution is beyond the scope of this chapter; there are a number of volumes available on the topic (e.g., Castro, 1972, 1975; Kirk & Paduras Fuentes, 2001; Pérez-Stable, 1999; Thomas, 1977). The programs promoted by the revolutionary government produced changes in the social, economic, and political structures of society. These changes, together with a U.S. economic blockade, produced dissatisfaction within sectors of Cuban society, which led to an extensive migration, primarily to the United States. The abruptness of the Cuban migration, its magnitude within a relatively brief period, and its predominantly middle- and upper-class composition (particularly during the earliest waves of migration) amplified its impact and created a unique situation in relation to other Latino populations in the United States.

CUBAN MIGRATION IN CONTEXT

Cubans have been migrating to the United States since the middle of the 19th century (Pérez, 2001). The two countries share a history that dates back almost 200 years. The Cuban wars of independence (1868–1878 and 1895–1898) resulted in many Cubans being exiled to the United States, where they often formed support communities for the pro-independence forces. Overall, there were perhaps 30,000 Cubans in the United States by 1958 (West, 1995). The largest Cuban immigration has occurred since the triumph of the Cuban revolution in 1959: More than 1.1 million Cubans have left their homeland since that year. Boswell (2002) used Census 2000 data and other sources to conduct the first study of 40 years of Cuban American demographics.

Although Cubans number only 3.7% of the U.S. Latino/Latina population, they have been singled out as a success story and viewed as a "model minority." The relative success of Cubans in the United States must be understood in terms of the sociohistorical context and its political meaning in the context of the Cold War (1945–1990) and U.S. foreign policy. The Cuban migration served U.S. interests, such as destabilizing Cuba, pointing to the dangers of communism, and highlighting a contemporary example of the rags-to-riches story of an immigrant group (Bernal, 1982; G. Bernal & Gutierrez, 1988; West, 1995).

Cuban success in the United States is associated with the nature of the Cuban migration and its historical context (Bernal, 1982; G. Bernal & Gutierrez, 1988; Pérez, 2001). For example, in contrast to the characteristics of Mexican and Puerto Rican immigrants (see Chapters 17 and 18), the Cuban migration of the 1960s—the first of four waves of modern migration—included primarily White, educated, upper- and middle-class professional groups that were less likely to experience racial barriers. In addition, these immigrants had educational and business know-how, shared U.S. cultural values, and received financial support from major federal programs (Bernal, 1982; G. Bernal & Gutierrez, 1988; Pérez, 2001). Arriving in large numbers within short periods, benefiting from these advantages, and believing that Castro's government would not last long, these immigrants created what Portes (1995) has called the "golden exile," a tightly knit community with economic and political power that made it possible for the unyielding ideologies of the first privileged exiles to dominate politically even as the community grew more diverse and complex with subsequent arrivals. Cuban exiles were also aided by the Cuban Adjustment Act of 1966, which helped them to legalize their status in the United States, and the Cuban Refugee Program, considered to be the most intensive refugee program in U.S. history (Szapocznik, Cohen, & Hernandez, 1985).

Scholars identify four phases of post-revolutionary migration (Pérez, 2001). The early phases of immigration, being primarily composed of Whites, females, and older individuals, did not represent the Cuban population as a whole (Bernal, 1982; Fagan, Brody, & O'Leary, 1968). The third phase of refugees exited Cuba via the port of Mariel; most were working class or unemployed and had a larger percentage of Afro-Cubans, as well as young men with no immediate kinship networks abroad. The United States and Cuba negotiated an orderly immigration policy after the 1980 Mariel incidents.

A fourth phase of migration began in 1989, when the Cuban economy entered into the *período especial* (special period) upon the disintegration of the Soviet Union and the subsequent end of aid to Cuba. With their difficulties compounded by the U.S. economic blockade, the years from 1991 to the present have been characterized by extraordinary economic hardship for the Cuban people, with an increased number willing to take great risks to reach the United States. This crisis reached its peak in the summer of 1994, when thousands of Cubans tried to elude the coastal police and attempted to cross the Straits of Florida on makeshift rafts. In July and August, when the flow of *balseros* (rafters) was becoming impossible to control, and in the absence of any U.S. interest in opening talks on immigration policy, Havana again declared that anyone wishing to leave Cuba could do so. More than 37,000 *balseros* attempted passage. About 20,000 were intercepted by the U.S. Coast Guard and sent to Guantánamo Bay (Ackerman & Clark, 1996; Castro, 2000; Eckstein & Barbieri, 2001).

We should note that the social and political dynamics in Miami are changing. The older, more emotionally politicized generation is being replaced by a more practical younger generation that has less difficulty in doing business with or even traveling to Cuba, despite the restrictions by the U.S Treasury. New Latin American immigrants are also helping to create a greater political balance between more politically diverse groups and the ideological hard-liners of the older Cuban American generation (Stepik & Stepik, 2002).

The political and economic situation in Cuba remains difficult. Although the recent legalization of the dollar and the diversification of the economy have improved Cubans' daily life, these measures have also polarized society between those who have, and those who do not have, access to U.S. dollars. The U.S. government continues its policy of economic blockade. As the two countries continue their polarized ideological battles, an increasing number of Cubans in both Cuba and the United States are softening political barriers and seeking greater contact between the two communities, which share an intense if embattled kinship (Task Force on Memory, Truth and Justice, 2003). These new transnational alliances are reflected in the $1 billion of remittances sent by Cuban Americans to the island, contributing to its gross national product, and in the 130,000 visits by Cuban Americans to the island every year. In contrast to the hard-liners' insistence on the "embargo" as a way to topple Fidel Castro, it is clear, as evidenced by the paths of other Communist regimes, that the most potent weapon is commerce, in both the economic and communicative sense. In the meantime, Fidel Castro, despite the erosion of his popularity in Cuba, Latin America, and elsewhere over the last decade, even among those on the left, remains a figure of historical value and respect, not only to Cubans on the island but to Latin Americans and Caribbean peoples throughout the region, who respect his success in standing up to U.S. dominance since the island is "too far from God and too close to the United States" (Castro, 2000).

CUBAN CULTURAL HERITAGE

The creative integration of many cultural threads, including those found in the new Cuban American context, characterizes the struggle of Cuban American families to define new identities while preserving continuity with, and retaining loyalty to, their culture of origin. This process of cultural transformation can best be understood in its intergenerational and developmental context (Bernal, 1982; G. Bernal & Gutierrez, 1988; Shapiro, 1994a, 1994b, 1996), as emphasized throughout the rest of this chapter.

Writers have described the Cuban and the Cuban American cultures as offering an example of "transculturation," in which cultures meet and transform one another. Anthropologist Fernando Ortíz first offered the term "transculturation" in the 1940s, in an effort to oppose the newly coined and still predominant anthropological term "acculturation," which Ortíz (1973) found too unabashed in its colonializing assumptions and inaccurate in describing the Cuban experience. Ortíz, followed by Afro-Cuban poet Nancy Morejón (1993) and many other scholars, views Cuban culture as the creative intermingling of indigenous Spanish, African, and Asian cultures, each newly arriving group contributing something to the *ajiaco*, or stew, whose ingredients are enriched by the presence of all the others.

If we follow Ortíz and Morejón to explore the implications of transculturation as an alternative to acculturation in the intergenerational experience of Cuban families, we find that the possibility for cultural creativity is enhanced. Pérez Firmat (1994) also makes this argument in his book *Life on the Hyphen*, even extending Ortíz's image of the Cuban *ajiaco* to a Cuban American tropical soup in Miami. Whereas acculturation implies the cultural loss of *cubanidad* as a primary source of individual and family identity, transculturation emphasizes continuity, mutual transformation, and cultural changes. American-style autonomy grants both men and women greater personal freedom for role inventiveness, as long as it is well balanced by the need for interdependence and family connections, which are an important contributions to Cuban cultural identity. Testimonials of Cuban Americans in the "one-and-a-half generation" describe their journey—as adults whose images of Cuba have frozen in time, and who have experienced politically motivated family cutoffs—to return and bring back living images of Cuba and restored family connections. These bridges to Cuba enrich families' ongoing development (Fusco, 1994, 1995; Gonzales-Mandri, 1994; Risech, 1994; Shapiro, 1994a, 1996; Torres, 1994; Troyano, 1995).

Researchers and clinicians have focused on an appreciation of cultural values in working with Cuban families (Bernal, 1982; Queralt, 1984; Rumbaut & Rumbaut, 1976; Szapocznik, Kurtines, & Hanna, 1979). Cubans share many Latin American and African cultural patterns (Bustamante & Santa Cruz, 1975; Ortíz, 1973), such as the value of the family, language, and social supports. At the same time, the creative transformation of culture that results from the dialogue between the culture of origin and the new circumstances, especially for new generations, is generating new forms of personal and cultural identity. New waves of immigrants are helping to re-Cubanize the newer generations by teaching them about Cuban culture. As the transnational traffic between Cuba and the United States transcends the current ideological divide, we may see even greater evolution in the creative connections between Cubans on the island and in the United States.

The Family

The role of the nuclear and extended family is central to Cubans. Ritual kinship, or *compadrazgo*, is important to many Cuban immigrants in the United States. *Familismo* is a cultural attitude and value that places the interests of the family over the interest of the individual and is the basis of the traditional Cuban family structure (Bernal, 1982; Queralt, 1984). The bonds of loyalty and unity, which include nuclear and extended family members, characterize the Cuban family. Maintaining a traditional family hierarchy with the man as provider depends on social and economic factors. *Respeto* (respect) is a means of reinforcing male authority over women and children. Conflicts may arise when the wife works, shifting the economic basis of the marriage. However, a characteristic of the Cuban "golden exile" has been its capacity to permit women to work outside the home within socially sanctioned gendered settings within family- and friend-owned businesses, supporting a slower gendered acculturation process. Moreover, as family members acculturate, conflicts emerge from the clash of values between generations (Bernal, 1982; G. Bernal & Gutierrez, 1988; Pérez, 2001; Szapocznik & Kurtines, 1993). As previously noted, the nature of Cuban marriages and family life is related to social class, degree of acculturation, migration stage, and Latino family values. The notions of *machismo* remain strong, although the traditional notion of female purity has been complicated by the long sojourn in a highly permissive, sexually open U.S. community. In contemporary Miami, where the "South Beach" area has become a magnet for the beauty and fashion industry, more acculturated Cuban American women struggle to bridge two very different worlds of body image, beauty, and sexuality. Cuban Americans also may be exposed to new ways of expressing alternative sexual orientations, such as gay, lesbian, and bisexual.

Family loyalty and cohesion are positive protective factors associated with resilience in immigrant families. For the Cuban families who were part of the earlier migrations, this dimension of family strength is often complicated by the rigid insistence on an ideology of punitive embargo and a fantasy that Castro's regime will be overturned, a very poor assessment of the prevailing realities. Bonnin and Brown (2000) conducted an intriguing study of family adaptability and cohesion as contributors to purpose in life and well-being among 104 recently exiled Cubans (who had arrived less than 3 weeks earlier) as compared with 98 Cuban Americans. Although the groups did not differ significantly in family cohesion, both groups reporting a high degree of cohesion, the most recently arrived Cuban Americans (those who had arrived within 3 weeks of participating in the study) scored significantly higher on family adaptability, purpose in life, and well-being. For Cuban Americans with a longer U.S. sojourn, increased transculturation was associated with higher purpose in life and better well-being. The authors note that unique characteristics of the Cuban American community in Miami, where they recruited their sample, permit Cuban Americans to acculturate while still preserving strong cultural and family ties within a cohesive community.

Language and Values

Although the preservation of their language has been, for the most part, possible among Cuban American families in the first and "one-and-a-half" generation, it has been much more difficult for children born in the United States to Cuban families. Miami public schools pioneered well-organized programs of bilingual education in the 1960s, but the "English only" movements have made bilingual education a much less supported program since the 1980s. The erosion of language as a rich resource of cultural heritage, especially in the face of hostile monolingualism reflected in the dominant North American culture, is a problem for most Latino families in the United States, whose ethnic socialization includes language as a key dimension of cultural continuity (M. Bernal & Knight, 1993). The intergenerational tensions created by the political cutoff between Cuban Americans and their culture and country of origin have resulted in families within which the parents protect a nostalgic image of the lost country. When older members of a family hold onto a lost and idealized Cuba, such static images imposed on the younger generation limit the children's access to developmental resources as they become adults in a new context. An understanding of the intergenerational and political dimensions of the loss of culture in overassimilation, "de-Cubanization," is critical. Such an understanding may make it possible for therapists to support the recapturing of language and the return to cultural roots, that is, to facilitate a "re-Cubanization" (Bernal, 1982), respecting the losses and memories of the elder generation while introducing greater flexibility and complexity into the dialogue on Cuban and U.S. family and political realities.

Cuban values have been studied by various clinicians and investigators (e.g., Bernal, 1982; Marín, Van Oss Marín, Sabogal, Otero-Sabogal, & Péres-Stable, 1986; Queralt, 1984; Szapocznik, Kurtines, & Hanna, 1979). Overall, Cubans value an interpersonal orientation over impersonal abstractions. *Personalismo* represents a preference for personal contacts and social situations. Perhaps *choteo* is the incarnation of Cuban *personalismo*. *Choteo* is a form of humor/ridicule directed at anything and anyone (Bernal, 1982). Mañach's (1929) early analysis (or *indagación*) of *choteo* characterizes this phenomenon as a uniquely Cuban trait that involves exaggeration, joking, and not taking things seriously (Ortíz, 1973). When combined with *tuteo*, the informal use of the pronoun *tú*, meaning "you," an even closer interpersonal contact is achieved.

However, Cuban Americans tend to endorse individualistic responses in problem solving more often than other groups. They also tend to prefer hierarchy and linearity in family relations. The value of action in the "here and now" is favored (Bernal, 1982; Marín et al., 1986; Szapocznick, Scopetta, Arnalde, & Kurtines, 1978). Clearly, in considering a treatment strategy, therapists who focus on the present and on problem solving, consider the family hierarchy, and involve the family are more likely to achieve effective results.

Social Supports

Traditional and nontraditional systems of support are firmly established in the Cuban community, especially in Miami. Religious, social, health, political, and neighborhood organizations are an important part of community life. One of the first organized systems of support—the Cuban Refugee Center—was established by the federal government to provide food, clothing, and shelter to Cuban immigrants. In fact, U.S. government loans and other financial assistance to Cuban families have been estimated to total between $2 and $3 billion, which is greater than the amount Washington spent on the entire Alliance for Progress program during the 1960s for all of Latin America. This financial and social support has enabled Cuban Americans, especially those in the first wave of migrations, to achieve a degree of social mobility that has been rare among foreign-born U.S. populations. The existence of economically successful Cuban American enclaves in Miami; West New York, New Jersey; and San Juan has created highly visible, politically organized, and powerful communities that have supported the successful preservation of a strong Cuban American presence with a distinct cultural identity (Lamphere, 1992). Religion, primarily Catholicism, is another instrument of support. Catholicism is the major religious preference, but the number of practicing Catholics has decreased (Cobas & Duany, 1995; Rogg & Cooney, 1980). A significant number of Cuban Protestants and Jews are also among the exiles. The formal structures for spiritual support may be an important resource in therapy, particularly for elderly Cubans. Less traditional forms of support are found in the folk-healing systems that are part of the Cuban heritage. *Botánicas* are visible in most Latino and Latina communities; these are stores that sell herbs, potions, and candles and are often operated by *santeros* or *espiritistas*. *Santeros* are priests from the Afro-Cuban Santeria religion that integrates Catholic and African Yoruba beliefs, which is described elsewhere (Bernal, 1982; G. Bernal & Gutierrez, 1988; Shapiro, 2000). Clinicians should be aware that mobilizing the support systems available through *santeros* and *espiritistas* can provide an important resource to the family in therapy.

CLINICAL CONSIDERATIONS

Cuban families have created distinctive intergenerational family relationships under the influence of the cultural, political, and historical forces described earlier, as they intersect with the evolving family life cycle (Carter & McGoldrick, 1999; Shapiro, 1994a, 1994b). Because the political circumstances of Cuban migration have caused family cutoffs and profound losses, strong tensions related to family ethics and loyalty obligations have characterized the evolving relationships of Cuban families in the United States and in Cuba as well. In the 1982 edition of this book, Bernal described cases in which members of the "one-and-a-half generation" voiced, at times directly, at times symptomatically, the burdens of immigration, hardship, and loss, as well as the desire to join the new culture while honoring a living, evolving image of the Cuba left behind. The danger in these families was an unacknowledged confrontation over the image of Cuba, which was idealized and frozen in time, yet represented a forbidden political territory.

As Cuban American families establish roots in the United States and face the reality that the myth of return is fading, they come to family therapy for various reasons. The birth of a new generation of children and grandchildren, the intermarriage of Cubans with Anglos (as well as with other ethnic groups), and the difficulty of maintaining their language in the U.S.-born generation all contribute to the evolving family life cycle relationships, which must still incorporate dialogue concerning cultural continuity as well as cultural creativity and change. Partly because of the many losses, and partly because of a strong Cuban presence in large enclave communities in Florida and New Jersey, Cuban families have tenaciously held onto, and have succeeded in preserving, their language, values, and culture, which creates dilemmas for a generation growing up exposed to North American values emphasizing individual strivings over family attachments. In our own work on family reconciliation, we found contextual therapy (Boszormenyi-Nagy & Krasner, 1986) useful, because of its emphasis on family loyalty, obligations, and appreciating the existential frameworks within which "destructive entitlements" emerge. Cuban families, like all immigrant families, experience dislocation, grief, and loss at the violent collision of the family life cycle with the arbitrary movements of politics and history in a particular context (Shapiro, 2002). With the aging of the generation that most acutely experienced the bitterness of losing the lives they had established, we have new responsibilities to respect their losses without sacrificing our ability to recognize changes in a changing world. We are close to a turning point as a maturing community in which second- and third-generation Cuban Americans will no longer be intoning "Next year in Havana."

Guidelines for the engagement and treatment of Cubans in therapy have been the focus of a number of chapters and volumes (Bernal, 1982; G. Bernal & Gutierrez, 1988; Szapocznik & Kurtines, 1989). In general, the clinician is required to have skills in family therapy, cultural competence, and sensitivity to cultural issues. More specifically, knowledge of the Spanish language is essential, at least in treatment of members of the first generation, as it is often through language that cultural issues are expressed. It is also important to appreciate the phases of migration and the connectedness to the culture of origin, and to evaluate the impact of the stress of migration, value conflicts, and developmental conflicts over gender issues and acculturation. Our focus here is on the interface between sociohistorical issues and cultural processes relevant to the family evaluation and treatment of Cubans in the United States.

The following examples are offered to illustrate issues faced by Cuban families in the United States.

The Dominguez Family

Carlos and Nancy Dominguez brought in their 8-year-old son, Bobby, for an assessment because his behavior was out of control at home and at school; they wondered if their child was hyperactive. Carlos, 42, was born in Cuba and had grown up in Queens, New York. He met Nancy Owens, 32, of a Boston Irish Catholic background, when he was completing his surgery residency and she was a student nurse. Although he had told her about his Cuban background, his lack of accent and physical distance from his family in Queens made their close-knit family habits a distant reality. She saw her own parents, who lived in Boston, once or twice a year, far less often than Carlos had been visiting his parents when they first met. As the family grew, first with Bobby and then Lindsay 3 years later, Carlos began to visit his parents less frequently. Upon evaluating Bobby, who was mildly distractible but quite responsive to consistent structure in school and at home, the therapist recommended family therapy as a way of exploring parental inconsistency and other family issues contributing to Bobby's behavior problems. In the family history that was collected, it emerged that Carlos's younger sister, Irma, had stayed close to home, attending Queens College and marrying the son of a Cuban refugee family.

When Irma's husband and 12-year-old son were killed in an automobile accident a year earlier, Carlos's family's needs and expectations for support increased enormously. Carlos felt terribly caught between his obligations to his sister and grieving parents, and his wife's expectations that their family would come first. He had attended his brother-in-law's and nephew's funeral and wake, but had then permitted work obligations to provide the justification for why he couldn't make regular return visits to his grieving sister and parents. In a poignant family session, Bobby expressed his sense of sadness and confusion at the death of his uncle and, especially, his cousin, who provided an understandable bilingual link to the more foreign world of his old-fashioned Dominguez grandparents, who still spoke Spanish at home and called him "Robertico" (little Robert).

Bobby's grief, and its reflection and resonance in his father's grief, had gone underground in the family because exposing their shared grief might push Carlos too far into the gravitational pull of his extended family obligations. When Nancy realized the burden of family grief that Bobby was carrying, she began to accept the importance of strengthening ties to the Dominguez family, as well as opening communication within their own family about Bobby's connections to his Cuban cultural identity. Carlos, too, needed to explore how he had used Nancy's more distant family style as a means of extricating himself from family connections he did not know how to negotiate in a more modulated way. His work hours had conspired with his parenting responsibilities to make it hard to travel to Queens and easy to lose contact with his parents. The crisis of death and grief in the Dominguez extended family renewed a family conversation concerning the preservation of family connections, and Carlos began to make more frequent weekend visits with both children, without Nancy, as well as visits in which she was included.

The Otero Family

Yvette, 24, was referred for treatment because of a major depression. She had migrated with her brother to Florida through a third country in early 1994 and had gone to live with their father, who had migrated to the United States about 5 years earlier. During a professional visit to the United States, her mother decided not to return to Cuba, shortly after the immigration agreement between the United States and Cuba in 1994. Although Yvette's parents had been divorced for more than 10 years, her mother now lived with her ex-husband and two children in a small studio apartment. During an initial interview, it became clear that Yvette and her brother had been pawns in their parents' marital struggle. During the economic hardships of the *periodo especial*, Yvette's father had persuaded her and her brother to migrate to the United States. Her mother had felt that life without her children lacked meaning and had taken the first opportunity to join them. However, the land of plenty was not what she had expected, as her ex-husband had painted a rosier economic picture than the exile reality. He held a professional job, but his means were limited. The mother, a professional in Cuba, now worked as a salesperson at a local flea market. Yvette and her brother, both college graduates and with professional degrees, were unemployed. Acknowledgment of Yvette's multiple losses (work, family, country), a validation of the complex family situation, in which the conditions they had lived with in Cuba had been recreated in the United States, and the mobilization of resources to deal with the crisis of migration were central in Yvette's treatment.

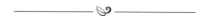

CONCLUSIONS

In this chapter we have proposed the integration of contextual, developmental, and cultural approaches consistent with the concept of transculturation as a way of describing creative cultural encounters and intergenerational dialogue that creates new cultural forms. Although at the international level, the Cold War has been over since 1989, it has remained a reality between the United States and Cuba. Thus, an in-depth consideration of political, social, and economic contexts remains an inseparable aspect of therapy work with Cuban families.

Despite the tensions of a continued Cold War rhetoric and the publicly perceived non-negotiation with Castro, privately, the Cuban community in the United States is undergoing an important transformation as it is "re-Cubanized" with the more recent waves of migrants. Individually, Cubans who have opted for an integration of U.S. and Cuban cultures (Szapocznik & Kurtines, 1989) and who have longed to be reunited with their families in their search for affirmation of their cultural heritage, have continued to do so despite the public anti-Cuba discourse. In his book *Next Year in Cuba*, Pérez Firmat (1995) offers powerful insights into the Cuban cultural experience and presents a testament of cultural affirmation:

> Although sometimes I have been unwilling to admit this, I can stop being Cuban no more than I can get out of my skin . . . unlike what I once thought, being Cuban does not depend on the pictures on your wall or the women in your bed or the food on your plate or the trees beyond your window. Because Cuba is my past, Cuba is my present and my future. I will never not be Cuban. Whether a burden or a blessing being Cuban in America is for me inescapable. (p. 259)

Recently, in *Bridges to Cuba* (Behar, 1995), and earlier in *Contra Viento y Marea* (Grupo Areito, 1978), the authors describe their own efforts to reconnect with their Cuban cultural roots. These efforts in facing losses, establishing reconnections with the culture of origin, and opening dialogue between families who migrated and those who chose to stay, are all encouraging signs of a reintegration among Cuban families (Task Force on Memory, Truth and Justice, 2003). The time may be near when it might be possible to go beyond bridging cultural, political, and generational rifts and toward a true integration among the different sectors of Cuban families outside, as well as inside, Cuba. Such integration is possible only if it is based on tolerance, acceptance, and respect for difference. We believe this process has begun.

REFERENCES

Ackerman, H., & Clark, J. (1996). *The Cuban balseros: Voyage of uncertainty*. Miami, FL: Policy Center of the Cuban American National Council.

Behar, R. (1995). *Bridges to Cuba/Puentes a Cuba*. Ann Arbor: University of Michigan Press.

Bernal, G. (1982). Cuban families. In M. McGoldrick, J. K. Pearce, & J. Giordano (Eds.), *Ethnicity and family therapy* (pp. 187–207). New York: Guilford Press.

Bernal, G., & Gutierrez, M. (1988). Cubans. In L. Comas-Díaz & E. E. H. Griffith (Eds.), *Clinical guidelines in cross-cultural mental health* (pp. 233–261). New York: Wiley.

Bernal, M., & Knight, G. (Eds.). (1993). *Ethnic identity: Formation and transmission among Hispanic and other minorities*. Albany: State University of New York Press.

Bonnin, R., & Brown, C. (2000). The Cuban diaspora: A comparative analysis of the search for meaning among recent Cuban exiles and Cuban Americans. *Hispanic Journal of Behavioral Sciences, 24,* 465–478.

Boswell, T. (2002). *A demographic profile of Cuban Americans*. Miami, FL: Cuban American National Council. Retrieved April 1, 2004, from www.cnc.org/demographicprofile.html

Boszormenyi-Nagy, I., & Krasner, B. (1986). *Between give and take: A clinical guide to contextual therapy*. New York: Brunner/Mazel.

Bustamante, J. A., & Santa Cruz, A. (1975). *Psiquiatria transcultural*. Havana, Cuba: Editorial Cientifico-Técnica.

Carter, E. A., & McGoldrick, M. (Eds.). (1999). *The expanded family life cycle: Individual, family and social perspectives* (3rd ed.). Boston: Allyn & Bacon.

Castro, F. (1972). *Revolutionary struggle*. Cambridge, MA: MIT Press.

Castro, F. (1975). *Discursos* (Vol. 1). Havana, Cuba: Editorial de Ciencias Sociales.

Castro, M. (2000). The trouble with collusion: Paradoxes of the Cuban-American way. In D. Fernandez & M. Betancourt (Eds.), *Cuba, the elusive nation: Interpretations of nation identity* (pp. 292–309). Gainesville: University of Florida Press.

Cobas, J., & Duany, J. (1995). *Los cubanos en Puerto Rico: Economia, étnia e identidad cultural*. San Juan, PR: Editorial de la Universidad de Puerto Rico.

Eire, C. (2003). *Waiting for snow in Havana: Confessions of a Cuban boy*. New York: Free Press.

Fagan, R. R., Brody, R. A., & O'Leary, T. J. (1968). *Cubans in exile: Disaffection and the revolution*. Palo Alto, CA: Stanford University Press.

Foner, P. S. (1962). *A history of Cuba and its relation to the United States* (Vol. 1). New York: International Publishers.

Fusco, C. (1994). El diario de Miranda/Miranda's diary. In R. Behar & J. Leon (Eds.), Bridges to Cuba/Puentes a Cuba. *Michigan Quarterly Review, 33,* 477–496.

Fusco, C. (1995). *English is broken here*. New York: New Press.

García, C. (1992). *Dreaming in Cuban*. New York: Ballantine.

Gonzales-Mandri, F. (1994). A house on shifting sands. In R. Behar & J. Leon (Eds.), Bridges to Cuba/ Puentes a Cuba. *Michigan Quarterly Review*, *33*, 553–556.

Grupo Areito. (1978). *Contra viento y Marea*. Havana, Cuba: Casa de las Américas.

Kirk, J., & Padura Fuentes, L. (2001). *Culture and the Cuban revolution: Conversations in Havana*. Gainesville: University of Florida Press.

Lamphere, L. (Ed.). (1992). *Structuring diversity: Ethnographic perspectives on the new immigration*. Chicago: University of Chicago Press.

Mañach, J. (1929). Indagación del choteo, *Revista de Avance*, La Habana.

Marín, G., VanOss Marín, B., Sabogal, F., Otero-Sabogal, R., & Pérez-Stable, E. J. (1986). *Subcultural differences in values among Hispanics: The role of acculturation*. San Francisco: University of California Hispanic Smoking Cessation Research Project.

Ortíz, F. (1973). *Contrapunteo Cubano de tabaco y el azúcar*. Barcelona: Editorial Ariel. (Also published in English by Duke University Press in 1995.)

Pérez Firmat, G. (1994). *Life on the hyphen*. Austin: University of Texas Press.

Pérez Firmat, G. (1995). *Next year in Cuba: A Cubano's coming of age in America*. New York: Anchor Books.

Pérez, L. (2001). Growing up in Cuban Miami: Immigration, the enclave and new generations. In R. Rumbaut & A. Portes (Eds.), *Ethnicities: Children of immigrants in America* (pp. 91–125). Berkeley: University of California Press.

Pérez-Stable, M. (1999). *The Cuban revolution: Origins, course, and legacy* (2nd ed.). New York: Oxford University Press.

Portes, A. (1995). *The economic sociology of immigration: Essays on networks, ethnicity and entrepreneurship*. New York: Russell Sage Foundation.

Queralt, M. (1984, March–April). Understanding Cuban immigrants: A cultural perspective. *Social Work*, 115–121.

Risech, F. (1994). Political and cultural cross-dressing: Negotiating a second generation Cuban-American identity. In R. Behar & J. Leon (Eds.), Bridges to Cuba/Puentes a Cuba. *Michigan Quarterly Review*, *33*, 526–540.

Rogg, E. M., & Cooney, R. S. (1980). *Adaptation and adjustment of Cubans: West New York, New Jersey*. New York: Hispanic Research Center.

Rumbaut, D. R., & Rumbaut, R. G. (1976). The family in exile: Cuban expatriates in the United States. *American Journal of Psychiatry*, *133*, 395–399.

Shapiro, E. (1994a). Finding what had been lost in plain view. In R. Behar & J. Leon (Eds.), Bridges to Cuba/Puentes a Cuba. *Michigan Quarterly Review*, *33*, 579–589.

Shapiro, E. (1994b). *Grief as a family process: A developmental approach to clinical practice*. New York: Guilford Press.

Shapiro, E. (1996). Exile and identity: On going back to Cuba. *Cultural Diversity and Mental Health*, *2*, 21–33.

Shapiro, E. (2000). Santeria as a healing practice: My Cuban Jewish journey with Oshun. In M. Fernandez-Olmos & L. Paravisine-Gerbert (Eds.), *Healing cultures: Art and religion as curative practices in the Caribbean and its diaspora* (pp. 69–88). New York: Palgrave Press.

Shapiro, E. (2002). Family bereavement after collective trauma: Private suffering, public meanings and cultural contexts. *Journal of Systemic Therapy*, *21*, 81–92.

Stepick, A., & Stepick, C. (2002). Power and identity: Miami Cubans. In M. Suarez-Orozco & M. Paez (Eds.), *Latinos: Remaking America* (pp. 75–92). Berkeley: University of California Press.

Szapocznik, J., Cohen, R., & Hernandez, R. E. (1985). *Coping with adolescent refugees: The Mariel boatlift*. New York: Praeger.

Szapocznik, J., & Kurtines, W. (1989). *Breakthroughs in family therapy with drug abusing and problem youth*. New York: Springer.

Szapocznik, J., & Kurtines, W. (1993). Family psychology and cultural diversity: Opportunities for theory, research and application. *American Psychologist*, *48*, 400–407.

Szapocznik, J., Kurtines, W., & Hanna, N. (1979). Comparison of Cuban and Anglo-American cultural values in a clinical population. *Journal of Consulting and Clinical Psychology, 47,* 623–624.

Szapocznik, J., Scopetta, M. A., Arnalde, M., & Kurtines, W. (1978). Cuban value structure: Treatment implications. *Journal of Consulting and Clinical Psychology, 46,* 961–970.

Task Force on Memory, Truth and Justice. (2003). *Cuban national reconciliation.* Miami: Florida International University. Retrieved April 11, 2004, from memoria.fiu.edu/memoria/documents/Book_English.pdf

Thomas, H. (1977). *The Cuban revolution.* New York: Harper & Row.

Torres, M. (1994). Beyond the rupture: Reconciling with our enemies, reconciling with ourselves. In R. Behar & J. Leon (Eds.), Bridges to Cuba/Puentes a Cuba. *Michigan Quarterly Review, 33,* 419–436.

Torres, M. (2003a). *By heart/De memoria: Cuban women's journeys in and out of exile.* Philadelphia: Temple University Press.

Torres, M. (2003b). *The Lost Apple: Operation Pedro Pan, Cuban children in the U.S., and the promise of a better future.* Boston: Beacon Press.

Troyano, A. (a.k.a. Tropicana, C.). (1995). Milk of amnesia/Leche de amnesia. *The Dream Review, 39,* 94–111.

West, A. (1995). Cuba and Cuban Americans: History, politics and culture. In F. Menchaca (Ed.), *American journey: The Hispanic American experience* [CD-ROM]. Woodbridge, CT: Primary Source Media.

CHAPTER 16

Dominican Families

Carmen Inoa Vazquez

There is no definition that encompasses family values that applies to all Dominicans. This chapter, however, describes some of the most salient characteristics of the Dominican family that can be useful to clinicians working with this population. For example, rural families with traditional middle-class values depend on each other for economic reasons, and they also have a strong sense of traditionalism, which includes the importance of the nuclear family. Yet this traditionalism is not always as prevalent in urban families in the Dominican Republic, where there are more opportunities for women to work or to live with their relatives in extended families, thus facilitating greater family stability for women who are separated from their mates. For couples and families who immigrate, the situation is somewhat different, as fewer of these families separate (Duarte & Tejada-Holguín, 1995).

HISTORICAL AND SOCIOPOLITICAL OVERVIEW

The Dominican Republic occupies two thirds of Hispaniola, which is shared with Haiti. In 1492, Christopher Columbus established a settlement and the island became the center of the Spanish colonialized region in the Western Hemisphere. Santo Domingo was called "the cradle of America" in the early colonial period because it had the first university and convent and was the first place where literature, theater, architecture, and art flourished.

When Christopher Columbus discovered America in 1492, the Antilles were inhabited by aborigines who had come from the Orinoco region in Venezuela and from Singu and Tapajos in the Guyanas. Different groups of aborigines occupied the area including the Caribes and the Tainos Indians (Moya Pons, 1984). The Taino family was monogamous, excluding chiefs and important men of the tribe, called *nitainos*, who practiced polygamy. Having several wives was a sign of power and success. The Tainos had a very structured society in which the rulers, or *caciques*, divided the island into five chiefdoms whose chiefs were Guarionex, Caonabo, Behechio, Goacanacari, and Cayacoa. Eventually, illnesses brought by the conquerors and forced hard labor annihilated the Indian population. From 1520 to 1607 the sugar cane industry brought African slaves into Hispaniola to make up for the lack of manpower.

The original name given by the indigenous populations to the island was Quisqueya (Mother of All Nations). The name was changed to Española (little Spain) by the Spaniards when they conquered the island, and later it was renamed Sainte Domingue, or Santo Domingo, by the French when they took the island from Spain in 1795 (Wiarda, 1969).

Other European groups, such as the British, were also interested in Hispaniola, including John Hawkins, who traded slaves and who supported the Dutch to undermine Spanish control; but Spain and France both retained the greatest interest in the island. Consequently, they fought to hold the territory and to control its vast natural resources. These wars determined the eventual split of the island between France and Spain (Moya Pons, 1984).

Toussaint Louverture, one of the leaders responsible for imposing order on the slaves for the White plantation owners, obtained the support of the slaves and played the competing European powers against each other. This revolt culminated in 1822 with the formation of a free Haitian nation. The entire island was governed by Haiti until the Dominican Republic obtained its independence from the Haitians on February 27, 1844. However, in 1861, at the request of the president of the republic, General Pedro Santana, Spain took possession and control of its former colony for 4 years until the Dominican Republic reestablished independence as a free nation in 1865.

The invasions by the French, and then by the Haitians, were an outcome of Spain's negligence; Spain was not invested in developing the island once its resources had been fully exploited. Spanish and French colonization brought severe economic hardship to the Dominican Republic. An occupation by U.S. marines, which lasted from 1916 until 1924, did not improve the economy. Six years later, Rafael Trujillo became president, staying in power as dictator for 31 years. In 1937, Trujillo ordered a Haitian massacre in the border region, particularly in the town of Dajabon (Bosch, 1984; Moya Pons, 1984; Ureña, 1966; Vazquez, 2001). Trujillo's regime lasted from 1930 until 1961, when he was assassinated. His regime was characterized by repression, torture, intimidation, tortures and assassination of his opponents.

The Post-Trujillo Era of Government

After Trujillo, there were a number of presidents and an invasion by the U.S. Marines, alleging that communists were in control of a political uprising. A year later Dr. Joaquin Balaguer was elected president and remained in office for a continuous period of 12 years, then followed by various other democratic presidents.

At present, the Dominican Republic is considered a free and democratic nation, where people are entitled to express their opinions without being censored. The media openly provides information for the people. Dominicans are very effusive when it comes to politics and quite involved in the political arena.

The Sequelae of the Haitian Occupation

Racism has been one of the consequences of the Haitian occupation in the Dominican Republic, particularly psychological animosity toward Haitians (what Ernesto Sagas, 2000, calls *antihaitianismo*), and is one of the main reasons Dominicans are mindful of skin color, but not the only one. Internalized racism can be seen in the many names Dominicans use to define themselves in their *cedulas* (identification card) and other official documents, such as *indio oscuro, indio claro, trigueña* (dark Indian, light Indian), but seldom Negro. Yet, paradoxically, terms of endearment such as *negrita* (blackie) and *morenita* (darkie) are used with children and esteemed people.

Another explanation for the continuation of racism among Dominicans is that it stems from their colonization experience. In this respect, the Dominican Republic is not different from other countries that were colonized by White Europeans and where white skin is preferred, because, historically, Whites have held more power and privilege. For example, in the Dominican Republic, children are told that they will have a career if they are White ("blancos"), and some families tend to favor the lighter child over the darker one. But at the same time, social and economic class seem to be important determinants as well. Intermarriage is accepted, particularly if the future mate is economically successful, regardless of skin color, especially for males.

FAMILY STRUCTURE

Extended and *compound* (including non-kin) households are predominant among Dominicans in urban areas, both in the Dominican Republic and in the United States. Nonetheless, it is important to realize that a family with a rural background may have lived for a significant period of time in the main city, Santo Domingo, and may have modified in some way its behavioral characteristics or traditional beliefs. An urban middle- to upper-class Dominican family that has been exposed to a more international world may have a different, less traditional worldview, but the clinician should always ask rather than assume absolutes.

The extended family is the most common family structure for Dominicans, which can include grandparents, parents, grandchildren, aunts, uncles, cousins, stepchildren, and the spouses of grown children. Other members of the extended family who may or may not live in the same household include *ahijados* (godchildren), *compadres* (godparents), and the *familia postiza*, non-kin who are considered part of the family. This family structure is common among families living in Santo Domingo as well as in New York City, which has the greatest concentration of Dominicans in the United States. (Duarte & Tejada-Holguín, 1995). Having non-kin living in the same household can increase the possibility of problems, such as infidelity and child abuse, for many Dominican families.

Couples

Dominicans usually marry early and have children early. Most couples come together through legal and religious marriages; however, consensual unions are still common both in the United States and in the Dominican Republic. Legal unions are more prevalent in the urban areas, whereas consensual relationships, or concubinage, are more frequent in the rural sections of the country. Interestingly, couples who immigrate to the United States stay longer within a legal marital relationship (Duarte & Tejada-Holguín, 1995). Yet it is also still a practice for some Dominican men, both in the United States and in the Dominican Republic, to have more than one partner and more than one household. This, however, is much less common in the United States, mostly because of economic realties, because of the long hours of work, and because of the more assertive position taken by women (Duarte & Tejada-Holguín, 1995).

Getting married and having children early can be psychologically taxing for couples. Many Dominicans find themselves in this situation, especially women who tend to marry before reaching the age of 20 (Duarte & Tejada-Holguín, 1995). They sacrifice their education, because once they have children they are expected to dedicate themselves entirely to child care. Although most Dominican men also marry very young, they feel entitled to go out with their friends and have a different sense of responsibility when it comes to caring for children. As long as they provide financially, they feel free to spend time outside the home. Men who divorce their wives tend to remarry much younger women, but divorced older women remarry men of their own age or older.

Because of their poverty, many couples are forced to divorce their Dominican spouses and marry American citizens in marriages of convenience in order to obtain legal residency in the United States, which can ensure better jobs and a better quality of life for the family.

Intermarriage

There is scarce information relating to intermarriage among Dominicans, but for Latinos in the United States the number of mixed-ethnicity marriages overall has doubled since 1980 (Aurbach, 1999; Suro, 1999). Dominicans prefer to marry Dominicans, or at least other Latinos, but this preference is less rigid among well-educated, high-income Dominicans. Clinically, a clash of cultural values begins to emerge when a couple has children. Differences in values related to child rearing, such as the extent of dependence that is fostered in children, or the level of respect and obedience that is expected from them, can lead to conflict between a couple. Dominican families expect the non-Dominican mate to follow traditional Dominican cultural values, which can put a great deal of pressure on the couple.

Dominican society is primarily traditional and conservative. The reasons probably include a combination of family and religious values that reflect specific beliefs, such as clear-cut gender roles, the continuation of the family, and old world traditions. These values reject homosexuality, which is considered a source of shame, particularly if a family adheres to *familismo*, *machismo*, and *marianismo*, all cultural values that cherish motherhood, manliness, and family. Many Dominican families still have a great deal of difficulty when a family member turns out to be gay or lesbian. The reactions range from denial, to shame and disappointment, to accusations of abnormality, to conditional acceptance: *"It is okay as long as nobody knows."* Fathers and male family members tend to have a harder time in accepting a gay, lesbian, or transgendered member than mothers or the women in a family.

However, for many Dominicans the pressure to adhere to cultural values such as *marianismo*, *machismo*, and *respeto* makes adaptation to life in the United States very difficult. In many cases the view held by Dominican parents is that North Americans are very permissive, especially when it comes to dealing with the behaviors and attitudes of women and children, who may be seen as disrespectful of their mates or parents. These discrepancies in values and beliefs between the old and young generations create conflicts within families, especially when the children have attained a different level of acculturation than their parents.

IMMIGRATION TO THE UNITED STATES

According to del Castillo (1987), immigration to the United States has replaced education as a road to social and economic mobility for Dominicans. However, adaptation to this country has not been easy. Once here, Dominicans face problems of unemployment, underemployment, poor housing, lack of knowledge of English, drugs, and lack of health services (Vazquez, 2001).

The Dominican population in the United States has grown significantly, as reported by the U.S. Bureau of the Census (2000; Logan, 2001), which showed an increase from 520,121 in 1990 to 1,040,910 in 2000, excluding the undocumented population. This figure makes Dominicans the fourth largest Latino group in the United States after Mexicans, Puerto Ricans, and Cubans. It is estimated that by 2010, Dominicans will be the third largest group in the United States, surpassing Cubans. This growth is still primarily due to immigration, although in the year 2000 there were 394,914 Dominicans born in the United States. The largest number of Dominicans reside in Washington Heights in New York City, but they are also located in New Jersey, Florida, Massachusetts, Rhode Island, Pennsylvania, and Connecticut (Hernandez & Rivera-Batiz, 2003).

At present the primary reason for Dominicans to leave their country is to search for a better life. Those who left prior to 1960 had a different reason; they came as a result of the political situation on the island. In those days, the political climate was very difficult for those who disagreed with Trujillo's regime. Some had a need to leave the country, mostly through self-exile, not only to seek democracy, but also to ensure safety. The *caliés* (informers), who reported on anyone who was not a friend of the government, posed a real threat to people's safety.

Today, women and men migrate in equal numbers and usually leave between the ages of 20 and 39. Parents often immigrate alone, leaving their children with relatives until they can send for them. This pattern makes it very difficult for the family members inasmuch as they may not be able to live together as a unit for long periods of time. Once in the United States, Dominicans tend to maintain ties to the Dominican Republic (Drachman, Kwohn-Ahn, & Paulino, 1996; Duany, 1994; Graham, 1996). They love to dance and gather with friends and continue to listen to Dominican music, including *merengue*, *bachata*, and *mangulina*, as well as other popular types of Latino music. They also prefer to meet and attend church with fellow Dominicans, shop in *colmados* that carry Dominican goods, and eat in Dominican restaurants, where they can get savory dishes such as *mangu* (mashed green plantains with sautéed shallots), *chicharrones de pollo* (small pieces of fried chicken), and *sancocho* (a stew with meats and vegetables).

The Dominican stay in the United States is considered to be "transnational," or characterized by a constant back-and-forth flow of individuals maintaining a dual sense of identity (Duany, 1994). This return pattern involves periodic visits, including special celebrations at Christmas, when family members and friends expect lavish gifts and meals in restaurants paid for by the visitor. It may also include a permanent return by those who have not adapted to life in the United States or by those who have achieved financial success (Hendricks, 1974). Most Dominicans dream of purchasing their own home back in the Dominican Republic, buying some land, and starting a business. However, many who return do not stay but remigrate to the United States because they face financial difficulties in the Dominican Republic or because they cannot readjust. The age of the immigrant is a factor in determining whether he or she will stay in the United States or return to the

Dominican Republic. It is easier for younger people to adapt to a new environment than for those who are older.

SOCIOECONOMIC FACTORS

The average income of Dominicans is the lowest per capita income in the United States, which may explain the need for extended family members to live together. The unemployment rate for Dominican men was 7.8% in the year 2000, in comparison to 3.9% for the United States as a whole. The Dominican unemployment rate for women was also much lower, 1.7%, as compared with 4.1%. Moreover, 38.2% of Dominican households in New York City that fall below the poverty line are headed by females without spouses, as compared with 22.1% for the city as a whole (Hernandez & Rivera-Batiz, 2003). This situation is compounded by the fact that many Dominicans have to provide financial support for relatives back home. However, when we look at U.S.-born Dominicans, we begin to see a different picture. They have made gains in education and a remarkable growth in human capital over the last 20 years, placing U.S.-born Dominicans at a higher level of education and capital growth than U.S.-born Mexicans and Puerto Ricans (Hernandez & Rivera-Batiz, 2003). The reasons for these gains are not clear; one could speculate that there is a great push by the families to obtain an education for their children and to work hard as the only way of "making it." It is also possible that the families instill in their children the need to succeed in order to take better care of their relatives. This gives meaning to the sacrifices the immigrant family has made for the children, who are then in turn expected to "pay back" their parents.

There is significant variability in the earnings of Dominicans in the United States ranging from an average of $12,866 per year in Florida, to $8,560 in Rhode Island, with a mean annual per capital income of $11,065 for the entire country (Hernandez & Rivera-Batiz, 2003). Language problems and adjustment to the new culture present barriers that limit Dominicans' earning potential in the United States upon their arrival.

CLINICAL CONSIDERATIONS

There are no clear markers to determine the level of acculturation for Dominican families living in the United States, because migration laws and remigration make full acculturation not only very difficult, but at times improbable, and quite different for each family member regardless of age, gender, or length of stay. Dominican families tend to migrate to the United States at different stages of life. This staggered pattern of migration, whereby parents may come first, not necessarily as a couple, but later sending for the partner left behind, followed by the children and then the grandparents and other relatives, can be a source of stress and conflict for Dominican families, which often require professional intervention. However, traditional Dominicans may see therapy as a waste of time, or a process that takes only a few sessions, or something needed only by people who are seriously disturbed. In this context, the "cure" for Dominican families may require a psychoeducational approach—offering an explanation of the process of therapy and stressing the importance of attending sessions regularly—and an understanding of the cultural values discussed here, such as *marianismo*, *machismo*, and *respeto*.

These values are all important, but the clinician must especially balance *respeto*, according to age and gender, among all the members of the family. This means that parents may have to be helped to recognize that adolescents require a certain amount of privacy to speak on the telephone with their friends and the ability to visit friends whom the parents trust. An example of *respeto* going both ways is a parent asking the child, rather than accusing, and communicating, rather than screaming, beating, or humiliating. It means parents not looking in their children's drawers behind their backs. *Marianismo* and *machismo* are also pivotal in helping parents in the rearing of their children overall, particularly in the family interaction in and execution of the daily chores each family member is expected to complete.

Parent–Child Relationships

Many Dominican parents are forced to separate from their children for long periods of time, primarily because of their undocumented immigration status when they arrive in the United States. For example, immigrating parents may leave a child back in the Dominican Republic; 5 years later, when the child joins them, he or she is an adolescent. Not only will they have to face the usual problems parents and children face in negotiating independence during adolescence, but this may be complicated by the resentment children feel when they have been left behind. This type of conflict can be even greater when Dominican parents remarry and start a new family in the United States before sending for the children. Often a child's or adolescent's negative and oppositional behavior toward the parents and new siblings brings the family to therapy.

While in therapy, Dominican parents usually complain that their children have become disobedient, disrespectful, and accusatory. Children complain that the parents do not love them, and consider their grandparents, or caretakers back home, to be their "real parents." Encouraging both parents and children to express their feelings about the separation and to understand the circumstances of the immigration experience is very helpful. The family members also need new avenues of communication to learn about each other.

Dominicans may also come to therapy when their children begin to acculturate and exhibit cultural values and expectations different from those of their parents. For instance, Dominican parents are generally very protective of their children and fearful about giving them too much independence. This inclination often clashes with the more liberal values and attitudes of other parents about children's independence and autonomy in the United States. A common example can be seen when a child asks a parent, "But why can't I go to see my friend Harry?" A traditional answer is, "Because I say so." This approach may result in children's rebelling and acting out, or being called hyperactive, when they are not allowed to play with friends in safe areas, when, in fact, they can just be reacting to imposed isolation and restraint.

In these situations a positive therapeutic intervention is to help the Dominican parents understand that it is much more productive to explain the reasons for saying no, rather than expecting their children to respect and obey without question. It is important to help parents recognize that their children's need for peer relationships is natural, and that blindly following old customs, such as refusing to allow them to visit friends or to socialize with peers, can be problematic. These reactions are often based on fears about a culture they don't understand, as well as real dangers in the neighborhoods where they live. Although parents tend to be more protective of their daughters, boys too are often not permitted to socialize and are kept isolated from peers. Validating the parents' traditional role as protectors of their children may open possibilities to renegotiate limits and privileges while the family adjusts to the new culture.

It may be difficult for parents to engage in therapeutic conversations with their children, because in traditional Dominican child-rearing patterns it is believed that including children's feelings in conflict resolution will harm or spoil them. In such cases psychoeducational interventions can help parents learn that the true purpose of discipline and obedience is to protect and provide safety for their children and to teach them the skills necessary for successful functioning in society, not to make them submissive or hostile (Vazquez, 2004).

Another value that may present conflict among family members is *simpatia*. There is no good translation for *simpatia* in English. It means that children should have good manners and common courtesy, but it goes further, indicating the expectation of conformity. *Simpatia* is a very important component of the socialization of a Dominican child, which can lead to cultural clashes for both parents and children (Vazquez, 2004). For instance, it may involve expecting a child, particularly a girl, not to assert herself, or a boy not to defend himself against abusive or disrespectful adults in the family or in the outside world.

Another area in which Dominican families may need help is in learning to understand their children's negative reactions when they are sent back to the Dominican Republic. Many Dominicans send their children back home for an entire summer, and in some cases, for longer periods of time. For many children this is a wonderful experience. There they can usually enjoy a freer environment, in terms of space, and have more opportunities to be with family and friends. However, some children, particularly younger ones, may react negatively. Explaining to parents the differences in children's needs and reactions, depending on their age, can very helpful. A very young child who may not know the relatives back home should not be sent alone. It would be better for the parents or another familiar person to accompany the child. Parents should prepare their children before they go to the Dominican Republic by showing pictures and talking about the wonderful experience they will have in what many Dominicans in New York City call "Camp Dominican Republic."

Although many Dominican youngsters report feeling loved and accepted when they return to the Dominican Republic, others feel that they "do not fit," either in the Dominican Republic or in the United States. The following is an example of such a situation.

Freddy was born in the United States and spoke primarily English. He was sent to the Dominican Republic at age 12 to spend the summer with his grandparents and improve his Spanish. But his cousins did not speak English, and Freddy's Spanish was very limited. They did not try very hard to incorporate him in their conversations, and he often felt left out. Freddy's grandmother did not allow him to go anywhere alone, because he did not know his way around and she felt very responsible for his welfare. Grandma was being stricter than Freddy's mother because, as she said, "I am responsible for you and must account to your mother if something happens to you." His traditional aunt and uncle scolded him for being disrespectful when he called everyone by the familiar *tu*, rather than the formal *usted*. He was teased by all the relatives because he did not speak Spanish well. At home in New York, Freddy also felt left out because his parents did not allow him to wear the trendy clothes he wanted or to visit friends.

As a result, he was left out of groups and did not get invited to birthday parties. Freddy's mother often said, "This is a Dominican house. Here we do things differently, and that is it; don't argue with me." In therapy Freddy said he did not feel he was "anything," meaning that he had no identity; he was neither a Dominican nor a New Yorker.

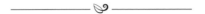

Freddy's experience in the Dominican Republic illustrates the dilemma of many Dominican children when they maneuver their two cultures and don't have the necessary command of these cultures. Language is an important factor in this process. Dominicans favor speaking Spanish, and for families in the United States language can create friction between children and parents. This is particularly true when adolescents refuse to speak Spanish or cannot speak it well. Parents feel embarrassed when family members back in the Dominican Republic bring to their attention that their child does not speak Spanish. But a more serious problem is the communication barrier that develops between parents and a child when the child does not speak Spanish and the parents do not speak English.

In therapy, when adolescents say that they speak better English than Spanish, it is important to help them communicate in their parents' primary and preferred language rather than translate for them. Of course, this is more difficult when the therapist is not able to speak Spanish. An interpreter who is familiar with the culture should be engaged in such cases. Many children's unwillingness to speak their parents' primary language may also be a way to create distance and an avoidance of the parents' values.

In general, Dominican parents tend to give their children advice and expect compliance without questioning and without receiving much explanation. There is typically little communication between Dominican parents and their children, particularly regarding sexual behavior. According to a survey conducted by Encuesta Nacional de Jovenes in 1992 (Holguín, 1995), most parents in the Dominican Republic do not talk to their children about sex. They found that 61.3% of mothers and more than 72.% of Dominican fathers do not talk to their children about sexuality (Duarte & Tejada-Holguín, 1995). This is troubling, because there are not many sources available to Dominican children to talk about these topics. In these situations a psychoeducational approach with the parents can be very helpful.

A common triangle that therapists need to avoid when working with Dominican families is created when parents want to know everything children say in private. They feel very strongly that they should have control over the healing process of their children (Paulino, 1994; Weiss, 1992) and that they are entitled to have this information. Therapists may feel drawn to comply with the parents' demands, or to collude with the children's secrecy, rather than encourage open communication between the two. This has important implications when older children are in treatment and parents ask questions that the therapist feels should not be answered, in order to maintain therapeutic rapport and trust. In these instances, again, using a psychoeducational approach that helps the parents understand adolescents' need for privacy within the therapeutic process is most helpful.

Couple Relationships

The immigration experience can cause significant stress for Dominican couples, leading to conflicts that bring the family to therapy. Many Dominican women experience immigration as a liberating force, finding that the values that were imposed back home are less rigid in the new country. Nonetheless, these changes can cause conflicts between the spouses and within the family.

The traditional gender-specific values in the Dominican family also create tension for couples living in the United States when women expect not only to experience greater equality with men, but to attain more independence. For example, women like to go out with their girlfriends and resent being told by their mates that they cannot dance with a male friend at a family gathering. This shift in behavior and expectations is due to women's attaining increased economic equality. It is also due to exposure to other Latinos who are at different stages of acculturation and exposure to media, and to educational and counseling opportunities. These factors help women to shift the balance of power and become more assertive and less tolerant of gender-specific values.

The return to the homeland is often another source of conflict for couples, in particular for women who do not want to return lest they lose their newly acquired status of independence. Women may also not want to separate from their grown children, who may not wish to return to the Dominican Republic.

Unemployment, or lowered occupational status as a result of immigration, particularly for professional men, is another cause of stress for couples. Such situations have the potential for increasing the possibility of domestic violence and alcoholism, as well as other problems between spouses, as exemplified in the following case.

Dario was very upset that after years of sacrificing to become a lawyer in the Dominican Republic, he was unable to get a job in Santo Domingo because he did not belong to the political party in power, and there were no other opportunities for employment in his field. The family decided to try their luck in the United States and moved to Rhode Island. Dario worked long hours as a clerk in a *bodega*. His symptoms of depression were mitigated by his drinking after coming home exhausted from a very long and unfulfilling day. Minerva, his wife, was working by cleaning other people's houses, whereas back home she used to have a maid. The couple's families stayed back in the Dominican Republic, and they had few friends in the United States. They found themselves isolated, fighting, screaming at each other, and accusing each other. Dario's drinking increased, and one day during an argument he threw a book at Minerva, hitting her in the eye. This incident finally led the couple to seek help.

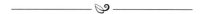

Therapy for this couple focused on helping the partners understand that their situation was caused by the stresses of immigration and the demands of acculturation. They were also encouraged to find a support system in which they could feel culturally accepted. Becoming part of a church community and meeting other Latinos was very helpful. However, finding a therapist who helped the couple understand that they were reacting to stressors created by the drastic changes in their lives as a result of immigration, made a significant difference. Many Dominican couples who face similar situations do not seek help, either because of their undocumented status and fear of deportation or because they feel they can resolve their problems on their own. A worse situation is faced by women with undocumented status who are victims of domestic violence, choosing to stay in abusive relationships because they do not know they have other choices. Clinicians must be very aware of these realities and make it a routine to ask about the legal status of clients and understand the possible ramifications of their being undocumented.

Although the overall socioeconomic status of many Dominicans in New York City has increased in recent years, families still experience severe economic hardships that require holding several jobs and working very long hours. These are variables that impact on the quality of time spent with the family and the quality of life of family members in general. Such conditions make it very difficult for families to attend therapy when needed, and traditional treatment approaches may not work. A treatment format that has worked with Dominicans is conducting family therapy sessions in the clients' home on weekends.

In Dominican middle-class families living in the United States, both the nuclear and the extended family structure is represented, and weekend family therapy can involve all the members in regularly scheduled family gatherings. Many Dominican middle-class families who own supermarkets, restaurants, taxi fleets, or other types of businesses in New York have found this arrangement beneficial. It is a format that has helped Dominican families to open up in a safe setting. The family typically expects the therapist to stay after a session for a celebratory meal, which is often a feast, including the succulent *pernil* (a pork roast), *moro* (a combination of rice and beans), or the famous *sancocho* (a wonderful mixture of meats and vegetables). When going to the house to visit the family is not feasible, the possibility of adjusting the schedule to have weekend sessions should be considered.

Religion and Spirituality

Clinicians working with traditional Dominicans can use religion or the religious community as a source of support for many families, as in the case of Dario and Minerva. There are certain religious beliefs specific to the Dominican culture that fall under what is called *religiosidad popular Dominicana* (popular Dominican religiosity). These beliefs are a mixture of mystical African beliefs and values with Catholicism. They include spiritism, Dominican voodoo, *curanderismo* (folk healing), and the messianic movement (Tejada-Ortiz, Sanchez-Martinez, & Rejias-Mella, 1993; Vazquez, 2001).

Religiosidad popular Dominicana includes *curaciones* (healings of illnesses, mental or physical) and other magical rituals (Vazquez, 2001; Zaglul, 1993) practiced by a *curandera*, or healer, who may offer special prayers or recommend baths with herbs or *agua de Florida* (eau de cologne), used to relieve aches and pains, or drinking *tizanas*, or curative teas. Applying the *toque de manos*, a form of magical healing may include a *santiguo* (blessing) and the rubbing of the hands until they get hot, which are then placed on the affected part of the body to provide healing. *Curacion divina* (divine healing) is also a healing practice using prayers either in groups or by a priest. The use of *resguardos* (amulets) is a practice carried out to guard against evil, especially with children who may suffer *alferecía*, a form of attack that is believed to be the result of a fright. In these cases the child stops breathing and becomes rigid. Amulets are used to protect a child from envy and bad thoughts. These amulets, made of black onyx, are called *azabaches*. Others are made out of *añil* (indigo) or camphor salts as a cure for some ailments.

Misunderstanding the meaning and importance of these beliefs and rituals can lead clinicians to misdiagnose clients, and clients to lose trust and terminate treatment prematurely. For example, a Dominican man in an inpatient unit was seen making the sign of the cross when he looked at the clock. It was deemed that he was delusional, when in fact he was blessing himself with a ritual that many traditional Dominicans practice at noon. Similarly, a mother may feel very guilty if she has not used a *resguardo* for her child and believe that problems may stem from this lack of protection. These beliefs are remnants of the African and Indian heritage and are not necessarily signs of pathology.

CONCLUSIONS

In closing, it is important to repeat that Dominican families are not all alike and that to make such an assumption can result in stereotyping. In general, Dominicans in the United States present a mixed picture, which at present is fraught with unemployment and other difficulties in adjusting to their new life. Yet the future is quite hopeful when we look at the gains of the second generation. To date, it seems that Dominicans' proximity to the United States and their economic vicissitudes are factors that make the Dominican population in this country a reality with which many clinicians will be faced in their daily work.

The clinician working with Dominican families is challenged to help, in a culturally competent manner that allows the maintenance of the Dominican heritage and ethnic pride, and at the same time teaches these families how to achieve a healthy adjustment to the North American culture, leading to a productively successful and fully functional family life.

REFERENCES

Aurbach, L. (1999). *Recent U.S immigration: Geography, assimilation and neighborhoods.* Available at users.rcn.com/aurbach/ImmigrantGeography.htm

Bosch, J. (1984). *Composicion social Dominicana, historia e interpretacion* (Decimocuarta ed.). Santo Domingo, Republic Dominicana: Alfa y Omega.

del Castillo, J. (1987). Balance de una migracion: Los Dominicanos en los Estados Unidos. In J. del Castillo & C. Mitchell (Eds.), *La imigracion Dominicana en los Estados Unidos* (pp. 19–67). Santo Domingo: Editorial Cenapec Republica Dominicana.

Drachman, D., Kwon-Ahn, Y. H., & Paulino, A. (1996). Migration and resettlement experiences of Dominican and Korean families. *Families in Society, 77,* 626–638.

Duany, J. (1994). *Quisqueya on the Hudson: The transnational identity of Dominicans in Washington Heights.* Dominican Research Monographs. New York: CUNY Dominican Studies Institute.

Duarte, I., & Tejada-Holguín, R. T. (1995). *Los hogares Dominicanos: El mito de la familia ideal y los tipos de jefaturas del hogar.* Santo Domingu, Repulica Dominiciana: Instituto de Estudios de Poblaciono y Desarrollo (IEPD) una entidad de PROFAMILIA.

Holguín, R. T. (1995). *Los hogares Dominicanos: El mito de la familia ideal y los tipos de jefaturas del hogar.* Santo Domingo, Republica Dominicana: Instituto de Estudios de Poblacion y Desarrollo (IEPD) una entidad de PROFAMILIA.

Graham, P. (1996). *re-imaging the nation and defining the district: The simultaneous political incorporation of Dominican transnational migrants.* Unpublished doctoral dissertation, University of North Carolina, Chapel Hill.

Hernandez, R., & Rivera-Batiz, F. (2003). *Dominicans in the United States: A socioeconomic profile, 2000* (Dominican Research Monographs). New York: CUNY Dominican Studies Institute.

Hendricks, G. (1974). *The Dominican diaspora: From the Dominican Republic to New York City—villagers in transition.* New York: Teachers College Press.

Logan, J. (2001). *The new Latinos, who they are, where they are.* Albany, NY: Lewis Mumford Center for Comparative Urban and Regional Research, University at Albany.

Moya Pons, R. (1984). *Manual de Historia Dominicana* (8th ed.). Santiago, Republica Dominicana: Universidad Catolica Madre y Maestra.

Paulino, A. (1994). Dominicans in the United States: Implications for practice and policies in the human services. *Journal of Multicultural Social Work, 3*(2), 53–65.

Sagas, E. (2000). *Race and politics in the Dominican Republic.* Gainesville: University Press of Florida.

Suro, R. (1999). *Mixed doubles: American demographics.* Available at www.demographics.com/publications/ad99 _ /9911_ad/ad991101.htm

Tejada Ortiz, D., Sanchez-Martinez, F., & Rejias-Mella, C. (1993). *Religiosidad popular y psiquiatria.* Santo Domingo, Republica Dominicana: Editora Corripio, C por A.

Ureña, H.M. (1966). *Panorama historico de la literatura Dominicana* (2nd ed.). Santo Domingo, Republica Dominicana: Coleccion Pensamiento Dominicana.

Vazquez, C. I. (2004). *Parenting with pride Latino style: How to help your child cherish your cultural values and succeed in today's world.* New York: HarperCollins.

Vazquez, C. I. (2001). Dominicans. In A. G. Lopez & E. Carrillo (Eds.), *The Latino psychiatric patient assessment and treatment.* Washington, DC: American Psychiatric Press.

Weiss, C. I. (1992). Controlling domestic life and mental illness: Spiritual and aftercare resources used by Dominican New Yorkers. *Culture, Medicine and Psychiatry, 16,* 237–271.

Wiarda, H. (1969). *The Dominican Republic, Nation in transition.* Frederick, MD: Praeger.

Zaglul, A. (1993). Prologo, in *Religosidad popular y psiquiatria.* Santo Domingo, Republica Dominicana: Editora Corripio, C por A.

CHAPTER 17

Mexican Families

Celia Jaes Falicov

This chapter focuses on four key parameters for understanding Mexican American families: migration/acculturation, ecological context, family organization, and family life cycle. A rationale for the use of these four parameters in culture and family therapy appears in several publications (Falicov, 1995, 1998, 2002b). My observations derive from extensive clinical work with Mexicans in the Midwestern and Western United States.

MIGRATION/ACCULTURATION

Descendants of Mexicans lived in several Southwestern states for several generations prior to the United States' appropriation of those lands, and increasing numbers of Mexicans are making the long journey from Mexico to the Northeastern states of this country. Because the majority of Mexican Americans are either born in Mexico, or the offspring of Mexican-born parents (Vega, 1990), Spanish is their native tongue or was spoken in their homes when they were children. They are primarily voluntary immigrants motivated to improve their economic situation.

Complementarity of economic needs between Mexico and the United States has resulted in a historical roller coaster, with periods when the United States recruits workers, encourages relocation, and legalizes migration, and periods of avoidance, when immigration is discouraged, made illegal, and punished with repatriation. Although, starting in the 1960s, Mexicans are no longer granted U.S. legal-alien status, immigration has risen steadily. Economic decline fueled antagonism toward immigrants and in 1994 led California voters to approve Proposition 187, which denies health care and education to nondocumented immigrants and compels employers to report them to government officials. Fear of detection discourages their use of mental health services (Falicov & Falicov, 1995; Ziv & Lo, 1995). In recent times, border apprehensions have multiplied as new immigrants have been lured by unclear government statements that promise legalization to temporary workers.

Meaning Systems

Perhaps the most fundamental dislocation of migration is the uprooting of a structure of physical, social, and cultural meanings, which have been likened to the roots that sustain and nourish a plant. With the disruption of lifelong attachments, many internal and external meanings are severely challenged (Marris, 1980). The uprooting of established values and exposure to new life constructs create various types of psychological distress, including culture shock; marginality, social alienation, and psychological conflict (Grinberg & Grinberg, 1989; Shuval, 1982); psychosomatic symptoms such as palpitations, dizziness, insomnia; and anxiety and depression (Warheit, Vega, Auth, & Meinhardt, 1985). Posttraumatic stress may occur if migration involved trauma, such as women who were raped and robbed when attempting to cross the border, often by men who had promised to help them (Zamichow, 1992).

New contexts slowly generate new meanings and accommodations. The observation that some stresses of cultural dissonance appear to decrease as the immigrant gains language and cultural competence, was based on acculturation theory. During the decades from 1950 through 1980, acculturation theory assumed that maintaining, rather than shedding, one's original culture and language could create mental health risks for immigrants. Nevertheless, in more recent decades the emphasis on acculturation as the solution to the immigrant's stress has been challenged (Griffith, 1983; Portes & Rambaut, 1990). Several studies indicate that Mexican Americans who try to "Americanize," or assimilate, actually have *more* psychological problems and drug use than those who retain the expression of their language, cultural ties, and rituals (Burnam, Hough, Karno, Escobar, & Teller, 1987; Falicov, 2002; Warheit et al., 1985) along with their instrumental acculturation.

A recent model, "alternation theory," assumes that it is possible to know two languages and two cultures and to appropriately use this knowledge in different contexts (Falicov, 2002b; La Framboise, Coleman, & Gerton, 1993; Rouse, 1992) without giving up one for the other. Among the factors that make this model particularly well suited to Mexican Americans are their concentration in border cities between Mexico and the United States, the availability of land transportation, and improved connections between the two countries, which create an active interchange of people, information, and goods that span "the here and the there." These connections concretize the circular, recursive nature of what has been called the two-home, transcontext lifestyle for Mexicans (Bustamante, 1995; Schiller, Basch, & Blanc-Szanton, 1992; Turner, 1991). Studying Mexicans in Redwood City, California, Rouse (1992) observed a "cultural bifocality," that is, the capacity to see the world through two different value lenses. Immigrant men maintained for many years their language and values within the family, while also learning English and the American work ethic. Most Mexican families today are transnational families because they maintain multiple relations (familial, economic, religious, organizational, and political) that span countries. Transmigrants take actions, make decisions, and feel concerns within a social field that links together their country of origin and their country of settlement (Schiller, Basch, & Blanc-Szanton, 1992).

Structural Dilemmas

Migration changes many family interactions, primarily because of recurrent separations and reunions between family members. A resilient adaptation may involve increased closeness between members of the nuclear family that cushions culture shock, but ultimately limits the reincorporation of other family members or curtails individual development.

When prolonged separation between nuclear family members occurs, it is usually the father who migrates first, and the mother may become a one-parent unit supported by relatives in Mexico. When the parents reunite, they undergo a second reorganization, analogous to the incorporation of a stepfather. Children may be left behind not only for practical reasons, but perhaps also for less conscious ones, such as loyalty to the family of origin. Reincorporation is often traumatic for all involved, especially children (Falicov, 1998; Suárez-Orozco, Todorova, & Louie, 2003). Recently, more women have begun migrating alone. They often become distant breadwinners who are peripheral to their childrens' lives, as compared with their substitute caretaker; ironically, they may become more attached to children whom they have been hired to take care of (Hondagnue-Sotelo, 2002).

Other gender and generational dilemmas occur when wives remain isolated in their homes and do not learn English, or when children serve as intermediaries with the institutions of the United States, situations that may eventually weaken parental authority and compound generational tensions having to do with language and culture.

Clinical Implications

Just as transnational families span countries, therapist's inquiries, and even interventions, should span the family's social fields in both countries. Obtaining a "migration narrative" provides the therapist an entrée into the family's cultural and migratory experiences. The clinician might ask how long the family has resided in the United States, who immigrated first, who was left behind, who came later or is yet to be reunited; what stresses and learnings were experienced by various family members here and there, and what strengths and resources they discovered.

The therapy should not become bogged down by conflicting testimony, dates, places, or events. The family's vagueness may be an attempt to conceal its undocumented status. More important, a migration narrative helps family members find meaning in their uprooting in terms of a unique personal history and continuity of personal outlook that can incorporate gains as well as losses. I previously explored family stressors and various therapeutic approaches for different immigrant generations (Falicov, 1988). Other helpful tools are Ho's (1987) cultural transition map, Comaz-Díaz's (1994) ethnocultural assessment, McGill's (1992) cultural story, and Hardy and Laszloffy's (1995) cultural genogram.

The alternation model and biculturalism model suggest that a therapist who quickly becomes an agent of adaptation to the new culture may create more rather than less emotional distress. I have illustrated in several clinical examples the importance of maintaining continuity and not overburdening an already unstable situation with more suggestions for "adaptive" change (i.e., the wisdom of "no change"; Falicov, 1993, 1998). Promoting acculturation goals may also in effect "impose" values without awareness of cultural biases as, for example, when the therapist supports the "Americanized" second generation against "old-fashioned" parents.

Separated nuclear families come to therapy with different challenges. Shortly after separation, there may be resistance to delving into feelings and revisiting the sadness or trauma of the separation, which often needs to be respected, acknowledging the value of cultural coping mechanisms of *no pensar* (not to think), *aguantar* (to endure), or *sobreponerse* (to overcome) (Shuval, 1982). At the time of reunion family members may feel like strangers to each other, and techniques such as developing a "catching-up life narrative" may be very helpful (Falicov, 1998).

ECOLOGICAL CONTEXT

Migration transports Mexican families to a new social terrain. Bombarded with differences, they attempt to recreate elements of the culture they left. Most Mexican Americans, including those of the second generation, live in urban *ethnic neighborhoods* that serve as buffers against culture shock and recreate a continuity of faces, voices, smells, and food (Falicov, 2002a). But the illusion of a safe haven is offset by the fear and loathing of discrimination and persecution. Precisely because of its homogeneity, the ethnic neighborhood is vulnerable to intrusion by the *migra*, the Immigration and Naturalization Service, which may suddenly approach, apprehend, and deport individuals—actions that are often witnessed by children (Rouse, 1992).

Relocation disrupts the structures of emotional support, advice, and material aid that *social networks* provide, which are so essential for physical and emotional well-being (Pilisuk & Hillier Parks, 1986). Enduring intimate relationships, whether husband–wife or parent–child, are taxed with many more requests for companionship and understanding than before (Sluzki, 1989). Lacking the watchful eye of nearby relatives, parents compensate with restrictions on adolescents' activities, which may aggravate intergenerational conflicts. Many Mexicans migrate into or quickly recover a supportive network of family and friends, but this network may lack the financial resources to change the stressful situations they are in (Valle & Bensussen, 1985).

Roman Catholicism provides continuity for a very large number of Mexican Americans. Guilt and shame about one's sinful acts or thoughts are common inner experiences. For many, religious values are private, centered on commitment to marriage, fertility, and the sanctity of mothers and the condemnation of premarital sex, abortion, contraception, and homosexuality. The church in the *barrio* also provides public support (e.g., sanctuaries for undocumented immigrants, crisis counseling, space for activist groups and community celebrations), and priests who officiate at such life cycle celebrations as baptisms, first communions, and weddings. Parochial schools, including Catholic colleges, decrease parents' and children's school anxiety, perhaps because of their attunement to Mexicans' religious culture.

It has been questioned whether the Roman Catholic Church is really attuned to its Mexican American members. Services are often in English and led by Anglo or Irish priests who may be ambivalent and condescending to Mexicans (Davis, 1990; Shorris, 1992). Many parishioners are leaving the Church, attracted by other evangelical religions such as Pentecostalism and Jehovah's Witnesses (Levitt, 2002).

Folk medicine and indigenous spirituality, which coexist with mainstream religion and medical practices, are embodied by "witches," those in charge of creating and diffusing goodness ("white witches"), and bad ones ("black witches"), who can inflict curses and personal harm. *Curanderos* (folk healers) are consulted for many maladies and are trusted the most for folk illnesses, physical manifestations that are believed to be caused by stress or other psychological issues, such as *susto* (fright), *mal de ojo* (evil eye), and *empacho* (indigestion). Another folk illness is *envidia* (envy); a feeling of envy in another person or oneself is believed to be affecting a relationship, for example, between two cousins, to the point of causing the symptoms of an illness, such as a nervous, anxious mood. Thus, Mexicans recognize the power of relationships to affect the individual psyche (Falicov, 1999b; Rumbaut, Chavez, Moser, Pickwell, & Wishile, 1988).

Most Mexican American immigrants are poor, working hard for little pay at jobs with low prestige. They are often exploited and have one of the highest unemployment rates (11.9%). However, Mexican American women's participation in the labor force has been increasing rapidly, and some census reports indicate that it may be near that of American women in general. Although some fulfill the immigrant's dream and others send money to their hometowns, many experience disappointment and depression at having to lower their expectations for a stable and moderate income. Some men cling to dreams of starting their own small businesses or owning their own homes, which is the model of progress in Mexico (Rouse, 1992).

Because most Mexicans are dark-skinned, they experience discrimination in housing, education, and jobs and are deported more readily than others. Although they make up only 18% of all undocumented immigrants, until recently they constituted 86% of all Immigration and Naturalization Service (INS) detentions (Bustamante, 1995). Internalized self-loathing (Shorris, 1992), is common because of racial discrimination in Mexico itself, which then is massively aggravated by discrimination in the United States. Disempowerment may lead to depression, low school achievement, learned helplessness, or dependence on mental health help (Korin, 1994). For example, the very high rate of school dropouts among Mexican American adolescents is due to a combination of language difficulties, ethnic discrimination, insensitive school reforms, and cultural dissonance (Suárez-Orozco & Suárez-Orozco, 2001).

Many social ills that affect minorities who have been discriminated against, such as drugs, alcohol, teen pregnancy, domestic violence, gangs, and AIDS, are visited upon Mexican immigrants, and they appear even more frequently in the second and third generations than in the first (Escobar, 1998; Padilla, 1995; Vega et al., 1998). The latter is a paradoxical finding in that the children and grandchildren of immigrants generally enjoy better economic conditions, are more educated and have better access to health care. A possible explanation is that there is a "protective" or "buffering" effect of traditional culture that may lead to more stable family households, healthier habits, and the supportive presence of extended or co-ethnic social networks.

Clinical Implications

Common problems of Mexican Americans in the social and cultural spheres are isolation, ignorance about community resources, and tensions between home norms and those of the school, peer group, or work situation. To inquire about such ecological issues, it is useful to explore the family's neighborhood (housing, safety, crime, gangs), the degree of racial acceptance, employment (income, occupation, job stability), extended family and friendship networks, and school and parent–teacher relationships. During this process it is possible to draw an *ecomap* with the family that depicts its social relationships (Hartman & Laird, 1983).

If ecological tensions are affecting the family's ability to cope, the therapist may need to become a "social intermediary" or "matchmaker" between the family and various communal institutions (Falicov, 1988; Minuchin, 1974). He or she can mobilize the family to use existing networks or facilitate building new reciprocal ones (Sluzki, 1989). If they are sensitive to the context of poverty, priests can offer spiritual support, particularly in dealing with physical illness, old age, and death. In addition, relatives can be advocates for a child and provide temporary relief for parents. The therapist often needs to help the family with larger systems and direct them to specialized mental health programs.

FAMILY ORGANIZATION

Mexican American families can be nuclear, extended, "blended," single-parent, or composed of never married, divorced, or widowed persons. Nuclear families usually live near, but separate from, extended family members. This preserves their boundaries and identity.

Families are usually large, consisting of the parents and four or more children. Birth rates among Mexican Americans are close to 20% higher than those of most other ethnic groups at all socioeconomic levels (Hamilton et al., 2003). However, family size is decreasing, probably due to changing norms and women's working outside the home.

Parent–child lifelong connectedness and respect for parental authority are valued over the husband–wife bond that is emphasized by the Western nuclear family. Certain dyads, such as mother–eldest son, are very strong. Important interactional aspects tied to the emphasis on the intergenerational bond can be discussed along several dimensions: (1) connectedness and separateness, (2) gender and generation hierarchies, and (3) communication styles and emotional expressivity. These preferences may remain over several generations, but can stir up dilemmas with Anglo American values reflected in social institutions, including therapy.

Connectedness and Separateness

Family collectivism and inclusiveness are central to Mexican Americans (Keefe, 1984; Vega, 1990). Family boundaries easily expand to include grandparents, uncles, aunts, or cousins. Children who are orphaned, or whose parents have migrated or divorced, may be incorporated in the family, along with adults who have remained single or become widowed or divorced.

Strong sibling ties are stressed from a young age and throughout life. Kinship ties, extending to third and fourth uncles and to cousins, are often close. Close friends of one's parents are often called "uncle" or "aunt." Extended family may provide a type of individual attention that is hard for parents in large families to provide.

Familismo, or family interdependence, involves extended family members sharing the nurturing and disciplining of children, financial responsibility, companionship for lonely or isolated members, and problem solving. Concomitantly, there is a low reliance on institutions and outsiders. The idea of a "familial self" (described by Roland (1988) in his psychoanalytic work in India and Japan), whereby the internalization of family as an integral part of one's individual identity is useful in understanding Mexicans' dedication to family unity and family honor. The process of separation/individuation, so highly regarded in American culture, is deemphasized in favor of close family ties, independent of age, gender, or social class.

Gender and Generational Hierarchies

Mexican American men and women, as well as parents and children, try to achieve *simpatia*, or smooth, pleasant relationships that avoid conflict. Both the mother and father are owed *respeto*, a word connoting more emotional dependence and dutifulness (Díaz-Guerrero, 1975) than is conveyed by the English "respect." In general, parents' status is high, whereas that of children, including adult offspring, is low. Most parents neither expect nor wish to be friends with their children, although they enjoy each other's company. Child-rearing practices reflect this stress on hierarchies. Punishment, shaming, belittling, deception, promises, and threats are sometimes used in response to children's misbehavior.

Although a patriarchal view of gender roles persists among Mexican Americans, more complex dynamics are evolving. For example, a double standard of gender socialization and sexuality persists (Falicov, 1992), yet decision making is often shared by the parents or involves a process in which the mother commands much authority (Kutsche, 1983; Ybarra, 1982). Increasingly, Mexican American family life is characterized by a wide range of structures and processes, from patriarchal to egalitarian, with many combinations in between (Vega, 1990). Acculturation toward more egalitarian gender relationships may stimulate marital conflict as husbands react to their loss of power while wives may be increasing their own economic opportunities (Flores, Tschann, Marin, & Pantoja, 2004).

Given the centrality of the parent–child dyad, romantic ties in the marital pair may fade soon after marriage. Women's status rises when they become mothers, for Mexican Americans believe that maternal love is greater and more sacred than spousal love. Often, the father disciplines the children and compels them to obey the mother, whereas she tends to defend and protect them. This dynamic sometimes generates father–mother–child triangulation, which should be seen contextually, rather than simply regarded as "pathological" (Falicov, 1998).

Although Mexican women usually initiate consultation, their husbands generally participate. Stereotypes about Mexican *machismo*, which emphasize a man's resistance to asking for help, may cause a therapist to be hesitant to engage the father. Instead, the therapist should take care to remember that *machismo* also involves a father's dedication to his children and his responsibility for the family's well-being. Thus, *machismo* may be a bridge, not an obstacle, to therapy (Mirande, 1997; Ramirez, 1979).

Communication and Emotional Expressivity

Indirect, implicit, or covert communication is consonant with Mexicans' emphasis on family harmony, on "getting along" and not making others uncomfortable. Conversely, assertiveness, open differences of opinion, and demands for clarification are seen as rude or insensitive to others' feelings.

The use of third-person ("One could be proud of . . . "), rather than first-person ("I am proud of . . . ") pronouns is a common pattern of indirectness and is viewed as a way of being selfless as opposed to self-serving. Thus, Mexican Americans are sometimes left guessing, rather than ask about the other's intentions; they often make use of allusions, proverbs, and parables to convey their viewpoints, which may give the American interlocutor an impression of guardedness, vagueness, obscurity, or excessive embellishment and obsequiousness.

Harmony is also obtained by curtailing public displays of anger within and outside the family ("The one who gets angry loses," a Mexican saying states) with the use of *indirectas*. These take the form of criticism by allusion rather than naming a person ("Some people just never change"), diminutives used in a sarcastic way, and belittlement. Yet positive emotional expressivity is also highly valued. Words of endearment and compliments about a person's appearance, dress, or smile, or support of his or her positive qualities, spice up conversations among intimates. These communication modes may be maintained even among acculturated families.

Clinical Implications

The nuclear family is embedded in a larger context of extended family relationships. These relationships need to be taken into account to understand the presenting problems and the possible solutions.

The therapist can assume the role of *family intermediary*, serving to clarify expectations, "translate" cultural behavior, justify conflict, encourage compromise and negotiation, or ameliorate imbalances in connectedness or hierarchies that occur as a result of migration (Falicov, 1988). It can further the therapeutic process to interview siblings and parents separately and then bring them together. Siblings can explore issues they are too inhibited to discuss with parents, such as violence, drug use, or sexual orientation, or rehearse how to present those issues in a respectful way. Parents usually value siblings' solidarity and opinions. A possible avenue of intervention is to start with siblings first and obtain their opinions or enlist their help in introducing the parents to issues that are very problematic in traditional family settings, such as a diverse sexual orientation. On this latter issue, families' acceptance differs widely, but a possible generalization may be that there is greater tolerance in urban families, in contrast to outright rejection in those that come from rural areas or small towns.

Language can also be a boundary strategy between parents and children. If the generational boundary is too rigid, young people can be asked to make the effort to speak in Spanish in the sessions. Alternating Spanish and English highlights intergenerational differences, while also being a metaphor for including bicultural and bilingual needs.

A therapeutic focus on individual over family needs is likely to run counter to cultural preferences. Communications that convey acceptance of inhibitions rather than pressuring for disclosure are desirable. Disclosure is easier when the therapist uses such culturally syntonic conversational modes as metaphors, proverbs, or humor that transmit an existential sense of the absurd, the impossibility of "winning the game," or life's propensity for sudden reversals.

An intense emotive tone is more appealing than an efficient, structured behavioral or contractual approach. When feelings are subtly elicited by the therapist, Mexican Americans respond much more openly than when they are directly asked to describe or explain their feelings and reactions. An experiential approach, with an emphasis on "telling it like it is" or "baring one's soul," and interpretations of nonverbal language, may well inhibit clients further.

Manifesting real interest in the client, rather than gaining data via referral sheets or obtaining many behavioral details about a problem, is essential, given the Mexican American emphasis on *personalism*, or building personal relationships. Similarly, a therapist who suggests an explicit contract about the number of sessions or treatment goals may be too task-oriented rather than person-oriented.

The therapist may assign "conditional homework," that is, asking the family to think about or to engage in a particular task should the occasion arise. Such a technique is consonant with a culture that values serendipity, chance, and spontaneity in interpersonal relationships. Conversely, Mexicans would not be comfortable with the idea of scheduling certain times to be intimate, express affection, or resolve problems.

Because of their culture's emphasis on cooperation and respect for authority, clients may feel that it is impolite to disagree with the therapist. Encouraging the family to express their reactions, both positive and negative, to the therapist's opinions helps to establish a tone of mutuality.

Externalizing conversations, that is, separating a client from a problem and stimulating personal agency or choice (White, 1989), may also be used, particularly in the form of "inner" rather than "outer" externalization. According to Tomm, Suzuki, and Suzuki (1990), an outer externalization involves talking about a problem as if it eventually could be defeated or escaped, and therefore, conversations about conflict and control prevail. An inner externalization, on the other hand, encourages talking about a problem as if it will be necessary to coexist with it. This latter formulation is more syntonic with the Mexican worldview that encourages accepting or being resigned to problems rather than confronting or struggling against them.

FAMILY LIFE CYCLE

The values of collectivism and respect for authority, the large family networks, and Roman Catholicism influence the definitions, stages, and rituals of the Mexican American family life cycle (Falicov, 1999a).

Examples of differences between the Mexican American life cycle and Anglo American norms include a longer state of interdependence between mother and children and a more relaxed attitude about children's achievement of self-reliance skills (often mistaken for overprotection); the absence of an independent living situation for most unmarried young adults; the absence of an "empty nest" syndrome, or a crisis and a refocusing on marital issues in middle age; and continuous involvement, a respected position, and the usefulness of parents and grandparents in the family. With increasing biculturalism, these developmental expectations persist alongside the new considerations of individual pursuits and romantic love espoused by the younger generations, sometimes causing intergenerational tensions.

Because leaving home occurs primarily through marriage, boundary or loyalty issues with families of origin are common, particularly because the second generation has begun to stress husband–wife exclusivity. Given the strong mother–son bond, a resolution of the relationship between the mother-in-law and daughter-in-law is crucial to marital success (Falicov, 1998).

Most Mexican families are led by two parents throughout their lifetimes. The number of divorces is considerably smaller for Mexicans than for Anglo populations (Becerra,

1988), as attested by statistics showing a high percentage of two-parent households throughout life. However, common-law marriages and desertions are common among the urban poor.

Godparents share financial and other duties at life cycle events. The two most important types of godparents are those "of baptism" and "of marriage" for the most important life cycle rituals. The former assume responsibilities throughout the child's lifetime; the latter contribute to the wedding costs and, at least in theory, can function as mediators during marital quarrels.

Some developmental impasses can be linked to the stresses of migration. Leaving home can become more problematic when parents have depended on their older children to be intermediaries with the larger culture. Younger siblings, too, may cling to older siblings who appear to be more understanding than the parents, and experience compounded difficulties of separation at the departure of these siblings (Falicov, 1997).

Because of their familistic orientation, family therapy usually is easily accepted by Mexican Americans. In fact, they tend to attribute their emotional problems largely to family conflicts and financial difficulties, which may be felt more intensely during life cycle transitions (Moll, Rueda, Reza, Herrera, & Vasquez, 1976). Many Mexican Americans believe that emotional problems are rooted in family interactions, particularly between the nuclear and the extended family. Even the folk illnesses described earlier (e.g., fright, indigestion, or nerves) are often attributed to interpersonal problems, such as infidelity or jealousy.

Clinical Implications

To deal with life cycle dilemmas, the therapist can assume the role of *family intermediary*. Acting as a "cultural mediator," he or she might encourage conversation between parents and offspring about developmental expectations and their loyalties to both Anglo American and Mexican culture.

Mexican culture prescribes many life cycle rituals that can be used to deal with developmental impasses. The maintenance of cultural rituals seems to be of particular importance for immigrant resilience (Falicov, 2002b). The therapist can encourage the family to perform "initiation rites" or fiestas at such life cycle transitions as engagements, weddings, baptisms, and graduations (from kindergarten on through graduate school). Sometimes the absence of such a ritual suggests uncertainty about whether a particular stage has been reached. For example, because many Mexican girls have a *quinceanera* (cotillion) at age 15 to announce their entrance into womanhood, and there is no equivalent ritual for boys, a family might be encouraged to invent an entrance-to-manhood ritual.

CONCLUSION

Quick perusal of the four parameters presented here may help therapists navigate the Mexican family's external and internal cultural landscape. This can facilitate decisions about which areas should be the focus of treatment.

Exploring the family's migration history and acculturation, as well as its environmental resources or constraints, will help "place" both family and therapist in the family's changed external landscape. Conversations about cultural values, particularly those related to family organization and life cycle markers, delineate the internal cultural landscape.

The therapist might note similarities and contrasts with dominant cultural meanings, and the possible dilemmas and enrichments precipitated by the meeting of the two sets of values. Among these contrasts are collectivism and individualism, hierarchy and egalitarianism, and communicative directness and indirectness. These explorations should set a tone of respect, curiosity, and collaboration in understanding the philosophical and behavioral consequences of a Mexican way of life in the midst of American society.

REFERENCES

Becerra, R. M. (1988). The Mexican American family. In C. H. Mindel, R.W. Habenstein & R. Wright Jr. (Eds.), *Ethnic families in America: Patterns and variations* (3rd ed., pp. 141–159). New York: Elsevier.

Burnam, M. A., Hough, R. L., Karno, M., Escobar, J. I., & Teller, C.H. (1987). Acculturation and lifetime prevalence of psychiatric disorders among Mexican Americans in Los Angeles. *Journal of Health and Social Behavior, 28,* 89–102.

Bustamante, J. (1995, Spring). *The socioeconomics of undocumented migration flood.* Paper presented at the Center for U.S.–Mexican Studies, University of California, San Diego.

Comaz-Díaz, L. (1994). An integrative approach. In L. Comaz-Díaz & B. Greene (Eds.), *Women of color: Integrating ethnic and gender identities in psychotherapy* (pp. 287–318). New York: Guilford Press.

Davis, M. P. (1990). *Mexican voices/American dreams.* New York: Henry Holt.

Díaz-Guerrero, R. (1975). *Psychology of the Mexican: Culture and personality.* Austin: University of Texas Press.

Escobar, J. I. (1998). Immigration and mental health: Why are immigrants better off? *Archives of General Psychiatry, 55,* 781–782.

Falicov, C. J. (1988). Learning to think culturally. In H. A. Liddle, D. C. Breunlin, & R. C. Schwartz (Eds.), *Handbook of family therapy training and supervision* (pp. 335–357). New York: Guilford Press.

Falicov, C. J. (1992, Summer). Love and gender in the Latino marriage. *American Family Association Newsletter, 48,* 30–36.

Falicov, C. J. (1993). Continuity and change: Lessons from immigrant families. *American Family Therapy Association Newsletter, 50,* 30–34.

Falicov, C. J. (1995). Training to think culturally: A multidimensional comparative framework. *Family Process, 34*(4), 373–388.

Falicov, C. J. (1997). So they don't need me anymore: Weaving migration, illness and coping. In S. Daniel, J. Hepworth, & W. Doherty (Eds.), *The shared experience of illness: Stories about patients, families and their Therapists* (pp. 231–246). New York: Basic Books.

Falicov, C. J. (1998). The cultural meaning of family triangles. In M. McGoldrick & R. J. Green (Eds.), *Re-visioning family therapy: Race, culture, and gender in clinical practice* (pp. 37–49). New York: Guilford Press.

Falicov, C. J. (1999a). Cultural variations in the family life cycle: The case of the Latino family. In B. Carter & M. McGoldrick (Eds.), *The changing family life cycle: A framework for family therapy* (3rd ed.). New York: Gardner Press.

Falicov, C. J. (1999b). Religion and spiritual folk traditions in immigrant families: Therapeutic resources with Latinos. In F. Walsh (Ed.), *Spirituality resources in family therapy* (pp. 104–120). New York: Guilford Press.

Falicov, C. J. (2002a). Ambiguous loss: Risk and resilience in Latino immigrant families. In M. Suárez-Orozco & M. Paez (Ed.), *Latinos: Remaking America* (pp. 274–288). Berkeley: University of California Press, 2002.

Falicov, C. J. (2002b). Immigrant family processes. In F. Walsh (Ed.), *Normal family processes: Growing diversity and complexity* (3rd ed., pp. 280–300). New York: Guilford Press.

Falicov, C. J. (2003). Culture in family therapy: New variations on a fundamental theme. In T. Sexton, G. Weeks, & M. Robbins (Eds.), *Handbook of family therapy: Theory, research and practice* (pp. 37–58). New York: Brunner-Routledge.

Falicov, C. J., & Falicov, Y. M. (1995, Spring). The effects of Proposition 187 on families: What therapists can do. *American Family Therapy Association Newsletter, 59,* 51–54.

Flores, E., Tschann, J. M., Marin, B., & Pantoja, P. (2004). Marital conflict and acculturation among Mexican American husbands and wives. *Cultural Diversity and Ethnic Minority Psychology, 10*(1), 39–52

Griffith, J. (1983). Relationship between acculturation and psychological impairment in adult Mexican Americans. *Hispanic Journal of Behavioral Sciences, 5*(4), 431–459.

Grinberg, L., & Grinberg, R. (1989). *Psychoanalytic perspectives on migration and exile.* New Haven, CT: Yale University Press.

Hamilton, B. E., Martin, J. A., Sutton, P. D., Ventura, S. J., Menacker, F., & Munson, M. L. (2003). Births: Final data for 2002. *National Vital Statistics Reports, 52*(10), 15–16. Hyattsville, MD: National Center for Health Statistics.

Hardy, K., & Laszloffy, T. (1995). The cultural genogram: Key to training culturally competent family therapists. *Journal of Marriage and Family Therapy, 21*(3), 227–237.

Hartman, A., & Laird, J. (1983). *Family-centered social work practice.* New York: Free Press.

Ho, M. K. (1987). *Family therapy with ethnic minorities.* Newbury Park, CA: Sage.

Hondagnue-Sotelo, P. (2002). From braceros in the field to braceras in the home. In M. Suárez-Orozco & M. Paez (Eds.), *Latinos remaking America* (pp. 259–273). Berkeley: University of California Press.

Keefe, S. (1984). Real and ideal extended familism among Mexican Americans and Anglo Americans: On the meaning of "close" family ties. *Human Organization, 43,* 65–70.

Korin, E. C. (1994). Social inequalities and therapeutic relationships: Applying Freire's ideas to clinical practice. *Journal of Feminist Family Therapy, 5*(3/4), 75–98.

Kutsche, P. (1983). Household and family in Hispanic northern New Mexico. *Journal of Comparative Family Studies, 14,* 151–165.

La Framboise, T., Coleman, H. L. K., & Gerton, J. (1993). Psychological impact of biculturalism: Evidence and theory. *Psychological Bulletin, 114*(3), 395–412.

Levitt, P. (2002). Two nations under God? Latino religious life in the United States. In M. Suárez-Orozco & M Paez (Eds.), *Latinos: Remaking America* (pp. 150–164). Berkeley: University of California Press.

Marris, P. (1980). The uprooting of meaning. In G. V. Coelho & P. I. Ahmed (Eds.), *Uprooting and development: Dilemmas of coping with modernization* (pp. 101–116). New York: Plenum Press.

McGill, D. (1992). The cultural story in multicultural family therapy. *Families in Society, 73,* 339–349.

Minuchin, S. (1974). *Families and family therapy.* Cambridge, MA: Harvard University Press.

Mirandé, A. (1997). *Hombres y machos: Masculinity and Latino culture.* Boulder, CO: Westview Press

Moll, L. C., Rueda, R. S., Reza, R., Herrera, J., & Vasquez, L. P. (1976). Mental health services in East Los Angeles: An urban community case study. In M. R. Miranda (Ed.), *Psychotherapy with the Spanish speaking: Issues in research and service delivery* (Monograph No. 3, pp. 52–65). Los Angeles: University of California, Spanish Speaking Mental Health Research Center.

Padilla, A. M. (Ed.). (1995). *Hispanic psychology: Critical issues in theory and research.* Thousand Oaks, CA: Sage.

Pilisuk, M., & Hillier Parks, S. (1986). *The healing web: Social networks and human survival.* Hanover, NH: University of New England Press.

Portes, A., & Rambaut, R. G. (1990). A foreign world: Immigration, mental health, and acculturation. In *Immigrant America: A portrait* (pp. 143–179). Berkeley: University of California Press.

Ramirez, R. (1979). Machismo: A bridge rather than a barrier to family counseling. In P. P. Martin (Ed.), *La Frontera perspective: Providing mental health services to Mexican Americans* (pp. 89–96). Tucson, AZ: La Frontera Center.

Roland, A. (1988). *In search of self in India and Japan: Toward a cross-cultural psychology.* Princeton, NJ: Princeton University Press.

Rouse, R. (1992). Making sense of settlement: Class transformation, cultural struggle, and transnationalism among Mexican migrants in the United States. In N. G. Schiller, L. Basch, & C. Blanc-Szanton (Eds.), *Towards a transnational perspective on migration: Race, class, ethnicity, and nationalism reconsidered.* New York: New York Academy of Sciences.

Rumbaut, R. G., Chávez, L. R., Moser, R. J., Pickwell, S. M., & Wishile, S. M. (1988). The politics of migrant health care: A comparative study of Mexican immigrants and Indochinese refugees. *Research in the Sociology of Health Care, 7,* 143–202.

Schiller, N. G., Basch, L., & Blanc-Szanton, C. (Eds.). (1992). *Towards a transnational perspective on migration: Race, class, ethnicity, and nationalism reconsidered.* New York: New York Academy of Sciences.

Shorris, E. (1992). *Latinos: A biography of the people.* New York: Norton.

Shuval, J. T. (1982). Migration and stress. In L. Goldberger & S. Breznitz (Eds.), *Handbook of stress: Theoretical and clinical aspects* (2nd ed., pp. 641–657). New York: Free Press.

Sluzki, C. E. (1989). Network disruption and network reconstruction in the process of migration/relocation. *The Bulletin: A Journal of the Berkshire Medical Center, 2*(3), 2–4.

Suárez-Orozco, C., & Suárez-Orozco, M. (2001). *Children of immigration.* Cambridge, MA: Harvard University Press.

Suárez-Orozco, C., Todorova, I., & Louie, J. (2003). Making up for lost time: The experience of separation and reunification among immigrant families. *Family Process, 41*(4), 625–644.

Tomm, K., Suzuki, K., & Suzuki, K. (1990). The Ka-No-Mushi: An inner externalization that enables compromise? *Australian and New Zealand Journal of Family Therapy, 11*(2), 104–107.

Turner, J. E. (1991). Migrants and their therapist: A trans-context approach. *Family Process, 30,* 407–419.

Valle, R., & Bensussen, G. (1985). Hispanic social networks, social supports, and mental health. In W. Vega & M. Miranda (Eds.), *Stress and Hispanic mental health* (pp. 147–173). Rockville, MD: National Institute of Mental Health.

Vega, W. A. (1990). Hispanic families in the 1980s: A decade of research. *Journal of Marriage and the Family, 52,* 1015–1024.

Vega, W. A., Kolody. B., Aguilar-Gaxiola, S., Aderete, E., Catalana, R., & Caraveo-Anduaga, J. (1998). Lifetime prevalence of DSMIII-R psychiatric disorders among urban and rural Mexican Americans in California. *Archives of General Psychiatry, 55,* 771–778.

Warheit, G., Vega, W., Auth, J., & Meinhardt, K. (1985). Mexican-American immigration and mental health: A comparative analysis of psychosocial stress and dysfunction. In W. Vega & M. Miranda (Eds.), *Stress and Hispanic mental health* (pp. 76–109). Rockville, MD: National Institute of Mental Health.

White, M. (1989). The externalizing of the problem and the re-authoring of lives and relationships. In M. White (Ed.), *Selected papers* (pp. 5–28). Adelaide, Australia: Dulwich Centre Publications.

Ybarra, L. (1982). Marital decision making and the role of machismo in the Chicano family. *De Colores, 6,* 32–47.

Zamichow, N. (1992, February 10). No way to escape the fear. *Los Angeles Times,* pp. B1–B3.

Ziv, T. A., & Lo, B. L. (1995). Denial of care to illegal immigrants: Proposition 187 in California. *New England Journal of Medicine, 332*(16), 1095–1098.

CHAPTER 18

Puerto Rican Families

Nydia Garcia-Preto

In times of stress, Puerto Ricans turn to their families for help. Their cultural expectation is that when a family member is in crisis or has a problem, others in the family will help, especially those who are in stable positions. Because Puerto Ricans rely on the family and their extended network of personal relationships, they will make use of social services only as a last resort (Comas-Díaz, 1989; Vazquez, 2000). They will also go to folk healers, or to medical doctors, rather than to therapists.

SOCIOPOLITICAL HISTORY

Borinquen was the name given to the island by the Taino Indians who populated Puerto Rico before it was colonized and settled by Spain in 1500 (Boas, 1940; Pane, 1973). It is believed that most of the Taino died of hunger, overwork, or suicide shortly after the Spanish invasion (Fernandez-Mendez, 1970). Of those who survived, the men worked for the Spaniards and the women became their consorts. Even though the Taino way of life soon faded, a few remnants of their culture are still visible. For instance, the value that Puerto Ricans place on preserving a peaceable demeanor is reminiscent of Taino tranquility, as well as the emphasis the culture places on kinship and dependence on the group. Some Puerto Rican physical characteristics, such as skin color, hair texture, and bone structure, have also been identified as Indian. The names of certain fruits and vegetables (e.g., *yuca*, *guineo*) are believed to be Indian, as are the names of a number of towns (e.g., Yabucoa and Humacao). In contrast, the Spanish influence is widely evident today. The Spaniards brought their language, literature, and food preferences to Puerto Rico, as well as the Roman Catholic religion and its rituals for birth, marriage, and death. Other Spanish legacies include the family's patriarchal structure and a double standard regarding

242

gender. Many aspects of Spanish culture, such as the Catholic devotion to saints and belief in an afterlife and the strong sense of family obligation, blended well with the Indian culture.

The Spaniards brought African slaves to the island to work in the production of sugar cane (Wagenheim & Wagenheim, 1973). The Africans, in turn, contributed their language, food, musical instruments, religion, and healing practices to the cultural and racial mix of the island. They also carried with them the acceptance, strength, and resilience of an enslaved race. Although there were fewer slaves in Puerto Rico than on other islands such as Haiti, Jamaica, or Cuba, Puerto Rican slaves suffered the same horrors as those elsewhere. Today there are neighborhoods on the island, such as Loiza Aldea, near San Juan, and San Anton, in Ponce, where larger concentrations of Blacks live and have maintained traditions that are distinctly African. These are usually characterized by music and dance, such as the celebration of Bomba in Ponce. Bomba is a type of dance in which the dancers compete by responding to each other with verses they spontaneously compose as they dance to the beat of African drum music.

In 1898, the United States colonized Puerto Rico after taking the island as war booty of the Spanish–American War. In 1900, a U.S. governor was appointed to head a civil government made up of island residents. The United States retained the power to veto laws they might pass, and the resident commissioner, who represented Puerto Rico in the U.S. House of Representatives, had no vote. The United States also mandated the use of English as the language of instruction in the public schools. Considering that few people on the island, not even the teachers, spoke English, this was perhaps the cruelest aberration imposed on the people of Puerto Rico. In 1917 the island's participation in its own government was increased. A Bill of Rights was established and U.S. citizenship was granted, and military service became obligatory for all eligible males. Puerto Rico elected its first governor in 1948, and in 1952 it became a commonwealth. With this latter change, Spanish was reinstituted as the language of instruction in public schools, with English becoming the second language.

Real political power over Puerto Rico, however, still rests in the U.S. House Committee on Insular Affairs and the Senate Committee on Territorial and Insular Affairs. Puerto Ricans continue to have little power over their fate, because they have no voting representative in Congress and do not vote for president. Puerto Rico is an *Estado Libre Asociado* (Free and Associated State), a territory of the United States with very limited self-rule. The sad joke among Puerto Ricans is that the designation is a grave misnomer: Puerto Rico is not a state and is not free. The status question has been a source of conflict in Congress, as well as for the three major political parties in the island, the Popular Democratic Party (commonwealth), the New Progressive Party (statehood), and the Independence Party. There have been a number of plebiscites to access the public's wish concerning status; however, whatever the results of the vote by the island's population, what has become clear is Washington's indifference to the issue. The most recent referendums (nonbinding advisory votes) are examples of that. Even after the Young Bill passed in Congress, making it clear that commonwealth status was not a permanent solution, no decision has been made. Puerto Ricans again voted statehood down in 1998, and in 2000 elected the Popular Democratic Party's candidate, Sila M. Calderon, who became the first female governor in the island. The Young Bill, although shelved by the Senate, was the first admission that colonialism must end (Gonzalez, 2000).

CULTURAL VALUES

Spirituality, Religion, and Folk Healers

Puerto Ricans celebrate life, and value being at peace with nature. Many will say that this spiritual goal is, ideally, more valuable than material possessions and social status. Living in the present and having a positive connection with both the material and the spiritual worlds is more important than the past or the future (Papajohn & Spiegel, 1975.) Although not resigned, they tend to accept fate, partly as a result of their colonial status, as well as their religious and spiritual beliefs. These beliefs give meaning to life and provide strength to cope with what life brings. Cultural sayings such as *Dios aprieta pero no ahoga* (God will squeeze, but will not choke you) and *No hay mal que por bien no venga* (Something good comes out of every evil) support this view. These spiritual values are reflective of Taino, African, and Roman Catholic religious beliefs.

Most Puerto Ricans are nominally Roman Catholics, although Protestant denominations and Pentecostal sects have been growing on the island since about 1900 (Fitzpatrick, 1976). Their methods of worship differ from those of U.S. Catholicism, which is strongly influenced by Irish customs. Many Puerto Ricans distrust the Catholic Church and the priest, believing that they are dispensable in making contact with God and the supernatural. They tend to personalize their relationship with God through special relationships with saints, who become their personal emissaries to God, again reflective of Taino and African beliefs. Promises and offerings are made, prayers said, and candles lit, all in attempts to show gratitude and faith. Puerto Ricans call on the church primarily for christenings, weddings, and funerals.

The inherent spiritual tendency in the culture has contributed to the rise of a strong belief in spiritism and in other religions, like Santeria, by many Puerto Ricans. Spiritism, or *espiritismo*, is a belief in an invisible world inhabited by good and evil spirits who influence human behavior (Delgado, 1978). Spirits can protect or harm, as well as prevent or cause illness. Everyone has spirits of protection, which can be increased by good deeds or decreased by evil ones. Spiritist beliefs also include the use of incense, candles, and powders, which are alleged to provide light for spirits, to gain their help, and to ward off the "evil eye." This belief is based on the writings of Allan Kardec, a French philosopher who was popular in the 1800s and believed that we are spiritual beings on a journey toward a state of purity and eternal light. Our souls and spirits move in the direction of that light, and their evolution depends on the life we live on earth. In times of stress Puerto Ricans may go to a spiritist, a medium who is able to communicate with the spirits of dead relatives or ancestors and to guide and give messages to them and receive answers (Garcia-Preto, 2004), or to santeras/os, who are priestesses or priests in the religion of Santeria. Santeria grew in the Caribbean, mainly in Cuba, and was practiced by African slaves, such as the Yorubas, who were forced to become Christians by the Catholic Church. They instead continued to practice their religion by disguising their gods as saints. Santeras/os have powers that can influence the spiritual world, and can also diagnose and treat illnesses that are considered to be spiritual in nature (Guarnaccia & Rodriguez, 1996).

Personalism and Respect

Puerto Ricans value personal and warm relationships with family and friends. These relationships tend to be defined by rules of respect that acknowledge the qualities that determine a person's worth. A person's worth is not always determined by material possessions or social status, but by his or her ability to relate to others in a personal and respectful way that earns their respect. Earning the respect of others is very important to Puerto Ricans, and one way of attaining it is by giving respect to others, especially those in authority, such as elders in the family. Asking for *la bendición* (a blessing) from parents, grandparents, and other elder relatives is a respectful, personal way of relating. This expectation can create problems for children and young adults who don't practice this behavior when they relate to older relatives here, or in the island, who are more traditional. Although this practice may not be as common now as it once was, even in Puerto Rico, for many it remains a tradition.

"Personalism" stems from the social situation that existed, and still exists, in many Latin American countries, former Spanish colonies where the rich and poor were fixed in their socioeconomic status with little chance for mobility. Focusing on inner qualities allows a person to experience self-worth regardless of worldly success, in clear contrast to American individualism, which values achievement above all. Respect for authority is first learned in the home and then expands to the outside society, especially when dealing with people in authority. Its rules are complex. For instance, some Puerto Ricans believe that a child who calls an adult by his or her first name without using "Dona," "Don," "Sr.," or "Sra." is disrespectful.

Familism

Familism refers to the value and expectations that Puerto Ricans, and most Latino groups, assign to the family. Traditionally, the family has provided emotional and economic support, protection, and caretaking for life, as long as a person stays in the system. Leaving it means taking a grave risk (Papajohn & Spiegel, 1975), and not meeting these mutual obligations can lead to anxiety and depression. Family is usually an extended system that encompasses not only those related by blood and marriage, but also *compadres* (godparents) and *hijos de crianza* (informally adopted children). *Compadrazgo* is the institution of *compadres and comadres* (coparents), a system of ritual kinship with binding mutual obligations for economic assistance, encouragement, and even personal correction (Mizio, 1974.) *Hijos de crianza* are children who are raised by relatives as their own, but are not necessarily legally adopted. They may live permanently with those relatives, or temporarily until their own parents are able to raise them. In Puerto Rico, transferring children from one nuclear family to another within the extended system in times of crisis is common and not necessarily seen as neglectful by the child, the parents, or the community. This doesn't mean that children and parents are not adversely affected psychologically or experience rejection and loss. It is good to inquire, but unless the family regards this as problematic, it is better for a therapist to support the family's strengths.

FAMILY STRUCTURE

Although extended families are still quite prevalent here and in Puerto Rico, their centrality as a support system has lessened. Marriage is still considered much more a union of two families in Puerto Rican culture than in America (Fitzpatrick, 1976). Traditionally,

Puerto Rican families have been patriarchal, a structure that gives men authority over women, as well as power and privilege to make decisions without consulting them. Men have been expected to protect and provide for the family, whereas women's responsibility has been to take care of the home and keep the family together. These gender roles have been rooted in Spanish culture and Western European tradition and have been reinforced by the constructs of *machismo*, *marianismo*, and *hembrismo*. However, these role expectations are changing as women gain more access to economic resources and are more aware of their personal power, and men are more collaborative and accountable for their caretaking responsibilities at home.

These changes have become quite evident in my work with Puerto Rican families and in conversations with friends and family, both here and in Puerto Rico. The constructs of *machismo* and *marianismo*, which traditionally have been so central in defining male and female behavior, are becoming more difused. This is not to say that they are not present, or that relationships between women and men are now egalitarian and power imbalances are not an issue. But what seems apparent is that the cultural expectations of *machismo* and *marianismo* are in transition, both here and in Puerto Rico, and that socioeconomic factors strongly influence the process. *Machismo*, which emphasizes self-respect and responsibility for protecting and providing for the family, continues to have a positive connotation except when it leads to possessive demands and an expectation that all decisions be made by the man. Similarly, *marianismo* continues to create cultural paradoxes for women who consider themselves morally and spiritually superior to men, yet continue to answer to male authority. This is especially true regarding the double standard for sexual behavior. Although Puerto Rican women enjoy considerably more sexual freedom now, both here and in Puerto Rico, the restrictions imposed on them are greater than those for men, or for "American" women. What continues to be characteristic of Puerto Rican women is their *hembrismo*, which means "femaleness" and connotes strength, perseverance, flexibility, and the ability to survive. It can be likened to the concept of a superwoman, that is, one who attempts to fulfill all female role expectations at home and at work (Comas-Díaz, 1989).

Traditionally, Puerto Ricans have married young and have many offspring; however, this trend has been changing recently (U.S. Bureau of the Census, 2000). Socioeconomic factors greatly contribute to this change, both here and on the island. During infancy, children are loved and enjoyed by all of the adults in the family, and as they grow, their parents, especially mothers, often make sacrifices for them. They are expected to be obedient and respectful and, as they mature, are taught to show gratitude by assuming responsibility for younger siblings and older parents. Unlike WASP or Jewish families, Puerto Ricans rarely encourage their children to join in adult conversations. Instead, children who talk back or interrupt are likely to be disciplined. Parents often speak harshly to them, demanding to know why they did something and then answering for them, or complaining about a child's refusal to answer before he or she has a chance to speak. They also view spankings as an acceptable form of discipline and often resort to it. Parents may be hesitant to reward good behavior for fear that children will lose their feelings of respect. This may cause familial tension and lead the child to act out feelings outside the home.

Although fathers are supposed to be the real enforcers, mothers have the major responsibility for disciplining children. This yields them a degree of power that is reflected in the alliances they often build with children against authoritarian fathers, who are perceived as lacking understanding of emotional issues. Relationships between sons and mothers are particularly close and mutually dependent. It is fairly common for a son to protect his mother against an abusive husband (Garcia-Preto, 1990). A family therapist working with this type of family may want to help the son to separate from the mother, who may be labeled passive and manipulative. However, the problem is not the mother–son bond, but the lack of power that women in such positions experience. Instead, a more useful approach is to empower women to stop the abuse. It is also important to challenge the dependence that mothers foster in sons, and to address the emotional distance between fathers and children when men are uninvolved or abusive at home. Mothers and daughters have more reciprocal relationships. Mothers teach their daughters how to be good women who deserve the respect of others, especially males, and who will make good wives and mothers. Daughters who take care of their elderly parents often take their widowed mothers into their homes. In turn, older women help out at home, enabling their daughters to attend school or work. Education is valued for both men and women and seen as the door to progress, especially by families of lower socioeconomic status.

Relationships between Puerto Rican women and their fathers vary greatly. In families where fathers assume an authoritarian position, there tends to be more distance and conflict. While attempting to be protective, fathers may become unreasonable, unapproachable, and highly critical of their daughters' behavior and friends. But in families where fathers are more submissive and dependent on mothers to make decisions, they may develop special alliances with their daughters, who may assume a nurturing role with them. With an increasing number of Puerto Rican families being headed by single women, children often grow up having memories of absent and distant fathers, whose behavior may have been abusive (Boyd-Franklin & Garcia-Preto, 1994).

IMMIGRATION TO THE UNITED STATES

Puerto Rican immigration to the United States began in the early 1900s. The granting of U.S. citizenship to Puerto Ricans in 1917 accelerated the process. They primarily moved to Northeastern cities in search of jobs, education, political refuge, and new opportunities. After World War II, the immigration rate increased, peaking in 1952, when the number of immigrants surpassed 52,000 (Rodriguez, Sanchez-Korrol, & Alers, 1980). Since then it has fluctuated, depending on economics and employment opportunities both in the United States and on the island (Gonzalez, 2000). According to the U.S. Census Bureau, in 2002 there were 3.2 million Puerto Ricans living in the United States mainland, as compared with 3,3,878,532 living in Puerto Rico (U.S. Bureau of the Census, 2002). They have settled throughout the United States, from New York to California, in Texas, and especially in Florida (Duany, 2004).

Because no visas are needed for travel, migration from the island to the mainland continues to be marked by a back-and-forth movement that has strongly influenced Puerto Rican family life. This phenomenon reinforces many links to the island, and it also reflects repeated ruptures and renewals of ties, dismantling and reconstructing familial and communal networks in old and new settings (Hernandez, 1000; Oritz, Simmons, & Hinton, 1999; Rodriguez et al., 1980). Some families immigrate to solve internal problems. For instance, a relative abroad may need help with child rearing, marital problems, or a sick relative. Other reasons are avoidance of difficult personal situations, such as the aftermath of a marital separation, legal difficulties, or the need for medical care. For Puerto Ricans, going back to the island also may represent a solution to the problems they face here, or an oasis from the prejudice, discrimination, and isolation that plague their lives.

The reality for most Puerto Ricans living here is that although they are U.S. citizens, they often are not acknowledged or received as citizens, and their legal status is always in question. Having to explain their citizenship every time their legal status is questioned is a constant reminder of the unresolved political status in the island and its effect on them. Not only are these immigrants affected by misperceptions about their citizenship status, but they also have to adjust to an experience of constant dissonance between the way they are perceived and the way they perceive themselves racially (Hernandez, 2000; Reinat-Pumarejo, 2001). Here they are identified as White or Black, whereas in Puerto Rico racial differences are seen as a continuum between the two polarities, with many words describing shades of color and physical characteristics (Rodriguez, 1990). This is not to say that racism doesn't exist in Puerto Rico. Like those in many Caribbean islands, Puerto Ricans are highly mixed racially and have internalized racism. This sad fact is made evident by the 2000 census results in which 84% of the population in Puerto Rico identified themselves as White and only 10.9% as Black (Reinat-Pumarejo, 2001). White skin represents power and privilege, and people with lighter skin and European features are considered more attractive, intelligent, and socially desirable than those with dark skin and African features. However, they identify themselves primarily in terms of ethnicity more than in terms of skin color, whereas the perception of Puerto Ricans by North Americans is based on race. Thus, the imposition of race on ethnocultural identity has created severe strains on Puerto Ricans living in the United States (Hernandez, 2000). It also has led to an emphasis on keeping strong ties to the culture, to building community, and to feeling proud of their heritage. However, a family's exposure to the racial dichotomy and prejudice in this country may lead to resentment, rejection, and family rifts when some members are perceived as White and others as Black (Comas-Díaz, 1994; Tomas, 1967).

For the majority of Puerto Rican families in the United States, however, socioeconomic factors are the most significant contributors to their experiencing pressure and stress. Most are relegated to a marginal existence as the poorest among all Latino groups. According to a special report on the Hispanic population by the U.S. Census in March 2002, 9.6% of the Puerto Ricans living in the United States in 2002 were unemployed, a higher percentage than that of any other Latino group (U.S. Bureau of the Census, March 2002). They also have a higher percentage of the population living below the poverty level. In 2002, one third of the 3.2 million Puerto Ricans in the United States lived in poverty. In 2000, there were 83, 000 Puerto Rican males and 52, 000 females unemployed (U.S. Bureau of the Census, 2000). The higher their social economic status and the more marketable skills they have, the better they do. In addition, Puerto Ricans who migrate to U. S. regions other than the Northeast seem to fare better economically than other Latinos in those areas. For example, only 6% of those who migrated to New York in 1994 had college degrees versus 24% of those who migrated to Texas (Novas, 1994). Proportionally, second-generation Puerto Ricans are closer to the national level in education and occupationally seem to be advancing steadily (U.S. Bureau of the Census, 2000).

EFFECTS OF IMMIGRATION AND ACCULTURATION ON FAMILY STRUCTURE

Puerto Ricans on the mainland quickly find that some of their cultural values and beliefs are frowned upon by the dominant culture, and when confronted with racism, ethnic prejudice, and socioeconomic oppression, they experience isolation and marginalization. The process of acculturation, or adapting to a new culture, is always accompanied by losses and feelings of isolation, especially when it becomes evident that their dream for a better life may not be attainable (Hernandez, 2000; Ortiz et al., 1999). Adjusting to a new environment, to speaking English, and to different expectations of behavior causes stress that often affects relationships in the family. This is especially true when support systems have been disrupted, as is often the case for Puerto Ricans because of the back-and-forth pattern of migration. For example, reliance on the extended family for emotional and economic support, which has been valued in Puerto Rico, may not be an option here. Relatives here may not be able to afford the emotional or economic help, or they may have adopted the values of independence and individualism that characterize the American culture. In an attempt to maintain family functioning, and consistent with the value of familism, members will tend to suppress their emotional needs and their experiences of oppression, racism, and prejudice (Hernandez, 2000). The effects of immigration and acculturation in families are mostly felt in the changes that take place in gender roles and relationships between men and women, and in the relationships between parents and their children. These changes often lead to difficulties and struggles within families, which bring them to the attention of therapists.

Gender Roles

Puerto Rican men tend to have significant difficulty in dealing with the stress caused by migration and acculturation because of the negative stereotypes associated with them in this culture. This, of course, depends on their social position and race. Unemployed, darker-skinned Puerto Rican men from a lower socioeconomic background are likely to experience the devastating effects of racism and oppression to a greater extent than White, upper- and middle-class, employed professional men who speak English. The more oppressed and helpless they feel, the greater risk there is for them to engage in alcoholism, addiction, and violence at home.

In contrast to that of men, the experience for Puerto Rican women tends to be more positive. Unlike men, they are not viewed as threatening, which eases acculturation. Joining the workforce, which is generally a necessity, accelerates the process. Whereas men have to contend with loss of social status, women are more likely to gain personal power by contributing financially to the home. Even women who do not work out of the home tend acculturate faster by interacting with other women through their children, shopping, and church (Hernandez, 2000).

Conflict in couples may erupt when traditional gender roles are reversed. Often, women are able to obtain employment more easily than men, and, if more acculturated, they may further their education, which increases their opportunity to access resources. Men may feel threatened by the change, particularly if not working and if expected to take care of the home and the children. This role reversal does not become problematic when women continue to accept their traditional role, which is common. The reason may be, in part, that in Puerto Rico a large percentage of women have always worked to supplement the family income. In 1920, women constituted 25% of the workforce in Puerto Rico (Fernandez & Quintero, 1974), which is also true in the present (U.S. Bureau of the Census, 2000). However, women who become main providers tend to feel more independent and self-confident and expect to have more decision-making power in the relationship, especially concerning money. Consequently, men may feel emasculated, particularly if their authority is openly challenged. If unable to regain their dominant position through employment, a man may experience panic and confusion. His spouse may, in turn, develop contempt for him when he no longer fulfills his macho role (Mizio, 1974). However, most women experience emotional pain and feelings of helplessness in such a situation. Marital discord and separation are common outcomes. According to the 2000 census, the number of Puerto Rican households headed by single females in the mainland is increasing, which reflects an increase in divorce and separations. Leaving home and breaking up the family is a very difficult decision for Puerto Rican women, who at some level may be still responding to the cultural rules of *marianismo* (Garcia-Preto, 1998; Hernandez, 2000).

Sonia, a 46-year-old Puerto Rican woman came to therapy because she was very depressed and was having extreme anxiety. She was unable to sleep or to concentrate at work. Married, with three daughters—two in college and the youngest a senior in high school—she was thinking about separating from her husband. He was a truck driver and worked many hours. She had gone back to college on a part-time basis when her daughters were first in school, while continuing to work as a school aide. She eventually achieved a master's degree in social work and was now working as a school social worker. Her husband, Daniel, had supported her decision, but was not interested in furthering his own education. During their 26 years of marriage, Sonia had been a devoted mother, housekeeper, and wife while working and going to school. Now she was questioning her role in the marriage and was very angry and sad about what she experienced as unfair, but did not feel entitled to make demands or to change the rules. She had lost respect for her husband who, according to her, was content with his life and had no interest in learning or being exposed to new ideas. She felt guilty about no longer wanting to be with Daniel, and worried about the effect that her leaving would have on him, her daughters, and others in her family who had come to love her husband.

   With my coaching she was able to sort out how she was caught in a cultural paradox that was contributing to her depression. She laughed and began to "wake up" when I joked about what a good *hembra* she was and how well she was performing as "Maria." Sonia had felt entitled to study and become a professional as long as her role at home didn't change, but didn't feel she had the right to ask her husband to take on more responsibility in the house, or to join her in interests such as attending a church that she found was meeting her spiritual needs. Traditionally, a good Puerto Rican wife knows that she is morally and spiritually superior to her husband, but will support his authority by not questioning or challenging him. I encouraged her to invite him to therapy so that he could begin to understand her depression and anxiety. With my help, the couple engaged in a conversation about their history of migration and about their dreams, what they liked and disliked about each other, how they experienced their lives here, their connections to Puerto Rico, what they liked and disliked about the two cultures, and the ways in which they had changed. It became easier for Sonia to talk to Daniel about her dissatisfaction and for Daniel to express his pride in all that she had accomplished

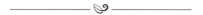

and how he did not want to lose what they had. He made some changes at home, but was not able to join her in her spiritual and intellectual pursuits. She became less depressed and anxious and more accepting of the differences between them, and stopped treatment.

———————— ❧ ————————

Puerto Rican gay men and lesbians may find that although similarly affected by all of the aforementioned forces, as well as subjected to homophobia, they have more freedom to be themselves here than in Puerto Rico, where they suffer much prejudice and marginalization. Coming out may also be easier here because they are more likely to have a support system outside the family. Coming out in their families is very difficult and has many implications in terms of status for both men and women. For men, it may mean that they are exposed to physical violence at home by their fathers and other males in the family (Garcia-Preto, 1999). Lesbians, however, are a greater threat to the culture because of the emphasis placed on motherhood (Garcia-Preto, 1998). Until recently, being lesbian meant that there would be no children. However, the increase in gay and lesbian activism in Puerto Rico and the movement here have begun to change those perceptions.

Parent–Child Relationships

Generally, children learn English and acculturate faster than parents, and as with most immigrant groups, the longer they live here the more they become identified with the new culture. There is, however, a high likelihood of Puerto Rican children becoming bilingual and bicultural, even when they are not born in Puerto Rico and have little connection to the island (Hernandez, 2000; U.S. Bureau of the Census, 2000). The back-and-forth pattern of migration contributes to the need and ability to speak both languages. For parents, this can become problematic if they are unable to speak English and have to depend on their children to interpret for them. Most Puerto Ricans, however, have some understanding of the language because they study English in school; however, they may feel embarrassed about their accent or intimidated by their lack of fluency. Depending on their children to express their wishes, concerns, and conflicts often puts Puerto Rican parents in an inferior, powerless position, which is particularly problematic in therapy. Asking a child to speak for his or her parents is also contrary to the cultural expectation that children should be quiet in front of strangers.

Children are often caught in cultural conflicts when at home they are expected to be quiet, to not talk back, and to be obedient and respectful, and at school they are expected to speak their minds, challenge, and debate. Parents, even when they are able to speak English, may find that advocating for their children at school is difficult because they do not know how to intervene in the system. The therapist's willingness to help parents become advocates is a crucial therapeutic intervention when working with Puerto Ricans (Aponte, 1976; Garcia-Preto, 1998; Hernandez, 2000; Mizio, 1974). The high dropout rate among Puerto Rican children, their involvement with substance abuse, and the high percentage of adolescent pregnancy are such critical issues that this becomes a necessity.

When parents don't know how to respond in the new culture, they often feel a loss of control and may give up. They usually react by imposing stricter rules, using corporal punishment, and, if necessary, appealing to the traditionally accepted values of respect and obedience. This is frequently true when children reach adolescence. Parents may become extremely strict and overprotective, especially with daughters who demand independence and sexual freedom, due to the conflict in cultural values and the realistic fears of crime, drug addiction, and different sexual mores (Badillo-Ghali, 1974; Boyd-Franklin & Garcia-Preto, 1994; Garcia-Preto, 1998). Without other adults in the extended family or in the community to help with discipline, their feelings of anxiety, loss, and isolation become overwhelming. Traditionally, the nuclear family was never expected to take care of all of their needs.

Mr. and Mrs. Rosa came to therapy after discovering that their 15-year-old, daughter, Jenny, had been having sex with her boyfriend, as well as drinking and smoking pot. Mr. Rosa was angry with Jenny, but seemed to be more worried about his wife, who was having a very difficult time functioning. Mr. Rosa worked as a machinist, and Mrs. Rosa was a secretary. They were both born in New York City, second-generation Puerto Ricans, whose parents had come with their families in the 1940s. Although quite acculturated, they were strongly identified as Puerto Ricans. They expected Jenny to live by their rules of no sex, no drinking, and no drugs. Mr. Rosa was disappointed by his daughter's behavior but saw it as something teenagers do; however, Mrs. Rosa felt that Jenny's life was ruined. I asked them about their experiences growing up, their adolescence, and about their parents' way of disciplining and setting limits. Their parents had instilled respect by fear; they had been expected to obey without answering back or else they would be hit. They had decided to raise their daughter differently, to be respectful but not fearful of them. They had encouraged her to speak her mind and be independent. Mrs. Rosa was regretful about trusting Jenny by giving her the freedom she had never had while growing up. She felt responsible for Jenny's mistake and that she was a failure as a mother. Conversations between mother and daughter about being responsible women and taking responsibility for one's body and spirit were very helpful. Jenny was able to talk to her parents about the pressure she felt at school from peers, and to express her regrets and plans to be more responsible.

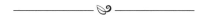

CLINICAL CONSIDERATIONS

Engaging Puerto Rican families in a warm and personal relationship during the first interview is critical to the outcome of therapy. They are more likely to respond to a therapist who is active, personal, and respectful of the family's structure and boundaries. Language is a major factor in therapy. When the family is unable to speak English, conducting the interview in Spanish is essential in engaging them. When the therapist is able to speak Spanish but is unfamiliar with the culture, he or she may miss important nuances about the family's perceptions of their situation (Guarnaccia & Rodriguez, 1996; Minsky, Vega, Miskimen, Gara, & Escobar, 2003). When there are no Spanish-speaking therapists, engaging professional interpreters is preferred to using family members to avoid distortions that result in limitations and frustrations for both therapist and client (Abad & Boyce, 1979).

Puerto Ricans underutilize mental health services (Guarnaccia et al., 2000; Vazquez, 2000), and when they come to therapy their expectations may be different from those of the therapist. Under stress, they are more likely to go to medical doctors for help than to mental health professionals and expect to be treated with medication, not psychotherapy. Their views about psychotherapy vary, depending on socioeconomic factors and level of acculturation, but the majority of Puerto Ricans are hesitant to discuss personal matters such as marital issues, domestic violence, or addictions. Using a genogram (Guerin, 1976; McGoldrick, Gerson, & Shellenberger, 1999) is very useful in engaging them and in assessing their family structure, determining their connections to relatives here and in the island, and in tracking their immigration pattern. This experience can be a powerful intervention that can help them identify unresolved losses and engage in conversations about how immigration, acculturation, oppression, racism, and prejudice have affected their lives and present situation.

Women are more likely to seek help than men, and usually come after being referred by a medical clinic, school, or another agency. They often exhibit depression and anxiety about having lost control of their children or about their husbands' drinking, abusive behavior, and general absence from the home. Although they may have attempted to change the situation at home by threatening to leave, their lack of resources makes carrying out this threat difficult. Because they are unable to change the situation at home, they experience themselves as failures. Their relatives and other women in the community often advise them to be strong and accepting. This advice reflects the cultural belief that it is a woman's role to hold the family together. There is a tendency among Puerto Ricans to admire a woman who "carries her cross." Women are likely to be ambivalent about accusing their partners in therapy. They feel disloyal, and yet betrayed. They try to clarify that their partners are basically good men and that their behavior is caused by alcohol, lack of job opportunities, friends, and this country's lifestyle. Mrs. Conde illustrates the bind in which some of these women find themselves. Women like her often drop out of therapy when the crisis is over and return when another arises.

Mrs. Conde has come to therapy on different occasions when the situation at home has reached a crisis. In therapy she claims to feel embarrassed about coming with the same problem and not taking steps to change. She wants to do things by herself but feels helpless. She wants the therapist to help her think clearly. She states that she wants to go away from her husband and her family of origin to a place where she can live in peace with her children. She holds back for fear that she will not be able to handle the children, especially her son, alone. She would prefer to stay home and help her husband. She does not want to talk about him behind his back, but he refuses to seek help.

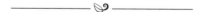

Generally, Puerto Rican men don't seek help. Abad, Ramos, and Boyce (1974) attributed this avoidance to their sensitivity to any situation that threatens their *machismo* image. I tend to agree more with the view that men have difficulty seeking help because they are already feeling oppressed and marginalized and seeking help is further proof of failure (Hernandez, 2000). In his work with Puerto Rican men, De La Cancela (1991) looks at the negative and positive aspects of *machismo* and tries to contextualize the definition, claiming that a dialectic view is more conducive to helping Puerto Rican men change when working with them in family therapy.

CONCLUSIONS

There seems to be a scarcity of studies that focus specifically on Puerto Rican families and mental health, much less on Puerto Ricans and family therapy. There is much more written under the misnomer "Hispanic/Latino." Considering that Puerto Ricans have U.S. citizenship, their overall socioeconomic status keeps dropping rather than flourishing. The 2000 census makes that very clear! Why, may we ask? I think that the island's sociopolitical reality and its marginalized status are powerful reasons. The majority of Puerto Ricans here struggle daily with little access to resources, yet many persevere in spite of the adversity. As a group, their spiritual beliefs seem to provide them with strength that, when tapped, can heal and give hope. Perhaps the most important intervention to keep in mind when working with Puerto Ricans is that as therapists we must keep that hope alive while helping them gain access to their rightful resources. For those who have access to resources, contextualizing their experience in terms of race, social class, gender, and ethnic identity is always necessary, for I think that most Puerto Ricans struggle at some level with an existential loss that is political. I agree with Herbert W. Brown, who writes for the *Miami Herald*, in his April 7, 2004, "Other Views" column, "Puerto Ricans need a way out of limbo. . . . Because of our nation's unresolved colonial relationship with Puerto Rico, the United States should be disqualified from pressuring other countries on civil rights" (Duany, 2004).

REFERENCES

Abad, V., & Boyce, E. (1979). Issues in psychiatric evaluations of Puerto Ricans: Socio-cultural perspective. *Journal of Operational Psychiatry, 10*(1), 28–30.

Abad, V., Ramos, J., & Boyce, E. (1974). A model for delivery of mental health services to Spanish speaking minorities. *American Journal of Orthopsychiatry, 44*(4), 584–595.

Aponte, H. (1976). The family–school interview: An eco-structural approach. *Family Process, 13*(3), 303–312.

Badillo-Ghali, S. (1974). Culture sensitivity and the Puerto Rican client. *Social Casework, 55*(1), 100–110.

Boas, F. (1940). *Puerto Rican archeology.* New York: Academy of Sciences.

Boyd-Franklin, N., & Garcia-Preto, N. (1994). Family therapy: A closer look at African American and Hispanic women. In L. Comas-Díaz & B. Greene (Eds.), *Women of color: Integrating ethnic and gender identities in psychotherapy* (pp. 239–264). New York: Guilford Press.

Comas-Díaz, L. (1989). Culturally relevant issues and treatment implications for Hispanics. In D. Koslow & E. P. Salett (Eds.), *Crossing cultures in mental health.* Washington, DC: Sietar.

Comas-Díaz, L. (1994). Lati Negra. *Journal of Feminist Family Therapy, 5*(3/4), 35–74.

De La Cancela, V. (1991). Working affirmatively with Puerto Rican men: Professional and personal reflections. In M. Bograd (Ed.), *Feminist approaches for men and women in family therapy* (pp. 195–211). New York: Harrington Park Press.

Delgado, M. (1978). Folk medicine in Puerto Rican culture. *International Social Work, 2*(2), 46–54.

Duany, R. (2004, April 18). Solve the colonial dilemma to gain the Puerto Rican vote. *Miami Herald*, p. 2.

Fernandez, C. C., & Quintero, R. M. (1974). Bases de la sociedad sexista en Puerto Rico. *Revista/Review Interamericana, 4*(2), 22–37.

Fernandez-Mendez, E. (1970). *La identidad y cultura.* San Juan, PR: Instituto de Cultura Puertorriquena.

Fitzpatrick, J. P. (1976). The Puerto Rican family. In R. W. Habenstein & C. H. Mindel (Eds.), *Ethnic families in America: Patterns and variations* (pp. 192–217). New York: Elsevier.

Garcia-Preto, N. (1990). Hispanic mothers. In Ethnicity and mothers [Special issue]. *Journal of Feminist Family Therapy, 2*(2), 1–65.

Garcia-Preto, N. (1998). Latinas in the United States: Bridging in two worlds. In M. McGoldrick (Ed.), *Re-visioning family therapy: Race, culture, and gender in clinical practice* (pp. 330–344). New York: Guilford Press.

Garcia-Preto, N. (1999). Transformation of the family system during adolescence. In M. McGoldrick & B. Carter (Eds.), *The expanded family life cycle* (pp. 274–286). New York: Allyn & Bacon.

Garcia-Preto, N. (2004). Their good spirits came to take them. In F. Walsh & M. McGoldrick (Eds.), *Living beyond loss* (pp. 419–423). New York: Norton.

Gonzalez, J. (1978). Language factors affecting treatment of schizophrenics. *Psychiatric Annals, 8,* 68–70.

Gonzalez, J. (2000). *Harvest of empire: A history of Latinos in America.* New York: Viking.

Guarnaccia, P., & Rodriguez, O. (1996, November). Concepts of culture and their role in the development of culturally competent mental health services. *Hispanic Journal of Behavioral Sciences, 18*(4), 419–443.

Guerin, P. J. (1976). Evaluation of family system and genogram. In P. J. Guerin (Ed.), *Family therapy* (pp. 449–450). New York: Gardner Press.

Hernandez, M. (2000). Puerto Rican families and substance abuse. In J. Krestan (Ed.), *Bridges to recovery: Addiction, family therapy, and multicultural treatment* (pp. 253–283). New York: Free Press.

McGoldrick, M., Gerson, R., & Shellenberger, S. (1999). *Genograms in family assessment.* New York: Norton.

Melendez, E., & Melendez, E. (1993). *Colonial dilemma: Critical perspectives on contemporary Puerto Rico.* Boston: South End Press.

Minsky, S., Vega, W., Miskimen, T., Gara, M., & Escobar, J. (2003). Diagnostic patterns in Latino, African American, and European American psychiatric patients. *Archives General Psychiatry, 60,* 637–644.

Mizio, E. (1974). Impact of external systems on the Puerto Rican family. *Social Casework, 55*(1), 76–83.

Novas, H. (1994). *Everything you need to know about Latino history.* New York: Plume/Penguin Books.

Ortiz, A., Simmons, J., & Hinton, W. H. (1999). Locations of remorse and homelands of resilience: Notes on grief and sense of loss of place of Latino and Irish-American caregivers of demented elders. *Culture, Medicine, and Psychiatry, 23,* 477–500.

Pane, F. R. (1973). Account of the antiquities or customs of the Indians. In K. Wagenheim & O. J. Wagenheim (Eds.), *The Puerto Ricans.* New York: Anchor Books.

Papajohn, J., & Spiegel, J. (1975). *Transactions in families.* San Francisco: Jossey-Bass.

Reinat-Pumarejo, M. (2001, May 8). *Raza y Racismo en Puerto Rico y en los Estados Unidos.* ILE., P.R.

Rodriguez, C. E. (1990). Racial classification among Puerto Rican men and women in New York. *Hispanic Journal of Behavioral Sciences, 12,* 266–380.

Rodriguez, E. E., Sanchez-Korrol, V., & Alers, J. O. (1980). *The Puerto Rican struggle: Essays on survival.* New York: Puerto Rican Migration Research Consortium.

Sluzki, C. E. (1982). The Latin loner revisited. In M. McGoldrick, J. K. Pearce, & J. Giordano (Eds.), *Ethnicity and family therapy* (pp. 492–498). New York: Guilford Press.

Tomas, P. (1967). *Down these mean streets.* New York: Knopf.

U.S. Bureau of the Census. (2000). *Statistical abstract.* Washington, DC: U.S. Government Printing Office.

U.S. Bureau of the Census. (2002). *The Hispanic population in U.S.* Washington, DC: U.S. Government Printing Office.

Vazquez, M. M. (2000, April). Puerto Rican family functioning, acculturation and attitudes toward family counseling. *Dissertation Abstracts International: Section B: The Sciences and Engineering, 60*(9-B), 4195.

Wagenheim, K., & Wagenheim, O. J. (Eds.). (1973). *The Puerto Ricans.* New York: Anchor Books.

CHAPTER 19

Salvadoran Families

Daniel Kusnir

This chapter offers a perspective on the multiple tensions, structural transformations, and dislocations experienced by Salvadoran immigrant families. It examines the contextual factors contributing to the decision to immigrate, the stresses of immigration itself, and the challenge of resettlement in the United States as these circumstances affect Salvadoran families. It then describes therapy that incorporates historical, political, social, and cultural perspectives.

IMMIGRATION TO THE UNITED STATES

El Salvador is the smallest and most densely populated continental country along the Pacific coast of Central America. It is south of Mexico and Guatemala and slightly smaller than the State of Massachusetts. Salvadoran immigrants are among the top ten foreign-born nationalities in the United States (Malone, Kaari, Baluja, & Davis, 2003). But considering the lack of cooperation with the U.S. census by undocumented populations, independent sources estimate the number of Salvadorans at one million or more, putting them among the top five foreign-born populations in this country (Menjivar, 2000; Ulloa, 1998).

The 1968 immigration reforms made it theoretically possible for more Salvadorans to immigrate than previously, but it was really during the civil war in El Salvador, from 1980 to 1992, that immigration rates dramatically accelerated. The fleeing population grew by 500% in the 10-year interval, from 94,447, as stated in the 1980 U.S. census, to 585,081 in 1990. Immigration levels rose again following natural disasters such as Hurricane Mitch in 1998 and the devastating earthquakes and landslides of 2001.

Patterns of Salvadoran emigration to this country over the last century have been influenced by economic and political relations with the United States, importation of indigo and, later, of coffee, and employment in the companies taking over the Panama Canal. Additional influences include employment in the shipbuilding industry during the

Second World War, as well as on passenger and cargo ships. The second wave of Salvadoran immigrants originated from all regions of the country and probably followed the initial settlements through informal networks of families and friends. In 1990, 60% of the Salvadoran-born population in the United States was living in California. The City and County of Los Angeles had the second largest urban population of Salvadoran nationality, surpassed only by the City of El Salvador.

Estimates are that 25% of Salvadoran nationals (6,122,515 in 2000) are living abroad, more than half of them in the United States. Only 2.3% of Salvadoran immigrants to this country were granted the status of "refugee." The rest have been classified as "economic immigrants"—in spite of the 75,000 casualties during the civil war. In contrast, of the Cuban immigrants admitted from 1981 to 1998, 77% were granted refugee status, allowing them to gain permanent residency and welfare benefits. The decision-making process in regard to immigration obviously involves economic and political factors and has been influenced by U.S. policies and the Cold War. These circumstances have been devastating to Salvadoran immigrants who are left without access to a permanent documented status in the United States. Some studies have found that in Los Angeles and San Francisco more than 50% of Salvadorans surveyed were undocumented (Menjivar, 2000).

HISTORICAL, SOCIAL, AND POLITICAL PERSPECTIVES

At the time of colonization in the 16th century, the Pipil, descendants of Toltecs and Aztecs with strong Mayan influences, dominated the country. They had a complex theocratic culture; they wrote in hieroglyphs, used mathematic concepts, and were cognizant of astronomy, applying it to farming and religious rites. They had a developed an agricultural economy centered on harvesting corn. After the Spanish conquest and colonization, a handful of Spanish families owned most of the property. Manpower was provided by enslaved indigenous people, who lived in poverty and were decimated by the new diseases introduced by the colonizers (Hernandez, 1996). Throughout the 17th century the colonizers introduced new crops, including balsam, indigo, and cotton for exportation to the metropolis. When the indigenous people offered resistance, they where brutally repressed and, at times, killed. El Salvador became independent from Spain in 1821, but this had little impact on the modalities of production or landownership. In 1833, Anastasio Aquino led a major indigenous uprising that was violently repressed. In 1841, El Salvador became independent when the Central American Federation dissolved. Synthetic dyes replaced indigo, and coffee became the main export, accounting for more than 90% of export income. At that time 2% of the population controlled most of the wealth.

The culture of El Salvador has been primarily agrarian, with peasant families working on communal lands, focused on subsistence farming and trading goods in the local market. There has been a gradual, although sometimes forced and violent move toward privatizing communal land with a few powerful colonizers owning most of the land, and local peasants being hired to work land they no longer owned. By the end of the 19th century the pressure of the big landowners was reflected in laws accelerating this process, abolishing all communal lands in 1882 (Browning, 1971).

Peasant families were forced into a progressive adaptation to a monoculture, abandoning the subsistence farming and accommodating the concentration of landownership in fewer and fewer hands. Small producers had increasingly less representation in the government, and the emerging policies further favored the powerful landowners. They repeatedly backed repressive military governments. Further mechanization and the growth of a capital-intensive agrarian industry accelerated the loss of the peasants' lands. This reality generated an expansion of the male workforce, including field workers, who were the hands hired wherever the next harvest occurred, and those who provided unskilled manpower in the cities. The loss of attachment to specific lands left families and communities impoverished, weakened, and brittle. Since the beginning of the century, more than one third of the rural population lived in common-law unions. The men became laborers, joined the military or the opposition, and frequently did not return to their families. This forced women to find ways to provide for their families, often selling goods in the market. More women than men were forced to migrate to the cities to live in crowded slums. (McGoldrick & Giordano, 1996). The history of peasant families in El Salvador is mostly one of poverty and instability, prompting them to change in organization and structure and, eventually, to migrate. After exhausting their ability to adapt and to overcome the progressively more demanding and violent circumstances, some of these families disorganized. They resorted to leaving some or all the children with their parents, other family members, or even friends.

The development and organization of a political force able to establish a dialogue with those in the government occurred in several instances, but critical moments led to bloody confrontations and, in some cases, to the extermination of thousands of people. This process was repeated several times and remains in the collective memory of Salvadoran families; one of the most well-known instances was *La mantanza*. It occurred in 1932 in the central western part of the country. Newly organized peasants reacted to the misery and heavy unemployment that followed the economic collapse of the Great Depression, and the falling of coffee prices by more than 60% between 1928 and 1932 on the international market. Peasants, students, and other groups struggled for social and economic reforms and for reinstatement of the expropriated communal lands. The insurrection culminating with the massacre of *La mantanza* was lead by Farabundo Martí. Its repression by the military was brutal: Within 2 months, 30,000 people were killed, which represented more than 1.5% of the country's total population. In the western and central region more than 28% of the people were exterminated, most of them indigenous peasants. Successive attempts to diversify the economy created small industries, while maintaining the progressive concentration of the ownership of the land, causing substantial impoverishment and displacement of workers. Hundreds of thousands migrated to the cities and to other countries, particularly Honduras. When Honduras passed laws redistributing the land, 300,000 Salvadorans were repatriated, which increased the rampant unemployment. The two countries had a brief armed confrontation that disrupted their abundant trade. Because the Honduran authorities closed the highway to Nicaragua, the Central American Common Market collapsed. In 1980 a civil war started, fueled by the Reagan Administration, which was worried that another Central American country was following the path of Nicaragua. What followed was divisive and cruel, as "low-intensity warfare" principles were applied (Kusnir, 1993). The polarization became extreme, and during the confrontation between the military and the FMNL (Farabundo Martí National Liberation Front), many atrocities were perpetrated by the death squads against political, religious and labor leaders, homosexuals, HIV/AIDS services, and in extreme cases complete small villages were exterminated as in *El*

Mozote (where hundreds of men, women, and children were killed and placed in a mass grave). Official estimates place the direct casualties of the 12 years of civil war at 75,000. The murdering of religious figures, among them Archbishop Oscar Romero in 1980, and the Jesuit and social psychologist Ignacio Martín Baró and five other priests and nuns in 1989 (Winn, 1992), gave rise to the Sanctuary movement in the United States. This cause generated institutions sensitive to the humanitarian needs of the Central American immigrants, creating opportunities for protecting those undocumented and in desperate need. Upon their arrival, personal conflicts reflecting the different political affiliations complicated conditions for the new immigrants, fragmenting informal networks of support and aggravating poverty. Undocumented status, overcrowded conditions, and the *migra* raids (raids performed by the Immigration and Naturalization Service [INS] to capture, imprison, and deport illegal immigrants) created a climate of persecution, interfering with an immigrant's chance of having a stable job and impeding the building of a supportive community.

THE CULTURAL PERSPECTIVE

In the broad sense, the Latino culture can be depicted as hierarchical, family-oriented, fatalistic, and emphasizing personalism, interdependence, and spiritualism (see Garcia-Preto, 1996; Ho, 1987). Among the immigrants there is a longing for familial ties, even though at times these ties may be perceived as oppressive. But, as Aimee Césaire (2000) has described, the dominant ideology imposed by the colonizers equated Christianity with civilization and paganism with savagery (Oboler, 1997). The first embodies power, refinement, and white skin, whereas the second is portrayed as embodying weakness, dark skin, vulgarity, and poverty. Many aspects of that initial proposition remain internalized in the culture of El Salvador today. Identification with those polarities was maintained through the political, social, and familial discourses. These divisions do not follow sharp social class boundaries, as the individuals internalize the discourses idiosyncratically and to different degrees. This polarization currently follows two main sets of beliefs (Lopez & Stanton-Salazar, 2001), which can be described as liberal and conservative in politics, religion, and ideology. People are loyal either to the insurgent movement, the FMLN, or to the government and the military. There is also some discordance between beliefs and social class in those polarities. On one hand, many individuals and families do not have a defined loyalty or even a defined political or ideological position. On the other hand, all members of a family may be galvanized toward one position, or they may be painfully disturbed by members taking opposing sides, sometimes along generational lines. The dislodging of families by immigration (Kusnir, 1995), economic conditions, the increase of the common-law unions, and the distancing of the male figures did not destroy the cultural archetype of the male role. Instead, the male was relegated to the role of "spokesperson" rather than a real leader. The concept of *Compadrazgo* (close friends of the family who take responsibilities for the protection and welfare of a newborn as godparents) and other forms of shared supervision and guidance of the children faded away (Kusnir, 1981).

Homosexuality is often strongly censored, particularly for the male. It is viewed as abnormal, degenerate, a perversion, or a "curable" psychological sickness, and often as the main cause of AIDS. Parents may strongly oppose some male body piercing and certain professions (i.e., nursing, fashion design, etc.) as effeminate. In urban settings individuals with open homosexual preferences, regardless of social position, may be beaten or even killed ("Mourning in," 2000). Within a few months in 1998, there were five murders and several beatings, generating reactions and demonstrations by the small homosexual community in San Salvador ("How Homosexuality," 1998). This level of persecution/rejection may explain the tendency for some homosexual Salvadorans to deny homosexual acts while maintaining heterosexual relations as a cover.

CLINICAL CONSIDERATIONS

Salvadoran families that come for consultation come from various paths of life, social classes, and cultural experience. They come with specific problems. Families appreciate a problem-focused approach, limited to the concerns they have brought, and this approach can increase their trust. Other pertinent dimensions to attend to may include basic needs such as food, clothing, shelter, access to work, health care, and child care. It is important for the clinician to take account of the family's strengths and resources such as kin support, language proficiency, education, and legal status (Rojano, 2004). Clients may have abilities such as self-employment or skill in conducing small enterprises. Other areas to be considered by the therapist include economic pressures, access to resources and information, and access to a community with sensitivity to political affiliation (Sapocznik, Hervis, & Schwartz, 2003). The therapist often becomes an intergenerational cultural broker and a resource for information and referral.

More specifically, at times family problems are intertwined with the context of their departure, involving the interplay of their personal and family history with the history of their community and country. At other times the problem is related to the ordeal of the migration process itself. Finally, the concerns of the family may be related to its misadventures in the process of resettling in the United States.

THE CONTEXT OF DEPARTURE

Maria is a shy 20-year-old monolingual Spanish-speaking woman, referred by a local religious organization because she suffered anxiety and intrusive memories of traumatic episodes that she experienced 7 years ago. Her parents were peasants, sympathizing with the FMNL. Seven years earlier, the family was living in their small village and receiving repeated threats, when suddenly a paramilitary group erupted into their home and killed Maria's 14-year-old sister, also shooting the father. Maria, then 13, witnessed the episode while hiding under a bed. The father barely recovered from his gunshot wounds in a hospital. The threats continued, so Maria was sent to another region to live with an aunt, where she remained confined to a bedroom for 5 years, having contact only with that aunt, in order to avoid detection by neighbors. With the support of a local priest, Maria's parents collected enough money to send her to San Francisco. During her interviews Maria focused on overcoming her fears, finding a job, and helping her parents. Just then an earthquake devastated the area where her family lived, and she became almost immobilized with anxiety. She focused herself on work, helping another woman who was a housecleaner. She was able to stay in contact with her family and started an ESL class to learn English, but had difficulties participating in the group. Responding to an urgent request from the religious organization that was sponsoring Maria, I wrote a report for the INS, and she was finally granted asylum status. Shortly later, Maria stopped attending therapy, letting me know before leaving that although I had helped her gain asylum and focus on her goals of work and learning English, our meetings had also increased her anxiety and for now she preferred to concentrate on work and not think about her past.

Although Maria came to therapy for individual treatment, her current situation is inextricably linked to the traumatic history of her family, her isolation, and hiding out before managing to emigrate, all of which were reexperienced with every new traumatic event, including the ongoing political news from her country. Maria's adaptive strategy, common among Salvadorans who come to the United States, was to throw herself into work, both to survive and to attempt to help her parents economically. Her choice of domestic work, although economically one of her few available options, may continue her history of isolation, a factor I would have wanted to help her reconsider if we had had time in our work together.

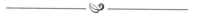

Maria's departure from her home was completely traumatic for her. It was instigated by her mother to save her life, but she had had no control over the decision to emigrate or to come to San Francisco. Most immigrants have at least a little more control in terms of weighing their emotional loss against their hopes for economic, personal, and political improvement. It is important for clinicians to be sensitive to the clients' sense of lacking control over their lives during the migration process. Feeling that they had a choice about immigrating will not diminish the enormous emotional cultural losses, but it can become a source of empowerment. Maria's losses included her sister's death, separation from her parents, confinement to a small room for 5 years, and finally being moved to a new country where she knew no one and could not speak the language. Coming from a deeply polarized society, with such a terrible history of massive killing, adds to the migration trauma for Salvadorans. Some patients will be unable to engage in therapy unless they sense that the therapist sympathizes with their political affiliation. At times, even a tactful reference to traumatic events must be postponed until the person's anxiety has diminished and he or she has, as Maria now has, some sense of mastery and control through knowledge of the language, job skills, and the security of making money. Trying to force the disclosure of secrets is never a prudent approach. Being sensitive to these areas was essential for joining with Maria and may be useful for joining with each member of a family. Her experience of support in our initial contact and her achieving asylum status will, it is hoped, enable her to return for help later if she needs it. My report provided concrete support for her economic empowerment in this country, her first priority for the moment. Although it also precipitated her leaving therapy for the time being, it also demonstrated to her that outside support can be helpful and that the trust she developed may enable her to turn to help again when she may be more ready to use emotional support to deal with other issues resulting from her traumatic history. An alternative that I was unable to use with Maria, which can be used in giving care to traumatized refugees, is to another therapist perform evaluations for the INS, leaving the original therapist to help the person deal with the anxieties triggered by the required narration of his or her immigration story. Fostering Maria's appreciation of her family's protecting her by hiding her and then sending her to a safe place may provide her with a source of strength. Seeing her family members as positive role models may increase her self-esteem and decrease her isolation. This goal needs to be balanced against the risk that family members could become rigidly idealized, making it difficult for her to find her own path.

THE CONTEXT OF THE IMMIGRATION ORDEAL

Nancy came for family therapy with her brother because of repeated conflicts she was having with him and his girlfriend. Oscar had been living in the United States for 4 years and was undocumented; Nancy joined him after 2 years, following several failed attempts to cross the border into Guatemala, where she was kidnapped for several months by a "coyote," the man whom she paid to arrange the border crossing. Later, in Mexico, she was raped and robbed, developing symptoms that led to a psychiatric hospitalization in that country. Her parents were peasants, and Nancy had been a street vendor in a small city in El Salvador, where Oscar had worked as a mechanic. Brother and sister had decided to immigrate for economic reasons.

Their consultation centered on the adjusting to their current situation and family structure, but it was clear that their difficulties, substantial as they were, had intensified because of their previous traumas along the way to this country, although many of the details of these experiences remained hidden. I had to approach Nancy gently at first, as she was clearly unwilling to include the most painful aspects of her life story in her presentation of who she was. Having separate interviews with her and her brother facilitated dealing with the history. In sessions alone with Oscar I was able to learn about the family history, because he was less reluctant to talk of it. Through re-storying the family history so that Oscar could appreciate the traumas they each had survived, I was able to encourage Oscar to continue to support his sister. I helped him to see that Nancy's sometimes erratic behavior was undoubtedly an effect of the trauma she had endured. I helped him to remember the closeness he and Nancy had as children, as well as the strength their family must have had to have survived at all. It would have been impossible to do this work with Nancy present, because the history was still too toxic for her to deal with. But knowing that history, I could help her brother to be less reactive to her moods and anxiety. In individual sessions with Nancy I was able to coach her to take advantage of her brother's support, while gradually encouraging her to examine some aspects of her traumatic history. This support enabled Nancy to be less frustrated with her brother and to accept his help until she was able to have a steady income. Of course, Nancy has still not fully recovered from her past trauma and periodically experiences depressive symptoms. She has not been able to find a job that offers insurance, a common problem for Salvadoran immigrants. Indeed, like many immigrants, she is in a catch-22. She does not qualify for the alternative insurance provided locally for the indigent population because her symptoms are not severe enough to qualify. This is because she has made so many efforts to function and support herself. Thus, her very success and efforts block her receiving the support she deserves.

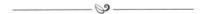

The ordeal of crossing the border by land may be traumatic in itself for Salvadorans or may revive old traumatic experiences. Salvadorans choose coming overland because they lack U.S. visas. This means that they have to first cross the border to Guatemala, and then the border between Guatemala and Mexico before crossing over to the United States. The crossing of the U.S.–Mexican border is dramatically depicted in the movie *El Norte*, but more immigrants are rejected at the Mexican–Guatemlan border than at the border between Mexico and the United States. For many Salvadoran migrants this journey takes months, and some spend years in the poor conditions of temporary refugee camps at the border between Mexico and Guatemala before they can cross, as in the case of Nancy. My observation has been that once they are here, Salvadorans, more than other Latino groups, tend to want to "start from scratch" and turn the page with the hope that what has happened will go away. Often, their inability to deal with their emotions results in broken relationships with family members. For Nancy the relationship with her brother continued and she was able to reconstruct it, but many families experience conflicts when new members arrive and those living here have no knowledge of the trauma that was experienced.

There are also conflicts about money. When Salvadorans arrive here, they usually find themselves with extraordinary debt. The initial amount they borrow often increases along the way, because additional money is needed to continue their journey, especially if they are blackmailed by the smuggler who brings them into the country. Those already living here may be feeling exploited, inasmuch as the trip is completely financed by relatives and friends in the United States (Menjivar, 2000). Relatives back in El Salvador are in such desperate conditions that they cannot contribute money, but those in the United States are themselves struggling and want to be paid. Adding to this stress is that upon arrival, the immigrants have unexpected difficulties in finding a job without a visa, which prevents them from paying their debts. Rather than ask for tolerance and patience, conflicts may increase and relationships can be broken. The therapist may find opportunities to enlarge the network of support by helping to reacquaint the parties in conflict.

Ms. Claudia Ruiz came to the United States on a temporary work visa 7 years ago, with her two youngest children, Heriberto, now 17, and Cecilia, now 15. Her visa will expire next year. She sought help because of difficulties with Cecilia, who failed in two schools and was about to fail again in ninth grade. Ms. Ruiz was working two jobs to keep the family going, spoke primarily Spanish, and complained about the difficulty she had in finding help at home. When she left El Salvador, she and her husband made a decision that he would remain because their older son, Carlos, had problems with alcohol and drugs; they used the influence of a local commander to get him into a military high school. Carlos did well and is currently planning to become a lawyer. Ms. Ruiz's husband became involved with another woman, had another child, and filed for divorce. Ms. Ruiz was entertaining the idea of sending Cecilia back to El Salvador, hoping that the solution that had proven effective with her older son, a boarding school, might now help her daughter. Ms. Ruiz is representative of many Salvadorans who are ambivalent about raising children in the United States.

Therapy for the Ruiz family focused first on their request for help, joining with each member to listen to his or her personal goals and expectations. In the interview, I explored the family process that had led to conflicts. Highlighting the positive affects and wishes underlying the blame, recrimination, and nagging facilitated more satisfying interactions. Another of my therapeutic functions was to act as a cultural broker in regard to the wishes of the youngsters. For example, Heriberto wanted to have an earring and his mother was adamantly opposed. Because of her anger, she was blocking an agreement for him to start work, which would help the family economically. As it was, Ms Ruiz had to work more hours and was less available without Heriberto's extra income. I discussed with them what they thought were the differences between personal life and family life. This conversation helped to validate Ms. Ruiz's right to have her own privacy and to develop broader relationships with friends, at the same time encouraging Heriberto's ability to have certain personal freedoms as long as he also took more adult responsibility in helping the family by working. Despite the importance of the transaction, Ms. Ruiz's inability to accept Heriberto's wish for an earring obstructed the therapeutic process. Her rigid position on this issue was probably related to intense feelings of homophobia. She may have thought that wearing an earring was a homosexual act, which she could not condone.

After migration, each segment of the family reconfigured itself and adjusted to its particular circumstances. In the United States, those who are younger usually acculturate more readily and obtain language proficiency more easily, which tends to make them unduly powerful in the family, acting as cultural brokers for the adults (Grinberg, 2003; Rumbaut & Ima, 1987). They may also view their Salvadoran heritage and culture as less valuable and powerful than the dominant culture. This weakens the parents' position, already undermined by other factors: the family's isolation, the lack of community connections that would traditionally help supervise children, lack of parental availability because they have to work more than one job, and the parents' lack of proficiency in English. Parents and children may get into cycles of mutual disillusionment, putting each other down, as children become acculturated to ideas that differ from parental expectations (Lopez & Stanton-Salazar, 2001). Paradoxically, the socioeconomic situation generating stress also prevents the family from having access to family therapy, because they lack money or time for sessions. This is often reflected in a premature interruption of treatment as soon as the precipitating crisis has shown any improvement. It may happen that despite the Salvadorans' wish to resolve family problems, they fall into blaming each other for their difficulties (Ho, 1987), unable to realize the power of the larger context against them. In such circumstances, the therapist tries to work with each family member, as illustrated in the case of Nancy and Oscar, to help diminish the blaming and increase the sense of commonality and mutual support.

Common problems to which these families are vulnerable include youth joining gangs; drug use; lack of access to scholarships, jobs, health care, and other social supports because of their undocumented status; and the parents' lack of experience in dealing with government agencies. Parents are often alienated or do not have access to natural support groups such as other parents or extended family.

CONCLUSION

Beyond attending to the language barrier when working with Salvadoran families in therapy, the clinician may often have to address other needs such as housing, clothing, food, personal safety, and immigration legal advice. This type of intervention, which can be labeled "cultural brokerage," may include helping the immigrant families to utilize human resources in their community to build social networks, and to understand that sometimes causes of stress are also sources of resilience.

Therapists must take into account that many of these families live in a very polarized milieu, depending on their religious and political affiliations. Therefore, it is crucial to balance the interest one expresses about their worldviews with respect for the their realistic needs for secrecy. This requires being sensitive to the family's pace, particularly for those who have been traumatized. Sometimes flexibility is needed regarding the time when sessions are held, the place, and the cost, primarily at the beginning of treatment. Paying attention to the families' hierarchical structure and leadership can help with successful joining. Taking into account the expectations of each family member when establishing goals in therapy will enhance the continuity of treatment. However, we must realize that although these clinical issues must be considered, many changes and interventions at a sociopolitical level are needed in addition to therapeutic interventions in order to make a difference.

REFERENCES

Browning, D. (1971). *El Salvador: Landscape and society.* Oxford, UK: Oxford University Press.

Césaire, A. (2000). *Discourse on colonialism* (J. Pikham, Trans.). New York: Monthly Review Press. (Original work published 1955)

Garcia-Preto, N. (1996). Latino families: An overview. In M. McGoldrick, J. K., Pearce, & J. Giordano (Eds.), *Ethnicity and family therapy* (2nd ed., pp. 141–154). New York: Guilford Press.

Grinberg, A. (2003). El Continente Perdido. Historia de una búsqueda. In M. I. Pazos & S. Gutkowski (Eds.), *Emigración, salud mental y cultura* (pp. 63–70). Buenos Aires: Ediciones Del Candil.

Hernandez, M. (1996). Central American families. In M. McGoldrick, J. K. Pearce, & J. Giordano (Eds.), *Ethnicity and family therapy* (2nd ed., pp. 214–224). New York: Guilford Press.

Ho, M. K. (1987). *Family therapy with ethnic minorities.* Newbury Park, CA: Sage.

How homosexuality is seen in El Salvador. (1998, July). *Proceso #813.* El Salvador: Universidad Centroamericana.

Kusnir, D. (1981). *De la convivencia en el hogar: El origen de la familia.* Mexico City, México: Dirección General de Publicaciones y Bibliotecas, Secretaría de Educación Pública.

Kusnir, D. (1993, October). The use of family therapy with victims of torture. In *Preventing torture and treating survivors.* Paper presented at the 121st annual meeting of the APHA, San Francisco.

Kusnir, D. (1995) Latino families coping with genetic disease and disabilities: A multilevel approach to therapy. *Diversity and Depth* (newsletter of the Multicultural Psychotherapy Training and Research Institute), *1,* 4–5.

Lopez, D., & Stanton-Salazar, R. (2001). Mexican Americans. In R. G. Rumbant & A. Portes (Eds.), *Ethnicities* (pp. 57–90). University of California Press.

Malone, N., Kaari F., Baluja, K., & Davis, C. (2003). *The foreign-born population: 2000* (2KBR-34, pp. 5, Table 2). Washington, DC: U.S. Bureau of the Census.

McGoldrick, M., & Giordano, J. (1996). Overview: Ethnicity and family therapy. In M. McGoldrick, J. K. Pearce, & J. Giordano (Eds.), *Ethnicity and family therapy* (2nd ed., pp. 1–27). New York: Guilford Press.

Menjívar, C. (2000). *Fragmented ties: Salvadoran immigrant networks in America.* Berkeley: University of California Press.

Mourning in the University of Central America. (2000, February). *Proceso #888.* El Salvador: Universidad Centroamericana.

Oboler, S. (1997). So far from God, so close to the United States. In M. Ronneno, P. Hondagneu-Sotelo, & V. Ortiz (Eds.), *Challenging Fronteras: An anthology of readings* (pp. 31–54). New York: Routledge.

Rojano, R. (2004). The practice of community family therapy. *Family Process, 43,* 59–77.

Rumbaut R., & Ima, K. (1987) *The adaptation of Southeast Asian refugee youth: A comparative study.* San Diego, CA: Department of Sociology, San Diego State University.

Szapocznik, J., Hervis, O., & Schwartz, S. (2003). *Brief strategic family therapy for adolescent drug abuse* (NIH Publication No. 03-4751). Bethesda, MD: National Institute on Drug Abuse.

Ulloa, R. (1998). *De indocumentados a ciudadanos: Características de los salvadoreños legalizados en Estados Unidos.* San Salvador: FLACSO.

Winn, P. (1992). *Americas.* Berkeley: University of California Press.

PART IV

❧

ASIAN FAMILIES

CHAPTER 20

Asian Families
An Overview

Evelyn Lee
Matthew R. Mock

Providing an overview of Asian American families poses some special challenges. In order to understand and work effectively with Asian American families, there must be an appreciation of the diversity and complexity contained in what it means to be Asian American. With more than five decades of combined wisdom gained in learning from and teaching others about Asian American families, we asked a number of questions in preparation for writing this chapter:

- What do we need to know about Asian American families' lives and values in order to work with them respectfully and effectively?
- What perspectives and resources have been most useful in working with them?
- How can we frame specific characteristics or cultural influences so they are not stereotypic or applied as a generality to fit all Asian American families?
- How can we pose a therapeutic framework for working with Asian American families that encourages hypothesis testing and rehypothesizing to fit the needs of the specific family in a culturally competent process?
- What therapeutic strategies may bring out the critical voices of Asian American family members themselves to inform the process?

Proceeding with these and other questions in mind, we offer a general snapshot of facts specific to Asian Americans and some common threads of the Asian American experience, followed by clinical recommendations.

ASIAN FAMILIES IN HISTORICAL AND CULTURAL CONTEXT

Terminology and Composition. The term "Asian American" has collectively referred to Americans whose families originated in many different Asian countries. Geographically, Asia includes countries encompassing the Far East, Southeast Asia, and the Indian sub-continent (including Cambodia, China, India, Japan, Korea, Malaysia, Pakistan, the Philippine Islands, Thailand, and Vietnam). In recent years, the U.S. census has referenced Pacific Islanders, that is, those people who are descendents of the original residents of the Pacific Islands, including Chamorro, Hawaii, Melanesia, Micronesia, Polynesia, and Samoa (Reeves & Bennett, 2003), with Asian Americans. There are 30 different groups listed as Asian American and 21 listed as Pacific Islander. The terms "Asian American" and "Asian American and Pacific Islander" (AAPI) came into use with the political activism of the 1960s replacing the outdated term "Oriental," which has been seen as offensive, insensitive, or, at best, socioculturally uninformed (Hong & Ham, 2001).

Population. As of the year 2000, it is estimated that there are almost 14 million people residing in the United States who list themselves as Asian American (13 million) or Pacific Islander (almost 1 million). This represents 5% of the total U.S. population. In terms of Asian Americans as a whole, the groups most numerous by percentage are Chinese (27%), Filipino (19%), Asian Indian (12%), Japanese (11%), Korean (11%) and Vietnamese (9%). The growth rate of the Asian American population has been one of the highest of all groups. In fact, if trends continue, by the year 2050 Asian Americans will make up 8% of the U.S. population (Barnes & Bennett, 2002).

Residency. A large majority of Asian Americans (95%) live in metropolitan or urban areas. Some 51% of the total population lives in the Western part of the United States. California, New York, and Hawaii have the largest concentrations of Asian Americans, with notable percentages also residing in Texas, New Jersey, Illinois, Washington, Florida, Virginia, and Massachusetts. Various groups may favor certain cities. For example, Chinese favor San Francisco, Boston, New York, and Washington, D.C. Japanese are drawn to Honolulu, Los Angeles, and Seattle. Filipinos favor San Diego, Daly City/San Francisco, and San Jose. The Vietnamese show concentrations in Orange County, San Jose, and the Central Valley area in California; Houston; and Minneapolis.

Birthplace and Immigration. Asian-born residents constitute one fourth of the nation's total foreign-born population. More than 8 million Americans were born in Asia, with 1.5 million tracing their birth to China. Next to Mexico, China is the leading country of birth for this country's foreign born. The Philippines, India, Vietnam, and Korea are four Asian countries among the top 10 around the world that contribute most to the American foreign-born population.

Size of Families and Ages. Almost three quarters of Asian American households are made up of families. Among these, 20% have five or more members; 26% of Asian Americans are under 18 years of age and 7% are 65 or older.

Languages. Among Asian American groups, there are at least 32 different primary languages spoken. Within each group (such as Chinese and Filipino), there are sometimes many dialects. An Asian language is spoken by 6.9 million Asian Americans, with proficiency and command of English varying among family members. A majority of foreign-born Asians still speak their root language at home and may still struggle with English to varying degrees. Next to Spanish, Chinese is the most widely spoken non-English language in this country. There are also notable numbers of individuals who still speak Taga-log, Vietnamese, and Korean.

Educational Attainment. Asian Americans, especially Asian Indians, Chinese, and Japanese, in the year 2000, were more likely than Whites to have earned at least a college degree. But they were also more likely to have less than a ninth-grade education, such as many Laotians and Cambodians. Therefore, although Asian Americans often stand out in terms college graduation rates and postgraduate training, there are also significant numbers of Asian Americans with little formal education.

Family Income. Parallel to their educational attainment, some Asian Americans have family incomes that are among the highest of all groups, yet others, such as Southeast Asians, are among the poorest. In 2001, 40% of Asian American families had incomes over $75,000 annually, whereas 10% lived below the poverty line, including 66% of Laotians, 49% of Cambodians, and 34% of Vietnamese (Reeves & Bennett, 2003). Asian Americans are also still known to pool their family economic resources and may have a larger number of individuals contributing to total family income.

Religion and Spiritual Backgrounds. Religious beliefs and spiritual practices vary greatly among the different Asian American groups. Among some Chinese Americans, the most popular religions include Buddhism and Christianity. More than 70% of Korean Americans are Protestant Christians and attend church regularly. Filipinos, under the earlier Spanish influence, are predominantly Catholic. Japanese Americans may follow Shintoism, Buddhism, or Christianity. Vietnamese practice Buddhism, and from their French colonial past, Catholicism. In addition to Buddhism, Cambodians and Laotians are strongly influenced by the religions of Brahmanism of the Hindus, and the Hmong and the Mien are usually animistic and believe strongly in supernatural causation. Religion, faith, and spirituality may impact child-rearing practices and family values both pre- and postmigration.

Common Threads among Asian American Groups

Centrality of the Family Unit

Asian family values are very different from Western family values. In contrast to Western cultures, in which the nuclear family stresses independence, autonomy, and self-sufficiency of the individual members, in Asian cultures the family unit is highly valued and emphasized throughout the life cycle. The teachings of Confucianism, Taoism, and Buddhism have a profound, lasting influence as Eastern philosophical approaches to life and family interactions even when they are not specifically articulated.

Rather than an "I" identity, Asians are taught to embrace a "we" identity. The individual does not stand alone, but is seen as the product of all the generations of his or her family and is therefore held in relation to them. The centrality of the family unit is reinforced by child-rearing practices, rituals, and customs such as family celebrations and meals, birth and death rites, the passing down of cultural metaphors and stories, and the sacredness of genealogy records.

Immigration Histories

Each Asian American group has a complex migration history in the United States. Chinese Americans were the first Asians to immigrate to the United States in large numbers and have come in three waves over a 150-year period. The 1965 Immigration Act brought a large number of Chinese, as well as Koreans and Filipinos. Most current Japanese Americans are descendants of Japanese who migrated to Hawaii or the U.S. mainland before 1924. With the end of the Vietnam War in 1975, a large number of Southeast Asian refugees arrived, initially mostly educated Vietnamese. Since 1978, a second wave came to the United States to escape persecution, including Vietnamese, Chinese Vietnamese, Cambodians, Lao, Hmong, and Mien. Worldwide events continue to impact migration and eventual resettlement patterns (Takaki, 1991).

Exposure to Trauma, War, and Political Upheaval

Many Asian countries suffered from war or political turmoil. As a result, different members of Asian American families were exposed to losses, separation, changes in health status, torture, or other forms of direct or secondary trauma before immigrating to the United States. Because the identity of Asian Americans is not just of those in the present but also those in the past and the future, trauma and loss may often be expressed and understood by Asian American families in different ways and to differing degrees. For some Chinese families, a traumatic experience may be viewed as preordained or a matter of fate. For traditional South Asian families, the notion of karma, suggesting that one endure current circumstances as part of life, can be important in understanding trauma. Among some Japanese communities, to withstand hardships or *gamman* is associated with maturity. Silence may be viewed as a virtue. Therefore, manifestations of posttraumatic stress disorder either pre- or postmigration, or even intergenerationally expressed, are significant to note (Westermeyer, 1989).

Stereotypes and the "Model Minority" Image

Asian Americans are still often held up to be the "model minority," particularly in relation to other ethnic groups. Despite facts to the contrary, Asian Americans are consistently viewed as high academic achievers and a group that does not create problems in society. Images of Asian women as passive, sexualized objects and Asian men as controlling and not being sexually attractive persist after a half century of media stereotyping. Diverse, more accurate images of Asian Americans are still highly lacking in contemporary, mainstream media. The lack of a range of realistic reflections of self may contribute to identity clashes. Mental health problems and social problems such as domestic violence, alcohol and substance abuse, gambling, gangs, and violence are often well known among Asian American communities. However, for those with limited exposure to this community, they must become aware of these salient issues that counter stereotypes. The persistent myth of the "model minority" may further contribute to family pressures and individual stresses.

Racism and Discrimination

Despite advances in society, Asian Americans may still be targets of racism, discrimination, and hate crimes. Even with a long legacy of contributions to the fabric of the United States, Asian Americans are still marginalized and regarded as foreigners to mainstream America. As the personal stories and struggles of famous Chinese Americans such as

Maya Lin, Chang-Lin Tien, Amy Tan, Michelle Kwan, Connie Chung, Gary Locke, and Wen Ho Le attest, subtle or overt racism toward Asian Americans still exists and anti-Asian sentiment can still rear its ugly head. After they have lived for several generations in America, the accents and cultural traditions of Asian American families may begin to fade, but skin tone and shape of eyes do not (Chang, 2003). Experiences of specific individual or community racism and discrimination can have profound effects on Asian American families, evidenced by the keeping of secrets to hide family shame, as well as stories of coping that strengthen their survival.

Mental Health and Psychopathology

Relative to the general American population, knowledge and awareness of the mental health needs of Asian Americans are thought to be limited. As reported in *Mental Health: Culture, Race and Ethnicity: A Report of the Surgeon General* (U.S. Department of Health and Human Services, 2001), the limited studies that are available have focused on Chinese Americans, Japanese Americans, and Southeast Asians. The available mental health studies suggest that the overall prevalence of mental health problems and psychological disorders does not differ significantly from that of other Americans. However, the distribution of disorders may be different for Asian American than for other groups. Asian Americans tend to show more symptoms of depression and depression-related syndromes and somatic complaints than White Americans.

The expression of mental health problems seems to depend on the family's level of acculturation. Those who remain more traditional tend to exhibit more culture-bound syndromes, defined as clusters of symptoms much more common in some cultural groups than others. For example, neurasthenia is a common diagnosis in China, characterized by fatigue, weakness, poor concentration, aches and pains, sleep disturbance, and so on. It is more closely related to a somatoform disorder than to mood disturbance and may be treated by changing the Chi energy, or life force, of the person.

There is some research that has underscored six predictors of mental health problems among Asian Americans: (1) employment or financial insecurity, (2) gender—Asian women seem more vulnerable, (3) older age, (4) social isolation, (5) relatively recent immigration, and (6) refugee premigration experiences and postmigration adjustment.

Utilization of Mental Health Services

Asian Americans continue to have the lowest rates of utilization of mental health services among ethnic populations regardless of gender, age, and geographic location. These low rates of utilization have been attributed to shame and stigma related to using the services, lack of financial resources, differing conceptions of illness and health, and lack of culturally competent services. Studies show that when Asian Americans seek mental health treatment, it is only when problems are very serious and have stretched the family system to its limit. Asian Americans may also turn to alternative resources within their communities, such as using alternative medicine, traditional healers, spiritual leaders, and the like. The Hmong, for example, often employ their *Hu Plig* (a calling back of the soul/spirit) ceremony and the related *Khi Tes* ritual (the tying of strings around each family member's wrists) for certain physical or mental illnesses (Fadiman, 1997).

Asian American Families and Interrelated Subsystems

The Family System

In traditionally influenced Asian American families, the family unit—rather than the individual—is most highly valued. The individual is seen as the sum of all the generations of his or her family. Because they are a part of this larger continuum, individual family members' personal actions reflect not only on themselves but also on their extended family and ancestors (Hong & Ham, 2001; Shon & Ja, 1982; Wong & Mock, 1997). Asian and Pacific cultures emphasize harmonious interpersonal relationships, interdependence, and mutual obligations or loyalty for achieving a state of psychological homeostasis or peaceful coexistence with family members or other fellow beings. Individuals are not usually encouraged to express directly how they are feeling. Indeed, the Chinese have a saying: "The nail that sticks up will be pounded down" (Hsu, 1971). Obligation, shame, and guilt are the mechanisms traditionally used to reinforce societal expectations and proper behavior. An individual is expected to function in his or her clearly defined role and position in the family hierarchy, in accordance with his or her age, gender, and social class.

The relative dominant influence of patriarchy still remains. In China, a woman's value historically was related to her giving birth to sons in order to preserve the family name. In 1979 the leadership in China instituted the "one-child family" policy whereby one-child families received better government benefits, and those who had more children could be penalized with burdensome fines or other harsh sanctions. To circumvent these one-child laws, Chinese couples who specifically decided to have sons would hide their daughters with relatives, would not even name their daughters (considering female life worthless), or, in some extreme situations, would engage in infanticide or abandonment. With orphanages being overwhelmed, in 1992 mainland China began facilitating large-scale international adoption. Between 1985 and 2002, Americans adopted more than 33,000 infants from the People's Republic of China, the largest number of children from any country (Chang, 2003).

The Marital Subsystem

In traditional Asian families, marriages are arranged by parents or grandparents to ensure the family prosperity and propagation of the husband's family line. The primary relationship is more likely to be the parent–child dyad, rather than that of the husband–wife. The husband assumes the role of leadership and authority and is the provider and protector of the family. The wife assumes the role of homemaker and childbearer. Physical and verbal expressions of love are uncommon. When things go wrong, the difficulties may be repaired by other adult mediators or confidants. Divorce is relatively uncommon. The wife is usually dominated by the authority of her husband, her father, her in-laws, and sometimes her oldest son. Traditionally, Asian women are often viewed in relation to men throughout their lifespan.

The Parent–Child Subsystem

The traditional role of a mother is to provide nurturance and support. The father's role is to discipline. These functions tend to be complementary, rather than symmetrical. The strongest emotional attachment for a woman is often to her children, especially her sons. Most parents demand filial piety, respect, and obedience from their children. In many extended families, children are raised by their parents but are cared for by a wide range of adults (grandparents, uncles, aunts, cousins, friends who have earned the status as an informal relative). Parents expect to be cared for in their old age. Elders are to be highly respected, revered, and cared for within families as part of the multigenerational family life cycle.

The Sibling Subsystem

Because of the large number of children in many Asian families, the parents usually delegate child-care functions to older siblings (especially the eldest daughter). Cooperation and sharing among siblings are expected. The emotional ties among siblings are especially strong for those who escaped and survived war in their homelands. Because of the tradition of sexism, sons are favored. If or when there is a conflict between siblings, it is not uncommon for a parent to admonish both: the younger child for not respecting the elder, and the older child for not being a good role model and setting a good example. In this reciprocal way of managing conflicts, the interrelated relationship between individuals is emphasized.

Asian American Families in Dynamic Transition

During the past 200 years many Asians families have migrated to the United States. Their contacts with American values over a prolonged period have changed their outlook on such issues as gender roles, child rearing, and family structure. The values, norms, and role behavior learned in the home country are modified when a family adjusts to the new culture. Many Asian American families are in transition from an extended family to a nuclear unit through the inevitable changes induced by migration, urbanization, and modernization. Family members struggle to hold onto the old way while also trying to develop new coping skills. Some are eventually successful, but others develop symptoms of stress in attempting to force a blend between two contradictory sets of rules (Lee, 1990). Where the stresses are extreme and the support systems are insufficient, a family may become isolated, enmeshed, or disengaged (Landau, 1982).

We may describe Asian American families in transition as fitting into several major types: traditional families, families in "cultural conflict," bicultural families, "Americanized" or highly acculturated families, and new millennium families (previously referred to as interracial). This typology is a construct that may help us understand the complexity of Asian American families. There are numerous variations within this typology, and some families may not fit into any specific type. There are also various dynamic aspects within these families to be noted, such as their degree of familiarity or affinity with their cultural roots (Mock, 1998a).

Traditional Families

Traditional families usually consist entirely of individuals born and raised in Asian countries. They include families from agricultural backgrounds, recent arrivals with limited exposure to Western culture, unacculturated immigrants who are deeply steeped in their home culture at the time of immigration, and families who live in ethnic Asian communities (e.g., Chinatown, Little Saigon, Koreatown, Japantown), havng limited contact with American mainstream society. Tending to be elders, these family members hold strong beliefs and traditional values and regularly speak in their native languages and dialects. Family members still practice traditional rituals and customs. Many may be members of family associations and social clubs consisting of people from a similar heritage, supporting adherence to traditional values.

Families in Culture Conflict

These families have either American-born children or children who were quite young when they arrived with their parents more than a decade ago. The family system usually experiences a great deal of cultural conflict between acculturated children and traditional parents or grandparents. Intergenerational conflicts and role confusion in which, for example, parents are reliant on their children to communicate with others in English, are common problems. Some families have conflicts because one spouse is more acculturated than the other. For instance, a husband may have lived in the United States for many years and eventually marries a wife from the home country who is not familiar with American culture. Conflicts may be caused not only by different degrees of acculturation, but also by religious, philosophical, or political differences. Differential command of the English language and abilities to negotiate the educational, governmental, social, or other systems in the family's life may be key stressors.

Bicultural Families

Bicultural families consist of well-acculturated parents who grew up in major Asian cities and were exposed to urbanization, industrialization, and Western influences. Many came to this country as young adults. Some were born in the United States but raised in traditional families. These parents often hold professional jobs, come from middle- or upper-class family backgrounds, and are bilingual and bicultural. In such families, the power structure has moved from a patriarchal to a more egalitarian relationship between the parents. Decision making is not solely the father's task; rather, there are "family discussions" between parents and children. These families typically do not live within their own ethnic neighborhoods. "Nuclear" family members may visit their close relatives, such as parents and grandparents, on weekends and holidays.

"Americanized" or Highly Acculturated Families

Some Asian families have become highly acculturated, adopting largely mainstream American ways. They usually consist of parents and children born and raised in the United States. As generations pass, the roots of the traditional Asian cultures slowly recede, and individual members may not express interest in or make any effort to maintain their ethnic identities. Family members communicate in English and may even adopt a more individualistic and egalitarian orientation. In many ways, they stress the American aspects of their identities and may not identify with their Asian roots or may do so only after deep consideration and exploration.

New Millennium Families

As a testimony to dynamic changes in cultural identity, new millennium families may be described as those going beyond any prior set norms or standards. Members of these families may call into question prior cultural expectations and are forging new identities. Lee (1997) previously described these families as "interracial families," noting the increasing number of multiracial Asian American families and interracial relationships, especially among Japanese, Filipino, Chinese, Vietnamese, and Korean Americans. Some multiracial families are able to integrate their multiple cultures with a high degree of success. Others may experience clashes in values, conflicts in communication styles, differences in managing societal pressures, and identity confusion. New millennium families are at the cutting edge of what it means to be an Asian American family, yet at the same time keep their cultural backgrounds in some perspective.

TREATMENT ISSUES

Family Assessment

Our proposed approaches to assessment are drawn from two major conceptual frameworks: social systems theory and its application to family therapy, and Eastern holistic concepts of health, wellness, and illness. This section offers a synopsis of a multilayered, complex assessment process described in other texts (Lee, 1997).

The family is a complex institution that can be investigated and understood from various perspectives. The clinician needs to assess (1) the internal family system, which includes understanding individual members and family subsystems, and (2) external factors, which include the impact of community and other environmental stressors. Because many Asian families undergo rapid social change and cultural transition, relevant background information and descriptive narratives on migration history, impact of war, cultural shock, racism, employment, and housing are extremely helpful. Although the Western psychological and biological understanding of emotional difficulties is important, incorporating the Eastern holistic way of thinking into clinical practice is also needed. The mind and body are integrally connected. We recommend taking into account psychological, social, biological, cultural, political, and spiritual influences on the lives of families. In addition to the traditional psychosocial assessment or mental health status examination, clinicians should adopt a holistic model in data collection and assessment (Lee, 1982). Beyond general demographic data collected in a genogram, the clinician should explore the family's ethnocultural heritage (both maternal and paternal lines), socioeconomic background (before and after migration), immigration status and history of each member (who came first, who was left behind, and why), basis of marriage (matched or romantic love), acculturation level of each family member, family leadership and decision making, sex role differentiation, child-rearing practices, forms of discipline, role expectations, family communication patterns, relationships with legal sponsors, and the like. Genogram information should be handled carefully and with strategic timing.

The clinician will need information on the neighborhood and larger community, including the availability of role models, housing conditions, economic climate and job availability, educational systems for children and adults, human service network and support systems, differential access to health care, and problems of crime, violence, drugs, racism, prejudice, and discrimination. In working with immigrant and refugee Asian families, the clinician should take time to conduct an in-depth assessment of the premigration history, the migration experience, and the postmigration experience and cultural shock (Lee, 1989). A systematic and longitudinal understanding of the migration experience and degree of war trauma is crucial. When taking a thorough migration history, the clinician can apply a chronological approach focusing on both premigration and immigration history. Genograms (McGoldrick, Gerson, & Schellenberger, 1998), oral history, cultural sayings and metaphors in the root language, use of media images or literature references (Mock, 1998a) and family photographs can be helpful. The clinician will need to discover the details of the premigration experience of the family: the city/village of origin, family composition, major political changes, socioeconomic status, employment status, support system, and other experiences and factors that influenced migration to the United States. The reasons for leaving, means of escape, hardships endured during the trip, types of loss, and the trauma experienced are also important to assess. In exploring postmigration experiences, the clinician should assess the degree of cultural shock and loss and the impact on each family member. When the stresses are extreme and the support system and prior methods used to cope are insufficient, the family in transition may be thrown into crisis. A member's failure to handle a particular problem may lead to dysfunction within the entire family system. The receiving environment of the new host culture is also important. In the case of ongoing discrimination, as in the internment of Japanese Americans during World War II, an entire generation of immigrants can be thrown into crisis. If not addressed, unresolved issues can persist in subsequent generations (Nagata, 1990).

The Impact of Migration on Individual and Family Life Cycles

The adjustment to a new culture is a prolonged developmental process that will affect many family members differently, depending on the individual and family life cycle phase they are in at the time of transition (Hernandez & McGoldrick, in press). For example, when families migrate at the same time when their children have grown and are leaving to establish their own lives, it is very difficult for the parents to break into new jobs, find new friends, and deal with the empty-nest syndrome simultaneously.

Differences in Rates of Acculturation of Family Members

Individual family members within a household may differ greatly in their rate of acculturation. In general, the degree of acculturation depends on years in the United States, age at time of migration, exposure to Western culture and people, professional affiliation, work environment, and English-speaking ability. Each family member may draw upon different resources for coping, including internal hardiness and resilience (Mock, 1998a).

Family Stresses Caused by Role Reversal

In many Asian American families, role reversals created by their migration cause serious strain. When monolingual adults depend on their English-speaking children as culture brokers and interpreters, the situation can cause anger and resentment. Prior power arrangements are thrown into chaos. Role reversals may also occur between husband and wife. Husbands, who are accustomed to male-dominated Asian cultures, find it difficult to accept wives who may find work more easily and become more independent and assertive, especially when the husbands have to find or accept work below their previous standing. This situation may contribute to domestic violence or other attempts to reassert power and control. Many immigrants and refugees have been raised by persons other than their biological parents because of the separation of family members. Family reunion in the United States after years of separation may trigger unresolved family conflicts, resentment, issues of guilt and shame, and loss of face.

Work and Financial Stresses

Asian American families value hard work, and economic stress has been significantly associated with depression (U.S. Department of Health and Human Services, 2001). Many Asian Americans immigrants experience unemployment and underemployment. "Downward mobility," not just economically but in social standing, may lead to low self-esteem, insecurity, and role reversal in families. For acculturated and professional Asian Americans, a "glass ceiling" (a term referring to barriers to success and upward mobility) and subtle discrimination at work sites often lead to frustration and job dissatisfaction. Family members' type of work and work hours also influence family dynamics. At one extreme, a typical Asian American small-business owner (e.g., laundry, grocery store) requires the whole family to spend long hours together, sometimes resulting in relationships that are intense and "too close." In other situations, such as at restaurants or engineering/research offices, parents may work extremely long hours. Family members seldom have sufficient time together to communicate. A phenomenon among these immigrants is the "astronaut" family, meaning that most of the family resides in the United States and one parent still conducts his or her business in the home country. Such families maintain their relationships by e-mail, phone, fax, and "frequent flyer" trips.

Neighborhood and Community Support

For Asian American families that live in ethnic communities that reflect and "mirror" their culture, the community support systems usually provide a cushion against the stresses of migration. Although those outside such communities may view Asians as cliquish, such Asian communities provide a sense of belonging, connectedness, and validation. Unfortunately, because of housing shortages, many recent immigrants and refugees have to live in poor neighborhoods, where they feel isolated from their ethnic communities and encounter problems of crime, violence, drugs, and substandard living conditions. Those who live in areas with relatively small Asian populations, such as in small towns and rural areas, generally have even more trouble adjusting and are pressured to assimilate more rapidly. The clinician should also explore the effect of racism, prejudice, and discrimination on family members especially during times of political unrest, when those who look different from the mainstream population are treated as "foreigners," outsiders who are not to be trusted.

Family's Religious and Spiritual Beliefs

Asian Americans come from a variety of religious backgrounds, including Christian, Buddhist, Shinto, and Muslim. Family behavior is often influenced by religious beliefs. In many Asian countries, religious organizations are highly respected. The priest, minister, or Buddhist monk is a key figure in the process of solving family problems. The clinician should determine whether the family belongs to a particular church or temple and the availability of emotional support or counseling from the particular organization. In many Asian American households, values that are shared by the grandparents or parents may be challenged by the younger generation, which is typically exposed to Western religions. The clinician should encourage the family members to share their spiritual beliefs in relation to the presenting problem and problem-solving strategies. Acknowledgement of differences in beliefs and other matters can allow clearer family decision making.

Family's Physical Health and Medication History

The clinician should explore the physical health of Asian clients, because they tend to express their emotional problems in somatic terms and usually come to treatment with many physical complaints. Many Asians, especially refugees, are in need of medical attention because of physical injuries, malnutrition, and lack of adequate medical treatment during times of conflict. They are often unfamiliar with Western medicine and may become confused by drug names, dosages, and side effects. Furthermore, for many Asian Americans, concurrent use of Western and traditional medicine is quite common. The family often appreciates the clinician's concern about these health and medication matters. In addition, networking with other skilled providers may facilitate critical aspects of the clinician being trusted as an effective healer and being a provider of tangible help. This has also been described as the clinician's "credibility" and "giving" (Sue & Zane, 1987).

Culturally Specific Responses to Mental Health Problems

Many traditional Asians do not accept Western biopsychological explanations of mental illness. A mental health problem may be conceptualized as a manifestation of organic disorders, hereditary weakness, an imbalance between yin and yang, a disturbance of chi energy, supernatural intervention, or emotional exhaustion caused by external environmental factors. In the assessment process, the clinician should encourage the client or family members to openly discuss their cultural and religious perspectives regarding the presenting problem, their past coping styles, their health-seeking behavior, and their treatment expectations. Questions to ask may include the following (Lee, 1990):

- What are the symptoms and problems as perceived by family members?
- What would be the diagnostic label given in the client's home country?
- What are the family's cultural explanations of the causes of the problem?
- What kind of treatment might the family get if they were back in their home country?
- Where did the family go for help before they came to see the clinician?
- What is the family's experience with herbal medicine, indigenous healers, and Asian healing exercises (such as tai chi, chi gong)?
- What were the family's previous experiences with health care and mental health care systems?
- What exposure has the family had to mental health professionals?

- What are the family's treatment expectations?
- What cultural metaphors or proverbs might be used to describe their symptoms or problems (i.e., are there phrases or stories in their root language that capture aspects of the presenting issues)?

Cultural Strengths

Along with assessment of family stresses and pathologies, an assessment is necessary with respect to individual and family strengths in adaptation, coping, and problem solving. Asian families may arrive in the United States with many challenges. But they are also strengthened by very highly developed cultures, religions and philosophies, as well as by powerful narratives of survival. Reintroducing family rituals can give voice to family connectedness across generations (Mock, 1998a). Asian cultures place great importance on hard work, education, family, friends, and others in the ethnic community. During a crisis, Asian families can usually rely on this network of support. The therapist should explore this with the client and encourage him or her to utilize community networks and organizations. Examining the current crisis may open new opportunities for the family.

Culturally Competent and Relevant Treatment Strategies

Traditional Western psychotherapeutic approaches based on the assumptions of individuation, independence, self-disclosure, verbal expression of feelings, and long-term insight-oriented therapy may go counter to Asian American values of interdependence, self-control, repression of most emotions, and short-term result-oriented solutions. A number of family therapists have offered valuable insights on how to respond to Asian Americans' cultural and expressive styles. Kim (1985) recommended an integrated family therapy orientation drawn from Haley's strategic and Minuchin's structural therapies. Ho (1987) suggested that Bowen's intergenerational perspective and Satir's cognitive approach might help teach the family's rules to its members. Paniagua (1994) suggested several effective treatment strategies, such as the therapist exhibiting expertise and authority, maintaining formality and conversational distance, providing concrete and tangible advice, and giving assurance that stress will be reduced as quickly as possible. Sue and Zane (1987) maintain two therapeutic processes to be critical: credibility and gift giving (i.e., seeing that the client receives a benefit early in the treatment process). Not only do clients need to have a strong belief that the therapist has the ability to be helpful throughout, but the adults also need to leave sessions with tangible evidence of hope, improved ability to problem solve, helpful suggestions to try at home, or potential for symptom relief in the foreseeable future. These are considered "gifts," manifested with the help of the therapist. Effective clinical strategies need to incorporate unique Asian cultural values and family characteristics. The following suggestions are divided into three distinct phases: beginning, problem solving, and termination (Ho, 1987).

Beginning Phase: Engaging the Family

Because Asian American clients are usually unfamiliar with family therapy, the clinician needs to pay special attention to the first contacts and beginning phase of therapy in order to avoid premature termination. The following suggestions may help establish rapport and deepen motivation for the family to continue treatment. Three areas are particularly important in this phase: engaging the family, assessing family readiness, and deciding which family members should be involved in therapy.

1. In view of the traditional family power structure, the initial appointment should be made with the family's "decision maker," often the father. Not respecting traditional lines of authority—for example, requesting the English-speaking children to inform the parents of an appointment—may reinforce a role reversal in the family. If necessary, ask an interpreter to make the arrangements. Be sure to set an appointment time that is convenient for working parents, because they typically value work more than therapy. Detailed explanations of the reasons for such an appointment and the location of your agency may be necessary.

2. Many immigrants do not understand the role of a mental health professional and may confuse him or her with a physician. A brief explanation of the clinician's role and training background may be helpful. Early inquiries about the therapist's degrees, publications, accomplishments, and other concrete testaments to his or her abilities, including where and how long the therapist has worked, may constitute polite probing into the therapist's credentials for effectiveness. Appropriately responding and acknowledging the newness of the process may facilitate therapeutic engagement.

3. During the first session, the clinician should address the family in a polite, somewhat formal manner. In addition, he or she needs to pay attention to "interpersonal grace" and offer warm expressions of acceptance, both verbally and nonverbally. Greeting each family member with a smile, hanging up his or her coat, offering a cup of tea, and providing comfortable chairs to older family members are examples of nonverbal ways of showing genuine respect, concern, and cultural sensitivity (Ho, 1987).

4. Many Asians are used to receiving help or advice from their friends or village elders. They may ask the clinician many personal questions, such as his or her country of origin, marital status, and number of children. The clinician must feel comfortable in answering such questions. Appropriate self-disclosure may facilitate a positive cultural alliance and a level of trust and confidence, as well as rapport across cultures. In fact, answering questions strategically and respectfully is not a boundary violation, but rather helps to build the cultural relationship and working alliance and establish credibility.

5. Forming a relational and cultural connection with the family during the initial session is very important. For the clinician who has lived in the Asian clients' home country or who has had extensive experience in working with Asians, it will be beneficial to disclose his or her familiarity with that culture to make the cultural connection. And for the clinician who is not familiar with the client's culture, it is important to show interest in and appreciation of it. Pictures of Asian countries and cultures on the office wall can also convey the clinician's interest. A therapeutic stance of naivete, along with knowledgeable curiosity, often facilitates a positive working relationship (Mock, 1998b).

6. Because many Asian family members are not used to verbal communications in therapy, asking nonthreatening personal questions can put the family at ease. Engaging the clients in small talk may help initiate the therapeutic process. To establish rapport, it is important to avoid direct confrontation, demands for greater emotional disclosure, or a discussion of culturally taboo subjects such as sex, death, or other emotionally charged topics.

7. For many Asians, publicly acknowledging mental health problems can bring intense shame and humiliation. The clinician may counter these emotions by empathizing with clients and encouraging them to verbalize such feelings. He or she should also assure family members about confidentiality and anonymity. A helpful technique is to reframe their courage in seeking help as love and concern for their family. If appropriate, mobilizing the family's sense of obligation to receive help in order to achieve family harmony, or for the sake of the children, can be very effective. Acknowledging strengths amid adversity and reframing their purposes can help to minimize blaming.

8. Many Asian clients come to treatment initially believing that the clinician is an authority who can tell them what is wrong and how to solve their problems. It is helpful for the clinician to establish credibility right away, to ensure that the client will return. Confidence, empathic understanding, maturity, and professionalism are all important ingredients. Other ways to establish credibility and authority include (a) using professional titles when making introductions; (b) displaying diplomas, awards, and licenses in the office; (c) obtaining sufficient information about the client and family before seeing them for the first time; (d) offering a possible explanation for the cause of the problem; (e) showing familiarity with the family's cultural background; (f) providing a set of cues that help the family judge the clinician's expertise (i.e., "According to my experience working with Asian families during the past 20 years . . . "); (g) acknowledging others (e.g., community elders) that give credence to the therapist's skills; and (h) sometimes utilizing a crisis intervention approach to offer some immediate relief from the stress being experienced by the family. It is important for the family members to feel that they are in good hands, and that there is a sense of hope, before they leave the first session.

9. Many Asian Americans do not comprehend the significance of the sometimes lengthy evaluation process. They may not be used to detailed history taking or may not understand the relationship between the questions and the presenting problems. Some clients may even suspect that such information will be put to political use, jeopardizing their immigration status. The clinician needs to help the client understand the reasons behind such questions. The therapist may decide to share his or her written information with the family in order to minimize suspicions of secrecy or the sense of being judged negatively.

10. Most Asian families come to the first interview only during a family crisis. The clinician should plan to allow more time than the usual 1-hour session, especially when an interpreter is utilized.

11. There may be may be some initially uncomfortable topics to discuss with Asian American clients. One such topic is sexual orientation and identity. It must be remembered that traditional Asian values do not support talking openly about sex, sexual intimacy, or related areas. In addition, it may be difficult to share stories of discrimination, prejudice, or oppression experienced by the family. The histories of most Asian Americans attest to the actual multiple social oppressions that impact and may be replicated by families. In setting a tenor for mutual work, it is recommended that the therapist take an affirmative stance early in the process to address areas of oppression, including sexual and ethnic identity (Aoki, 1997). After credibility is established, the therapist may acknowledge that there may be challenging areas to be discussed, but that they will be handled with expertise and with the essential commitment of the family. Psychoeducation can also help normalize more open discussion. Strategically exploring sexual identity can actually relieve some sources of individual and family stress (Wong & Mock, 1997).

ASSESSING FAMILY READINESS FOR THERAPY

Even though family therapy can be highly effective with Asian Americans, they are generally quite reluctant to seek treatment and are mostly unfamiliar with the concept of therapy or the role of the clinician. They usually do not see individual problems as family related. They rarely agree to the suggestion that the problem is the group's instead of the identified client's. Because of the traditional hierarchical and vertical structure of Asian American families prohibiting free verbal expression of emotions, especially true thoughts and negative feelings, family members may not be equipped with the communication skills to discuss problems and to express themselves openly in a family group setting. For example, for parents to discuss their "adult" problems or to express sadness in front of the children is considered highly inappropriate and is viewed as losing control.

Because of long years of separation within immigrant and refugee families, there may be family secrets and unresolved grief that members are not ready to share openly with each other. A "conspiracy of silence" is a common way to cope with unpleasant events. Premature interventions that bring out the "ghosts" from the past can be very overwhelming, and at times damaging, to the family's relationships. A careful balance must be maintained between protecting members from hurtful information and the power of secrets leading to dysfunction. Traditional Asian husbands and fathers are quite resistant to attending family sessions or allowing the therapist to enter into the family system. Admitting emotional problems and receiving help from outside the family network may be interpreted as a sign of weakness and "losing face" for many traditional Asian men. In the event that their children are in trouble and the parents are forced to receive treatment, husbands usually send their wives to be the family representatives in dealing with service agencies. It is very difficult to conduct family therapy without the cooperation and participation of the male adult figure.

For some, family therapy may be neither feasible nor desirable. However, if the clinician believes that family therapy will be the most effective treatment strategy, family members (especially the decision makers) should be told why it could be helpful. Even though the whole family may not be available, it may still be possible to work with one person, keeping the family context in mind.

INVOLVING FAMILY MEMBERS IN THERAPY

The definition of "family" in traditional Asian cultures may include a wide kinship network, not always fitting the traditional definitions of family ties. For example, a Vietnamese teenager who left his homeland with his aunt when he was an infant may have more emotional ties to his aunt and her family than to his own biological parents. In many Filipino families, trusted friends and allies serve as godparents to children and play an important role in their growth and development. The clinician can, if appropriate, ask the identified client to define his or her own concept of family members and discuss who should be included in therapy. In many cases it is advisable to encourage all family members to come to the first session so that the family dynamics among members can be observed. However, in many instances, family members are either unready emotionally or physically unavailable to participate in treatment.

Therapy for Asian families does not always require all-encompassing family involvement. A flexible subfamily system approach in the establishment of therapeutic relationships with family members at the beginning phase can be very helpful. For example, an effective method is for the clinician to interview the parents first, then the identified client, and then the siblings. The parents can discuss their adult concerns or express their emotions freely in the absence of the children. The children, usually more acculturated and fluent in English, can negotiate issues they might not bring up with their parents present. When all parties feel "safe" and have more control over what will be discussed in the family group, they may be more willing and ready to accept family therapy. This "staging" process requires skill in establishing trust, credibility, and relationships with each family member at the initial phase of treatment.

MUTUAL GOAL SETTING

Many Asian Americans find it difficult to admit to having family problems or psychological difficulties. They usually present themselves as victims of some unfortunate environmental events or "impersonal" physical discomfort. The clinician should take their presenting problems seriously and respond immediately to the "concrete" needs of the clients. Goals may be best mutually stated in terms of external resolution or symptom reduction. Many clients find loosely targeted and emotion-oriented goals incomprehensible, unreachable, and impractical (Ho, 1987). A problem-focused, goal-oriented, and symptom-relieving approach is highly recommended in the beginning phase of treatment. Providing between-sessions homework or assignments can also be productive. In addition, long-term goals are best broken down into a series of easy-to-understand, achievable, measurable, short-term goals laid out as one path for resolving issues. Once the family is engaged in the therapeutic relationship and gains a sense of success, which is very reassuring, the clinician can gradually introduce other, more insight-oriented goals and renegotiate with the family members.

Problem-Solving Phase

Asian American families often come to counseling with a physical or behavioral problem and expect the clinician to "fix it" with immediate results. Therefore, the problem-solving approach seems to be more appropriate. A brief strategic approach may be helpful with the family (Soo-Hoo, 1999). Adaptations of other family therapy approaches, taking into account both Eastern and Western perspectives, have also been shown to be useful (Hong & Ham, 2001; Jung, 1998). The following eight techniques have generally been found to be useful across several approaches (Lee, 1997).

FOCUSING ON THE PROBLEMS AS PRESENTED BY THE FAMILY

In order to engage the family in therapy, it is important for the clinician to (1) acknowledge the family's feeling that the identified patient has problems, (2) verbalize the family pain caused by the difficulties, (3) assist the family to shift from a person-focus to a problem-focus in order to minimize scapegoating, (4) focus on the effect of the problem on each family member, and (5) reinforce the sense of family obligation and the importance of solving the problem together. At times it may be helpful to encourage family members to elaborate on previous attempts to deal with the problem. The realization of their coping failure, and the unpleasant consequences if the problem is uncorrected, may motivate the family to continue in treatment. In some instances the clinician may use the family's sense of guilt to get hesitant members to participate for no other reason than to uphold the family name (Lee, 1990).

APPLYING A PSYCHOEDUCATIONAL APPROACH

Education is highly valued in Asian cultures. Many Asians consider the clinician as "doctor," "teacher," or "expert." The psychoeducational approach based on social learning principles is compatible with Asian values and beliefs. Such intervention focuses on five major areas: (1) education about the illness (or problem), (2) communication training, (3) problem-solving training, (4) behavioral management strategies (McGill & Lee, 1986), and (5) conflict resolution techniques. In addition to providing education on the individual and family levels, psychoeducational programs dedicated to multiple families in the Asian community can be very effective.

ASSUMING MULTIPLE HELPING ROLES

Flexibility and willingness of the clinician to assume multiple helping roles enhance the therapeutic relationship, especially in working with multiproblem families. In addition to being the counselor, the clinician should be comfortable in playing the roles of teacher, advocate, intermediary, and interpreter, and show investment and care by "doing" and "being there" when the family needs help.

INDIRECTNESS IN PROBLEM SOLVING

Most Asians view confrontation as disrespectful and lacking in moderation. Many take criticism as a personal attack or rejection. The clinician is advised to use an "indirect" means to address sources of conflict. For example, in the case of a Japanese mother-in-law who might be considered intrusive and overbearing, it may be useful to ask her how and in what ways she wants to have a lasting positive impact on the family.

EMPLOYING THE REFRAMING TECHNIQUE

Haley's and Minuchin's reframing technique can be very helpful. Using this technique, the clinician capitalizes on the pragmatics of Asian American cultures by emphasizing the positive aspects of behavior, redefining negative behavior as positive (Ho, 1987). Reinforcing mutuality can reinforce the importance of relatedness that is culturally syntonic. For example, an elder's nagging of an adult daughter can be viewed as concern about being cared for in later years. Or the daughter's inability to move out of oppressive circumstances can be viewed as acknowledging the need to maintain cultural continuity across generations.

CAPITALIZING ON FAMILY STRENGTHS AND COMMUNITY SUPPORTS

In many circumstances, especially when family members are coping with death, loss, or unpredictable changes, one of the functions of therapy is to mobilize the family's cultural strengths. Such strengths include support from the extended family, a strong sense of obligation and family loyalty, parental sacrifice for the children's future, filial piety, a strong focus on educational achievement, the work ethic, and support from their religious and ethnic communities. Strengthening the family's sense of cultural pride can also be very therapeutic.

UTILIZING INTERMEDIARY/GO-BETWEEN FUNCTIONS

In some situations, when there is a large gap between certain family members, the clinician may be able to bridge the gap by using an intermediary who can serve the function of linking the two uncommunicative members (Kim, 1985). Such intermediaries can include a trusted uncle, a good family friend, a leader from the family association, or a cultural healer, monk, or minister.

UNDERSTANDING THE FAMILY'S COMMUNICATION STYLE

There is a lack of "common" language spoken in many Asian American households, especially in families with "Westernized" adolescents who do not speak their parents' and grandparents' native dialects. It is quite difficult to conduct therapy in two or three different dialects and different communication styles. English-speaking clinicians should avoid using bilingual children as interpreters, particularly when the presenting problem involves parent–child issues. To place children in this role may replicate some of the very dynamics that contribute to family problems. The bilingualism of a child can reinforce the problem of role reversal and the monolingual parents' sense of helplessness. Clinicians should also avoid the use of relatives and friends as interpreters, but should try instead to use trained interpreters who match the Asian dialects and cultural background.

In addition to determining the preferred language and dialect to be used in therapy, the clinician must understand a family's communication style, which may include indirect communication and avoidance of direct confrontations. The clinician is expected to read between the lines in order to grasp the major issue; otherwise, he or she may be perceived as being blunt, pushy, and insensitive. Asian clients often speak in an oblique, understated way, with little overt emotion, implying that the problem is milder than it really is (Hong, 1989). Negative emotions such as anger, grief, and depression may be expressed in an indirect way. A culturally naive clinician may mistake this style for denial, lack of affect, a person's lack of awareness of his or her own feelings, deceptiveness, or resistance (Sue, 1990). Even positive feelings, such as care or love, are frequently not expressed openly. Care should taken not to mistake Asian parents' inexpressiveness as lack of caring. Love may be expressed more often by hard work within or outside the home.

Termination Phase

In this final phase, it is unrealistic for the clinician to expect an Asian client to verbalize anger or separation anxiety. Moreover, a client may not be able to comment on the progress achieved to someone outside the family. In showing appreciation, he or she may invite the clinician for dinner or present him or her with a gift. If clinically appropriate, the clinician should accept such gestures with genuine appreciation. Many Asian Americans went through many losses because of war and migration. A good relationship with the clinician is a permanent one that is to be treasured. A client may want the clinician to continue as a friend after termination (an "interminable termination") and may include him or her in family celebrations. Such culturally appropriate behavior should not be interpreted as pathological. With relatedness and family relationships as the cornerstone of Asian cultures, treating the therapist as an extended family member may be a great compliment.

CONCLUSION

Asian Americans are a heterogeneous group reflecting a diversity of educational, political, socioeconomic, and religious backgrounds, as well as different migration histories. This chapter has presented a practical assessment guide and treatment strategies that take into account the physical, psychological, social, spiritual, and cultural backgrounds of Asian American and Pacific Islander (AAPI) families. Many Asian immigrants and refugees are survivors of war, political upheavals, and cultural transitions. They deserve our compassion, respect, cultural responsiveness, and the best we can offer as culturally competent mental health professionals.

REFERENCES

Aoki, B. K. (1997). Gay and lesbian Asian Americans in psychotherapy. In E. Lee (Ed.), *Working with Asian Americans: A guide for clinicians* (pp. 411–419). New York: Guilford Press.

Barnes, J. S., & Bennett, C. E. (2002, February). *The Asian Population: 2000* (Census 2000 Brief). Washington, DC: U.S. Census Bureau.

Chang, I. (2003). *The Chinese in America: A narrative history.* New York: Viking.

Fadiman, A. (1997). *The spirit catches you and you fall down.* New York: Farrar, Straus & Giroux.

Hernandez, M., & McGoldrick, M. (in press). Migration and the family life cycle. In B. Carter & M. McGoldrick (Eds.), *The expanded family life cycle: Individual, family and social perspectives* (Classic ed.). Boston: Allyn & Bacon.

Ho, M. K. (1987). *Family therapy with ethnic minorities.* Newbury Park, CA: Sage.

Hong, G. (1989). Application of cultural and environmental issues in family therapy with immigrant Chinese Americans. *Journal of Strategic and Systemic Therapies, 8,* 14–21.

Hong, G., & Domokos-Cheng Ham, M. (2001). *Psychotherapy and counseling with Asian American clients.* Thousand Oaks, CA: Sage.

Hsu, F. L. K. (1971). *Under the ancestor's shadow: Kinship, personality, and social mobility in China.* Stanford, CA: Stanford University Press.

Jung, M. (1998). *Chinese American family therapy.* San Francisco: Jossey-Bass.

Kim, S. (1985). Family therapy for Asian Americans: A strategic–structral framework. *Psychotherapy, 22*(2), 342–348.

Landau, J. (1982). Therapy with families in cultural transition. In M. McGoldrick, J. K. Pearce, & J. Giordano (Eds.), *Ethnicity and family therapy* (pp. 552–572). New York: Guilford Press.

Lee, E. (1982). A social systems approach to assessment and treatment for Chinese American families. In M. McGoldrick, J. K. Pearce, & J. Giordano (Eds.), *Ethnicity and family therapy* (pp. 527–551). New York: Guilford Press.

Lee, E. (1989). Assessment and treatment of Chinese-American immigrant families. *Journal of Psychotherapy and the Family, 6*(1/2), 99–122.

Lee, E. (1990). Family therapy with Southeast Asian refugees. In M. P. Mirkin (Ed.), *The social and political contexts of family therapy* (pp. 331–354). Needham Heights, MA: Allyn & Bacon.

Lee, E. (1997). *Working with Asian Americans: A guide for clinicians.* New York: Guilford Press.

McGill, C., & Lee, E. (1986). Family psychoeducation intervention in the treatment of schizophrenia. *Bulletin of the Menninger Clinic, 50*(3), 269–286.

McGoldrick, M., Gerson, R. & Schellenberger, S. (1998). *Genograms: Assessment and intervention.* New York: Norton.

Mock, M. R. (1998a). Clinical reflections on refugee families: Transforming crises into opportunities. In M. McGoldrick (Ed.), *Re-visioning family therapy: Race, culture, and gender in clinical practice* (pp. 347–359). New York: Guilford Press.

Mock, M. R. (1998b). Developing cultural proficiency in clinical practice. In M. Mock, L. Hill, & D. Tucker (Eds.), *Breaking barriers: Psychology in the public interest.* Sacramento: California Psychological Association.

Nagata, D. (1990). The Japanese American internment: Exploring the transgenerational consequences of traumatic stress. *Journal of Traumatic Stress, 3,* 47–69.

Paniagua, F. A. (1994). *Assessing and treating culturally diverse clients.* Thousand Oaks, CA: Sage.

Reeves, T., & Bennett, C. (2003, May). *The Asian Pacific Islander Population in the United States: March 2002* (Current Population Reports, P20-540). Washington, DC: U.S. Census Bureau.

Shon, S., & Ja, D. (1982). Asian families. In M. McGoldrick, J. K. Pearce, & J. Giordano (Eds.), *Ethnicity and family therapy* (pp. 208–228). New York: Guilford Press.

Soo-Hoo, T. (1999). Brief strategic family therapy with Chinese-Americans. *American Journal of Family Therapy, 27,* 163–179.

Sue, D. W. (1990). Culture-specific strategies in counseling: A conceptual framework. *Professional Psychology: Research and Practice, 21*(6), 424–433.

Sue, S., & Zane, N. (1987). The role of culture and cultural techniques in psychotherapy: A critique and reformulation. *American Psychologist, 42,* 37–45.

Takaki, R. (1991). *Strangers from a different shore: A history of Asian Americans.* Boston: Little, Brown.

Uba, L. (1993). *Asian Americans: Personality patterns, identity, and mental health.* New York: Guilford Press.

U.S. Department of Health and Human Services. (2001). *Mental health: Culture, race and ethnicity—A supplement to mental health: A report of the Surgeon General.* Rockville, MD: Author.

Westermeyer, J. (1989). *Psychiatric care of migrants: A clinical guide.* Washington, DC: American Psychiatric Press.

Wong, L., & Mock, M. R. (1997). Asian American young adults. In E. Lee (Ed.), *Working with Asian Americans: A guide for clinicians* (pp. 196–207). New York: Guilford Press.

CHAPTER 21

Cambodian Families

Lorna McKenzie-Pollock

OVERVIEW OF HISTORY AND CULTURE

Violent displacement as a result of armed conflict has been the experience of vast numbers of people. United Nations' figures indicate that more than 15 million people currently meet the criteria for refugee status. Among them, Cambodian refugees have suffered devastating losses, destruction, and brutality. Yet their story is one of courage, resilience, and transformation, as well as vulnerability, as illustrated by a Cambodian man who sought treatment at a Boston area clinic:

> "When I woke up I was under a pile of bodies. I climbed out from under the body of my younger brother. The Khmer Rouge had gone by then, but the bodies of my relatives were all around me. They killed 39 people that day, and now I was the only one in my family alive."

Cambodia is bordered by Thailand, Laos, and Vietnam. The Khmer are the country's principal ethnic group, accounting for about 94% of the population. The rest of the population consists of a combination of small ethnic minorities, mostly Chinese and Cham (a Muslim group), Vietnamese, Lao, and Thai. Theravada Buddhists make up 95% of the population. One of the two major forms of Buddhism, Theravada Buddhism, is the predominant religion of continental Southeast Asia (Thailand, Myanmar, Cambodia, Laos, and Sri Lanka.). The other form, known as Mahanaya Buddhism, is practiced in China and Tibet. (Zen Buddhism, more widely known in the West, is a variant of the Mahayana tradition). Buddhism originated in India and was based on the teachings of Gautama Buddha, who lived around 600 B.C. Theravada Buddhism is based on the texts of the *Pali Canon*, the earliest surviving record of the Buddha's teachings. The language of worship is Pali, an ancient language related to Sanskrit. (Bullitt, 2002; Robinson & Johnson, 1997). Interestingly, although the people of Cambodia are Theravada Buddhists, the monarch and his family have always practiced Mahayana Buddhism.

Cambodia has been a monarchy for most of its history. Between the 6th and 15th centuries, the Khmer controlled a vast empire, with Angkor as its capital. During subsequent periods the country was attacked by neighboring Vietnam and Thailand. In 1863, Cambodia became a French protectorate. During the 1940s an independence movement gathered strength, and in 1953 Cambodia gained its independence from France. Until 1970, the country was ruled by Prince Norodim Sihanouk. During the 1960s, as the war in neighboring Vietnam escalated, Cambodia took a neutral stance, although part of eastern Cambodia was utilized as a section of the "Ho Chi Minh trail," a route bringing arms and personnel from North to South Vietnam to fight in the war. In late 1969, American saturation bombing in the eastern part of Cambodia, which was intended to stop the flow of supplies and personnel along the Ho Chi Minh trail, threw the country into turmoil. There were heavy casualties and many people were left homeless. Considerable political destabilization ensued with the overthrow of Prince Sihanouk and the installation of a short-lived pro-American government led by Lon Nol. There was widespread corruption in this government, as well as civil war in the countryside.

In April 1975, just 2 months after the fall of Saigon, the government of Cambodia fell under the control of the Khmer Rouge, a Maoist-inspired group led by Pol Pot. The Khmer Rouge declared the "Year Zero," a radical new beginning, and embarked on a program to rid Cambodia of all Western influences. What followed has been called the Cambodian holocaust. The Khmer Rouge forced people out of the cities and sent them by foot or by train to rural labor camps. All wealthy, educated, and professional people were hunted and executed. Teachers, doctors, and soldiers were killed or had to disguise their identity in order to survive. The Khmer Rouge embarked on a systematic program of thought control. Compulsory nightly meetings were held in the labor camps, in which Khmer Rouge cadres made speeches about the new social order and people who had been accused of disloyalty to the party were publicly castigated or, in some cases, tortured and killed. Children were separated from their parents and sent to children's labor camps. Adults were made to work long hours in the rice paddies and other agrarian projects. The people who had been sent out from the city and were suspected of being members of the upper class were given the most taxing jobs and were systematically starved. *Chhlops*, or spies, would hide next to houses and listen for people making statements disloyal to the party. With the dismantling of the old social order, the once prosperous country experienced social and economic collapse, so that famine and disease became endemic. Conditions in the labor camps became even more nightmarish. The Khmer Rouge maintained control by mass public torture and execution of all dissidents or suspected dissidents. Family members, neighbors, and coworkers were forced to watch the most horrific atrocities without showing emotion. Any outpouring of emotion was punished by further acts of brutality. It is estimated that more than 2 million Cambodians died during the Pol Pot regime.

In 1978, the Vietnamese army invaded Cambodia. At this point people became able to move about freely and thus discovered the full extent of their losses. Amid the mass confusion, people began pouring over the border on foot into neighboring Thailand, a long and dangerous journey through a mine-studded border region, where many died or lost limbs. A series of refugee camps were set up along the border region of Thailand.

Cambodian refugee families spent anywhere from 1 to 12 years in these camps, in austere, overcrowded, and often unsafe conditions, awaiting resettlement in a third country. Most Cambodians currently in the United States came here from one of these refugee camps.

Upon arrival in the United States, refugee families were generally resettled in poor urban areas, where, as the newest group, they were often preyed upon by other minority and immigrant groups. The word got around that these new arrivals kept cash and gold in their homes, and robberies, home invasions, and muggings were common. Many Cambodians became symptomatic and were referred for therapy after a violent incident in the neighborhood revived memories of events back home.

DEMOGRAPHICS

Most Cambodians came to this country between 1980 and 1989. Prior to coming to the United States, about 80% were small rice farmers from rural areas. Most of the men had only a few years of schooling provided by the Buddhist monks. The majority of women from rural backgrounds were illiterate at the time of their arrival in the United States.

According to the 2000 census, there are 171,937 Cambodians residing in the United States. This figure probably represents an undercount. The largest number live in California, where the majority reside in the Long Beach area. There is also a smaller community in the Oakland area. There are 19,696 Cambodians living in Massachusetts—next to California, the second largest number in the United States. It is reported that 17,301 live in the Greater Boston area, with the greatest concentrations in Lowell, Revere, and Lynn. Many Cambodians live in ethnic enclaves with their own neighborhood stores, groceries, and restaurants. Many older Cambodians have little contact with people outside their community. Although a number of Cambodians in the greater Boston area have become highly successful, and in some cases prominent members of society, there is a high degree of poverty and disability in the community. Most of such problems are related to chronic posttraumatic stress disorder symptoms and to health issues resulting from prolonged starvation, malnutrition, and lack of health care during the war and the period of genocide.

FAMILY STRUCTURE

The extended family formed the core of the traditional Khmer social structure. Kuoch and colleagues state, "The role of the family is central to the survival of the individual. One's sense of wholeness comes from belonging to a family. Buddhism and Brahmanism reinforce the importance of family with age-old rituals which provide meaning and comfort in times of change or distress" (Kuoch, Miller, & Scully, 1992, p. 193). Traditionally, the social order was highly stratified; social relations were clearly defined, so people knew what to expect from each other. This hierarchical nature of the society is revealed even in the Khmer language. For example, different words for eating are used, depending on the rank of the person being addressed.

Relationships within the family were also stratified. The husband, as head of household, expected to be deferred to on all matters. The eldest son had a special position in the family. He was treated with additional respect by both the parents and other siblings, and he was expected to take responsibility for the younger siblings. In female-headed households in this country, he is expected to be responsible for the family. Much of this structure has endured in this country. Siblings refer to each other as older or younger brother or sister. This familial ranking still carries over to social relationships in all spheres. For example, a Khmer counselor will address a client as *bong* (older sister) or *pu'on* (younger sister), depending on her relative age. The terms *older* and *younger* do not only convey age. Because of the respect accorded to elders, someone may be referred to as *bong* when that person is actually chronologically younger than the speaker, if he or she is highly respected in the community. People in the community all refer to each other by familial terms, such as "sister" or "uncle."

One of the most devastating aspects of the Pol Pot regime was that, in an attempt to impose a new social order, a systematic effort was made to destroy the family. Children were separated from, and encouraged to spy on, their parents. Women were tortured to make them report on their husbands. Large numbers of men were led off and executed because of alleged involvement with the old regime. A major consequence of the genocide is that many Cambodian families are now headed by women, many of them illiterate and without job skills transferable to an industrialized society. Their stories are often ones of great hardship and emotional strength.

Central values in Khmer society are harmony and balance. Conflict is to be avoided at all costs (Ebihara, 1968). To the American observer, the Cambodian style of communication often appears elliptical and indirect. This sometimes causes confusion and miscommunication, as Cambodians experience confrontation or direct questioning as very rude and threatening. In a clinical setting this means that if clients are angry or upset with something a therapist said, they will not indicate this directly. Instead, they may tell the therapist, very politely and pleasantly, that it is simply not possible to come in for another session because their hours at work are about to change or transportation is too difficult. Alternatively, they will simply not show up for the next session. Cambodian clients expect this same indirectness from an American therapist and experience confrontation or direct questioning by a therapist as very rude and frightening. For example, a Cambodian widow came to see me for help in dealing with recurrent depression. She told me about an experience she had had with a psychiatrist 2 years earlier, whom she described as conducting an interrogation, which she said felt like a torture session. Curious, I sent for her records and found that the psychiatrist in question, a female resident, had simply been conducting a mental status exam as part of a medication evaluation. There was no indication in the record that she was aware that the client was upset. Direct questioning can also trigger traumatic memories of the Pol Pot period, when people were subject to interrogation as part of "re-education" and were often tortured and killed if they gave the wrong answer.

TREATMENT ISSUES

Trauma and Loss

Trauma and loss are, understandably, the most common treatment issues in Cambodian families. Clinicians therefore need to be familiar with the symptoms and treatment of posttraumatic stress disorder. Anyone working with Cambodian families should be aware of the magnitude of the destruction of the Khmer Rouge period. Not only did millions of people die, but the two key organizing institutions in Cambodian life—the family and the Buddhist religion—were systematically destroyed.

Savuth was referred by a physician to my Cambodian cotherapist, Svang Tor, and me for an evaluation because he was not complying with medication he had been prescribed for suspected tuberculosis. When we met with him and asked him about his family, he told us he was married and had three daughters, ages 3, 4, and 6. When he informed us that his 6-year-old had not yet started attending school, even though it was a month into the school year, we brought in the whole family. On meeting his wife, Saroeun, I immediately became concerned. She was a thin, attractive woman in her mid-30s, whose face wore a blank, frozen stare. The three daughters ran around my office, and she barely appeared to notice them. The oldest daughter looked out for the younger ones, and their father would set limits periodically. Saroeun hardly spoke.

Svang, my Cambodian cotherapist, suggested we set up an individual meeting with Sarouen. We first asked her about her physical symptoms, an approach we had found helpful in connecting with Cambodians about their distress. She told us she could sleep for only a half-hour at a time before being woken up by terrifying nightmares. She would then spend hours shaking violently, sweating, her heart pounding. In the nightmares she would hear the cries of her three young children who had died. As she began to tell her story, she became intensely distressed and sobbed uncontrollably.

When the Khmer Rouge came to Saroeun's village they lined people up and began shooting. Eighteen people died. They put her in prison and starved and tortured her for 6 months because they suspected her brother had been a soldier. Although she said she did not tell on him, they executed him anyway. During her imprisonment, her three young children would be repeatedly brought to her, then taken away. She watched them deteriorate, and eventually two died of starvation. The third died of typhoid in a Thai refugee camp.

We had a series of individual meetings with both Sarouen and Savuth in which they each recounted their trauma stories, hers with intense outpourings of emotion, his with quiet sadness. The cotherapy team experienced these sessions as disturbing and exhausting. We also felt what Kinzie (2001) describes as "an increased empathic intensity—the sense of being much closer to each other, of sharing a unique experience" (p. 479).

We arranged a consultation with a psychiatrist, who prescribed medication for their severe sleep disturbances and depression. We then began meeting with them as a couple, and they began to talk about these events that they had never discussed together. Sometimes these meetings were emotional and sorrowful, at other times the couple were able to use humor in talking about their situation. In one session they jokingly portrayed a typical night in their household, with alternating episodes of nightmares and flashbacks, humorously pantomiming how each would awake shaking and terrified. We then began talking about the children and had several meetings with them present. By this time Saroeun was much more actively involved with the children.

At one point Saroeun announced that she did not want to come in more than once a month because the nightmares had mostly gone, returning only on on the nights before she came to meet with us. We scheduled the meetings in accordance with her wishes. About 6 months later, Saroeun came in with a gift for me, a tapestry in startlingly bright fluorescent colors. She said she was feeling better and that this was to thank me. By this time I was familiar enough with the Cambodian culture to know that this meant she would not be coming in any more.

——————— ∾ ———————

Intergenerational Conflict

Danieli (1985) has described the intergenerational effects of traumatizaton continuing into the third generation. One way this manifests itself in Cambodian families is through difficulties when members of the younger generation try to separate in some way or go off to form their own nuclear families. Members of the older generation, deprived of the companionship of spouse, extended kin, or peers whom they would have enjoyed in Cambodia, sometimes experience these attempts to leave as total abandonment. Given the tradition of close extended family relationships, the distress of the older generation can cause the younger people enormous pain. Because families have endured so much together, there is a tremendous loyalty that can sometimes result in families accepting extremely difficult and even out-of-control situations.

An elderly Cambodian widow was brought in by her two married sons, ages 32 and 28, who were very concerned about her multiple somatic complaints. The older son told us, "When she hurts, I feel pain too." When this son went on a vacation to another city, with the intention of looking into moving there, the mother developed such terrible aches and pains that the son had to be summoned back immediately to perform coin rubbing (a traditional healing practice). She began attending regular biweekly sessions with us, sometimes with the sons and sometimes alone, and this became a place for her to talk about her aches and pains, complain about her daughters-in-law, and talk about her loneliness. In time, her aches lessened and the emergency calls to her son decreased. Trips to the emergency room stopped. She became very active in a local Buddhist temple, at times spending all day there meditating and chatting with other women. At this point her symptoms improved dramatically. The older son also reported that his life was going more smoothly. He was no longer torn between his wife and his mother.

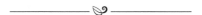

There are often major communication problems between older Cambodians and the children who were raised in this country. In recent years the most frequent presenting complaints of clients at the Southeast Asian Community Clinic in Revere (in addition to distress secondary to posttraumatic symptoms) has been concern about their adolescent and young adult children. Because so many of the parents speak little or no English and often are illiterate, they are unable to assist their children in negotiating the school system. Communication from the school comes in English, and the child is often the one translating.

American social mores concerning relationships with the opposite sex are incomprehensible to older Cambodians. Traditionally, there were strict rules of conduct for young women. They were not allowed to be alone with members of the opposite sex, and adherence to the rules brought honor to a family's name. Most Cambodian parents are vehemently opposed to their children dating. The idea of a girl going away to college and living in a dormitory is often unacceptable to them.

Setting limits and disciplining children is often problematic for Cambodian parents. Traditionally, corporal punishment was acceptable, but word has spread in the community that Social Services would take away their children if they hit them, and so some have become fearful of all limit setting. The Cambodian norm is to be indulgent with younger children and to set stricter rules when they reach adolescence (Ebihara, 1968), a practice at odds with American norms. Because members of the older generation were raised in a tradition of reverence and respect for elders, they become completely over-whelmed when their children talk back and disrespect them.

In addition, Cambodian families often live in violent inner-city neighborhoods. Gang violence mars some of the Cambodian enclaves in the Boston area. A significant number of older Cambodian clients report living in fear of their adolescent children; others are worried that their children will be killed or end up in jail. This is particularly terrifying now that an agreement has been reached between the Cambodian and American governments allowing deportation of Cambodians convicted of crimes. Recently a number of young men, who had never lived in Cambodia, have been deported. Many were born in a Thai refugee camp or left Cambodia as infants. Most speak only rudimentary Khmer. Their fate in Cambodia is a source of tremendous worry for the parents.

Children and young adults are often under tremendous pressure. They are frequently the translators for their parents, entrusted with taking them to medical and social service appointments, and assisting them in reading mail and paying bills. At times these responsibilities involve missing school or work. I have frequently been struck by the high level of anxiety among young Cambodian men, brought in by their families, who often show many of the symptoms of posttraumatic stress disorder. Frequently, those of the older generation have never told their children about the trauma and losses they suffered in Cambodia, and the children are confused about their parents' distress. A 12-year-old girl told me that she did not know why her mother cried every day. She assumed it was because she was a "bad daughter."

Kheav came into therapy in great distress over the oldest of her two teenage sons. He had been skipping school and had stolen money from her. She had come to Massachusetts after leaving her abusive husband in California. This was her second marriage. Her first husband and many members of her family had died during a Khmer Rouge massacre, during which she had been severely beaten. After the Khmer Rouge were overthrown, she and her mother made their way on foot to Thailand, where she met her second husband in a refugee camp. They were resettled in Oakland, California, and there they had two children. Her husband became increasingly violent, and she became fearful that he was going to kill her. She therefore fled with her two children to Massachusetts, where she had a brother. When she arrived at the clinic, she was in a great deal of distress with nightmares, headaches, spells of terror, and frequent suicidal thoughts. After several meetings with her, we asked her to bring in the sons, but they refused. I contacted them directly, and they reluctantly agreed to participate in sessions. When they came in, the older son, who seemed extremely anxious, admitted to being afraid of being scolded or punished. When he told us that he was having trouble in school, we contacted the guidance counselor and set up a meeting; we also contacted the teacher to discuss his academic difficulties. We continued to alternate seeing Kheav individually and with her sons. She worked on learning relaxation and grounding techniques for coping with her trauma symptoms and began to see the clinic as a haven of safety and support. She became less symptomatic, and it was then that the son was able to tell us that an older boy at school had been threatening him and had demanded that he give him money. He had been afraid to tell his mother before, as he was fearful that she would "lose it."

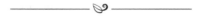

Kheav's story illustrates the importance of assisting the family in dealing with outside stresses. Therapy with Cambodian families, of necessity, involves doing a great deal of outreach, case management and advocacy. Because there are often so many pressing external problems, a traditional model of sitting in the office doing "talk therapy" is often ineffective and frustrating for both client and therapist.

Trust

Establishing trust is a major issue in working with the Cambodian community. During the Khmer Rouge period people learned that telling the truth could cost them their lives. There was systematic brainwashing. Meetings were held at night, in which people were lectured about the "correct" way to think, and people were publicly tortured and killed as an example of what would happen to those who did not obey the party line. Later, during the immigration processing, word spread that it was necessary to hide and fabricate information in order to gain entry into the United States. In addition, as mentioned earlier, the mode of communication in Cambodian culture is often elliptical and indirect. The Cambodian word *kohok*, which is literally translated "tell a lie," does not have the same negative connotation as its English linguistic equivalent. High value is placed on harmony and keeping the peace, in contrast to the American value of confronting issues directly. For all these reasons, stories unfold in a circuitous and multilayered fashion in work with Cambodians. The issue of trust is an important element to consider in doing outreach to the community. If a bilingual, bicultural team approach is being used, the Khmer worker needs to have ties to the community and to be respected and trusted by the community. It is also important to work with key community agencies and institutions such as the local Mutual Assistance Association and the local Buddhist monks. The Cambodian community is small, and information is largely passed on through word of mouth.

The Need for Community-wide Healing

The destruction of the genocide in Cambodia went beyond the death of two million people. It also involved the destruction of the religious institutions, the people's culture, and traditions. Healing the wounds resulting from a tragedy of this magnitude needs to go beyond individual and family healing. There is a need for a rebuilding of the entire culture. Community-wide rituals and festivals are an important part of this process. Many Cambodian communities have raised money to buy a building, turn it into a Buddhist temple, and bring over monks from Cambodia. The temple quickly becomes a powerful focus for the community. Women gather there every morning to prepare food for the monks, and traditional festivals are observed there. At the Southeast Asian Clinic we recognized the importance of interfacing with the monks. Our Cambodian outreach worker would assist women who were depressed or otherwise disabled, in participating in the food preparation at the temple, and in turn they would enjoy the support of the other women in the group. In addition, a celebration of the *chol chnam*, the Cambodian New Year, has become an important annual feature of the clinic, with all of the clients participating in preparing and eating food and receiving the blessings of the monks.

Mind–Body Connection

Cambodian people do not make a distinction between physical and emotional pain. Emotional distress is almost never a presenting problem. People generally come in with somatic complaints, very commonly headache, dizziness, and weakness. Clients sometimes report episodes of blindness with no organic basis. When telling their stories, however, people readily connect their physical symptoms with painful events in their past and the intense and painful feelings that accompanied them.

TREATMENT MODEL

The most important first step in meeting with a Cambodian family, or with any refugee or immigrant family for that matter, is to ensure linguistic access for all family members. Many older Cambodians have been unable to learn English. A common complaint is that since their Pol Pot experiences they have been unable to retain new information. The level of trauma they experienced may in fact have interfered with their capacity to learn language. Recent neuroimaging studies have shown that people exposed to high levels of trauma undergo changes in the brain involving decreased hippocampus volume, and that the subjects performed significantly worse on tests of verbal memory than did controls (van der Kolk, 1966). Lack of literacy or formal education also makes the learning process foreign and more difficult.

If the therapist is a non–Khmer speaker, it is critical that he or she works with a Khmer speaker from outside the family. The clinician should not use family members to translate, for three reasons: First, the inability of elders to learn the language and negotiate the culture relative to their children has already eroded the traditional authority of the elders, and putting the children in charge of the session further disempowers the parents. Second, making the children translate for the parents can put additional stress on an already overstressed system. Third, family members will often edit out information they consider shameful or embarrassing. A tragic example of this happened a few years ago when a family brought their mother to the emergency room. The doctor asked the children to ask their mother if she was suicidal. Because suicide is considered sinful by Buddhists, they denied that she was. She subsequently went home and killed herself.

Clearly, it is preferable to have a Cambodian therapist working with the family; however, when I first began working with Cambodians, few mental health or social service people who spoke the Khmer language were available. Various interim treatment models therefore had to be devised to meet the need for services in this community.

The model I have used to work with Cambodian families involves a bilingual cotherapy team consisting of a bilingual Cambodian paraprofessional working together with an American clinician. The trio of the bilingual worker, the American clinician, and the family or individual client are in the room at all times. This triadic cotherapy model can be confusing and difficult to get used to. It can present two traps for the unwary. The first is the danger of a struggle for control between the bilingual worker and the English-speaking clinician. Sometimes English-speaking clinicians try to take control by insisting that the bilingual person be nothing more than a mouthpiece for them by doing direct translation. This results in discomfort and loss of face for the bilingual worker, who feels disempowered, especially if asked to make culturally inappropriate interventions. It also robs the English-speaking clinician of the insights and expertise of the bilingual person and does not make effective use of the empathic ethnic connection between bilingual worker and client. A frequent outcome of this model is that the bilingual worker resorts to what has been called the "ten-to-one phenomenon," in which he or she and the client engage in lengthy animated exchanges, and when the English-speaking clinician asks for clarification, the bilingual worker responds with a short or uninformative response (e.g., "he said yes").

Another trap is that of the disengaged American clinician who remains detached from the details of the case by busying him- or herself with taking notes, writing prescriptions, or going in and out of the room, supervising other cases. This results in the bilingual worker's feeling unsupported and overwhelmed by having to pick up all the details of follow-up for what are often complex and demanding cases, including negotiating the unfamiliar maze of the American social service system alone. This tactic is often resorted to because it protects the American clinician from having to experience the discomfort of working in an unfamiliar language and culture, and of hearing overwhelming stories of sadness and loss, and leaves the bilingual worker, frequently a trauma survivor him- or herself, to sit with the stories alone.

The model I use (McKenzie-Pollock, 1987) is adapted from the Milan systemic model (Palazzoli, Boscolo, Cecchin, & Prata, 1981). The Cambodian staff person and I meet before each session to clarify our goals and make sure we are headed in the same direction. We attempt to resolve differences in how we see the issues before meeting with the family. Because the families and I did not speak the same language when I first began this work, it felt comfortable to sit back slightly and mentally assume the position of a coach behind a one-way mirror (formed in this case by the language barrier). In this way I have removed myself from the temptation to vie for control and can make use of my particular vantage point to be an effective coach or advisor.

Throughout the session I observe the family interactions very closely. I maintain close contact with the bilingual worker, who frequently stops (at his or her discretion) and tells me in English what is being said. I also periodically share my observations with my coworker. Because our communications are in English, we are usually not understood by everyone in the family. I therefore frequently ask the bilingual person to fill the family in on what we have discussed. Sometimes, if the situation is particularly sensitive or complex, or if a split is developing in the team, the bilingual staff person and I leave the room and confer.

At the end of the session we confer and give the family our impressions and, frequently, a task to work on. This kind of directive approach tends to be acceptable and reassuring to Cambodian families. I find it helpful for both team members to keep a model of triadic communication in mind at all times. The effectiveness of the therapy breaks down if avenues of communication are not constantly kept open between the three points of the triangle, namely, the American clinician, the bilingual clinician, and the family.

The model can be seen as one of "bridging" between the two cultures. For families in cultural transition, this can be particularly powerful. Westermeyer and Williams (1986) state that in order to "regain a stable sense of self," refugees need to both "re-establish a foothold in their culture" and "develop a new foothold in the receiving culture" (p. 242). This model is a means of facilitating such a process.

Today, fortunately, a new generation of Khmer mental health professionals is available to provide treatment, though still not enough to fill the demand for services. Cambodian service providers need to continue to use the "bridging model" and to be both respectful of the traditional values of the older generation and able to guide the family through the maze of American values and expectations.

In trying to understand a Cambodian family's presentation, I often find myself dealing with two or three levels of reality or "explanatory models" (Kleinman, 1980) simultaneously.

A 35-year-old married Cambodian woman was referred because of depression and marital conflict. She was extremely withdrawn, avoided interacting with her neighbors, and had angry outbursts. Her husband told her, her children, and her neighbors that she was crazy. He spent much time out of the house and had had several affairs.

The family's explanation of the problem was that a spell had been put on the wife. She dated the onset of the spell to 5 years earlier, when in a refugee camp in Thailand she was hospitalized as a result of complications following childbirth. The woman was given an intravenous drip and believed that this was how the spell had entered her body. The psychiatric/biomedical explanation appeared to be a major affective disorder, probably originating in a postpartum depression. The systems explanation would be that her symptoms were a response to her husband's behavior. A treatment plan should address all of these levels to be effective. In this case the plan included attempts to find a *kru Khmer*, or shaman, who would remove the spell, couple therapy to explore family's difficulties, and a trial of an antidepressant medication.

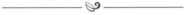

ACKNOWLEDGMENTS

The material presented here is based on 19 years of clinical work with Cambodian families. The work was conducted at the Indochinese Psychiatry Clinic, Brighton, Massachusetts; Harvard Vanguard Medical Associates, Chelmsford, Massachusetts; the Southeast Asian Community Clinic, Revere, Massachusetts; my private practice in Brookline, Massachusetts; and in consultation to clinics and agencies throughout New England. I would like to express my gratitude to my Cambodian colleagues, friends and teachers Phalnarith Ba, Svang Tor, Audria Chea, Sunnary Uk, Saly Pin-Riebe, Bounthay Phath-Reth, Bou Lim, and Diane Kay—my windows into Cambodian culture. Working with them has provided some of the most wonderful and enriching moments of my career as a therapist. I am also indebted to Thang Pham, Dr. Nancy McDonnell, Dr. Richard Mollica, and James Lavelle, whose dedication to providing specialized treatment for Southeast Asian refugees allowed this work to be done.

REFERENCES

Bullitt, J. (2002). *What is Theravada Buddhism?* Available at www.accesstoinsight.org/theravada.html

Danieli, Y. (1985). The treatment and prevention of long-term effects and intergenerational transmission of victimization: A lesson from Holocaust survivors and their children. In C. Figley (Ed.), *Trauma and its wake*. New York: Brunner/Mazel.

Ebihara, M. (1968). *A Khmer village in Cambodia*. Unpublished doctoral dissertation, University of Michigan, Ann Arbor.

Kinzie, J. D. (2001). Psychotherapy for massively traumatized refugees: The therapist variable. *American Journal of Psychotherapy, 55*(4), 475–490.

Kleinman, A. (1980). *Patients and healers in the context of culture*. Berkeley: University of California Press.

Kuoch, T., Miller, R. A., & Scully, M. F. (1992). Healing the wounds of the Mahantdori. In E. Cole, O.

M. Espin, & E. Rothblum (Eds.), *Refugee women and their mental health: Shattered societies, shattered lives*. Binghamton, NY: Haworth Press.

McKenzie-Pollock, L. (1987). *A model for bilingual bicultural therapy*. Unpublished manuscript.

Mollica, R., Wyshak, G., & Lavelle, J. (1987, December). The psychosocial impact of war trauma and torture on Southeast Asian Refugees. *American Journal of Psychiatry, 144*(12), 1567–1572.

Palazzoli, M. S., Boscolo, L., Cecchin, G., & Prata, G. (1981). The treatment of children through brief therapy of their parents. In R. J. Green & J. Framo (Eds.), *Family therapy: Major contributions*. New York: International Universities Press.

Robinson, R. H., & Johnson, W. L. (1997). *The Buddhist religion: A historical introduction* (4th ed.). Belmont, CA: Wadsworth.

van der Kolk, B. (1996). The body keeps the score. In B. van der Kolk, A. McFarlane, & L. Weisaeth (Eds.), *Traumatic stress: The effects of overwhelming experience on mind, body and society*. New York: Guilford Press.

Westermeyer, J., & Williams, C. L. (1986). Planning mental health services for refugees. In C. Williams & J. Westermeyer (Eds.), *Refugee mental health in resettlement countries*. Washington, DC: Hemisphere.

CHAPTER 22

Chinese Families

Evelyn Lee
Matthew R. Mock

In Chinese culture, the family, rather than the individual, is the major unit of society. The sense of the family's importance and its contribution to the individual's core identity have been molded by cultural norms and values over 4,000 years of Chinese history. In the oldest Chinese dictionary, there are more than 500 terms describing different family relationships. For many Chinese Americans, particularly for immigrants and refugees, the family often provides the sole means of support, validation, and stabilization. In order to provide a culturally relevant clinical intervention for Chinese Americans, it is essential to understand the cultural aspects of Chinese family systems, functions, and their unique life experiences.

CHINESE AMERICANS: A DIVERSE POPULATION

According to the 2000 U.S. Census figures, a total of 2.7 million people reported being Chinese, alone (2.3) or in combination with one or more races or Asian groups (0.4)—the largest Asian Pacific American group, making up close to 23% of the Asian Pacific American population. Between 1980 and 1990, the Chinese American population doubled as a result of the new influx of immigrants and emerged as one of the most diverse Asian American groups. Similar growth was seen between 1990 and 2000. The diversity of the Chinese American population can be examined in terms of country of origin, generations, language, economic background, residential preferences, and religion. Most Chinese Americans reside in California, followed next by New York and then Hawaii. More than 63% of Chinese Americans were foreign-born (Barnes & Bennett, 2002), 23% did not speak English well, and 53% lived in the Western United States. There were 542,000 Chinese Americans residing in California; 147,250 in New York; and 55,900 in Hawaii. It was estimated that 13.3% of Chinese Americans live below the poverty level, 69.4% are high school graduates, and 72.5% speak a language other than English at home (Asian American Health Forum, 1990).

LANGUAGE

There is no single "Chinese language." The major dialects are Cantonese (most commonly used in Chinatowns), Mandarin (spoken by most Chinese from China and Taiwan), Toishanese, Chiuchow, Shanghainese, Taiwanese, Fukien, and Hakka. The written Chinese characters are less complicated than the variety of Chinese spoken dialects. Generally, there are two major styles: the "traditional" style, practiced by the majority of Chinese from Hong Kong, Taiwan, and Southeast Asian countries, and the "simplified" style of writing, developed by the People's Republic of China.

MIGRATION HISTORY

The history of Chinese migration to the United States tells a complex yet fascinating story of change, adaptation, and survival. It also reveals how the Chinese family system is affected by the immense power of political, legal, social, and economic forces. The Chinese have been residing in the United States in significant numbers for more than 150 years. Data have been collected on the Chinese population since the 1860 census. Major national immigration policies and economic upheavals in the United States and in Asian countries have resulted in different waves of immigration and different types of family systems.

The First Wave: The Pioneer Family (1850–1919)

Although there were Chinese residing in the United States as early as 1785, the impetus for large-scale immigration to this country did not occur until the discovery of gold in California in 1848 and the need for manual labor for the construction of railroads. Many Chinese migrants, mostly peasant farmers, left their villages in China to pursue their dreams in *Gam Saan*, the "Gold Mountain." The Chinese Exclusion Act of 1882 barred Chinese laborers and their relatives, most notably their wives, from entering the United States. This type of "sojourner" family pattern had profound consequences on the personal and social development of the family life of early Chinese immigrants.

The Second Wave: The Small Business Family (1920–1942)

As a result of the discriminatory Immigration Act of 1924, it was impossible for American citizens of Chinese ancestry to bring their wives and families to the United States. With a change in the law in 1930, there was eventual allowance of wives of Chinese merchants and Chinese wives who were married to American citizens before 1924 to immigrate to the United States. This was sometimes easier said than done, given the years of separation (Chang, 2003). However, when reunifications did happen, sizable family units with second-generation American-born Chinese were emerging in Chinatowns. At the same time, many first-wave laborers began to leave the mines and railroads, using their savings to start their own small businesses, such as laundry shops or fishing, either alone or with partners. The small-producer families emerged during this period. This family type consisted of the immigrant and first-generation American-born family members, functioning as a productive unit (Chang, 2003).

The Third Wave: The Reunited Family (1943–1964)

During the period from 1943 to the repeal of the quota law in 1965, Chinese immigrants were largely female. After years, or sometimes decades, of separation from their husbands, many wives were reunited with them for the first time. When they finally arrived in the United States, these women and their children had already established very powerful bonds that were far more intense than the marital tie. Reform in immigration policies also encouraged Chinese men to return to Hong Kong to find wives. These trans-Pacific marriages, with wives who were 10–20 years younger than their husbands, were usually arranged by matchmakers or relatives.

The Fourth Wave: The Chinatown and Dual-Worker Family (1965–1977)

Unlike the pre-1965 immigrants who came to this country individually, most Chinese immigrants who arrived under the Immigration Act of 1965 came as families. Many of them chose to settle in or close to established Chinatowns in major metropolitan areas. Most adults sought employment in labor-intensive, low-capital services such as garment sweatshops and restaurants. Economic survival was the priority. The long work hours often meant little family time together.

The Fifth Wave: The New Immigrant, Refugee, and Astronaut Family (1978–Present)

For over two decades, there has been a tremendous influx of Chinese immigrants from China, Hong Kong, Taiwan, and Vietnam. The reestablishment of diplomatic relations between the United States and the People's Republic of China in 1978 also provided an opportunity for students and professionals from China to study in this country, and many elected to stay. Another group of immigrants, who came from Hong Kong, worried about the 1997 transfer of British sovereignty to China. The recent political climate in Taiwan and the desire to seek higher education for their children also created an impetus for many Chinese to come to this country.

Adding to the diversity of the community, many of the refugees from Vietnam, Laos, and Cambodia were ethnic Chinese. They constituted the second wave of Southeast Asian refugees. A significant number of them were survivors of hunger, rape, incarceration, forced migration, and torture. There are also "overseas Chinese" from countries such as Japan, Korea, the Philippines, Singapore, Malaysia, Thailand, Mexico, Canada, and many other countries of South America and Europe.

Another recent phenomenon is the emergence of "astronaut families." This term refers to the "frequent flier" families, who set up two households: one for the children in the United States and one for the adults who work back in their home country after they have received their green cards. The increased number of such families was due to the economic boom of the Pacific Rim and the sometimes challenging task of finding suitable employment in the United States. More recently, this phenomenon has included not only new immigrants, but also many Chinese American families who have lived in the United States for many years.

In the 1990s, the "Internet revolution" gave another boost to immigration. For "high-tech" Chinese, it has been said that the 1990s resembled the gold rush days, except that the fortune seekers were no longer mining for gold nuggets but for silicon chips (Chang, 2003). Overall, the influx of immigrants and refugees from many parts of Asia and many different socioeconomic and political backgrounds has contributed to the complexity of the existing Chinese American communities.

THE TRADITIONAL CHINESE FAMILY

The unique characteristics of the traditional family in China stemmed from the primary influence of Confucianism. Confucian teachings emphasize harmonious interpersonal relationships and interdependence. Family interactions were governed by prescribed roles defined by family hierarchy, obligation, and duties. Independent behavior or expression of emotions that might disrupt familial harmony were discouraged. The family was patriarchal. Males, particularly fathers and eldest sons, had dominant roles. Marriages were commonly arranged, and it was socially acceptable for influential men to have concubines. Husbands dealt with the outside world and provided for the family. The spousal relationship was secondary to the parent–child relationship. Filial piety was highly cherished. Respect, shame, and face saving were measures used by parents as means of control. The father usually played the role of a stern disciplinarian, whereas the mother was affectionate and caring. The eldest son was expected to carry on the family name and enjoyed special privileges, and the eldest daughter was taught to assist the mother with household chores and attend to younger siblings. The most elevated family dyad was the father–son dyad.

Throughout history, Chinese mothers have been portrayed as self-sacrificing, suffering, overbearing, guilt inducing, and overinvolved with their children. Throughout their lifespan, women were to be seen in relation to men (fathers, brothers, sons, husbands). Traditionally, in accordance with the custom of "thrice obeying," women were expected to comply with their fathers or elder brothers in youth, their husbands in marriage, and their sons after their husbands' death. The value of wives was judged by their ability to produce male heirs and to serve their in-laws. Grandparents and other extended family members also had a significant influence on family life. Because of the strong bond and the intense sense of obligation, many sons never left their parents in their adult lives. Parents expected to be taken care of in their old age and never experienced the "empty-nest" period in their family life cycle.

CONTEMPORARY CHINESE AMERICAN FAMILIES

Chinese families have been historically molded by economic, political, and sociocultural factors (Tseng & Hsu, 1991), and, as discussed earlier, their structure and composition have been heavily influenced by U.S. immigration policy as well. In the past generation, the traditional Chinese family has undergone tremendous transformation due to economic and political forces in the United States and Asia. As indicated previously, with the large number of Chinese immigrants from China, Hong Kong, and Taiwan, the massive economic and political changes in those countries have had a dramatic impact on Chinese families in the United States. Since the Communist takeover of China in 1949, Confucian thought and religions have largely been banned. A one-child family system has replaced the traditional extended family system. During the 10 years of the Cultural Revolution period, many families suffered forced separation. Red Guard youths openly challenged their parents and teachers; filial piety and respect for the elderly no longer dominate life in China. In recent years the economic boom in China has brought another wave of Western influence and urbanization.

After World War II, both Hong Kong and Taiwan underwent rapid growth in light industry and exports. The forces of industrialization, Westernization, urbanization, and economic affluence brought huge changes in Chinese social and family structure. Although older Chinese still embody some traditional beliefs, the younger generation has shown some rejection of conservatism and traditionalism. Political history has also influenced traditional Chinese family values. In Hong Kong, the British colonial past has produced profound effects on the education, legal, and social systems. In Taiwan, the long period of Japanese occupation, lasting until the end of World War II, has had a large impact on the society, especially among the older generation.

In recent years, Chinese American writers such as Amy Tan, Gus Lee, Gish Jen, Chang-rae Lee, Helen Zia, and Eric Liu have presented rich, textured views of the contemporary Asian American experience, including issues of contemporary racism, continued discrimination, the search for cultural identity, consumerism, political strife, and the experiences of the baby boomers and members of Generation X. Writings about relationships, intimacy, and sexuality have also begun to appear.

Shifts in contemporary Chinese American families include the following: (1) The traditional Chinese extended family has gradually yielded to a more nuclear family; (2) the traditional patriarchal family has transformed, in many cases, into a system in which a mother shares decision making with the father; (3) the parent–child dyad has diminished in importance, and importance of the husband–wife relationship has increased; (4) the favoring of sons has slowly decreased; daughters now attain comparable education and careers and can be counted on to take care of aged parents; (5) there has been a change in the family life cycle from arranged marriages to marriages preceded by romantic love; (6) adult children now leave the home, when previously, there was no empty-nest phase; (7) successful child rearing is now measured mostly by the children's academic and career achievements; and (8) earning power is no longer solely the father's responsibility, but is shared with other adult family members.

MENTAL HEALTH NEEDS AND COMMON DIAGNOSES AMONG CHINESE AMERICANS

It is difficult to specify the rates of mental health needs for this population, because our overall knowledge of the mental health needs of Asians is very limited (U.S. Department of Health and Human Services, 2001). The studies that have been conducted have been criticized for their small sample size and failure to be conducted in the languages of the Asian American groups being researched. However, research findings strongly suggest that Chinese Americans do have major mental health problems, contrary to the widespread belief that they are a well-adjusted "model minority."

The large-scale Chinese American Psychiatric Epidemiological Study (CAPES), conducted in the mid-1990s in Mandarin, Cantonese, and English, concluded that Chinese Americans had moderate levels of depression (Sue, Sue, Sue, & Takeuchi, 1995; Takeuchi et al., 1998). Some researchers have discussed the frequency of culture-specific syndromes, such as neurasthenia, in China and in the United States. Sometimes resembling a somatoform disorder, neurasthenia is characterized by such symptoms as loss of energy, inability to sleep or concentrate, and aches and pains without significantly persisting depressive moods. Studies of Chinese American students have reported that they have high rates of anxiety (Sue & Zane, 1985). Overall, although Chinese Americans seem to have mental health needs similar to those of other groups, specifics have been difficult to clarify; it is hoped that future research will improve our understanding.

CLINICAL CONSIDERATIONS IN TREATING CHINESE AMERICAN FAMILIES

Western-trained clinicians have paid great attention to either the intrapsychic influences or the biological explanations of the causes of mental illness. But many Chinese are still highly influenced by their religious and spiritual beliefs and by concepts of health and disease in traditional Chinese medicine. The Chinese have several common explanations for the development of mental illness and emotional problems.

1. *Imbalance of* yin *and* yang *and disharmony in the flow of* chi. In traditional Chinese medicine, humankind is viewed as a microcosm within a macrocosm. The energy in each human being interrelates with the energy of the universe. *Chi* (energy) and *jing* (sexual energy) are both considered vital life energies that are kept in balance by the dual polarities of yin and yang. If there is an imbalance of the *yin* and *yang*, then the immunity of the body is disturbed and the body is susceptible to illness. According to Chinese philosophy, the five elements metal, water, wood, fire, and earth make up all matter and influence everything and everyone. It is important to keep these core elements in balance for health and well-being. Too much or too little of one or more elements may lead to problems that are physically manifested.

2. *Supernatural intervention.* Mental illness is seen as a form of spiritual unrest meted out to the individual through the agency of a "ghost" or vengeful spirit. It is a sign of punishment caused by the transgression of family dictates (Lin & Lin, 1981).

3. *Religious beliefs.* Mental illness is viewed as negative karma, caused by deeds from past lives or punishment from God.

4. *Genetic vulnerability or hereditary defects* caused by bad genes passed down or a tainted hereditary lineage.

5. *Physical and emotional strain and exhaustion* caused by external stresses such as failing in a business, ending a love affair, death of a family member, and so on.

6. *Organic disorders.* Mental illness is conceptualized as a manifestation of physical disease, especially brain disorders, diseases of the liver, hormonal imbalance, and so on.

7. *Character weakness.* Mental health is achieved through self-discipline, exercise of will power, and the avoidance of morbid thoughts. Persons who are born with weak character will not be able to practice these disciplines and are more vulnerable to emotional problems.

Indigenous Healing Practices in the Chinese Community

Despite the existence of an advanced, highly institutionalized U.S. medical system and the availability of mental health professionals, many traditional healing methods are still utilized by Chinese clients for physical or emotional problems. Various indigenous healing practices are available in major Chinatowns and refugee communities, the most popular being herbal medicine, acupuncture, and therapeutic massage. Ritual or faith healing is also perceived to be helpful. Other practices such as "coining," "cupping," or fortune-telling are also used to prevent or to remove "bad spirits." Indeed, Chinese healing practices such as acupuncture and the use of herbal medicines have been gaining broad popularity among Americans in general.

The Chinese are usually very conscious of good nutrition and view it as an important factor in restoring health. Traditional Chinese medicine categorizes foods into five groups: "hot," "cold," "allergic," "moderate," and "nutrient." Therapeutic cuisine that gives "good *chi*" or contributes positively to the "life force" is very popular in treating health and emotional problems. In addition, many Chinese practice health exercises such as *tai chi chuan* and *chi gong* to bring harmony to the body and mind. Relaxing the mind through meditation and breathing exercises is also expected to positively impact the flow of *chi*.

Dealing with Psychological Problems

Most Chinese Americans try to deal with their psychological problems without seeking professional mental health counseling. Traditional families usually seek help from family members first, because it is considered the collective responsibility of the family to take care of the disturbed member as long as possible. Such problems are kept from outsiders for fear of the shame, guilt, and stigma that this knowledge might bring upon the family. The family often tries to deal with the problem by denying the seriousness of the illness or by exhorting or reasoning with the patient to "correct" his or her behaviors (Lin & Lin, 1981). When the family and the troubled person are not able to resolve the problem, they still have been found to turn to certain trusted outsiders and helpers within the ethnic community, such as community elders, spiritual leaders, indigenous healers, and physicians (Sue & Morishima, 1982; U.S. Department of Health and Human Services, 2001). When these efforts fail, assistance from other agencies and providers, including psychiatrists and other mental health professionals, is sought while the troubled family member is kept at home. Family members usually resist hospitalization until all other efforts have failed and utilization of resources outside the family system is of absolute necessity.

Treatment Expectations

For many clinicians, the success of a case is measured by the emotional growth of the client or the psychological understanding of the problem. Although some acculturated Chinese may expect "insight" therapy, the majority of Chinese immigrants and refugees expect more concrete help and the immediate alleviation of tangible symptoms.

Process of Healing

Many Chinese Americans seek help from mental health professionals only as a last resort, after they have exhausted all other resources, and usually come in for help in a state of crisis, with the expectation of an immediate "cure." They are used to the traditional Chinese healing practice, which usually includes a brief physical observation, diagnosis, and prescription writing—all in one session. They expect a rapid diagnosis and do not understand the purpose of lengthy evaluation and the apparent lack of treatment in the initial session. They may also become upset with initial interviews that probe into their family and personal backgrounds, which in their view have nothing to do with the presenting problem. To reveal family secrets to an outsider also evokes a sense of guilt. Consequently, many Chinese clients may drop out of treatment (Lee, 1982). Brief treatment or episodic brief treatments may be indicated (Soo-Hoo, 1999).

Perception of the Mental Health Professional Role

Many mental health disciplines are not widely recognized in Asian countries. Many Chinese do not have the same worldview or knowledge base to understand the role of clinicians or their specific professional orientations. Because the role of a physician is more clearly understood and respected, Chinese patients may expect clinicians to conduct themselves in the traditional role of physicians who prescribe medication. Therefore, especially in the initial stage of the therapeutic relationship, it is very important for clinicians to explore their clients' experiences with mental health professionals in the past. It may be important to acknowledge generational or language differences. Intentional brokerage and collaboration with other respected professionals can add to credibility in the initial engagement process.

FAMILY ASSESSMENT OF IMMIGRANT CHINESE FAMILIES

Effective assessment of Chinese families must take into consideration their holistic views of health and illness and culturally specific ways of coping with emotional difficulties. The assessment must include information beyond traditional intake data. Relevant personal, familial, and community information, as well as cultural mapping, are extremely helpful in the assessment of Chinese families who have undergone rapid social change and major cultural upheaval (Ho, 1987). As in any assessment, it is vital for clinicians to base their evaluation on (1) the physical: constitutional or somatic organization, (2) the psychological: the ego or self-concept as an organizing force, and (3) the sociocultural: the organizing response to the rules and expectations of society and culture (Lee, 1982).

The assessment guidelines discussed here for Chinese American families follow those presented in Chapter 20, the overview on Asian American families, and discussed elsewhere (Lee, 1982, 1989, 1990).

Migration and Relocation History

As a result of the major political changes in China during the past several decades, many Chinese have been exposed to international conflict, such as the Sino-Japanese War and the civil war between the Nationalists and the Communists. Many families also endured hardships during the Cultural Revolution. It is helpful to understand how much energy clients have spent in coping with their losses and separations, and how much energy they have left to cope with new demands. Questions to ask include the following: How many times did the family move in the past? From where to where did they move? Who left, and with whom? What were the reasons? Who made the decision? Which family members are still left behind? What was the order of migration? Were these voluntary or involuntary migrations? To what political and economic systems was the family exposed? When did family members come to the United States? Who is the sponsor? What kind of relationship does the family have with the sponsor? If their root language is Chinese, what are the words, phrases, folktales, or stories in their dialect that might be used to capture some of the aspects of transition? These culturally based conceptualizations, when viewed as metaphors, may provide useful insights into their experiences (Mock, 1998).

In view of the long history of losses and separation in many Chinese families, it is common for the pain and unresolved conflicts of one generation to be suppressed or denied and then passed on and expressed in the next generation. It is very important for clinicians to view the pain an individual brings to the session as pain experienced by the total family, including parents and grandparents.

Adjustment Problems and Cultural Shock

Many new immigrants arrive in the United States with losses, separations, and unresolved grief. At the same time, they are placed in a strange and unpredictable new environment. As minority members, they have to learn and get used to the behavioral and value orientation of American culture. The problems encountered, such as language, transportation, employment, housing, child care, and racism, can be overwhelming.

Impact of Migration on Individual and Family Life Cycle

In addition to the overall impact of relocation, migration disrupts both the individual and the family life cycle. How does an ethnic Chinese Vietnamese child growing up in a refugee camp with no provision for substitute mothering establish a basic sense of trust? How does an adolescent from mainland China integrate old values with the new ones learned from the media, school, and peer groups? How does a Chinese housewife deal with new values in regard to gender role, sexual orientation, independence, achievement, and work? How does a newly arrived elderly Chinese man who expects to be supported by his children and grandchildren deal with his loneliness in a housing project for the elderly or in a nursing home?

From a life cycle perspective, families that migrate with young children are perhaps strengthened by having each other, but they are vulnerable to the reversal of parent–child hierarchies. Families migrating when their children are adolescents may have more difficulties because they will have less time together as a unit before the children move out on their own. Thus, the family must struggle simultaneously with multiple transitions and generational conflicts (Hernandez & McGoldrick, in press).

Differences in Rate of Acculturation

Given the great diversity of languages, norms, and immigration status among the Chinese in the United States, clinicians are advised to assess a client's acculturation in the United States very carefully. A non-Chinese-speaking, third-generation Chinese American may be very "Westernized" and have a different value orientation from a non-English-speaking, newly arrived immigrant. However, length of time in the United States is not an absolute yardstick to measure the degree of acculturation. Many older Chinese, who came to the United States before the Cultural Revolution, still try to preserve their heritage by "freezing traditions" and may be more "Chinese" than newly arrived immigrants from Hong Kong or Taiwan.

The country of origin and its relationship to Western values also influence the rate of acculturation. A professional from Singapore may absorb American culture much more easily than an adult from China, because Singaporeans have rapidly adopted many Western practices, whereas mainland Chinese are only beginning to do so.

Professional affiliation is also a factor in acculturation. An English-speaking Chinese doctor from Hong Kong who works in an American hospital is exposed to many more American practices than a Chinese cook who works in the kitchen of a Chinese restaurant with other non-English-speaking Chinese.

Age at time of immigration is another factor. A 10-year-old child who immediately enters the public school system is more easily assimilated than an 80-year-old man who lives in Chinatown.

Family Stress Caused by Role Reversal

Many monolingual Chinese parents and grandparents depend on their English-speaking children as cultural brokers and interpreters. Such dependency can cause resentment and anger (Lee, 1988). Role reversal may also occur between spouses when one is more acculturated than the other. Many Chinese women, for the first time, earn more than their husbands, demand more rights than before, and may have more lifestyle options than previously socially sanctioned.

Work and Financial Stress

For the Chinese, the work environment and work roles contribute greatly to individuals' self-definition and self-esteem. Work can be a facilitator or a barrier to life adjustment. Hope of improving the family's financial status is one of the major reasons Chinese immigrate to the United States. However, language barriers and other factors have trapped many Chinese in restaurant work, garment factory work, or other manual labor with no alternatives. "Status inconsistency," created by underemployment, is one of the major stresses for Chinese in this country. In addition, the demands of work have caused drastic changes in the Chinese family system. Because of long working hours, many Chinese men find it difficult to maintain the traditional family role as husband and father. Women, especially those who were not employed outside their homes before they came to the United States, find it very stressful to be working mothers with little support from their husbands. Becoming the breadwinner is devastating for one who has not faced that responsibility before. For Chinese American professionals, economic downturns, "glass ceiling" barriers, and the stress of continually being treated as the "foreign other" also cause discouragement.

Neighborhood and Community Support

Enclaves of Chinese Americans living in Chinatowns across the United States represent a psychological and physical sense of community. To many Chinese Americans, especially recent immigrants, the community provides the psychological significance of an extended family. In place of the support available in their home village, the community provides the family with an informal support network for socialization into the behaviors needed for survival and adaptation. Chinese depend on other Chinese to learn about their "new world." Community groups such as family associations and social/cultural clubs provide much needed support. The community may have a much more important psychological meaning for Chinese families than it does for many Western families.

Because Chinese communities tend to be cohesive, with strong informal communication networks, the clinician must assess the constraints any particular Chinese community places on a particular family or person. Therapeutic problems may arise because of a sense of losing face, attributable to the community's stigmatization of emotional problems; cross-ethnic relationship conflicts involving racism; conflicts within the Chinese community; lack of service alternatives; and the poor reputation of the treatment system in handling Chinese family issues and confidentiality. Many Chinese live in urban neighborhoods with crime, violence, and the perniciousness of overt or covert stereotyping. Special attention should be given to the effects of these stressors on family systems.

Religious, Spiritual, and Cultural Beliefs

Among Chinese Americans, Christianity, Buddhism, Taoism, and ancestor worship are the most prevalent religions or teachings underlying their worldviews. The clinician should respect the spiritual perspective of the family. For example, the concepts of *karma*, reincarnation, and compassion are effective in working with Buddhist clients. The Confucian teaching of "the middle way," the Buddhist teaching of *karma*, and the Taoist teaching of "the way" are examples of how religious and philosophical teachings can be helpful in coping with life stresses. In addition, the support of extended family members and the strong focus on harmony and interpersonal relationships in Chinese families should be utilized. The clinician should encourage family members to share their cultural beliefs on the causes of their problems, their past coping style, their help-seeking behavior, and their treatment expectations. (See Chapter 20 for a list of questions that may be helpful.)

Family Physical Health and Medication History

Because of the holistic view of health and illness in Chinese culture, it is important to pay attention to the physical as well as the emotional state of the client. Gathering information on physical health, nutrition, and medication history is vital. Many Chinese patients take herbal medicines and receive treatment from indigenous healers. Such practices need to be respected and taken into account. A blended East–West bicultural approach may offer the best of both worlds.

Relationship Issues, Intimacy, and Sexuality

Chinese cultural worldviews may initially create awkwardness in discussing relationship issues in depth. However, like a thorough examination performed by a good physician, timely probing or inquiring can be acceptably received. By laying out the array of potential topics to be covered in therapeutic conversations, such as sexual or racial identity, discrimination and violence, or ways in which couples and families converge or diverge, the clinician can ensure that such hard-to-discuss and essential topics can later be explored for optimal family functioning.

TREATMENT STRATEGIES

The treatment strategies discussed in the overview of Asian American families, Chapter 20, can be applied in working with Chinese American families. Specific strategies that continue to be effective (Lee, 1982, 1997) are summarized here:

1. The clinician should convey expertise and use caution in establishing an initial egalitarian therapeutic relationship. Chinese family members view the clinician as the "problem solver" and expect that person to behave in a direct manner, applying his or her expertise.

2. Clinicians need to convey an air of confidence. Clients need to know that the clinician is more "powerful" than their illness and will "cure" them with competence and know-how. The potential gains from going to therapy must be greater than the underlying potential shame if others should know the client is in therapy.

3. It is not unusual for Chinese clients to ask the clinician many personal questions about his or her family background, marital status, number of children, and so on. The clinician will need to feel comfortable about answering some select personal questions about credentials or background in order to gain the client's trust and to establish rapport.

4. Active engagement and problem solving may be useful. Nonjudgmental listening and neutrality of the clinician's responses may be viewed as lack of interest, not caring, or lack of confidence.

5. Flexibility and willingness to assume multiple helping roles enhance the therapeutic relationship. Assuming the various roles of advocate, educator, consultant, and broker to other services, especially for Chinese families that are limited in resources or knowledge, can be very therapeutic. With the therapist flexibly taking on these appropriate roles, the family may feel relieved that a core person understands their multiple sources of stress.

6. Clients often need demonstrations of caring and empathy. Among Chinese clients with a long history of separation from their loved ones, there is a yearning for an actively empathic parental figure. Clinicians who exhibit warmth and a desire to do something concretely to relieve symptoms or reduce problems are more able to gain the trust of their clients.

7. Chinese clients may expect to have a dependent role at the outset of the therapeutic relationship. The clinician should encourage initial "healthy dependency" and set up a therapy plan that will foster future independence, anticipating the client's readiness.

8. It is very important for the clinician to identify the decision makers in the Chinese family and gain their support for the treatment plan. Their active participation in the implementation of the plan can be very effective. In the early stages of therapy, individual sessions (some Chinese families refer to these as "secret meetings") can foster unnecessary guilt and isolation within the family and increase the family's resistance to involvement in therapy. It is preferable to establish relationships with multiple family members through family therapy.

9. Flexibility and some informality in regard to clinical entry and exit are essential. Some Chinese clients come to an agency for help not by formal referral, but by word of mouth. Unduly formal evaluation sessions with rigid time frames may create barriers.

10. It is important to acknowledge and work with the clients' inherent ambivalence. The family may want the clinician's help but feel shame or experience pain and not want to share their feelings because they worry that others might find out and they will "lose face." Validating their feelings, that sharing family secrets with an outsider may feel uncomfortable yet be a powerful action that will be treated with all respect, trust, and confidentiality, can be very reassuring and uplifting.

11. Creative use of the family's cultural strengths is encouraged. Strengths such as support from extended family members and siblings, the strong sense of obligation, the strong focus on educational achievement, the work ethic, the high tolerance for loneliness and separation, and the loyalties of extended relationships should be respected and used creatively in the therapeutic process.

12. There may be certain topics that should be addressed with sensitivity, such as intimacy and sexuality. It is our experience, however, that avoiding certain topics such as homosexuality can collude with the keeping of family secrets and increase pressure. Strategic psychoeducation can help to normalize discussions. The therapist's introducing such topics as racism, heterosexism, discrimination, and violence in a timely manner to Chinese families can be initially difficult but in the end may actually be a relief, opening up new ways of relating and creating perspectives to strengthen relationships (Mock, 1999).

13. Special caution is advised for clinicians who share similar cultural backgrounds with their Chinese clients. Those with the same cultural background may have particular difficulties and blind spots. For example, a young Chinese clinician who is still struggling with his or her own cultural identity and dependency in regard to parents may overidentify with the teenagers in a family. Transference and countertransference issues should be explored and handled appropriately to best work with the Chinese family.

14. Termination is another area requiring special attention. The Chinese concepts of time and space in relationships can be quite different from the clinician's. Chinese families invest a great deal of energy in trusting their clinician and in allowing him or her to be part of the family. They may want to maintain periodic contact even after the successful achievement of treatment goals. Upon being presented the "gifts of improvement," Chinese families may want to give back or show gratitude by providing the clinician with updates about family members' progress or reaching other milestones.

CASE EXAMPLE

The C. family (David and Mai, in their mid-40s, and their son Jason, 10), who had immigrated to the United States from China, were referred by their family physician, who had seen David for complaints of debilitating headaches. Recently, there had been increased family stress, focusing on their son. The physician thought the couple could benefit from a helper who could understand their culture and family expectations.

The C. family arrived punctually for the initial session. As I (MRM) invited them to my consultation area, I asked if the directions, parking, and so forth, had been clear. This attention to their initial comfort seemed to put them at ease. Coming into my office, they took notice of my degrees, asking politely if I had worked successfully with many children and families. Mai asked whether my family was originally from China and referred to a prominent Chinese American community leader. I strategically answered these questions in order to establish rapport, credibility, and trust. I acknowledged my Cantonese background and familiarity with several community leaders during my many years of work. Taking this as an additional cue regarding privacy, I asserted that all that we would discuss would be kept confidential unless they gave specific consent otherwise. Engaging in this culturally syntonic initial discussion helped establish a bond for framing our work together.

I commended the family for being so invested in each other that they took time off from work and school to come see me. The three major problems they openly related were (1) David's headaches, which did not seem to have a medical cause. David also mentioned his increased stress at work as an electrician, having to work more hours to stay in the good graces of his boss; (2) Jason, although he did well academically, had recently been in two school fights, after which his father was called to take him home; and (3) Mai was experiencing pressure from members of her family who were still in China. They were saying that she needed to take better care of her family. Both Mai and David had also experienced shame that they were not good parents, because they had had to meet with school administrators about Jason.

I conveyed to the family that by their seeking help so quickly, we had a good opportunity to address these problems. I also gave them between-session homework. David, with his family's help, was to keep track of when his headaches occurred and what was going on at the time. If they wished, they could consult with a specialist I knew. Although they did not take me up on this, they seemed to appreciate that I had linkages to other reputable professionals. As I would later find out, most of David's migraines happened during the beginning of his week's work assignments.

During subsequent sessions, Mai, who was the primary spokesman for the family, indirectly revealed that there had been increased conflict within the parental dyad. While working such long and hard hours, David had been more impatient and demanding at home. Eventually, Mai related three incidents in which he had become verbally angry, but not violent or threatening. One of these outbursts had come after Mai had spoken with her parents in China. They had asked her if she needed financial help and encouraged her to be more involved as a wife and mother. When asked how she experienced her parents' comments, Mai was initially at a loss for words. I asked her to think about how she might describe her feelings in Chinese. She told a story about a wife of a Chinese emperor, who had attempted to fend off some attacking warlords. Mai said that it was her duty to fend off others, including her parents' criticism of David. She said that Jason missed David, who was away at work a great deal even though the family was financially stable. Attempting to show empathy to each of them, I validated them in their substantial efforts to pay attention to the family's well-being, both materially and in terms of others' respect. Even Jason perked up. We helped him to realize that he too was contributing through his interactions at school.

While unraveling further family history, David revealed that his family of origin was from a working class background and that, as the eldest son, he had immigrated from China to this country on his own. The expectation was for him to pave the way for other family members to come. Mai, in contrast, the middle child of three, had come from a rather well-to-do family and had been sent to the United States for school. She had been able to travel back and forth several times to China during her studies, deciding after school to stay in the United States. Her family had supported her as the favored only daughter of her family.

From a cultural perspective, several issues were noteworthy: (1) David, from a typical patriarchal family, felt responsible for taking care of the needs of the family, especially economically; (2) he felt guilty for not being able to provide adequately for his family, as he concluded from Mai's parents' criticism and suggestions to Mai to do more; and (3) both parents felt shame and loss of face by having to go to school to talk about Jason's fights.

From the outset, I sensed that family loyalty was a key issue. I empathized with their struggle and having to go it alone as the "launched pioneers" of their families and commented on the obvious strengths they both possessed. David played the role passed down from his father, to work and prove himself by working long hours. If David were to show distress, he would be viewed as "weak" or "inadequate" in his role as head of the family. Instead, I facilitated his sharing his thoughts and problem-solving abilities.

In observing the couple's communication patterns, I noticed that as emotional subjects arose, David would defer to his wife to speak for him. I eventually changed this pattern and invited him to share his thoughts equally in the sessions. We also talked about the contrasting perspectives here in America about the role of elders. For example, when Mai's family heard about Jason's school difficulties, they attributed them to his general disposition and how Mai mothered him. This only created additional pressures for David and Mai. As we considered alternative possibilities and discussed their immigration stresses, economic challenges, and "wanting to live the American dream," David and Mai felt relieved that they were not at fault. These discussions about extended family with traditional ideas also revealed that David and Mai had seldom spoken about their families of origin.

Subsequent sessions revealed that there were important life cycle issues relating to migration. David had actually used staying in America, in part, to get away from family. I asked him if he could share what he might have otherwise keep private. He described his father as being tyrannical, sometimes drinking and "being harsh" when he had had a hard day at his factory job. David recalled trying hard to prove his worth to his father, even to the point of overachieving and being a "workaholic." Mai also shared that her family had been hesitant to approve of her marrying David. Their main concern seemed be their different class backgrounds, questioning how David could provide for the family. While openly discussing this subject, David and Mai became more animated with each other. David was able to share his worries and anxieties that he was not living up to expectations as the head of the family, with Mai listening attentively.

I encouraged David to break from his usual pattern and to spend special time just with Jason. Taking the initiative, David turned down a weekend overtime opportunity and took a fishing trip with his son. At the next session, Jason came bounding up the stairs with increased energy. He talked excitedly about the weekend fishing trip. His dad chimed in, describing how Jason had caught two small fish, which they had returned to the water. David proudly announced, "Jason was able to cast his line out better than I ever could at his age." This focus on changing interactions seemed to have positive residual effects. The week after this trip, Jason's teacher reported that he had been more actively engaged with peers.

Over time, each member of the C. family became more comfortable in speaking about his or her accumulated pressures. The parents shared their migration stories and how their experiences had affected them in the past and in their current family. Even Jason took interest, asking how David related to his own father. This led to validating David and Jason's father–son relationship, and they were given an opportunity to write down their wishes for their future legacies. Mai talked more directly with her family in China about things she was proud of, her current family's strengths. She also spoke to Jason's teacher about her volunteering in the classroom. In this way, she maintained loyalties with her own family of origin but also articulated her allegiance to her husband. David took on less overtime work and was given "nonmonetary pay" through verbal recognition by Mai and Jason. His headaches diminished in both frequency and intensity. He was able to talk through some of his personal self-doubts and identify his contributions to the family. We worked with Jason to find alternatives to his frustrations, and eventually he made more friendships at school. Mai felt less conflicted loyalties, becoming able to negotiate and balance the pulls between her family of origin and her husband. As we ended, the C. family announced that Jason would be graduating successfully from the fifth grade.

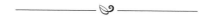

CONCLUSIONS

This chapter provides a historical background of the migration of Chinese American families. Cultural issues and clinical considerations are presented. Practical guidelines are offered for family assessment and treatment. From the pioneer family to the "astronaut" family, diverse Chinese American families have undergone numerous changes and are continuing to evolve. With the changing political and economic climates in the United States and Asia, Chinese American families may undergo more changes in their composition, size, and family dynamics. Clinicians need to stay in tune with these rapid changes and must be flexible in designing treatment strategies.

Effective cross-cultural family therapy requires not only the knowledge of cultural differences, but also the professional skills necessary to achieve about positive changes and effective treatment outcomes. The establishment of a therapeutic relationship is based not only on mutual trust, but also on the clinician's ability to empathize with compassion. A culturally competent clinician should also have a clear understanding of his or her cultural identity, cross-cultural communication style, and countertransference issues while working with Chinese American families. The most challenging task is, however, to take advantage of the long and rich cultural strengths (such as philosophy, religion, historical survival, and a holistic approach to health) of Chinese culture and families and integrate them with the best that modern Western medicine and psychology can offer. We believe that such an integrated model will not only benefit the treatment of Chinese Americans, but will also enhance overall American society in appreciating its multicultural riches.

REFERENCES

Asian American Health Forum. (1990). *Asian and Pacific Islander American population statistics.* (Monograph Series 1). San Francisco: Author.

Barnes, J. S., & Bennett, C. E. (2002, February). *The Asian population: 2000* (Census 2000 Brief). Washington, DC: U.S. Census Bureau.

Chang, I. (2003). *The Chinese in America: A narrative history.* New York: Penguin Group.

Hernandez, M., & McGoldrick, M. (in press). Migration and the family life cycle. In B. Carter & M. McGoldrick (Eds.), *The expanded family life cycle: Individual, family and social perspectives.* Boston: Allyn & Bacon.

Ho, M. K. (1987). *Family therapy with ethnic minorities.* Newbury Park, CA: Sage.

Lee, E. (1982). A social system approach to assessment and treatment for Chinese American families. In M. McGoldrick, J. K. Pearce, & J. Giordano (Eds.), *Ethnicity and family therapy* (pp. 527–551). New York: Guilford Press.

Lee, E. (1988). Cultural factors in working with Southeast Asian refugee adolescents. *Journal of Adolescence, 11,* 167–179.

Lee, E. (1989). Assessment and treatment of Chinese-American immigrant families. *Journal of Psychotherapy and the Family*, 6(1/2), 99–122.

Lee, E. (1990). Family therapy with Southeast Asian refugees. In M. P. Mirkin (Ed.), *The social and political contexts of family therapy* (pp. 331–354). Needham Heights, MA: Allyn & Bacon.

Lee, E. (1997). *Working with Asian Americans: A guide for clinicians*. New York: Guilford Press.

Lin, T., & Lin, M. (1981). Love, denial and rejection: Responses of Chinese families to mental illness. In A. Kleinman & T. Lin (Eds.), *Normal and abnormal behavior in Chinese culture* (pp. 387–401). Dordrecht, The Netherlands: D. Reidel.

Mock, M. R. (1998). Clinical reflections on refugee families: Transforming crises into opportunities. In M. McGoldrick (Ed.), *Re-visioning family therapy: Race, culture, and gender in clinical practice* (pp. 347–359). New York: Guilford Press.

Mock, M. R. (1999, Spring). Cultural competency: Acts of justice in community mental health. *Community Psychologist*, 1–3.

Soo-Hoo, T. (1999) Brief strategic family therapy with Chinese-Americans. *American Journal of Family Therapy*, 27, 163–179.

Sue, S., & Morishima, J. (1982). *The mental health of Asian Americans*. San Francisco: Jossey-Bass.

Sue, S., Sue, D. W., Sue, L., & Takeuchi, D. T. (1995). Psychopathology among Asian Americans: A model minority? *Cultural Diversity and Mental Health*, 1(1), 39–54.

Sue, S., & Zane, N. (1985) Academic achievement and socioemotional adjustment among Chinese university students. *Journal of Counseling Psychology*, 32, 570–579.

Takeuchi, D. T., Chung, R. C., Lin, K. M., Shen, H., Kurasaki, K., Chun, C., & Sue, S. (1998). Lifetime and twelve-month prevalence rates of major depressive episodes and dysthymia among Chinese Americans in Los Angeles. *American Journal of Psychiatry*, 16, 237–245.

Tseng, W. S., & Hsu, J. (1991). *Culture and family: Problems and therapy*. Binghamton, NY: Haworth Press.

U.S. Department of Health and Human Services. (2001). *Mental health: Culture, race and ethnicity—A supplement to mental health: A report of the Surgeon General*. Rockville, MD: Author.

CHAPTER 23

Filipino Families

Maria P. P. Root

Because a complex sociopolitical history has shaped Filipino culture, effective assessment of a family requires understanding the complex tapestry of influences. Filipinos are the second largest Asian-descent group in the United States, at almost 2.4 million, constituting 18.3% of the Asian population (see www.asian-nation.org/population.shtml). More than half of all Asian Americans live in six metropolitan areas: Los Angeles, New York, San Francisco, Honolulu, Washington, D.C.–Baltimore, and Chicago (U.S. Bureau of the Census, 1999). Among the various groups of Asian origin, Filipinos are comparable to Pacific Islanders in having the highest rates of English proficiency. A constellation of variables, including multigenerational households, sharing of resources, language proficiency, and education, results in one of the highest median family incomes and lowest number of people living in poverty (6.9% for Asian groups; see www.asian-nation.org/demographics.shtml).

Filipinos, by definition, are a multicultural people with Chinese, Spanish, Malayan, Indonesian, South Asian, American, and, in the south, Muslim cultural influences. The result of these influences emphasizes a shared identity and connectedness, the centrality of the family, acceptance of uncertainty, ability to relate to others, respect offered according to the individual's place in the structure of hierarchical relations, adaptability, and religiosity (Enriquez, 1994).

Only in recent years has an informed, insider description of Filipino American families appeared (Agbayani-Siewert & Enrile, 2003; Agbayani-Siewert & Revilla, 1995; Chan, 1998; Santa Rita, 1996). This chapter provides a foundation for understanding Filipino families and kinship patterns so that the therapist may intervene more effectively with them.

A therapist increases his or her credibility with a family by respecting and understanding the differences between Filipino and assimilated American notions of kinship, boundaries, causality, individuality, communalism, and social means of control. Therapy with families almost always means there will be at least two generations, and often three, involved, even if one does not live in the particular family's household. Given the continued immigration of Filipinos to the United States, many families include someone who is an immigrant, holding many original cultural values even if acculturated. In times of crisis this duality surfaces.

There are many Filipino family constellations, driven by economic, political, and historical factors. The common *multiple-generation household* allows for pooling of resources provided by income earners, which contributes to the high-ranking economic standing of Filipino Americans among Asian Americans (Lott, 1997; see also www.asian-nation.org/demographics.shtml). *Transnational family arrangements*, with one spouse living in the United States and the other in another country, are driven by the need for income not available in the Philippines. Sometimes these arrangements are a face-saving way of marital separation in a country that does not allow divorce. Growing out of this arrangement may be the situation of *multiple families in different countries*, driven by loneliness and economics. Both men and women create additional families in this way. *Correspondence marriages*, new for Filipinas (Ordonez, 1997), are usually interracial marriages, a choice shaped by the economic devastation after the Marcos regime, which ended in the early 1980s. Contrary to stereotypes, these marriages can have significant levels of satisfaction (Lin, 1991). *Cross-cultural families* and *domestic interracial marriages* are common for Filipino Americans, who have one of the highest rates of intermarriage of all Asian-descent groups, for both men and women (Kitano, Fujino, & Sato, 1998). These marriages are driven by the influences of colonization and sex ratio differences (Lott, 1997). *Undocumented families* result from immigration laws (Montoya, 1997), expired visas, and the need for economic survival. The emergence of t*eenage families* (Tiongson, 1997) is driven by the restrictiveness of families (Galang, 1997), lack of sex education (Tiongson, 1997), and conflicting values at home between restrictive sexual values and permissive sexual mores in the broader culture (Tiongson, 1997). These families are often embedded in multigenerational households. *Lesbian and gay couples and families* pose a challenge to Filipino extended families for reasons that are similar across ethnic groups. The challenges arise from stereotypes, parochial religiosity, parental self-blame (which may interface with notions of causality), and worry that such a proclamation and lifestyle eliminate the possibility of children (Lipat, Ordona, Stewart, & Ubado, 1997; Singco-Holmes, 1993). Manalansan (1997) notes that the socialized expression of being gay differs cross-culturally. Thus, Filipino Americans raised in the United States, versus the Philippines, may express themselves in some critically different ways.

HISTORY AND WAVES OF IMMIGRATION

Little is known or documented about the second largest group of people of Asian descent in the United States, whose origins are melded from traders, visitors, and colonists from China, India, Spain, the United States, Malaysia, and the Middle East (Root, 1997). The Philippines is a country viewed as Catholic with a significant Protestant presence. It is further divided between the north and south, with perpetual attempts at establishment by a small but separate Muslim population in the south. Carlos Bulosan (1995) has observed of Filipinos, "Our outward guise is more deceptive than our history. . . . Our history has many strands of fear and hope that snarl and converge at several points in time and space" (p. 131).

Colonization for 400 years, first by the Spanish and then by the Americans, starting after the Spanish-American War in the late 1800s, has made Filipino identity and culture complex (Enriquez, 1994; Pido, 1986; Tompar-Tiu & Sustento-Seneriches, 1995). U.S. colonization reinforced many of the attitudes of the previous Spanish colonists. Many Filipino and Filipino American scholars and activists suggest that there is a complex interaction between the history of colonization by Spain and the United States and self-mastery and survival (Pido, 1986; San Juan, 1998). Pido (1997) suggests that the nationwide system of schools patterned after American education, often taught in English, contributed to "inculcating Pilipinos to American values and the Coca-Cola culture" (p. 24). Thus, the colonist's imprint is evidenced by the unifying language, which is English, more than the national language (Chan, 1998). The internalization of Western values and customs facilitates a cultural fluidity and code switching within the larger American culture that are less common among families of other Asian origins.

Colonialism enters into some family dynamics by way of colorism, the valuing of lighter skin color and European features over indigenous features and color, such as brown skin, broad nose, slanted eyes. It is important for the therapist to recognize the influence of this irrational preference on family dynamics, as it may be the only explanation of preferential treatment of lighter-skinned children in a family.

The impact of colonization on Philippine economic development and the country's dependence on the United States catalyzed distinct waves of Filipino immigration from the islands to Hawai'i and then to the U.S. mainland. Filipino immigration has been viewed as occurring in three waves, generally agreed upon by Filipino American historians (Pido, 1986; Vallangca, 1987). Cordova (1983) documented the Filipino presence in the United States as beginning 300 years prior to these waves. Chan (1998) conceptualized a fourth wave.

The first wave, composed primarily of men hired for farm labor, occurred from the end of the Spanish-American War in the late 1880s to the time of official independence of the Philippines from the United States in 1946. This wave also included a small group of men sent over for education by missionaries, the *pensionados* (Pido, 1986). The second wave took place from the end of World War II until the enactment of the revised immigration laws in the mid-1960s. It reflected the Philippine's instrumentality to the needs of the U.S. military and the physical devastation that World War II wreaked upon the Philippines, leading men and women to leave the war-torn country. Women married U.S. servicemen, families emigrated, relatives came in search of new beginnings, and Filipinos were scattered throughout the United States (Vallangca, 1987). Because professional degrees from the Philippines were not honored, women went to work for the survival of their families, which changed the traditional roles in families. The third wave of immigration started with the amended Immigration and Nationality Act of 1965, which removed restrictive quotas, and has lasted to the present time. More equal numbers of women and men and families from wealthier strata, many of whom settled on the East Coast, were included in this wave. Chan (1998) described a fourth wave made up of political exiles from the Marcos regime, which started in 1972 after his election in 1965 and continued for approximately 10 years after his overthrow in 1986. One might consider that this fourth wave includes more than political exiles, as the economic devastation of this political era catalyzed a Filipino diaspora that drastically altered family lives. Wives and husbands, in search of work for survival of the family and betterment of their children's futures, endured family constellations heretofore nonexistent or rare. Children were left with relatives for years, increasingly alienated from their parents. Long-separated wives and husbands created new families in the United States.

Simultaneously, the numbers of Filipino Americans in the United States have increased with each generation. The grandchildren and great-grandchildren of the *pensionados* and farmworkers are quite acculturated.

UNDERSTANDING IMMIGRATION STRESSES AND FAMILY KINSHIP AND GENDER ROLES

As in many cultures and ethnic groups, the Filipino family is the cornerstone of social relations and identity. The welfare of the family is valued over that of the individual, although cultural values would assert that the well-being of the family would contribute to the happiness and well-being of the individual. For people closer to immigrant Filipino cultural values, there is an orientation to the present that is adaptive, recognizing a certain lack of control over the future, that may allow for some risk taking (*bahala na*), which is often misunderstood as fatalism (Enriquez, 1994). This orientation allows for moments of happiness even during times of tragedy. In Filipino families, difficult-to-translate values or concepts such as *hiya* (dignity/self-respect/face/shame), *utang nang loob* (debt of gratitude for meaningful action taken on behalf of a loved one). *amor propryo* (self-esteem/pride), *pakikisama* (esteem/deference to a respected one or to the needs of the majority) explain some relational dynamics and reactions regarding disappointments, decisions, actions and inactions, and admonishments (Bulatao, 1966/1992; Enriquez, 1994).

For immigrant families, hopes and stresses are always present in cultural transition. Immigration carries hope for bettering a person's economic situation, providing options for his or her children, and sending money to relatives in the Philippines to ease their financial stresses. Families maintain hope that additional relatives, particularly parents, can be sent for. Immigration also imposes stresses, particularly in regard to language, homesickness, gender roles, isolation from extended family, and acculturation. The immigrant Filipino may speak English, but native English speakers may have difficulty understanding him or her. The immigrant has to adjust to the culture, which is often a shock; daily life in America is much more stressful than families have usually imagined. Changes in sex roles because of the lack of recognition of professional degrees, as well as lower status, in the United States stress a marital relationship. Equalization of income-earning power or reversal of traditional roles also creates stress. Whereas there is a tradition of maintaining relationships through reciprocal action, service, and loyalty in the Philippines, it may not operate constructively in a new culture with these additional stresses (Agbayani-Siewert & Revilla, 1995).

Conflict emerges from a generation gap widened by acculturation. Children acculturate more readily than parents do. They become more direct and may challenge their parents, as do other American children, in a way that is experienced by parents as disrespectful (Agbayani-Siewert & Revilla, 1995). This behavior, which may be experienced by parents or grandparents as shameful, disrespectful, ungrateful, and out of place, results in a tremendous culture gap in the core values described earlier. Whereas the parents may understand their children and try to adapt to new ways of communicating with them, grandparents may direct them to discipline their children more harshly.

Kinship patterns may confuse the family therapist who sets out to make a family genogram, initially listening to more people described as grandparent (e.g., *lolo*, *lola*), older sister or brother (e.g., *ate*, *kuya*, *manong*), aunt or uncle, or cousin than makes sense by European-derived standards. Because Filipino families' affiliations are conceived as tribal or as connections to the clan, *family* is construed very broadly. A household many consist of multiple generations, and this pattern is carried over to the United States. But even this definition has been changing, driven by geographic displacement, economic hardship, acquisition of values of materialism, and a shift in strategies for survival. The traditional family includes elders and cousins (Dearing, 1997). The kinship system does not differentiate specifically between first and second cousins or cousins once or twice removed. Fictive kin may become family, and these ties are further cemented by marriage and by a system of godparenting as part of baptism and marriage (Jocano, 1998). Because the Philippines does not recognize divorce, sometimes multiple families exist in different countries because of economic hardships, which forces prolonged separations.

Although externally patriarchal, much evidence demonstrates differentiated and shared authority in the family with some overlapping of roles (Jocano, 1998; Medina, 1991). Regional folklore has various origin stories that usually revolve around either the simultaneous emergence of man and woman from sections of bamboo, or the emergence of man first. Despite what many Americans interpret as oppression of women, it is important to understand and interpret the nuances in which women are respected and powerful. This is a country that has had two women presidents in the last 20 years, as compared with none in the United States. Women are held in high regard for their ability to manage money and a household, which often includes a helping staff in the Philippines. Ironically, movement to the United States often leads to exaggerated role differentiation and the reinforcement of patriarchal patterns of authority.

In contrast to strong patriarchal structures and power, there are interesting ways in which women are recognized in the culture that are evident in the family. Evidence from folktales and historians suggests that there were some matriarchal tribes and clans, but that this was not universal throughout the Philippines. Precolonial history suggests that women were able to be village chieftesses (Tompar-Tiu & Sustento-Seneriches, 1995). A family that does not have respect for women violates some intrinsic cultural values. Kinship is bilineal, rather than patrilineal as in other Asian cultures (Jocano, 1998; Medina, 1991). For example, in traditional naming, a child carries a middle name that is his or her mother's maiden name (e.g., Cruz); the child's last name derives from the father (e.g., Manalansan). Thus, Felice de la Cruz Manalansan provides a bilateral tracing of kinship. Mary, the mother of Jesus, is revered and viewed as a central figure in the lives of Catholics, again, a mark of respect for and centrality of women.

Nevertheless, gender roles impose stress. For women, being both physically attractive and intelligent is encouraged and valued. However, in being beautiful, a woman is not to act on her sexual desires before marriage (Galang, 1997). Women have been encouraged to seek education similar to their brothers'. However, if there are not enough resources for all, young women may sacrifice their educational opportunities in order to send brothers and younger siblings, both female and male, to school. A woman is expected to support a man publicly and not undermine his masculinity. However, she must also continue to strive to be competent in many areas of her life so that she may be an advisor or equal partner to her spouse. There are pressures for young men as well. The role of hard worker and successful provider is highly valued. They are expected to be responsible and to express their masculinity in physical style and sexuality. Masculinity does carry proscriptions against a broad range of behaviors, such as crying and expressing certain types of emotions.

When relationships are strained, members of a couple may seek consultation outside the family. Over the last 20 years, Philippine studies demonstrate that women are less willing to put up with strain, with many filing for annulment, petitions against husbands for mistreatment, and legal separation (cf. Medina, 1991, p. 180). Because divorce is against Philippine law, some couples obtain divorces in other countries, often after having lived separately for an extended period of time.

Status is an important part of Filipino culture and family. Within the family, status is predicated on age and relational position in the family. Outside the family, status is derived from a person's ability to influence important decisions, education, and economic status (Jocano, 1998; Santos, 1983). Education prevails over economics as a status predictor (Jocano, 1998, p. 36). Honorific titles are used for those outside the family and even within the family (Chan, 1998; Santos, 1983). For example, a physician or professor, even if not practicing in the United States or retired, may be initially greeted as "Doctor" or "Professora." It is important for the therapist to use these titles unless directed to use a first name or another title.

Hierarchical relationships by age and generation determine patterns of respect and conflict resolution. Age is traditionally revered and respected, as life experience and survival yield wisdom. Cultural values that esteem age still respect the individual openly, despite physical ability or cognitive decline. However, if elders do not fulfill their roles at expected times when they are capable, they may not be accorded genuine elder status. One of the difficulties immigrants face as they age in American society is the lack of reverence for age. Invisibility accompanies old age. In all of the dialects there are terms a person uses to convey respect to an older person even if they are not related. Those of the same generation, even if not related, may be referred to respectfully with terms that connote "older brother" (*kuya, manong*) or "older sister" (*ate, manang*). A term connoting respect, *po*, may be used in the course of speaking (in place of the person's name) to a person with status derived from age, relational status, or achievement. A traditional gesture from children to parents, aunts, uncles, grandparents, or another elder, is to take the elder's hand and bring it up to one's forehead while bowing one's head. This is sometimes a point of contention when older relatives come to visit and the children have been born and/or raised in America, or when Filipino Americans go to visit older relatives in the Philippines, and the greeting is absent.

In addition to what has been observed already about authority, it is important to know that authority is used to be persuasive. The child's responsibility and obligation to parents is to trust and see them as the authority so that he or she is predisposed to be persuaded.

Communal thinking about resources may conflict with therapists' conventional values. It is not unusual for a family to strain its resources for family members even when this creates a heavy burden of stress. However, acculturation and a departure from this sense of taking care of extended family members can become a source of conflict within families. Likewise, if a therapist supports a family member in withholding these resources from another family member, she or he may be met with tremendous resistance. For example, it is not unusual for 30-year-old unmarried family members to live with their parents. No one thinks that this is necessarily a situation of freeloading or lack of differentiation. A mother less well off than her grown children may still host the extended family lunch on Sundays and send her children and siblings away with food. In order to offer this sharing, she may ration her portions of food between visits. A gift sent to an individual, particularly if it is perceived that the person needs it more than the original recipient, especially if the gift is food, will be seen as a communal gift. Thus, the boundaries are different for immigrant generations and American-raised generations.

COMMUNICATION, EXPECTATIONS, AND SOCIAL CONTROL

The combination of kinship patterns and communication styles has significant implications for conflict resolution, whether the conflicts are about bridging generation gaps between immigrant parents and their children who have grown up in the United States or about expectations and standards of sex role behavior. The latter surface in dating expectations, career aspirations, and taking care of parents and younger siblings. The relationships involved are maintained through reciprocal action, service, and loyalty (Agbayani-Siewert & Revilla, 1995).

Shared identity is important (Enriquez, 1994). Family members typically seek to avoid competitiveness, particularly with other family members (Santa Rita, 1996). To this end the family takes precedence over the individual, and shared visions and goals may be asserted. Such values may lead the therapist to interpret a family's behaviors as enmeshed or undifferentiated, when they are part of the way in which strength is mutually exchanged between the group and the individual. For members of many generations, even in the United States, the importance of the collective often supersedes the needs of the individual. Eventually, in multigenerational households, the importance of the collective before the individual becomes a point of conflict. Regardless, most families have some rules for balancing the recognition of the collective with the needs of the individual.

Although Filipino and Filipino American communication is viewed as indirect, this perspective is contextual. Much communication is very direct as understood within the culture. Phrasing is key. To complicate this, it is expected that in close relationships, a person will develop a perceptiveness in regard to another family member's needs or feelings. The inability of American children to do this and the expectation that they should by Filipino American parents can be a source of conflict and miscommunication.

Respect that derives from hierarchical relationships commonly employs "go-betweens" or informal mediators to resolve conflict and to avoid embarrassing confrontations. It is important to understand the pervasiveness of the use of messengers, go-betweens, or mediators, which otherwise looks like triangulation. Falicov and Brudner-White (1983) stress the importance of understanding the meaning of triangular patterns in a cultural context before assuming they are pathological. Chan (1998) observes that the initial contact with an agency or therapist may be by the mediator or high-status person rather than a family member who will be directly involved in the therapy. In more traditional families, this has significant bearing on how family therapy interventions are conducted and their effectiveness.

Many studies by outsiders have misinterpreted the value placed on smooth relationships (Enriquez, 1994; Santa Rita, 1996) in the Filipino value system. In order not to disappoint or hurt, people may agree to do things, but without having an intention to do them. Rather than thinking of this as noncompliance, the therapist should understand that there is a value of accommodation to prevent hurting and humiliating people. This value has both a social and a moral base. The therapist may seek consultation with someone with an insider's knowledge of the culture to help determine when this is a cultural pattern or something else.

The families a therapist encounters generally embody both the desire to keep relationships smooth and the use of humiliation and shame for social control of family members. These values are also socially and morally rooted. What is complex, particularly in cross-cultural families and multigenerational households, is that what one culture may consider direct and hurtful, may not be deemed as such by a person from another culture.

At its heart, Filipino culture values sincerity underscored by behavioral congruence with words. For example, apologies and remorse are expressed in corrected action. This is the most sincere form of apology. Whereas children may be expected to apologize both verbally and with corrected action, the hierarchical nature of the culture does not expect parents to apologize. However, this same propensity for action may pose difficulty in the realm of expressions of love. Although parents may be affectionate, they may not say "I love you." Parents may also work multiple jobs to provide extra material goods and opportunities for their children, at the expense of time, because they love them.

The pressure to achieve is a point of contention that sets up familial conflict in regard to education, dating, and sexual behavior. In accord with cultural norms, parents may refrain from giving praise directly. Good to excellent school achievement, social courtesy, civility, and upstanding moral values are expected of children. For example, a child's fear of disappointing his or her parents, who have sacrificed to send the child to private school, may result in cheating on an exam so as not to let the parents down (Bulatao, 1966/1992). The pressure to achieve has been documented by Heras and Patactsil (2001) as a source of suicidal ideation and attempts among older school-age youth and young adults. Such pressure to achieve can create difficulties, particularly in immigrant families when the time needed to accomplish an educational objective may compete with other time commitments, such as obligations to family and friends.

RELIGION, SPIRITUALITY, AND CAUSALITY

Spiritual and religious values are embedded in Filipino cultural practices. The nation is 85% Catholic; the rest of the population is affiliated with the Philippine Independent Church, the Protestant churches, Iglesia Ni Cristo, Jehovah's Witnesses, and the Church of Latter-Day Saints (Burgonio-Watson, 1997). Missionaries brought all of these religions to the islands. In the southern Philippines, the Muslim religion dominates. This small population constitutes a very small number of immigrants. Evidence suggests that all of these religions have been enculturated to some degree to accommodate the original customs and beliefs. Thus, Filipino Catholics can pray to God, but at some level believe in different types of ghosts and spirits in line with the original polytheistic spiritual base in which notions of cause and effect are rooted. Spirituality is linked to health. Mental and physical health are interrelated and often thought to be linked to the state of a person's spiritual life.

The therapist's notions of causality must take into account religious, spiritual, and cultural values in order for him or her to have credibility. Montepio (1986/1987) notes that illness is divided between natural and unnatural causes. This belief would direct help seeking toward different sources. Whereas educated Filipinos may overtly deny their belief in the spirits of folklore, at times of crisis they may make attributions of causality or may seek relief from healers outside the conventional medical system. The centrality of their faith may be seen in their approach to healing. Consider the following example:

A 60-year-old educated Filipino American, born in the Philippines, and living in the United States for 30 years, has been diagnosed with prostrate cancer that his doctors believe is curable with conventional medical treatment. He refuses treatment and asks family, friends, and the priests and nuns to form prayer groups to pray for him. Although the family may like him to seek medical treatment and a person of status may be asked to persuade him to reconsider treatment, the family may also believe that it is reasonable to pray for a cure. When he dies, many family members will not dwell on the possibility that he might have been cured with conventional medicine, but will remember that they accepted his choice and joined in offering him what he thought might heal him.

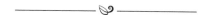

When a Filipino family comes to therapy, usually as a last resort, it is important to ask what means of "natural help" they have employed—priest or other religious figures, herbalists, faith healers, or psychics. If the therapist does not offer examples after priests or nuns or physicians have been suggested, the family may not reveal what they have tried. The value of this question is in asking about the family's sense of causality. Bulatao (1986) notes that it might be helpful for the therapist to conceptualize notions of "possession," poltergeists, or spirits in terms of "as if someone was possessed." This can be a way of gathering information to explore what other healers a family has consulted, what they thought was the cause of the problem, and what the family thinks of the explanation.

The blending of religion and cultural values identifies sharing and hospitality as significant expressions of being a good person. Burgonio-Watson (1997) observes that the Christian influence is seen in the reminder "We were once strangers in the land of Egypt," thereby directing people to be hospitable to one another. This is a value that opposes the mainstream value "Every man for himself" (p. 330). Therefore, if members of a poor family—that is, those who at times do not have enough food for themselves—come into some extra money or a supply of extra food, they may choose to throw a party with a spread of food to be shared with other families and neighbors.

MENTAL HEALTH ISSUES

The immigration experience challenges the mental health of many immigrants. Emigration may result in the loss of authority that is tied to reverence for age, wealth, education, titles, and accomplishments (Santos, 1983). What a person has achieved in the Philippines may disappear or be discredited, because degrees may not be recognized, leading to under- or unemployment and lack of status. Family immigration that takes place in stages poses stresses resulting from separation and later reunification. Culture shock, homesickness, and isolation from social support networks add further stress (Tompar-Tiu & Sustento-Sereniches, 1995), as do racism and the changed dynamics of gender roles pose. The possibility of physical and mental abuse are heightened by the loss of control inherent in the stress of immigration and the disparate value systems between cultures and generations.

Therapy is not a well-known healing practice in the Philippines. The culture allows for idiosyncratic behavior without labeling it truly mental illness, which may delay necessary intervention. Immigrant families usually do not enter therapy unless sent by the courts, a priest or minister, or a person they trust.

Many significant problems among adolescents in various Filipino American communities are hidden from the larger community. These difficulties include high pregnancy rates (cf. Tiongsen, 1997), significant high school dropout rates (cf. Tompar-Tiu & Sustento-Seneriches, 1995), and high rates of suicidal ideation and attempted suicide (cf. Heras & Patactsil, 2001; Tompar-Tiu & Sustento-Seneriches, 1995). Isolation and boredom contribute to substance abuse in immigrant men (cf. Tompar-Tiu & Sustento-Seneriches, 1995). Gambling poses a significant problem in some families. AIDS is a concern. In a San Francisco study conducted in the 1990s, Filipino Americans had the highest rate of AIDS among both Asians and Pacific Islanders (cf. Tompar-Tiu & Sustento-Seneriches, 1995).

THE FAMILY THERAPIST

Ideally, the therapist must engage in consciousness raising about his or her own racial biases and ethnocentrism and seek cultural knowledge. For example, a couple who has come together as a result of their correspondence may enter therapy defensively, prepared to be stigmatized, dismissed, or judged, based on media depictions of such relationships. It is important to reflect on stereotypes one might hold in terms of accommodation, compliance, and nonconfrontativeness. Cultural knowledge will allow the therapist to establish credibility more quickly. Likewise, with cultural knowledge, the therapist can provide a certain educational or decoding role, particularly between generations, which will be appreciated and congruent with what a family expects from therapy.

Personal style is important, especially if older family members are involved. Casual dress, such as jeans and tight or revealing tops or T-shirts, should be avoided. The way the therapist dresses will be interpreted as reflecting his or her success and achievement and respect for the family. Education is important to credibility, so the therapist should speak of his or her training and experience.

Rapport is extremely important in the Filipino culture. The degree to which the therapist extends him- or herself is meaningful. Assessing who is the private, versus public, head of household facilitates intervention. The therapist who is willing to "shoot the breeze" (make small talk) will facilitate the family's revealing itself. Shooting the breeze is a way in which many serious communications take place in Filipino culture. This may include being prepared for the family to ask questions about the therapist's family of origin and training. They may want to know if the therapist's family lives nearby and how often they see each other. Although these questions may seem intrusive, they are meant to establish connections and assess the therapist's values. The therapist may also gain respect from the family if he or she does not resist being somewhat "adopted" over time. The therapist may be invited to weddings and funerals. Such an invitation is often an expression of appreciation. Learning how to turn down invitations and to know which of them are extended out of politeness so as not to hurt the therapist, versus invitations that, if refused, may hurt the family and the therapy process, may require consultation with someone who has insider cultural knowledge.

The way the therapist interacts with family members who have lost their titles and their status in this country may be a healing intervention. Using titles, such as Doctor or

Professor, provides a measure of courtesy to counteract the losses. Adopting the convention of referring to an older immigrant person as *manong* or *manang* facilitates credibility. Furthermore, respect paid by the therapist may confer some status to family members who have been devalued in the eyes of younger family members. Using such titles may also bring up sadness, which may be useful to address.

Food is extremely central and important to Filipino culture. In more traditional families, it may seem that people are eating all the time or always offering food. The therapist's bringing gifts of food (which should not be expensive, because the family may wish to reciprocate) or suggesting an outing a family might enjoy are ways of expressing concern for the family and its well-being. Therapists should be mindful that if they offer food, it needs to be in an amount that can be shared. Although the family may offer to share it during the session, it is usually important to assure them that you have given this so that they can share it at home among the family, which may include more people than those who appear for sessions. If the family brings food, the therapist should accept it. If the family meets with the therapist mid- to late afternoon, it would be a traditional time for *merienda* or a snack. It would be important to participate in eating some of the snack. Much business is conducted over food.

Code switching is a shift in value system, from American to Filipino, that the therapist must track and, at times, decode between family members. A mother who immigrated as a 10-year-old may appear very acculturated. However, in addressing some issues she might "switch" to more traditional values. These switches are very idiosyncratic and are sometimes at the heart of family misunderstandings, but usually consistent within the person. For example, this mother may allow her daughter to date and accept her son's wish to pierce his ears, but may have no tolerance for her children being disrespectful to her. Her definition of disrespect is more traditional: Her children contradicting her or "back talking" or questioning her publicly may have much more meaning for her and cause much more distress than for American-born mothers. Likewise, a mother who is very independent in personality and spirit may have a difficult time denying extended family members money or a place to stay indefinitely if they are in need. This latter type of code switching is often a point of contention in cross-cultural marriages if one of the partners is of European descent.

Although these guidelines may be helpful for therapists working with more traditional families composed of older generations, they must also be aware of some of the code switching that unconsciously occurs among those of younger generations. The therapist has a respected role, and thus young people may bring gifts or act in certain respectful ways because this is how they initially interact with elders even if they are American raised. Nuclear families that seek help and have been born and raised in the United States will not differ much from other families in their expectations of therapy.

SUMMARY

There is no monolithic Filipino or Filipino American family. Family constellations have arisen out of economic, social, and political conditions. The values of Filipino culture have changed through emigration and immigration, as well as religiosity and spirituality, and because of coexisting and sometimes conflicting values. The result is our appreciation for how resilient individuals and families can be in balancing communal and individual needs. Filipinos and Filipino Americans have a unique history that leads to the coexistence of seemingly disjointed value systems and behaviors. This can be an advantage to family therapists, because it suggests some flexibility and adaptability that have allowed the survival of Filipino families. However, interventions must take into account the level of acculturation, who heads the family or household, and how the therapist can gain credibility with the family.

REFERENCES

Agbayani-Siewert, P., & Enrile, A. V. (2003). Filipino American children and adolescents. In J. T. Gibbs (Ed.), *Children of color: Psychological interventions with culturally diverse youth* (2nd rev. ed., pp. 229–264). New York: Jossey-Bass.

Agbayani-Siewert, P., & Revilla, L. (1995). Filipino Americans. In P. G. Min (Ed.), *Asian Americans: Contemporary trends and issues* (pp. 134–168). Thousand Oaks, CA: Sage.

Bulatao, J. C. (1966). *Split-level Christianity.* Quezon City, Philippines: Ateneo de Manila University Press. Reprinted in Bulatao, J. C. (1992). *Phenomena and their interepretation: Landmark essays 1957–1989.* Quezon City, Philippines: Ateneo de Manila University Press.

Bulatao, J. C. (1986). A note on Philippine possession and poltergeists. *Philippine Studies, 34,* 86–101. Reprinted in Bulatao, J. C. (1992). *Phenomena and their interpretation: Landmark essays 1957–1989.* Quezon City, Philippines: Ateneo de Manila University Press.

Bulosan, C. (1995). Freedom from want. In E. San Juan, Jr. (Ed.), *On becoming Filipino: Selected writings of Carlos Bulosan.* Reprinted from the *Saturday Evening Post* (1943, March 6).

Burgonio-Watson, T. B. (1997). Filipino spirituality: An immigrant's perspective. In M. P. P. Root (Ed.), *Filipino Americans: Transformation and identity* (pp. 324–332). Thousand Oaks, CA: Sage.

Chan, S. (1998). Families with Pilipino roots. In E. W. Lynch & M. J. Hanson (Eds.), *Developing cross-cultural competence: A guide for working with children and their families* (2nd ed., pp. 355–400). Baltimore: Paul H. Brookes.

Cordova, F. (1983). *Filipinos: Forgotten Asian Americans.* Seattle, WA: Demonstration Project for Asians.

Dearing, E. G. (1997). The family tree: Discovering oneself. In M. P. P. Root (Ed.), *Filipino Americans: Transformation and identity* (pp. 287–298). Thousand Oaks, CA: Sage.

Enriquez, V. G. (1994). *From colonial to liberation psychology: The Philippine experience.* Manila, Philippines: De Salle University Press.

Galang, M. E. (1997). Deflowering the Sampaguita. In M. P. P. Root (Ed.), *Filipino Americans: Transformation and identity* (pp. 219–229). Thousand Oaks, CA: Sage.

Falicov, C. J., & Brudner-White, L. (1983). The shifting family triangle: The issue of cultural and contextual relativity. In J. C. Hansen & C. J. Falicov (Eds.), *Cultural perspectives in family therapy* (pp. 51–67). Rockville, MD: Aspen Systems Corporation.

Heras, P., & Patactsil, J. (2001). *Silent sacrifices: Voices of the Filipino American Family, a Documentary.* San Diego, CA: Health and Human Services.

Jocano, F. L. (1998). *Filipino social organization: Traditional kinship and family organization.* Manila, Philippines: Punlad Research House.

Kitano, H. H. L., Fujino, D. C., & Sato, J. T. (1998). Interracial marriages: Where are the Asian Americans and where are they going? In L. C. Lee & N. W. S. Zane (Eds.), *Handbook of Asian American psychology* (pp. 233–260). Thousand Oaks, CA: Sage.

Lin, J. (1991). *Marital satisfaction and conflict in intercultural correspondence marriage.* Unpublished doctoral dissertation, University of Washington, Seattle.

Lipat, C. T., Ordona, T. A., Stewart, C. P., & Ubaldo, M. A. (1997). Tomboy, dyke, lezzie, and bi:

Filipina lesbian and bisexual women speak out. In M. P. P. Root (Ed.), *Filipino Americans: Transformation and identity* (pp. 230–246). Thousand Oaks, CA: Sage.

Lott, J. T. (1997). Demographic changes transforming the Filipino American community. In M. P. P. Root (Ed.), *Filipino Americans: Transformation and identity* (pp. 11–20). Thousand Oaks, CA: Sage.

Manalansan IV, M. F. (1997). At the frontiers of narrative: The mapping of Fiipino gay men's lives in the United States. In M. P. P. Root (Ed.), *Filipino Americans: Transformation and identity* (pp. 247–256). Thousand Oaks, CA: Sage.

Medina, B. T. G. (1991). *The Filipino family: A text with selected readings.* Quezon City, Philippines: University of the Philippines Press.

Montepio, S. N. (1986/1987). Folk medicine in the Filipino American experience. *Amerasia Journal, 13,* 151–162.

Montoya, C. A. (1997). Living in the shadows: The undocumented immigrant experience of Filipinos. In M. P. P. Root (Ed.), *Filipino Americans: Transformation and identity* (pp. 112–120). Thousand Oaks, CA: Sage.

Ordonez, R. Z. (1997). Mail-order brides: An emerging community. In M. P. P. Root (Ed.), *Filipino Americans: Transformation and identity* (pp. 121–142). Thousand Oaks, CA: Sage.

Pido, A. J. A. (1986). *The Pilipinos in America: Macro/micro dimensions of immigration and integration.* New York: Center for Migration Studies.

Pido, A. J. A. (1997). Macro/micro dimensions of Filipino immigration to the United States. In M. P. P. Root (Ed.), *Filipino Americans: Transformation and identity* (pp. 21–38). Thousand Oaks, CA: Sage.

Root, M. P. P. (1997). Contemporary mixed-heritage Filipino Americans: Fighting colonized identities. In M. P. P. Root (Ed.), *Filipino Americans: Transformation and identity* (pp. 80–94). Thousand Oaks, CA: Sage.

San Juan, E., Jr. (1998). *From exile to diaspora: Versions of the Filipino experience in the United States.* Boulder, CO: Westview Press.

Santa Rita, E. (1996). Pilipino families. In M. McGoldrick, J. Giordano, & J. K. Pearce (Eds.), *Ethnicity and family therapy* (2nd ed., pp. 324–330). New York: Guilford Press.

Santos, R. A. (1983). The social and emotional development of Filipino-American children. In G. J. Powell (Ed.), *The psychosocial development of minority group children* (pp. 131–146). New York: Brunner/Mazel.

Singco-Holmes, M. G. (1993). *A different love: Being gay in the Philippines.* Manila, Philippines: Anvil.

Tiongson, A. T. (1997). Throwing the baby out with the bathwater: Situating young Filipino mother and fathers beyond the dominant discourse on adolescent pregnancy. In M. P. P. Root (Ed.), *Filipino Americans: Transformation and identity* (pp. 257–271). Thousand Oaks, CA: Sage.

Tompar-Tiu, A., & Sustento-Senemiches, J. (1995). *Depression and other mental health issues: The Filipino American experience.* New York: Jossey-Bass.

U.S. Bureau of the Census. (1999). *1997–1998 State and metropolitan area data book.* Washington, DC: Author.

Vallangca, C. C. (1987). *The second wave: Pinay and Pinoy.* San Francisco: Strawberry Hill Press.

CHAPTER 24

Indonesian Families

Fred P. Piercy
Adriana Soekandar
Catherine D. M. Limansubroto
Sean D. Davis

Indonesia, formerly known as the Dutch East Indies, is a developing country in Southeast Asia with more than 234 million people. The world's fourth most populous country (after China, India, and the United States), it stretches over 3,200 miles of tropical ocean and spans 17,508 islands (6,000 of them inhabited). Indonesia is the land of the Spice Islands, boogeymen (pirates), Bali, and Komodo dragons. It has a rich history of artistic, religious, and cultural diversity.

Indonesia is also the world's largest Muslim nation, with almost 90% of the population identified as Muslim. However, the Muslim faith practiced here is less doctrinal than that found in many other countries (Guest, 1992). Indeed, in many Indonesians' belief systems, one can see the influences of animism (e.g., the belief that spirits are within objects) and Hinduism (e.g., reincarnation).

One "tall tale" highlights, through humor and exaggeration, Indonesia's cultural diversity. The story says that, on a crowded bus, if you were to accidentally step on an Indonesian's foot, the way the Indonesian would respond depends on where he or she is from. If from East Java, the tale goes, the Indonesian might speak to you in a convoluted, respectful way about the bus being crowded, in the hope that you would realize that you are standing on his or her foot. If from Central Java, the person whose foot you're stepping on might simply smile at you and say, "I'm sorry." If from Bali, he or she might silently pray for your enlightenment. If from North Sumatra, the person might shout and push you away.

Although each description stretches the truth (like claiming that all New Yorkers would shoot you), the tale's underlying truth is that not all Indonesians are alike. With such wide cultural differences, American family therapists must learn as much as they can about their Indonesian client families. What part of the country is the family from? What is the *adat*, or custom, of their ethnic group or community? How do economic class and religion influence values and beliefs? What is their level of acculturation or acceptance of Western values? How do family members feel about coming to therapy, and what do their parents or other relatives think about their problems?

In this chapter, we give a broad-brushed overview of several Indonesian social, cultural, political, and class issues that may relate to the presenting problems of some of the approximately 65,000 Indonesians presently living in the United States, and how best to address them. However, because of the differences among Indonesians, the reader should think of these as issues worth exploring, rather than rigid formulas for intervention.

ISSUES TO CONSIDER

Family Closeness

Indonesians value family closeness, loyalty, obligation, and respect. Children must obey their parents, and all must preserve the family's honor. Collective obligation is reflected in the traditional practice of parents approving whom their children will marry. Until they wed, most young Indonesian adults live with their parents and extended families. Indonesians don't understand why so many Americans are in such a hurry to move out of their parents' homes after high school. Of course, Western values of independence will influence Indonesian youth who grow up in America. When this Western worldview clashes with the more traditional Indonesian values of family togetherness, sparks can fly (Piercy, 1991).

One of us (A. S.) recently conducted therapy with an Indonesian family in Los Angeles in which the adult female expressed concern that her mother-in-law criticized her, and that her husband never intervened to stop her. Clearly, extended family loyalties can create problems in a person's immediate family. Surprisingly, the couple's relationship improved dramatically in four sessions. The wife found it particularly helpful for me to listen to her complaints and support her in front of her husband. He began to understand her concerns and became more supportive of his spouse in the process.

Hierarchy

Hierarchy in Indonesian families is important. The wife should respect and obey her husband (although there is more variation in gender roles across Indonesia than in other Asian countries), and children should respect and obey their parents. Younger people should defer to elder grandparents, aunts, and uncles. Again, problems can occur when clashes arise between these values and the egalitarian ones of American culture.

Because hierarchy is important, and because Indonesian adults may be uncomfortable—even ashamed—to be in treatment, the therapist should show respect to all family members. For example, he or she should speak first to the older family members and should not call adults by their first names until asked to do so.

In certain Indonesian subcultures, such as among traditional Javanese or Chinese Indonesians, children are not allowed to talk about their fathers and mothers to outsiders, at least when their parents are present, inasmuch as this may result in the parents losing face. It may be better with such families for the therapist to meet separately with the children.

Parenting

Indonesian child rearing may appear strange to Western therapists. Parents sometimes pamper young children in an effort to make them happy and secure (M. Morgan, personal communication, March 8, 2004). For example, it is fairly common to see Indonesian mothers in restaurants endlessly coaxing their young children to eat. What Americans might see as coddling a child appears to foster a culturally desirable dependence, but not discipline problems. Somehow, when it is time for the children to be more observant of family hierarchy and to follow the rules at school, they do so. Thus, the American family therapist should not apply traditional Western developmental expectations to Indonesian children and parents. To do so could potentially pathologize an Indonesian parenting behavior that is culturally appropriate and healthy.

Difficulty in Being Direct

In many areas of Indonesia, it is considered more polite to "talk around" sensitive issues than to discuss them directly; being too direct is impolite. The therapist should take time for small talk and follow the lead of the Indonesian client in what may be a rather circuitous discussion. The therapist should also realize that, spoken by an Indonesian, "maybe," "sometime," and "yes, but" may all mean "no" or "never." Some Indonesians believe that it is better not to say what one means than to utter something that might cause the therapist or family member to lose face.

Shame

Scheper-Hughes (1992) states that "without our cultures, we simply would not know how to feel" (p. 431). Indeed, culture both defines and shapes emotions. For example, the concept of shame assumes different shapes across cultures. Americans often feel shame about getting or looking older, or about experiencing the infirmities of age, but these are not reasons for shame among Indonesians. Instead, many Indonesians feel shame (*malu*) about anything that calls undue attention to them—a loud laugh, a misbehaving child, or a comment that could be seen as bragging. Similarly, many Indonesians feel shyness (*sungkan*) in the presence of higher-status people.

Malu can play a role in the problems that bring an Indonesian into therapy. Collins and Bahar (1995) report a case in which an Indonesian woman was brought to a psychiatric facility because her husband had found her compulsively rocking back and forth in her home. In later discussions with a doctor, the woman stated that she had lost 25 pounds over the last few months. She also revealed that she lived in a small, three-bedroom house with 14 other family members, did most of the laundry and cooking, and was worried about expenses.

The doctor privately told the husband that he believed that the wife's strange behavior resulted from the exhaustion, depression, and irritation related to these living conditions. The husband was surprised, for his wife had never complained to him. Although she did admit to the doctor (in private) that he was right, she still could not express her feelings to her husband, because it would not be proper (*kurang pantas*) for her to complain. She wanted to protect her husband from feeling *malu*. Thus, she could express herself through her symptoms. Fortunately, the husband listened to the doctor and asked several of his brothers to move from the house.

Indonesian men who are made to feel *malu* may become aggressive. An extreme example of this is seen in the syndrome known as *amok*, which is specific to Malay culture (Azhar & Varma, 2000; Mohamed, 1997). In amok, the person dissociates in reaction to extreme frustration, anger, or an affront to his honor and literally "runs amok," committing random acts of homicidal violence. However, this behavior is rare among Indonesians today.

For many Indonesians, the problems that bring them into therapy, as well as therapy itself, may cause *malu*. For example, divorce is a great source of family shame. And because admitting marital problems to strangers is a source of *malu*, Indonesians are more likely to seek therapy for child-related problems.

The Aftermath of September 11, 2001

The tragedies of 9/11 may bring a vague sense of *malu* to Indonesian Americans, who run the risk of being perceived as Muslim extremists. Even when Americans do not believe this, their real or alleged perceptions may lead to stress among Indonesian Americans and a need to prove themselves to their American peers.

Gender Roles and Homosexuality

Indonesian men are expected to marry and be the providers and leaders of their families. Women (in most areas of Indonesia) are expected to defer to their husbands and are responsible for tasks related to home and family life—cooking, housekeeping, and child care. Ideally, each member of a couple takes pride in his or her prescribed gender role. For American therapists who value both cultural sensitivity and egalitarianism, dealing with rigid gender roles may be a challenge. However, Indonesians also value fairness. If rigid roles are part of the presenting problem, they should be open to discussion and renegotiation, just as when an American therapist is working with a religiously conservative American family.

What about Indonesians who are gay or lesbian? Because a heterosexual marriage is expected, some gay Indonesian men marry but seek sex with other men outside of marriage (Stevenson, 1995). Other gay men and lesbians remain single but keep their sexual orientation hidden. The many cultural sanctions against homosexuality make it difficult for them to "come out," much less develop a gay or lesbian identity (Gerard & Jackson, 2001; Stevenson, 1995; Tien & Olson, 2003). Thus, they face the choice of keeping their same-sex sexual relationships secret and sharing their sexual orientation with only a select few, or developing a more open gay or lesbian identity. Any of these choices is legitimate, given the cultural sanctions—Indoneian and American—they may face. However, each involves challenges that will require the therapist's support and understanding.

Social Class

For Indonesian Americans, class—whether wealthy, middle class, or poor—brings its own challenges. For the wealthy Indonesian who has immigrated to America for a better life, the challenges may relate to the different levels of acculturation. For example, they may have very different ideas about working hard in school, courtship, and parental respect. That is, second-generation Indonesians born and raised in America may reflect values more representative of American norms than those of their Indonesian-born parents.

Indonesians in the United States on scholarships to study for a few years face a different set of problems. For example, because they are graduate students, they are often separated from close family and friends. In addition, they may make less money upon returning to Indonesia with their PhDs and work longer hours than they did in their university assistantships. For example, most of the colleagues of one of us (F. P. P.) at the University of Indonesia make less than $2,000 per year, which is still higher than the mean income in Indonesia.

Political Influences

More than 300 years of Dutch domination and the strong nationalism that exists today in Indonesia contribute to Indonesians' sensitivity to forms of foreign domination. Thus, they may distrust American experts who do not try to understand or appreciate their way of doing things. Margaret Morgan, an American who lived a number of years in Indonesia, states, "I often experienced a dual phenomenon of extreme deference toward Westerners on the one hand, and an underlying resentment of having to defer to them on the other. A therapist might find an Indonesian client to be extremely polite, yet sense that the deference is a bit forced or resented" (M. Morgan, personal communication, March 8, 2004).

Because Indonesians are sensitive to being "colonized" (subjected to Western norms) in therapy, the clinician would do well to look for ways to appreciate and empower Indonesian family members, and to provide options rather than directives. For example, instead of assigning homework, one of us (A. S.) usually suggests tasks that his Indonesian clients "might like to try" at home. Rather than directing clients older than the therapist to do a particular task, he always lets them decide whether to do it or not.

Length of Therapy

Indonesians generally seek short-term advice in therapy. At the psychology clinic at Udayana University, in Bali, the average number of sessions is two. The American therapist may need to discuss the concept, purpose, and process of therapy in order to broaden the Indonesian client's conception of what can take place in a therapy session.

HOW INDONESIAN CLIENTS DIFFER FROM OTHER ASIAN CLIENTS

In the preceding discussion, we suggest a number of ways Indonesian culture differs from ours in America (political, religious, and familial). We also asked Indonesian family therapist Andrew Bratawidjaja (personal communication, March 9, 2004) about the differences between Indonesians and other Asians. He responded:

"One critical aspect . . . is the HUGE ECONOMIC GAP between the rich and the poor [in Indonesia] . . . because it has a ripple effect to other areas of life for Indonesians. The separation between the powerful and the powerless; those who 'have' and those who 'don't have'; those who are 'privileged' and those who are 'underprivileged' is sharp and obvious. This leads to corruption. Corruption leads to injustice. Injustice leads to hatred. Hatred poisons one ethnic group against another, one religion against another, . . . separates Indonesians from other Asians . . . [and] significantly impacts the culture, society and the family life. Even though the corruption and status gap happens in other Asian nations, I think Indonesia has gone through a worse experience, especially after the riots of 1998."

In these riots, the Indonesian president, Suharto, was ousted, the economy collapsed, and many conservative Muslims set fire to Christian churches and brutally attacked thousands in the Chinese Indonesian minority. This experience was akin to the attempted coup in 1965 that led to the killing of 300,000 "communists." Some say that many poor, oppressed Indonesians used the coup as an excuse to rid the country of intellectuals and wealthy minorities. An Indonesian told one of us (F. P. P.) that he still remembers, as a child, seeing the river near Jakarta being red from the blood of dead bodies.

Although there is a beauty and gentleness to the Indonesian culture, there also exists a backdrop of colonialization and oppression, and a very wide gulf between the rich and the poor, to which American family therapists must be sensitive.

FAMILY THERAPY CONSIDERATIONS

Family therapy needs to be modified to fit Indonesian families (Limansubroto, 1993; Soekandar, 1993). For example, because extended family members are central to the lives of Indonesians, therapists should consider inviting them to sessions. At the same time, many Indonesian clients do not want others, even those close to them, to know about their problems. They would rather solve them privately and may feel shame at being unable to do so. Therefore, the family therapist must present therapy as something that capable, caring people engage in, should foster respect for the clients, and, when appropriate, invite extended family members into the therapeutic process (but perhaps not in the same session as the primary client).

Many Indonesians appreciate direct advice. One of us (A. S.) recently sent a questionnaire to her clients asking them what they need from therapy. Most responded that they need books and articles about their problems, practical suggestions, homework assignments, and solutions. One suggested that advice could be given over the telephone.

A therapy appropriate to Indonesians will also be consistent with, and makes use of, their religious faith, their commitment to family, and their rich culture and customs. The family therapist needs to be a good listener and collaborative partner in the change process. For example, it would be more helpful to ask a devoutly Muslim family, "How can Islam help you face this issue?" rather than to either assume or ignore the personal meaning of religion in their lives.

Certain family therapy techniques seem particularly helpful with Indonesians. For example, we like to use genograms to help client families see their problems in a wider context. Because some Indonesian families are enmeshed in ways that disadvantage certain family members, Bowen's (1982) ideas about differentiation and taking "I positions" can be useful. Feminist discussions about differential power, exploitation, and personal agency will benefit some clients, although some Indonesians may resist them if the therapist labels them as "feminist."

The respectful nature of many social-constructionist family therapies based on co-constructing reality through conversation seem to fit Indonesian cultural values. Reflecting teams, by which teams of observers respectfully share multiple reflections or suggestions, leave the Indonesian client to choose which ideas fit with him or her. Such therapy provides a context in which the Indonesian client does not feel lectured to or colonized. Similarly, narrative and solution-focused therapies (which focus on what the client does well) recognize and amplify an Indonesian's strengths. Home-based family therapy may also be appropriate because it allows the therapist to involve all family members, especially fathers and extended family, on nonthreatening turf.

Finally, particularly important will be the therapist's curiosity and deep respect for Indonesian clients, characterized by sensitivity to their world, and a willingness to learn more about that world.

REFERENCES

Azhar, M. Z., & Varma, S. L. (2000). Mental illness and its treatment in Malaysia. In A. Ihsan (Ed.), *Al-Junun: Mental illness in the Islamic world* (pp. 163–186). Madison, CT: Psychological Press.

Bowen, M. (1982). *Family therapy in clinical practice*. New York: Aronson.

Collins, E. F., & Bahar, E. (1995). *Malu: Shame, gender, hierarchy, and sexuality*. Unpublished manuscript, Ohio University, Athens.

Gerard, S., & Jackson, P. A. (2001). *Gay and lesbian Asia: Culture, identity, community*. New York: Haworth Press.

Guest, P. (1992). Marital dissolution and development in Indonesia. *Journal of Comparative Family Studies, 23*, 94–112.

Limansubroto, C. (1993). *A compilation and organization of a family therapy teaching curriculum for Indonesian university students*. Unpublished master's thesis, Purdue University, West Lafayette, Indiana.

Mohamed, S. H. (1997). A Malay crosscultural worldview and forensic review of amok. *Australian and New Zealand Journal of Psychiatry, 30*, 505–510.

Piercy, F. (1991, November/December). Of progress and palm trees: Indonesian families feel the strains of modernization. *Family Therapy Networker*, pp. 57–62.

Scheper-Hughes, N. (1992). *Death without weeping: The violence of everyday life in Brazil*. Berkeley: University of California Press.

Soekandar, A. (1993). *Selected family therapy interventions and their application in Indonesia*. Unpublished master's thesis, Purdue University, West Lafayette, Indiana.

Stevenson, M. (1995). Searching for a gay identity in Indonesia. *Journal of Men's Studies, 4*, 93–110.

Tien, L., & Olson, K. (2003). Confucian past, conflicted present: Working with Asian American families. In L. B. Silverstein & T. J. Goodrich (Eds.), *Feminist family therapy: Empowerment in social context* (pp. 135–146). Washington, DC: American Psychological Association.

CHAPTER 25

Japanese Families

Tazuko Shibusawa

The lives of Japanese American families have been shaped by the culture and values of their country of origin as well as the social and political conditions of the United States. The majority of Japanese Americans are descendants of Japanese who immigrated to the United States in the late 1800s and early 1900s. Others include post–World War II immigrants such as Japanese wives of U.S. servicemen. There is also a sizeable population of expatriate overseas Japanese families who are in the United States to work for Japanese businesses. The purpose of the chapter is to provide the historical background of Japanese in the United States, outline common cultural values among Japanese Americans, and offer clinical considerations for working with Japanese American families.

HISTORICAL BACKGROUND

Japanese immigration to the United States began in the late 19th century. The first Japanese immigrants were single men who had been recruited in response to the shortage of cheap labor, which was brought about by the Chinese Exclusion Act of 1882. Although Japanese men came to the United States as short-term laborers, many eventually settled down and started families. As antimiscegenation laws barred Japanese from marrying outside their race, the men either returned to Japan to find wives willing to return with them to the United States or had their families arrange a marriage. The women who came without ever meeting their husbands were known as *shashin hanayome*, or "picture brides." Members of the first generation left an important legacy in the United States by raising their families and establishing Japanese American communities while enduring harsh labor and living conditions.

Most Japanese, except for those who immigrated to Hawai'i, settled on the West Coast during an era of intense anti-Asian sentiment. Japanese were prohibited from becoming U.S. citizens because the Naturalization Act extended only to the White race.

The Japanese were also prohibited from owning the land on which they toiled because of Alien Land Laws. Exclusionary laws, such as those mandating the segregation of Japanese children from public schools, resulted in the formation of small ethnic enclaves in California, Oregon, and Washington. Pressure from White labor leaders in California led to the passage of the 1924 Immigration Exclusion Act, which banned all immigration from Japan (Ichioka, 1988).

Because immigration from Japan took place within a brief period of time, Japanese Americans are identified by distinct generational cohorts. The first generation who migrated from Japan are known as *Issei*, or first generation. The children of the *Issei* are known as *Nisei*, or second generation. A subgroup of *Nisei* are known as *Kibei Nisei*, "return to the United States," because they were sent back to Japan to be educated and later returned to the United States. The children of *Nisei* are known as *Sansei*, or third generation. Their offspring are *Yonsei* (fourth generation), and their grandchildren are *Gosei* (fifth generation).

The ban on immigration to the United States from Japan was not lifted until 1952 for relatives of U.S. citizens, and 1965 for all others. Japanese who migrated to the United States after 1952 and 1965 are known as *Shin-Issei* or *new-Issei*.

WORLD WAR II

Anti-Japanese sentiment culminated with the outbreak of World War II. More than 110,000 Japanese Americans living on the West Coast, including children who had U.S. citizenship, were classified as "enemy aliens," uprooted from their communities, and forced into 10 different concentration camps in desolate areas of Arizona, Arkansas, California, Colorado, Idaho, Utah, and Wyoming under Executive Order 9066.

Internment during World War II had devastating effects on Japanese American families (Nagata, 1993). Men who held leadership positions in the community were rounded up following the attacks on Pearl Harbor and imprisoned in POW camps. Families lost their homes, businesses, savings, and personal belongings. Some families were themselves divided when members were sent to different internment camps. Others were scarred by divided loyalties between Japan and the United States. The second generation (*Nisei*), who were adolescents or young adults during internment, faced shame and humiliation regarding their ethnic heritage, and pressure to prove their loyalty to the United States by becoming "super American" (Mass, 1991; Nagata, 1993). This is evident in the way *Nisei* who were U.S. citizens enlisted in the American army and suffered heavy casualties fighting in Europe.

Following World War II, and after being released from camp, some Japanese Americans moved to the East Coast because of the lingering anti-Japanese sentiment on the West Coast. This shift in population led to the development of small Japanese American communities in cities such as Chicago and New York.

Most second-generation *Nisei* kept silent about the internment experience for many years and did not talk about it with their children (Nagata 1993). It was not until the 1980 Redress Hearings[1] that the *Nisei* voices became public (Maki, Kitano, & Berthold, 1999). The *Nisei* also put an emphasis on "Americanizing" their *Sansei* children as much as possible out of fear of discrimination and racism.

Many Japanese Americans continue to feel that they are vulnerable to acts of racism and discrimination based on racial-ethnic identity (Mass, 1991; Nagata, 1993). The treatment of Arab and Muslim Americans following the September 11, 2001, terrorist attacks are chilling reminders of World War II for many Japanese Americans. Furthermore, post-9/11 attempts by Conservatives to justify the World War II internment of Japanese Americans and racial profiling, despite the Civil Liberties Act of 1988, which yielded a presidential letter of apology and $1.65 billion in reparations, indicates to Japanese Americans that the discriminatory attitudes that led to internment are still alive and well.

DEMOGRAPHIC CHARACTERISTICS

Although most Asian American groups include a sizable number of recent immigrants, the majority of Japanese Americans are U.S.-born, with an increasing number who are multiethnic and multiracial. According to the 2000 census, there are 796,700 Japanese Americans[2] (U.S. Department of Commerce, 2002). Although the Asian American population, as a whole, increased by 48% between 1990 and 2000, the Japanese population decreased by 6% (Asian American Federation, 2001), which can be attributed to low immigration rates, aging of the population, and growing rates of interracial marriages. Nearly one third of the Japanese[3] reported being of one or more other Asian groups or race(s), the highest percentage of the six Asian American groups in the United States (Asian Indian, Chinese, Filipino, Japanese, Korean, and Vietnamese (U.S. Department of Commerce, 2002).

CULTURAL VALUES

The first generation of Japanese immigrants (*Issei*) migrated to the United States during the Meiji era (1868–1919), in which family norms were heavily influenced by Confucianism. Marriage was seen as a union of two households, rather than two individuals, and women were expected to sever ties with their own families of origin when marrying into the husband's family. Family relationships were strictly hierarchical, with a male (grandfather or father) as the head of the household governing family interactions, which were determined by prescribed roles. Confucian ethics of filial obligation emphasized respect for parents.

Japanese American families have retained aspects of their culture of origin despite acculturation into the dominant culture. Differences in parenting have been observed between Japanese Americans and European Americans in the areas of developmental goals, educational expectations, child rearing, and communication patterns (Shibusawa, 2001). Some of the key differences between Japanese and European cultural values are observed in the areas of (1) concept and presentation of self, (2) group identity, (3) coping methods, and (4) expression of emotions.

Individuation and autonomy are generally considered the main goals of child development in European American/White families (Hess & Hess, 2001). Emphasis is placed on fostering "self-determination" and "self-sufficiency," and children are expected to grow out of a dependent state to acquire a sense of independence. Japanese culture, however, does not consider autonomy and independence developmental goals. Instead, parents try to instill in their children what Johnson (1993) refers to as a "non-egocentric conception of self," which helps children adapt to group norms and function as social beings. Japanese American parents stress "good behavior" and prioritize social expectations over "self-directed behavior" (Reilly, cited in Yee, Huang, & Lew, 1998). Verbal humiliation and disapproval of parents occurring in childhood are themes that frequently come up among Japanese American adults in psychotherapy (Shibusawa, 2001). The emphasis on interdependence in family relationships can also pose challenges when children reach adolescence or adulthood. Parents can experience their children's attempts toward separation/individuation as rejection or betrayal (Shiozaki-Lee, personal communication, October 3, 2004).

The emphasis on interdependence in human relationships can also been seen in the way Japanese act in groups. Japanese children are discouraged from showing off their competence because this prevents them from being threatening or offensive toward others. Studies have found that in comparison to their European American cohorts, third- and fourth-generation Japanese Americans demonstrate a greater need for affiliation, sensitivity toward the attitudes of others, tendency for self-abnegation, and avoidance of conflicts (Akimoto & Sanbonmatsu, 1999).

The ways in which Japanese and Western cultures cope with problems and adversity also differ. The Japanese way of adapting to unfavorable circumstances is known as *gaman*, a term that has been translated as "endurance," "perseverance," or "bearing the unbearable" (Tomita, 1998). Whereas some Western therapies view this silent suffering as an act of repression and denial (Itai & McRae, 1994), *gaman* is viewed by the Japanese as strength of character and capacity to endure difficulties posed by the environment, including interpersonal relationships. Suppressing one's dissatisfaction and not acting on one's desires are viewed as culturally determined coping strategies (Johnson, 1993). Tolerance of adversity stems from the Buddhist notion of fatalism and the importance of accepting reality. This is evident in another common attitude,—*shikataganai* (things can't be helped), which emphasizes the importance of a person's accepting things that he or she cannot change.

Nonverbal, rather than verbal, communication is valued in Japanese culture. Japanese are taught to infer what others are trying to communicate from the context and the way in which it is being communicated. Japanese also place more emphasis on what is not said, than on what is said (Doi, 1986), partly because they feel that emotions and sentiments cannot necessarily be captured or communicated by words. The extent to which affection is displayed in Japanese American families varies according to the degree to which they have incorporated the communication patterns of mainstream culture. In traditional Japanese culture affection is not expressed physically. Parents do not display physical intimacy toward each other in front of their children, nor do they demonstrate physical affection toward their children.

CLINICAL CONSIDERATIONS

Japanese Americans, in general, are reluctant to seek mental health services because of the culturally fostered stigma attributed to mental illness (Kitano, 1976; Uomoto &

Gorsuch, 1984). Traditionally, mental illness was thought to be "in the blood" and hereditary, thus leaving families with a sense of disgrace about having a mentally ill family member. Mental illness was also attributed to a "lack of will power" (Sue & Morishima, 1982). In general, Japanese Americans try to resolve problems on their own and do not seek outside help until the situation has worsened. Because therapy may be a new concept for many Japanese American clients, therapists need to explain the process to the families. In addition, normalizing and universalizing the presenting problem will help diminish the stigma and shame.

In order to work effectively with Japanese American clients, therapists need to be aware of Western values inherent in family therapy so as not to impose their own cultural values on their clients. The following paragraphs discuss some of the value-laden assumptions that are found in family therapy.

Assumptions about Problem Solving

There are two assumptions about problem solving implicit in Western psychotherapy: first, that problems *can* be solved, and second, that they can be solved by talking about them. Japanese do not necessarily believe that problems can be solved, nor do they think that talking about problems will bring about resolutions. As Chung (1992) notes, although Westerners "believe in freedom of speech, East Asians believe in freedom of silence." Clients may feel threatened if a therapist suggests a family meeting at which everyone will be asked to talk about problems. In the initial stages of therapy, it is important for clinicians to solicit information about the presenting problem in a nonthreatening way. In family sessions, the therapist should take the lead in soliciting information from each family member. Giving directives to family members to talk to each other can hinder communication. Nonverbal activities, such as family sculpting and drawing, can be effective in working with Japanese families, especially with children (Shibusawa, 2001). Conducting genogram interviews is also a nonthreatening way to begin exploring family issues. When families have a clear presenting problem, it is important for clinicians to offer suggestions and concrete advice, rather than delving into the issues that may be contributing to the problem.

Assumptions about Secrets

In family therapy, there is an assumption that the keeping of secrets tends to promote dysfunction because it prevents family members from communicating with each other directly. In Japanese culture, secrets are not necessarily viewed as negative. In fact, there is a Japanese phrase, *fumon ni fusu*, which means, "keeping things unquestioned." In interactions with Japanese clients, the therapist can acknowledge that there is a secret, but does not need to ferret out details unless the situation warrants legal intervention. Secrets that clients keep from the therapist include events from the past such as suicides, adoption, affairs, family conflicts, and alcohol addiction. The acknowledgement that there is a secret itself can, at times, be sufficient for the family to begin therapeutic work. If there is therapeutic value in exploring the secret, the clinician should first make sure that he or she is not viewing the family's reticence to disclose and discuss the secret as resistance. Otherwise, the family may sense this, and it can create distrust in the therapeutic relationship.

Assumptions about Emotional Expression and Communication

When Japanese clients do not express their emotions, it is important for therapists to refrain from assuming that their clients are "denying" or "repressing" their feelings. Just because Japanese clients do not express their affect does not mean that they are not experiencing emotions. When asked about their feelings, Japanese may feel as if they are being asked to expose rather than express their emotions (Shibusawa, 1996). Asking Japanese clients to discuss their emotions can put them on the spot, inasmuch as they may not be accustomed to talking about them. It is important not to press clients to express their feelings or to be eager to elicit emotional responses.

In Western psychotherapy, therapists try to encourage direct communication among family members. They often encourage clients to use "I statements" to convey their feelings and desires by taking ownership of what they say. Given the emphasis on the "nonegocentric nature of the self," soliciting "I statements" is not necessarily effective in working with Japanese clients.

Therapists also need to respect the hierarchical structure of the family when encouraging communication among family members. Encouraging egalitarian communication patterns can make parents feel that they are losing face in front of their children. Therapists need to be deferential to parents in family therapy even when working with third-generation Japanese Americans who are very acculturated to the mainstream culture (Shiozaki-Lee, personal communication, October 4, 2004).

Japanese, in general, avoid conflict (Tomita, 1998). Because of the emphasis on politeness and observance of social protocol in Japanese culture, clients may not be very communicative with therapists, especially when there are negative opinions about the therapist. Because therapists are viewed as expert authority figures, Japanese clients may not communicate their disagreement with them. Instead of trying to work out the differences, clients may drop out of therapy. Therefore, it is important for therapists to address, beforehand, the need for clients to share differences of opinion in therapy sessions.

Assumptions about Culture

When considering Japanese American culture, it is easy for therapists to get trapped into the notion of culture as a static entity devoid of social context. It is important to understand culture as an evolving entity, and that families change according to the changing historical circumstances. In addition, ethnic culture cannot be separated from the sociopolitical conditions of a given ethnic group in the United States. A large number of Japanese in the United States are third- and fourth-generation Americans. They may be more acculturated than second-generation European Americans, but their attitudes may differ because of their experiences as people of color. It is therefore important for clinicians to consider the geographic and sociopolitical contexts in which Japanese identity development has occurred.

Furthermore, an increasing number of Japanese are part Japanese–part Asian, part Japanese–part White, and part Japanese–part other races (Root, 1996). It is important for therapists to understand issues involving identity development when working with Japanese Americans who are biracial and multiracial (Fukuyama, 1999; King & DaCosta, 1996; Stephan & Stephan, 1989; Williams & Thornton, 1998).

Derrick is an 18-year-old Japanese American freshman at a prestigious private college on the East Coast. He was referred by the Student Health Services for counseling because he had been suffering from anxiety attacks and depression. Derrick grew up on the West Coast, and this is the first time that he is living on the East Coast. His parents are both third-generation Japanese Americans. Both are successful professionals: His mother is an opthalmologist, and his father is partner in an accounting firm. Derrick has always done well academically, but has been failing since entering college. He does not feel comfortable in his new environment. Nor does he feel comfortable with his White and Asian American classmates and would like to transfer to a state university on the West Coast. Derrick attended a predominantly White private high school and never felt that he fit in. However, he has never discussed his experiences as a Japanese American with his parents. His parents grew up in upwardly mobile communities where they socialized mostly with other Japanese and Asian Americans. Derrick's father has no inkling that his son is having a difficult time fitting into his new environment. His mother senses that something is wrong and is concerned, but has had problems in communicating with Derrick ever since he reached adolescence.

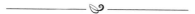

Before working with clients like Derrick and his family, therapists need to consider a variety of issues, including the following. Researchers find that many Asian American adolescents, as compared with their European American cohorts, grow up with a poorer body image and self-image (Pang, Mizokawa, Morishima, & Olstad, 1985; Yee et al., 1998). Many Japanese American youth also prefer belonging to either Japanese or Asian American groups rather than racially heterogeneous groups (Kitano & Daniels, 1988). Third- and later-generation Japanese Americans, with the exception of those who live in Hawai'i or on the West Coast, are often asked by Whites about their country of origin. Questions such as, "Where are you from? California? No, I mean where are you *really* from?" are not addressed to a third- or fourth-generation European American. Japanese Americans, no matter how much they "feel American, speak American, act American, and think American," can never "be American" in the eyes of the dominant American culture (Henkin, 1985, p. 502).

As Nagata (1993) notes, traumas related to racism are situated within historical contexts across generations. Although each generation needs to teach its children how to survive in hostile environments, many Japanese American families do not discuss racial bias and discrimination with their children. The reasons for this may include the cultural values of *gaman* (endurance), the belief that to talk about such difficulties would be a sign of weakness. Another is the "model minority" myth that pervades the dominant culture, in which the educational achievements of Japanese Americans and other Asian Americans are used to denigrate other people of color. This myth can at times hinder Japanese Americans from acknowledging micro-insults against them as racism. A young person like Derrick may have a difficult time placing his experiences in a broader context because of intergenerational patterns in which parents and grandparents have not discussed the way in which they have dealt with discrimination and racism, including the internment during World War II.

Japanese American parents typically hold higher educational expectations for their children than do European American parents (Goyette & Xie, 1999; Schneider, Hieshima, Lee, & Plank, 1994). This is attributed to two factors: a cultural tradition that places value on education for its own sake, and the belief that educational achievement will improve occupational opportunities and help counteract racial discrimination. Helping Derrick and his parents to discuss and understand how each generation in his family has coped with racism and micro-insults may assist Derrick in having a better understanding of what he perceives as his internal conflicts.

CONCLUSIONS

This chapter has provided an overview of the historical background and traditional cultural values, as well as contemporary issues, that affect Japanese American families. Japanese American families are diverse, and it is important for therapists to be aware of their assumptions about their clients. Some Japanese Americans are well acculturated to the dominant society, whereas others retain more traditional cultural values. Families also differ in terms of their relationship with their culture of origin, in which some value their traditions and others try to minimize them. One of the main tasks for therapists is to assess the dynamic interplay of cultural issues and the presenting problems. Family members may be at different levels of acculturation, which triggers various intergenerational conflicts.

When seeing Japanese American families in therapy, therapists may be tempted to judge what the family is like based on its apparent level of acculturation (i.e., generation, educational background, and social status). It is important to know that no matter how acculturated and "successful" in terms of socioeconomic status, Japanese Americans experience micro-aggressions and insults as people of color. For White therapists, it is important to be aware of how their privileged status as members of the dominant culture may act as blinders to the challenges that Japanese Americans continue to face as members of a minority group. Therapists of color also need to be aware of the way in which Western assumptions inherent in family therapy may have influenced their clinical views in working with Japanese American families.

ACKNOWLEDGMENTS

I would like to thank Laura Shiozaki-Lee, LCSW, Vivian Matsushige, LCSW, and James Runsdorf, PhD, for their helpful comments in preparing this chapter.

NOTES

1. In 1980, the Commission on Wartime Relocation and Internment of Civilians (CWRIC), which was established to review Executive Order 9066 and make recommendations for redress, held a series of testimonial hearings.
2. Japanese who responded as being of one category in the 2000 census.
3. According to the 2000 census, 852,237 reported as being Japanese alone or in combination with one or more other categories of the same race (i.e., biethnic or biracial), and 1,148,932 reported as being Japanese alone or in combination with one or more other categories of the same race (biethnic or biracial), or in combination with any other race group (i.e., multiracial).

REFERENCES

Akimoto, S. A., & Sanbonmatsu, D. M. (1999). Differences in self-effacing behavior between European and Japanese Americans: Effect on competence evaluations. *Journal of Cross-Cultural Psychology, 30*(2), 159–177.

Asian American Federation of New York. (2001). *Census 2000: Detailed Asian groups in the United States.* Available at www.aafny.org/cic/table/ust.asp

Chung, D. K. (1992). Asian cultural commonalities: A comparison with mainstream American culture. In S. M. Furuto, R. Biswas, D. K. Chung, K. Murase, & F. Ross-Sheriff (Eds.), *Social work practice with Asian Americans* (pp. 27–44). Newbury Park, CA: Sage.

Doi, T. (1986). *The anatomy of self: The individual versus society* (M. A. Harbison, Trans.). Tokyo: Kodansha International.

Fukuyama, M. A. (1999). Personal narrative: Growing up biracial. *Journal of Counseling and Development, 77*(1), 12–14.

Goyette, K., & Xie, Y. (1999). Educational expectations of Asian American youths: Determinants of ethnic differences. *Sociology of Education, 72*(1), 22–36.

Henkin, W. A. (1985). Toward counseling the Japanese in America: A cross-cultural primer. *Journal of Counseling and Development, 63,* 500–503.

Hess, P. M., & Hess, H. J. (2001). Parenting in European American/White families. In N. B. Webb (Ed.), *Culturally diverse parent–child and family relationships: A guide for social workers and other practitioners* (pp. 307–333). New York: Columbia University Press.

Ichioka, Y. (1988). *The Issei: The world of the first generation Japanese immigrants: 1885–1924.* New York: Free Press.

Itai, G., & McRae, C. (1994). Counseling older Japanese American clients: An overview and observations. *Journal of Counseling and Development, 72*(4), 373–378.

Johnson, F. A. (1993). *Dependency and Japanese socialization.* New York: New York University Press.

King, R. C., & DaCosta, K. M. (1996). Changing face, changing race: The remaking of race in the Japanese American and African American communities. In M. P. P. Root (Ed.), *The multiracial experience: Racial borders as the new frontier* (pp. 227–244). Thousand Oaks, CA: Sage.

Kitano, H. H. L. (1976). *Japanese Americans: The evolution of a subculture* (2nd ed.). Englewood Cliffs, NJ: Prentice-Hall.

Kitano, H. H. L., & Daniels, R. (1988). *Asian Americans: Emerging minorities.* Englewood Cliffs, NJ: Prentice Hall.

Maki, M. T., Kitano, H. H. L., & Berthold, S. M. (1999). *Achieving the impossible dream: How Japanese Americans obtained redress.* Urbana: University of Illinois Press.

Mass, A. (1991). Psychological effects of the camps on the Japanese Americans. In R. Daniels, S. C. Taylor, & H. H. L. Kitano (Eds.), *Japanese Americans: From relocation to redress* (pp. 159–162). Seattle: University of Washington Press.

Nagata, D. K. (1993). *Legacy of silence: Exploring the long-term effects of the Japanese American internment.* New York: Plenum Press.

Nagata, D. K., & Cheng, J. Y. (2003). Intergenerational communication of race-related trauma by Japanese American former internees. *American Journal of Orthopsychiatry, 73*(3), 266–278.

Pang, V. O., Mizokawa, D. T., Morishima, J. K., & Olstad, R. G. (1985). Self-concepts of Japanese American children. *Journal of Cross-Cultural Psychology, 16*(1), 99–109.

Root, M. P. P. (1996). The multiracial experience: Racial borders as a significant frontier in race relations. In M. P. P. Root (Ed.), *The multiracial experience: Racial borders as the new frontier* (pp. xiii–xxxvii). Thousand Oaks, CA: Sage.

Schneider, B., Hieshima, J. A., Lee, S., & Plank, S. (1994). East-Asian academic success in the United States: Family, school, and community explanations. In P. M. Greenfield & R. R. Cocking (Eds.), *Cross-cultural roots of minority child development* (pp. 323–350). Hillsdale, NJ: Erlbaum.

Shibusawa, T. (1996). Espressione dei sentimenti: Prospettive dall' Orient [Expressions of emotions: Eastern perspectives]. In M. Andolfi, C. Angelo, & M. DiNichilo (Eds.), *Sentimenti e sistemi* [Feelings and systems] (pp. 137–149). Milano: Rafaella Cortina.

Shibusawa, T. (2001). Japanese American parenting. In N. B. Webb (Ed.), *Culturally diverse parent–child and family relationships: A guide for social workers and other practitioners* (pp. 283–303). New York: Columbia University Press.

Stephan, C. W., & Stephan, W. G. (1989). After intermarriage: Ethnic identity among mixed-heritage Japanese-Americans and Hispanics. *Journal of Marriage and the Family, 51*, 507–519.

Sue, S., & Morishima, J. K. (1982). *The mental health of Asian Americans.* San Francisco: Jossey-Bass.

Tomita, S. K. (1998). The consequences of belonging: Conflict management techniques among Japanese Americans. *Journal of Elder Abuse and Neglect, 9*(3), 41–68.

Uomoto, J. M., & Gorsuch, R. L. (1984). Japanese American response to psychological disorder: Referral patterns, attitudes, and subjective norms. *American Journal of Community Psychology, 12*(5), 537–550

U.S. Department of Commerce. (2002). *The Asian population: 2000.* Census 2000 brief. Available at www.census.gov/prod/2002pubs/c2kbr01-16.pdf

Williams, T. K., & Thornton, M. C. (1998). Social construction of ethnicity versus personal experience: The case of Afro-Amerasians. *Journal of Comparative Family Studies, 29*(2), 255–267.

Yee, B. W. K., Huang, L. N., & Lew, A. (1998). Families: Life-span socialization in a cultural context. In L. C. Lee & N. W. S. Zane (Eds.), *Handbook of Asian American psychology* (pp. 83–135). Thousand Oaks, CA: Sage.

CHAPTER 26

Korean Families

Bok-Lim C. Kim
Eunjung Ryu

For centuries, pragmatism, perseverance, and a hierarchical family structure with rules and prescribed role relationships have all served to sustain Koreans through famine, political and social upheaval, foreign domination, and war (Choy, 1971). Although pragmatism and perseverance have persisted, the tumultuous events of the 20th century have drastically altered traditional family organization. In the early 20th century, the Japanese colonized Korea, exploiting its natural and human resources and attempting to eradicate the Korean language and culture (Nahm, 1973). These experiences have made Koreans mistrustful of foreigners and cynical, as well as rebellious, toward government and authorities in general. The division of Korea along the 38th parallel in 1945 and the Korean War in 1950 created cataclysmic sociopolitical upheaval. Mass destruction of its people and its land challenged the strength and stamina of Korean individuals and families. The traditionally strong sense of loyalty and allegiance to the extended family was weakened through lifelong separation, and the accompanying anxiety and grief amid the confusion generated by the uncertainties of social upheaval. Allegiance to different political ideologies and governments divided families, spawning tragedies such as sons turning against fathers, brothers against brothers.

During this time the founding of women's high schools and universities increased the accessibility of education for women (Kim, 1976). These educated women became a major force in abolishing gender-based discriminatory laws and modernizing the education of the Korean masses—women as well as men. Urbanization and industrialization of the past four decades so greatly increased the demand for skilled labor that unmarried women for the first time broke with tradition, left home, and became a part of the labor force (Kim, 1990).

Theses changes in women's education as well as their participation in the workforce resulted in greater respect for women and increased their status. However, gender discrimination and class stratification have remained in different forms. Money and academic credentials have replaced inherited class as markers of status, and although women are not barred from higher education or business, their success is still measured by marriage, rather than by professional success. No matter what a woman has accomplished, she is measured by her husband's status and the achievements of her children (Mintz, 1990).

IMMIGRATION TO THE UNITED STATES

Korean immigration to the United States occurred in three distinct waves. The first consisted of only 7,000 desperately poor farmers, who came to Hawai'i between 1903 and 1905 as contract laborers (Yang, 1982), followed by their "picture brides" (Chai, 1987). The second wave began around 1950, when significant numbers of Korean war orphans and Amerasian children arrived as transracially adopted children of American parents (D. S. Kim, 1978). At about this time, Korean women married to U.S. servicemen began to immigrate in large numbers (Kim, 1981).

The third wave of Korean immigration began with the passage of the 1965 Amendment to the Immigration and Naturalization Service Act of 1955 (Public Law 89-236, 79 Stat. 911), which ushered in a new era of racial and ethnic equality in American immigration policy (Kim & Kim, 1977; Takaki, 1998). The amendment opened the floodgates for Koreans and other Asian groups severely restricted by previous quotas. In the past two decades, more than 30,000 Koreans have immigrated annually, accounting for the tenfold increase in the Korean American population between 1970 and 1990. This rapid increase has made Korean Americans visible to the American public as a distinct group, different from the Chinese or Japanese.

The third wave of Korean immigrants differed from those who came earlier in a number of ways. Although they are better educated than the first wave of immigrants, they come from a wider range of socioeconomic and educational levels. Most Koreans are emigrating as nuclear families rather than as single adults. Close to three fourths of them have relatives or close friends already living in the United States, who assist with their initial adjustment. Most cities in the United States now have Korean resident associations, ethnic churches and temples, and businesses that offer practical help and ongoing support for ethnic identification. Immigrants in this third wave are coming to a society that has become less prejudiced and more tolerant of minority groups. Emigrating from a country that is modern, industrialized, and relatively affluent, they no longer see the United States as superior. Koreans simply see America as a place that offers better business and career opportunities, as well as superior education for their children. The third-wave population is the major focus of this chapter.

KOREAN AMERICANS IN THE UNITED STATES

Family patterns and cultural values of the third-wave Koreans in the United States and those in Korea are remarkably similar. The immigrants' recent history in the United States, daily contact with Korea through newspapers, radio, television, telephone, and frequent transpacific travel account for the congruence of values. In this chapter, for these reasons, no distinction is made except when there are marked differences.

Korean Americans numbered over 1 million in the year 2000, a 34% increase from 1990 (U.S. Census Bureau, 2000a). As a group, they are an adventurous, upwardly mobile people who are willing to move wherever education, employment, and business opportunities beckon them. They are widely dispersed throughout the United States, primarily in urban centers of the Northeast (22.8%) and Western states (44.4%). Seventy-eight percent of Koreans are foreign born and use Korean at home, and 21.7% use only English, which seems to suggest that this latter percentage is composed of either native-born Korean Americans or intermarried couples. The census data of 2000 indicate that 59% of all Korean Americans 15 years old and over are married, as opposed to the 84% reported in 1990. This low percentage in 2000, however, seems to be the function of including 15-year-olds in the calculation. Twenty-one percent of Koreans are 21 years old and younger, and about 10% are 60 years old and older (U.S. Census Bureau, 2000b). Most Korean households in the year 2000 consisted of immigrant parents and American-born or -raised children, where two cultures and two languages collide and individual members reflect different stages of acculturation, as well as different life cycle phases.

Korean Americans are well-educated people; 51% have college or graduate degrees, either from Korea or the United States. The remaining 49% have high school and/or trade school diplomas (U.S. Census Bureau, 2000a). Such high educational achievement, however, does not necessarily translate into high status and high-paying occupations.

Because the majority of Koreans are relatively recent immigrants, their English proficiency level is low, whereas their unfamiliarity and functional discomfort with American social structures are high (Hurh & Kim, 1984; B.-L. C. Kim, 1978). Most college graduates educated in Korea find that differences in job market requirements make the transfer of their education and work experience to the American situation difficult and uncertain.

Koreans have been willing to take skilled and semiskilled jobs that do not reflect their education and experience. Thus, their participation in the labor force has been high. More than four fifths of men and three fourths of women work outside the home on a full-time basis (B.-L. C. Kim, 1978; Min, 1988). The shrinking job market has turned these people toward labor-intensive small businesses that require long hours of work, such as convenience stores, groceries, and laundries.

FAMILY PATTERNS AND VALUES

Hierarchies by gender, generation, age, and class have long been a "given" in Korean society. Although the situation has largely changed on the surface, hierarchy remains a lingering and sometimes powerful force determining thinking and behavior. Strict segregation between the sexes has largely disappeared, as have traditionally prescribed role differentiation and work division based on gender, particularly among the young adults. Throughout life, the generational boundary between parents and children has remained firm. Parents are to support and guide, and children of all ages are to obey and respect, although their opinions are now being given more consideration than before.

The legacy of hierarchical relationships can be seen in age stratification within the family as well as in social and business intercourse. The Korean language, with more than three classes of nouns and verbs signifying the ranking orders of relationships, reinforces this way of thinking (B.-L. C. Kim, 1978). The absence of this kind of differentiation in English creates much discomfort in social interactions with Americans and has special implications for parent–child relationships. Tension and ill feelings are often generated between Korean immigrant parents and their American-raised children, who lack the appreciation of and fluency in Korean to properly observe the hierarchical protocol.

Korean families have a clear boundary as to who is "in" and who is "out." The term *jip-an* means literally "within the house" and identifies family membership, values, and traditions practiced within a particular family. *Ka-moon* means "the family gate" and refers to family standing and reputation within the community. This boundary also determines what information needs to be kept *jip-an* and what can be shared. Although it is common in most societies to conceal family problems and boast about successes, Koreans attach an unusually high level of shame to such a wide range of problems that they are highly selective about what is revealed. This boundary tends to be quite rigid among more traditional families and less so among rural people. This may partially account for the rigid, often hostile and agonized, reactions of Korean immigrant parents to interracial dating and marriage. To label such reactions merely as ethnocentric or racist (as Korean American children are likely to do) often blocks avenues for conflict resolution through cross-cultural understanding.

As for the issue of gay and lesbian relationships, Koreans are highly homophobic, hostile, and rejecting. Most even deny the possibility of gays and lesbians among Koreans. Yet they exist. The experiences of the first author (B.-L. C. K.) on university campuses and in clinical practice reveal the extent to which traditional Korean attitudes make it difficult for Korean gays and lesbians to work through pervasive feelings of low self-esteem, depression, fear of exposure, and anger. When these problems are not identified, it is impossible to solve them. As a beginning step, public education is urgently needed.

Although Korean American family boundaries remain rigid in terms of the larger society, within the immigrant community boundaries are porous and permeable because of the absence of an extended kinship network. Nevertheless, harmony and connection between geographically dispersed extended family members is maintained through frequent telephone calls as well as transpacific travel. Korean immigrants make extraordinary sacrifices of time and money to participate in events such as *han-kap*, the special celebration of the 60th birthday, and *chae-sa*, the ancestor-worship ceremony honoring deceased parents and grandparents for six generations past (Janelli & Janelli, 1982).

MARRIAGE

Marriage is still considered to be the joining of two families rather than merely of two individuals. Each family's status in the community, as well as the couple's academic credentials and health, are discretely but thoroughly checked before a decision is reached. Either romantic love or formal matchmaking can lead to marriage, but mutual investigation by the two families and the consent of both sets of parents and the bride and groom are a must.

WIFE–HUSBAND AND IN-LAW RELATIONSHIPS

Most Korean American couples expect faithfulness, mutual respect, and joint decision making. Money management is usually the wife's responsibility. The gender-ordered rule for the three obediences of women—obediece to her father before marriage, to her husband after she is married, and to her son in old age—is no longer strictly adhered to. The power relationship and division of work for the couple depend on how close in age they are, their educational levels, and their commitment to traditional values. Among older couples and more traditional families, the unequal division of responsibilities and rights remains. It is not uncommon for an unemployed husband to expect his wife to prepare family meals after returning from her job.

It is among such couples that domestic violence occurs (physical and verbal abuse). A husband who is either unemployed or disabled, feeling marginalized by his limited earning power and limited English proficiency, tries to compensate such lack by employing violent means to control and dominate his wife. Unfortunately, such behavior is often condoned by Korean communities, while the victimized wife's pain and needs are ignored. It is important to note that systemic and institutional oppression of women in Korea has decreased dramatically in the past 30 years, thanks to persistent, hardworking, courageous women who managed to change the laws and public attitude. Korean women today, whether in Korea or in the United States, nevertheless encounter more subtle discrimination. Women's capacity to surmount such discrimination depends largely on family and community support as well as their socioeconomic status. Public response to domestic violence and gender inequality in Korean society is far from ideal. Today, however, as compared with the early 1950s, the situation has improved; for instance, legal remedies and protection services are available. Even more significant is that many Korean women today, with the support of their families, will not tolerate such abuse whether from a husband or from in-laws. Korea ranks fourth in the divorce rate among the industrialized nations (National Statistical Office, 2003; "Nearly half of married couples," 2003). Among the many contributing factors, women's increasing independence and intolerance for abuse seem clear.

There are many forces that impinge on the marital relationship. The Korean Family Legal Center estimates that 70–80% of marital problems involve the in-laws of the wife (Lee, personal communication, 1992). Geographic distances protect most Korean Americans from the intricate network of daily obligations to their in-laws. However, even when families live far apart, the influence and interference of in-laws are ever present. They are involved in all major and many minor decisions, ranging from the type of car or housing a couple may choose, to number of children they might have. Their influence decreases considerably as the couple's economic independence increases and, especially, with the birth of children.

Problems between mother-in-law and daughter-in-law are most common and can be quite intense. The mother-in-law is generally possessive of her son and critical of the daughter-in-law. The daughter-in-law frequently perceives her mother-in-law's "helpfulness" as controlling. Changing expectations in the relationship between these two further exacerbates their differences. Because the issue of in-laws is such a central one, it is important for the therapist to inquire about the couple's in-law relationships with every Korean American family, regardless of the presenting problems. In contrast, the husband's relationship with his in-laws is less conflictual because less is expected from him. As long as he is a good provider for the family and a faithful husband, the obligation to his in-laws is fulfilled.

Korean couples are typically inexperienced in conflict management and resolution. They tend to see a problem as a matter of right or wrong, to be resolved by proving the other person wrong. Men also tend to invoke male superiority to win their points, and frustration is often handled with alcohol. Even though this behavior is culturally condoned, the immigrant wife feels she does not have to tolerate it, and the conflict can easily escalate to violence.

There are a number of acculturation problems that provide fertile ground for stress and conflict. All studies of Korean immigrant families have listed limited English proficiency as the number one stressor (Hurh & Kim, 1984; B.-L. C. Kim, 1978, 1980, 1988). For "face-saving" or appearance-conscious Korean adults, the inability to express oneself and be understood is a major blow to self-esteem.

The limited English proficiency of many immigrant adults, particularly men, causes them to feel exposed and humiliated in the English-speaking world. One man related his despair by saying, "Overnight I became deaf and mute when I came to America." Underemployment and long working hours in unsafe neighborhoods are also highly stressful and constitute a major source of family conflicts.

An important resource for dissipating stress is the ethnic church, where this struggle is tacitly understood and those experiencing it are supported. Church membership among Korean Americans is between 70% and 80% (Hurh & Kim, 1984; B.-L. C. Kim, 1978) as compared with 47% in Korea (Korean Overseas Information Service, 1990). It is clear that the Korean ethnic church not only administers to spiritual needs but, more important, also provides support and a sense of belonging (Hurh & Kim, 1984). As Hurh and Kim (1984) pointed out, the church is both an acculturation agent and a resource for preserving culture and ethnic identity. Although Korean Buddhist temples in the United States are fewer in number than the churches, they also provide a similar service and refuge for their members.

PARENT–CHILD RELATIONSHIPS

Male children have been very important to Korean families in order to carry on the family lineage and ensure continuity of the generations. Female children have been viewed as a burden because of the exorbitant expenses incurred in marrying them off and their subsequent joining with their husband's family (Min, 1988). Such discriminatory attitudes are slowly disappearing as increasing numbers of married daughters maintain close contact with parents and even care for them in their old age.

The traditional Korean primacy of the father–son dyad, maintained from one generation to the next, has recently been replaced with the development of the husband–wife dyad, though this may be challenged again when the oldest child enters first grade, and then superseded by the mother–child dyad as the key relationship. Koreans place such a high value on *hak-bul*, academic credentials, that the parents' self-esteem is intimately tied to the academic success or failure of their children. The fiercely competitive nature of the Korean educational system has made successful education of children an all-consuming enterprise for most families, requiring much time, energy, and money, with the mother assigned to this task full-time. This system is not needed in the United States, and the mothers who work outside the home are not available to enforce it. Nonetheless, immigrant parents deprived of traditional sources of self-esteem and feeling undervalued by American culture, insist even more strongly that their children excel in school, as well as gain admittance to prestigious universities.

The hierarchical relationship is extremely stressful for Korean American children who wish to have their feelings heard and opinions respected, whereas the parents who feel they are losing their children to the "selfish" American culture cannot appreciate their children's wishes. Parents and children are further handicapped because each is using a translated language for communication. Just as the parents' English lacks an American cultural context and mindset, the children's Korean lacks Korean cultural context and social norms. An American-born, English-speaking 13-year-old boy said to his father, "You are crazy!" during their humorous exchange of funny stories, whereupon the immigrant father was offended and got angry.

Immigrant parents' limited appreciation of the wide difference between American and Korean cultures and their ambivalence about their children's acculturation may cause them to make incongruent demands on their children (Kim, 1980). They want them to be successful in school but to be obedient, respectful, and humble at home, not realizing that the attributes needed to succeed in American schools are assertiveness, initiative, and independent thinking. They want their children to be proficient in English and to retain fluency in Korean. They restrict after-school activities with English-speaking peers, but expect their children to be socially popular. They profess no prejudice toward other racial and ethnic groups, yet resist interracial dating and marriage and justify this in terms of the importance of compatibility between the two families.

On the positive side, we found that parents had nondiscriminatory career goals for male and female children, and that there was remarkable agreement between the generations about the children's future goals. The children also recognized their parents' hard work and sacrifice for them and shared their parents' dream of success in America (Kim, 1980).

AFFECT MANAGEMENT

Westerners are often surprised when Koreans, who are usually very reserved and reticent, express themselves more spontaneously. Koreans are most spontaneous among their peers and social equals, and they are reserved and deferential in the presence of superiors and during official occasions. Educated and cultured persons tend to be more controlled and selective in expressing feelings and usually express negative feelings only to their immediate families. Teaching children about appropriate affect management is too important to be left to chance, and children learn from parents and teachers by both lecture and example.

Koreans are variously described as hot-tempered, easily offended, generous, gregarious, and humorous. It is safe to say that Koreans are an emotional people whose overriding concern in all human interaction is the issue of respect. The non-Korean therapist needs to know about several key Korean qualities that orchestrate the expression of respect in all social relationships.

First, there is *jeong*, a unique Korean concept that has no English equivalent (Kim, 1990). It expresses a combination of empathy, sympathy, compassion, emotional attachment, and tenderness, in varying degrees, according to the social context. *Jeong* enriches and humanizes social relationships and makes life meaningful. It is expressed by attention to the small but important details that show concern for another person's comfort and well-being. The Korean equivalent of "How are you?" is "Are you at ease?" Without *jeong*, a person loses his or her humanity. Korean clients will observe whether the therapist has *jeong*, and if they do not perceive it, treatment is doomed. *Jeong* is easy to miss in cross-cultural encounters, and the therapist needs to be especially careful to demonstrate human qualities, despite the professional nature of the contact. This can be done with small talk, such as asking whether the client had any difficulty finding the office or locating a parking space.

Hahn is a pervasive sentiment, referring to an unexpressed mixture of grievance and regret, with resulting heartache. This condition is commonly experienced by the oppressed and abused person who feels there is no recourse to rectify the wrong. Koreans experienced a lot of *hahn* during the Japanese rule and the Korean War. Korean women, who for many centuries had been oppressed by the patriarchal family system, have accumulated much *hahn*. The resulting condition is now listed in DSM-IV (American Psychiatric Association, 1994) as *hwa-byung* under "Culture-Bound Syndromes." *Hwa-byung* is predominantly seen among middle-aged Korean women. In contrast with Korean men, who can relieve their *hahn* by drinking, these women have no culturally sanctioned outlets other than physical symptoms. In working with this group, it is important not to see *hahn* in a pejorative sense as learned helplessness or somatization, but rather to appreciate its cultural roots. The therapist can label the client's immigrant status as an opportunity to leave behind old practices and learn new ways of active mastery that are more appropriate for this country.

Noon-chi and *boon-soo* are closely related concepts born out of the necessity of surviving as a subordinate in a hierarchically ordered family and society. *Noon-chi* literally means "measuring with the eyes," learning to pick up external cues in order to choose a course of action that is both nonoffensive and appropriate. Once they are in America, Korean immigrants have found that these *noon-chi* skills cannot be practiced in such a different society with a whole different set of cues and meanings. Until they become highly acculturated, Koreans will be extremely uncomfortable and anxious in social interactions with Americans. The therapist must communicate concern for the client's discomfort and anxiety about the therapeutic situation by showing the client that the need for help in no way diminishes the therapist's respect for the client as a human being. Clients will feel less need to rely on their *noon-chi* when the therapist makes the context and purpose of the treatment as explicit as possible.

Boon-soo refers to knowing and accepting one's status, regardless of the advantage or disadvantage accorded to that status—in short, knowing one's place. The highly stratified social class of the past relied on each person to persevere in their *boon-soo* to preserve the status quo. When a person's expectations or demands are excessive, that person is said not to know his or her *boon-soo*. The therapist needs to appreciate that the Korean client, trying to act within his or her *boon-soo*, might express such low expectations that in an American context, this would suggest serious problems with low self-esteem.

Chae-myun is face-saving, a concept familiar to many Asians. Making a good impression is very important to all Koreans in all relationships outside the immediate family. Maintaining *chae-myun* protects the dignity, honor, and self-respect of the individual and the family. The therapist should anticipate that clients will be reluctant to reveal vital information if this will cause loss of *chae-myun*. Respect for the therapist's *chae-myun* may stop them from correcting or disagreeing with the therapist. This needs to be differentiated from passive aggressive or subservient behavior. Protecting the client's *chae-myun*, especially that of male clients, is important. The therapist must be very careful about any comments or gestures that could be construed as criticism, put-downs, or indifference. There is no room for error, because just as with *jeong*, loss of *chae-myun* is absolute. The client who loses *chae-myun* probably will not return.

TREATMENT CONSIDERATIONS

The difficulty in writing this section stems from the significant differences among Koreans in terms of their values, affect management, and problem-solving strategies. Such differences are related to variances in the levels of acculturation, foreign versus native birth, length of stay in the United States, language used at home, age, socioeconomic and educational level, occupational status, and availability of a social network. The model chosen here is one of the most culturally sensitive situations: an immigrant family household in which the parents' references are Korean and the children's are American.

Traditionally, Koreans have resolved conflict with the help of a mediator chosen for his or her fairness and wisdom. This worked well as long as there was trust and respect for the mediator. For other Koreans, the help of shamans (*moo-dang*) and fortune-tellers, superb listeners and astute observers of people, has been valuable. Shamans exorcise evil spirits with elaborate and often costly ceremonies (Covell, 1983), whereas fortune-tellers console and prescribe a course of action, which may include inaction and patience as well. Faith healing by the Christian clergy has also entered the field of problem resolution.

Deprived of most of these resources in the United States, Korean immigrants are turning to relatives, close friends, clergy, and lawyers for help with emotional, psychological, and relational problems (Kim & Condon, 1975). They seldom seek professional help from mental health workers because they define both the problems and the remedies so differently from Americans (Sue, 1977; Sue & McKinney, 1975; Tien & Olson, 2003). They consider some of the worry caused by relational, financial, or health problems as *pal-ja*, immutable destiny, which must be endured without complaint. University students and employment assistance program (EAP)–referred clients are the only groups that seek help voluntarily.

Most Korean Americans are ignorant of available mental health services, and even when they are willing to consider them, most do not meet the language and cultural requisites of this population (B.-L. C. Kim, 1978). As a result, involvement with mental health services usually comes by way of mandatory counseling when schools, courts, or child protective agencies require it.

Involuntary clients are difficult to engage and treat even when their race, language, and culture are the same as those of the clinician. Korean Americans, already very anxious, defensive, and deeply shamed by their encounter with the system, do not expect understanding or help with their problems and assume that the therapist will be critical, punitive, and authoritative. Because clients entering the mental health system are likely to perceive themselves as occupying an inferior position within the system, therapists must take into consideration the question of the individual clients' and/or family's experience of hierarchy within the Korean context. This will aid in devising the most effective strategy for easing the client's fears.

Korean notions of hierarchy are based on the Confucian system, which defines five key relationships as the basis for a harmonious family and society: first, between king and subject; second, between teacher and student; third, between parents and children (or, more specifically, between father and son); fourth, between husband and wife; and fifth, between peers (Tien & Olson, 2003). All these relationships are hierarchically structured, with gender and age playing predominant roles (Ahn-Toupin, 1980; Chung, 1992). Each relationship involves reciprocal obligations and responsibilities. In a given family, the head of the household (*hoju*)—usually the eldest son—is responsible for providing for the family's material needs and protection and for making major decisions. He is to be respected and obeyed by the family members. Ideally, his authority requires him to be wise and benevolent in the discharge of his responsibilities so that harmony and prosperity can prevail.

However, there is no traditional provision for remedies when the *hoju* fails to fulfill his responsibilities, and in practice, misuse and abuse of the *hoju*'s authority have been frequent. When his responsibility to provide wise guidance and care is neglected, the result is that the wife and children suffer. During the 500 years of the Yi dynasty, which embraced the Confucian ideology, gender- and age-based inequality was codified in the legal, institutional, and ethical spheres. Thus, the second-class status and oppression of women and male dominance and privilege became entrenched in all aspects of Korean society until the mid-20th century. However, in recent years, industrialization, democratic ideals, and the availability of education have all nurtured an environment in which strong female leadership could flourish. As mentioned elsewhere, women have gained equality in legal status, educational opportunities, and social participation. Still, in the sphere of family life, strong patriarchal attitudes may remain and when applied rigidly to a dysfunctional family situation, they can wreak considerable havoc.

Among the clinical population of Koreans in the United States, many individuals and families still adhere to the values of a conservative patriarchal family system. Locked into these rigid and inflexible values, they experience great difficulty in adapting to changing times and new cultural situations, as they are highly insecure and fearful of losing the roles defined by the traditional relationships that granted them their identity and a modicum of security in the homeland. Because these cherished beliefs are not shared by the majority of Koreans and because the family system that supported these beliefs is no longer functional, either in Korea or in the United States, the resulting disconnect can lead to highly dysfunctional behavior. The following anecdote concerning a Child Protective Service referral may illustrate this point.

The couple had two grade-school-age children. The husband had just been released from a 3-day detention in jail for a violent attack on the wife, which had been reported to the police by a neighbor. In spite of the couple's strong desire to be seen together, the first joint session proved unproductive, as predicted, with the wife sobbing throughout and the husband remaining stoically silent with frequent sighs. Tension and anguish were palpable. Because the session was nonproductive and the couple could see that, they agreed on separate sessions. The first step was to explain the confidentiality of the interviews and their purpose: safety of the wife and children and reconciliation if desired, rather than punishment. The therapist explained to the couple that each had his or her own story that needed to be heard, and this could be done best in individual sessions. The therapist then asked each, in great detail, how they had resolved their conflicts in Korea. This was followed by an inquiry as to how their situation here in the United States differed from that in Korea. Evasions and generalities were slowly overcome by a matter-of-fact, step-by-step inquiry into the specifics of their conflict and how they attempted to resolve them. The therapist's assumption was twofold: one, that both had good intentions but lacked the skills needed to identify the problem and to develop behavior that would aid in resolving conflicts; and two, that people resort to extreme behavior usually because they are fearful of losing something valuable.

Individual sessions for both partners became productive when they began to recognize and articulate the fears underlying their anger and aggressive behavior, and to accept the challenge to their role expectations in the present environment. The emphasis was on labeling behavior as functional or dysfunctional, rather than right or wrong. The therapist focused on highlighting their shared goal of raising happy, productive children. The exploration of how each dealt with conflicts and stress in Korea, as compared with the current situation, helped them recognize how changed circumstances required new strategies and skills, as well as a critical appraisal of unexamined belief and patterns of interaction brought over from their homeland.

The therapist's approach of asking the couple about their understanding of the way things were done in Korea illustrates what is probably the most important general rule for a therapist dealing with Korean clients: Do not assume that all Koreans have picked up the same message from their home culture, or that they have brought the entirety of their traditional culture along with them to the United States.

Therapists who can acknowledge ignorance about the Korean American experience and who take time to read or talk with people will gain familiarity and appreciation for the client's mindset. On a more practical level, the therapist needs to find out about the client's level of English proficiency and acculturation before the first appointment. Having a well-trained interpreter available on an on-call basis is ideal. If clients bring their own interpreter, the therapist must be prepared to screen for bias and English competency to minimize the risk of editing, censorship, or mistakes. Engaging family members as interpreters has the advantage of convenience but is fraught with problems related to family hierarchy or *chae-myun* and family secrets.

As in all clinical situations, assessment is an ongoing process and particularly essential when working with Korean American clients who begin by presenting their problems in a highly disorganized and inconsistent manner. They are vague about dates and the specifics of problems, and they become ever more evasive about their reactions and feelings. It is difficult to determine whether they are deliberately making themselves unintelligible or are just confused and upset. It is usually better to postpone obtaining factual information and to concentrate on the client's immediate concern. The therapist needs to appreciate the client's high anxiety and fear of being accused or misunderstood. Explanation about how legal, social service, and mental health systems function and how the therapist can make the system work for the client establish what Sue and Zane (1987) refer to as therapist's credibility. Once clients clearly perceive the therapist's role and sincere desire to help, they can commit to therapy (Kim, 1985).

Problem-solving and psychoeducational approaches are most effective because Korean Americans are not particularly introspective. Framing problems as acculturation issues common to other immigrant groups may also remove their sense of "blame" and decrease their shame (Szapocznik, Santisban, Kurtines, Perez-Vidal, & Hervis, 1984). Parent–child conflicts and problems can be reframed as cultural conflicts requiring mutual Korean–Americn acculturation. New or alternative perspectives and methods of problem solving can be offered as "doing things differently in a new country," as in the proverb "When in Rome, do as the Romans do." The therapist can take the dual position of being a teacher of American ways and a student of Korean ways, thus empowering the client and bridging the distance between therapist and client.

Once the therapist gains their trust, Korean American clients are remarkably open with their feelings and opinions and will expect something of the same from the therapist. They will want to know about the therapist's marital status, age, number of children, and academic credentials. Most American therapists consider such personal questions to be intrusive, but questioning motives will only embarrass and offend. It is best to answer factually without getting too personal. Gift giving is a normal expression of appreciation after the therapist's help, and an invitation for dinner, a family birthday, or holiday celebration is not uncommon. As with personal information, a good rule of thumb is to maintain professionalism, with politeness, and to accept gifts gracefully, if they are not expensive, and decline invitations to meals.

CONCLUSION

Korean Americans as recent immigrants are experiencing a variety of adjustment and acculturation difficulties they could never have anticipated. Although they are used to major changes, they have no precedent for learning to live in a foreign culture that in itself is undergoing rapid change. Further, the majority of immigrants are ill equipped for the monumental job of acquiring English competence and other social skills needed to survive. Neither these new immigrants nor the American public in general can begin to appreciate the great difficulty of trying to become grounded in a society where extreme change has become the norm. Under these circumstances, we can expect exaggerated expression of individual and family dysfunction complicated by cultural stress. The task of the therapist is to discriminate between inner conflicts or weaknesses in personality or family structure and those that are primarily situational and culture generated (Falicov, 1988). The therapist needs to recognize that therapy alone is not the answer. The therapeutic mission must include working with specialized ethnic resources as well as sensitizing mainstream institutions to be responsive to the needs of new immigrants.

REFERENCES

Ahn-Toupin, E. S. W. (1980). Counseling Asians: Psychotherapy in the context of racism and Asian-American history. *American Journal of Orthopsychiatry, 50*(1), 76–86.

American Psychiatry Association. (1994). *Diagnostic and statistical manual of mental disorders* (4th ed.). Washington, DC: Author.

Chai, A. (1987). *Feminist analysis of life history of early immigrant women from Japan, Okinawa, and Korea.* Unpublished manuscript, University of Hawaii, Women's Studies Program, Honolulu.

Choy, B. Y. (1971). *Korea: A history.* Rutland, VT: Charles E. Tuttle.

Chung, D. K. (1992). *Asian cultural commonalities: A comparison with mainstream American culture.* In S. M. Furuto, R. Biswas, D. K. Chung, K. Murase, & F. Ross-Sheriff (Eds.), *Social work practice with Asian Americans.* Thousand Oaks, CA: Sage.

Covell, A. C. (1983). *Ecstasy: Shamanism in Korea.* Elizabeth, NJ: Hollym International.

Falicov, C. J. (1988). Learning to think culturally. In H. Liddle, D. C. Breunlin, & R. C. Schwartz (Eds.), *Handbook of family therapy training and supervision*. New York: Guilford Press.

Hurh, W. M., & Kim, K. C. (1984). *Korean immigrants in America: A structural analysis of ethnic confinement and adhesive adaption*. London: Fairleigh Dickinson University Press.

Janelli, R. L., & Janelli, D. Y. (1982). *Ancestor worship in Korean society*. Stanford, CA: Stanford University Press.

Kim, A. S. (1990). Economic status and labor conditions. *Koreana, 4*(2), 24–33.

Kim, B.-L. C. (1978). The Korean sample. In *The Asian Americans: Changing patterns, changing needs*. Montclair, NJ: Association of Korean Christian Scholars in North America.

Kim, B.-L. C. (1980). *The Korean-American child at school and at home* (Project Report [09-30-78-06-30-80], Administration on Child, Youth, and Families, U.S. DHEW, Grant No. 90-C-1335 [01]). Washington, DC: U.S. Department of Health, Education and Welfare.

Kim, B.-L. C. (1981). *Women in shadows: A handbook for service providers working with Asian wives of U.S. military personnel*. La Jolla, CA: National Committee Concerned with Asian Wives of U.S. Servicemen.

Kim, B.-L. C. (1988). The language situation of Korean Americans. In S. L. McKay & S.-L. Wong (Eds.), *Language diversity: Problems or resource?* New York: Newbury House.

Kim, B.-L. C., & Condon, M. E. (1975). *A study of Asian Americans in Chicago: Their socio-economic characteristics, problems and service needs* (Final Research Report, NIMH, U.S. DHEW, Grant No. 1, R01 MH 23993-01). Washington, DC: National Institute of Mental Health.

Kim, C., & Kim, B.-L. C. (1977). Asian immigrants in American law: A look at the past and the challenge which remains. *American University Law Review, 26*(2), 373–407.

Kim, D. S. (1978). From women to women with painful love: A study of maternal motivation in intercountry adoption processes. In H. H. Sunoo & D. S. Kim (Eds.), *Korean women in a struggle for humanization*. Montclair, NJ: Association of Korean Christian Scholars in North America.

Kim, L. (1990). *The concept of* jeong *and other Korean ethos*. Paper presented at the meeting of the American Academy of Psychoanalysis, San Antonio, TX.

Kim, S. C. (1985). Family therapy for Asian Americans: A strategic–structral framework. *Psychotherapy, 22*(2), 342–348.

Kim, Y. C. (1976). Modern education. In Y. C. Kim (Ed.), *Women of Korea: A history from ancient time to 1945*. Seoul, Korea: Ewha Women's University Press.

Korean Overseas Information Service. (1990). *A handbook of Korea*. Seoul, Korea: Ministry of Public Information, Republic of Korea.

Min, B. G. (1988). The Korean American family. In D. H. Mindel, R. W. Habenstein, & R. Wright, Jr. (Eds.), *Ethnic families in America: Patterns and variations* (3rd ed.). Elsevier Science.

Mintz, B. R. (1990). Changing—for better or worse? *Koreana, 4*(2), 69–73.

Nahm, A. C. (Ed.). (1973). *Korea under Japanese colonial rule—Study of the policies and techniques of Japanese colonization*. Grand Rapids: Center for Korean Studies, Institute of International and Area Studies, Western Michigan University.

National Statistical Office. (2003). *Marriage and divorce statistics*. Retrieved June, 15, 2004, from www.nso.go.kr

Nearly half of married couples divorce last year. (2003, December 28). Retrieved September 19, 2004, from www.hankooki.com

Sue, S. (1977). Community mental health services to minority groups: Some optimism, some pessimism. *American Psychologist, 42*(1), 37–45.

Sue, S., & McKinney, H. (1975). Asian Americans in the community mental health care system. *American Journal of Orthopsychiatry, 45*, 111–118.

Sue, S., & Zane, N. (1987). The role of culture and cultural techniques in psychotherapy: A critique and reformulation. *American Psychologist, 42*(1), 37–45.

Szapocznik, J., Santisban, D., Kurtines, W., Perez-Vidal, A., & Hervis, O. (1984). Bicultural effectiveness training: A treatment intervention for enhancing intercultural adjustment in Cuban American families. *Hispanic Journal of Behavioral Science*, 6(4), 317–344.

Takaki, R. (1998). *Strangers from a different shore: A history of Asian Americans.* Boston: Back Bay Books.

Tien, L., & Olson, K. (2003). Confusion past, conflicted present: Working with Asian American families. In L. B. Silverstein & T. J. Goodrich, *Feminist family therapy: Empowerment in social context* (pp. 135–145). Washington, DC: American Psychological Association.

U.S. Census Bureau. (2000a). *2000 census of population: Asians and Pacific Islanders in the United States.* Washington, DC: U.S. Department of Commerce, Economics and Statistics Administration.

U.S. Census Bureau. (2000b). *Census 2000 Supplementary PUMS data set.* Los Angeles: Author.

Yang, E. S. (1982). Koreans in America, 1903–1945. In E. Y. Yu, E. H. Phillips, & E. S. Yang (Eds.), *Koreans in Los Angeles: Prospects and promises.* Los Angeles: Koryo Research Institutes, Center for Korean-American and Korean Studies.

CHAPTER 27

Vietnamese Families

Paul K. Leung
James K. Boehnlein

Thirty years ago we witnessed the beginning of the forced exodus of the people of Vietnam from a homeland that was lost to a repressive regime. Toward the second half of the previous two decades, Vietnamese had also come as legal immigrants because of the sponsorship of financially secure family members who had arrived earlier and had successfully assimilated into the United States. In the meantime, a whole new generation of Vietnamese Americans born in the United States has come to adulthood with only a minimal emotional tie to the "old country" way of life that their parents so dearly cherish.

Since 1975, many authors have focused on the health and mental health issues facing individual Vietnamese refugees (Frisbie, Cho, & Hummer, 2001; Hinton, Tiet, Tran, & Chesney, 1997; Ito, 1999; Kinzie et al., 1988; Kinzie & Manson, 1983; Nemeto et al., 1999; Ta, Westermeyer, & Neider, 1996). Several studies have discussed the practice of folk medicine among this population and its impact on contemporary medical treatment (Golden & Duster, 1977; Kinzie & Leung, 1993; Muecke, 1983; Mull, Nguyen, & Mull, 2001). It has repeatedly been pointed out that although the prevalence rates of various mental health problems are higher among the Vietnamese than among the general U.S. population (Gong-Guy, 1987), they have underutilized mainstream mental health resources (Nguyen, 1985). Rarely has the Vietnamese family been the focal point of mental health surveys or research studies (Boehnlein et al., 1995); however, many authors have pointed out the importance of involving the family in the treatment process (Kinzie & Fleck, 1987; Lee, 1988). In fact, one study has noted the phenomenon of unrelated individual refugees forming a "pseudo family" for the purpose of mutual emotional support and survival (Lin, Tazuma, & Masuda, 1979).

In this chapter we examine the traditional Vietnamese family and its values and the changes that have evolved in America. Unique considerations in the treatment setting are illustrated with case histories.

THE TRADITIONAL FAMILY

Vietnamese society has gone through tremendous changes since the turn of the century, and especially since World War II. These changes are due to French colonial rule, Japanese occupation during World War II, and the period of struggle of the Vietnamese people for freedom and reunification. Throughout this turmoil, the family as an institution has adapted itself and endured in the midst of great social change.

TRADITIONAL VIETNAMESE CULTURE

Vietnamese culture and history have long been influenced by China (Frieze, 1986). In the middle of the 10th century, Vietnam gained independent sovereignty from China, but it continues to maintain close ties with its bigger and richer northern neighbor. People from all walks of life have traveled between the two countries, ensuring a steady stream of mutual influence on their societies. Trade flourished for centuries, and it was an honor for a family to send its favorite son to be schooled in China. Vietnam has adopted Chinese Confucianism with open arms, and this code of conduct has governed its society for centuries. Confucius, a philosopher who 3,500 years ago was regarded as the greatest teacher in the history of China, set forth a code of conduct that still influences Chinese society. In a larger sense, Confucianism demands that an individual revere heaven, earth, the emperor, parents, and his or her teachers, in that order. It defines the relationships of an individual with other people and his or her obligations to them. Loyalty and forgiveness are always emphasized in any interpersonal relationship. The "self" is to be minimized for the good of the family and the society. One is to seek a harmonious existence with the environment and with other people.

The worshiping of ancestors is important in the Vietnamese culture, as it is for the Chinese. The practice is pervasive and commonly found even among the converts to religions rooted in the Judeo-Christian tradition. On important anniversaries, dates, festivals, or significant individual or family events, the presentation of offerings to ancestors is often the first act of the celebration. This is usually conducted by the elderly figures in the family, with active participation expected of the younger members. Children are raised with the constant reminder of the importance of never bringing shame to the ancestors.

Roles of the Old and Young

Traditional Vietnamese society follows other Asian cultures, especially those influenced by Confucianism, regarding attitudes toward elders, who are to be respected and not openly disagreed with. Elders are often called in to resolve conflicts and crises among members of the family. Young people are frequently reminded to remain quiet when in the midst of elders. Age may not be the only factor determining one's status as an elder. One's generation in the family tree and birth order are other factors.

Little Tuan N. was born in America. He was accompanying his parents to a wedding. At the banquet his parents began to instruct Tuan to greet people around the table. The elderly lady sitting across the table should be addressed as "Grandma," the young lady next to her would be "Aunt Ngoc," and the young man next to her was "Brother Thanh." Such formality was repeated for the rest of the evening. Finally, after greeting the 20th "relative," Tuan commented to his parents that he had met so many uncles, aunts, and cousins, he wondered where they had been prior to the occasion. His parents replied that these people were not really his relatives and that he was not to ask any more "embarrassing" questions in front of the guests.

The issue of eye contact is also important as part of the process of communication between different generations. As a rule, a person of a lower position in the hierarchy does not maintain direct eye contact with elders or those in a higher social position, which would be interpreted as a sign of disrespect.

Roles of Husband and Wife

In a traditional family, spouses are governed by a set of rules of etiquette. The spouses may have married as a result of a prearrangement by the respective parents rather than on their own initiative. Before agreeing to the union, the parents usually want to be assured that the two families are compatible in social status, cultural background, and religious beliefs. Once a couple is married, the bond is regarded as permanent and breakable only if adultery is committed by the woman—but not by the man. Prior to World War II, divorce was exceedingly rare in Vietnamese society. However, it was quite acceptable for a man to take on a second or even a third wife and to have a mistress on the side as well. This situation changed after the 1950s with the institution of laws forbidding polygamy, but the practice of a man "entertaining" or "enjoying" in a "leisure-oriented environment" is still looked upon as somewhat acceptable. The wife usually would overlook the issue as long as her position in the extended family was secure and the provisions for her children had been satisfied.

Mr. Quang D., a man from a very affluent family, was in his 60s when Vietnam was under the colonial government of France. He had taken a wife before he was sent to Paris for his higher education in the late 1940s. Within 7 years, he earned his engineering degree. Throughout those years, as a student in the university, he was known more for his reputation as a drinker and a womanizer than as a student. In the middle of the 1950s, because of changes in the Vietnamese political situation, Mr. D.'s family followed the refugee tide south and resettled in the city of Saigon. At this time, Mr. D. also returned to Vietnam and was reunited with his family. However, it was not long afterward that he began staying overnight frequently in a woman's house. He often commented to friends that this woman was attractive to him because she was more "Westernized, capable of new thinking." He remained faithful in providing for his wife and children. Later in his life, he took on another wife while remaining married to the first one. In 1975, he came to America as a refugee along with his two wives and seven children. Not long after, each of his wives demanded to have her own place, saying that he should go to stay with the other one, because neither had time for him. At present, neither of the wives, nor any of the children, is living with him.

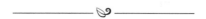

As for financial matters, the husband is expected to be the main provider of the family, but he does not discourage his wife from having a small business on the side, which can sometimes indeed bring in a handsome supplement for the family. Before the fall of Saigon in 1975, it was common to see men holding jobs in offices and women running ships and businesses in the local markets.

Roles of Sons and Daughters

Even now, children are regarded as property by their parents, although this belief has loosened gradually since World War II as the culture has become more Westernized. Parents have the responsibility to provide for their children and be accountable for their actions. Children are expected to follow their parents' advice in all aspects of life, including matters relating to marriage and career selection. From a very young age, they are taught the concepts of obligation and shame. For instance, children learn that they have an obligation to provide for their elderly parents. There will be reminders throughout life that they have a duty to fulfill the dreams of their parents, often presented in the name of the "family." Failing to carry out these obligations can only bring shame to a person's life and may even cause the individual to become an outcast within the extended family and the community.

The firstborn of a family holds a special position; this is especially true for a son. In the absence of the father, the eldest child can assume leadership among the siblings and is regarded as the head of the household. The eldest child, especially if that child is a son, is expected to provide good modeling for the rest of the children and to take the blame for the wrongdoings of his siblings. Parents most likely favor the oldest son, but also expect to be taken care of by him. The oldest son is expected to carry on the name of the family.

Trinh L., while a sophomore majoring in business administration, had his heart set on studying for an MBA degree after his undergraduate years. Trinh's father, a hardworking man who had to struggle in order to provide for the family after their resettlement in the United States, went to the son one day and said, "We need a doctor in the family. You are my eldest son, and it is my wish for you to pursue this career in order to bring honor to the family." Trinh took his father's words seriously and changed his career goal. This decision did not come without great struggle for Trinh. He discussed the matter at length with his counselors at college and in church, and finally accepted the challenge. Eventually Trinh graduated from medical school and is now a successful practitioner in his community. Very often, in his private moments, Trinh wonders when he will have an opportunity to return to school for the degree he had to cast aside for the sake of the family honor and the fulfillment of his father's wishes.

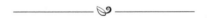

THE FAMILY IN TRANSITION

Historical Facts

To appreciate the changes that the traditional Vietnamese family has endured, we have to first understand the forces behind them. As we begin to examine the disruption of the traditional family system in Vietnam, we find that the root of the problems really started prior to the Indochinese conflict. As early as the turn of the 20th century, the struggle to gain independence from the French colonial government had already pitted members of families against each other because of differences in political ideology. In 1954, at the signing of the agreement in Geneva, two Vietnams were created. This separation brought about an exodus from the north of people seeking to flee communist rule. As a result, many families were broken up, with their members unable to see each other for the following 20 years, and in some cases, never again. Throughout the Indochinese conflict, the breakup of Vietnamese families continued because of the very destructive and disruptive nature of the war. Although they had to endure this turmoil, these families were still able to maintain their integrity because they could draw upon the support of their innate cultural environment. However, for the group of Vietnamese who left the country after the collapse of the Saigon government in 1975, the devastation of the family system was nearly complete. This group consisted of millions who had gone to foreign lands under overwhelming stress. For them, a way of life that treasured harmonic living among people related by blood and marriage had largely disappeared.

Statistics

The most recent national census review in 2003 showed that at the time of the survey, 1,122,528 Vietnamese had made America their home. The top five ranking states for the settlement of most Vietnamese/Vietnamese Americans were California (447,032), Texas (143,352), Washington (50,697), Virginia (40,500), and Massachusetts (33,962). The top five metropolitan areas were Los Angeles-Riverside-Orange County (233,573), San Francisco-Oakland-San Jose (146,613), Houston-Galveston (63,924), Dallas-Fort Worth (47,090), and Seattle-Tacoma (40,001). The age distribution for the Vietnamese population was as follows: 18 and under (27.8%), 18–24 (10.6%), 25–44 (37.1%), 45–64 (19.5%), and 65 and above (5%). Although no recent data are available, we believe that the age distribution should remain basically unchanged or may show a slight aging of the population, given an obvious trend of a much smaller family size in the younger generation both here and in Vietnam.

Changes in the Family Structure

For the Vietnamese who live in America, one of the biggest changes has been the loss of the extended family structure. In Vietnam, they would expect to live within a network of family and relatives, which sometimes would encompass many layers of relationships. As they sought refuge in foreign lands, some were fortunate to have their nuclear families with them, but others remained separated. For those who came at the beginning of the influx of Indochinese refugees into America, assimilation was complicated by the stresses associated with upward mobility. Many Vietnamese parents were shocked to see their children moving away for better job opportunities after finishing their education. The loss of this extended family structure meant the loss of a natural and familiar supportive system and an associated identity that one could attain only while living within a network of related people.

The Confusion of Roles

In the traditional society, the roles were always clear. The husband was the head of the family, he was the chief provider for the family, and the rest of the family looked to him for guidance. The wife was the caregiver and comforter of the family, and she was not required to deal with the outside world unless she chose to. Children were always under the protective wings of the parents, and they were not expected to provide leadership for the family. Often, once the family was transplanted outside its natural environment, the roles of its members were altered.

Most Vietnamese have discovered in America, as well as in most Western countries, that it is a matter of survival for all able family members to participate in the workforce. As women have increased their contribution to the family's financial well-being, they have become increasingly forceful in demanding that their status in the family, and in the society, be elevated. Sometimes the wife becomes the primary wage earner for the family because of her age or because of employment options available in the community favoring low-paid female workers. The husband may lose his leadership role if his ability to contribute to the family's finances is the only gauge of his status. Children are also encouraged to be financially independent as soon as they can, further eroding the leadership base of the parents. In addition, children who grow up in America become more proficient in English and often act as bridges to the outside world for non-English-speaking parents. This has further contributed to role confusion for many members of the family.

Mr. Phuoc V., a 57-year-old former South Vietnam Army intelligence officer who was released from a reeducation camp after an incarceration of 12 years, came to America several years ago to be reunited with his wife and three children; they had come to the United States in the late 1970s. The wife had been working as a housekeeper in a motel and was able to get by with her English. The three children had completed their formal education, and each had been working in a high-technology industry. Mr. Phuoc was referred to the mental health clinic for treatment of depression and previous trauma-related symptoms. In the course of therapy it was discovered that Mr. Phuoc had developed severely low self-esteem since his arrival in the United States. Mr. Phuoc said, "I feel so useless now because I have to rely on my wife to support me. My children have changed; they are too Westernized, they do not listen to me, they do not honor me any more. I am just a dumb old man who cannot even speak or understand the language here." Mr. Phuoc engaged in treatment. At the beginning he was receptive only to medication therapy and resisted attempts by the counselor to engage in talk therapy. The psychiatrist and the counselor continued to meet with him together for management of his medication and gradually enticed him to talk about his family problems. Eventually, Mr. Phuoc became increasingly comfortable with this way of meeting, beyond just talking about medications. The frequency of meeting with the psychiatrist was gradually reduced, while the time and frequency of meeting with the counselor alone were increased. Through a process of active education, explanation, and refocusing, he began to understand the need to reshape the structure of his value system. He accepted his wife as an equal partner in providing for the family and agreed that it was equally fair for him to stay home to attend to the chores. As for his children, he realized that it is different in America, the children have their lives to live, and he could not expect them to behave as if they were in Vietnam. Mr. Phuoc's favorite quote was, "The world has to change too."

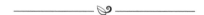

Another identity issue affected by contemporary acculturative change is sexual orientation. Homosexuality has always been acknowledged as a reality of life within Vietnamese families, but it never has been an issue that was outwardly discussed in society. In fact, the professional literature dealing with homosexuality in Vietnamese families is virtually nonexistent. However, as younger generations of Vietnamese refugees and immigrants come in greater contact with a broader range of groups, including sexual minorities, families are being forced more frequently to confront the issue of homosexuality among their sons and daughters. Therefore, this issue will likely be presented more frequently to therapists in the coming years.

TREATMENT CONSIDERATIONS
Resistance to Seeking Help

Studies have repeatedly shown that Asians underutilize mental health treatment facilities (Brown, Stein, Huang, & Harris, 1973; Pham, 2000; Sue & Sue, 1974). Some authors have attributed this to the inability of mainstream providers to meet the needs of Asian patients (Chien & Yamamoto, 1982; Stephenson, 1995; Sue & Morishima, 1985), but others have identified different factors (Kinzie et al, 2003; Kleinman, Eisenberg, & Good, 1978; McKelvey, Baldassar, Sang, & Roberts, 1999; Ngo-Metzger et al., 2003). For instance, when working with Vietnamese families, it is important for the clinician to remember that they reserve outside intervention as the last resource, to be utilized only when all internal family options have failed. Like other Asians, Vietnamese prefer to resolve problems among family members by dealing with them within the family circle. Sometimes a respected relative or an elderly friend of the family is invited to play the role of referee to help with settling differences. Going to a total stranger for advice and discussion about family or personal problems is an alien concept to most Vietnamese. It is important for the family therapist to recognize that the step taken by a Vietnamese family to seek help is itself a significant and stressful event and needs to be handled with patience, respect, and gentleness.

The Therapeutic Alliance

It is vitally important for the therapist to gain the trust of the Vietnamese family. With the exception of some urban areas, most of the communities where Vietnamese families have congregated are relatively small. One issue that concerns Vietnamese clients is confidentiality. There must be reassurance that the matters brought to the therapist will not be spread in the community. It often takes more than a few visits before the client can feel reassured and comfortable with the therapist. It is necessary to repeatedly educate the client about the professional obligation of upholding confidentiality.

Once trust has been established, the therapist may need to take an active role in the therapeutic process rather than the traditional passive and facilitatory position favored by most Western-trained therapists. Vietnamese clients are likely to see the therapist in the role of teacher, adviser, and someone who is there to give guidance in a time of trouble.

Huyen H. was 23 years old when she was referred to the mental health clinic by a caseworker in the community, who had noted Huyen's extremely withdrawn behavior and her sad affect. During the evaluation it was obvious that the young lady was severely depressed, with vegetative signs and symptoms. However, the patient was quiet and passive and denied having any problems. In subsequent months she was asked to return to the clinic for follow-up care. Although Huyen came back faithfully, she persistently refused to take part in any group therapy or activity. It was determined that the therapist would see her for individual treatment. Huyen remained passive and quiet and took her medicines as instructed. The therapist met with the patient regularly, engaged her actively in conversation, and educated her about the new country. Five months into the process, Huyen asked for permission to tell the therapist about the ordeal she went through when she had escaped from Vietnam. The therapist subsequently learned that Huyen was raped by Thai pirates seven times on three separate occasions and twice by guards when she was jailed on an island somewhere in Malay. Huyen remained in treatment 8 years after her initial evaluation. In the beginning, she was seen by the psychiatrist and a Vietnamese counselor for medication and engaged in talk therapy when the opportunity presented itself. As time passed, Huyen began to meet with the counselor for therapy, with more time between visits with the psychiatrist. She then began attending a group that focused on depression and posttraumatic stress disorder issues, and she joined a work group as part of a vocational rehabilitation job-training program.

For Indochinese parents in general, regardless of their length of stay in America or the stage of assimilation into American culture, one of the biggest challenges arises when the therapist puts all family members on the same level in open and "equal" discussion of family problems. Therapists often encourage children "to speak their minds" with the parents listening in. This is no doubt useful when all parties involved know the rules of the game. But unless Vietnamese parents have been thoroughly prepared, this style of therapy may undermine their sense of parental authority and immediately discredit the counselor.

Another major issue in therapy is the use of interpreters. Although many have written about the importance of using trained interpreters to reach non-English-speaking clients (Kinzie, 1981; Monroe & Shiranzian, 2004), it is still very common to see those well-tested principles being violated. Many service providers make the fundamental mistake of equating an interpreter simply with someone who can speak the language of the client and some English. In many situations a family member with some English capability, who may even be the client's child, is drafted into the role of interpreter. Sometimes a friend, or even a bystander who happens to be present, is asked to be the interpreter. There is often little regard for the training and professionalism of the person who does the interpreting. In reality, no effort should be spared to have a person who has professional training in medical and mental health interpretation, and preferably with credentials recognized by the public, to assist the therapist or counselor in bridging the gaps of language and culture in the treatment process. It is better if ethnic professional therapists or counselors can be recruited to provide such services in their respective communities. The Intercultural Psychiatric Program in Oregon over the last 26 years has successfully trained a group of highly experienced ethnic mental health professionals who can provide services to clients of all Southeast Asian ethnic groups.

High Prevalence of Severe Mental Illnesses

Over the past two decades an accumulated body of data has revealed that there are high levels of distress and mental illness among traumatized refugees, including those from Southeast Asia (Gong-Guy, 1987; Kinzie et al., 1990; Steel, Silove, Pham, & Bauman,

2002). Depression and posttraumatic stress disorder (PTSD) are the most prevalent problems, although other major psychiatric illnesses are common among this population (Kinzie & Manson, 1983; Mollica, Wyshak, & Lavelle, 1987; Ton-That, 1998). Studies involving nonpatient Southeast Asian high school students have also shown high rates of both depression and PTSD (Kinzie & Sack, 1991; Sack, Him, & Dickason, 1999; Ton-That, 1998). Furthermore, other studies have shown that parents with chronic mental illnesses can adversely affect the development of the interpersonal skills of their children, as well as foster a sense of distrust of the outside world (Anthony & Cohler, 1987; Westermeyer, 1991). It is therefore important to keep in mind the dual effects of mental illness and the stress of being a refugee on the integrity of the family.

CONCLUSION

Providing mental health care for Southeast Asian families, including the Vietnamese, will continue to pose a tremendous challenge to professionals for a number of reasons. These include language barriers, different expectations of treatment resulting from different cultural perspectives, and a shortage of adequately trained professionals in the field. The development of human resources in the areas of health, mental health, and other human services is an urgent issue that needs to be addressed in order for care to be effective. Working with families of various ethnicities, like the Vietnamese, should also receive more attention from family researchers and from health care providers.

REFERENCES

Anthony, E. J., & Cohler, B. J. (Eds.). (1987). *The invulnerable child*. New York: Guilford Press.

Boehnlein, J. K., Tran, H. D., Riley, C., Vu, K. C., Tan, S., & Leung, P. K. (1995). A comparative study of family functioning among Vietnamese and Cambodian refugees. *Journal of Nervous and Mental Disease, 183*, 768–773.

Brown, T., Stein, K., Huang, K., & Harris, D. (1973). Mental illness and the role of mental health facilities in Chinatown. In S. Sue & N. Wagner (Eds.), *Asian Americans: Psychological perspectives*. Palo Alto, CA: Science and Behavior Books.

Chien, C. P., & Yamamoto, J. (1982). Asian-American and Pacific-Islander patients. In F. X. Acosta, J. Yamamoto, & L. A. Evans (Eds.), *Effective psychotherapy for low-income and minority patients*. New York: Plenum Press.

Frieze, R. (1986). The Indochinese refugee crisis. In J. Krupinsk & G. Burrows (Eds.), *The price of freedom*. New York: Pergamon Press.

Frisbie, W. P., Cho, Y., & Hummer, R. A. (2001). Immigration and the health of Asian and Pacific Islander adults in the United States. *American Journal of Epidemiology, 153*, 372–380.

Golden, J. M., & Duster, M. C. (1977). Hazards of misdiagnosis due to Vietnamese folk medicine. *Clinical Pediatrics, 16*, 949–950.

Gong-Guy, E. (1987). *The California Southeast Asians' Mental Health Needs Assessment* (California State Department Mental Health Contract #85-7628-2A-2). Oakland, CA: Asian Community Mental Health Services.

Hinton, W. L., Tiet, Q., Tran, C. G., & Chesney, M. (1997). Predictors of depression among refugees from Vietnam: A longitudinal study of new arrivals. *Journal of Nervous and Mental Disease, 185*, 39–45.

Ito, K. L. (1999). Health culture and the chemical encounter: Vietnamese refugees' responses to preventive drug treatment of inactive tuberculosis. *Medical Anthropology Quarterly, 13,* 338–364.

Kinzie, J. D. (1981). The evaluation and psychotherapy of Indochinese refugee patients. *American Journal of Psychotherapy, 35,* 251–261.

Kinzie, J. D., Boehnlein, J. K., Leung, P. K., Moore, L., Riley, C., & Smith, D. (1990). The high prevalence rate of PTSD and its clinical significance among Southeast Asian refugees. *American Journal of Psychiatry, 41,* 813–917.

Kinzie, J. D., & Fleck, J. (1987). Psychotherapy with severely traumatized refugees. *American Journal of Psychotherapy, 41,* 82–94.

Kinzie, J. D., & Leung, P. K. (1993). Psychiatric care of Indochinese Americans. In A. C. Gaw (Ed.), *Culture, ethnicity, and mental illness.* Washington, DC: American Psychiatric Press.

Kinzie, J. D., Leung, P. K., Bui, A., Rath, B., Keopraseuth, K., Riley, C., et al. (1988). Group therapy with Southeast Asian refugees. *Community Mental Health Journal, 24,* 157–166.

Kinzie, J. D., & Manson, S. (1983). Five years' experience with Indochinese refugee psychiatric patients. *Journal of Operational Psychiatry, 14,* 105–111.

Kinzie, J. D., & Sack, W. (1991). Severely traumatized Cambodian children: Research findings and clinical implications. In F. L. Ahearn Jr. (Ed.), *Refugee children traumatized by war.* Baltimore: Johns Hopkins University Press.

Kleinman, A. M., Eisenberg, L., & Good, B. (1978). Culture, illness and care: Clinical lessons from anthropological and cross-cultural research. *Annals of Internal Medicine, 88,* 251–258.

Lee, E. (1988). Cultural factors in working with Southeast Asian refugee adolescents. *Journal of Adolescence, 11,* 167–169.

McKelvey, R. S., Baldassar, L. V., Sang, D. L., & Roberts L. (1999). Vietnamese parental perceptions of child and adolescent mental illness. *Journal of the American Academy of Child and Adolescent Psychiatry, 38,* 1302–1309.

Mollica, R. F., Wyshak, G., & Lavelle, J. (1987). The psychosocial impact of war trauma and torture on Southeast Asian refugees. *American Journal of Psychiatry, 144,* 1507–1572.

Monroe, A. D., & Shiranzian, T. (2004). Challenging linguistic barriers to health care: Students as medical interpreters. *Academic Medicine, 79,* 118–122.

Muecke, M. A. (1983). In search of healers—Southest Asian refugees in the American health care system [Special issue]. *Western Journal of Medicine, 139*(6), 835–840.

Mull, D. S., Nguyen, N., & Mull, J. D. (2001). Vietnamese diabetic patients and their physicians: What ethnography can teach us. *Western Journal of Medicine, 175,* 307–311.

Nemoto, T., Aoki, B., Huang, K., Morris, A., Nguyen, H., & Wong, W. (1999). Drug use behaviors among Asian drug users in San Francisco. *Addictive Behaviors, 24,* 823–838.

Ngo-Metzger, Q., Massozli, M. P., Clarridge, B. R., Manocchia, M., Davis, R. B., Iezzoni, L. I., & Phillips, R. S. (2003). Linguistic and cultural barriers to care. *Journal of General Internal Medicine, 18,* 44–52.

Nguyen, S. D. (1985). Mental health services for refugees and immigrants in Canada. In T. C. Owan (Ed.), *Southeast Asian mental health: Treatment, prevention, services, training, and research.* Washington, DC: U.S. Department of Health and Human Services.

Pham, T. (2000). Investigating the use of services for Vietnamese with mental illness. *Journal of Community Health, 25,* 411–425.

Sack, W. H., Him, C., & Dickason, D. (1999). Twelve-year follow-up study of Khmer youths who suffered massive war trauma as children. *Journal of the American Academy of Child and Adolescent Psychiatry, 38,* 1173–1179.

Steel, Z., Silove, D., Pham, T., & Bauman, A. (2002). Long-term effect of psychological trauma on the mental health of Vietnamese refugees resettled in Australia: A population-based study. *Lancet, 360,* 1056–1062.

Stephenson, P. H. (1995). Vietnamese refugees in Victoria, B.C.: An overview of immigrant and refugee health care in a medium-sized Canadian urban centre. *Social Science and Medicine, 40,* 1591–1596.

Sue, S., & Morishima, J. (1985). *The mental health of Asian Americans*. San Francisco: Jossey-Bass.

Sue S., & Sue, D. (1974). MMPI comparisons between Asian-American and non-Asian students utilizing a student health psychiatric clinic. *Journal of Counseling Psychology, 21*, 423–427.

Ta, K., Westermeyer, J., & Neider, J. (1996). Physical disorders among Southeast Asian refugee outpatients with psychiatric disorders. *Psychiatric Services, 47*, 975–979.

Ton-That, N. (1998). Post-traumatic stress disorder in Asian refugees. *Psychiatry and Clinical Neuroscience, 52*(Suppl.), S377–S379.

Westermeyer, J. (1991). Psychiatry services for refugees' children: An overview. In F. L. Ahearn Jr. & J. L. Athey (Eds.), *Refugee children: Theory, research, and services*. Baltimore: Johns Hopkins University Press.

PART V

❧

ASIAN INDIAN
AND PAKISTANI FAMILIES

CHAPTER 28

Asian Indian Families

An Overview

Rhea Almeida

> When I despair, I remember that all through history the way of truth and love has always won. There have been tyrants, and murderers, and for a time they can seem invincible, but in the end they always fall, always.
>
> —Mahatma Gandhi

This chapter presents an overview of the Asian Indian culture and discusses some differences between Hindus, Muslims, and Christians of Indian origin. Historically, Indians have been tolerant toward cultural and religious diversity, with many different religious groups migrating to India, including the Jews and Parsis. India's greatest historical intolerance is toward women and harijans (untouchable caste). The current raging conflict between Hindus and Muslims is a reflection of both contemporary fundamentalism and the unresolved tensions created by colonial partition.

ASIAN INDIAN FAMILIES
IN A HISTORICAL AND CULTURAL CONTEXT

The relation of India to the global context is tied to its history and to its location in the global path of trade and migration. It has always been an invader's paradise. No matter how many Persians, Greeks, Chinese nomads, Arabs, Portuguese, British, and other conquerors marauded this land, local Hindu kingdoms survived. These dynasties, built on the roots of a culture established for 5,000 years,[1] had a written language and were highly sophisticated.

The first groups to invade India were the Aryans, who came out of the north in about 1500 B.C. They brought strong cultural traditions that, miraculously, remain in force today. They spoke, wrote, and later used Sanskrit in the first documentation of the Vedas. Though they were warriors and conquerors, the Aryans lived alongside Indus, introducing them to the caste system and establishing the basis of the Indian religions. The Aryans inhabited the northern regions for about 700 years, then moved farther south and east when they developed iron tools and weapons. They eventually settled the Ganges valley and built large kingdoms throughout much of northern India.

Originating in the south as early as 3,000 B.C., they built complex, mathematically planned cities, some of which were almost 3 miles in diameter and contained 30,000 residents, along with granaries, citadels, and even household toilets. India's long history of survival has been due largely to its people's tolerance of diversity and their ability to integrate the best from the host culture, while expanding to absorb the invaders' strengths.

European colonization began with the Portuguese, trading in Goa as early as 1510 and later founding three colonies on the west coast in Diu, Bassein, and Mangalore. In 1610, the British, with their East India Company, created their own outpost at Surat. This marked the beginning of a remarkable presence that lasted over 300 years, eventually controlling the entire subcontinent.

The British dominated more than 300 million people through a highly organized system called the Raj. They lost no time in competing with the Portuguese, the Dutch, and the French. Through a combination of combat and deft alliances with local princes, by 1769 the East India Company controlled all European trade in India. The Raj constructed the infrastructure and trained natives for its own military, although in theory these were for India's own defense.

Finally, in 1858, claiming to be interested primarily in trade, the Raj established a seamless imperialism, with the princes ruling in name only. The current patterns of globalization are glaringly similar to this imperialist control of resources.

The Raj's demise was partially a result of its remarkable success. India had become a profitable venture, and the British were loath to allow the Indian population *any* power in a system that they viewed as their own accomplishment. As the 20th century dawned, there were increasing discontent and movements toward self-rule.

Prior to British colonization, Muslims and Hindus had lived harmoniously from about the 8th century (Nanda, 1990), with many Hindus converting to Islam. Over 1,200 years, Islam offered a kinder fate than the caste system. Numerous Hindus and Muslims were equals in social, political, and legal status.

Arab traders had visited the western coast since 712, but it was not until 1001 that the influence of Muslim world began to make itself keenly felt. Turkish kings ruled the Muslim acquisition until 1397, when the Mongols invaded under Timur Lang (Tamerlane) and ravaged the entire region. Islamic India fragmented after the brutal devastation that Timur Lane left in Delhi, and it was every Muslim strongman for himself. The situation changed, however, in 1527, when the Mughal (Persian for *Mongol*) monarch Babur came into power. Babur was a complicated, enlightened ruler from Kabul who wrote cultural treatises on the Hindus he conquered. He loved poetry and gardening and even took elaborate notes on the local flora and fauna. Babur conquered the Punjab (the northern region of India) and quickly asserted his own claim over them by taking Delhi. This was the foundation of the Mughal dynasty, whose six emperors ruled the most influential of all the Muslim dynasties in India.

Babur died in 1530, leaving behind his grandson, Akbar, the greatest Mughal ruler of all. Unlike his grandfather, Akbar, more warrior than scholar, extended the empire as far south as the Krishna river. Akbar tolerated local religions and married a Hindu princess, establishing a tradition of cultural acceptance that would contribute greatly to the success of the Mughal rule. In 1605, his son Jahangir, who passed the expanding empire along to his own son Shah Jahan in 1627, succeeded Akbar. One of the colossal monuments of his era was the Taj Majal, a tomb built in memory of his wife. The Mughal Empire crumbled, just as the Europeans were about to launch their own imperialistic maneuvers. The Portuguese held Goa until the 1950s, when Nehru regained it militarily.

The desire for independence, coupled with the challenge to colonial rule, heightened tensions between Hindus and Muslims. The Muslims, a minority, were wary of an exclusively Hindu government, resisting the Raj. Mohammed Al Jinnah, a Muslim leader, playing to the fears engendered by the forces of colonization, advocated the partition of India into two states: Muslim and Hindu.

In 1915, Mohandas Karamchand Gandhi emerged, calling for unity between the two groups (Gandhi, 1983). The profound impact Gandhi had on India and his ability to gain independence through a totally nonviolent mass movement, made him one of the most remarkable leaders the world has ever known. However, many scholars of liberation in India today question the authenticity and wisdom of Gandhi's contributions. It is quite widely known that Gandhi saw the British as India's savior for many years. As a British sympathizer in World War II, he urged the Indian troops to fight with the British. His activism came late in life.

Many wonder whether some of Gandhi's compromises contributed to the adversarial separation of the subcontinent. Certainly, independence came at a great cost. There is also a growing body of criticism in regard to his abusive treatment of his wife, while publicly pledging to liberate women and harijans.

Muslims: The Myths and Facts about Islam

In a tumultuous world that struggles with multiple forms of terrorism and oppression, it is crucial to remember the traditions within Christianity, Judaism, Islam, and other faiths that oppose terrorizing and killing others. Furthermore, it is essential to provide children and families with critical knowledge.

The spiritual practice of Islam has existed in the United States since the late 19th century. The tragic deaths of thousands of Americans and multinationals on September 11, 2001, created a curiosity about Islam and Muslim communities. Unfortunately, it also refueled the undercurrent of hate and bias that is a part of many Americans' intolerance of difference.

Before examining some of the myths and facts about Islam, it is necessary to situate the current interest in Islam within the larger context of this country's attitude toward difference.

The question asked by a number of politicians, news media, and many Americans following 9/11 was "Who are they?" and, more recently, "How can we root them out of all civilized cultures?" These questions stem from intolerance and a lack of critical knowledge. According to FBI statistics, although 40% of hate crimes target Blacks, and 13% are anti-White, the greatest increase in hate crimes in recent years is against Asians (indiscriminate targeting of brown-skinned people) and homosexuals.

The indiscriminate incarceration of thousands of South Asians after 9/11 is similar to what occurred prior to the Japanese internment following Pearl Harbor. The recent massive outsourcing of jobs to India, and the loss/lack of jobs for many Americans, is bound to heighten racial tensions with respect to South Asians in general. More than ever, a deeper knowledge of the other, the Asian Indian, is needed.

An examination of some widely held myths about Muslims and Islam, and some facts about this ancient religion and its diverse practitioners, can be helpful:

Myths

- Muslim families are more male-dominated than families from other cultures.
- Islam encourages the veiling, or *purdah*, of women.
- All Muslims originate from the Middle East.
- All Muslims are radical fundamentalists.
- All Muslims are terrorists.
- All Muslims are willing to commit suicide to fight a holy war for their cause.
- All Muslims hate Western culture, democracy, and freedom.

Facts

- Muslims are an enormously heterogeneous group. Their beliefs are based on a broad continuum of cultural, spiritual, ethnic, and political principles and influences. Because Muslims live in many parts of the world, the level of acculturation within the host countries also affects the "purity" of the Islamic beliefs and practices. (Almeida, 1997).
- The male domination of women in families varies from group to group and within groups.[2]
- Islam is the fastest growing religion in the United States and in the world.
- Not all Arabs are Muslims.[3] About 85% of the world's Muslims are *not* Arabs.
- Muslims believe in nonviolence; the Qur'an teaches peace.
- Islamic beliefs range widely, from extreme fundamentalism to conservatism and progressive theology.

Islam, a religion practiced by Muslims, is based on the holy book, the Qur'an. *Islam*, from the term *salaam*, means peace, and was preached by the prophet Muhammad, who appeared in Mecca about 1,400 years ago. Muhammad is the "final prophet," completing the earlier revelations from God (in Arabic, *Allah*) that were intended to correct the discrepancies found in the practices of Christianity and Judaism. Although the universal norm of viewing women as lesser beings is often laid at the door of Islamic theology, Muhammad's wife, Khadija, is actually credited with being the first person to believe and accept the message from God, and the first convert to Islam. Muhammad became fearful after a visit from the angel Gabriel. Khadija encouraged her husband to accept the word of God and the role of the messenger (El Saadawi, 1999). Embraced by her story, feminist writers consider Khadija to be a significant participant in the founding of Islam. Furthermore, Muhammad had only daughters, and he used his political power to ensure that all of them would be cared for. Years before his death, he bestowed on his wives the title "Mother of Believers."

The Qu'ran describes five major tenets by which Muslim men and women should conduct themselves. These are the Five Pillars of Islam:

- *Shahada*—to believe in one God, Allah, and Muhammad as his messenger.
- *Salat*—to pray five times a day facing Mecca (rapid exercise in intense meditation).
- *Ramadan*—to fast from sunrise to sunset, for 28 days, during the month of Ramadan.
- *Zakat*—to give generously to poor and disadvantaged people.
- *Haj*—to go, at least once, on a pilgrimage to Mecca (the birthplace of Muhammad)

The primary teaching of the Qur'an is the value of piety and moral responsibility: *taqwa*. Literally, *taqwa* means, "to protect oneself" against moral dangers. Taqwa enables a follower of the Qur'an to discern right from wrong and to be the judge of his or her own actions.

At the societal level, Islamic states govern on the principles of the Qur'an, which prohibits slavery; emphasizes charity toward those in need; places great importance on education, regardless of sex, age, and race; and prioritizes family life and collective values. A Muslim does not "own" his or her life and hence cannot end it. A Muslim can give and take life "in the path of Allah," as a martyr in *jihad*, or holy war. Martyrs are those who die defending themselves, their families, community, or country against aggression. Suicide in the Muslim community is rare, and the current association of suicide bombers with Islam cannot be analyzed solely within a cultural/religious framework, but rather within the larger contemporary discourse of global oppression and genocide (Pilger, 2002; Roy, 2003).

As stated earlier, Muslims are as heterogeneous in their expression of customs, religious practices, and beliefs as the cultures and societies in which they live. An exploration of these subtle and broad differences is essential (Khalidi, 1991).

For example, Muslim tradition incorporated veiling, a form of purdah, or gender segregation, which originated as a Byzantine practice. It ranges from totally covering a woman's face, head, and body, to a partial covering, to the wearing of the Salwar Kameese (pajama pants with a tunic top) as many Indian and Pakistani women do, with a thin chiffon shawl thrown around the shoulders or head.

Western feminists often view this covering one-dimensionally, as oppressive. In contrast, Muslim feminists, defend veiling (*hijab*) as a cultural symbol of collectivity aimed at countering individualism, a Western ideal, which is often a source of conflict at various points in the life cycle. Writers such as Saha Farah and Taslima Nasrin, who have been outspoken critics of Islamic fundamentalism and its impact on women and children, assert that although veiling maintains boundaries that separate women, it also organizes family and community life in Muslim societies, ensuring the control by men over women's sexual lives (Mernissi, 1982). Such segregation, paradoxically, allows women to excel in female education systems (Mernissi, 1992). Segregated Muslim women have pointed out that they feel safer from rape and attack than women who live in integrated societies.

For instance, Islamic law (*Shari'a*, or personal law) is inherently incompatible with a secular democracy because it determines religious, social, and political standards that Muslims must follow. Today, however, Pakistan has secular laws, which do not infringe on the *Shari'a*, and religious laws. Marriage, divorce, family relationships, and inheritance, however, remain areas of religious law, frequently respected by U.S. courts even though the ruling would be unjust according to secular law (Saijwani, 1989).

The Qur'an also contains certain moral and legal ordinances, forbidding activities such as drinking, gambling, and eating pork. It defines penalties for crimes and sets forth rules for marriage, divorce, and inheritance (Cooper, 1993). Nevertheless, these practices receive varying degrees of social recognition in different countries, according to the educational level, economics, societal influences, immigration patterns, and acculturation influences that dictate the level of observance.

Another challenge for therapists is the tendency to view Muslim women as representing the epitome of disempowerment and patriarchal control. Without a thorough examination of the complex historical, class, and religious differences within the larger group, one may assume that women experience intolerably inferior status, citing polygamy, divorce by repudiation, the wearing of the veil, segregation, imprisonment in household tasks, strict dependence on their husbands, and a lack of legal rights (Arkoun, 1994).

Between 1937 and 1986, Muslim women gained legal rights regarding their consent to marriage, inheritance, polygamy, and divorce. Although it is true that these rights are enforced in India to varying degrees, depending on the region (Lateef, 1990) and the particular sect (Al-Hibri, 1982; Baffoun, 1982), many Muslim feminists consider the segregation of women to be a less serious problem than class inequality.

Poverty has enormous implications for children, girls in particular, who receive little education and few societal protections (Mernissi, 1982, 1992). This class schism is profoundly impacted by the way other cultures, including the United States, relate to Muslim societies, exploiting the poor and promoting the elite through which their interests, but not necessarily Muslim interests, are served. (The oil resources of the Middle East are a good example of such interests.)

Unequal access to knowledge further divides the Muslim world, creating animosity between classes, as well as polarization between traditional religious practices and modern Western ideas. The resulting violence of today is certainly, in part, a reflection of this situation.

Asian Indian Muslims and Christians, like other Asian Indians, consider marriage the most important life cycle transition (Ahmad, 1976; Almeida, 1997). Parents often plan for this event from the time their children are very young. In Muslim practice, marriage brings together two families rather than two individuals. Although intermarriage is prevalent, it continues to be viewed as a threat to the integrity of the family, culture, and faith. There are great challenges confronting young men and women who revere many aspects of their culture, but also embrace what the host culture offers, a view that is in sharp contrast to their religious and familial beliefs.

Like Hindus, Muslim families are likely to live in a hierarchical, joint (extended) family system of three or four generations, which demands respect and obedience toward elders, while encouraging interdependence and conformity (Rizvi, 1989; Williams, 1991). This often creates a formidable barrier for women and adolescents in challenging the hierarchy in an effort to reshape family life.

Adolescence, young adulthood, and marriage are often sources of conflict. Neither adolescence nor leaving home is part of the extended life cycle stage within Muslim and Hindu families, and either can have a dynamic effect on an already embattled immigrant family. Explaining the normalcy of these transitions can be greatly reassuring to Muslim clients. Marriages, whether arranged or not, bring many unresolved conflicts surrounding the issue of leaving home (Almeida, 1997; Vaidyanathan & Naidoo, 1991).

In many marriages between individuals from India or Pakistan, and those of the United States, the couples have a difficult time adjusting to intimate life with a "stranger," one of them with the values of friendship from the homeland and the other with the friendship values of this country. Men in these marriages frequently resort to violence in order to gain the status expected in traditional marriages.

Women, however, keep the code of silence for fear of shaming their families within the community. A lot is at stake when two individuals across two continents bring their families together in marriage.

Many of these dilemmas bring Asian Indians to therapy. Although highly literate, they are often quite naïve about sexual and emotional issues. There is a gap between their emotions and their intellect. Offering them a critical consciousness and ideas for empowerment and accountability is usually well received (Almeida, Parker, & Dolan-Delvecchio, 2005; Hernandez, Almeida, & Dolan-Delvecchio, in press).

India has a culture consisting of highly educated and technologically advanced people, as well as those who are illiterate and do not fit the model minority profile. Therapists see this range of immigrants today in this country.

Hindus

The culture of Asian Indians exists within a context of contradictions. Heavenly icons such as Shiva and Shakti represent the *yin* and *yang*, or the male and female aspects of spirituality. They embody the strength and power of resistance, together with love and compassion for self and others. The Day of Goddess Gouri (Goddess of Knowledge and Enlightenment) and the Day of God Ganesha (God of Learning and God of Obstacles) are High Holy Days celebrated in most Hindu homes. Women, revered in the scriptures, are nevertheless devalued in everyday life (Bumiller, 1990; Mitter, 1991). (The goddess Durga/Kali is sought after as well as feared by men, who feel powerless before her.)

However, despite this antiquated cultural phenomenon, the Indian constitution provides for equality between the sexes. With a population of 800 million people, India is the largest democracy in the world. Tolerance and diversity are central to the Asian Indian culture, and significantly embodied in Hindu beliefs (Almeida, 1990).[4] Indians believe in the connectedness of all living things and in immortality maintained by reincarnation. This belief is reflected in the notion that when we die, the soul is born again into another human being or animal. Thus, patience and compassion toward all beings and the universe are essential human qualities. These values are embodied in the concepts of *karma* (destiny), caste (a hierarchical organization of human beings), and *dharma* (living life in accordance with the principles that order the universe), essential ideas for understanding the worldview of Asian Indian families, whether they are Hindu, Christian, Muslim, or Parsi.

An individual belongs to the caste of his or her parents and cannot change from one caste to another. Castes are usually associated with traditional occupations. There are distinct boundaries between castes and prohibitions against intermarriage, members of different castes eating together, and other customs of spatial purity and accordance of pollution.

Although the Indian constitution specifically outlaws the demeaning and oppressive aspects of the caste system—particlarly those that limit the full participation of the lowest caste, the untouchables (now called scheduled castes)—caste consciousness and hierarchical relations based on caste distinctions have not disappeared from the modern political and social scene (Lynch, 1969; Malayala, Kamaraju, & Ramana, 1984; Nanda, 1990, p. 144).

Asian Indians have greater affiliation across religious lines than across caste lines. Sikhs (a sect of Hinduism) Muslims, Christians, Jews, Buddhists, and Parsis or Zoroastrians (a Persian sect) constitute 20% of India's population, but the overarching Hindu beliefs of caste and *karma* structure Indian society. Although Sanskrit words such as *varna* and *suklatva* refer to standards and classes of things, the European racist ideology of whiteness and darkness has come to inform the caste system, which is now strongly associated with skin color. Much is written about the fair-skinned Aryan versus the Black Dravidian.

In the context of Asian colonial history, religious writings about the forces of lightness and darkness in the universe are interpreted literally to refer to skin color: Dark skin denotes evil, and light skin denotes rebirth and fairness. Matrimonial advertisements in Indian newspapers, as well as *India Abroad*, use a complex color code reflecting the demand for women with whitish or fair skin color and light eyes. For men, the demand is for handsome and well-educated individuals, as well as those of particular castes (skin color not defined) and religions.

Hinduism is secular in its spirituality, in that worship at a temple is not necessary to practice Hindu beliefs. Indian society acts as a sanctioning system for Hindu beliefs. Indian families in the United States must maintain their beliefs within the privacy of their homes, with no societal support, unlike members of Christian faiths who enjoy both private and public practice of their beliefs.

This responsibility for maintaining its spirituality frequently skews the adaptability of a family toward inflexibility. Therapists must assess acculturation within this context (Sodowsky & Carey, 1988). The high level of education and professional skills of many Asian Indians, as well as their language fluency, has enabled them to achieve a privileged status in the United States. However, since September 11, 2001, and with the current trend toward outsourcing, this situation is changing.

Christians

Missionaries, arriving in the wake of Portuguese, French, Dutch, and English colonization, brought Christianity to India, resulting in the establishment of Catholicism and various Protestant denominations. As is common in the colonial experience, converts to Christianity in India integrated their new religion with their original indigenous beliefs, which arose primarily out of Hinduism.

Asian Christians tend to be more flexible than Hindus in regard to their adolescent children, allowing both boys and girls to attend church and to engage in other social activities, including dating. Unlike their Hindu and Muslim counterparts, they have no dietary or dress restrictions. Although they may acculturate more rapidly, like other Asian Indian immigrants Asian Christians struggle with family transitions and cultural adjustment (Misumi, 1993).

The influence of Hindu beliefs, even in an acculturated Christian family, is clear. Girls learn from an early age that their sexuality is tied to family honor, so any violation of sexual purity before marriage brings disgrace to the family. Boys are also constrained by taboos about premarital sex, but are also expected to be "Don Juans" when they marry. In spite of these taboos, mixed-youth parties, dances, and music are central to the culture of Christian families.

FAMILY ISSUES

Acculturation

Within the pedagogy of acculturation, assimilation is a process whereby members of a newly arrived group subordinate to the host culture, in lieu of emphasizing their own cultural identity. White racial identity is the preferred norm. Acculturation is the process of maintaining an identity with one's culture of origin, *while* adapting to the host culture.

Obscured in the literature is the reciprocal experience that occurs when two cultures integrate. Through contact and connection, marginal cultures have a strong and positive impact on the mainstream culture (Visram, 1986). This is evidenced notably in jazz and rap—an African American art form—clothig styles, food, music by Indian classicists like Ravi Shankar, who was popularized by the Beatles, and various forms of mysticism and spirituality derived from Hinduism. Except for skin color, Asian Indians are seen by the host culture as fitting in smoothly[5] ("passing") because of their language competence and Caucasian likeness.

Further impacting acculturation is the fact that Hindus were romanticized during the 1960s. The Hare Krishna movement, which promoted belief in other-world natural powers and rejection of material values, was in alignment with a general quest for Indian spirituality by children of the 1960s This altered the primitive view of Asian Indians as polytheists (i.e., spiritually depraved).

Prashad (2000) is critical of how "godmen" like Deepak Chopra have exploited the stereotype of inherent spirituality. Asian Indians and Pakistanis of Muslim faith have not experienced the same measure of acceptance

The challenge of maintaining one's identity, versus acquiescing to colonial socialization, continues to be a struggle. Prashad (2000, p. ix) quotes Du Bois (1996) when he decries India's

> temptation to stand apart from the darker peoples and seek her affinities among whites. She has long wished to regard herself as "Aryan," rather than "colored" and to think of herself as much nearer physically and spiritually to Germany and England than to Africa, China or the South Seas.
>
> Yet, the history of the modern world shows the futility of this thought. European exploitation desires the black slave, the Chinese coolies, and the Indian laborer for the same ends and the same purposes, and calls them all "niggers."[6]

For Asian Indian families in the United States, acculturation varies, depending on education, class, caste, family size, economic support, connections to their traditional culture, degree of religiosity, past migration history, and other factors. The levels of stress that families endure depend on these factors (Almeida, 1997; Krishna & Berry, 1992). Sikhs were one of the first groups of Indians to enter the United States as migrant workers

386 eg V. ASIAN INDIAN AND PAKISTANI FAMILIES

in California in the early 1900s. Many of them married Mexican women (Takaki, 1989). Although the American Dream continues to elude some, Asian Indians on the whole are the wealthiest ethnic group in the United States today (Papadimitriou, 1994).

Women who work in their homes acculturate later than their male counterparts. Many women do, however, participate in the labor force and demonstrate greater role flexibility (Gune, 1994). Men continue to enjoy the privileged status of the work world, while maintaining traditional expectations in the home. Their wives, mothers, and daughters honor their expectations. However, women who work outside the home acculturate at rates similar to those of men, often demonstrating even greater role flexibility.[7]

Women who contribute to their families' earnings enjoy greater decision making about spending than their mothers-in-law had in either India or the United States. This has encouraged elderly parents to visit and live with their sons *and* their daughters, rather than seeking the traditional arrangement of living with sons.

The higher the social class and the longer the time since immigration, the weaker the allegiance to traditional gender roles and the greater the tolerance for balancing individual and family loyalties (Dhruvarjan, 1993). Thus, women are launching their careers before marriage, negotiating the completion of their educational dreams with arranged marriages, and successfully leaving abusive marriages. There is also a growing gay and lesbian community among these Asian immigrants.

Life Cycle

Indians expect to follow a life course, referred to as *dharma*, that presents separate patterns for men and women. Traditionally, men had four life stages: studentship, householder, forest dweller, and homeless wanderer. As householders and forest dwellers, men marry and fulfill family responsibilities. During the studentship and wandering stages, they live as single individuals, free of any worldly desires. Although few Hindu men achieve all stages, they are supported in their quest for study, marriage, children, and spiritual self-fulfillment.

As "good Hindus," women expect to marry early and produce sons. When families do educate their daughters, it is usually with the goal of making them more marketable as brides, as opposed to any commitment to their personal development (Almeida, 1997; Roland, 1988).[8]

Asian Indian families have an elaborate network of relationships, determined by male lineage (Ayakar, 1994; Kolenda, 1993). Families will embrace daughters when there are one or more sons. Concerning higher education and dating, girls are subject to lower standards than their brothers. When a woman marries, she typically leaves her family of origin and moves into the home of her husband's family. There are some regional differences in this practice.

In some regions, a new bride may make a long visit to her own parents' home until the birth of the first child. A new bride's measure of purity (tolerance) rests in her ability to adjust to all of the women in her husband's family and to honorably accept the numerous tasks delegated to her. In this country, this adjustment may be required all year round, or periodically when the family visits. During the early years of marriage, she visits her husband briefly at night. These practices continue until the children, preferably sons, provide status to the wife in the in-laws' home.

Although women in general have low status, mothers-in-law have a tremendous amount of power over their daughters-in-law, increasing their desire to have sons. A mother-in-law may be involved in many aspects of a couple's relationship, even their intimate sex life, asking the son if he is being pleasured in the way a good wife ought to pleasure him, offering her opinion about the number of children the couple should have, their preferred sex, child care, second-shift responsibilities, money, work, child rearing, and social activities. Abusive behaviors, ranging from emotional intimidation and harassment to domestic violence, arise from dissatisfaction with dowries, women who refuse subjugation, and the sex of the grandchildren.

This conjoint home physically and economically supports the sons, their families, unmarried sisters, and paternal aunts (single or widowed), as well as the parents. Men expect to care financially for this entire family system. As immigrants, they support family members who arrive on student visas, as well as siblings and *their* families back in India or Pakistan.

In general, everyone, including older siblings and extended family, pampers children. A 4- or 5-year-old child is often less independent than children of European background. Sibling roles vary, depending on the region of origin in India (Kolenda, 1993; Nuckolls, 1993). Brothers expect to live and cooperate with one another.

In many regions, a sister must leave at marriage to join her husband's family. In others, she returns to her parents' home after the marriage, sometimes until the children are of school age. Brothers are responsible for the general welfare of sisters, including their marriages. After marriage, they turn responsibility for their sisters over to the husbands. This frequently results in a relationship cutoff.

Anthropological studies have shown a positive relationship between inheritance rights that favor the brothers in family, large dowries paid for a sister, and lifelong connections between brothers and their sisters. Noteworthy here is the fact that large dowries for sisters are included in the male inheritance rights, thereby reducing the emotional conflicts that occur in families in which sisters have no rights to family inheritance.

Brothers, however, seem to cultivate stronger bonds with one another in the interest of preserving the family legacy, often guided by economics. Like many other family patterns, immigration, economics, and acculturation can alter this legacy. It is not uncommon for older siblings to assume parental responsibilities for their younger siblings as early as age 9 or 10.

In northern India, there is a particular celebration of the brother–sister dyad, called *raki*. This celebration consists of a ritual whereby sisters give bracelets and cook a meal for their brothers. Brothers, in turn, bring gifts and money for their sisters, whether they are single or married. The common term *cousin brother*, which describes first and second cousins, is used to extend the loyalty between sibling dyads to cousins.

Parenting for most mainstream Americans is complex, given the current context of violence in schools and little to no support for mothers in the workforce. Added to these stressors for Indian parents is their desire to maintain traditional family patterns while upholding high expectations for their children. Lack of knowledge about developmental changes as they pertain to setting limits, for a child, differentiating between the positive and the harmful sources of information gathered from the Internet, music, TV, and the like, and the various ways in which children can socialize (sports for girls, sleepovers for all children) are among the many challenges they face. "Philosophical talks" are favored over behavioral consequences. Because of the collective psychology, single interventions such as time-out procedures, or rewards for positive behaviors, are not consistent with cultural and family values.

Adolescent sexuality is defined within the value structure of purity and pollution, and therefore free expression of sexuality is regarded as incongruent with spirituality. Masturbation is discouraged; rather, boys are encouraged to meditate. Asian Indian adolescents living in the United States often feel caught between two worlds: their family and culture versus the prevalent values in the United States. Then there is the gay issue.

For young gay and lesbian adults, identity confusion may develop in regard to the coming-out process. The notion of a third gender, or *hijra*, appears in the scriptures. *Hijras* worship the Mother goddess, saying, "It is the Mata who gives us life, we live only in her power" (Nanda, 1990, p. 26). Historically they held powerful roles in the community by performing at weddings and births, bringing good *karma* to the event and enjoyed support in communal living. However, as with other paradoxes in Indian culture, homosexuality is not culturally sanctioned (Nanda, 1990).[9]

Gays and lesbians in the United States struggle between the pressures to marry and retain the support and buffering of their communities against racism, or to leave their communities and choose an alternate lifestyle. A gay lifestyle can only flourish outside of the ethnic enclave.

There is, however, a steadily growing activist Indian movement, named *Shakti*. In Urdu *Shakti*, the potency of female strength is represented through the creation of life. *Shakti* as an organization is critical to the transitional process, which solidifies the sexual orientation of gays and lesbians in the Asian Indian community in the United States. Contrary to Western male norms, the culture of India and Pakistan encourage close emotional bonding and physical affection between male friends (Schmitt & Sofer, 1992).

Although men have embraced these connections, and relationships between women are commonplace, Muslims tend to view gay and lesbian relationships through the prism of procreation and therefore community good. According to Dynes and Donaldson (1992, p. 27), "Islamic law and tradition tend to relate sexuality to the maintenance of the social order rather than taking the Judeo-Christian approach of treating it as a matter of individual morality." The Qur'an explicitly condemns homosexual behavior: "Whenever a male mounts a male, the throne of God trembles" (Khan, 1992, p. 27).[10]

Given their beliefs about *karma* and destiny, death is a particularly potent symbolic event for Hindus (McGoldrick et al., 2004). It is expected that widows will perform many rituals of sacrifice glorifying the family, whereas widowers and other family members are not required to perform such rites (McGoldrick et al., 2004).[11]

Family life cycle transitions can be particularly difficult when they collide with karmic values of passivity, obedience, and sacrifice. The acceptance of life's difficulties with expectations for rewards in the next life is at odds with Western constructs of pursuing one's dreams.

Treatment Strategies

Therapy remains controversial within this community. Their apparently effortless immigration, obscured by economic power, reinforces the notion that only the unsuccessful need therapy. Consultation with religious leaders such as priests, imams, and yogis is more acceptable (Musmi, 1993). This creates many ethical complications in the area of couple conflicts, domestic violence, and child abuse (Hernandez et al., in press).

The priests uphold traditional family values, therefore much of the counseling is done within the structural hierarchy of the male-centered family, rather than challenging the very structure that perpetuates many of these problems.

Muslim Christian and Hindu families come to therapy for many reasons, such as child-related difficulties; conflicts with parents regarding dating, socializing, and sexuality; domestic violence and incest; and the courtship difficulties encountered by young men. In addition, there is the increasing burden of caring for elderly family members, a huge problem facing the "sandwich generation." Depression is a common mask for mother-in-law issues, couple difficulties, problems of adolescence and launching into independence, and work-related difficulties. Men are particularly conflicted around this dilemma. The distinction between acculturation and assimilation must be clear to families and therapists. Although the scholarship on acculturation tends to present a one-sided view of adaptation, it is a reciprocal and multidimensional process. The positive influences of these immigrants on U.S. culture ought to be celebrated and central to the therapeutic process (Hutnik, 1986; Jiobu, 1988; U.S. Department of Commerce, 1993).

Even when individuals come alone for treatment, the focus of treatment for Asian Indians and Pakistanis must be connected to familial and cultural issues. Embedded within a collective psychology, the social and familial contexts are central to individual development. The following are among the problems presented by both children and adults:

- Issues of racial and cultural identity masked as somatic complaints.
- Extended family dilemmas, expressed through school-related difficulties with children who have little privacy or structural support for school, friendships, or social life.
- Family issues of violence expressed by girls with academic difficulties, depression, and suicidal thoughts. Boys sometimes exhibit arrogant behavior toward their parents and teachers, and, more recently, substance-abuse problems, while trying to fit into the mainstream culture.
- Couples with violence issues (Almeida & Dolan-Delvecchio, 1999) and those with more normative issues concerning the boundaries of intimacy within the hierarchy of the extended family. The mother–son tie can create particular conflicts for the young wife, her husband, and his mother.[12]
- Extramarital affairs.
- Issues related to loss through immigration, death, illness, and sexual orientation.

Concrete and time-limited interventions within the complex familial and cultural issues are most appropriate.[13] Therapeutic solutions should include definitions of success and happiness: If a person believes that his problem is connected to something bad he did in a past life, then some ritual about karmic fate must be created to absolve him of this bad "past" deed. Focusing on the future with an open heart and good deeds bring strong, positive life forces. With Muslim families, attention to the proper codes of behavior as defined by the Qur'an is crucial.

The following intersecting influences exacerbate family difficulties:

- Immigration and acculturation
- Adaptation to a racist culture and the identity and economic issues inherent within this context of adaptation

- The struggle of balancing autonomy and separation with collective familial and cultural loyalties
- The hierarchy of the age- and male-centered family system

The development of a strong racial/cultural identity is critical to intergenerational resilience. A "whitening" of identity is likely to be hazardous. Thus, it is crucial that the therapist empower the parents and cultural experiences while bridging these with progressive values from the dominant culture. A therapeutic endeavor that symbolizes liberation is one that weaves together progressive legacies from a specific culture and that of the host culture. For example, cultural traditions that promote equity for all members of a family regardless of whether they are old or female are progressive. Similarly, promoting violence as a hallmark of strength would be antithetical to liberation.

CONCLUSION

When treating Asian Indian families, as in treating families of all ethnic, cultural, and racial groups, therapists cannot assume that the clients are homogeneous in their backgrounds or preferences for treatment. A therapist must also be cognizant of the fact that Indian families in the United States often maintain rigid cultural boundaries as a bulwark against assimilation and racism. Such buffering is often evident in authoritarian family roles. The following are suggestions for determining the experiences of family members when they enter treatment:

1. Explore the connections of family members to one another and their economic investments in these connections.
2. Ask questions that clarify the family's cultural beliefs and traditions.
3. Because there are enormous regional differences that influence family patterns, religious values, and inheritance rights, it is important to determined which part of India or Pakistan the family is from.

    a. Assess the family's social location (class *and* caste).
    b. Explore its members' experience with Western colonization.
    c. Explore their migration history.

4. Offer direct suggestions with respect to differences in the family role structure in comparison with that of dominant nuclear families (i.e., consider the importance of a mother-in-law to the marital dyad, which may involve the couple's negotiation of money and child care while considering the mother-in-law's contributions in this marital negotiation; coach the husband to differentiate between control and inclusion; coach the husband to be generous to his wife while maintaining loyalty to his mother; acknowledge the husband's/father's importance, while offering suggestions of empowerment to the wife/mother). All of these apparently competing life trajectories can coexist in harmony.
5. Shift the structure *carefully*, empowering alliances between father and sons, fathers and daughters, and mother and children, while strengthening the marital dyad, economically, emotionally and socially.
6. Pay special attention to the life stage of the family's culture vis-à-vis mainstream

culture, so that the anxiety about loss of cultural identity is lessened—such as in the life stages of leaving home or launching, young adulthood, and anticipation of an arranged marriage.

NOTES

1. The second great invasion into India occurred around 500 B.C., when the Persian kings Cyrus and Darius, pushing their empire eastward, conquered the ever-prized Indus Valley and occupied the region for a relatively brief period, about 150 years.

   In the 5th century B.C., Siddhartha Gautama founded Buddhism, a profoundly influential work of human thought still espoused by much of the world. The Greeks conquered the Punjab in 150 B.C., and by this time Buddhism was becoming so influential that the Greek king Menander became a Buddhist himself. The local kingdoms enjoyed relative autonomy for the next few hundred years, occasionally fighting (and often losing to) invaders from the north and China, who seemed to come and go like the monsoons. (Unlike the Greeks, the Romans never made it to India, preferring to expand westward instead.) In A.D. 319, Chandragupta II founded the imperial Guptas dynasty, which conquered and consolidated the entire north and extended as far south as the Vindya Mountains. When the Guptas diminished, a golden age of six thriving and separate kingdoms ensued, and at this time, some of the most incredible temples constructed were in Bhubaneshwar, Konarak, and Khahurajo. It was a time of relative stability, and cultural developments progressed on all fronts for hundreds of years, until the dawn of the Muslim era.

   Arab traders had visited the western coast since 712, but it was not until 1001 that the Muslim world began to make itself keenly felt. Led by Mahmud of Ghazi, they raided the area just about every other year for 26 years. Then the Arab traders vanished behind the mountains for nearly 150 years.

   They returned in 1192 under Mohammed of Ghor, this time determined to stay. Ghor's armies laid waste to the Buddhist temples of Bihar, and by 1202 he had conquered the most powerful Hindu kingdoms along the Ganges. When Ghor died in 1206, one of his generals, Qutb-ud-din, ruled the far north from the sultanate of Delhi, while the southern area of India was free from the invaders. Turkish kings ruled the Muslim acquisition until 1397, when the Mongols invaded under Timur Lang (Tamerlane) and ravaged the entire region. One historian wrote that the lightning speed with which Tamerlane's armies struck Delhi was prompted by their desire to escape the stench of the rotting corpses they were leaving behind them.

2. There were strong female-centered movements even within Taliban-ruled Afghanistan, and they still exist throughout the Muslim world. El Sadaawi, an Egyptian American scholar of the Qur'an, has spent much of her life educating Americans about the compassionate and humanistic side of Islam. She is also known for taking on the *imams* (male spiritual leaders) in the United States for promoting their sexist beliefs about men and women and ascribing them to knowledge gained from the Qur'an (El Sadaawi, 1999).

3. Twelve million Arabs are Christians and thousands are Jewish (www.adc.org).

4. Some of the most important beliefs are embraced in the teachings of Mahatma Gandhi: "Not to hurt any living thing is no doubt a part of Ahimsa. However, it is its least expression. The principle of Ahimsa is hurt by every evil thought, by undue haste, by lying, by hatred, by wishing ill to anybody. It is also violated by our holding on to what the world needs" (Gandhi, 1983, p. 4). Ahimsa is the philosophy of nonviolence toward all living things, the avoidance of killing any living being for good or other purposes. It also embodies the notion of strength in diversity.

5. The notion that Asian Indians have adapted smoothly to American life is showing signs of

unraveling. Although the findings are questionable, as most of the research focuses on middle-class, educated immigrants, the trend of current data taken from domestic violence and juvenile justice statistics reveals that Asian Indians as a group are experiencing many of the difficulties that other immigrant groups face. Most important, they too are fast becoming a part of the criminal justice system (Prashad, 2000).

6. For instance, the Indian League of America has not wanted Indians to be given "minority" or non-Caucasian status out of concern that it will place them at a disadvantage. At the same time, the *Hindu Times* (which most Indians in the United States read regularly) reports efforts in India to halt globalization. One story tells of a high school teacher encouraging his students to examine the insidious and harmful effects of globalization, as he points them toward the rebuilding of India's own resources.

7. In California, for instance, women were found to have highly visible roles as grocery store and motel managers, clerks, restaurant managers, and in other professional positions.

8. Although the scriptures may revere women, in everyday life their value is not equal to that of men. They are not socialized to be independent in any facet of their lives. In dual-career households, money earned by the wife is considered, with few exceptions, to be the property of the husband and his family. A woman's identity comes from marriage, childbearing, and her status as a mother-in-law, wherein she wields tremendous power over her daughter-in-law. Being a mother of sons is celebrated more than being a mother of daughters. Female infanticide and abandoning girl babies to missionary adoption homes are especially common among poor, uneducated families. Within the United States, given the economic bounty of most families, girls are less prone to such practices. Daughters are groomed to be married; their dowries are a burden that every father and brother must carry. In a family that has only daughters, especially if it is economically disadvantaged, both mothers and daughters are vulnerable to abuse by the husband's family. They are likely to develop a myriad of somatic and psychological symptoms. Clearly, the possibility of having a lesbian or unmarried daughter is unheard of, unless in the Christian faith she responds to God's calling by becoming a nun. This is true for men as well, who might be gay, and choose God's calling as priests. Boys are highly valued, and having many sons is a way for women to gain power economically and spiritually. Even well-educated families seem to accept this prejudice.

9. *Hijras* worship the Mother goddess, saying, "It is the Mata who gives us life, we live only in her power" (Nanda, 1990, p. 26). They have historically held powerful roles in the community by performing for weddings and births, bringing good *karma* to such an event and embraced and supported in communal living.

10. Because Muslims prize family life so highly, it is not uncommon for a homosexual person to live a gay or lesbian lifestyle until marriage, then marry and have children, while continuing to have a separate homosexual partner. Homosexuals find that having a family within the boundaries of tradition and maintaining a gay lifestyle is preferable to risking alienation by pursuing an exclusively homosexual lifestyle.

11. *Sati* is a practice of burning a widow on her husband's funeral pyre. This practice was outlawed during the British Raj, but was still practiced as recently as 1987 in the state of Rajasthan. The underlying belief is that by this glorified sacrifice, a widow brings good luck to her husband, his entire family, and herself. Women defending the honor of their husbands from invading armies, and preventing through suicide the rape and capture of women and children, describe *sati* as an act of political protest. Through time, this practice is sanctioned by patriarchal notions of how widows should behave in the event of their husbands' death, the lack of appropriate status for widows, and economic difficulties. This practice attached new religious meaning to enforced suicide. There is a huge difference between the origin of Sati, a political protest act, and the evolution of Sati, as a death required and sanctioned by the culture.

12. Couples, men in particular, need a lot of help detriangling from the husband's mother and extended family, while simultaneously maintaining connections with them, and building a

structure of intimacy with the new partner. Men are strongly bonded to the idea of the mother–son connection, expecting the wife/daughter-in-law to subordinate to them and meet the expectations of this familial order.

13. For instance, Asians Indians prefer to attend a session that lasts several hours rather than weekly sessions for a single hour. This is a direct contradiction to the reimbursed therapeutic hour; however, efforts should be made to accommodate this culture's experience with *time*.

REFERENCES

Ahmad, I. (1976). *Family, kinship and marriage among Muslims in India*. New Delhi: South Asia Books.

Al-Hibri, A. (1982). *Women and Islam*. Elmsford, NY: Pergamon Press.

Almeida, R. (1990). Asian Indian mothers. *Journal of Feminist Family Therapy*, 33–40.

Almeida, R. (1996). Hindu, Muslim, and Christian families. In M. McGoldrick, J. Giordano, & J. K. Pierce (Eds.), *Ethnicity and family therapy* (2nd ed., pp. 395–424). New York: Guilford Press.

Almeida, R., & Dolan-Delvecchio, K. (1999). Addressing culture in batterer's intervention: South Asian communities as an illustrative example. *Violence Against Women*, 5(6), 654–683.

Almeida, R., Parker, L., & Dolan-Delvecchio, K. (2005). Foundation concepts for social justice based therapy: Critical consciousness, accountability, and empowerment. In E. Aldorando (Ed.), *Promoting social justice through mental health practice* Mahwah, NJ: Erlbaum.

Arkoun, M. (1994). *Rethinking Islam*. Boulder, CO: Westview Press.

Baffoun, A. (1982). Women and social change in the Muslim Arab world. In A. Al-Hibri (Ed.), *Women and Islam* (pp. 227–241). Elmsford, NY: Pergamon Press.

Bumiller, E. (1990). *May you be the mother of a hundred sons: A journey among the women of India*. New York: Random House

Cooper, M. H. (1993). Muslims in America. *CQ Researcher*, 3(16), 373–380.

Du Bois, W. E. B. (1996). *The souls of Black folk*. New York: Modern Library.

Dhruvarajan, V. (1993). Ethnic cultural retention and transmission among first generation Hindu Asian Indians in a Canadian prairie city. *Journal of Comparative Family Studies*, 24(1), 63–79.

Dynes, W., & Donaldson, S. (1992). *Asian homosexuality*. New York: Garland.

El Saadawi, N. (1999). *The hidden force of Eve: Women in the Arab world*. London: Zed Books.

Gandhi, M. K. (1983). *Autobiography*. New York: Dover.

Gune, R. (1994, October 28). Problems of South Asian women. *India Abroad*, p. 31.

Hernandez, P., Almeida, R. V., & Dolan-Delvecchio, D. (in press). Critical consciousness, empowerment and accountability. *Family Process*.

Hutnik, N. (1986). Patterns of ethnic minority identification and modes of social adaptation, *Ethnic and Racial Studies*, 9(2), 150–167.

Jayakar, K. (1994). Women of the Indian subcontinent. In L. Comas-Dias & B. Greene (Eds.), *Women of color: Integrating ethnic and gender identities in psychotherapy* (pp. 161–181). New York: Guilford Press.

Jiobu, R. M. (1988). *Ethnicity and assimilation*. Albany: State University of New York Press.

Khalidi, U. (1991). Minority role in the U.S.: A model for Muslim Indians. In U. Khalidi (Ed.), *Indian Muslims in North America* (pp. 60–63). Watertown, MA: South Asia Press.

Khan B. (1992). Not-so-gay life in Karachi: A view of a Pakistani living in Toronto. In A. Schmitt & J. Sofer (Eds.), *Sexuality and eroticism among males in Moslem societies* (pp. 79–91). New York: Harrington Park Press.

Kolenda, P. (1993). Sibling relations and marriage practices: A comparison of North, Central and South India. In C. W. Nuckolls (Ed.), *Siblings in South Asia: Brothers and sisters in cultural context* (pp. 103–142). New York: Guilford Press.

Krishna, A., & Berry, J. W. (1992). Acculturative stress and acculturation attitudes among Indian immigrants to the United States. *Psychology and Developing Societies, 4*(2), 187–212.

Lateef, S. (1990). *Muslim women in India: Political and private realities.* London and Atlantic Highlands, NJ: Zed Books.

Lynch, O. (1969). *The politics of untouchability: Social mobility and social change in a city in India.* New York: Columbia University Press.

Malayala, S., Kamaraju, S., & Ramana, K. V. (1984). Untouchability—Need for a new approach. *Indian Journal of Social Work, 45,* 361–369.

McGoldrick, M., Almeida, R., Hines, P. M., Rosen, E., Garcia-Preto, N., & Lee, E. (2004). Mourning in different cultures. In F. Walsh & M. McGoldrick (Eds.), *Living beyond loss: Death in the family* (2nd ed., pp. 86–89). New York: Norton.

Mernissi, F. (1982). Virginity and patriarchy. In A. Al-Hibri (Ed.), *Women and Islam* (pp. 183–191). Elmsford, NY: Pergamon Press.

Mernissi, F. (1992). *Islam and democracy* (M. J. Lakeland, Trans.). Reading, MA: Addison-Wesley.

Misumi, D. M. (1993). Asian-American Christian attitudes towards counseling. *Journal of Psychology and Christianity, 12*(3), 214–224.

Mitter, S. S. (1991). *Dharma's daughters—Contemorary Indian women and Hindu culture.* New Brunswick, NJ: Rutgers University Press.

Nanda, S. (1990). *Neither man nor woman: The hijras of India.* Belmont, CA: Wadsworth.

Nuckolls, C. W. (Ed.). (1993). *Siblings in South Asia: Brothers and sisters in cultural context.* New York: Guilford Press.

Papadimitriou, D. (1994). *Aspects of distribution of wealth and income.* New York: St. Marin's Press.

Pilger, J. (2002). *New rulers of the world.* London: Verso.

Prashad, V. (2000). *The karma of brown folk.* Minneapolis: University of Minnesota Press.

Rizvi, S. A. A. (1989). *Muslim tradition in psychotherapy and modern trends.* Lahore, Pakistan: Institute of Islamic Culture.

Roland, A. (1988). *In search of self in India and Japan.* Princeton, NJ: Princeton University Press.

Roy, A. (2003). *War talk.* New York: South End Press.

Saijwani, V. (1989). *The law reporter* (Vol. 5). New Brunswick, NJ: Rutgers University Press.

Schmitt, A., & Sofer, J. (Eds.). (1992). *Sexuality and eroticism among males in Moslem societies.* Binghamton, NY: Harrington Park Press.

Sodowsky, G. R., & Carey, J. C. (1988). Relationships between acculturation-related demographics and cultural attitudes of an Asian-Indian immigrant group. *Journal of Multicultural Counseling and Development, 16*(3), 117–136.

Takaki, R. (1989). Asian Indians in Southern California: Occupations and ethnicity. In I. Light & P. Bhachu (Eds.), *Immigration and entrepreneurship: Culture, capital, and ethnic networks* (pp. 96–98). New Brunswick, NJ: Transaction.

U.S. Department of Commerce. (1993). *We the American Asians.* Washington, DC: Economics and Statistics Administration, Bureau of the Census.

Vaidyanathan, P., & Naidoo, J. (1991). Asian Indians in Western countries: Cultural identity and the arranged marriage. In N. Bleichrodt & P. J. D. Drenth (Eds.), *Contemporary issues in cross-cultural psychology* (pp. 34–79). Amsterdam: Swets & Zeitlinger.

Visram, R. (1986). *Ayahs, iascars and princes: Indians in Britain 1700–1947.* London: Pluto Press.

Williams, R. (1991). Asian-Indian Muslim in the United States. In O. Khalidi (Ed.), *Indian Muslims in North America* (pp. 17–25). Watertown, MA: South Asia Press.

CHAPTER 29

Indian Hindu Families

Vimala Pillari

India represents a vast diversity, springing from an ancient civilization dating back 4,000 years. Historically, regional expansion produced India's high population density, as well as many social, economic, and cultural complexities.

India has had its share of conquerors. Starting with the arrival of the Aryans in 1500 B.C., various peoples settled in the region until some degree of unification of the entire country was reached in the 17th century under the Moguls. The Moguls expanded the agricultural economy and instituted new cultural norms of religions such as Islam. The Europeans, mainly the English, came in force in the early 17th century; for the first time, under the British, India was placed in a subordinate role within a system based on industrial production, which affected many aspects of Indian life. For example, cottage industries had long attracted foreigners to India. But with the competition of mass production, such industries became unimportant. A country that was a magnet of trade in the 18th century was, by the 20th century, an underdeveloped, overpopulated country groaning under foreign rule. In 1947, India obtained independence from foreign domination through a movement of civil disobedience and nonviolent resistance promoted by Gandhi.

The British had united India under one official language: English. However, today there are 18 official languages, including English, and about 1,652 mother tongues/dialects. Migration has caused a substantial degree of assimilation, acculturation, and intermarriage. Thus, people in India vary from the very fair-skinned to the very dark-skinned, with eye colors ranging from blue and green to the more common brown and black, with hair varying from straight to very curly and colors ranging from brown and black to lighter shades, depending on the people's historical backgrounds. By 2004, the Indian population was classified as 83% Hindus, 12% Muslims, 2.3% Christains, 1.9% Sikhs, and 0.8% others (India Election Statistics, 2004).

HINDUISM

Hinduism is the religion most associated with India by the West. But what is Hinduism? For one thing, Hinduism does not attach the same religious significance to historical events that Judaism, Christianity, and Islam do. A great deal of controversy remains over Hinduism's historical origins. It has no single founder, no central authority or fixed creed. There is evidence to show that the Hinduism of the Vedas goes back to at least 1200 B.C.

The word *Hinduism* was originally a name that the British gave to part of the Indian subcontinent and that later came to represent to the West a set of traditions, beliefs, and practices. Historically, in Vedic Hindu perception, "Truth is one; sages call it variously." The basis of Hindu philosophy is found in the four Vedas. In 800 B.C., Vedic Hinduism started with the *Rig Veda*, which is the earliest and the holiest text. It contains hymns of praise to various deities, called *devas*. These hymns were passed on orally until 1200 B.C., after which the Vedas were written down. However, this transcription took hundreds of years to complete. The other three Vedas include the *Sama Veda*, the *Yajur Veda*, and the *Atharva Veda*. Another holy text, the *Upanishads* (600 B.C.) explores the philosophical theme about the knowledge of the inner self. The *Upanishads* are not dogmas but a set of recollections and records of experiences (Sharma, 2004).

The aim of Hinduism is to enlighten rather than to convert. The Hindu worldview of pluralism (many religions) and respect for many paths has pointed to at least one way for the reconciliation of religious conflicts without calling for conversion to any one creed; Hinduism expects each religion to maintain its unique identity and practice (Sharma, 2004). The expression of Hinduism in India is itself varied and complex, although many common ideas run through it. These include *reincarnation*, a type of rebirth that depends on the kind of life a person has led in this birth. There are also four goals in life: *Moksha* represents the ultimate goal, that is, for the soul to overcome the cycle of rebirths. *Dharma* is a code for leading one's life; that is, an individual has to perform duties, and these duties depend on the age and position of a person's life. *Artha* is the pursuit of material gains through lawful means. Finally, *karma* says that through the use of positive action, knowledge, and devotion, a person can be reincarnated at a higher level.

CASTES

The caste system is a way of separating people, resulting in thousands of groups who, at birth, are automatically associated with a particular occupation, status, social class, and language. Scholars who debate the origins of the caste system argue that the agricultural systems over the millennia, or occupational stratification within emerging class societies, created the system (Heitzman & Worden, 1996). Like race in the United States, the caste system is a matter of birth. Even if you change jobs, you cannot change your caste. Change comes through rebirth, and the caste you are reborn into depends on the acts you committed in your previous lives. The caste system divides people into four broad categories: the *Brahmins*—the priests or intelligentsia; the *Kshatriyas*—the administrators and the military; the *Vaishyas*—the shopkeepers, traders, and farmers; and the *Sudras*—the laborers and service workers. There are a large number of subclassifications in every group. The structure is much like Protestantism, which comprises many denominations of Christianity, each with its own rules and dogma.

With independence from Britain, the Indian government sought to eradicate discrimination on the basis of caste. Today it is impossible to identify caste by a person's occupation. However, in many homes marriages are still dictated by the caste system. Because there are such diverse groups of Hindu Indians, it is no surprise that they present themselves differently, depending on their family histories and backgrounds. To help therapists understand and serve Hindu Indian families, in this chapter I review the history of Indian immigration to the United States, current demographics, practices of their families, and, finally, some specific counseling strategies.

HISTORY OF HINDU IMMIGRATION TO THE UNITED STATES

The Hindu Indians who have come to the United States represent many classes, castes, colors, and family histories. In the first phase of immigration (between 1899 and 1908), about 6,800 Indians arrived in California. Most of these Indians were from the Province of Punjab in the northwest part of India, which consisted mostly of Sikhs and some Hindus. The majority of these people were illiterate or semiliterate and had agricultural and military backgrounds. A very small number constituted an educated, elite group of professionals and students.

Who are the Sikhs? Hindus, Sikhs, Buddhists, and Jains have the same origin. The Sikh sect was founded by Guru Nanak Dev (A.D. 1469–1538) and promoted by the gurus. Guru Nanak was born in a Vaishnava family when the sword of the Islamic invaders in India was causing immeasurable damage to temples and symbols of Hinduism and demoralizing the Hindu people. Hindu warriors fought in the battles while another group of Hindu saints and sages created a country-wide spiritual surge called the *bakthi* (holy) movement, and it was at this time that Sikhism came into being. Guru Nanak preached the equality of all people (Goel & Swarup, 2003) and described God as *Sat*, true, pure, or essential reality; he saw the divine as being both *sakar* and *nirakar*, both form and formless. It is humankind's duty to mediate on God's name to reach *nirvana* (heavenly bliss). The *Shri Guru Granth Sahib* is the holy book of the Sikh people. It is divided into 10 *granths*, each reflecting the teachings, beliefs, and views of one of the 10 gurus of the Sikh faith. The guru was the guide through whom one could attain salvation. The *Gurubani* (*Guru ki bani*), or teachings of the guru, were to be given the same reverence as the presence of the guru. Meditation on these teachings was considered the best form of worship (Chauhan, 1999). The Sikh name *singh* is adopted from the Rajputs (a martial race of the Hindus, identified with Aryan ancestry), and the turban is a common headdress of the Hindu people of India and is not exclusively Sikh. The concept of uncut hair was introduced by the 10th guru and was unknown before that. Hindus and Sikhs have intermarried since Guru Nanak's time, as this did not present a loss of identity. Sikhs have never accepted intermarriage with Muslims, however (Chauhan, 1999). The Hindus accepted such intermarriage because Sikhism was considered part of Hinduism and marriage for Sikhs was performed by *pundits* (Hindu priests) until the beginning of the 20th century.

The second phase of the Indian immigration to the United States took place in the 1960s, when upper-class, usually wealthy, well-educated, and professionally advanced Indians came to the United States (Williams, 1998).

Many came in the 1960s to enter well-known universities or work in reputable companies. Other reasons for coming included the wish to experience the American dream of a better life. Some also came to escape the lack of personal freedom in India, where family desires often overshadowed individual wishes. In privileged families in India, many responsibilities were placed on its members, including carrying out assigned roles. If the father was a businessman, for instance, the son was expected to carry on the family business tradition and fulfill his parents' desires in marrying the woman they had chosen for him, as well as accept other imposed responsibilities. In contrast, the United States represented freedom of choice and a good place to call home.

In the 1990s, with the passage of the Family Reunification Act, many Indians were admitted to the United States under the family sponsorship program. The newer arrivals were not as well educated as their predecessors and faced more challenges in adjusting to their new home, such as the inability to access services and social networks.

Starting in the late 1980s, and increasingly in the 21st century, the United States saw another influx of highly skilled Indian professionals, especially those who worked with computers (Duleep, 1988). A large number of these Indians settled in California, New York, Massachusetts, New Jersey, and Illinois. This particular group of people have relatively close ties to India and are highly mobile.

U.S. HINDU INDIANS TODAY

The groups of Hindu Indians living in the United States today can be categorized in many ways, such as by their differing relationships to U.S. culture. First are the Hindus who come from the upper castes and classes who, while growing up, were exposed to Western culture, including exposure to American lifestyles through the media. Such people enter the United States with the idea of becoming part of the U.S. culture. They fit in comfortably because they accept the cultural way of life in the United States. Acceptance of the vast American culture includes acceptance of both its positives and its negatives.

The second type of Hindus are also well educated and accept the American culture cautiously. They harmonize while they are at their workplaces and appear to "fit in," but once they are back in their family environment in the United States they tend to be more tied to the cultural traditions of the Indian group to which they belong.

The third type, the newest immigrants, who are sponsored by relatives, tend to be completely entrenched and tied to their Indian home culture. They fit in only for the purposes of earning a salary, which is used to support their families in the United States as well as in India.

Many more distinctions can be added when we consider factors such as ethnicity, language, caste and class subgroups, socioeconomic status, family upbringing, educational qualifications, and attitudes toward women. But perhaps the most fundamental factor in understanding Indian immigrants lies in the values and beliefs associated with Hinduism. This factor is now considered, along with demographics and family structure, and then the practical matter of how counselors can best help Hindu immigrants cope with their new setting.

Hinduism differs from the Western worldview, which emphasizes individualism and human rationality (Crocker, 1997; Hodge, 2004; Jafari, 1993). In the Hindu worldview, the concepts of personal autonomy, materialism, and secularism so integral to U.S. culture are subordinated to the concepts of community, interdependence, and divinity. These Hindu concepts are implicitly embedded in the Hindu way of life and thus pose a direct contrast to the American way of living (Shweder, Much, Mahapatra, & Park, 1997).

As practiced in India, Hinduism is best described as a way of life rather than an organized religion. People go to the temples when they wish to, and there is no organized way of belonging. However, as a relatively small ethnic group in the United States, Hindus have built temples and conduct classes and lectures to attract the younger generation to be part of the religion. Religion also serves to sustain families and individuals through difficult times.

To an outsider, the Hindu religion is confusing, with its large number of deities and ways of praying, which may be evaluated negatively when viewed from a linear Euro-American perspective. The Hindu belief is that most people are easily distracted from prayer when they cannot focus on a physical object; therefore, these objects are presented in the form of gods and goddesses. These deities help Hindus to move toward prayer, rituals, concentration, and meditation, all of which may eventually lead a person to become a better human being.

To support the growing Hindu populations, the number of Hindu institutions has mushroomed. Since 1976, 412 Hindu centers have been established in the United States, such as the Maharishi University (an accredited university in Fairfield, Iowa) and about 50 temples (Hodge, 2004). These organizations offer a wide variety of programs and provide social support for Hindu immigrants (Miller, 1995).

DEMOGRAPHICS IN THE UNITED STATES

There is only limited demographic information on Hindu immigrants. However, the available data have been concisely and well documented by Hodge (2004) as follows: Hindus ranked 10th in terms of annual income among U.S. religious groups, placing ahead of Catholics, Lutherans, and Baptists. In education, Hindus were second after Unitarians. About 47% of Hindus were college graduates—more than the national average. On average, 64% reported full-time employment (Kosmin & Lachman, 1993), and roughly 95% of Hindus in multiple-adult households lived in settings where adults were of the same religion.

FAMILY ISSUES

Hindu Indians face many different issues within their own families. In India, the culture supports large extended families, and relatives tend to drop by. Family members converse easily with each other about their family problems, particularly within their own related large family networks. There is no stigma associated with such family discussions. However, families living in the United States often do not have this problem-solving network available to them. Without their built-in family networks, many Hindu families in the United States feel restricted and isolated in a culture where closed doors are a way of life. Indeed, most Hindu American families depend solely on each other. Many create a network of friends who become like their families. It is only within this group that problems and issues are discussed and shared.

Even so, as Kurien (2001) so aptly writes, immigration for many Indians has been a disruptive experience. Indian immigrants to the United States are uprooted from the social and cultural context with which they are familiar and thrust into a radically new and alien environment. Although they are quick to appreciate the economic and educational benefits they obtain from immigration, they also often end up highly critical of many aspects of U.S. culture. They may view U.S. culture and society as having unstable and uncaring families, lacking close community ties, and allowing sexual promiscuity, violence, drug and alcohol abuse, and delinquency among young people. Furthermore, when children are born in the United States or immigrate when they are very young and assimilate into the culture through peers, school, and the media, they begin to think and behave differently from their parents and thus create intergenerational cultural problems.

Again, kinship is an important aspect of Indian Hindu life. Family life is generally stable, and families discuss everything from philosophical matters, to which university a child should attend, to how to help someone find a spouse. Marriages of entering immigrants are often arranged between two family systems; arranged marriages are still the norm.

As in other parts of the world, relationships in India have changed and evolved according to the changing norms in society. Sriram (1993) writes that the family is the basic and essential unit of society because of the role it plays in generating human capital resources and the power that is vested in it to influence individual, household, and community behavior. Sonawat (2001) specifies that the family is the first line of defense for children and an essential factor in their survival, health, development, education, and protection. Desai (1995) indicates that the family is an important source of nurturance, emotional bonding, and socialization, as well as a link between continuity and change. He adds that an enriched family life enhances healthy human growth.

Sonawat (2001) indicates that more recently, the husband–wife relationship is the basic and most important among the network of relationships in which a family evolves. Couples' healthy relationships provide the support system necessary to perform their roles effectively and promote the proper socialization of children. As in the rest of the United States' population, marital conflicts lead to family disorganization and negatively affect the upbringing of children. Patterns of emotional support among siblings are established in their early years. However, sibling relationships are surrounded by conflict and disharmony when paternal authority is weak or absent. Sibling violence is more prevalent among boys than girls (Sonawat, 2001). That is, brothers may fight with each other, rather than with their sisters. Unlike any other culture, Hindu Indians celebrate a festival centered on the brother–sister relationship—the *rakhi* festival. *Rakhi* literally means "bond of protection," and sisters tie colorful pieces of art with silken threads on the right wrists of their brothers for good health, wealth, happiness, and success. This festival establishes and reinforces the bond of love and affection between siblings. Women can also tie the threads on the wrists of men they consider to be like brothers to them. Once the thread is tied, the bond between them can grow more like that of a brother and sister. Rituals such as *rakhi* ease social strains, open channels of communication between siblings, and offer an opportunity to rework issues, if any, and, more important, bring joy to each other. This annual bonding can also be used effectively in therapy if there are problems between a brother and sister.

Most of the time, in a Hindu Indian American home the roles within the family overlap, depending on the traditions and tasks in a particular home. Such functions can also vary because of the influence of the Euro-American culture, the socioeconomic status of the family, and so forth. For instance, Indian traditions of authority diminish when couples who both work raise their children together, which is becoming the most common type of lifestyle in the United States.

According to Hinduism, women are to be respected and given equal rights with men (Kurien, 2001). Specifically, in terms of religious, cultural, social, and individual aspects, a woman has the same rights as a man in Hindu society. "Where women are honored, Gods are pleased," declare the Hindu scriptures. Hindus have elevated women to the level of divinity. Only Hindus worship God in the form of the Divine Mother. Even so, women in many Hindu homes are subordinate to men. Violence against women has been part of world history for many centuries. As in the Euro-American culture, any domestic violence among Hindu Indians is generally kept secret until the woman realizes there can be a way out. Often, her secrecy is a way of protecting herself, particularly if she is unable to reach out and receive help. Consider the following example.

Meena, an educated young woman, was married to an Indian American through an arranged marriage. This young bride came from India and landed in a vastly different culture, complete with apartment living. Her husband, Arun, had lived with his widowed mother for about 10 years before his marriage. Soon there were issues between the mother-in-law and daughter-in-law in regard to food preparation, folding clothes, and cleaning the house. The mother-in-law had the upper hand, as her son was used to her ways. The two women constantly engaged in verbal battles. Luckily, Meena found a minor job outside the home, but coming home became more and more unbearable. One day the mother-in-law struck her in anger and was supported by Arun, who felt that his wife had to be respectful to his mother. That was only the beginning; Arun and his mother had the advantage, and the verbal, emotional, and physical mistreatment became unbearable. Rather timid and new to everything around her, Meena started inquiring about help; when she could, she secretly left home and went to an Indian shelter. At the shelter she got in touch with her parents in India, who were horrified at the abuse their daughter had suffered. Although divorce was considered taboo in their family, they agreed with their daughter that divorce was a better solution to her problems. They offered her wholehearted nurturing support to help through this painful crisis. This love and support were necessary for her healing. She chose not to return to India, but served her husband with divorce papers.

Clinicians need to be aware that seeking out family relationships that support healing and caring is common in most Hindu families.

Hindu couple relationships in the United States are as varied as the different subcultures they come from. For the purposes of therapy, the various types of marriages can be classified. There are egalitarian marriages, in which each partner participates in taking care of family responsibilities. In patriarchal family situations, the man is the dominant person who makes the family decisions. Finally, there are families in which the woman is more in charge. This happens when the husband sees his marriage as permanent and is completely devoted to his wife, and the couple has a loving, caring relationship. Under these circumstances, the wife is given complete control over finances and family decisions; again, it must be emphasized that this occurs through the couple's nurturing and commitment to each other.

There are two small groups in India in which women have power through a truly matrilineal system. First, among the Nairs of Kerala, who live in southwestern India, inheritance is passed through women. Yet even in these families, patriarchy is present in the form of power held by the brother, not by the women themselves. Second, among the Khasis of Meghalay, power, wealth, and rights of inheritance are vested in women. However, the matrilineal system overall has undergone several changes because of politics, education, and technology. Members of the younger generation often question the matrilineal system, and they show a desire to be similar to the rest of India and move toward some form of patrilineal system, although the elders feel the existing matrilineal system should continue (Sonawat, 2001). If such families are to be seen in therapy, therapists should ask questions in order to understand and learn about this culture.

Often, partners' roles are interchanged out of understanding and affection. Although arranged marriages are common, divorce in the United States is comparatively rare among Hindus (Mullatti, 1995).

The parent–child relationship is generally built on love and some degree of discipline (Gupta & Gupta, 1985). Love and caring are often the binding forces that eventually help parents and children to accommodate, assimilate, and accept differences in behaviors and points of view regarding lifestyle and choice of partner, as shown in the following example.

A 16-year-old teenager, Veena, a Hindu, fell in love with her brother's best friend, 23-year-old Tom, a Christian. Veena was already betrothed to another man through a family arrangement, and the marriage was to take place in a few years after Veena had completed her schooling. However, she was adamant and wanted to marry Tom. There were constant fights between her parents—her father, Raj, a surgeon, and her mother, Sheila, a homemaker—about this issue. Tom was forbidden to enter their home. Secretly, Veena and Tom planned to elope, and eventually they did. As Veena was still a minor, the worried parents reported the situation to the police. Within 2 days, Veena and Tom were found in another town about 200 miles from home. The police called Raj to let him know that his daughter had been found. Tom was taken into custody and Veena was sent to a juvenile detention center. At that point, late in the evening, Raj started to cry because he could not bear to see his daughter in a detention center and worried about what would happen. He quickly made several phone calls, trying to prevent his daughter from being placed in detention. In a quick change of heart, he wanted to withdraw the case and have the police release Tom. He got in his car and drove until the wee hours of the morning to reach his daughter; he was accompanied by his just-awakened lawyer friend. The father wept and, in a repentant manner, held his daughter in his arms, saying that she should marry Tom after her schooling and that he, Raj, had been foolish to interfere in love and that Tom was welcome in their home. He and Sheila would explain the situation to the betrothed's family.

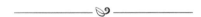

Why did the father, Raj, change so dramatically? This is a good example of how love and caring in Hindu Indian homes can transform and transcend cultural norms. Because love took over, the emotional cutoff that could have happened never did. It is important for therapists to understand the importance of family relationships and how cultural norms will be broken to keep the family together. In crisis, particularly, love and caring often transcend other emotions.

Adolescent rebellion is often a reaction to the contrast between the wide variety of choices available to youth in the United States and the restrictions the family places on them in terms of expectations and requirements. In regard to marriage, some families allow and encourage their children to choose their own spouses, irrespective of who the partner is, as long as their child is happy. Some offer restricted freedom, allowing the child to marry another Indian but not an American. Others allow their children to marry Euro-Americans, but only after a great deal of debate and discussion. Children who defy these boundaries face a great deal of grief and, at times, rejection from their families. Such rejection may be short-lived, as seen in the preceding case, or may last longer until love and caring eventually transcend the grief (V. Arora, personal communication, 2004).

Regardless of where they grew up, Hindu immigrants function from a perspective of interdependence. Generally, when they marry, they are committed to their spouses and their families; among young people there is limited dating, some acceptance of arranged marriages, heterosexuality, role distinctions for women and men, and modesty as a way of life (Miller, 1995).

Whereas the three-generation family relationship is honored in India, in which the oldest person receives a great deal of respect, this is not true of all families who live in the United States. In India, the mother-in-law has a dominant status and an important role in the life of her daughter-in-law. As Sonawat (2001) indicates, there have been very few research studies on this topic. An old study by Srivastava (1974) of two folk cultures in Rajasthan and Uttar Pradesh (Central India) reveals that in both cultures the mother-in-law has strict control over her daughter-in-law. As the earlier case example implies, the mother-in-law may view the daughter-in-law as an intrusion in her family and often finds that the young daughter-in-law disrupts unity among the brothers. At the same time, the daughter-in-law may find the mother-in-law to be intolerably demanding and domineering.

However, in the United States, a young couple who have children or who have many responsibilities outside their home may bring their parents to live with them. Often a widowed mother will be trusted as the built-in help and family baby-sitter. Grandparents generally enjoy the young children and may be satisfied with the role they play. However, friction between the mother-in-law and the daughter-in-law can become detrimental to all family members. For the grandmother, problems may arise if she is isolated, because she does not know the language or culture of the United States. In this situation, she cannot communicate with neighbors or anyone else outside the home about her problems. Often, the husband of the young woman is caught in the middle of a perpetual net of conflicts, unless the older parent is sent back to India or solutions are worked out for the family conflicts.

Many older Hindu immigrants have adult children who, in turn, have children. The issue of three generations growing up and living in the United States has yet to be explored fully. However, in almost all homes, placing an older person in a nursing home is considered totally unacceptable.

The gay and lesbian community in India is marginalized to the point of virtual invisibility. Sexuality is considered an inappropriate topic for public discussion. Until recently, in spite of their significant numbers, gays and lesbians have been ignored in the national political arena and in community-planning programs in India (Kavi, 2004).

As in India, homosexuality among Hindus in the United States is shrouded in secrecy and remains underground. For most people the obligatory arranged marriage is inevitable, and the gay life is left to be expressed outside the family (Sairah, 2003).

Because the family is considered to be very important, individual family members may cover up their issues rather than discuss them with an outsider. Taking problems outside the home is generally considered an act of betrayal. However, because their networks are less available in the United States, family members, after a conscious effort to work their issues (and if the situation worsens), may find themselves visiting a clinician.

COUNSELING HINDUS

As noted earlier, Hindu Indian Americans consider it shameful to discuss family issues outside the family. How conflict is dealt with varies greatly. Some confront and deal with it, others ignore it and hope it will go away, and still others deal with it minimally to keep peace in the family. The understanding of a social worker is usually restricted to those issues the family is willing to bring up, limiting his or her ability to help.

Often, practitioners in the United States do not understand how to counsel Hindu Indians. At times, counselors maintain exaggerated and conflicting images of a fictionally homogenous Hindu Indian community. As discussed previously, there are many differences based on language, caste and subcaste, socioeconomic class, ways of raising children, region from which a family emigrated, and the value systems of the family. However, in terms of intervention, the most important factor is that the family comes first. This idea differs greatly from the concept of individualism, which emphasizes the growth and well-being of a person. Instead, Hindus believe in interdependence and the philosophy that the family is more important than the individual.

Mental health issues in this population are often not recognized by practitioners. Adding to the confusion in the United States are the misconceptions of practitioners who have not been exposed to Hindu culture. For example, I recently received a frantic call from a practitioner who had a Hindu Indian couple in therapy. The wife constantly criticized her husband's parents, particularly his mother, and the husband would end up so frustrated that he would begin to beat on himself. The therapist asked me, "Why he is so upset about his wife criticizing his mother? Is beating himself a common way for Asian Indian men to deal with their problems?" I responded with caution, saying that this was perhaps how this particular man was dealing with his frustration, but surely it was not common for Indian men. The clinician was advised to ask questions about this particular family so that she could better help the couple. This sort of caution is an important aspect of counseling, especially counseling people of different cultures. However, it is also important, as Chandras (1997) says, for counselors to have an awareness of their own sociocultural backgrounds, assumptions, biases, values, and perceptions. They must take care to avoid imposing their own values on clients and to be aware that Hindu clients come from various subcultures.

Conflicts often arise in regard to issues of intergenerational relationships concerning who is in charge at home. In the early days, when roles are not clearly designated, clearly redefining roles and responsibilities with respect and care can create less friction. When opportunities are created for quality time between mother-in-law and daughter-in-law, such as shopping, taking care of grandchildren, and exchanging recipes, any relevant common interests can lead to more congenial relationships.

Another aspect of Hindu culture that counselors need to be aware of is that Hindus tend to combine spirituality with their everyday living. In particular, the concepts of *karma* and *dharma* are often integral to their dealing with the problems that all families face, such as loss, anguish, and pain. For example, a Hindu father who is laid off can take action (*karma*) by finding a job and performing his duty/responsibility (*dharma*) by being a productive member of the family.

Spirituality and Hinduism are closely entwined (Hodge, 2004). Many Hindu homes, even in the United States, have a quiet place of prayer and meditation where images of Hindu deities are located. These places are called *puja* (prayer) rooms. They are places to which a person can retreat, where he or she can connect with God. Prayer generally eases anxiety, fears, and loneliness, cultivates a sense of security, and establishes a sense of being loved (Levin, 1994). Hinduism is rich in ritual. Performing a prayer, or *puja*, every morning and evening may be a way of life. Praying reinforces a person's connection with the Absolute (Jacobs, 1992). Meditation and yoga are also used to ameliorate various problems and anxiety.

Many Asian Indian social service organizations have been formed in the United States to provide services to Asian Indians in distress. They accommodate various Indian languages and act with sensitivity toward the different Hindu Indian subcultures. These organizations address issues such as family violence, divorce, children's welfare, problems concerning the elderly, and assimilation problems faced by Indians entering the country. They also provide confidential referrals to other social agencies (Chandras, 1997).

CONCLUSION

This chapter presents some thoughts on how therapists can best work with Hindu Indian American clients. Almost all problems presented by a Hindu family are unique to their family situation, and understanding the family's degree of assimilation as well as their sociocultural, educational, economic, and regional status is important for understanding the family issues. The therapist needs to understand that there are many facets to this culture and to the person/family presenting the problem. Listening carefully and asking relevant questions will open the door to meaningful therapy. Finally, even Hindu Indian therapists may find some areas of a family difficult to understand, because of family customs. It is generally true that once a Hindu family has accepted a therapist, he or she finds it easier to ask questions, give advice, or offer explanations. Once the channels of communication are open, Hindus tend to be open and congenial and especially ready to offer information when the therapist needs it. This chapter is merely a beginning; there is a continuing need for more research and writings as Hindu Indians find their place in U.S. society.

REFERENCES

Chandras, K. V. (1997). Training multiculturally competent counselors to work with Asian Indian Americans. *Counselor Education and Supervision, 37*, 10–50.

Chauhan, S. S. (1999). Common heritage of the Sikhs, Hindus, Buddhists, Jains. In *Common heritage of the Sikhs, Hindus, Buddhists, jains*. Retrieved July 2004 at www.geocities.com

Crocker, L. G. (1997). Enlightment. In M. Cummings (Ed.), *Encyclopedia Americana* (Vol. 10, pp. 468–471). Danbury, CT: Grolier.

Desai, M. (1995). Towards family policy research. *Indian Journal of Social Work, 56*, 225–231.

Duleep, H. O. (1988). *The economic status of Americans of Asian descent*. Washington, DC: Commission on Civil Rights.

Goel, S. S. R., & Swarup, S. R. (2003). *Hindu–Sikh relationship*. Retrieved July 2004 at www. Hinduweb.org

Gupta, O. K., & Gupta, S. O. (1985). A study of the influence of American culture on the child-rearing of Indian mothers. *Indian Journal of Social Work*, 46(1), 5–104.

Heitzman, J., & Worden, R. L. (1996). *History of India*. Retrieved August 2004 at www.indianchild. com/history_of_india.htm

Hodge, D. R. (2004). Working with Hindu clients in a spiritually sensitive manner. *Social Work*, 49, 27–38.

India Election Statistics. (2004). *Indian demographics*. Retrieved August 2004 at www.Hinduism, India, statistics.htm

Jacobs, J. L. (1992). Religious rituals and mental health. In J. Schumaker (Ed.), *Religion and mental health* (pp. 291–299). New York: Oxford University Press.

Jafari, M. F. (1993). Counseling values and objectives: A comparison of Western and Islamic perspectives. *American Journal of Islamic Social Sciences*, 10, 326–339.

Kavi, A. R. (2004). Ashoka regional web sites. India: *Humsafar Trust Publications*. Retrieved July 2004 at www.Humsafar.org

Kosmin, B. A., & Lachman, S. (1993). *One nation under God*. New York: Harmony Books.

Kurien, P. (2001). Religion, ethnicity and politics: Hindu and Muslim Indian immigrants in the United States. *Ethnic and Racial Studies*, 24(2), 263–293.

Levin J. S. (1994). Investigating the epidemiologic effects of religious experience. In J. S. Levin (Ed.), *Religion in aging and health: Theoretical foundations and methodological frontiers* (pp. 3–17). Thousand Oaks, CA: Sage.

Miller, B. D. (1995). Precepts and practices: Researching identity formation among Indian Hindu adolescents in the United States. In W. Damon (Ed.), *Cultural practices as contexts for development* (pp. 71–85). San Francisco: Jossey-Bass.

Mullatti, L. (1995). Families in India: Beliefs and practices. *Journal of Comparative Family Studies*, 26(1), 11–26.

Sairah. (2003). Homophobia within India. *Write words. Organization UK Writers' Community*, pp. 1–7.

Sharma, A. P. (2004). *Hinduism redefined*. New Delhi: Vedam Books.

Shweder, R. A., Much, N. C., Mahapatra, M., & Park, L. (1997). The "big three" of morality (autonomy, community, divinity) and the "big three" explanations of suffering. In A. M. Brandt & P. Rozin (Eds.), *Morality and health* (pp. 119–169). New York: Routledge.

Sonawat, R. (2001, May). Understanding families in India: A reflection of societal changes. *Psicologia: Teoria e Pesquisa*, 17(2), 177–186.

Sriram, R. (1993). Family studies in India: Appraisal and new directions. In T. S. Saraswati & B. Kaur (Eds.), *Human development and family studies in India: An agenda for research and policy* (pp. 122–128). New Delhi: Sage.

Srivastava, S. L. (1974). *Folk culture and oral tradition*. New Delhi: Abhinav Publications.

Williams, R. B. (1998). Asian Indian and Pakistani religions in the United States. In W. W. Heston (Ed.), *The annals of the American Academy of Political and Social Sciences* (Vol. 558, pp. 178–195). Thousand Oaks, CA: Sage.

CHAPTER 30

Pakistani Families

Shivani Nath

Pakistan was born in torment more than a half century ago in 1947. It appears to be in constant pursuit of its own identity; at the same time it has become a pivotal player in global politics. Its short existence has witnessed an extraordinary variety of events: coups d' état in 1969, 1977, and 1999, the rise of Islam as a power, tensions between ethnic and religious groups, the Kashmir conflict and near-constant war footing with India, the rapid establishment of separatist movements such as that which lead to the establishment of Bangladesh, and its own increasingly important position at the axis of the Middle East, central Asia, and China. Furthermore, the ongoing issues surrounding Afghanistan and the fact that the most recent coup that leaves Pakistan the sixth most populous country in the world and the only nuclear power governed by the military, make the study of this country's history crucial in terms of understanding modern international relations, politics, religion, economics, and global military strategy.

HISTORICAL PERSPECTIVE

When Pakistan came into existence in 1947, it was the realization of a yearning by a section of India's Muslims, who feared domination by the Hindu majority in a postcolonial India. The tensions between Hindus and Muslims on the Indian subcontinent were recognized by Great Britain, and the British made their final plans to surrender the "Jewel in the Crown" of their empire after 90 years—their "Two Nations Theory"—premised on the notion of a separate homeland for the subcontinent's Muslim minority. This evolved into a collective vision championed by Muslims, who broke ranks from their nationalist counterparts of all backgrounds. The partition of the Indian subcontinent at the time of independence from colonial rule in August 1947 entailed the creation of two new sovereign states—India and Pakistan, with the latter composed of areas where Muslims were in a numerical majority. Partition involved not only the institution of separate administrative and political structures for the two newly independent states, but also a momentous upheaval of population migration, as well as unanticipated bloodshed and brutality among Hindus and Muslims on a unimaginable and inexplicable scale. Twelve to 14 million people were caught up in this process of mass migration; more than a million were killed in violent encounters, and an estimated 75,000 women were abducted and subjected to sexual violence (Butalia, 2000). In 1946 and 1947 the subcontinent was torn by Hindu–Muslim riots in an atmosphere of religious hatred inflamed by the emerging reality of partition (Gooptu, 2002).

The partition of India and Pakistan had separate meanings and identities for both countries. As Gooptu (2002) further postulates, on the Indian side, partition was portrayed as an aberration in India's heroic struggle for independence and her triumphant march to nationhood; partition was projected as the product of an act of betrayal of the national cause by so-called separatist Muslims. On the Pakistani side, partition was seen as a necessary step toward the realization of nationhood and a safe homeland for South Asian Muslims. The lived experience of partition and the trauma of death and destruction, hardship and dislocation, misery and debasement has been shrouded in what some have recently called a tyranny of silence. The history of loss, suffering, and uprootedness, which is how the people of the subcontinent actually experienced partition, was hardly ever aired in public in the first 40 years following partition. Collective amnesia and denial appear to have been the ways in which this catastrophic experience of violence and displacement was psychologically and culturally negotiated.

After independence, the decision as to what system of government the new nation should adopt was never fully reached. In the decades following independence, this irresolution contributed to a recurrent pattern of crisis: repeated coups and extended periods during which martial law replaced civilian government, violent deaths of several national leaders, periodic strife among ethnic groups, and, most traumatically, a civil war in 1971 involving linguistic and cultural issues that divided the East and West parts of the country in two. After India intervened, East Pakistan seceded and renamed itself Bangladesh.

IMMIGRATION TO THE UNITED STATES
AFTER SEPTEMBER 11, 2001

The 2000 census data reported 200,000 Pakistanis in the United States, with the majority living in the New York and New Jersey areas. This trend of consistent immigration has, however, been impacted by the recent sociopolitical issues in the United States in the wake of the September 11, 2001, attacks. U.S. immigration law has been under constant revision and scrutiny after the World Trade Center attacks. According to a *Daily Times* news report (Hasan, 2003), Pakistanis have borne the brunt of new restrictive immigration legislation; of the 2,760 people deported by U.S. authorities in 2002, as many as 961, or more than 34%, were Pakistanis. Citing the 2001 U.S. immigration and deportation data on Muslims, the July 29, 2003, report states that in 2001, of the 1,264 deported, 375 were Pakistanis, the highest number from any of the 24 Muslim countries whose nationals have been required to register with the immigration authorities and on whom the finger of suspicion has rested since the World Trade Center attacks. In both 2001 and 2002, Pakistanis remained on top of the list of those deported. Other Muslim countries had fewer of their nationals deported, one reason being that they were fewer in number. According to Ibrahim Hooper of the Council on American-Islamic Relations, the policy (on mass deportation) "is causing a lot of fear and apprehension." It is therefore imperative to explore such emotions with Pakistani clients in therapy.

A growing number of Pakistanis who have been living in the United States are crossing the border and seeking asylum in Canada for fear that they will be jailed or deported if they register with a new U.S. Justice Department tracking program, according to Canadian officials (Donohue, 2003). Under a program enacted in response to the 9/11 attacks, about 24,200 men, age 16 and older, from 20 countries are required to register at local Immigration and Naturalization Service (INS) offices to be photographed, fingerprinted, and show certain documents. The registration requirement is part of the National Security Entry–Exit Registration System (NSEERS), a program created after the attacks of September 11, 2001, to better track foreigners entering the country and flag potential terrorists. Testimonials from some Pakistanis migrating to Canada cite "fear of being framed for some terrorism-related activity, racial profiling in the United States, as in reported cases in New Jersey, New York, and California, or simply apprehension" as some of the reasons that these families are undertaking mass migration from the United States to Canada. This action has created uncertainty in families residing legally in the United States. Furthermore, families have trepidation about seeking medical services for a sick member. Even when mental health services are offered to "undocumented" families, the number of Pakistani and Islamic families seeking such services is extremely low.

PEOPLE AND GOVERNMENT

Pakistan has one of the world's most rapidly growing populations. Its people are a mixture of many ethnic groups, a result of the occupation of the region by groups passing through on their way to India. The pathans (Pashtuns) of the northwest are a large indigenous group that has long resisted advances by invaders and has, at times, sought to establish an autonomous state within Pakistan. Baluchis, who live mainly in the southwest, have also pressed for the creation of a state that would incorporate parts of Afghanistan and Iran. Punjabis reside mainly in the northeast, and Sindhis in the southeast. Sindhis and Pashtuns form the majority. Since 1978, Pakistan has been home to Afghan refugees who fled their country's civil war. At one time more than 3 million refugees were living in Pakistan; now they are estimated at just over 1 million, many of them living in officially designated camps. The two largest cities are Karachi and Lahore. The capital city is Islamabad. Pakistan is an overwhelmingly (about 97%) Muslim country, of which about three quarters of the people are Sunni Muslim and another one fifth are Shiite Muslim. Christians, Hindus and others constitute 3% of the population. The population of Pakistan is almost 150 million (Murray, 2002). Urdu is the official language, but Punjabi, Sindhi, Pashto, Baluchi, and Brahui are also spoken; English is commonly used among the upper classes and in the government.

Until October 1999, when the Constitution was suspended, Pakistan was governed by the Constitution of 1973 as amended in 1985, which provides for a federal parliamentary form of government. Constitutional government was restored in 2002, although Pervez Musharraf, who seized power in 1999, remained president, as well as the chief of army staff, by unilaterally amending the Constitution.

RELIGION

Muslims believe their destiny is subject to the will of Allah, and their religion is based on the "Five Pillars of Islam." The Five Pillars of Islam consist of certain beliefs and acts to which a Muslim must adhere to affirm membership in the community (see Chapter 28 for details).

A number of other elements contribute to a sense of social membership, whereby Muslims see themselves as distinct from non-Muslims, including a prohibition against the consumption of pork and alcohol, the requirement that animals be slaughtered in a ritual manner, and the obligation to circumcise sons. Another element is *jihad*, the "striving." *Jihad* is often misunderstood in the West, where people think of it as a fanatical holy war. There are two kinds of *jihad*: The far more important inner one is the battle each Muslim wages with his or her lower self; the outer one is the battle that each Muslim must wage to preserve the faith and its followers. People who fight the outer *jihad* are *mujahidin*. The concept of predestination in Islam is different from that in Christianity. Islam posits the existence of an all-powerful force (Allah) who rules the universe and knows all things. Something will happen—*inshaallah*—if it is God's will. The concept is not purely fatalistic, for although people are responsible to God for their actions, these actions are not predestined. Instead, God has shown the world the right way to live as revealed through the Qur'an; then it is up to individual believers to choose how to live. There are two major sects in Islam, the Sunnis and the Shia. They are differentiated by Sunni acceptance of the temporal authority of the Rashudin Caliphate (Abu Bakr, Omar, Usman, and Ali) after the death of the Prophet, and the Shia acceptance solely of Ali, the Prophet's cousin and husband of his daughter, Fatima, and his descendants. Over time, the Sunni sect divided into four major schools of jurisprudence; of these, the Hanafi school is predominant in Pakistan. The Shia sect split over the matter of succession, resulting in two major groups: The majority Twelve Imam Shia believe that there are twelve rightful imams, Ali and his eleven direct descendants. A second Shia group, the numerically smaller Ismaili community, known also as Seveners, follows a line of imams that originally challenged the Seventh Imam and supported a younger brother, Ismail. The Ismaili line of leaders has been continuous down to the present day.

EDUCATION

The level of adult literacy is low, but improving. The rate of improvement is highlighted by the 50% literacy achieved among 15- to 19-year-olds in 1990. School enrollment has also increased, to 24% in 1990. However the population over age 25 still has, on average, less than 2 years of schooling. This fact explains the minimal criteria for being considered literate: having the ability to both read and write (with understanding) a short, simple statement on everyday life. The government is spending an increasing percentage of its funds on education, but, like the United States, Pakistan spends 10 times as much on the military as on education. In 1990, Pakistan was tied for fourth place in the world in the ratio of military expenditures to health and education expenditures. Furthermore, there is a significant disparity in educational attainment between men and women. In 1992, only 22% of women over age 15 were literate, as compared with 49% of men.

HEALTH CARE, MENTAL HEALTH, AND INDIGENOUS FORMS OF TREATMENT

National health planning began with the second Five-Year Plan (1960–1965) and continued through the eighth Five-Year Plan (1993–1998). Provision of health care for the rural populace has long been a stated priority, but efforts to provide such care continue to be hampered by administrative problems and difficulties in staffing rural clinics. In the early 1970s, a decentralized system was developed in which basic health units provided primary care for a surrounding population of 6,000–10,000 people, rural health centers offered support and more comprehensive services to local units, and both the basic units and the health centers could refer patients to larger urban hospitals.

In the early 1990s the orientation of the country's medical system, including medical education, favored the elite. There has been a marked boom in private clinics and hospitals since the late 1980s and a corresponding, unfortunate deterioration in services provided by nationalized hospitals. In 1992 there was only one physician for every 2,127 persons, one nurse for every 6,626 persons, and only one hospital for every 131,274 persons. There was only one dentist for every 67,757 persons.

In addition, the indigenous forms of treatment are quite popular. For example, *Unani Tibb* (Arabic for Greek medicine), also called *Islami-Tibb*, is galenic medicine resystematized and augmented by Muslim scholars. Herbal treatments are used to balance bodily humors. Practitioners, or *hakims*, are trained in medical colleges or learn the skill from family members who pass it down through the generations. Some manufactured remedies are also available in certain pharmacies. Homeopathy, thought by some to be the "poor man's Western medicine," is also taught and practiced in Pakistan. Several forms of religious healing are common as well. Prophetic healing is based largely on the *hadith* of the Prophet, pertaining to hygiene and moral and physical health, and simple treatments are used, such as honey, a few herbs, and prayer. Some religious conservatives argue that reliance on anything but prayer suggests lack of faith, whereas others point out that the Prophet remarked that Allah had created medicines in order that humans should avail themselves of their benefits. Popular forms of religious healing, at least protection from malign influences, are common in most of the country. The use of *tawiz*, or amulets, containing Qur'anic verses, or the intervention of a *pir* (spiritual leader or healer), living or dead, is generally relied upon to direct the healing.

Mental illness is widespread in Pakistan, with some 20% of the population affected by depression, drug abuse, personality disorders and obsessive–compulive disorders, and schizophrenia. During a 2-year study in 1996–1997 (Khan & Reza, 2000), 306 suicides were reported. The most common reason for suicide was "domestic problems" (e.g., problems in spousal relationships, problems with extended family members living in the household, financial difficulties, problems related to career choice, etc.), as reported in 78% of cases. This was followed by unemployment in 11%, "parents' refusal to let their child marry a person of his or her choice" in 8%, financial difficulties in 4%, and mental illness in 3% (rates of mental illness seem to be underreported in Pakistani families because of the stigma attached to any label pertaining to mental distress). A small number (three men and one woman) committed the act because of "failure in a love affair," and in five males and two females "failure in exams" was given as the reason for suicide.

There are very few resources in Pakistan to deal with problems relating to mental health (Khan, 2004). Doctors see between 15 and 20 patients per hour, and no more than 300 psychiatrists are treating a population of 140 million people. There are also many myths surrounding mental illness in this deeply traditional Islamic society. The best form of treatment for patients would be a combination of medical care (medication plus spirituality) in familiar settings, preferably with the family (Kahn, 2004). The social fabric in Asian countries is better suited to supporting mentally ill patients than the society in the United States because of the availability of the extended family network. Immigrant families don't have this additional support, and it is very difficult for them to look after their relatives. In the sometimes unwelcoming context of the United States, it often happens that the love, care, and attention that are crucial for the recovery process are absent and people don't have the time or resources to care for mentally ill relatives; that is why they are institutionalized.

The perception of positive mental health in Pakistan encompasses all aspects of a person's life. This positivity enables him or her to lead a fulfilling life while helping others to do the same. Mental illness is defined as a state of arrested or incomplete development of the mind that results in impaired intelligence and social functioning and is associated with aggressive or seriously irresponsible conduct. Similarly, a personality disorder is defined as a persistent disorder or disability of the mind, which can result in abnormally aggressive or seriously irresponsible conduct. Mental illness is believed to be caused by supernatural forces such as spirit possession, black magic or exaltation, or testing by God as punishment for one's sins. Some people believe that mental illness can be caused by a bodily dysfunction such as a gastrointestinal upset, and others believe that it can be caused by taking a lot of "Western" drugs. Modern education, especially in urban areas, has affected these perceptions and changed attitudes toward the origins of mental illness.

An important consideration is the reaction of family members of a mentally ill individual. There is a huge stigma attached to mental illness, and although some family members may try to hide the illness, others may become overinvolved in caring for their relative or may not seek help because they believe the illness is a sign that God has granted him or her "special status" (Karim et al., 2004), meaning that because it was God's will that the person got sick, they believe that God is looking out for that person.

Psychological practice in Pakistan is based on the Western model (Murray, 2002). U.S.- and European-trained psychologists brought the practice to the universities in the 1960s, and many Pakistani psychologists continue to be trained in the West. But over the past 10 years, Pakistani psychology practice and research have been increasingly interested in, and shaped by, indigenous culture, wherein prayer is an essential component in healing. Pakistani psychologists recognize the pervasive influence of religion and believe that "indigenized" psychology (a treatment plan involving facets of religion and spirituality) is more helpful to clients. To accomplish such a change, and to overcome culture clashes, the mental health field in Pakistan is increasingly accommodating Muslim ideals and Pakistani culture. Religious healers are usually the first health care contacts for all sick people and their families, particularly for the mentally ill. Pakistani people have strong faith in religious healers and the Qur'anic texts used by them, which puts these healers in a strong position to help people solve their psychosocial problems. For this reason, religious healers often identify mental illness early—a very useful contribution to Pakistani mental health care (Karim et al., 2004).

Practitioners also take into account their clients' family constraints, particularly the fact that most women live with the husband's family and are beholden to their in-laws' wishes (Zaman, 1992, quoted in Murray, 2002). Dr. Zaman, a woman psychologist in Pakistan also states that with so few outlets and choices, Pakistani women commonly suffer depression and somatoform disorders such as headaches, ulcers, aches, and pains. And where Western psychologists might help steer such women toward self-sufficiency, in Pakistan "you mostly help women work as best they can with the marriage they are in," says Zaman (as quoted by Murray, 2002). Such an approach can be viewed as a pragmatic moderation of therapeutic goals, inasmuch as working in a society where women have limited rights and their identity depends on the intricate family network, the support of the marital structure is seen as practical. Dr. Zaman therefore favors using a family systems approach with her clients, in which therapists focus on couple and family dynamics and interpersonal skills, and make interventions by exploring the presenting problems within the context in which they occur. This approach also helps men, who often find themselves caught in the crossfire between their wives and parents. In addition, just as other classically trained psychologists do, Zaman uses her clients' religious faith in their treatment (Murray, 2002).

Murray (2002) postulates that some Pakistani psychologists believe that religious healing *ought* to be part of practitioners' training. Murray states that Syed Azhar Ali Rizvi, a founder of the Society for the Advancement of Muslim Psychology, has pioneered training in Islamic counseling at the Institute of Muslim Psychology at Al-Khair University in Lahore. Trainees learn to assign religious readings to clients and help them "fight negative thinking (pessimism, distrust in others, selfishness) that leads to abnormality." Murray also reports that because of Rizvi's influence, 9 of Pakistan's 16 postgraduate psychology departments require students to take at least one course in Muslim psychology. And even though Pakistani psychologists use Western research methodology, they increasingly study issues and problems specific to their own culture. For example, Rizvi researches the academic and emotional development of children born into polygamy, a fairly common practice in Pakistan.

Murray (2002) also reported that psychology has gained increasing respect relative to psychiatry over the past 20 years. More psychologists hold top jobs in such areas as drug addiction and rehabilitation of schizophrenics. In addition, Punjab University's Center for Clinical Psychology has set up a popular hot line for Pakistani citizens anxious about September 11 and the ensuing war. However, the lingering stigma and suspicions about the field's Western origins, along with a lack of professional regulations and a largely poor, uninsured population, hurts the practice of this discipline. Psychological research is also underdeveloped, as funding is scarce, and only two journals are published for the field in Pakinstan.

SOCIALIZATION AND CULTURAL NUANCES

A handshake is the most common greeting in Pakistan, although close friends may embrace if meeting after a long absence. Women may greet each other with a handshake or a hug. It is not appropriate for a man to shake hands with or to touch a woman in public, but he may greet another man's wife verbally without looking directly at her. Greetings often include inquiries about a person's health and family, which can take some time. The most common greeting is *Assalaam alaikum* ("May peace be upon you"). The reply is *Waalaikum assalaam* ("And peace also upon you"). "Good-bye" is *Allah haafiz*. Male friends may walk hand in hand or with their arms over each other's shoulders (Society, 1997).

There is a long tradition of hospitality in Pakistani families. Friends and relatives visit each other frequently. Hosts take pride in making guests feel welcome and, whenever possible, will greet each person individually. Unless told not to, a person normally removes his or her shoes when entering a home. Visitors are usually offered coffee, tea, or soft drinks and may be invited to eat a meal. If well acquainted with the host or if the occasion is special, guests often bring fruit, sweets, or a gift for the children or the home. It is customary to socialize primarily before a meal and then to stay at least a half hour after the meal is finished. In traditional homes, men and women do not socialize together, which includes the practice of not eating together as well. This may also be true in traditional or first-generation Pakistani families residing in the United States; girls might also not "hang out" with boys in school cafeterias. Women tend to serve the food at a meal, as all male members of the household eat first (Society, 1997). Again, one might see such patterns of custom in newly immigrated or extremely traditional families.

Islamic holidays are scheduled by the lunar calendar and fall on different days each year. The most important of these include the Feast of the Giving, or *Eid-ul-Fitr*, the three-day feast at the end of the month of *Ramzan* (Ramadan); *Eid-ul-Azha* (Feast of the Sacrifice), which commemorates Abraham's willingness to sacrifice his son, as well as the pilgrimage (*hajj*) to Mecca , and *Eid-i-Milad-un-Nabi*, the birth of the Prophet Muhammad. On evenings during *Ramzan*, many towns sponsor fairs and other celebrations. During *Shab-e-Barat*, which precedes *Ramzan*, Pakistani Muslims ask Allah to forgive their deceased loved ones. This is a night for prayer in mosques, reading the Qur'an, and visiting graveyards. It is believed that this is the time at which Allah decides people's fates for the coming year. People also set off fireworks, light up the exteriors of mosques, and donate food to the needy.

MARRIAGE, FAMILY, AND LIFE-CYCLE DYNAMICS

The family is the fundamental unit of Pakistani society. Individual choice of a marriage partner has traditionally played a small role in the marriage process, and arranged marriages are still the standard. Formal engagements may last from a few months to many years, depending on the age of the couple. In some cases, the bride and groom meet for the first time on their wedding day. Pakistanis view marriage as a union of two families as much as a union of two people. Both families participate in the wedding preparations. A Muslim holy man or priest, usually called a *qazi*, completes the marriage contract between the two families. Muslim marriage is a civil contract, and a financial consideration (*mahr*) and the consummation of the marriage are its two vital points; in the absence of these two prerequisites, a marriage is considered invalid. Islamic law permits a man to have as many as four wives if he can care for them equally. To be sure, the usual difference between religious doctrine and actual practice remains prevalent in this regard. How the practice is transported across cultures among Pakistani families living abroad is also intriguing. Although no hard data seem to be available, there is anecdotal evidence that certain Pakistani Americans in the United States, especially those who are more ethnocentric, occasionally do marry more than one woman at the same time. Usually such a practice involves a Pakistani woman and a Caucasian American woman of lower socioeconomic status. Or a man might be "legally married" to one woman but still have ongoing relationships with as many as three other women, openly or secretively. However, the situation mostly remains clandestine. This, again, makes it imperative that the therapist explore the "marriage dynamic" with every Pakistani client/family.

In the Shia Muslim school of jurisprudence, contract marriages (*mutaa'h*) are also permissible, whereby a marriage between man and a woman is allowed for any specific period of time and, upon completion of the contractual period, the marriage is ended. Originally, this institution was evolved to meet the erotic and anaclitic needs of merchants, diplomats, and those belonging to other professions requiring extended out-of-town/country stays. It is noted that people might go in for such an arrangement for financial reasons, a need to explore their sexuality (inasmuch as premarital sexual relationships are not allowed), and for traveling (for example, to a foreign country when it is difficult to get a visa if one is single), and so forth.

Pakistani nuclear families are generally large, with the average woman bearing seven children in her lifetime (Society, 1997). In Islam, women do not generally inherit agricultural or business assets of the deceased. These assets are distributed to the linear descendant in the male line of descendancy. Wedding rituals are elaborate, and men and women celebrate separately. Although increased modernization has brought many women into public life, the male is considered head of the home. It is common for the extended family—a father and mother, children and their families—to live together in the same household. Therefore, it is not uncommon to have three generations living under one roof or in close proximity to each other. It is not unusual for children, particularly sons, to continue to live with their parents following marriage, which produces strong vertical, intergenerational relationships (Moazam, 2000).

Personal identity takes second place to the collective family identity and consciousness, and obligations as well as harmonious living are considered moral imperatives, second in importance only to submission to the will of God. According to Moazam (2000), discourses about the rights of individual members in a family, including what one "owes" another or the issue of "rights" between parents and their children, are alien. It has been further noted that "medical ethics," such as confidentiality, are incomprehensible to most Pakistanis (Kuczewski, 2000), inasmuch as the family plays a pivotal role in analyzing and addressing a problem at hand. Keeping secrets can be characteristic of a Pakistani family, in the view of the fact that most family members avoid disclosure of terminal diseases (like cancer) to patients so as to avoid "burdening" them further and to allow them to "die in peace." This is perceived as a form of caring, particularly toward elderly members (Moazam, 2000). Nursing homes for those who are aged, terminally ill, or incompetent are unknown in Pakistan; such individuals are cared for at home by the family. Members of the extended family with whom a patient resides generally undertake decisions regarding terminal care for the patient, whether he or she is competent or incompetent. Although affluent families may hire nurses for home care of a member who is ill, caregiving in most cases is a shared responsibility of the female members of the extended family system. These may include a wife, unmarried daughters, and/or daughters-in-law. Pakistani families are both hierarchical and patrilineal, and the presiding male of the family has significant influence over the lives of all family members, although women are becoming more active in decision making.

HOMOSEXUALITY

Homosexuality is illegal and a crime punishable by whipping, imprisonment, or even death, in Pakistan. In villages throughout the country, young boys are often forcibly "taken" by older men, starting a cycle of abuse and revenge that social activists and observers say is the common pattern of homosexual sex in Pakistan. Often these boys move to the cities and become prostitutes. Most people know this happens—from the police to the wives of the men involved (Kennedy, 2004). There are no known reports on female homosexuals, however, because "women in Pakistan inhabit, for the most part, a strictly private realm" (Kennedy, 2004). Even though such reports are missing from the mental health literature, Pakistani fiction and poetry are not devoid of allusions to such liaisons.

Although illegal in some areas, homosexual sex is accepted as long as it doesn't threaten traditional marriage. In the Northwest Frontier Province (NWFP), which shares many tribal and cultural links with neighboring Afghanistan, the ethnic Pashtun men who dominate the region are renowned for taking young boys as lovers. No one has been executed for sodomy in Pakistan's recent history, but across the border in Afghanistan, the Taliban (who are also overwhelmingly Pashtun) executed three men for sodomy in 1998 by bulldozing a brick wall over them and burying two of them alive (Kennedy, 2004).

Furthermore, according to a *Boston Globe* news report (Kennedy, 2004), Pakistani gay men usually succumb to family pressure to marry, and those who are brave or rich enough to refuse to marry live under constant threat. Human rights workers say that the dearth of Pakistani gay rights and community groups heightens the isolation and fear of those who identify themselves and live as homosexuals. There are groups working against the spread of AIDS in Pakistan, but their work is often impeded by the cultural disapproval of homosexual sex. It is noted, however, in literature pertaining to immigration and homosexuality (e.g., Akhtar, 1999; Knafo & Yaari, 1997) that homosexual individuals tend to migrate in greater proportions than would otherwise be demographically expected, and individuals who have kept their homosexuality a secret from others may become more covert in their sexual preferences after migration to a more accepting culture. This dynamic is important to explore in therapy when working with a Pakistani client who might be gay. The client may look for validation of his homosexuality from a therapist rather than presenting it as a problem. In my experience in working with a Pakistani family in which a child's homosexuality was of utmost concern for the parents, it was helpful to explore the cultural dynamics of the United States and Pakistan and help them to dispel the notion of "pathology" in regard to homosexuality, especially in light of the U.S. mainstream culture. It was helpful for the family in question to look at the literature on homosexuality and the resources available for the lesbian, gay, bisexual, and transgender (LGBT) community. In all, it was helpful for the family to move away from the perception that their gay child would be isolated and left out of all social circles.

CASE EXAMPLE

The following case highlights some of the cultural aspects of a Pakistani family in New York. Therapeutic interventions are provided as well.

Samira is a 32-year-old Pakistani American woman who immigrated to the United States in 2000. She is a mother of two teenage boys: Riyaz, 14, and Jahaan, 13. Samira is currently separated from her husband, Shahid, who lives in Pakistan. Samira sought political asylum in the United States because her life was in danger in Pakistan. Shahid had threatened to kill her when Samira announced she wanted a separation. The marriage was "extremely abusive," according to Samira, wherein her husband "banned" any "outside contact" for her and did not "allow" her to call her family members or friends. Samira took her boys to her aunt's house in Pakistan one night and did not plan to return to Shahid. Upon learning of his wife's "running away," Shahid had Samira's mother, Mrs. Razia, kidnapped by local goons and threatened to have her family killed if his wife didn't come back. Faced with this dilemma, Samira called her younger sister who lived in New York City, who suggested that Samira, her sons, her brother, and her parents seek asylum in the United States.

By a terrible coincidence, on the day they were scheduled to fly to New York, Samira's mother and father both had heart attacks. The father died, but the mother survived. This became a very traumatic issue for the family, who were faced with the dilemma of having a funeral for the father or working toward their escape. On the advice of their extended family, the fleeing family members took their assigned flight and left the funeral arrangements to the extended family.

Samira came for therapy for her sons, whose school counselor had referred them. According to reports from the teacher and other school personnel, Riyaz and Jahaan had gotten involved in various situations including "acts of aggression." On one occasion, Riyaz had taken a knife to school and "threatened to hurt a Caucasian boy." He was suspended for 30 days, after which the principal mandated that he receive "anger management counseling." Similarly, Jahaan was evaluated by the child study team shortly after the incidents of September 11, 2001, and was classified with having attention-deficit/hyperactivity disorder (ADHD). Again, on the school's recommendation, Jahaan was taken to see a pediatric neurologist who prescribed Wellbutrin for him.

Samira's sister Nida brought the boys and Samira to the clinic because Samira did not have a driver's license. After the initial introduction, Samira asked to excuse herself so that I could work with the boys alone. I asked if she would be interested in joining us as well so that we could talk about the presenting problems. Samira appeared quite pleased at the idea and stated, "This is the first time I will be sitting with my sons in a formal setting; I asked to speak with the school counselor, but they probably don't work with parents."

Samira remarked on being "happy to talk to someone who speaks the same language, and someone who knows the culture fairly well." My Indian American ethnicity was of interest to her. Interestingly, the Italian intake worker who first saw the family had noted that the "mother and the boys barely talked and had a constricted, flat, and depressed affect." He also noted the boys' "lack of eye contact" with him, recommending a "complete psychiatric evaluation to rule out psychosis." Coming from a culture where men and women have such separate roles, Samira had probably felt uncomfortable talking personally with a man. From my perspective, her affect was probably quite natural under the circumstances. Pakistani American families stress the importance of children treating their elders with respect, and maintaining eye contact is seen as disrespectful.

It is of prime importance to take into account the immigration history of the client/family and look for the patterns of acculturation and assimilation. Interestingly, even though Samira was fairly new to the United States, she was dressed in Western garb. When I inquired about that, she stated, "I hate to say it, but I don't want to dress in Pakistani outfits. I really miss that . . . but I don't want people to think that I am a Pakistani Muslim. I want to be like them and I know I am not. I don't want to be killed like many Islamic people after 9/11." The events of 9/11, of course, impacted immigrants from Islamic countries, and many families either were deported or chose to leave the United States due to fear and apprehension. Many families who chose to stay in this country changed their traditional patterns of dress; Indian women gave up wearing the dot (*bindi*) on the forehead, and Pakistani women gave up wearing the *hijab* (head scarf) *or salwar-kameez* (traditional pants suit with a long shirt).

Including parents in therapy with the identified patient is deemed appropriate in working with a Pakistani American family. Riyaz and Jahaan were quite comfortable in the family therapy setting as well, especially when Nida and her children were also included in "family meetings." The boys were able to voice their anger toward their father, as well as their frustration at the "helplessness" of their mother, because she didn't know how to drive and it made them dependent on their aunt Nida. Similarly, the whole family was able to discuss the events of 9/11 with me and how much they feared being portrayed as *jihadis* in school and society. I made every effort to validate their concerns and make them feel safe in my presence.

Another construct to work with was the trauma of the coincidental death of Samira's father and its impact on the family system. Earlier in the therapy, Samira presented herself as "bad luck" to her family; in her (and her extended family's) view, she was the only one having a tumultuous relationship with her husband, and the only person who wanted to disentangle herself from an abusive marriage. For instance, while living in the same household in New York, Mrs. Razia had cut herself off emotionally from her daughter and her grandsons Riyaz and Jahaan. Samira was portrayed as someone who had caused upheaval in her family. For her kids, the trauma of losing their birthplace, coupled with losing their grandfather in the midst of a parental separation, was overwhelming, and their grandmother's "cold behavior" certainly added a catalyst. This, of course, was an important issue in this family's treatment. Individual sessions were undertaken with Samira to work through her feelings of guilt and remorse about her immigration ordeal. Mrs. Razia was also invited to a session; she didn't agree to it at first, stating that she was "all right." I then asked Samira and Nida if it would be okay for me to conduct in-home sessions twice a month. That was a good arrangement, as I was able to successfully work with all three generations of this family in their home environment. The process was extremely profound in that Mrs. Razia was encouraged to tell her life stories, which included vignettes of struggle, upheaval, and emergence as a survivor. Such experiences were validated in therapy, as was the family's belief that Allah was "looking out" for them. For the first time, Samira was also able to voice her opinions on women's empowerment and how she wanted to set a good example for her kids. Interestingly, her ideas coincided with her mother's, which I was able to highlight time and again. This, indeed, helped Mrs. Razia and her daughters to travel a path toward reconciliation.

I also incorporated the idea of spiritualism into my work with this family. Samira and Nida were able to discuss "Allah's wishes for a person's life" in therapy and the kids were able to work on their unresolved anger toward their father and about the loss of their home, immigration, and being portrayed as terrorists. Bibliotherapy also proved effective with this family: Samira brought in literature on empowerment and newspaper cuttings on the media's acknowledgement of Islam as a religion of peace and universality. Samira and her kids also joined a local group of South Asian immigrants in the United States and made positive contacts. Gaining the family's consent, I had a meeting with the school's principal, the teacher, and the counselor and elaborated on my observations and culture-specific recommendations. This was quite positive for the school personnel and the family, as they started to look at the context from which the boys' behavior had emerged, to the extent that the teacher appreciation night (to which students and their parents are invited), incorporated presentations by counselors on working with ethnic minority students. Moreover, as Samira became more self-

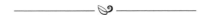

assured in the various aspects of her life, and as the boys were able to verbalize their feelings, their school reports improved.

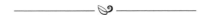

OTHER TREATMENT ISSUES

For a therapist working with a Pakistani family, there are also a number of other issues of concern.

Clients may bring up matters related to unresolved feelings of loss associated with immigration. Of prime importance for the therapist is to explore the history and circumstances of the client's immigration to the United States. This is critical in the light of the fact that the majority of Pakistani families were affected by the 1947 partition between Pakistan and India. The therapist should look into the themes of intergenerational migration, inasmuch as a family seen in the United States may have had multiple immigration experiences. Especially in the post-9/11 period (as stated earlier in this chapter), many Pakistani families in the United States have relocated to or are planning to move to Canada or back to Pakistan. Therefore, it is crucial to evaluate presenting problems in the context of a person's immigration and acculturation experience. As shown earlier in the case example, the academic difficulties and behavioral problems of children and adolescents should be explored systemically. Recently, substance abuse problems have also appeared in Pakistani families, as well as domestic violence and child abuse. It is important to note the Pakistani cultural practices to discipline children, which may be more evident in "recent immigrants" or "nonacculturated" families. Issues related to the extended family are also seen in working with Pakistani families, wherein matters related to loyalties and keeping secrets are prevalent, as stated earlier in this chapter. In all, as Almieda (Chapter 28, this volume) indicates, mental illnesses and emotional difficulties can be exacerbated by the stresses of immigration acculturation, as well as the male-dominated family system hierarchy. It is crucial for therapists to validate, encourage, and respect the experiences of Pakistani clients within the context of Pakistani culture, norms, nuances, and cultural practices. Failure to do so may indeed be detrimental to the process of psychotherapy.

REFERENCES

Akhtar, S. (1999). *Immigration and identity: Turmoil, treatment, and transformation.* Northvale, NY: Jason Aronson.

Butalia, U. (2000). *The other side of silence: Voices from the partition of India.* Durham, NC: Duke University Press.

Donohue, B. (2003, January 8). Pakistanis seeking haven in Canada. *New Jersey Star Ledger.* Available: Why-War.com/Pakistanis seeking haven in Canada.htm

Gooptu, N. (2002, December 12). *India and partition.* Available at www.sant.ox.ac.uk/areastudies

Hasan, K. (2003, July 29). Pakistanis bear brunt of immigration swoop. *Daily Times.* Available: notinourname.net/detections/habi-bear-brunt.juhtm

Karim, S., Saeed, K., Hussain, R. M., Hussain, M., Mubbashar, M. H., & Jenkins, R. (2004). Pakistan mental health country profile. *International Review of Psychiatry, 16*(1–2), 83–92.

Kennedy, M. (2004). Open secrets. Retrieved July 17, 2004, from www.boston.com/news/globe/ideas/articles/2004/07/11/open_secrets

Khan, M. M. (2004). The NMS International Fellowship scheme in psychiatry: Robbing the poor to pay the rich? *Psychiatric Bulletin, 28*, 435–437.

Khan, M. M., & Reza, H. (2000). The pattern of suicide in Pakistan. *Journal of Crisis Intervention and Suicide Prevention, 21*(1), 31–35.

Knafo, D., & Yaari, A. (1997). Leaving the Promised Land: Israeli immigrants in the United States. In P. H. Elovitz & C. Kahn (Eds.), *Immigrant Experiences: personal Narrative and Psychological Analysis* (pp. 221–240). Cranbury, NJ: Associated University Press.

Kuczewski, M. (2000). Informed consent: Does it take a village? The problem of culture and truth telling. *Cambridge Quarterly of Healthcare Ethics, 10*(1), 34–46.

Moazam, F. (2000). Families, patients, and physicians in medical decision making: A Pakistani perspective. *Hastings Center Report, 30*(6), 28–37.

Murray, B. (2002). Psychology takes a tenuous hold in Pakistan. *Monitor on Psychology.* Available: ana.org/monitor.jan

Society magazine. (1997). Pakistan: Society. Available at www.pakistan2000.8m.com

Zaman, R. M. (1992). Psychotherapy in the Third World: Some impressions from Pakistan. In U. P. Gielen, L. L. Adler, & N. A. Milgram (Eds.), *Psychology in internal perspective* (pp. 314–320). Amsterdam: Swets & Zeitlinger.

PART VI

MIDDLE EASTERN
FAMILIES

❧

CHAPTER 31

Arab Families
An Overview

Nuha Abudabbeh

Americans of Arab heritage have been described as one of the "most misunderstood ethnic groups in the United States, frequently misrepresented and vilified" (Erickson & Tamimi, 2001). This vilification and negative stereotyping has been more pronounced in the United States than in other Western countries even prior to the tragedy of September 11, 2001. The reasons for the negative stereotyping and the most recent justification for vilification are complex and not the subject of this chapter. Instead, this chapter attempts to dispel some of the negative stereotypes about Arab Americans and Arabs by describing their history, their cultural values, and their mental health problems, drawing on a growing number of articles and chapters as well as the author's own clinical experience.

If asked to define who Arabs are, most Arabs would say they include all peoples who speak the Arabic language and claim a link with the nomadic tribes of Arabia, whether by descent, by affiliation, or by appropriating the traditional ideals of human excellence and standards of beauty. This definition includes reference to a historical process that began with the preaching by Mohammed of a religion called Islam, a process in which all Arabs play a leading part and by virtue of which they can claim a unique role in the history of humankind (Hourani, 1970). More than 170 million Arabs live in 18 countries located in the Middle East (Palestine, Jordan, Lebanon, Syria, and Iraq), the Gulf region (Saudi Arabia, Kuwait, Oman, Qatar, United Arab Emirates, and Yemen), and North Africa (Morocco, Algeria, Tunisia, Libya, Egypt, and Sudan.

ARAB FAMILIES IN A HISTORICAL AND CULTURAL CONTEXT

The cultural traits of modern Arabs have been impacted by several significant historical events. The period between the 7th and 10th centuries A.D. witnessed the emergence of one of the most profound and influential historical changes in the Arab world: the growth and spread of the religion of Islam. In the early 7th century, the Prophet Moham-med called upon the people of the Arabian Peninsula to submit to the will of God as expressed in a book called the Qur'an. Uniting the tribes in the name of Islam, Moham-med guided them to the conquest of the surrounding countries. By the end of the century, this new empire, called the Caliphate, extended from central Asia in the east and to Spain in the west. This era saw the spread of both Islam and the Arabic language and the build-ing of an urban civilization.

The Arab world was dominated by the Ottoman Empire for the next four centuries (15th–19th). Upon the conclusion of World War I, it was divided among the European victors. In this latter period, Muslim states were forced to adopt new systems of govern-ment and law to face the new developing realities as first Egypt, and then Tunisia, fell under European control and were eventually followed by Morocco and Libya.

Islam's legal practices were preserved, but new thought emerged to incorporate the strength of Europe and to promote the merit of adopting European ideas without being untrue to Islamic beliefs and culture. A new class of Arab "intelligentsia" was created, one that was convinced of the need to adopt European ideas to improve living conditions in Arab countries. Its ideas provided the foundation for the crystallization of 19th-century Arab nationalism.

The partition of Palestine in 1948 and the creation of the state of Israel ignited a political reaction that led to the fall of most of the old regimes in Arab countries. The new regimes were committed to nationalism that aspired to the close union of all Arab countries, independence from the superpowers, and social reform in the direction of greater equality. These ideas were embodied throughout the 1960s in the persona of Egyptian president Gamal Abdel Nasser. The defeat of Syria, Egypt, and Jordan in the 1967 Arab–Israeli war halted the advance of these goals and led to a period of disunity and increasing dependence by Arab countries on one or the other of the two superpow-ers, Russia or the United States.

In the 1980s, the Arab world witnessed the reemergence and strong expression of Islamic feelings and loyalties. This filled an identity vacuum for the uprooted urban pop-ulation, providing a solid base for their lives and filling a need for their own traditions and customs, as opposed to adopting those of the Western world. The 1991 Gulf War, which provoked conflict among the Arabs, was a historical event that further alienated the Arabs from the West. More recently, the bombing of the Twin Towers of the World Trade Center on September 11, 2001, the invasion of Iraq, and the continued violation of the Palestinians' human rights have ushered in one of the lowest periods in the history of Arabs and Arab Americans.

Religion

Islam

The essence of Islam, as preached by the Prophet Mohammed, was transmitted through the Qur'an, which is believed to be the literal word of God. In addition to the Qur'an were the laws of society, elaborated on by adding the Prophet's own traditional sayings (*hadith*) and his practices (*sunna*). A fourth dimension was also added, taking into account certain pre-Islamic traditions and integrating other existing societal norms and customs.

Except by implication, the Qur'an does not contain explicit doctrines or instructions; basically, it provides guidance. The *hadith* and *sunna*, however, contain some specific commands on issues such as marriage and the division of property. They also address such daily habits as how often the believer should worship God and how all people should treat each other.

Based on the general guidance of the Qur'an, five basic obligations of Muslims emerged in the form of the "Pillars of Islam." These consist of (1) oral testimony that there is only one God and that Mohammed is his prophet, (2) ritual prayer practiced five times a day with certain words and certain postures of the body, (3) the giving of alms, (4) keeping a strict fast, including no liquid or food from sunrise to sundown, during the month of Ramadan, and (5) a holy pilgrimage to Mecca (*hajj*) once in a lifetime at a specific time of the year. A general injunction was added, *jihad*, which carries the universal meaning that every Muslim must exercise strenuous intellectual, physical, and spiritual efforts for the good of all. (For a more detailed description of Islam, see Chapter 28.)

Christianity

Approximately 14 million Arabs follow the Christian faith. Lebanon contains the largest Christian population, which constitutes almost 50% of the overall population. Christians remain a minority in all other Arab countries, with the highest percentage in Sudan, followed by Syria, Egypt, Jordan, and Palestine. The largest Christian denomination in the Middle East is the Coptic Orthodox Church, numbering nearly 6 million believers, most of them in Egypt. Other Christian denominations include the Assyrian Church of the East, the Syrian Orthodox Church, the Eastern Greek Orthodox Church, and the Eastern Rite Catholic Church, that is, the Maronite Church (predominantly in Lebanon).

Although Christians make up only 10% of the overall Arab population, Arab Christians are described as having played a disproportionate part in the post–World War II political activities of Arab countries. This is especially true in the nationalist movement in the Middle East and in the Palestinian movement (Carmichael, 1977).

Christians often impress outsiders as being more "Arab" than Muslim Arabs in their Arab nationalist position. Among Arab Americans it is not uncommon to find Arab Christians holding traditional and conventional attitudes toward a variety of issues synonymous to those held by Muslim Arab Americans. After World War II, Christian Arabs led most Arab nationalist movements. Christian Arabs in the United States are very active in fighting to dispel the negative image of Arabs in the United States and the West. Some of the most prominent spokespersons for Arabs are Christians (e.g., Professor Edward Said and Dr. Hanan Ashrawi). Christian Arabs often become quite irate about any hint of their not being seen as part of the Arab community.

When the first major split in Christianity occurred (5th century), Western church leaders affirmed the dual nature of Christ (Christ was both spirit and body) in contrast to Middle Eastern Christians, who adhered to a Monophysite definition of Christ—that he was of a single nature, divine and spiritual. The Arab Christians belonged to the Monophysites.

The Assyrians are unique in that they use neither paintings nor sculpture in worship, but simply a plain cross above the altar. Prayer and worship are conducted in Aramaic, the language of Christ, and are led by laymen.

The Coptic Orthodox, located primarily in Egypt but also found in Ethiopia, believe that their church originated from St. Mark the Evangelist. Today the Coptic Cathedral is located in Cairo, Egypt, and the head of the church has the title of Pope and is revered as the successor to St. Mark.

The Syrian Orthodox Church is also known as the West Syrian Church to distinguish its members from those of the East Syrian Church; its members are also referred to as the Jacobites, after Bishop Jacob Baradaeus. Numbering about 160,000, members of the Syrian Orthodox Church consider the Patriarch of Antioch in Damascus as their spiritual leader. Worship is conducted in Syriac (a dialect of Aramaic), and the sign of the cross is made with one finger, signifying their Monophysite belief.

Eastern Rite Catholics are Arab Christians who maintained their ancient languages of worship and continue their tradition and rites but have split from the rest of the Arab Christians by accepting papal supremacy and returning to the Catholic Church. Unlike Eastern Rite Catholics, the Maronites claim never to have been outside the Catholic Church. The Maronite Church became the first Eastern church to accept papal supremacy in 1180. The Maronites have preserved their ancient Syriac liturgy, although most of their worship is conducted in Arabic (Shabbas & Al-Qazzaz, 1989).

Language

Albert Hourani (1970), in describing the relationship between Arabs and their language, said that they were "more conscious of their language than any people in the world, seeing it not only as the greatest of their arts but also as their common good."

Arabic today is spoken by 130 million people. It was named the sixth official language of the United Nations and is ranked as the fourth most widely spoken language in the world (tied with Bengali). Spoken Arabic differs significantly from one Arab country to the other. It can be separated into five dialects, related to the different geographical regions: (1) the Middle Eastern dialect spoken by Palestinians, Syrians, and Lebanese; (2) the Gulf dialect; (3) the Egyptian dialect; (4) the North African dialect; and (5) the Iraqi dialect. The most familiar of these dialects is the Egyptian dialect, which has historically dominated the film industry as well as artistic expression. Although spoken Arabic is as varied as the different parts of the Arab world, classical Arabic is used for formal speech and in broadcasting and writing.

The Arabic language is extremely difficult and grammatically complex, with its structure lending itself to rhyme and rhythm. Although many other people feel an affection for their native languages, Arabs' feeling for their language is much more intense. The Arabic language is one of the greatest Arab cultural treasures and achievements (Nydell, 1987). Because it is difficult to achieve, a good command of the Arabic language is highly admired.

Family Structure

If the Qur'an is the soul of Islam, then the family can be described as the body. Whereas pre-Islamic Arabs found their strength in tribes, Islam emphasized the extension beyond the tribe, focusing on the *umma* and considering all Muslims as brothers and sisters belonging to the same *umma*. *Umma* is the Arabic translation for the word *nation* in English (Stowasser, 1987). Within the *umma*, families are given importance as units. Men are given specific duties toward their wives and children, wives are given instructions as to how to treat their husbands, and children are advised to honor their mothers. The empowerment of the family unit reassures women of economic and emotional support in regard to their social position in the world. Both men and women are expected to contribute to the support and maintenance of the family unit according to the traditional codes of family and honor and are responsible for the rearing of children. In crisis, both are also expected to view the good of the family above the fulfillment of individual wishes and self-satisfaction. The concept of honor goes beyond the simplistic interpretation of sexual misconduct, encompassing such values as hard work, conservatism, educational and economic advancement, and avoidance of criminal involvement or other unacceptable conduct (Abudabbeh & Aseel, 1999).

There are today many signs of strain on the family system due to factors such as industrialization, urbanization, war and conflict, and Westernization. Despite these pressures, however, the family remains the main system of support throughout the Arab world and for Arabs living elsewhere. For the majority of Arabs, as for virtually all other cultural groups, no institution has replaced the family as a system of support (Fernea, 1985).

The Arab family can be described as patriarchal, pyramidically hierarchal with regard to age and sex, and extended. Despite movements toward a more Westernized nuclear family, the extended family remains important. Although families may have established their own households, they nevertheless maintain the concept of extension by considering their own kin as being worthy of the most attention, of being confided in, and of their allegiance.

Bedouins are the part of Arab society that came mostly from the Arabian Peninsula and migrated to other parts of the Arab world with the spread of Islam. Unlike city people, Bedouins are a migrant, tribal society. The Bedouin family, in both rural and urban areas, constitutes the dominant social institution through which persons inherit their religion, social class, and identity. Whatever befalls one member of the family can bring either honor or shame to the whole family. Family dynamics involve a great deal of self-sacrifice and also provide satisfaction based on the happiness of others or by vicarious living through others.

Another feature of the Arab family is its style of communication, which is described by both Sharabi (1988) and Barakat (1985) as hierarchal, creating vertical as opposed to horizontal communication between those in authority and those subservient to that authority. This relationship, according to Barakat, leads to styles of communication between parents and children in which parents use anger and punishment and the children respond by crying, self-censorship, covering up, or deception.

Marriage

The focus of this chapter on Islamic regulations governing marriage derives from the fact that the majority of Arabs are Muslim, which establishes an undeniable Islamic influence on the entire society. Islam considers marriage an important duty of every Muslim and a safeguard for chastity. Marriage (*nikah*) is recognized as a highly religious, sacred ceremony and is regarded as central to the growth and stability of the basic units of society (having moved away from the pre-Islamic tribalistic emphasis on kinship and blood relation). In Islamic law marriage is a contract legalizing intercourse and the procreation of children. Under Hanafi law, a Muslim man is allowed to marry a non-Muslim woman as long as she belongs to the "people of the Book," meaning that she is either Jewish or Christian. Women, however, are not allowed to marry non-Muslims (Esposito, 1982).

Marriage is seen as a family affair, in which a partner is chosen by a person's family and not based on the Western concept of romantic love. However, despite some changes in this regard, this method of marriage remains the rule and romantic marriage an exception. Although the woman's opinion is supposed to be respected in accepting or rejecting a certain suitor, this is seldom practiced. In Islam, when the marriage contract is drawn, some Sunni sects allow the inclusion of clauses that would give women the power to terminate a marriage. Despite changes in family laws in some Arab countries, women continue to be shortchanged because of the long-standing traditional pre-Islamic and persisting post-Islamic attitudes toward women's role in society.

Practices such as endogamy continue to occur in many Arab countries where marriage within the same lineage (cousins) is still a norm. This is another indication that the family and the tribe, rather than individuals, form the basis of a community. The reasoning behind this type of marriage remains rooted in tribal tradition, which is pre-Islamic. Marriage to close kin ensures the kind of economic and blood kinship needed to continue and enhance the position of the tribe. However, studies conducted in several communities indicate that endogamy constitutes only 3–8% of all marriages and is more prevalent among the more traditional and conventional Arab groups (Barakat, 1985).

Muslim law allows a woman to be contracted for marriage by her guardian (in most countries, this is her father). This is the case at all age levels, unless the woman has been married before. Several Arab countries, however, have enacted laws more favorable to women in this respect, allowing adult women to draw their own marriage contracts. The minimum age for marriage for a Muslim girl is 15 in most Arab countries, and 18 for boys. The more education a woman has, the more likely she is to marry at an older age (Barakat, 1985).

Traditional Islamic law allows men four wives. Although the Qur'an qualifies the multiplicity of wives by stating that a man should not marry more than one unless he is able to treat them equally, the choice is left to him to determine whether to marry more than one. In recent years, some Arab countries have forbidden the practice of polygyny (Tunisia), whereas others have required that a husband must obtain a court's permission prior to taking a second wife (Iraq). In others (Lebanon and Morocco), a wife can insist on a clause in the premarital contract, giving her the option of divorcing her husband in the event he decides to take a second wife (Beck & Keddie, 1978). In practice, polygyny is rare in modern Arab societies.

Most Arab Christians belong to denominations that do not allow divorce. Among Muslims, it is permitted with certain legal stipulations. Mohammed is reported to have said, "Of all permitted things, divorce is the most abominable to God." Many verses in the Qur'an were intended to limit the frequency and facility of divorce that existed in pre-Islamic Arabia (Esposito, 1982).

Barakat (1985) describes the divorce rate as having risen in Arab countries, attributing it to the pressures of modern life. In analyzing the divorce trend, however, it was noted that most divorces occurred in the "engagement" period or during the first 2 years of marriage. This is probably related to the nature of these marriages (i.e., arranged marriages). It may be that what Western couples are able to discover in each other before marriage is possible for Arab couples to discover only after "engagement" (which in Islam is usually a binding contract) or during the early period of marriage.

Children

Children are raised to perpetuate the customs and traditions of the family. Methods of discipline vacillate between mild punishment for unacceptable behavior and putting fear in the child with warnings of what happens to those who do bad things. This is often accompanied by a great deal of unconditional love, especially toward sons.

Differential treatment of boys is not uncommon, and the instilling of traditional expectations in girls is common practice. Although these trends are changing, Arab children are encouraged to maintain close ties with their families and are not encouraged, as Westerners are, to be individuated and separate from their parents. Children who disobey and or shame their parents are likely to be disowned by them (Abudabbeh & Hamid, 2001).

In the event of divorce, a woman retains custody of her children for only a limited period of time and then places them, usually, with the father or the closest male relative as guardian. The age at which the mother relinquishes custody of her children varies according to the Muslim sect to which she belongs.

As the Arab family is more likely to use an authoritarian style in interaction with their children, it is not uncommon to observe that parents are more likely to lecture children than to engage them in discussion or dialogue. It is also common for the children to respect the father's authority, and they are encouraged to obey orders, as opposed to exploring ideas with him. It is likely that the children will spend more time with their mother, and they are more likely to be open with her, at times using her as a messenger or go-between with their father. Therefore, there is a greater likelihood of acting out on the part of the children, and of triangulation, as opposed to open communication among all members of the family.

ARAB AMERICANS TODAY

Arab Americans arrived in the United States in three distinct waves. The first wave, which came between 1890 and 1940, consisted mostly of merchants and farmers who emigrated for economic reasons from regions that were then part of the Ottoman Empire. Ninety percent of this first-wave immigrant population was Christian and originated from the regions known today as Syria and Lebanon. They seem to have assimilated in their new country with a good deal of ease.

The second wave of Arab immigrants began after World War II (after the creation of the State of Israel). Unlike its predecessor, this wave consisted mostly of people with college degrees or those seeking to earn them. It also differed in that its people came from regions of post-European colonization and from sovereign Arab nations. Dominated by Palestinians and Muslims, this wave arrived with an "Arab identity" that was absent in the first. The third wave of immigration occurred after the 1967 Arab–Israeli war. This group came from a variety of Arab countries, seeking refuge to escape the political unrest in their countries of origin. A disproportionate number of these people included Lebanese immigrants, fleeing the civil war in their country, and Iraqis following the Gulf War. With the crystallization of an Arab identity also came the practice of traditions and customs that affected either a hyphenated identity as "Arab Americans" and cultural separateness from the majority of Americans (Abudabbeh & Hays, in press).

Since 1991 several recent historical events, culminating with the tragedy of September 11, 2001, have put Arab Americans in an exceedingly difficult position. The commonplace negative stereotyping of Arabs prior to 9/11 (Mansfield, 1990; Suleiman, 1988) has now become significantly more pronounced, and hate crimes against them has increased 500% (Zoghby, 2003). Following the passage of the Patriot Act, Arab Americans have faced increased scrutiny, possible questioning, arrest, and deportation. This has impacted thousands of Arab American families, whose lives have been disrupted by the deportation or incarceration of their members.

Today Arab Americans can be described as a heterogeneous, multicultural, multiracial, and multiethnic group, currently estimated at nearly 3.5 million people (U.S. Census Bureau, 2000). The largest concentrations of Arab Americans are in Detroit, Los Angeles, New York, New Jersey, Chicago, and the Washington, D.C., area. The majority of Arab Americans are Christian (Catholic 42%, Protestant 12%, Orthodox 23%), and 23% are Muslims (Arab American Institute, 2003).

Approximately 85% of Arab Americans have a high school diploma, more than 4 out of 10 hold a bachelor's or higher degree (as compared with 24% of the American average). Twice as many Arab Americans as Americans have postgraduate degrees. Occupationally, 64% of Arab Americans are in the labor force, mostly in professional and managerial posts, with only 12% in government jobs. The median income for Arab Americans (1999 statistics) was $47,000 in comparison to the American median of $42,000. Close to 30% of Americans have an income of $75,000, in contrast to 22% of Arab Americans (Arab American Institute, 2003).

Cultural Values and Beliefs

Regardless of its country of origin, the family is the cornerstone of the Arab American culture. There may be differences from one country to another in the intensity of the centrality of the family, but not in its impact on the dynamics of the family. Final authority rests with the father or, in his absence, with the oldest male in the family. Within this paradigm, what are considered to be normal individualistic pursuits according to Western values, are often regarded as selfish and are therefore discouraged. Major decisions, such as the choice of a partner and/or a career, are impacted by family expectations.

Privacy is of primary significance, as it is connected to maintaining the honor and good name of the family.

The elders of a family are expected to be cared for by the other family members. Their place in the family requires respect and payback for their roles as good parents. Talking negatively about a parent is unacceptable and regarded almost as a sin.

Sexuality is a taboo subject, rarely if ever discussed openly between parents and children, which presents a dilemma for a large number of immigrant Arab families. Sexual inappropriateness can bring shame to a family; thus, there is little tolerance for homosexuality. Struggling with issues related to sexual identity or making such a choice is usually kept secret from the family. The following case vignette is an example of this type of struggle.

A Syrian college student was referred for an assessment of his eligibility for accommodations for attention-deficit/hyperactivity disorder (ADHD). Suhail had had difficulties with his academic work prior to his arrival in the United States. His struggle with education had affected the family dynamics, as it made him more of a target for criticism by the males in the family, thus pushing his mother to become ever more protective. Suhail, unbeknownst to his family, had been struggling with issue of gender identity and homosexual tendencies. Growing up in a society that would not allow for such a lifestyle or the questioning of his identify, Suhail had kept his struggle a secret from the family, leaving them with concerns about the issue of ADHD only. His contact with a therapist in the United States was Suhail's's first opportunity to reveal his struggles, and he was assured that they would be kept confidential.

There is some variation in attitude from one Arab country to the other on this issue; Morocco and Lebanon are among those described as more tolerant of homosexuality. Abdallah, a young Moroccan male was a self-referral because of his intention to change his major in college. His dilemma of disobeying his family was secondary to his homosexuality. Unlike Suhail, Abdallah had been able to reveal his sexual preference to at least some Moroccans.

Relationships with those outside a person's family are often regarded as crucial for the person's safety and well-being, but never as significant as the relationships within a person's own family. Central to maintaining the strength of those relationships is adherence to certain social obligations, expressing specific verbal responses for particular occasions, and, above all, speaking in a manner that is always respectful of the person being addressed. Openness and directness can be interpreted as rudeness. Dwairy (1998) describes this style of communication as *musyara*. The power of the spoken word is a two-edged sword, capable of maintaining a "good" relationship by using the appropriate phrases, or causing irreparable damage by uttering the wrong ones. Thus, openness and directness are avoided for the sake of keeping a relationship intact. This style of communication inevitably creates a fertile ground for what Dwairy calls *istigaba*, which implies saying what you really mean about a person only in his or her absence. Thus, one of the most important elements in building intimacy with others is significantly impacted.

In addition to being proud of their language, Arabs take a great deal of pride in their generosity and hospitality. One of the greatest characteristics that can be attributed to a person is generosity, and the most dreaded is stinginess, as illustrated by the following Arabic saying: "Generosity conceals a thousand shortcomings."

TREATMENT IMPLICATIONS FOR ARAB AMERICANS

The emphasis on family as the source of support, as well as the concept of the *umma* in Islam, discourage Arabs from seeking professional help for their emotional problems. Dwairy (1998) describes Arabs as less likely than Westerners to seek help from mental health providers because of their higher tolerance for mental illness and their attribution of mental illness to outside factors. In recent years the combined loss of support systems and proliferation of Arabic and Islamic community resources has led to a documented increase in the number of Arab Americans seeking professional help.

According to information from the Naim Foundation, a nonprofit mental health clinic in Washington (1982–2001) and a call-in mental health radio program in Arabic (1990–2001), Arab Americans seeking help were more likely to telephone than to come in person. The majority of the callers were females, most probably because of to their inability to drive or to ensure anonymity. Those seeking help in person were likely to come for only one visit, seeking advice for a specific situation, or at times asking for information for someone else. This approach is probably akin to asking advice from a learned person or a trusted friend to assist in decision making. For example, a Sudanese female who was unwilling to accept her husband's word that her test results from a physical examination were negative, was brought by the husband to the therapist to convince his wife that he was telling her the truth about the results of her examination. The wife was apprehensive of the test results, fearing that she might have cancer. This consultation illustrates (1) the esteem in which a therapist is held, (2) the suspiciousness aroused because of the custom of keeping bad news from family members to protect them from the psychological harm it may cause, and (3) the need to keep such a situation secret even from those who are close.

Arab men were as likely as women to seek help from a female therapist, including Arab men from such conservative backgrounds as Saudi Arabia. Common problems presented include the following:

- Obsessive–compulive disorder, depression, posttraumatic stress disorder, and generalized anxiety. The increase in the number of Arab Americans diagnosed with posttraumatic stress disorder has been documented in recent surveys of Iraqi and Lebanese immigrants (Abudabbeh and Hays, in press).
- Generational conflict, gender-related conflict, and challenges presented by the forging of a hyphenated identity.
- College students with learning disability and attention-deficit disorder.
- Marital discord.
- Legal problems leading to placement on probationary requirements, as well as evaluations to assist the courts with a variety of legal charges.

The experience of the Naim Foundation is that, unlike other ethnic groups, Arabs were more likely to seek help for couple problems than for family problems. Although families have had to be "lured" into treatment, couples presented a steady stream of patients. This is likely due to the motivation to keep a marriage going, inasmuch as divorce is frowned upon and keeping the family intact is paramount.

Problems presented by couples are as follows:

- Emotional or physical abuse by the spouse, most often the husband.
- Cross-cultural marriages impacted by religious differences.
- Within-culture differences between Arab Americans and Arabs and between Arab Americans from different Arab countries.
- Problems in dealing with a partner with mental illness.
- Premarital counseling.

In contrast to couple therapy, family therapy with Arabs can be more challenging because of their fear of exposing the shaming behavior of family members, along with the possible undermining of the authority of the father. However, the situation is ameliorated by most Arabs' attitude toward a therapist whom they respect as knowing more than they do and often approaching the therapeutic intervention as a learning experience.

The following cases illustrate the complexity of working with Arab American families whose adherence to societal norms at times supersedes the welfare of the individual in the family.

The therapist received a call from a young man who wished to refer his brother, Kader, to therapy. Kader's family is a well-known Israeli Arab family in the community, described as conservative with traditional expectations of their children. The men were expected to achieve academically and marry women chosen by the parents. All the children were born in the United States, but spoke Arabic fluently and remained in close contact with the country of origin. Kader had fulfilled one of his obligations by becoming a physician. However, unlike his siblings, he "failed " his family by not complying with their wishes to accept the chosen bride. Although he was able to complete a preliminary part of this obligation, he was unable to go through with the latter part of it. Having obliged his parents by marrying in the country of origin and fulfilling other associated rituals, upon return to the United States he adamantly refused to have his bride come to live with him. Kader was further described as having had emotional problems as a child and having always been in conflict with his father. Kader had been the one to challenge the authority of his father, who was a strict disciplinarian. Kader had disciplinary problems in school as well. None of these issues were ever discussed in a mental health context prior to Kader's reaching adulthood. There was tension between Kader and his father, who perceived him as a failure, thus exacerbating his problems further. The mother, an illiterate woman, realized that her son's problems were serious. As she was the only member of the family with this awareness, she had no choice but to become his protector. Later, as Kader's emotional problems began to manifest themselves in a variety of ways, such as in his isolation from others, he became more paranoid and conservative in his religious practices and beliefs. His siblings urged him to seek help, but he refused. Based on the description given by his brother, the hypothesis was that Kader might be suffering from depression with paranoid features. The therapist recommended that his brother, as well as his parents, accompany Kader, explaining that his likelihood of coming would be highly enhanced if the whole family came. The challenges presented were typical of those presented by other Arab American family members. A child is seen to have problems, which are either denied or ignored for fear of revealing a family secret. Eventually, the problem child becomes an adult and a particular situation reveals the secret of the family. In this case the parents were forced to deal with their son's emotional problems as they became exposed to the community at large because of the marriage. The secret in this family was having a son with a mental illness or an emotional disorder that had needed attention during childhood. The emotional disturbance was seen as disobedience to the authority of the father and treated accordingly. The mother's intuitive understanding of the vulnerability of her son was interpreted as spoiling him and never given the weight it deserved because of her secondary role in this particular family.

Anticipating the first session to be the only visit the family would be making, the therapist scheduled the session accordingly. First complimenting the father on his willingness to come to therapy, and acknowledging it as a sign of his caring for his son, attended to Arab family dynamics and cultural values. The mother was given credit for her supporting role within the constraints of these particular family dynamics. The son was given a great deal of support by the therapist's congratulating him on his accomplishments. There followed a description of what other Arab immigrant families experience in their struggle to find a balance between the values of two cultures. The session ended with concrete advice given to each member of the family to help them improve their communication and interaction, as follows:

- The father was asked to accept the realities of Kader's emotional status and to also appreciate how much his son had been able to accomplish despite his problems. He was also told that his son's accomplishments were in part due to (the father's) input. This reassured the father of his role as the authority figure and prepared the way to improve his relationship with the "failing" son.

- The mother was told about her very significant role in protecting her son, as that may have given him the inner strength to go on to earn a degree despite his depression.
- The therapist focused on Kader mostly by validating his difficult position, and his guilt about having disappointed his parents was alleviated by the therapist pointing out that he had done exceptionally well under his specific circumstances, by educating the whole family about depression.

A 16-year-old Jordanian American girl, Sana, was referred by Child Protective Services for therapy after running away from her home. She was the younger of two sisters who were born in Jordan. The father was a successful businessman who had divorced the mother and remarried when he immigrated to the United States. The two daughters had never met their mother, nor were they ever given much information about her. The sisters, who were 1 year apart, were very close. Sana described her father as a caring man, who was American in "certain ways" but remained Arab in others. Although Sana could dress like any other teenager in her school, she was not allowed to date. The stepmother was described as caring and basically close to both of the girls. Sana, who described her home situation as "confusing," especially when it came to boys, began acting out, initially by smoking marijuana and, eventually, sexually. In contrast to Sana, the older sister, who was academically successful, did not exhibit similar behavioral problems. She had initially smoked marijuana with Sana and had sneaked out of the house with her. Their father became aware of the problems when Sana's academic performance began to deteriorate. When called for a conference with the school, he discovered that Sana had missed school on many occasions and had also forged her father's signature.

Untraditional approaches in dealing with Sana and the family included the therapist's paying a visit to the family's home, with the knowledge that hospitality is of utmost importance and a visit by a therapist would not be rejected. Initially, the father was reluctant to participate in family therapy, especially when Sana was unwilling to return home, because he insisted on maintaining strict rules and regulations about outings. Family therapy was adapted to meet the needs of this particular situation by seeing Sana individually while continuing to meet with the rest of the family at home. The therapeutic intervention included the following:

- Sana was helped to understand her father's position in the community, his cultural constraints—that is, his need to "save face," meaning to redeem his reputation before his own family and friends. The father's contradictory positions on various issues, such as ways of dressing and sexuality, were explained to Sana within the context of her father's own challenges in bringing up his children in a milieu that was totally different from that in which he was brought up.
- Sana was taught how to take better care of herself and was engaged in trying to understand her possible reasons for acting out. She was able to look at her anger about her mother's abandonment, and at her father for leaving her mother.
- The father was given advice as to what might be more effective in working with Sana. The discrepancy in the two daughters' behavior was explained as possibly resulting from early attachment issues that may have affected the two daughters differently. Sana, the younger of the two, may have been more affected by the separation from her biological mother and, consequently, had more anger at her father.
- The father was advised to challenge his traditional inclination to remain angry with his daughter for having left the home and having "shamed" the family. This might take a while, but he was advised to keep the "door open" to reconciling by talking to Sana when she called the house and to eventually bring himself to visit with her. He was also told not to prevent the sister from keeping in touch with Sana.

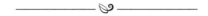

Treatment ended with Sana's acting out behavior having subsided significantly, the father's position improved by agreeing to talk to Sana on the telephone, and options remaining open to accept future sessions for family therapy.

———————— ❧ ————————

Treatment can be enhanced if the therapist relinquishes traditional approaches, such as the most formalized aspects of conducting psychotherapy:

- To facilitate treatment, the therapist should use didactic and structured therapies, rather than in-depth or insight therapy, which is contraindicated.
- In the event that family members refuse to come for therapy, calling them personally and inviting them might work. This fits with the Arab response to those who make an effort, in contrast to the negative reaction to formalized relationships with caretakers.
- A family's giving of gifts and invitations to their home is a common experience, done as a gesture of appreciation. A therapist's refusal may be interpreted as an insult.
- The hierarchical and patriarchal nature of the family should be kept in mind while helping the parents work through new norms for the family. In dealing with Arab families, the definition of *family* should be expanded to include any other persons designated by them. As in the cases described earlier, therapeutic intervention should always take into account the authoritarian position of the father while integrating the protective role of the mother in the process.
- In dealing with taboo issues such as homosexuality or sexual problems, the therapist has to consider the traumatic implications of these problems in the family within the community. The treatment approach in dealing with Suhail and Abdallah involved exploring with them strategies for dealing with their families' views about homosexuality, and their families' response to such a choice. In Suhail's situation, even with the therapist's support, he was unable to tell his family.
- Scheduling and timing should be sufficiently flexible to accommodate the expectations and needs of this population, as was done with Kader's family.
- There should be openness to providing family therapy even when family members cannot all be in one physical space, as was the case with Sana's family.

CONCLUSION

Like other minorities or culturally diverse groups, Arabs are newcomers to the benefits of psychotherapy. Seeking psychotherapy is not an instinctual behavior; it is a learned behavior. The benefit of psychotherapy or psychological intervention as we see it today is the outcome of at least a half century of ongoing research and education in this country. Our sensitivities to incorporating other cultural norms into the delivery of services are even more recent. Ensuring the delivery of optimal services to non-Western people calls for educating both the service providers and those who receive the services. To provide the appropriate services, the emphasis should be on education. The experience to date supports the impression that when Arab families, like others, become aware of the benefits of psychotherapy as an essential tool in achieving a better or less stressful life, they are good candidates for psychotherapy. Like other non-Western populations, Arabs can benefit from changes in the approach used in the delivery of service, changes that incorporate some of the expectations of Arabs in seeking a therapist. Given the pervasive anti-Arab sentiment in the United States today, therapists are urged to examine their own attitudes and biases before treating Arab clients. To familiarize themselves with this population, Western-educated therapists are encouraged to seek various resources to enhance their understanding of Arabs. In addition to self-educating, it is suggested that direct consultation with those who are familiar with this population be initiated.

REFERENCES

Arab American Institute, CIC. (2003). *Arab American demographics*. Washington, DC: Author.

Abudabbeh, N., & Aseel, H. A. (1999). Transcultural counseling and Arab Americans. In J. McFadden (Ed.), *Transcultural counseling* (2nd ed., pp. 283–296). Alexandria, VA: American Counseling Association.

Abudabbeh, N., & Hamid, A. (2001). Substance use among Arabs and Arab Americans. In S. L. A. Straussner (Ed.), *Etnocultural factors in substance abuse treatment* (pp. 275–290). New York: Guilford Press.

Barakat, H. (1985). Arab families. In E. Fernea (Ed.), *Women and the family in the Middle East: New voices of change* (pp. 27—48). Austin: University of Texas Press.

Beck, L., & Keddie, N. (Eds.). (1978). *Women in the Muslim world*. Cambridge, MA: Harvard University Press.

Carmichael, J. (1977). *Arabs today*. New York: Anchor Books.

Dwairy, M. A. (1998). *Cross-cultural counseling: The Arab-Palestinian case*. Binghampton, NY: Haworth Press.

Erickson, C. D., & Al-Tamimi, N. R. (2001, November). Providing mental health services to Arab Americans: Recommendations and considerations." *Cultural Diversity and Ethnic Minority Psychology*, 7(4), 308–327.

Esposito, J. L. (1982). *Women in Muslim family law*. Syracuse, NY: Syracuse University Press.

Fernea, E. (Ed.). (1985). *Women and the family in the Middle East*. Austin: University of Texas Press.

Hourani, A. (1970). *Arabic thought in the liberal age: 1798–1939*. London: Oxford University Press.

Mansfield, P. (1990). *The Arabs*. New York: Penguin Books.

Nydell, M. K. (1987). *Understanding Arabs: A guide for Westerners*. Yarmouth, ME: Intercultural Press.

Shabbas, A., & Al-Qazzaz, A. (Eds.). (1989). *Arab world notebook*. Berkeley, CA: Najda.

Sharabi, H. (1988). *Neopatriarchy*. New York: Oxford University Press.

Stowasser, B. F. (1987). *the Islamic impulse*. Washington, DC: Center for Contemporary Arab Studies, Georgetown University.

Suleiman, M. W. (1999). *Arabs in America: Building a new future*. Philadelphia: Temple University Press.

U. S. Census Bureau. (2000). 2000 Summary, File 4. Washington, DC: Author.

Zoghby, J. (2003). *Report on survey of Arab American households*. Washington, DC: Zoghby International.

CHAPTER 32

Armenian Families

Steve Dagirmanjian

Many times, when meeting people, I am asked the origin of my name. After I identify myself as Armenian, the questioner often responds by telling me a story of a favorite neighbor, a close friend from college, or a helpful coworker who was Armenian. This may then be followed by a fond recounting of the various Armenian culinary delicacies that he or she has sampled by way of the friend. Sometimes the truly initiated will even recite an Armenian phrase or two, almost as if delivering the secret handshake of some esoteric fraternal organization–which, in effect, is exactly what that person is doing.

Living at the crossroads of competing civilizations, Armenians were perpetually overrun by powerful outside groups. For centuries they have struggled to maintain their unique identity while living side by side with people they considered outsiders at best or, more often, enemies.

In environments such as this, there are certain adaptive benefits in assessing quickly a new acquaintance's hostile, friendly, or neutral posture. For many Armenians, such a "sizing up" of outsiders is almost reflexive—as basic as looking both ways before crossing the street. It is something therapists attempting to work with Armenian families would be wise to recognize. Given Armenians' ancient cultural narrative of survival, their acute wariness of outsiders, and their attention to the ethnic origins of new acquaintances, it seems ironic when someone asks an Armenian the origin of his or her name (i.e., "sizing" him or her up).

A counterpoint to the hypervigilance Armenians may exhibit before getting to know someone is the warmth and affection they typically shower on people whom they accept as friends. Friends visiting an Armenian family's home for the first time are often surprised by the red carpet treatment and the "one-of-the-family" kind of acceptance they instantly receive. Sam, an Armenian college student, described how touched his best friend was by the hugs he received the first time he met Sam's parents, when the two students were home for a holiday break. The friend was received more like a member of the extended family than as a guest.

The paradox of wariness versus emotional warmth and openness suggested by this brief example is one of several contradictory images that appear to characterize Armenian Americans. These contrasting currents of identity are explored throughout this chapter, along with their historical antecedents and some possible clinical responses.

HISTORY

Historically, the lands of Greater Armenia are located northeast of the Euphrates River on the high Eastern Anatolian Plateau of Asia Minor. Mount Ararat (17,000 feet), located at the eastern edge of modern-day Turkey, is considered by many Armenians to be the spiritual, as well as geographical, center of their homeland. It is here that the Bible says Noah's ark landed. Ancient Armenian legend claims that the Armenian people are descended from Japheth, one of Noah's sons (Bournoutian, 2003).

Located in the midst of major caravan routes linking the West with the East and Middle East, Armenia was a battleground throughout most of its history, as powerful neighbors (Greeks, Romans, and Byzantines to the west, and Persians, Arabs, and Turks to the east) vied for control of its strategic territory. Regardless of who were the political rulers of the regions of Armenia in the centuries following the birth of Christ, local control was essentially dominated by feudal lords. Whether paying tribute to Romans, Persians, or other rulers, the local Armenian feudal lords (*nakharans*) remained fiercely independent. Local rivalries abounded, so that the *nakharans* were constantly fighting with each other. So great was the jockeying for power that it was not uncommon for these Armenian feudal lords to ally with Arab or Greek forces if it might gain them an advantage over a nearby Armenian rival. As a result, Armenians never presented a unified front to outside aggressors (Der Nersessian, 1945). However, this lack of centralization may have ultimately aided Armenian survival. Outsiders could conquer its armies, but could not assimilate its people (Bournoutian, 2003).

This parochialism was further exaggerated by Armenia's inaccessible geography and the "excessive individuality" (Der Nersessian, 1945) of its inhabitants. The Armenian nature, including self-reliance and mistrust of authority, did not lend itself to coalition building. The skillful exploitation of regional rivalries by both Arab and Greek interlopers added to the divisiveness of an already fractious people.

The "excessive individuality" is amusingly reflected in my grandfather's comment that Armenians were fierce fighters but lousy soldiers, because every private in the army thought that he knew more than the generals. Apparently, the Armenians' narrowly focused egocentrism has not always served them well. By the 15th century, Armenians were subjects of the Ottoman Empire. In an attempt to find a mechanism that allowed the Muslim Turkish majority to peacefully coexist with the various ethnic minorities (e.g., Armenians, Jews, Greeks) living within the empire while still maintaining governmental control, the Ottomans created the millet system. Essentially, the Armenian millet was a semi-independent religious, political administrative entity that functioned within the Ottoman Empire, while still under the ultimate authority of the sultans (rulers). Although this structure allowed Armenians cultural and religious autonomy, it also added to the political inequality and social distance between Armenians and the Turkish majority. It was a separate, but not so equal governmental structure, which institutionalized the preferential treatment of the Turkish majority in any interethnic matters. The oppression and prejudice this system nurtured eventually led to genocide early in the 20th century (Bakalian, 1993).

An early historical event in which Armenians take great pride is the establishment of Christianity as its state religion. King Tiridates was converted by St. Gregory in A.D. 301, making Armenia the first country to adopt Christianity as its official religion (Der Nersessian, 1945). However, Armenians carved out their own independent path. Rather than ally themselves with the larger Greek Orthodox Church, they maintained their own church doctrine and hierarchy. This further accentuated their separateness (for better or worse) from neighboring peoples and cultures.

A final critical element in the maintenance and development of Armenian culture as a distinct entity was the invention of the Armenian alphabet in the 5th century by the monk Menob Mashtots. His translation of the Bible paved the way for a burst of intellectual expansion that established Armenians "as part of the civilized world and consolidated their Christian identity" (Bakalian, 1993). The Armenian language and the Armenian Orthodox Church can be said to have provided the backbone of the people's identity throughout centuries of living under outside domination. Many Armenians hold their language in the same kind of reverence as they do their church.

Following World War I, an independent Republic of Armenia existed for a short time (1918–1920) before being partitioned by its powerful neighbors, Turkey and the Soviet Union. For many years, the only "Armenia" was the Soviet Socialist Republic of Armenia. In 1991, with the dissolution of the Soviet Union, Soviet Armenia declared its independence and joined the world community as an independent nation. Today's Armenian Republic faces geopolitical challenges to its survival that are no less hazardous than those faced by the *nakharans* 2,000 years ago. Because of economic hardships, significant numbers of Armenians have been immigrating to Russia (see the later section, "Immigration to the United States"). Armenia's present population is little more than two million (Bournoutian, 2003).

GENOCIDE

The single most defining element of 20th-century Armenian identity is the Genocide of the Armenian people perpetrated by the Turkish government during the early part of the last century. Large-scale massacres began in the 1890s at the direction of the Ottoman sultan Abdul-Hamid and culminated in the Genocide of 1915, in which the new government of the Young Turks orchestrated the slaughter of 1.5 million Armenians. The impact of such a horror on a group who presently number approximately 6 million, worldwide, is incalculable. It is a rare Armenian family who has been untouched by these events (e.g., each of my four grandparents was the sole surviving sibling in his or her family). However, what keeps the Genocide alive in the hearts and minds of most Armenians today is the unyielding denial of its occurrence, maintained by the present Turkish government.

When the Young Turk government came to power in 1908, few Armenians could have imagined the implications of the new rulers' xenophobic vision of a pan-Turkic empire, one which excluded non-Turkic minorities such as Christian Armenians. Early in 1915, using the pressures of World War I to justify suppressing "subversive" Armenian activities, the Young Turk government set in motion a simple yet startlingly effective plan of mass murder. Men of fighting age were arrested, removed from their villages, and, far away from populated areas, killed by military troops. The rest of the defenseless population of women, children, and elderly people were collected and deported from their homelands. These "deportations" were nothing more than death marches into the desert, where the Armenians were stripped of their possessions, even their clothing, denied food and water, and subjected to attacks by marauding bandits (Miller & Miller, 1993).

The Genocide resulted in the death of approximately 1.5 million Armenians, one quarter of the total Armenian population, worldwide. It cut through all strata of Armenian society, rending the fabric of Armenian life in unimaginable ways and imprinting its terrible effects on subsequent generations. Every year on April 24, Armenian Martyrs Day, Armenians around the world take time to remember the events of 1915.

RESPONSES TO THE GENOCIDE

Responses to the Genocide are varied and complex. Miller and Miller (1993), in their collection of oral histories from 100 survivors of the Genocide, have categorized their responses into six types: (1) avoidance and repression, (2) outrage and anger, (3) revenge and restitution, (4) reconciliation and forgiveness, (5) resignation and despair, (6) explanation and rationalization. The range of responses reflects, perhaps, the difficulty inherent in attempting to move beyond an event of such enormous proportions. Herein lies another Armenian paradox. The Genocide, more than any other single aspect of being Armenian, can muster feelings of solidarity and unity among broadly disparate subgroups of Armenians. Yet it creates intolerable dissonance for a self-reliant, industrious, and vibrant people to be identified primarily by a generations-old tragedy.

Although survivors' responses may vary according to the degree to which they were directly exposed to atrocities and are not limited to simply one category, a dominant response among many has been avoidance and repression. Apparently, many surviving children raised in Turkish families or in orphanages were discouraged from speaking about what they had seen (Miller & Miller, 1993.) Unless questioned directly about it, survivors I have known rarely mention the Genocide and then only to state in rather matter-of-fact, dismissive terms, "My father and brothers were killed by the Turks"—end of story. My maternal grandmother simply would not discuss how she came to have the tattooed cross on her wrist. Apparently, Hitler's Germany was inspired by the Turks in more than one way.

Miller and Miller (1993) also state that survivors were more likely to say positive things about the Turkish people than subsequent generations of Armenian Americans. For some survivors, Turks had been instrumental in their survival, some even reporting acts of courage by Turkish citizens to resist the official policies of the government. However, in general, reconciliation and forgiveness seem to be least common among the responses, particularly among second- and third-generation Armenian Americans, primarily because of the Turkish government's continuing denial of the Genocide.

Non-Armenian therapists may be surprised by how deeply resistant contemporary Armenians may be to feelings of forgiveness for the Genocide. For example, many years ago, I treated a Harvard-educated hippie client in a drug program, whose speech was full of love and peace and brotherhood. But when I happened to mention the assassination of a Turkish government official by a militant group of Armenians, he said he was glad, adding, "It's paying the Karmic debt, man."

The story of victimization and its subtle ripple through the generations is not unlike that reported by adult survivors of sexual abuse. Life has moved on, and the survivors can be functionally quite successful, but an irrational undertow of guilt and shame seems to blight their self-esteem like an oil slick untouched by the tides of time.

Boyajian and Grigorian (1986) describe a "survivor syndrome" in which individuals feel apologetic for being alive while the "good" family members died. However, a subtler form of shame may be lingering with subsequent generations of Armenians. This shame, again, is more like that of the incest survivor's and may be described as the unassimilated debris of the abject humiliation of the Genocide. The survivor has an ongoing, if irrational, feeling that there is something irreparably wrong with him or her for having experienced such heinous crimes. As a result of the perpetrators' denial of responsibility and the unwillingness of the world community, due to political expediency, to recognize the crimes (e.g., the U.S. Congress has failed to pass several resolutions acknowledging the Armenian Genocide; the *New York Times* now uses terms like "ethnic conflict"). (In 2004, *New York Times* editorial policy changed to allow journalists use of the term "genocide" if they so choose.) when referring to the Genocide, despite its detailed coverage of the massacres when they occurred), the victim's shame may burrow farther within, to remain hidden and unaltered.

Bruno Bettelheim (1979) described a similar avoidance response among Jewish survivors of the Holocaust. The memories of endured atrocities do not fade, and the survivors seem to fear that if they were to talk about the past, they would once again become crushed and consumed by the horrors lurking in the shadows of their present lives. Yet talking is the "cure" Bettelheim prescribes. This may be true of the descendants of survivors as well, as the story of Katchi illustrates.

At the time she sought therapy Katchi was a 44-year-old, third-generation Armenian, whose second marriage was foundering. She felt overwhelmed by the demands of her two children and burnt out by the routine of nearly 20 years of teaching. On the face of it, her problem appeared to be a familiar one: Overresponsible, caretaking wife is unable to satisfy or engage with her emotionally aloof and exacting husband. Therapeutic efforts involving the husband yielded some early positive changes, which eased the crisis in the marriage. However, Katchi remained depressed and listless. A new therapeutic avenue presented itself when the therapist noticed that her depression seemed to coincide with her mother's hospitalization for emphysema. As this was explored further, Katchi, who had openly expressed pride in her Armenian heritage at the outset of therapy, now revealed more contradictory feelings. Her mother's illness had stirred memories of her grandmother, who had lived with Katchi's family when she was a child. Her grandmother, a survivor of the Genocide, was beset with multiple health problems—many quite real, some seemingly imagined. Katchi recalled how she felt embarrassed and smothered by the infirm old woman's neediness and fears, and by how she was different from the American-born grandmothers of her friends. Katchi was ashamed of her grandmother's broken body and spirit and hated herself for feeling so. It was not until she allowed herself to talk about how oppressed she felt by her grandmother's painful existence that she recognized the historical origins of her own despair. As she considered the grotesque ways in which the Genocide had twisted her grandmother's life, Katchi became less ashamed and more accepting of her grandmother and herself. Concurrently, her depression dissipated and eventually disappeared.

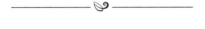

CHURCH AND POLITICS

As mentioned earlier, Armenia was the first country to adopt Christianity as its state religion. As in many ancient cultures, church and state were not separate. The church served as the hub of cultural and political activities almost as much as it served as a religious center.

In the early 19th century, because of the proselytizing efforts of Roman Catholic and New England Protestant missionaries (Bakalian, 1993), some Armenians left the "mother church" (the Armenian Apostolic Church) to become Catholics and Protestants. Armenians remain active in three different denominations, Apostolic, Catholic, and Protestant, with Apostolics being by far the largest group, and Catholics the smallest.

Armenians were also divided by political affiliations. Through much of the 20th century, Armenian politics had largely been defined by the conflict between militant proponents of Armenian nationalism (the Tashnag Party) and advocates of accommodation with the Soviet Union (the Ramgavar and Hunchag Parties. The Tashnags' primary focus had been to establish a free and independent Armenia, including the use of violence toward this end. The Tashnag revolutionary doctrine effectively polarized the Armenian political arena. The Ramgavars, Hunchags, and other minor political groups, although having different political ideologies themselves, were united in their anti-Tashnag, anti-militancy position. They believed that allying with a powerful, friendlier neighbor, the Soviet Union, offered the best solution for preservation and growth of the Armenian people (Bakalian, 1993). Tashnag versus anti-Tashnag feelings ran deep and were evident wherever Armenians lived in the world.

This heated political schism was punctuated by periodic outbreaks of violence, the most infamous being the assassination of the Armenian Archbishop Tourian of New York on Christmas Eve, 1933, by members of the Tashnag Party. The Armenian Apostolic Church claimed Archbishop Tourian to be the spiritual leader of all Armenians living in North America. The Tashnags disapproved of what they perceived as the church being unduly compromising with Soviet authorities, and the assassination of the archbishop served as exclamation mark to their position. This resulted in the expulsion of all Tashnags from the church and the establishment of a separate Tashnag division of the Armenian Apostolic Church.

For first- and second-generation Armenian Americans, these religious and political divisions maintained enough emotional charge to influence their choices of which churches or clubs to attend. This factionalism is much less influential today. Perhaps because of assimilation and/or the reality of the Republic of Armenia's existence, the religio-political feuding of the past is not as likely today to stop a family of the original Armenian church from attending church services of the Tashnag wing of the church.

Another significant aspect of the Apostolic Church is its flexibility in regard to doctrinal beliefs. Again, individuality is encouraged. The church does not strictly enforce rules of observance. This religious tolerance seems to be balanced by quite conservative moral values (particularly in regard to sexual mores) among the families of the church community (Bakalian, 1993). Behavior that dishonors the family is likely to be more strongly censured than the religious implications of a "sin." For example, a family would likely be more disturbed by friends and acquaintances knowing that a son or daughter was living out of wedlock with someone than by its simply being against church teachings. A paradox emerges again—Armenins are religiously liberal while being morally conservative.

IMMIGRATION TO THE UNITED STATES

Despite the presence of Malcolm the Armenian in the Jamestown Colony in 1619, the first significant influx of Armenian immigrants to the United States did not occur until the 1890s, when the first wave of massacres in the Ottoman Empire began. From that time until 1924, when an immigration quota system was instituted, tens of thousands of Armenians immigrated to the United States (Bakalian, 1993). The great majority of immigrants were survivors, directly or indirectly, of the Genocide and the deportations.

In addition to the personal tragedies the newcomers brought with them, they were ill prepared for the demands of a complex, industrialized society, coming as they did from a largely agrarian culture. Their integration into their new home was further hindered by the intense intolerance for differences prevailing at the time. Yet most Armenian immigrants felt enormous gratitude for their host country and attempted to demonstrate their appreciation by working hard and becoming good citizens.

The second significant wave of Armenian immigrants arrived after World War II. Another spurt came in 1965, when the quota law was liberalized. Unlike the first immigrants, these Armenians were not survivors of the Genocide and were not coming from the ancestral homeland. Instead, they immigrated from a variety of the Armenian diaspora communities in Syria, Lebanon, Greece, France, and elsewhere. These immigrants were generally better prepared to face the exigencies of life in their new home than the earlier Armenian immigrants (Bakalian, 1993).

The hardships of settling in a new country and culture are obvious. Nevertheless, Armenians were quick to establish their own connections with each other apart from the majority American culture. Accustomed as they were to preserving their ethnic identity while coexisting with alien cultures, Armenians quickly established fraternal organizations, built churches, and created schools to teach the Armenian language and history in a formalized way to their children. The strong Armenian community became and remains testimony to Armenian cultural pride, as well as being a resource for sustaining it.

The most recent groups of Armenians to arrive in the United States came following the earthquakes in Soviet Armenia in 1988 and after the conflict between Soviet Armenia and Soviet Azerbajian over the Nagarno-Karabagh region, where the Muslim majority massacred Armenians in Baku in January 1990 (Bakalian, 1993). These refugees tended to be middle- to upper-middle-class businesspeople and professionals.

All too predictably, the new arrivals have not been entirely well received by the established Armenian American community. The older community disapproves of what it sees as the newcomers' arrogant and pushy behaviors. They are viewed as often disdainful of the established community's degree of Americanization. Although the Armenian Church has attempted to foster integration between the groups, relations remain strained between them (Sungarian & Guglielmo, personal communication, September 15, 1994).

The earlier immigrants settled primarily in the urban industrial centers of the Northeast and the Midwest, where the jobs were, and a small percentage settled in California. Now 600,000–800,000 Armenians are more widely distributed throughout the United States. Today, Los Angeles is clearly the favorite location of newcomers.

The early immigrants tended to be better educated than immigrants from other countries arriving at the time. Many were skilled artisans or experienced businesspeople. Armenians have been referred to as "middlemen minorities" (Bakalian, 1993) because their economic pursuits have been in activities that are liquid and transportable, typical of a merchant class.

Armenians were quickly recognized in their new country for their intelligence and industriousness. For this reason, they escaped the standard ethnic slurs of the time, pointing to ignorance and laziness, that were applied to many other ethnic groups in the early 20th century. Instead, a pejorative stereotype of the wily, self-serving, overambitious Armenian was created to account for the group's relative economic successes (Bakalian, 1993). Ironically, these are some of the same criticisms that Armenian Americans have directed at more recent Armenian immigrants from the Middle East and the former Soviet Union (Sungarian & Guglielmo, personal communication, September 15, 1994). Being hardworking and self-sufficient are clearly cornerstone values for most Armenians. A story common to many Armenian families is how they managed to get through the Great Depression without relying on public assistance.

THE FAMILY

The traditional, pre-Genocide family structure usually consisted of several generations living together often within one room. The family was strongly patriarchal, with the elder males dominating the affairs of the family. Marriages were arranged, and a new bride was expected to live with the husband's family, where she was clearly subservient to the eldest female in the household (Miller & Miller, 1993). The eldest female could often be a formidable figure within the family, because of her accrued authority over household matters within the overarching patriarchal structure.

After the Genocide, widows sometimes filled the void as the family elder, because so many of the men had been killed. Yet the family remained patriarchal, and the eldest males' authority was not challenged, although there were more instances of family situations in which female voices held sway. Stories abound among latter-generation Armenians about the centrality of beloved grandmothers in their childhood households (Bakalian, 1993).

One second-generation Armenian woman recognized the roots of her own precocious feminism, as she warmly recalled days spent with her grandmother as a child. Her grandmother's household was among the poorest in a neighborhood of poor families. The meagerness of what she had to give to her children and grandchildren was further limited by her autocratic husband's selfishness. His allowance to his wife for food and clothing for the family often was given only after he had reserved sufficient money for cigars and gambling (cards and backgammon) at the local Armenian club.

This grandmother, who had nothing of her own, would share whatever she did have with neighbors, even temporarily taking in people who had become homeless. The woman recalled wanting to spend all her time with her grandmother. She also recognized, as she told her story, that kindness such as her grandmother's, in that male-dominated culture, reflected an entire life given over to personal sacrifice. Her grandmother had no life of her own by today's standards, and yet she left an indelible mark on many of those who knew her. The storyteller realized that her own quiet resistance to what was traditionally expected of her in her role as an Armenian woman owed much to what her grandmother "gave" her. She had, for example, been earning her own income for more than 40 years.

The close-knit nature of contemporary Armenian families has not diminished much from the days of their ancestors, when the evening's activity consisted of sitting around the circular fireplace (*tonir*) eating and talking (Miller & Miller, 1993). Family needs always took precedence over individual needs, and the importance of maintaining a strong sense of family honor was continually reinforced. Armenian children were taught not to bring shame (*amot*) upon the family name.

The precedence of family over individual needs is maintained among present-day Armenians as well. Given the statement, "A person should always consider the needs of his family as a whole more important than his own," a large majority of Armenians agreed, although the sentiment was less pronounced with each newer generation (Bakalian, 1993). Clinicians most often see these values reflected when young adult children have difficulty separating from their parents, as in the example of David, whose case is discussed later in this section.

Living among hostile majority cultures for many, many years, Armenians developed strong prohibitions against marrying non-Armenians. The commitment to in-marriage was a significant aspect of preserving their distinctive culture against the forces of assimilation. This value has not been preserved among subsequent generations of Armenian Americans, for whom marrying outside the group is now quite common. In Soviet Armenia, where there was little church influence, marrying non-Christian ethnics, unheard of in the past, has become prevalent.

As Armenians have become more assimilated in mainstream American culture, the formerly almost universal aspects of ethnicity, such as language spoken or church attended, are no longer universally common. A survey of Armenian Americans revealed that the higher their income or educational level, the less likely they were to speak Armenian (Bakalian, 1993). External expressions of ethnicity, such as language or religion, are no longer automatically predetermined but are now much more a matter of choice. Bakalian (1993) refers to this phenomenon as "symbolic ethnicity." She explains that it is the middle and upper-middle classes of Armenian Americans who are the chief arbiters of these chosen expressions of ethnicity, whether it be through black-tie fund-raisers, the food served at church bazaars, or the scholarships and grants awarded to Armenian American scholars.

Historically, Armenian attitudes regarding sexual mores have been quite conservative and consistent with the familiar male–female double standard. Part of maintaining family honor involved ensuring the "purity" of the women in the family. Women who had "been around" were not considered good marriage material. In general, however, both men and women tend to be "shy" when interacting with the opposite sex (Bakalian, 1993).

Views about homosexuality among Armenian Americans are expected to vary according to generation, with older people being less accepting than younger ones. In this way, Armenian attitudes are similar to popular American cultural values. However, in a family in which there are negative biases against homosexuality, it would likely encourage secrecy in a gay family member. The main motive would be preserving the family honor rather than personal biases for or against homosexuality itself. A gay family member willing to maintain secrecy about his or her homosexuality could still be regarded as a loved, although misguided, part of the family by members having negative biases. In all probability, an Armenian choosing to be open about his or her homosexuality would encounter much more conflict within the family than one who is secretive.

Armenians have shown the greatest affinity with those ethnic groups to whom they have the widest exposure and with whom they have the most in common. Social-distance indicators show that Armenian Americans are closest by friendship or marriage to White Americans of European ancestry. Bakalian's social-distance survey revealed the closest links with Italian Americans and American Jews, with Irish Americans and Anglo Saxons following close behind. Despite Armenians' own experiences with bigotry, they are no less racist as a group than other Whites (Bakalian, 1993).

As one might expect within a culture in which great respect was afforded elders, families traditionally tended to be adult-centered, with children conforming to the needs of parents. Nevertheless, children have always been highly valued members of the family, and especially so following the Genocide. Children came to be seen as "special," in the sense that they carried the hopes and dreams of a ravaged generation into the future. In this light, life is seen by these children as "serious business" and comes with an implicit sadness (Boyajian & Grigorian, 1986).

Housom, the Armenian word for a deep feeling of sorrow and sadness, seems to be an unarticulated legacy that many of these "special children" unconsciously assimilate. As one of my boyhood Armenian friends put it when asked why he, who was usually so boisterous and joyous, seemed so sad, "The sadness is as much a part of being Armenian as breathing."

Bettelheim (1979) noted a similar vein of emotional intensity among Holocaust survivors. This intensity seems to potentiate the expectable ebb and flow of feelings occurring during the course of living one's life. The resulting surge of emotions can sometimes become unmanageable. This is evident in Armenian families in which the usual kinds of ambivalent feelings about individual members, or struggles between generations or among siblings, are experienced in enormously powerful ways, and small differences are often played out as if major stakes were in the balance.

THERAPY WITH ARMENIAN FAMILIES

The recent postmodern trend toward a narrative style of family therapy seems to lend itself well to incorporating elements of ethnicity into the therapeutic dialogue. Narrative approaches assume that personal meaning emerges from the intersubjective crucible of one's social environment. The therapeutic conversation, therefore, is oriented toward recognizing the context of values and meaning within which a client's self-narrative takes form. As the client's own attributions of meaning are encouraged, themes with ethnic origins can be noticed and developed.

In our group at the Catskill Family Institute in Kingston, New York, we emphasize client narratives that are consistent with what we call the client's preferred view of self.

People are, of course, more at ease when their preferred views (or ideal sense of self) are consistent with how they think others see them. It is when their preferred views and others' views are contradictory that problems tend to develop (Eron & Lund, 1993). This is obviously a major issue with Armenians when they sense that others do not acknowledge their history. When therapists acknowledge clients' preferred views, problems seem to diminish; when their comments conflict with these views, problems intensify. We find this a helpful guide in conducting therapeutic conversations that are sensitive to our clients' sense of their ethnic identity.

Not surprisingly, Armenians are unlikely to see psychotherapy as a way of dealing with their problems. The idea of paying someone for "advice" runs counter to centuries of self-reliant individualism and may even be considered shameful or dishonorable. When Armenians come into therapy, it is probably because they are in extreme distress or because of some external pressure. They often present themselves as being in better shape than they actually are. An assumption of a viable therapeutic contract should not be made simply because an appointment has been made, as the case with Arikel will show.

Arikel was a maintenance man for the county's administrative offices and the only son of Genocide survivors. He was approaching retirement after 28 years of valued service to the county, when he suddenly began to demonstrate erratic behavior. He was missing work frequently, his work was sloppy and incomplete, and his attitude toward coworkers and the public had become increasingly belligerent. When he had a screaming match with one of his bosses, he knew he had gone too far. This always irascible but beloved employee was given the ultimatum of going to an Employee Assistance Program counselor or losing his job. After Arikel stomped out of the counselor's office, his boss gave him one last chance, and he reluctantly agreed to try a second therapist.

The second therapist's questioning did not start with the assumption that Arikel ("Call me Ace") had a "problem." Instead, he expressed curiosity about the circumstances that brought Arikel to the office. This elicited a diatribe, recounting 28 years of county governmental incompetence and how his division head was a phony son of a _____. The therapist took pains to acknowledge Ace's references to what a hard worker he had always been, even when most of his coworkers didn't do half of what he did. Only after the therapist asked how someone as obviously savvy as Ace was about the civil service game could have upset his boss enough to draw a referral for counseling, did Ace say that he hadn't been himself at work for months. Inquiring further about what he meant by "not being himself," the therapist learned that Ace had always lived with his mother (he had never married) and that she had died about a year earlier.

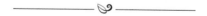

Ace could not tolerate being considered needy or incompetent. It was only after the therapist joined with his preferred view of himself as a savvy, hardworking person that he could acknowledge the incongruities of the picture he was presenting. Only then could a meaningful treatment contract about his unresolved grief be established and a constructive course of therapy be started. Like many Armenians, Arikel was not going to allow just anyone to be a witness to his grieving for his mother, whom he regarded as an almost saintly figure. Further exploration revealed that Arikel and his mother had been the only survivors of their village in Armenia, and that his pride in himself as a worker, a son, and an Armenian were all part of the same intense life experience.

Armenian preferred views were also threaded throughout the course of therapy in the following case:

Mary, a legal secretary, made a panicked phone call for help after her 19-year-old son, David, had revealed to her that he had been having suicidal thoughts. David had recently dropped out of college and returned home, where he was working part-time at a local sporting goods store, feeling defeated and depressed. In the first session the therapist faced a sullen David, a worried Mary, and her testy husband, Mike, a manager for IBM. Clearly, the men, who were used to getting their own way, did not want to be there, but in a matter of such gravity, Mary would not take "no" for an answer and insisted they come.

David had been an excellent student and athlete in high school. He had been Mike and Mary's pride and joy. Initially, he seemed happy at the prestigious college he attended, although a bit bothered by the more modest nature of his achievements. However, over time his dissatisfaction grew, and with it the intensity of his parents' advice to him, until he abruptly dropped out of school, to everyone's great dismay.

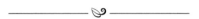

To these second-generation Armenian parents, this turn of events represented a failure of their entire family. All three family members felt out of place as they sat stiffly in my office—confused, hurt, and angry. Recognizing that family pride and closeness of the family were highly regarded virtues in this Armenian family, I chose a conversational path that accentuated the strengths of this close-knit unit, rather than assuming, as some therapists might, that David's problem stemmed from the family's being too enmeshed.

While in college, David had perceived his parents' worry about how he was doing as disappointment in him. As he came to believe he was failing them, he withdrew further into himself and did worse. David's parents perceived his withdrawal as lack of caring about them and what they had taught him. In separate meetings with the parents and with David, I developed a narrative of a young man who had lost confidence, rather than someone who had stopped caring for his family. I described to the parents how much David respected their achievements and how he feared that he could not do nearly as well. With David, I commented on the ambitious plans he had loosely formulated to move away and try another school as evidence that the family ethos of achievement had not left him, rather than dwelling on his frustration with his low-paying job.

Fortified with the understanding that they were the best people to be boosting David's confidence when he doubted himself, the parents were able to calmly encourage him to finish the semester at his new school when he again wavered in his belief in himself. This supportive nudge was enough for David to overcome his crisis in confidence and move forward in his life.

By respecting the family's high regard for closeness and utilizing it rather than trying to circumvent it, I was able to help its members help themselves. This allowed his parents to address David's problem in a manner that remained consistent with their ethnically preferred value of self-reliance.

A final example is of a young, fourth-generation Armenian American woman and her Italian American husband. Again, recognizing preferred ethnic qualities suggested a productive avenue for the therapeutic dialogue.

Ani came into therapy with her husband, Anthony, because she feared that her marriage of 3 years was in jeopardy. Although she and Anthony readily professed their continued love for each other, their arguments had become more frequent and increasingly vehement. Ani was mortified at how quickly she would say things that she knew would hurt Anthony. Anthony, a strong, silent type, indicated his refusal to capitulate to his wife's tactics by stubbornly withdrawing into silence. Ani had come to fear that Anthony did not care about her, whereas he believed that Ani had to have things her way.

In reviewing how they had become a couple, I learned that the quality to which each of them was most attracted in the other was a willingness to state frankly what was on his or her mind. Ani, like her ancestors before her, put great stock in her own counsel and did not want to be a deferring wife as her mother was with her father. Anthony knew he was strong willed and believed he would be unhappy if he had a wife he could dominate as his father had dominated his mother. They quickly got their fighting under control when I observed that they had not made mistakes about each other as they had feared, but that sparks were the inevitable consequences of choosing strong-minded partners. Ani and Anthony then acknowledged that their goals usually were the same, but their approaches differed.

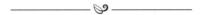

Identifying ethnically preferred views of self pointed the way to a common ground, around which the rest of the couple's therapy was organized (Dagirmanjian, Eron, & Lund, 1993). After all, both Ani and Anthony had learned from their parents' marriages that it was not good for one partner to customarily defer to the other; they agreed that this was not what they wanted. When they recognized that their bickering was the by-product of what they preferred in each other and not the result of a flaw in either of them, they were able to address their expectable differences with each other more collaboratively and less confrontationally. As these preferred elements of their ethnic identities (i.e., pro-independent thinking and anti-inequality) were respectfully identified, accentuated, and threaded through a mutually acceptable narrative of the marriage, solutions began to emerge.

CONCLUSION

Probably the single most difficult obstacle to achieving a successful therapeutic experience with Armenian families is getting beyond their heightened wariness of outsiders, coupled with their reflexive self-reliance. It is essential for the therapist to establish meaningful reasons to meet. Even if a therapist is able to demonstrate his or her trustworthiness, it may be hard for Armenian families to believe that the therapist could tell them something they did not already know about themselves. The therapist who successfully engages Armenians in therapy, more often than not, has been "reminding" them of what they already know but may have overlooked in the midst of life's exigencies. In essence, that is what was done in each of the case examples in this chapter. Arikel would not reveal the pain of his loss to a therapist until his knowledge and competence had been acknowledged. David and his parents interacted more constructively in regard to his leaving-home difficulties only after their closeness as a family was emphasized as a strength and a resource on which they could draw. Katchi was unable to move forward in her life before she realized that her feelings of shameful ambivalence about being Armenian were an unwanted and unnecessary legacy of the Genocide. By noticing aspects of the clients that were consistent with their preferred ethnic values, the therapists were able to foster feelings of agency that allowed the clients to try alternative solutions to their problems.

As wary as Armenians may often be, there are no people warmer and more devoted to those whom they have accepted into their lives. Sometimes, however, the ways in which these sentiments are manifested may not be easily recognized. As Ace was leaving my office at the end of his final session, and after he had emotionally expressed his gratitude for my help, he turned, showed an expression of genuine puzzlement, and stated with total sincerity, "You know, you're a lot smarter than you look."

REFERENCES

Bakalian, A. (1993). *Armenian-Americans: From being to feeling Armenian.* New Brunswick, NJ: Transaction Publishers.

Bettelheim, B. (1979). Afterword. In C. Vegh, *I didn't say goodbye* (pp. 161–178). New York: Dutton. (Translated by R. Schwartz, 1984)

Bournoutian, G. A. (2003). *A concise history of the Armenian people.* Costa Mesa, CA: Mazda Publishers.

Boyajian, L., & Grigorian, H. (1986). Psychological sequelae of the Armenian Genocide. In R. Hovannisian (Ed.), *The Armenian Genocide in perspective* (pp. 177–185). New Brunswick, NJ: Transaction Publishers.

Dagirmanjian, S., Eron, J., & Lund, T. (1993, August). *Mapping the path to narrative common ground with couples.* Paper presented at 101st annual convention of the American Psychological Association, Toronto, Canada.

Der Nersessian, S. (1945). *Armenia and the Byzantine Empire.* Cambridge, MA: Harvard University Press.

Eron, J., & Lund, T. (1993). How problems evolve and dissolve: Integrating narrative and strategic concepts. *Family Process, 32,* 291–309.

Miller, D., & Miller, L. T. (1993). *Survivors: An oral history of the Armenian Genocide.* Berkeley: University of California Press.

CHAPTER 33

Iranian Families

Behnaz Jalali

Iranian immigrants constitute a steadily growing ethnic group in the United States. Many Iranian families in the United States are first-generation immigrants, as new immigrants keep arriving, and thus many families have characteristics similar to those of families in their homeland. However, a second generation is now emerging as well, with different cultural characteristics and increased adaptation to Western culture, coming from several specific socioeconomic groups. Because social class is a central factor in Iranian society, especially in regard to their level of contact with Western values and culture, it greatly influences the nature of migration to the United States.

Social class is more clearly defined in Iran than in the United States, comprising distinct, identifiable elements (Bill, 1972). Therapists should be sensitive to these important distinctions among Iranian families and should not assume that all Iranians identify with each other's experience. For example, the therapist should not assume that financial circumstances alone signify Iranian families' class distinctions, and they should inquire about the family background, belief in traditional values, and exposure to Western lifestyles.

Most of the initial Iranian immigrants to the United States were from the elite, Westernized, educated, and business classes. They reflected, in fact, a relatively small portion of the Iranian population, which was primarily either rural and agrarian or lower middle class. However, since the Iranian revolution, immigrants from various social backgrounds began to flow out of the country. I focus here on basic Iranian cultural characteristics that influence each person, irrespective of social class.

WAVES OF IRANIAN MIGRATION TO THE UNITED STATES

There have been four waves of Iranian immigrants to the United States. The first (1950–1970) were mostly from large Iranian cities. The migrants generally had an understanding of Western culture, were highly educated and affluent, and belonged primarily to the elite and professional middle-class groups. Most were engineers, doctors, dentists, teachers, or scientists, and their skills allowed them to adapt well to the new culture (Adams, 1968; Baldwin, 1963).

Those who came in the second wave (1970–1978) were both affluent and city oriented and came from various social classes which, during these years of economic boom and rapid growth, had become wealthy. Like those in the first wave, most were professionals in a good position for gaining employment and were thus usually able to remain in the social class they had enjoyed in Iran. Of the 14,500 Iranian immigrants who came between 1970 and 1975, 30% held advanced degrees, including 10% who were physicians (Askari, Cummings, & Izbudak, 1977). Some were from less Westernized families, more rooted in the traditional culture and thus not as well prepared to manage cultural change (Bill, 1973).

Although economics was still a major factor in this group's immigration, they also came for professional possibilities and to provide opportunities for their children (National Science Foundation, 1973) or for political reasons, such as opposition to the ruling political regime. Second-wave immigrants are scattered all over the United States, with the highest concentrations in the Northern, Eastern, and West Coast urban centers.

Those in the third wave (1978–1984) came immediately before and after the Iranian revolution, largely for personal, economic, or political security. This was a more heterogeneous group in terms of education and age, although, again, most were affluent. Some had exposure to Western culture, others did not. Unlike those in the first two waves, many were forced to flee Iran. Like people from any culture who are forced to leave for political or economic reasons, they experienced extreme cultural shock, alienation, frustration, and depression in adjusting to life in the United States. Some had to break ties with their families, at least temporarily. Their future remained uncertain; many had lost their social positions and power and could not practice their professions; their strong ties to their homeland made them reluctant to settle and acculturate. This group probably had the highest incidence of symptoms.

Since 1984, an even more heterogeneous group of immigrants than those in the third wave have continued to arrive in the United States (the fourth wave). They are mostly very disillusioned about the conditions in their country because of the increased inflation, insecurity, and lack of religious freedom and educational opportunities for their children. There is a population explosion of young people under the age of 30 in Iran, and economic and educational opportunities have not caught up with the sheer number of young people.

Within a few years, many Iranians in the United States were able to acquire the necessary education, licenses, or other qualifications to either continue in their professions or begin new ones. Many businesses were set up, with entrepreneurs hiring other Iranian employees or seeking Iranian partners. Iranian newspapers, TV and radio stations, and Yellow Pages have been created. Most of these immigrants settled where they had family members or friends who could help them with the transition and provide financial and psychological support.

Cultural characteristics are interwoven into Iranians' everyday lives and interactions with family members, friends, fellow workers, and authority figures (e.g., a therapist). Given the regional and ethnic diversity among them (there are several regions in Iran that have their own ethnic characteristics, including their own dialect of the language), any collective profile has only limited applicability (Banuazizi, 1977).

Iranians have assumed several cultural characteristics to ensure their self-preservation and to cope with political instability and turmoil over the centuries. They tend to be individualistic, fatalistic, and nostalgically tied to the past (Haas, 1946). Iranians are proud people who believe deeply in their uniqueness, which is rooted in their history. They survived several foreign invasions and repeated internal turmoil. Time and again Iran has managed to absorb cultural influences without losing its own identity and continuity. Thus, when the Arabs invaded, Islam was assimilated into Iranian culture; in fact, most of the rules of this religion became the governing laws of Iran. However, Iranians opted for a new branch of Islam, called Shiism. This differentiates them from most of the Muslim world, who are Sunnis. (Currently, 98% of Iran's population is Muslim, and 93% of these are Shiites.) Shiism, a highly emotional, mystical form of Islam, focuses on a series of martyrs: the 12 divinely designated, martyred descendants of the Prophet, the Imams.

Iran's spoken language is Persian (Farsi), which has Indo-European roots. Although the Arabic alphabet has been integrated into Persian writing, the language is distinctive from the Arabic spoken by Lebanese, Jordanians, and Iraqis. Individuality and nonconformity are especially evident in the diversity of Iranians' opinions and behavior (Arasteh, 1964). Iranians' sense of individuality has always been so powerful that authoritarian controls were needed to ensure their allegiance and support. Rulers are authoritarian in order to guarantee the submission and respect of their subjects. Iranians simultaneously accept authority and indirectly resist it, or they may passively accept authoritarian treatment from their superiors and act in the same authoritarian manner toward their inferiors. Iranians also express their individuality through creativity in their art, poetry, literature, and philosophy. Iranians' cultural, historical, and individual pride may account for their boastfulness, impatience with learning, and difficulty in admitting mistakes (Zonis, 1976).

Basic to the culture is the belief that this world and its material belongings are not worthwhile, a worldview evident in the Sufi philosophy common in Iran that started to grow in the beginning of the 9th century. Its doctrine has some links with Islam, but it was influenced by such other philosophies and religions as Zoroastrianism, Buddhism, Christianity, and Neoplatonism, which it views as shadows of the central truth that it seeks. Sufism essentially seeks to give the individual a spiritual union with God, devoid of the rituals and intermediaries of a religious hierarchy. Through self-renunciation, spiritual realization, and concentration, the individual may reach a stage of unity with God (Arasteh, 1964). Iranian epicurean poets, such as Omar Khayyam, also express the worldview that, because life is short, we should enjoy the present; this has become part of the Iranian philosophy of life.

Iranians' greatest concern is to extract the most from the present. Plans are not necessary, as the future is either uncertain or preordained (Gable, 1959). Iranians may work 5 to 6 days a week, only to spend all of their earnings on the 7th by having fun. Because of rapidly changing political circumstances, they have learned to live with uncertainty, distrust, and cynicism (Zonis, 1976). They also manifest mistrust in interpersonal relationships. Individuals must always be on guard to protect themselves; they fear that others will take advantage of them. Trusting relationships exist mainly with family members and lifelong friends.

Iranians usually believe deeply in fate, or *Taghdir*; they are expected to accept with grace the outcome of their lives. Their respect for strength and submission to superior forces is part of this concept (Vreeland, 1957). However, this fatalism has decreased visibly among educated Iranians over the past 30 years, as their experience has led them to believe instead that it is up to the individual to change his or her own life.

Iranians are very hospitable; guests are treated with unusual courtesy and generosity. They also tolerate verbal exaggeration (Gastil, 1958). Because Iranians try to avoid publicly criticizing or embarrassing one another, truthfulness is avoided if it hurts another (Arasteh, 1964). Rather, they express disagreement through socially acceptable humor and wit.

Friendships, which often begin in school and are close, intimate, and of long duration, are very important in Iranian culture. Friends remain loyal and are likely to meet regularly, make mutual demands, exchange favors, and have high expectations of each other. There is also a large circle of less intimate friends and acquaintances, who are an important part of an Iranian's social and professional life. Iranians of both sexes are emotionally expressive people. Both men and women show their pain, anger, and affection easily. Kissing and hugging as a way of greeting are common for both men and women, but are less socially acceptable between a man and a woman. Iranians' social code prescribes correct behavioral patterns with those in each position in the hierarchy. People of a lower rank respond to those of higher rank with deference, politeness, and respect, even though they may harbor resentment and hostility toward them. Because pride in and identification with one's occupation are more important than material rewards, Iranians will not perform a job that they consider beneath them. For example, they usually do not perform well on assembly lines.

Iranians have a predictable pattern for resolving conflicts in families and among friends; fighting ensues and overt communication stops for days, weeks, or months. Eventually, a mediator (a family member of authority, a powerful and persuasive friend, or a wise elder) may be engaged to reconcile the parties. Such mediators are extremely important, because they facilitate compromise while allowing each party to save face by not "giving in." They arrange separate negotiations with each party and try to reach a compromise. Afterward, the two parties will meet and make up.

As far as cultural prejudices are concerned, Iran has historically always been in interaction with many different cultures and races and has tended to show a tolerance of the various races and cultures.

FAMILY STRUCTURE AND RELATIONSHIPS

My view here is based largely on personal and cultural interactions and my experience in treating Iranian families, inasmuch as little formal research on these families is available. In Iran the individual's total life is dominated by the family and family relationships (Gable, 1959). People rely on family connections for position, security, influence, and power. The importance of the family as a social unit for Iranians dates back to Zoroastrian times (the pre-Islam period), when rearing children and the duties of children to their parents were considered sacred.

The extended family has traditionally been the basic social unit, as befits the society's predominantly agrarian nature. In villages and tribes this pattern is crucial for survival in hard times. However, in urban areas, the geographical dispersion of the extended family and the differences in status and material holdings diminish the extended family's significance. Still, it has preserved its significance as an important psychological and bonding entity. Iranian society's hierarchical organization is apparent in the ascending order from family, to village, to tribe, and finally, to country (Wilber, 1963).

The Traditional Family Structure

The traditional Iranian family unit is patriarchal: The father is the undisputed family head. Sons and their wives may live in his household or compound. Old Iranian houses were built to accommodate extended families. A wall surrounded the home to ensure privacy, and each nuclear family had its own sleeping quarters. Many extended families continue to maintain close ties, which frequent marriages between relatives serve to strengthen.

The father has authority over his wife, children, and grandchildren; others hesitate to question his decisions openly. The patriarch's responsibility is to unify the group and to resolve internal conflicts. Religious laws define a wife's relationship to her husband as one of submission. He expects her to take care of the home and children, and her actions at home and in public should enhance his and the family's status. He is expected to be a strict disciplinarian, but is also a provider of affection and love. At times he may make decisions for his children even when they are adults. When the father dies, the eldest son inherits the authority and accepts responsibility for his mother and any unmarried brothers and sisters.

The mother's authority and power, which are more subtle and indirect, depend in part on the relationship she has built over time with her husband, sons, brothers, and the other women in the family. The mother never openly disagrees with the father, but may prevail on other relatives, such as her children or mother-in-law, to intervene on her behalf as she expresses her opinions or requests. Iranian women are particularly close to their children and devote much time to them. When conflict arises between father and children, the mother tries to intervene and mediate (Nyrop, 1978).

Mothers are also very affectionate toward their children, especially their sons. Sons may show great love and devotion toward their mothers and, when married, encourage their wives to be friendly with them. If the relationship between mother-in-law and daughter-in-law becomes conflictual, as frequently happens, the son/husband serves as mediator, a role fraught with difficulty inasmuch as he is pressured to take sides and must behave wisely and diplomatically.

Relationships between brothers and sisters are complex, stemming from both their bonding and their mutual responsibility. A brother assumes the role of supporting his sister, but if she behaves inappropriately, his disapproval is as powerful as a husband's. Should a woman lose her husband, her brother automatically becomes her protector.

The most difficult relationship may be that between fathers and sons. The father continuously dominates his son but also encourages him to assume more responsibility. A son's identification with the father is strongly encouraged, because it is assumed that he will someday not only take on his father's role, but also become the head of his own nuclear family and possibly the patriarch of an extended family. This pattern stimulates conflict, as both submission and competition are expected.

Marriage

Women are often 10–15 years younger than their spouses. In traditional families they marry at about age 16–18, although among modern urban families the age may be 22–25 or older, particularly among the most Westernized families, in which men try to develop economic independence before marriage. Financial demands are made on the man by the woman's family prior to marriage, which depend on the family's wealth and social status. When marriage occurs, the two families become united; they join their wealth and increase their power and influence.

Generally, the woman goes to live among her husband's relatives; however, she maintains close ties with her own family. Conflicts among in-laws are a common source of stress. To marry, women must obtain their fathers' agreement, whereas men do not have this legal prerequisite, although it may be a moral one. Depending on the family's social class and tradition, premarital sex for women may be viewed with disdain and contempt, whereas for the man it is tolerated.

In traditional rural and urban families, parents choose the ideal young woman for their son, arrange meetings, and undertake negotiations with her family. If these go well, a time is set for the wedding, at which time a sum of money, or *mehr*, is guaranteed to the wife if her husband dies or divorces her. Very few meetings occur between the man and the woman until they officially marry. Their meetings are usually in the presence of the family. Although the number of arranged marriages is declining, they still occur.

A woman gains status when she gets married, which increases further when she has a child, especially a boy (Arasteh, 1964). Sons are regarded as economic assets. Men may be allowed to have as many as four wives, yet with some restrictions. Polygamous marriages, although very infrequent, invariably lead to rivalries and jealousies among the wives as each competes for her husband's attention and favor. However, the first and oldest wife maintains a senior position. A Muslim man may marry a non-Muslim woman, but a Muslim woman cannot marry a non-Muslim man unless he converts. Moreover, men can divorce their wives, but the reverse is not true unless there is an exceptional situation. The father is the legal custodian of the children, and he retains custody after a divorce. Once divorced, a woman has less chance of remarrying than does a divorced man, and particularly of marrying one who has not been married before.

Wealthier families may also have servants and nannies, who take a very active role in rearing their children, and with whom a child may have a very special relationship, at times even closer than that with the mother (Arasteh, 1964).

The mother receives guidance and advice in rearing children from her mother, mother-in-law, and other relatives. She may fear losing her children, as expressed in the old belief in the evil eye, which is still maintained by some. The evil eye, which explains misfortunes due to envy or the hostility of outsiders, has both supernatural and personalized aspects. Consequently, people refrain from commenting on a child's health and beauty for fear that it may make the child vulnerable to the evil eye (Arasteh, 1964).

Child Rearing

Children, especially young boys, are the focus of attention and affection from both the nuclear and extended family and may be spoiled by aunts, uncles, and grandparents. As they grow older, they are expected to be polite and respectful toward adults. The Iranian child is typically well mannered and can sit quietly for hours in an adult's presence.

Boys learn to respect their fathers' authority and dominance, yet are also encouraged to be assertive and independent. They tend to bully their sisters and sometimes tyrannize their mothers, but their misbehavior and aggressiveness are often affectionately praised even while they are scolded. The controlling overprotection of sisters by brothers has been exaggerated within the lower social class since the revolution, and any perceived moral infraction by a sister increases this control. Thus, there are many reports of physical abuse by brothers in some sections of the society. Both parents are more permissive with their sons than their daughters. Boys grow up believing themselves superior to girls.

Fathers maintain discipline, which may consist of scolding or slapping. There is no specific pattern to the punishment; depending on the father's mood, a child may be punished for a trivial act of misbehavior; at other times, a more serious act may be laughed off or overlooked. A child may be slapped if he or she misbehaves in public or in front of a family guest, yet in private the same misbehavior might only merit a scolding. Western methods of disciplining, such as withholding favorite foods or sending children to their rooms, are rarely used.

Child training involves many prohibitions that parents express repeatedly. For example, children are told to be obedient, to behave like adults, and to be quiet.

LIFE CYCLE AND TRADITION

Parents gain more respect and power as they get older. In old age, they may retain their own residence and be cared for by the children, or may live with one of them. In Iran there are no nursing homes. When death occurs, mourning ceremonies are an important function for the family and the neighborhood where the person has lived. Mourning is expressed quite openly, especially by women, who sometimes faint from extreme grief. The neighborhood and community are very much involved in supporting the bereaved, soothing them, bringing food, visiting, and talking with them about the deceased person. Mourning for men and women is arranged in separate rooms.

No formal funeral homes exist in Iran, and the dead body may remain in the home for 1–2 days in a secluded area of the house in the presence of a clergyman reciting prayers. Then the body is taken to the cemetery. Mourning lasts for 3 days; the family holds a memorial for the deceased on the 7th and 40th days and the first-year anniversary. When the extended family, friends, and community visit the mourners, they remember the deceased. It is generally believed that a person is judged after death and, depending on his or her behavior in life, is sent to hell or heaven (Nyrop, 1978).

Inheritances pass from husband to wife and children, but the shares are unequal: Sons receive a full share, daughters a half share, and the wife even less, although she can own property in her own name.

The traditional family's structure is relatively immune to conflict and tension. Although to an outside observer this structure may appear as a source of conflict, the values and roles are internalized and accepted as norms, and conflicts are at a minimum. Women generally accept their husbands' dominance, at least on the surface; however, that practice is changing rapidly.

MODERN IRANIAN FAMILIES

Upper- and middle-class families in urban areas of Iran are caught between the pull of traditional religion and culture and an acceptance of more Western family relationships. The mass media and modern schools have changed urban children's attitudes toward traditional values. However, these developments have not penetrated all levels of society, and traditional forces remain strong. In fact, they have grown since the mid-1970s.

Industrialization and urbanization have weakened parental authority and increased the ability of young adults to choose their marriage partners. Young people in particular often experience conflict between their desires for independence and their strong sense of duty to their fathers.

Among the upper and middle classes, married men tend to establish households separate from their families of origin, perhaps even in different neighborhoods. But ties remain strong and visits frequent. The attitudes toward women remain conservative, and premarital sex is uncommon. A spouse is usually chosen from the same social group, although often with parental interference.

Western education and travel abroad have profoundly changed women's roles and have resulted in demands for change in family relationships. More women are seeking higher education, and many have begun working outside the home. Modern Iranian women marry later than their traditional counterparts; with no servants, child caretakers, or housekeepers, they also have fewer children. However, although some women have entered the workforce, traditional culture retains a strong grip, and sex roles have been enormously difficult to change. A pilot study done in Iran (Kurzman, 2002) revealed the presence of a generation of educated and strong-willed women in high numbers who are present in all professions, yet careers are sometimes hindered by family priorities. Today women outnumber men in some colleges in Iran.

Western influences have also caused families to become more oriented toward the nuclear family, which has led to a partial breakdown of the extended family. Consequently, family members have become conflicted about their obligations and sense of responsibility toward elders.

Immigrant families' stability is threatened by the many stresses they encounter, and they may abandon cultural standards of behavior in favor of Western norms and greater freedom of expression. There is a striving and competition to achieve more status and wealth. A father may resent his children's not respecting his authority as much as he respected his parents'. He may also have ambivalent feelings toward his professional wife.

Like other immigrants who have emigrated from patriarchal societies, Iranian women have gained more familial power and equality after living in the United States for several years. Iranian men, on the other hand, have not enjoyed the powerful role they held in the family prior to immigration. Several recent studies confirm this clinical finding (Hanassab & Tidewell, 1994; Hojat et al., 1999; Moghissi, 1999; Sundquist, Bayard-Burfield, Johansson, & Johansson, 2000). They confirm poorer adjustment in the Iranian male immigrant and greater cultural resistance to change among men than among women, who show a more flexible attitude regarding sexual values. Another study (Hojat et al., 2000) concluded that the gender difference in adopting new values may explain the higher rate of divorce among Iranians in the United States. The extended family network is usually no longer available to either intervene when conflicts arise or to provide a context for diluting relationship conflicts.

All of these factors have contributed to an increase in the separation and divorce rate among Iranian immigrant couples, as compared with their incidence in the homeland. The generation gap between parents who grew up in Iran and their children who grew up in the United States has widened. Families express a great deal of conflict and ambivalence regarding adolescents and young adults, especially with respect to their daughters' dating. Hardest hit with adaptive difficulties are older Iranian immigrants who lack English fluency.

The combination of the loss of their social network status, position, and friends, plus cultural alienation between them and their children and grandchildren, has added to the immigrants' feelings of isolation and loneliness. There is a better chance of cultural adjustment for the children if the family has a strong and positive sense of its cultural identity and heritage, as well as an openness and flexibility to add on new values. A study of Iranian refugees in the Netherlands showed that there is an association between higher cultural self-esteem and better coping with the stress of acculturation (Verkuyten & Nekuee, 2001).

ADAPTATION TO IMMIGRATION

Iranian families' adaptation to American culture vacillates between acculturation and holding onto the old culture (Jalali & Boyce, 1980). At times, Iranians preserve aspects of their culture no matter how Westernized they are in appearance, mode of thinking, and behavior. Because Iranian immigration to this country is so recent, it is unclear how these patterns will develop over several generations. Several recent studies have attempted to look at patterns of acculturation and its variables among Iranian immigrants (Kheirkhah, 2003; Ostovar, 1997; Safdar, 2003). The most common modes of adaptation are as follows.

1. *Denigrating the old culture.* Some families sever the old ties, avoid other Iranians, and denounce the old traditions and beliefs. This amounts to an effort to deny their cultural origin by adopting the external features of American culture, including, especially, materialistic habits and values.

2. *Denying the new culture.* The new becomes so frightening that the old cannot be abandoned. Families turn inward, associating only with Iranians and attempting to reproduce a micro-culture similar to that in Iran. They eat the same foods they ate in Iran, follow the same traditions, and criticize Western values and beliefs. However, their children become acculturated through schools and friends and frequently develop conflicts with their parents.

3. *Biculturation.* The family attempts to integrate the two cultures and tolerates the conflict and anxiety of crossing cultural boundaries. Important attachments to the old culture are maintained, along with a productive assimilation of the new culture. Therefore, they can integrate without disrupting their basic sense of identity.

Often, some family members adhere to one mode, whereas others follow another, which leaves the family prone to internal intergenerational conflicts. In the United States, family relationships remain important, although they have undergone significant transformation, with family ties less close, mainly because the extended family is not available. The father retains some of his authority; the mother, although having more social freedom, maintains many traditional patterns. The trick is to juggle career and family and maintain a dual role to the point of being a superwoman.

Decision making lies with the nuclear family. The extended family is informed after decisions are made, although at times its members may be consulted for their special expertise. The sense of obligation to the family exists, but is ambivalent.

The first wave of Iranian immigrants, because of their prior exposure to the West through education, the media, and travel abroad, adjusted easily to the new culture. They also had marketable skills and were affluent, which allowed them to survive the insecurities of a new environment. Many married Americans, which also facilitated acculturation. However, because of cultural differences, the American spouse often became a source of conflict, especially when not accepted by the Iranian spouse's extended family. Conflicts would erupt, especially when the extended family members arrived for long visits. The extended family felt resentful and resented; the Western spouse found it difficult to grasp the intricate system of the Iranian extended family.

Immigrant Iranians who married Iranian spouses did better, particularly if well educated. Less educated and more traditional Iranian spouses were less employable and did not speak English as well. They often retreated from the new experiences, whereas their partners were employed and fully exposed to the new environment. American-born children usually grew up with very little command of the Persian language, even if both parents were first-generation Iranian Americans. (This was even more likely if one parent was American.) Children strongly influence the behavior of their parents through school and peer relationships. Children become a vehicle to acculturate their parents to the details of the new culture. Initially, many second-wave families were enthusiastic and excited about immigration. But later they began to miss their extended families, neighborhoods, and communities and felt isolated and alienated in the new culture. Families of the second wave are particularly prone to intergenerational conflicts. Their children may attempt to dissociate themselves from the old culture, ridicule their parents, and reject ethnic food. Fathers, in particular, are threatened by these changes in their children; they may blame the new culture and criticize its values. These families are also prone to developing marital conflicts as wives welcome more social freedom, which further threatens their husbands.

The third wave of Iranian immigrant families is very prone to develop psychosocial stresses and psychological symptoms. The family's integrity and unity has been disrupted by political, ideological, and physical separation. Some fled their homeland but hope to return to it. This subgroup's traumatic entry into American culture has often been marked by disappointments, failures, and a sense of hopelessness.

When such immigrants cannot use their skills or professions, they also have financial worries, worry about their extended families back home, and difficulty in merging with their subgroup. These factors may contribute to a resistance to becoming acculturated, which makes them feel alienated from their surroundings. Several recent studies of Iranian immigrants showed a direct relationship between cultural resistance and level of depression, anxiety, somatization, and stress (Ghaffarian, 1998; Kadkhoda, 2001; Rouhparvar, 2001). Women, overall, appear to have an easier time in adjustment than men and show more successful adaptation to their new culture (Ziabakhsh, 2002).

Children's ability to cope with their new environment depends considerably on their parents' ability to adapt, in spite of their conflicting loyalties and anxiety. They may feel unaccepted and shy, avoid peer relationships, or may develop school problems or delay learning the new language, which makes adaptation even more difficult. Most of these families suffer cultural, physical, and emotional isolation with concomitant anxiety and depression.

TREATMENT ISSUES

An American therapist's lack of familiarity with Iranians' cultural expression of psychological stress and mistrust of outside helpers often leads to misunderstandings. This may result in problems in the therapist–patient relationship. There is a more holistic attitude toward health—that is, that health can be disrupted in the absence of illness and can be achieved despite the presence of illness (Emami, Benner, Lipson, & Eckman, 2000). The following paragraphs highlight some of the issues involved.

The self is divided into the outer self, which the individual presents to the outside world, and the inner self, which guards strongly against strangers and is revealed only to intimates and very close friends. The outer self may appear very well adjusted while the inner self is not (Hoffman, 1991).

Among Iranians, sadness and melancholy are seen as indicating inner depth (Good, Good, & Moradi, 1985); however, dysphoric affect, *narahati*, is experienced as distress. It must be guarded and masked for fear of exposing powerlessness (Pliskin, 1987). It may be experienced in various verbal forms as well as physical ones and includes such symptoms as worry, anxiety, sadness, and distress. Some may even avoid sharing it with their intimates because of fearing that they may make those close to them *narahat* (Pliskin, 1987).

Problems are frequently expressed through somatization and projection. Heart symptoms such as aching, pounding, fluttering, rapid beating, pain, or discomfort, almost always reflect anxiety that can be traced to interpersonal problems, work, or worry (Good, 1976). Heart-related symptoms that reflect depressed moods are evident in comments such as "My heart is closed in" and in requests for the therapist or doctor to "open it up," which, in essence, is a request for sympathy and listening. The brain is the center of the mind, but the heart is the center of emotions (Good, 1976).

Weak nerves, tired nerves, shaking hands, lack of sensation, and numbness may indicate neurological problems, but can also be psychosomatic equivalents of depression and anxiety. General body pain (especially pain in the limbs), exhaustion, and lack of strength are also somatic symptoms, as are complaints of upper gastrointestinal pains, a weak stomach or liver, digestive problems, heart-related symptoms, and vitamin deficiency. Some of these symptom presentations lead to incorrect diagnoses by mental health professionals who are not familiar with Iranian culture.

Physical symptoms are more acceptable and less stigmatized than psychological ones. Symptomatic individuals can make demands of the family for special privileges, caretaking, or other changes in family behavior. It is thus difficult to convince them that they may have psychological problems, and therefore it may be important not to confront them directly about the meaning of the symptoms but to accept the presenting complaint and use more subtle interventions.

Problems are also explained by outside events, people, or forces, such as grief, school failure, or heartbreak. Usually the precipitating stress is seen by the family as the sole cause of a problem; they may not talk about larger cultural factors unless questioned in detail about their situation. Iranians with problems usually turn to same-sex friends or relatives for advice and support. Younger people turn to parents or older relatives, and friends gossip about problems to other relatives or friends. Only as a last resort do they turn to an outside "helper" or "doctor." By this time a whole network of people are aware of the problem, even though the confidants have all been sworn to secrecy.

THERAPIST–PATIENT RELATIONSHIPS

To understand the complex nature of the doctor–patient relationship in treating Iranians, we must appreciate its roots. Iranians are ambivalent, even mistrustful of a "helper's" expertise, although in specific instances a person may have a trusting relationship with one physician, assigning him or her special healing powers. Iranians are also "doctor shoppers," going from one specialist to another, requesting medication and demanding quick results, particularly if the illness is serious or difficult to diagnose. If a cure is not imminent, the patient will visit another doctor, hoping that he or she will express a different opinion, which only increases the patient's mistrust of the previous physician.

Ensuring family support is essential, because families take an active part in decisions about which specialist to consult, or which course to follow (Good, 1976). If satisfaction is not achieved, the family will consider sending the ill member elsewhere, even abroad, although it may also disagree with the foreign physician's diagnosis. Nonmedical health care professionals may be treated with particular mistrust, for in Iran nonphysician professionals are not involved in direct patient care; even the nurse's role is based on a purely medical model. Noncompliance with physicians' orders is common and does not necessarily indicate rejection of a particular physician. Iranian doctors often view their patients as exaggerating symptoms and holding unscientific beliefs; thus, they frequently prescribe vitamins, minor tranquilizers, and intramuscular medications to partially satisfy the patients. Iranians may have more trust in American physicians, but still seek prescriptions for vitamins and laboratory tests. Special diets that avoid certain foods, herbs, or spices have constituted a basic therapeutic element in traditional Iranian medicine, and patients often expect their doctors to prescribe such regimens. Indeed, when they do not do so, a patient may feel that an incorrect diagnosis has been made. In addition, Iranians may be embarrassed to provide personal information (e.g., about sexual problems) and may screen the information they give.

Many American therapists complain that they cannot get to know their Iranian patients. Because the inner self is preserved for intimates and very close friends, it may take a therapist much longer before he or she is trusted enough to gain entry to the inner self of a patient. For the same reason, Iranians are not very accurate research subjects, because they will reveal only the outer self in questioning. The therapist also has to be aware of the limits of the cross-cultural validity of psychological testing (Aposhian, 1995). Iranian immigrants in general are not very responsive to group therapy because of their lack of trust of strangers and suppression of the inner self.

A study shows that Iranian male immigrants with more culturally identified male roles had more negative attitudes toward psychotherapy (Khoi, 2002). There also appears to be a significant inverse relationship between less family support and increased rate of depression (Elia, 2002).

FAMILY THERAPY WITH IRANIAN FAMILIES

Reluctant about psychotherapy, Iranian families are almost always referred by an internist or family physician but do respond positively to a call for a family interview, because it deemphasizes the identified patient. The family expects the therapist to address the father first, as the head of the family, and he or she should proceed with respect and caution in challenging patriarchal power hierarchies or role patterns to avoid alienating the family.

Every attempt should be made to involve extended family members in therapy if they are available. Most often, such invitations are readily accepted. Extended family members may act as experts on family matters during sessions; it requires therapeutic skill to ally with them and, when possible, use them as cotherapists.

As compared with Westerners, Iranians are neither conforming nor obedient patients. Although seeming to follow a therapist's suggestions and orders, they often modify suggestions to suit their own evaluation of a situation. Iranian men, in particular, have difficulty following a female therapist's directions and recommendations and sometimes avoid discussing painful feelings, personal concerns, weaknesses, vulnerabilities, and sexual matters with her. Women patients use the same avoidances with a male therapist. Therefore, the therapist should address marital issues with utmost tact and scrutiny, preferably in a man and woman cotherapy team if at all possible.

A difficult bicultural situation involves therapy with an Iranian husband and an American wife. Conflictual situations include the Iranian husband's closeness to his friends and extended family, while the American wife is comfortable with greater distance and wishes to be more independent of them. They may also clash about male–female roles and child-rearing practices. Therapists should recognize that for a successful bicultural marriage, they should help the couple to communicate across their differences so that cultural identity does not become threatened (Bateson, 1994).

A 42-year-old first-generation Iranian physician who immigrated 12 years earlier from a middle-class family was referred with his 38-year-old American spouse because of chronic marital conflicts. They had a son, age 8, and a daughter, age 5.

The couple's relationship had been fraught with difficulty because the husband was chronically ambivalent about making a commitment to stay in the United States. He occasionally entertained serious thoughts of leaving his job and home here and returning to Iran. The husband's extended family still lived in Iran, and four or five of them at a time periodically visited the couple for months at a time, which was always a source of stress for the couple. The wife never felt accepted by her husband's relatives and resented the intrusion into their lives.

The couple also disagreed about child rearing, male–female roles, socializing, and other cultural issues. Each ridiculed aspects of the other's culture to assert his or her own values. Their son was repeatedly triangulated as each tried to bring him up in his or her own way. The husband insisted on frequent entertaining and would spend several evenings a week with his Iranian friends. The wife wanted more time together as a family and as a couple. Even though the husband was quite open and Western in his thinking, he repeatedly accused his wife of being aggressive and demanded more traditional and submissive behavior from her. She insisted that he share in domestic tasks and decisions. When his extended family visited, he reverted to the old ways, refusing to share any domestic tasks and attempting to dominate his wife.

The therapist attempted to focus the couple on their marital problems, highlighting their similarities and encouraging them to accept the differences. The husband was encouraged to teach his wife Farsi so that she could communicate better with him and his extended family. She was urged to resolve conflicts with her in-laws on a one-to-one basis, instead of pressuring her husband. Surprisingly, his sister responded quite positively to her sister-in-law's request for privacy and control of household affairs. The wife was encouraged to ask her in-laws about recipes for ethnic food and sources of ethnic herbs and spices, to which the extended family's response was overwhelmingly positive.

The husband was instructed to support his wife when she needed it, but generally to let her work out her own relationship with his family. The extended family then began to accept her more and actually to brag about her new talents. No attempts were made to decrease the number and length of the extended family's visits, but arrangements were made for their relatives to visit other members of the extended family during their stays. As the two families got along better, the husband's focus on the integrity of his nuclear family became evident.

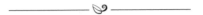

Cultural family patterns, such as a mother's closeness to her children, especially to boys, and her permissive attitude toward them, should not be confronted directly. Instead, the therapist should try to strengthen the child's sibling, peer, and father–child relationships, rather than weaken the mother–child bonds. Similarly, the mother may be encouraged to present a united front with the father when disciplining a child. The therapist might be a mediator and use his or her power and authority to resolve conflict and unify the family group.

The most effective family therapy technique with Iranian families is either the structural or the strategic problem-oriented approach, possibly because the power-hierarchical orientation matches the culture. An Iranian family usually responds positively to directives and may actually request them.

Finally, therapists can help by encouraging their Iranian patients to ventilate their feelings, listening to them with empathy and compassion, developing an appreciation of their cultural isolation, and treating real symptoms as they emerge.

CHANGES OVER THE PAST 20 YEARS

Iranian American immigrants have proved to be very resilient in adjusting and accommodating to their new culture and its nuances. Biculturalization is the most common and preferred mode of adjustment, as Western and traditional Persia show two different sets of behavior and own two sets of value systems simultaneously. According to Mostashari and Khodamhosseini (2004), Iranian Americans are among the most educated immigrant groups in the United States; among the 67 ethnic groups studied, Iranians have the highest rate of education, as one in four Iranian immigrants has a doctoral or master's degree. Therefore, they make a substantial contribution to the U.S. economy. They also surveyed Fortune 500 companies and found at least 50 Iranian Americans to be in the senior leadership positions at companies with more than $200 million of assets. Iranian Americans have also become prominent members of academic institutions including Yale, Harvard, MIT, the University of California system, Stanford, and many others. They are also represented in all professional, business, and white-collar segments of society; however, they remain underrepresented in the political process of their new country.

The emerging second-generation offspring of the third- and fourth-wave Iranian immigrants have flocked in large numbers to colleges and universities. For many ethnic immigrants, higher education is a source of pride and accomplishment, but especially for Iranians.

Iranians have a strong negative attitude toward substance abuse; however, because of peer pressure, availability of drugs, and desire for pleasure seeking, some young Iranian adults and adolescents struggle with substance abuse. This is a source of shame and loss of face for the parents in the community and is often hidden and not shared with family and friends.

Family ties remain close, and contact and relationships with extended family members are strong. Many members of extended families live in the same city or in close proximity with each other, and frequent visitation and contact are the norm. There are no clear statistics comparing the rate of divorce between Iranian Americans living in the United States and Iranians in Iran, but divorce does appear to be more common and more acceptable in the United States. Clinical evidence suggests that the majority of divorces among Iranian immigrants living in the United States are initiated by women. The men suffer the loss of pride and spousal role more than the women, although both must deal with the stigma of divorce and the ensuing isolation and loneliness.

There is currently a higher rate of cross-cultural marriage than there was 20 years ago, and families are adjusting to them now more easily than in the past. Many people have been able to travel back and forth to Iran to visit or settle their affairs, and this has decreased their sense of isolation and separation from other family members who still live there. Several Persian TV and radio stations, some of them playing continuously, have been a great source of entertainment and comfort, especially for older Iranian immigrants. There are also multiple daily, weekly, and monthly newspapers and magazines published regularly and countrywide. They include news, poetry, literature, and political commentaries and articles. The various religious denominations have become better organized and established in their communities. As far as mental health care is concerned, Iranians' attitudes toward mental illness and psychological problems are changing, and Iranians are becoming much more comfortable in seeking mental health services and requesting counseling when the need arises. But they are still much more receptive to educational and self-help programs. As a result, there is a proliferation of such programs, which have attracted hundreds of Iranian Americans. This type of education has helped them to become more knowledgeable about and receptive to psychotherapy, counseling, and family/couple therapy. There are now a large number of Iranian psychologists, therapists, and psychiatrists in the community in each city in the United States, allowing patients to select a therapist much more easily if they choose to.

REFERENCES

Adams, W. (1968). *The brain drain.* New York: Macmillan.

Aposhian, M. A. (1995). Iranian archetypes; Toward the principal integration of core Iranian belief systems. *Dissertation Abstracts International, 56*(6-A).

Arasteh, A. R. (1964). *Man and society in Iran.* Leiden, the Netherlands: E. J. Brill.

Askari, H., Cummings, J. T., & Izbudak, M. (1977). Iran's migration of skilled labor to the United States. *Iranian Studies, 10,* 3–35.

Baldwin, G. B. (1963). The foreign-educated Iranian: A profile. *Middle East Journal, 17,* 264–270.

Banuazizi, A. (1977). Iranian "national character": A critique of some Western perspectives. In L. C. Brown & N. Itkowitz (Eds.), *Psychological dimensions of Near Eastern studies.* Princeton, NJ: Darwin Press.

Bateson, M. C. (1994). *Peripheral visions: Learning along the way.* New York: HarperCollins.

Bill, J. A. (1972). *The politics of Iran: Groups, classes and modernization.* Columbus, OH: Merrill.

Bill, J. A. (1973). The plasticity of informal politics: The case of Iran. *Middle East Journal, 27,* 131–151.

Elia, C. (2002). The relationship between depression, percieved social support, family conflict and acculturation among Iranian young adults. *Dissertation Abstracts International. Section B: the Sciences and Engineering, 62*(10-B).

Emami, A., Benner, P. E., Lipson, J. G., & Eckman, S.-L. (2000). Health as continuity and balance in life. *Western Journal of Nursing Research, 22*(7), 812–825.

Gable, R. W. (1959). Culture and administration in Iran. *Middle East Journal, 13,* 407–421.

Gastil, R. D. (1958). Middle-class impediments to Iranian modernization. *Public Opinion Quarterly, 22*(3), 325–329.

Ghaffarian, S. (1998). The acculturation of Iranian immigrants in the United States and the implications for mental health. *Journal of Social Psychology, 138*(5), 648–654.

Good, B. J. (1976). Medical change and the doctor–patient relationship in an Iranian provincial town. In K. Farmanfarmaian (Ed.), *The social sciences and problems of development.* Princeton, NJ: Princeton University Press.

Good, B. J., Good, M.-J. D., & Moradi, R. (1985). The interpretation of Iranian depressive illness and dysphoric affect. In A. Kleinman & B. Good (Eds.), *Culture and depression: Studies in the anthropology and cross-cultural psychiatry of affect and disorder.* Berkeley: University of California Press.

Haas, W. S. (1946). *Iran.* New York: Columbia University Press.

Hanassab, S., & Tidewell, R. (1994). Changes in the premarital behavior and sexual attitudes of young Iranian women: From Tehran to Los Angeles. *Counseling Psychology Quarterly, 6*(4), 281–289.

Hoffman, D. M. (1991). Beyond conflict: Culture, self, and intercultural learning among Iranians in the U.S. *International Journal of Intercultural Relations, 14*(3), 275–299.

Hojat, M., Shapurian, R., Foroughi, D., Nayerahmadi, H., Farzaneh, M., Shafieyan, M., & Parsi, M. (2000). Gender differences in the traditional attidudes towards marriage and the family: An empirical study of Iranian immigrants in the United States. *Journal of Family Issues, 21*(4), 419–434.

Hojat, M., Shapurian, R., Nayerahmadi, H., Farzaneh, M., Foroughi, D., Parsi, M., & Azizi, M. (1999). Premarital sexual, child rearing, and family attitudes of Iranian men and women in the United States and in Iran. *Journal of Psychology, 133*(1), 19–31.

Jalali, B., & Boyce, E. (1980). Multicultural families in treatment. *International Journal of Family Psychiatry, 4,* 475–484.

Kadkhoda, B. (2001). Acculturation and acculturative stress as related to level of depression and anxiety in Iranian immigrants. *Dissertation Abstracts International. Section B: The Sciences and Engineering, 62*(2-B).

Kheirkhah, S. P. (2003). Acculturation among Iranian immigrants in America: A phenomenological inquiry. *Dissertation Abstract International. Section B: The Sciences and Engineering, 64*(2-B).

Khoi, K. (2002). Predictors of attitudes of Iranian males seeking psychological help. *Dissertation Abstracts International. Section B: The Sciences and Engineering, 63*(2-B).

Kurzman, C. (2002). *Iranian family attitudes project: Global view.* Chapel Hill: University of North Carolina Press (University Center for International Studies).

Moghissi, H. (1999). Away from home: Iranian women, displacement, cultural resistance and change. *Journal of Comparative Family Studies, 30*(2), 207–217.

Mostashari, A., & Khodamhosseini, A. (2004). *An overview of socioeconomic characteristics of the Iranian-American community based on the 2000 U.S. census.* Iranian Studies Group at MIT. Available at www.mit.edu/isg

National Science Foundation. (1973). *Immigrant scientists and engineers in the United States.* Washington, DC: Author.

Nyrop, R. F. (1978). *Iran: A country study.* Washington, DC: American University Press.

Ostovar, R. (1997). Predictors of acculturation among Iranian immigrant adults living in the United States. *Dissertation Abstracts International. Section B: The Sciences and Engineering, 58*(3-B).

Pliskin, K. L. (1987). *Silent boundaries: Cultural constraints on sickness and diagnosis of Iranians in Israel*. New Haven, CT: Yale University Press.

Rouhparvar, A. (2001). Acculturation, gender and age as related to somatization in Iranians. *Dissertation Abstracts International. Section B: The Sciences and Engineering, 61*(8-B).

Safdar, S. (2003). Understanding the patterns of acculturation in different societies: A confirmation of a pan-cultural model. *Dissertation Abstracts International. Section B: The Sciences and Engineering, 64*(1-B).

Sundquist, J., Bayard-Burfield, L., Johansson, L. M., & Johansson, S. E. (2000). Impact of ethnicity, violence and acculturation on displaced migrants: Psychological distress and psychosomatic complaints among refugees in Sweden. *Journal of Nervous and Mental Disease, 188*(6), 357–365.

Verkuyten, M., & Nekuee, S. (2001). Self-esteem, discrimination and coping among refugees: The moderating role of self-categorization. *Journal of Applied Social Psychology, 31*(5), 1058–1075.

Vreeland, M. M. (1957). *Iran*. New Haven, CT: Human Relations, Area Files.

Wilber, D. N. (1963). *Contemporary Iran*. New York: Praeger.

Ziabakhsh, S. (2002). The relationship between the "Iranian self" and the acculturation patterns of Iranian immigrant women. *Dissertation Abstracts International. Section B: The Sciences and Engineering, 62*(9-B).

Zonis, M. (1976). *The political elite of Iran*. Princeton, NJ: Princeton University Press.

CHAPTER 34

Lebanese and Syrian Families

Karen L. Haboush

I believe that you have inherited from your forefathers an ancient dream, a song, a prophecy, which you can proudly lay as a gift of gratitude upon the lap of America. I believe you can say to the founders of this great nation, "Here I am, a youth, a young tree whose roots were plucked from the hills of Lebanon, yet I am deeply rooted here and I would be fruitful."

—KAHLIL GIBRAN, "I Believe in You" (1965)

An understanding of clinical work with Lebanese and Syrian families begins with an appreciation of both histories. Although present-day boundaries exist between the two countries, these boundaries are relatively new, having been drawn only in the early 20th century. Thus, historically, what is today referred to as Lebanon was actually part of Greater Syria. Furthermore, Syria continues to play an important role in present-day Lebanese politics. Yet, despite areas of historical, cultural, and religious overlap, there are differences between the two countries as well as within the subgroups that inhabit each country. This chapter first provides some brief historical context necessary for understanding each country. Next, topics of relevance for conducting clinical work with families, and their application to case examples, are discussed. Case examples, modified to protect confidentiality, are included to illustrate certain clinical points.

The following sections provide a general overview of relevant cultural considerations, in light of the variability both within and between the various subgroups that inhabit the two countries. In writing about Lebanese and Syrian families, I have primarily drawn on scholarly sources, supplementing such information with anecdotal comments from Lebanese and Syrian Americans, as well as clinical observations of practicing psychotherapists. Written information on Lebanon is easier to find because of Lebanon's greater political openness and stronger ties to the West and the presence of Western universities. In Syria, the media is under goverment control and outside journalistic access is restricted. Additionally, English is not taught until college, which further limits the publication of articles in English.

The key decision point in determining how best to approach clinical work with Lebanese and Syrian families involves examining the extent of acculturation to either Western or Arabic societies. Given that in Arabic culture there is heavy emphasis on solving problems within the family unit, family therapy constitutes a good "fit" with traditional cultural values. However, the family therapist still needs to assess issues of acculturation and cultural identity prior to formulating interventions. Modifications in technique are indicated for families that are more closely identified with Arabic, rather than Western/ Euro-American, cultural values. In general, these families will respond best to interventions that maintain family cohesiveness. As family members become more acculturated within Western societies, treatment can also incorporate insight-oriented interventions and support greater autonomy among family members.

HISTORICAL OVERVIEW: SYRIA AND LEBANON

The boundaries of modern-day Lebanon and Syria were established during the 1920s. Previously, this region, known as Greater Syria, had been under Ottoman rule since 1517. Lebanon originally consisted of a much smaller area, including Mount Lebanon, which was primarily inhabited by Christians (Chamie, 1981). Following World War I, Turkey lost her rule of Greater Syria to France. During World War II, both Lebanon and Syria overthrew the French mandate and became separate, independent countries.

Syria

Historically, Syria was the center of one of the oldest civilizations, with Damascus dating back to at least 2500 B.C. Damascus fell under Muslim rule in A.D. 636. Syria was occupied by many groups, including the Phoenicians, Hebrews, Persians, Greeks, Romans, and Byzantines. In 1517, it fell under Ottoman rule. Following the overthrow of the French in the 1940s, Syria underwent various political changes. Syria has been under a "state of emergency," declared by the Ba'athists, since 1963. Today, Syria is supposed to be run as a democratic country, although its president, President Asad, ran unopposed in 2000. The leading party is the Ba'ath Party, which is socialist, emphasizes Arabism, and is secular, even though more than 90% of Syrians are Muslims, most of whom are Sunnis (U.S. Department of State, 2003c). Other Muslim groups include the Shiite, Druze, and Alawi. The dominance of Muslims within Syria makes Syria more like other Arab countries than Lebanon, which has a large Christian population. The Ba'ath Party is dominated by the Alawis, of which President Asad is a member. As in other Arab countries, there have been clashes among the various Muslim groups; however, there is presently limited opportunity for dissenting opinions within Syria. The Kurds, which comprise 9% of the population, speak Kurdish as well as Arabic. There are also small Syrian Christian (Catholic, non-Catholic, and Orthodox) and Jewish populations. Syrian Jews are part of the group of Jews referred to as Sephardic; they also constitute part of the Syrian community that migrated to the United States. Finally, about 400,000 Palestinian refugees also reside in Syria (U.S. Department of State, 2003c).

Military service is compulsory for all Syrian men over the age of 18. Syria became involved in Lebanon's civil war on behalf of the Maronite Christians, beginning in 1976 and then again in 1982. About 16,000 Syrian troops are still deployed in Lebanon (U.S. Department of State, 2003c). Syria has argued that the presence of troops in Lebanon, and use of martial law in Syria, are necessary because of ongoing conflict with Israel.

Lebanon

Lebanese society is characterized by a much greater degree of personal freedom than other Arabic countries. Although it is an Arabic country, Lebanon differs from the surrounding countries because of its large Christian population and relatively strong ties to the West. Historically, sources of Western influence have included the presence of Western and European schools, Western businesses in Lebanon, and France's mandate in the early 20th century, which dominated cultural life. This influence was most strongly felt within Beirut, "the Paris of the East," by members of Lebanon's upper class prior to Lebanon's 16-year civil war, which began in 1975. Even today it is not uncommon to hear French interspersed with English and Arabic within the same sentence

Many Maronite Christians, the country's largest Christian population, prefer to identify themselves as descendants of the Phoenicians, rather than Arabs (Gibran, 1965; Mackey, 1991). The Phoenicians, who settled in this area at about 2800 B.C., were skilled traders who used sophisticated bookkeeping practices. Their legacy is important in terms of the long-standing emphasis within Lebanese culture on trade, family-owned businesses, and a strong work ethic (Mackey, 1991).

Although the West has held a cosmopolitan image of Lebanese life, based on perceptions of Beirut, family therapists should be aware that this image largely represented the upper classes, who were predominantly Christian. However, the number of Muslims grew in the 20th century, owing, in part, to the settlement of Palestinian refugees in camps. Both government representation and the distribution of resources throughout the country tended to favor the Maronite Christians, who were originally in the majority. Eventually, this unevenness in representation and resources and the country's divided identity (Western/Christian and Arab/Muslim) contributed to Lebanon's civil war (Mackey, 1991; Pintak, 1988; Reed & Ajami, 1988). Although the Lebanese civil war has ended, there are still tensions and deep divisions. Today, in an attempt to ensure greater representation of the most prominent religious groups, Lebanon has a Christian president, a Sunni Muslim prime minister, and a Shiite Muslim president of the National Assembly (U.S. Department of State, 2003a)

RELIGION AND IDENTITY

Of key importance in understanding Lebanese and Syrian culture is an understanding of the different cultural and religious groups that make up the country's population. Thus, despite a common Arabic heritage, when a person claims to be of Lebanese or Syrian ancestry, he or she may be a descendant of any number of subgroups residing within Lebanon and Syria. It is important for family therapists to understand the differences between these groups, as group membership influences certain values, including openness to psychotherapy. Especially in Lebanon, personal identity is much more closely linked to family and religion than to a sense of nationalism (Haddad, 2002; Hofman & Shahin, 1989).

One of the major dimensions in which various subgroups differ is the extent to which they are more closely identified with either the Western/Christian or Arab/Islamic world. In turn, neither the Christians nor the Muslims constitute a homogeneous group, and differences within the subgroups have been as strong as those between the two main religious groups (Chamie, 1981). For instance, the Christians are composed of Catholic (Maronites, Greek Catholics, Armenian Catholics, Syrian Catholics) and non-Catholic

(Greek Orthodox, Armenian Orthodox, Protestant, and Syrian Orthodox) groups (Chamie, 1981; Mackey, 1991). My memories of childhood include attending a Greek Catholic (Melkite) church in Brooklyn, where a strong Eastern influence was conveyed through the use of incense, chanting, and golden mosaics.

Unlike other Catholic groups whose membership extends across countries (i.e., one can be a Roman Catholic living in Poland, Italy, Ireland, or any of a number of other countries), the Maronite church is exclusively a Lebanese church. The Maronites originally lived in present-day Syria but migrated to the Lebanese mountain range in the 7th century, seeking protection from religious persecution. Fearing ongoing persecution from the Muslims, the Maronites were the only group within the Arab Middle East to support the Crusades. However, after the Crusades ended, many Maronites remained fearful of being overtaken by Muslim rule. Ultimately, support for the Crusades, as well as France's protection of the Maronites in the 18th and 19th centuries, contributed to the Maronites' greater identification with the West rather than with Arabic countries. Because they originally constituted the largest percentage of Lebanon's population, the Maronites held the greatest political power within the country until the time of Lebanon's civil war. They continue to maintain a separate sense of their identity as non-Arabs (Khashan, 1990; Mackey, 1991; Reed & Ajami, 1988).

Among the Muslims are the Sunnis, the Druze, the Shiites, and (in Syria) the Alawi (Mackey, 1991). As in other parts of the Arab world, the Sunnis were originally the largest group of Muslims within Lebanon prior to the civil war. The Shiites were originally most concentrated in the southern part of Lebanon, where resources were least developed and fighting occurred between Israel and the Palestinians. Many Shiites adhere to *Shari'a*, or Muslim law, and are more closely identified with the Shiite movement in Iran than with a sense of Lebanese or Syrian nationalism. The Druze are another subgroup within Islam whose beliefs are characterized by an emphasis on mysticism. Finally, the Alawis (12%), including President Assad, although fewer in number than the Sunnis (74%), hold most of Syria's political power (U.S. Department of State, 2003c). The Sunnis object to the predominance of the Alawis in the Ba'athist secular government because they view the Alawis as less religious.

As a result of differences in beliefs, intermarriage between members of the various Muslim groups is as unacceptable, as is marriage between Christians and Muslims. As much fighting occurred among the various Muslim factions during the Lebanese civil war as occurred between Christians and Muslims. In Syria, although 90% of the population is Arabic, ethnic, religious, and regional alliances remain evident despite the government's attempt to emphasize nationalism and an Arabic identity (U.S. Department of State, 2003c). Therefore, the family therapist needs to inquire carefully about religious affiliation and degree of religious observance, inasmuch as husbands and wives who marry across religious lines may lack extended family support, which can increase isolation, depression, and anxiety.

A word about other ethnic groups within Lebanon and Syria, such as the Armenians, Jews, and Palestinians, is warranted. Many Armenians immigrated to Lebanon and Syria between 1915 and 1922 following the Genocide in Turkey. Armenians presently make up approximately 6% of Lebanon's population (U.S. Department of State, 2003d). In Lebanon, the Armenians were widely accepted into Lebanese society, owing to the fact that the majority were Christian and many had emigrated with skilled trades. In contrast, the settlement of Palestinian refugees into Lebanese camps was resented by the Christians because most Palestinians were Muslim. The difficult living conditions endured in the refugee camps ultimately contributed to the rise of Palestinian militarism and the Lebanese civil war (Fernea & Fernea, 1985; Pintak, 1988). Today, more than 160,000 Palestinian refugees still have no political rights, are not considered citizens of Lebanon, and generally hold the least skilled jobs. Although Jewish families constitute less than 1% of the population in both Lebanon and Syria, many Syrian Jewish families have been involved in successful businesses, which they have continued to pursue upon immigrating to the United States. Only a handful of Jewish families remain in Syria.

In summary, although the Lebanese are ethnic Arabs, many Lebanese, especially the Maronite Christians, have rejected identification with their Arab ancestry. For many Lebanese Christians, Arab nationalism has historically been perceived as a threat, in terms of engulfment by large numbers of Muslims both within Lebanon and from other Arab countries (Fernea & Fernea, 1985; Khashan, 1990; Mackey, 1991). These fears are deeply rooted in historical events (e.g., the Crusades), which have left their marks, evident in the age-old tensions between Christians and Muslims and their fear of being overthrown by each other. There is a deep cultural mistrust that permeates different religious groups. Because of years of infighting among various groups, both prior to and during the Lebanese civil war, there can be a high level of anxiety and guardedness within families as well. These feelings are often extended to the family therapist. A psychologist recently commented on the clinical sense that Lebanese clients "continually feel under siege," referring to the internalized sense of mistrust and fear of attack that have permeated the Lebanese psyche. These fears may sometimes be masked by a defensive "bravado" or sense of superiority (Mackey, 1991). Thus, in family therapy, the therapist must assess the trust level of the family in working with an "outsider." For American-born family therapists, this challenge may be heightened by the fact that America has generally not been perceived as supportive of either Lebanon or Syria. The family therapist should also be aware that because of a prevailing cultural emphasis on hospitality and respect for authority, Lebanese and Syrian families may behave in an outwardly gracious manner that serves to conceal their fears in regard to trust (Mackey, 1991; Rugh, 1997). Thus, the therapist must carefully assess a family's actual level of compliance with therapeutic interventions inasmuch as disagreement with the therapist may not be directly expressed (Dwairy & Van Sickle, 1996). Providing education and a rationale for particular interventions, which can lessen ambiguity, may be helpful in reducing a family's guardedness.

For Syrian families, the lack of political openness within present-day Syria may also contribute to generalized feelings of mistrust and suspiciousness. In addition, the United States and Syria currently have strained diplomatic relations (U.S. Department of State, 2003b, 2003c, 2003d), partially related to Syria's continued military presence in Lebanon. In 2003, Syria was added to the United States' lists of countries believed to be harboring weapons of mass destruction as well as Iraqi leaders who fled Iraq following the United States' invasion (U.S. Department of State, 2003c).

PATTERNS OF IMMIGRATION

The largest number of Arabic immigrants currently residing within the United States are Lebanese (Ajrouch, 2000). Both Syrians and Lebanese immigrated to the United States (as well as Africa, Europe, South America, and Australia) in several waves. Earlier immigrants primarily migrated for economic reasons after the creation of the Suez Canal in

1869 lessened opportunities for trade (Gibran, 1965). The majority of these immigrants were farmers or laborers, who tended to settle in small communities (i.e., "Little Syria") in various regions, including Manhattan, Brooklyn, Detroit, Boston, Pittsburgh, Atlanta, Rhode Island, and New Jersey. They were predominantly Christian (Khater, 2003).

Many Arabic names were anglicized by using the father's first name as a new last name (Solomon & Gostomski, 2001). These immigrants tended to maintain an identification with their "Arabness." Because of a historically strong mercantile influence, owing to the tradition of their occupation in the markets of the Middle East and the Phoenicians' legacy as traders, many early immigrants, including women, became involved in sales, peddling, and other mercantile pursuits (Khater, 2003). My own Lebanese *giddu* (grandfather) owned a linens business and traveled with his wares throughout New York and New Jersey. Family therapists working in different parts of the United States may encounter regional variations in the immigrant experience of Lebanese and Syrian Americans. Although large numbers of Lebanese and Syrians initially settled in the Northeast, many eventually moved farther South, seeking the kind of climate that was more familiar to them. Lebanese and Syrians growing up in the southern United States may have experienced more racism because of the historical legacy of African slavery and the darker skin color of many Arab Americans.

Following World War I, many Arabic immigrants to the United States were listed as Syrian Nationals, even if they came from Lebanon (Gibran, 1965). In fact, more than 90% of Arab immigrants during this period were from Lebanon and Syria (Abudabbeh, 1996), with the majority being Christian. A second wave of Lebanese immigrants arrived during the mid-1960s, when the Immigration Act of 1965 stressed opportunities for family reunification (Ajrouch, 2000). A third wave of immigration occurred once the Lebanese civil war began in 1975 (Fernea & Fernea, 1985; Mackey, 1991) and then again following the 1982 Israeli occupation (Ajrouch, 2000). These immigrants were predominantly Christians, especially Maronites, seeking to flee the country and, to some extent, to distance themselves from the rise of Arab nationalism (Mackey, 1991). However, the number of Muslim (Syrian and Lebanese) immigrants also increased in the second half of the 20th century. Unlike the earlier waves of immigrants, this later wave of Christian and Muslim immigrants included many well-educated professionals and business owners (Solomon & Gostomski, 2001). Currently, much of Lebanon's current income still derives from immigrants living abroad who send money back to family members. This practice reflects a strong belief about the responsibility of family members to help the extended family, a value that is widely held by both Christian and Muslim families (Fernea & Fernea, 1985; Mackey, 1991).

As a rule, the family therapist should assess the recency of immigration status, as well as the circumstances under which family members migrated (e.g., war, economic hardship). Related to immigration issues, the family therapist will also need to determine how acculturated family members have become in their new country and the extent to which they identify themselves as more Western or Arab.

WAR, TRAUMA, AND MENTAL HEALTH ISSUES

In working with Lebanese and Syrian families, the family therapist should assess their exposure to war, including the Lebanese civil war and occupation of Southern Lebanon.

Fighting in the Lebanese civil war permeated all religious and socioeconomic groups, and women sometimes fought in paramilitary combat (Karam et al., 1998). Therefore, assessment for war trauma should not be limited to inquiring about formal military service. Furthermore, because military service is compulsory for Syrian men over the age of 18, Syrian families may include members, both male and female, who have been involved in combat, such as in the Gulf War.

Despite noting that many Lebanese are proud of their "resiliency" and may thus be reticent to acknowledge emotional difficulties, Karam and colleagues (1998) found that symptoms of major depression occurred with the highest frequency (41.9%) in communities with greatest direct exposure to the civil war. These authors also found that 49% of their adult sample had consulted with a physician or specialist and/or had taken medication for depression. Given that many Lebanese are reluctant to acknowledge emotional problems, these figures probably underestimate the percentage of individuals affected by the civil war.

Therapists should also evaluate family members for possible symptoms of posttraumatic stress disorder (PTSD). Because intergroup tensions and divisions remain, lingering feelings of mistrust, suspiciousness, and hypervigilance, all symptoms of PTSD, may be encountered in working with Lebanese and Syrian families. Anxiety may be more readily reported than depression (Abdel-Khalek, 1998).

A number of authors have noted a tendency toward somatization in Arabic cultures, consistent with the decreased emphasis on the outward expression of one's feelings (Dwairy & Van Sickle, 1996; Erickson & Al-Timimi, 2001). Thus, family members may be more likely to present physical complaints to physicians rather than seek mental health treatment. The family therapist should be attentive to the family's discussion of physical complaints, as this may be the "language" its members use to convey their emotions. A Lebanese American psychotherapist has commented on the tendency for depression to be referred to as " a dark life" and for fear to be described as "my heart fell down."

As with many other individuals of Arabic descent, many Lebanese and Syrians do not to want to be seen as having psychological problems. Traditional sources of help for mental health issues include religious and community leaders. If the family therapist can establish that such figures are supportive of a family's decision to seek therapy, this can greatly enhance the acceptability of treatment. Many Lebanese and Syrians may be more likely to consult with physicians than with therapists, yet cultural norms in which the physician's authority is respected and he or she is often deferred to when discussing symptoms may in fact diminish the likelihood that emotional problems will be disclosed (Adib & Hamadeh, 1999; Kabakian-Khasolian, Campbell, Shediac-Rizkallah, & Ghorayeb, 2000).

In general, there is greater openness regarding mental health treatment in Lebanon, owing to its stronger ties to the West and its educational system (Nassar-McMillan & Hakim-Larson, 2003). The overall development of psychological services has been slow in Arabic countries and is strongly influenced by Western and European models of diagnoses and treatment (Abou-Hatab, 1997; Soliman, 1987). However, increasing interest in the "development of an Arabic theoretical frame of counseling" (Soliman, 1987, p. 141) has slowly been emerging. In particular, interest in developing psychological models that are influenced by Islamic beliefs appears to be increasing (Abdelkarim, 1987; Abou-Hatab, 1997).

FAMILY

Clinical work with Lebanese and Syrian families must recognize the centrality of the family unit. This point cannot be overstated. Syrian and Lebanese cultures are considered "collectivist" rather than "individualistic" (Bierbrauer, 1992; Hofman & Shahin, 1989), in that individuals define their identities based on group membership. Greater importance is placed on the consequences of one's actions for the group, whereas individual needs (autonomy, achievement, independence) are secondary. As in other Arabic countries, the family is the primary unit with which the Lebanese or Syrian identifies (Fernea & Fernea, 1985; Kibbi, 1995; Mackey, 1991). This identification cuts across different religious groups and even precedes identification with one's religion.

Ahl, or kin, refers to the concept of the extended family, and Lebanese and Syrians maintain a strong sense of responsibility to their extended family members (Kibbi, 1995). Financial, medical, and child-rearing support are all provided to family members. Much socializing occurs within the family, and, historically, marriages between relatives have been preferred (Chamie, 1981; Mackey, 1991; Starr & Alamuddin, 1990). Boundaries are typically very enmeshed by Western standards (Mackey, 1991), and this is considered more appropriate than striving for greater separateness and independence. Thus, family therapists who encourage greater separation and individuation of children will likely encounter opposition from family members, possibly resulting in early termination (Dwairy & Van Sickle, 1996). Instead, family therapists need to convey the expectation that therapeutic solutions can be found that will not threaten the family's stability.

As subsequent generations become more acculturated, greater conflict may arise within Lebanese American and Syrian American families. In studying Lebanese immigrants in an ethnic Michigan community, Ajrouch (2000) found that the children, although retaining many traditional values, also wanted to assimilate aspects of American culture. Girls viewed leaving for college as one of the few means available for achieving greater separateness from their families, outside of marriage. Thus, for the family therapist working with different generations, conflict arising from issues of acculturation is likely to emerge. He or she may need to provide education and normalize this conflict as an inevitable by-product of immigration. Underlying fears about loss of traditions and the importance of the family should be discussed. The therapist may wish to point out that greater independence does not have to be mutually exclusive with maintaining family ties and traditions. Ajrouch found that although Lebanese adolescents wished to acquire power and prestige, which they associated with an American lifestyle, they also felt positively about maintaining a strong sense of community support and identification.

Family therapists need to be careful not to view these family systems necessarily as pathological, and to recognize that the extended family provides considerable emotional, financial, and other support. The family therapist needs to make direct statements, during sessions, attesting to his or her recognition of the importance of family. Interventions that build on the strength of the family (e.g., acknowledging the positive aspects of parents' concerns for their children) are likely to be more acceptable to more recently immigrated, traditional families.

Hospitality is another central value among Lebanese and Syrian families (Mackey, 1991; Rugh, 1997; Simon, 1996). More than just serving the function of providing nourishment, meals serve to enhance family ties (Rugh, 1997). Like many other Lebanese Americans, I recall with great fondness the elaborate Lebanese meals shared with my family: *tabouli*, *hummus*, and *baba ghanough* prepared by my *situ* (grandmother) and *umti* (aunt). Because it is considered impolite to refuse food, the family therapist should accept food or *shahy* (tea) if offered. I offer a clinical observation: Perhaps such graciousness, a long-standing tradition relating to maintaining family honor, has more recently served to compensate for the losses resulting from the Lebanese civil war and annexation of Syrian and Lebanese lands. Such graciousness may also cover a deeper level of cautiousness toward outsiders (Rugh, 1997).

GENDER ROLES

Although Arabic countries, including Lebanon and Syria, are largely patriarchal (Wehbi, 2002; Yared, 2001), women have a certain measure of power within the family (Erickson & Al-Timimi, 2001; Fernea & Fernea, 1985; Rugh, 1997) because of their role in maintaining family ties. As Simon (1996) has noted, mothers play a central part in family life. Although women in Beirut and Damascus are more likely to pursue professional occupations, many still face traditional expectations regarding their "proper" role as wife and mother (Wehbi, 2002; Yared, 2001). Furthermore, within Islam the importance of the family unit, and therefore the role of women inside the home, has been strengthened (Wehbi, 2002). Education and employment for women are encouraged in Islam, but the primary aim is to strengthen the family unit, not to advance women.

In both Syria and Lebanon, girls are encouraged to attend school and achieve at high levels (El Hassan, 2001); however, fairly traditional sex role expectations continue to shape socialization experiences for children (Ajrouch, 2000). Girls' responsibility to male family members includes brothers as well as fathers. Brothers often exert considerable control over their sisters, and these practices within the family help to prepare males and females for their traditional sex roles as adults (Joseph, 1994). As families become more acculturated within Western countries, girls are likely to achieve greater independence and to fulfill less traditional roles. A Lebanese American psychotherapist has noted that an adaptive outcome of girls caring for male family members is the development of a strong sense of personal responsibility in Lebanese girls. *Oweah* is a descriptive term referring to a capable, sharp female. In certain communities, including ethnic communities of Lebanese immigrants living in the United States, there is still some gender segregation of adolescents in terms of socializing (Ajrouch, 2000).

In the public sector in Syria, women remain underrepresented in government and professional arenas even though the Syrian constitution provides for equality between men and women and equal pay for equal work (Women's International Network News, 1998). Both government and religious laws continue to discriminate against women. The punishment for women for adultery is stricter than it is for men. If they divorce, women may not receive child support and may also lose their rights to their children (boys at age 9, girls at age 12). Fathers must grant permission for children under 18 to leave Syria, even if the parents are divorced, and husbands, fathers, and brothers can take legal action to prevent female relatives from leaving Syria (Women's International Network News, 1998). Some Shiite women in both Syria and Lebanon have fewer rights under Islamic law (*Shari'a*). Women are usually granted half of the share of an inheritance that male heirs receive, but males are expected to take care of female relatives.

Muslim men in Syria may legally take as many as four wives as long as they can provide financially for them. However, the majority of Muslim men marry one woman (Women's International Network News, 1998). Unlike other Muslim groups, the Druze are monogamous. Marriage contracts within the Druze and other groups are intended to provide financial protection for the female (Starr & Alamuddin, 1990). Unmarried women are frequently expected to remain within their parents' home, with the result that they are often seen as a financial burden (Wehbi, 2002).

Consistent with its greater openness, Lebanon has various advocacy groups for women (Wehbi, 2002). In Syria, there are no reliable figures for the incidence of domestic violence (Women's International Network News, 1998). Although battered women have the right to press charges, few do because of the accompanying social stigma. In dealing with these issues, the family therapist must recognize that neither a wife nor her husband will likely volunteer that domestic abuse is occurring within their marriage. In addition, women may lack family and social supports for leaving a marriage. In light of these considerations, the family therapist should not push for separation or divorce early on, if he or she suspects domestic violence, because such a suggestion is usually counter to the prevailing cultural attitudes. Divorce is generally not encouraged by either Muslim or Christian groups. A more productive approach may involve working to enhance family ties, cohesiveness, and sound functioning. For example, the family therapist may incorporate statements pertaining to religious beliefs that reflect the dignity of women. Within the United States, some Arab American community groups have begun to address domestic violence; these groups may provide the family therapist with additional resources for dealing with this issue (see, e.g., the Arab-American Family Support Center's website at www.aafscny.org).

Since women traditionally have less opportunity for emotional expression, the family therapist may anticipate seeing larger numbers of Lebanese and Syrian females coming to therapy with internalizing disorders. In addition to somatic features, internalizing disorders include depression and anxiety. The strong influence of the father within a family may mean that many daughters often feel unprotected by their mothers. The following case example illustrates the strong patriarchal emphasis within Lebanese families, traditional sex roles, the tradition of family-owned businesses, and prevalence of internalizing symptoms.

A Lebanese mother and her adult Lebanese American daughter were seen in family therapy. The mother sought treatment because of increased anxiety and depression regarding her relationship with her adult daughter. These feelings were prevalent when she attempted to speak with her daughter about their relationship. Her anxiety prevented her from speaking, as did certain medical problems affecting her vocal cords. The mother feared that she would incur her daughter's anger and criticism if she attempted to speak with her.

The origin of this anger was her daughter's long-standing resentment because her college savings had been used to pay various debts left by her father when he passed away. Although the daughter had planned to attend college, her mother urged her to work in the family business to pay off the family debt. In family therapy, the daughter expressed her hurt and anger toward her mother for not protecting her interests. Her mother acknowledged her passivity in the face of a demanding husband and ultimately expressed regret that she had not acted on her daughter's behalf. In time, it became possible for the daughter to understand that her mother's actions did not reflect a lack of caring for her, the source of her hurt feelings. The therapist helped the dyad to understand the mother's actions as upholding very traditional cultural expectations regarding deference to the father, the passive nature of a wife's role, and the responsibility of daughters to the family. This reframing was helped by the fact that the therapist disclosed his own Lebanese American heritage in order to facilitate the establishment of an empathic connection with the dyad. As the daughter was better able to understand her mother's actions within this cultural context, her hurt lessened, resulting in diminished feelings of anger and improved communication.

SEXUALITY

Sexuality also reflects the patriarchal aspects of Lebanese and Syrian cultures. Although female attractiveness may be emphasized as being important in terms of pleasing a man, men are accorded more sexual freedom than women, which results in a double standard (Yared, 2001). Sex outside of marriage is still more acceptable for men than for women (Wehbi, 2002). The emphasis on protecting women's virginity in order to ensure their desirability as marriage partners (women's main social role), and the emphasis on preserving family honor, contribute to this value. Enjoyment of sex within marriage is sanctioned for women under the *Qur'an* (Mynti, Ballan, Dewachi, El-Kak, & Deeb, 2002; Wehbi, 2002).

Socioeconomic status also has implications for sexuality. Underscoring the importance of virginity and family honor is the fact that affluent women in Lebanon sometimes undergo surgery for hymen reconstruction in order to "prove" their suitability for marriage (Wehbi, 2002). Although infrequent and more common in rural villages, "honor killings," performed to preserve family honor if a female relative has engaged in sex outside of marriage, do occur. In Lebanon, the penal code carries lighter penalties for a man who kills a family member without premeditation if he does so to preserve the family honor (Wehbi, 2002). These points are included here to further illustrate cultural attitudes toward the importance of female virginity.

In Syria, AIDS tests are required for foreigners between the ages of 15 and 60 who wish to reside in Syria and/or marry Syrian nationals (U.S. Department of State, 2003a). In both Lebanon and Syria, homosexuality tends not to be openly acknowledged, owing to the central role of religion and the importance of maintaining family honor. Because of strong family pressures, many gays and lesbians marry heterosexual partners. A family therapist may encounter couples who come for treatment in regard to "marital problems." Over time, the therapist may sense that one partner has not acknowledged his or her homosexuality.

CHILDREN

Because of the emphasis on family, the Lebanese and Syrian child is raised to look to parents for solutions and advice rather than encouraged to obtain greater independence and autonomy (Goodnow, Cashmore, Cotton, & Knight, 1984). The idea of giving children choices, which is more common in Western societies, reflects a recognition of individual determination and is therefore less commonly observed in Lebanese and Syrian families (Rugh, 1997).

Although families are frequently very loving and affectionate, they also rely on punishment and verbal criticism in disciplining their children (Dwairy & Van Sickle, 1996; Joseph, 1994; Mackey, 1991). Parents may have high expectations for their children, related to the importance of preserving family honor. In conducting family therapy, it may be helpful for the therapist to first establish an alliance based on the parents' good intentions for their children, in order to enhance the parents' openness to reconsidering their parenting style. Dwairy and Van Sickle (1996) discuss acknowledging parents' love and care for their children underlying other parental behavior, such as criticism and holding high expectations. This aspect of parenting is covered further in a later section, "Shame, Honor, Identity, and Self-Esteem."

In both Lebanon and Syria, schools are viewed as places where teachers have the same authoritarian control accorded to parents (Goodnow et al., 1984; Kibbi, 1995; Rugh, 1997). Education is highly valued in Lebanon and Syria for both girls and boys, and teachers are given considerable respect (Kibbi, 1995). Parents view education as helping to ensure their child's occupational success later in life. Therefore, in working with recently immigrated families, the family therapist may need to provide information regarding the differences in Arabic and Western schools, especially if the family is seeking treatment for problems concerning their children. A higher level of assertiveness is required in American schools, and the Lebanese or Syrian child may be unaccustomed to asking teachers for help and engaging in more critical thinking (Kibbi, 1995). Parents may also be unaccustomed to challenging a school system on issues of advocacy for their children (e.g., regarding special education eligibility). Moreover, Lebanese parents may not believe that their role should include the active "teaching" of their children, which many American parents adopt as a cultural norm (Goodnow et al., 1984).

The following case example illustrates the emphasis on family ties and the challenges presented by greater acculturation within Western society. Second- and third-generation Lebanese Americans and Syrian Americans may be more likely to come for individual therapy, including insight-oriented approaches, especially in attempting to establish greater separation from their families of origin.

A Syrian American female college student sought treatment for anxiety, depression, and various somatic problems. These symptoms had intensified after her decision to live on campus while attending college. Her family wanted her to commute from home. As a result of the client's decision, her family cut off almost all financial support and her father refused to speak to her for a period of time. Therapy initially focused on helping the client to problem solve on how to function on a daily basis, given the limited financial and emotional support she was receiving from her family. In time, the client was able to find work while taking classes and slowly saved enough money to purchase a car. An informal network of support eventually emerged from within her family; her mother began to meet her without her father's knowledge, and her siblings phoned her. The therapist acknowledged the cultural importance of family by not pushing the client too strongly to separate from her family. Instead, the therapist recognized that the client wished to become more independent while continuing to maintain a relationship with her family. The therapist reaffirmed that these goals did not have to be mutually exclusive. Over time, the period of no contact with her father allowed the client to consolidate some gains in establishing her personal identity and developing her coping resources. Eventually, the client began to rejoin the family for holiday celebrations and resumed phone contact with her father. At termination, the client had established herself as more independent from her family by continuing to reside outside of the family home, but also maintained a connection through attending family events.

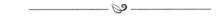

COMMUNICATION AND EMOTION

Arabic is the national language of both Syria and Lebanon, although English and French are also spoken. Traditionally, written language, such as the poetry of Kahlil Gibran, has been honored; thus, there is a tradition involving the use of language to convey strong emotion (Fernea & Fernea, 1985; Gibran, 1965). More recently, contemporary women authors have been gaining prominence in Lebanon (Yared, 2001). Children learn English in school. In Lebanon, many Maronites pride themselves on speaking French and English for business (Mackey, 1991). In contrast, following Syria's independence from France, Arabic has been the primary language taught in schools (U.S. Department of State, 2003c). Students learn English in college. An implication for recently immigrated Syrian families is that their children may face greater difficulty in school because of the English-language curriculum. Unlike English, Arabic is written from right to left.

In conducting family therapy, it is important to recognize the contradictions that exist regarding affective expression. Some writers have noted that affective expression, especially in public, remains very constricted because of the importance of preserving honor and the cultural tendency to discourage introspection into one's feelings. Dwairy and Van Sickle (1996) have suggested that the lack of emphasis on emotional insight is consistent with the importance of family; greater awareness of one's feelings can lead to greater conflict with the family. However, especially for males, expressions of anger can be strong and somewhat dramatic, inasmuch as aggressiveness is valued (Joseph, 1994; Rugh, 1997). At the same time, displays of affection and expressions of endearment are also common and can quickly follow an angry outburst (Mackey, 1991). Despite more open expression of frustration, direct expression of other emotions may be less common in public situations, including therapy sessions; this is further complicated by the emphasis on graciousness and hospitality, which can also serve to mask more honest emotional expression.

The family therapist needs to anticipate these communication patterns (i.e., either a high level of affective expression or a more constricted emotional style), and understand that encouraging more direct communication among family members will be a challenge. This is especially the case for more traditional families, inasmuch as such shifts may be perceived as a challenge to the father's authority (Dwairy & Van Sickle, 1996). Early on, the family therapist should ensure that he or she has established a good working alliance with the father. A female therapist may have to be especially sensitive to not challenging the traditional power hierarchy within families. The use of "why" questions, which are often asked by therapists, may also increase a family's defensiveness and a reluctance to disclose information (Dwairy & Van Sickle, 1996). Instead, the use of metaphors and analogies, religious references (when appropriate), and Arabic words is recommended. Initially, rapport can be enhanced if the therapist approaches the family members as though socializing with them, rather than assuming a more formal stance. This is consistent with the strong cultural emphasis on hospitality and the preference for less direct emotional communication. Home visits and sharing food/beverages, when possible, may facilitate rapport building. A traditional Arabic greeting is *Salaam* ("peace").

Because family boundaries are so intertwined, communication between family members is often indirect and messages are conveyed through other family members (i.e., triangulating a third party). As this is commonplace, family members do not perceive such patterns as problematic. Although Western forms of psychotherapy encourage individuals to speak directly for themselves, the family therapist may actually need to encourage members of the extended family to impart messages to other family members. Many Lebanese and Syrians are accustomed to expecting that family problems can be solved when powerful individuals in the community exert their "influence" (Mackey, 1991; Rugh, 1997).

The family therapist may consider reframing the emphasis on family in terms of need for affiliation, rather than "dependency." The latter term assumes a more negative connotation in Western-influenced psychotherapy. Thus, acknowledging the importance of family cohesiveness, bonding, closeness, and caring will be more acceptable than discussing how family enmeshment results in less independence and autonomy. In attempting to join with the family, the family therapist should convey the understanding that the cohesiveness of the family is crucial and has probably been highly adaptive in terms of survival, given the extensive history of conflict among subgroups in Lebanon and Syria.

In terms of psychotherapy, both Lebanese and Syrian societies have operated from the perspective in which personal intervention and family influence are the means by which matters are resolved (Mackey, 1991; Rugh, 1997). Culturally, respect for authority is valued. Given the combination of these perspectives, Lebanese and Syrian families may be likely to expect the family therapist to "solve the problem." Adding to this tendency to demonstrate a greater external, rather than internal, locus of control (Abouchedid & Nasser, 2002; Rugh, 1997), is the strong influence of religion. The family therapist may notice that family members often make statements referring to *Allah's* (God's) role in determining fate (i.e., "*Allah rad*" meaning, "If God wills it"). The influence of religion further contributes to Lebanese and Syrian family members being unaccustomed to the family therapist's expectation that they will have to assume a more active role in solving their problems (Dwairy & Van Sickle, 1996). Thus, a nondirective or more neutral stance on the part of the family therapist (such as is typical of more psychodynamic therapies) will be unfamiliar for the traditional Arabic family and will not enhance the establishment of a therapeutic alliance. Providing education about the family therapy process may help family members to better understand their roles and maintain appropriate expectations. As with many other non-Western families, it has been suggested that a short-term, solution-focused approach, in which the therapist assumes a more active role, will be more comfortable for traditional Lebanese and Syrian families (Dwairy & Van Sickle, 1996; Erickson & Al-Timimi, 2001).

A Syrian American family sought treatment for their two children, a boy and a girl, both of whom were under 10 years of age. Both children manifested considerable anxiety when separated from their parents. The older child, the boy, also had difficulty regulating his emotions when frustrated by limits. Some of the initial therapeutic interventions involved the therapist and parents exploring the degree to which their own upbringing in fairly traditional Syrian homes had shaped their parenting style. The parents gave preferential treatment to their son, while expecting their daughter to be "a good girl." The family therapist provided psychoeducation regarding the need to set firmer limits with the son. Further work with the family, however, suggested that some of the children's anxiety was related to their awareness of underlying marital conflict between the parents. Both parents were Muslim but differed as to how strongly they felt about practicing their religion. Couple work to address the marital issues ultimately constituted the focus of treatment.

―――――― ❧ ――――――

SHAME, HONOR, IDENTITY, AND SELF-ESTEEM

Sharaf (honor) and shame are important concepts within Arabic countries, and, by extension, within Lebanese and Syrian families (Bierbrauer, 1992; Mackey, 1991). In part, the collectivist emphasis is believed to intensify a propensity toward shame, rather than guilt, because of the greater importance of exposure in front of others (Bierbrauer, 1992). The greater emphasis on the group, rather than the individual, increases the likelihood for one to feel ashamed (which connotes public exposure of failure), rather than feel guilty (a more internal sense that one has not lived up to one's standards).

In addition to religious influences, the cultural importance of the family may heighten the propensity toward shaming as a means of behavioral control. Among young children, for example, despite the lovingness and close attachments in their families, one may observe a strong reliance on criticism, comparisons with other children, and shaming as a means of parenting (Mackey, 1991). The intent of shaming in child rearing is to preserve family honor, not to injure the self-esteem of children. Even schools in Lebanon have been noted to rely more heavily on shaming and reprimanding, rather than the use of positive reinforcement, to enhance desired behaviors (Saigh, 1980).

In working with families, it is important for the therapist to understand that family members are unlikely to perceive their actions as harmful to their children but, rather, to construe such a parenting style as necessary for the child and, more important, for the family's benefit. Rugh (1997) has noted, "Parents should do the right thing by their children, doing the right thing . . . [is], first of all, right for the whole family, not a single child" (p. 181). Thus, the family therapist needs to convey his or her understanding that parental actions are aimed at preserving family honor. As these patterns are so culturally embedded, parents are unlikely to consider the effects of criticism on their children. In turn, children may cope with underlying feelings of shame by becoming angry. In family sessions, this process often seems to account for the quick flare-up of frustration and anger sometimes observed in Lebanese and Syrian clients. Furthermore, there is likely to be an intergenerational transmission of shame, because parents tend to parent in the same way they were raised. More psychodynamically oriented therapists would likely refer to these injuries to self-esteem as narcissistic injuries (McWilliams, 1994). Although family therapists may not conceptualize this process in terms of a psychodynamic framework, understanding the intergenerational transmission of affect is highly consistent with family therapy approaches (McGoldrick, Giordano, & Pearce, 1996).

Because of the importance of family honor, therapists should avoid interventions that may be construed as shaming family members. Therefore, confrontation of an individual in front of other family members should be avoided. Second, the family therapist can join with parents regarding their concerns for a child's "inappropriate behavior" but then model alternative response styles that rely less heavily on criticism. This may include using praise to reinforce appropriate behavior, as opposed to criticism. The family therapist may also attend to expressions of anger as a signal that underlying feelings of shame have been triggered. If possible, helping family members to acknowledge these feelings may reduce the intensity of affect; however, in more traditional families, this may be difficult and the family therapist may instead choose to reaffirm the family's honor and dignity.

The following case example illustrates the transmission of shame to children, the overall importance of the family rather than individual needs, and the importance of traditional male–female roles in Lebanese families.

A Lebanese American adolescent was brought to treatment by her mother, who was concerned that her daughter was becoming increasingly depressed. The daughter also acknowledged feeling depressed. A discussion of these feelings suggested that the daughter was especially troubled by her mother's criticism of her. She felt that she could never please her mother, and this was contributing to a view of herself as *haram* (Arabic, connoting a pathethic case). In speaking with the mother over time, it became apparent that she was overburdened and resentful about her ongoing responsibility for an aging, but nevertheless demanding, father. The mother, who was first-generation Lebanese American, felt a great sense of responsibility toward her aged father, consistent with cultural expectations. At the same time, she was also resentful of his failure to recognize that she had her own family to care for. Much of the mother's anger was displaced onto her daughter. Over time, it was possible to reframe the mother's seemingly critical rejection of her daughter as reflecting her unspoken frustration toward her father. As the mother began to understand the damaging effects of this pattern, she began to praise her daughter more.

A discussion of these cultural expectations also allowed the mother to acknowledge her own unspoken cultural belief that her daughter should happily submit to her mother's treatment of her. The mother eventually lessened the extent of her involvement with her father, in order to create a better balance, in terms of responsibility, between her current family and her family of origin. To help the daughter feel less personally rejected by her mother, the therapist spoke directly with the adolescent and the mother about their understanding of traditional Lebanese expectations for daughters. This allowed the daughter to begin to reframe the problem in terms of cultural expectations rather than a personal rejection by her mother.

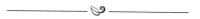

Perhaps on a broader cultural level, this reliance on anger to manage feelings of shame can also be understood as a response to the many losses that have been sustained by the Lebanese and Syrians. Fernea and Fernea (1985) discuss the sense of rage and accompanying feelings of powerlessness that many in Arab countries experienced as a result of Western colonization and denigration of Arab culture. Family therapists need to understand that many Arab Americans do not perceive the United States as sympathetic to, or even interested in understanding, the worldview of Arab Americans. This view may heighten the difficulty of an American-born family therapist in establishing trust within the therapeutic relationship. Thus, the therapist may consider normalizing the family's wariness in working with an "outsider" as a useful survival mechanism in attempting to establish a working alliance with family members. In this vein, the therapist can acknowledge the history of colonization by European countries and the accompanying devaluing of Arabic culture (Fernea & Fernea, 1985). The losses encountered upon immigrating to other countries can also be acknowledged (Khater, 2003).

In addition to the devaluing of Arabic culture, the loss of Lebanese and Syrians territories, and the increased racism directed at Arab Americans following September 11, 2001, have all intensified the feelings of powerlessness and shame. Images within the popular media, including the Walt Disney cartoon movie *Aladdin*, which was ultimately revised, typically portray individuals of Arabic descent in a negative light. Because of such racism, Lebanese and Syrian Americans are likely to internalize many of the negative images presented within Western societies and to anticipate further discrimination. Ambivalence regarding the degree to which one's appearance is visibly "Arabic," especially in regard to the darkness of skin color, may emerge in family therapy, particularly for children. Families may present concerns about their visibility as Arab Americans and their fear of encountering discriminatory treatment. A Lebanese American psychotherapist recently discussed how a Lebanese American male allowed his hair to turn gray, rather than continuing to dye it black, because he bore such a strong resemblance to Saddam Hussein. There is evidence that more recent immigrants have encountered greater discrimination than earlier immigrants and have responded to this by creating Muslim schools with Arabic language classes (Erickson & Al-Timimi, 2001). Individuals residing within the more closed communities may be especially wary of family therapists from different backgrounds. By acknowledging the reality of increased racism against Arab Americans following the tragic September 11 terrorist attacks (Abdelkarim, 2003; Nassar-McMillan & Hakim-Larson, 2003), the American-born family therapist can convey genuine interest in understanding the experience of Lebanese and Syrian families in America.

CONCLUSION

In conducting clinical work with Lebanese and Syrian families, the most critical decision involves determining the extent of acculturation to either Western or Arabic societies. Given the centrality of the family, the therapist must determine the degree to which greater independence among family members should be encouraged. Failing to consider this issue may contribute to early terminations. Because insight-oriented interventions may bring individuals into greater conflict with the family, these approaches should be avoided with more traditional families. Instead, therapeutic interventions that recognize the centrality of family, incorporate an understanding of religious beliefs, and include education regarding the family's role in the therapeutic process are recommended.

ACKNOWLEDGMENTS

I wish to acknowledge, with deep appreciation, the contributions of my research assistants, Julie Callaghan and Scott Roth. The following individuals graciously reviewed earlier drafts and/or provided commentary regarding various aspects of this chapter: Mary Aun, MA, MSW; Rita J. Basile, BA; Maureen Hudak, PsyD; Meline Karakashian, PhD; Joshua Landis, PhD; Saliba Sabah; and Kathryn Stratton, PsyD.

REFERENCES

Abdelkarim, A. M. (1987). Status, rationale and development of counseling in the Arab countries: Views of participants in a counseling conference. *International Journal for the Advancement of Counseling, 10,* 131–141.

Abdelkarim, R. Z. (2003, May). Arab and Muslim Americans: Collateral damage in the wars on terrorism, Iraq. *Washington Report on Middle East Affairs, 22,* 55–56.

Abdel-Khalek, A. M. (1998). Death, anxiety, and depression in Lebanese undergraduates. *Journal of Death and Dying, 37,* 289–305.

Abouchedid, K., & Nasser, R. (2002). Attributions of responsibility for poverty among Lebanese and Portugese university students: A cross-cultural comparison. *Social Behavior and Personality: An International Journal, 30,* 25–37.

Abou-Hatab, Fouad A-L. H. (1997). Psychology from Egyptian, Arab, and Islamic perspectives: Unfufilled hopes and hopeful fufillment. *European Psychologist, 2,* 356–365.

Abudabbeh, A. (1996). Arab families. In M. McGoldrick, J. Giordano, & J. K. Pearce (Eds.), *Ethnicity and family therapy* (2nd ed., pp. 333–346). New York: Guilford Press.

Adib, S., & Hamadeh, G. N. (1999). Attitudes of the Lebanese public regarding disclosure of serious illness. *Journal of Medical Ethics, 25,* 399–404.

Ajrouch, K. J. (2000). Place, age, and culture: Community living and ethnic identity among Lebanese American adolescents. *Small Group Research, 31,* 447–469.

Bierbrauer, G. (1992). Reactions to violation of normative standards: A cross-cultural analysis of shame and guilt. *International Journal of Psychology, 27,* 181–194.

Chamie, J. (1981). *Religion and fertility: Arab Christian–Muslim differentials.* New York: Cambridge University Press.

Dwairy, M., & Van Sickle, T. D. (1996). Western psychotherapy in traditional Arabic societies. *Clinical Psychology Review, 16,* 231–249.

El Hassan, K. (2001). Gender issues and achievement in Lebanon. *Social Behavior and Personality: An International Journal, 29,* 113–124.

Erickson, C. D., & Al-Timimi, N. R. (2001). Providing mental health services to Arab Americans: Recommendations and considerations. *Cultural Diversity and Ethnic Minority Psychology, 7,* 308–327.

Fernea, E. W., & Fernea, R. A. (1985). *The Arab world: Personal encounters.* New York: Doubleday.

Gibran, K. (1965). I believe in you. In *Mirrors of the soul.* New York: Philosophical Library.

Goodnow, J. J., Cashmore, J., Cotton, S., & Knight, R. (1984). Mothers' developmental timetables in two cultural groups. *International Journal of Psychology, 19,* 193–206.

Haddad, S. (2002). Cultural diversity and sectarian attitudes in postwar Lebanon. *Journal of Ethnic and Migration Studies, 28,* 291–317.

Hofman, J. E., & Shahin, E. (1989). Arab communal identity in Israel and Lebanon. *Journal of Social Psychology, 129,* 27–36.

Joseph, S. (1994). Brother/sister relationships: Connectivity, love, and power in the reproduction of patriarchy in Lebanon. *American Ethnologist, 21,* 50–73.

Kabakian-Khasolian, T., Campbell, O., Shediac-Rizkallah, M., & Ghorayeb, F. (2000). Women's experience of maternity care: Satisfaction or passivity? *Social Science and Medicine, 51,* 103–113.

Karam, E. G., Howard, D. B., Karam, A. N., Ashkar, A., Shaaya, M., Melhem, N., & El-Khoury, N. (1998). Major depression and external stressors: The Lebanon wars. *European Archives of Psychiatry and Clinical Neuroscience, 24,* 225–231.

Khashan, H. (1990). The political values of Lebanese Maronite college students. *Journal of Conflict Resolution, 34,* 22–32.

Khater, A. F. (2003). "Queen of the house?" Making immigrant Lebanese families in the *Mahjar.* In B. Doumani (Ed.), *Family history in the Middle East: Household, property, and gender* (pp. 271–299). Albany: State University of New York Press.

Kibbi, I. (1995). Lebanese and American educational differences: A comparison. *Education, 115,* 441–445.

Mackey, S. (1991). *Lebanon: Death of a nation.* New York: Doubleday.

McGoldrick, M., Giordano, J., & Pearce, J. K. (1996). *Ethnicity and family therapy* (2nd ed.). New York: Guilford Press.

McWilliams, N. (1994). *Psychoanalytic diagnosis: Understanding personality structure in the clinical process.* New York: Guilford Press.

Mynti, C., Ballan, A., Dewachi, O., El-Kak, F., & Deeb, M. (2002). Challenging the stereotypes: Men, withdrawal, and reproductive health in Lebanon. *Contraception, 65,* 165–170.

Nassar-McMillan, S., & Hakim-Larson, J. (2003). Counseling considerations among Arab-Americans. *Journal of Counseling and Development, 81,* 150–160.

Pintak, L. (1988). *Beirut outtakes: A TV correspondent's portrait of America's encounter with terror.* Lexington, MA: Lexington Books.

Reed, E., & Ajami, F. (1988). *Beirut: City of regrets.* New York: Norton.

Rugh, A. (1997). *Within the circle: Parents and children in an Arab village.* New York: Columbia University Press.

Saigh, P. A. (1980). The effects of positive reinforcement on the behavior of Lebanese school children. *Journal of Social Psychology, 110,* 287–289.

Simon, J. P. (1996). Lebanese families. In M. McGoldrick, J. Giordano, & J. K. Pearce (Eds.), *Ethnicity and family therapy* (2nd ed., pp. 364–375). New York: Guilford Press.

Soliman, A. M. (1987). Status, rationale and development of counseling in the Arab countries: Views of participants in a counseling conference. *International Journal for the Advancement of Counseling, 10,* 131–141.

Solomon, W. E., & Gostomski, C. (2001, November). *Identity.* Retrieved June 19, 2003, from www.mcall.com

Starr, P. D., & Alamuddin, N. S. (1990). Marriage—Lebanese style. *Natural History, 90,* 8–11.

U.S. Department of State. (2003a, May). *Syria—Consular information sheet.* Retrieved June 10, 2003, from travel.state.gov/syria.html

U.S. Department of State. (2003b, September). *Syria's weapons of mass destruction and missile development programs.* Retrieved April 10, 2004, from www.state.gov/t/us/rm/24135.htm

U.S. Department of State. (2003c, October). *Background note: Syria.* Retrieved April 10, 2004, from www.state.gov

U.S. Department of State. (2003d, November). *Background note: Lebanon.* Retrieved April 10, 2004, from www.state.gov

Wehbi, S. (2002). "Women with nothing to lose": Marriageability and women's perceptions of rape and consent in contemporary Beirut. *Women's Studies International Forum, 25,* 287–300.

Women's International Network News. (1998, Spring). *Syria.* Retrieved June 7, 2003, from web15.epnet.com

Yared, N. S. (2001). Identity and conflict in the novels of contemporary Lebanese women novelists. *Edebiyat: Journal of Middle Eastern Literatures, 12,* 215–229.

CHAPTER 35

Palestinian Families

Nuha Abudabbeh

Palestinians American clients present a challenge to American therapists because of the complexity of their political situation with the Israelis. This is an intensely emotional and highly charged conflict. Regardless of personal feelings about this conflict, to treat this particular population, it is important for therapists to understand how Palestinians think and feel about their history, and to know their current experiences. The history of the conflict, as well as the current situation, is a significant contributor to the psychological makeup of Palestinian Americans, influencing their perceptions of the world, their values, and their attitudes.

HISTORY

The title of Kathleen Christison's book *The Wound of Dispossession* (2001) tells the Palestinian story succinctly. This state of dispossession is well represented by two Palestinians. One is a young Palestinian American who stated that whenever someone asked where he came from he had to "go into 20 minutes of history" (Christison, 2001, p. 1). The late Edward Said (1966), a prominent Palestinian American, in response to the same question wrote: " I feel compelled to bring logic, history and rhetoric to my aid, at tedious length. We need to retell our story from scratch every time, or so we feel." To present a historical account of the Palestinian American version of this intensely emotional and highly charged history is a daunting task for anyone on either side of the conflict. The following is a chronology of the history of Palestinians as taught and passed on from one generation to the next (Jayyusi, 1992).

• In the 19th century under the Ottoman rule, landowning was created, ushering in the modern era, in Palestine. New rules during this period permitted foreigners to own property, and the first Jewish colony was founded near Jaffa in 1878. By 1924 three additional Jewish colonies were founded, raising the percentage of the Jewish population to10%.

• In the 20th century formal nationalistic opposition to Jewish settlement began simultaneously with other nationalist movements in other Arab countries.

• During World War I, the Ottoman Empire (Turks) formed an alliance with Germany against Britain. In 1916 the British, French, and Russians agreed secretly to divide the Arab world under different spheres of domination. The British, with the assistance of Arabs, drove the Ottomans out of the Arabian Peninsula, with the understanding that this alliance would allow for the formation of independent Arab states. In the meanwhile, in return for financial support in World War I, the British secretary of state sent a secret letter to Baron Rothschild (a British Zionist), promising a national home for Jews in Palestine.

• In 1918, Britain occupied Palestine and was subsequently awarded the mandate for Palestine by the League of Nations. Among the mandate's provisions was the facilitation of Jewish immigration and settlement in Palestine. In response, Palestinians began rioting. The British attempted to balance the conflicting aims of the promises made to the Jews and the Palestinians by establishing immigration quotas.

• Between 1924 and 1929 a third wave of Jewish immigration took place. This triggered a surge of riots and protests, leading to deaths and casualties on both sides.

• Between 1931and 1938 a fourth wave of immigration led to the establishment of 64 more Jewish colonies, raising the percentage of the Jewish population to 30%.

• Between 1932 and 1939, Palestinians organized into political parties and approached the British, asking them to change their policies of immigration, thus signaling the creation of armed rebellion.

• In 1939, the Great Rebellion, sparked partly by unemployment and by the British refusal to hold elections, began; it lasted 3 years. Following the killing of several Jews and Palestinians, a commission was set up by the British, recommending the partition of Palestine into three states; Arab, Jewish, and British. This was accepted by the Zionists but rejected by Palestinians. The British, in the meanwhile, continued their crackdown on Palestinian rebellion. More than 1,000 Palestinians were killed during this period and most of their leaders were exiled. In May of the same year the British offered a new 10-year plan to reunite Jews and Palestinians under a single independent state. Both rejected this plan.

• Between 1944 and 1947, the Zionists began guerilla warfare against the British, undertaking assassinations and terrorist raids, which were followed by British reprisals.

• In February 1947, the British announced their plan to withdraw from Palestine (subsequent to the bombing of their headquarters by the Zionists), leaving the responsibility for the country's future to the United Nations.

• On November 29, 1947, Partition Day, the United Nations voted to partition Palestine into Jewish and Palestinian states.

• In 1948 fighting between Palestinians and Zionists escalated into war, with 1,974 killed on both sides by January 1948. That same year Arab volunteers entered Palestine to join the fighting. In April 1948, Palestinian villagers were massacred in Dair Yasin. The news of the massacre reached many parts of the country. More than 10,000 Palestinians fled their homes, leading to the Zionists' takeover of several cities and areas near Jerusalem. On May 15, 1948, the British left, and the Jewish state, Israel, was proclaimed. The United States recognized the State of Israel, fighting continued, many villages were razed, and properties belonging to those who fled were transferred to the Israeli government. By December 1948 there were nearly one million Palestinian refugees.

- In 1950, Jordan annexed what remained of Palestine, absorbing more than 600,000 refugees and residents of what came to be known as the West Bank. In the late 1950s a commando group, the Palestine Liberation Organization (PLO), was organized and recognized by the United Nations (October 1974) as the legitimate representative of the Palestinians.

- In 1967, Israel attacked Egypt and occupied parts of Egypt, Syria, and the rest of Palestine.

- In 1970 a civil war, triggered by the Palestinians in Jordan, led to the massacre of many Palestinians and to their expulsion from Jordan. This event became known as "Black September."

- The Palestinians relocated in Lebanon. Between 1975 and 1987 civil war broke out in Lebanon, and the Palestinians were drawn into the hostilities.

- In 1976, the Tal al-Zaatar Palestinian refugee camp massacre occurred, forcing its inhabitants to flee to the Sabra and Shatilah refugee camp in Lebanon.

- In 1982, the Palestinians were expelled from Lebanon and relocated in Tunis. Christian militias massacred 1,700 civilians in Sabra and Shatilah under Israeli protection.

- In 1987 the first intifada took place, killing and wounding thousands of Palestinians and preparing the ground for the return of the PLO to the West Bank and Gaza.

- The PLO moved into parts of Palestine, beginning several futile attempts at gaining sovereignty.

- In 2000 the second *intifada*, triggered by Sharon's visit to the Palestinian quarter of Jerusalem, began, leading to the most recent developments in Gaza and the West Bank.

- In 2000–2004, during the second Intifada, 3,000 Palestinians were killed and thousands more injured and/or imprisoned. In addition, more homes were demolished and properties seized. The September 11, 2001, attack on the United States led to Israel's successful repression of any Palestinian aspiration for independence by labeling their struggle as a terrorist activity.

- In 2004, Arafat dies in Paris, ending a significant phase in the history of the Palestinian struggle for independence.

- In 2005, efforts for peace between Palestinians and Israelis become possible.

DEFINITION AND DEMOGRAPHICS

A Palestinian is anyone whose ancestors originated in Palestine prior to the establishment of the State of Israel (1948). Palestinians identify themselves as Arabs and speak a dialect of Arabic they share with Syria and Lebanon. The majority of Palestinians are Muslims of the Sunni sect. The majority of Christian Palestinians are Orthodox. There are several ethnic minorities among the Palestinians, such as Armenians and Cirkasians. Unlike those in other Arab countries where Christians and Muslims were and are in conflict, Palestinian Arabs have historically lived in harmony. Some of the most outspoken defenders of Palestinian rights are Christian Palestinians such as the late Edward Said and Hanan Ashrawi.

Of the estimated 3.5 million Arab Americans, 12–15% are Palestinians. They are concentrated mostly in Detroit, Chicago, and Los Angeles. Most of the pre–World War I immigrants to the United States were from villages (Seikaly, 1999). This first wave of immigrants were mainly sojourners; they made their living by peddling goods and were minimally involved in the American lifestyle. Settlement that began with one village led to a succession of other villages, thus beginning what was called a chain migration. The chain referred to the arrival of one generation after the other from specific villages. This immigrant population lived between the two cultures, with parts of their families remaining in the Palestinian village while the father worked in the United States.

A second wave of Palestinian immigrants arrived in 1948, followed by another in 1967, who were markedly different from their predecessors. This wave tended to be better educated and more politically motivated and had immigrated because of the loss of their homeland. The next wave of Palestinian immigration occurred after the expulsion of the Palestinians from Jordan (1970). In 1982, Palestinians emigrated from Lebanon following the expulsion of the PLO from Lebanon and the Sabra and Shatilah massacre. The Gulf War triggered the most recent immigration, when Palestinians in Kuwait and the Gulf area were expelled because of the PLO's support of Iraq during the Gulf War.

Most Palestinian immigrants were better educated than other Arab immigrants. They were more invested in their Palestinian identity because of the loss of their homeland and became instrumental in leading the Arab American community toward political activism in the United States (Said, 1995).

Seikaly (1999) studied a group of Palestinians in the Detroit area, describing them as emphatically attached to their Palestinian identity and ethnic culture. The entire group emphasized the continuation of their cultural norms. This was the grounding for a group whose lives had been in constant upheaval as they were forced into exile more than once and expected to survive under unfamiliar conditions. The intensity with which this attachment was expressed differed by socioeconomic class and sectarian and generational factors. Muslim men who were older, of lower economic class, with little education, and whose origins were primarily the villages, expressed the most conservative and traditional point of view. The women of this class held the same view. In contrast, the attitudes of Christians and middle-class educated Muslims were more flexible and moderate.

The Palestinian village remains alive in the memory of the Palestinian American. Most homes are decorated with Palestinian embroidery and other reminders of the culture. Those of the older generation consider themselves transplants in exile and continue to dream of returning "home," either alive or in a casket. This yearning for return is often a psychological necessity that helps Palestinians to protect their shattered selfhood. In contrast to the first generation of immigrants, the second generation has forged a "hyphenated" identity to accommodate their Palestinian culture within an American one. The hyphenated identities are expressed in a multitude of ways as impacted by their family's level of acculturation, socioeconomic class, and level of education.

Palestinian families have been socialized within a patriarchal system to some degree (Seikaly, 1999). Families have undergone many changes resulting from their geographic location and their history of dislocation. The less familiar and alien the new surroundings were, the more the Palestinians were likely to be entrenched in their customs and traditions. Those who grew up in different Arab countries prior to their immigration to United Sates may have acquired the customs of those countries. For example, Palestinians who grew up in Saudi Arabia tend to be more conservative and traditional, in contrast to those who grew up in Lebanon, who are more liberal and westernized. Another contrasting difference is between those who grew up in large cities and those who grew up in refugee camps. Regardless of the location of the camp, Palestinians who grew up in a camp were more likely to be conservative, more nationalistic, and continued to maintain cultural norms that were closest to their ancestral roots. Those who grew up in refugee camps were the ones who primarily led the fight for regaining Palestinian sovereignty.

PSYCHOLOGICAL SEQUELAE OF DISPOSESSION

The loss of Palestine, for many Palestinian Americans, is a traumatic loss. For a Palestinian American to maintain psychological stability as an American continues to present a challenge. "In trauma, terror overwhelms not just the self, but the ground of the self, which is to say our trust in the world. In this way trauma is an injury not just to the central system or to the psyche, but to the culture which sustains body and soul"(Farrell, 1998, p. xii). In his book, *Post Traumatic Culture*, Farrell (1998) describes one person's transgenerational trauma as follows:

> In part my experience was a contagious effect of trauma in parent's early lives, and in a nation that had been maimed by the Great Depression: an America still mourning its dead from WWII and Korea and spooked by the new Soviet H-bomb and by Spectral Communist spies. . . . Like a shaken war veteran, the nation reassured the neighbors that it felt on top of the world, yet it slept badly, with the light on, one eye open, and a pistol under the pillow.

To fully understand the Palestinian American's trauma one has to simply change the historic American events. The Great Depression can be replaced with the Palestinian Great Catastrophe (*al-karitha*), followed by subsequent events of expulsion, deportations, and a continued state of hypervigilance for survival. The impact of these traumatic events on Palestinians remains a question of much needed epidemiological studies that have yet to be conducted. In contrast to the multiplicity of studies on the traumatic effects of war on Israelis, there is a dearth of studies on the effects of the traumatic events on Palestinians. Attempts to study the effects of these traumatic events on Palestinians have been conducted primarily by Palestinians themselves (Awwad, 1989; Baker, 1991; El Sarraj, Punamaki, Salmi, & Summerfield, 1996; Kevorkian, 1988; Khamis, 1990; Mahjoub, Leyens, & Yzerbyt, 1989; Masalha, 1993). Non-Palestinians who have studied this population include Garbarino, Kostelney, and Dubrow (1991), Volkan (1990), Punamaki (1988), and Punamaki and Sulieman (1990).

The traumatic events endured by Palestinians are crystallized in several historical events that have impacted the collective consciousness of most Palestinians. These events began with the creation of a country that negated their existence, followed by decades of struggle to affirm their existence while living as refugees and/or an unwelcome entity in a number of countries. Researchers have focused their attention on Palestinian trauma after the first *intifada* (1987). A substantial number (40%) of the casualties among the Palestinians in Gaza and the West Bank were under the age of 15. The majority of these children were shot, detained, arrested, and beaten (Raundalen & Melton, 1994). Baker (1990) found that the level of psychological distress among Palestinians post-*intifada* had increased 15–26% from its prior level. A more recent study, conducted in four countries between 1997 and 1999 among survivors of war or mass violence, ages 16 or less, reported a 17.8% prevalence of posttraumatic stress disorder among children in Gaza. (De Jong et al., 2001). This percentage was lower than that reported in two of the four countries studied (Algeria, 28.4%, and Cambodia, 28.4%.) The results of this study offer very compelling reasons for continued interest in studying cultural differences in resilience. The differences between the Algerian and Palestinian samples raise several questions that are worth pursuing. A very obvious difference between the two groups is the cause of the trauma or its context. In the Palestinian situation, the trauma is inflicted by a well-defined enemy, an outsider and an occupier, but in the Algerian situation, it is inflicted by an Algerian against another Algerian (Abudabbeh, 2002).

Unlike other traumas, the Palestinian trauma has had to "compete" with the trauma of the Holocaust. The incompatibility of the two traumas has led not only to the minimization of the Palestinian trauma but also to its neglect and more recently to its vilification as it continues to be associated with terrorism in the United States. Mainstream trauma experts rarely if ever address the Palestinian trauma. For example, in *Ethnocultural Aspects of Posttraumatic Stress Disorder* (Marsala, Friedman, Geritty, & Scurfield, 1996), in a chart summarizing the prevalence of posttraumatic stress disorder in different ethnic groups (13 pages), listing approximately 130 studies, not a single study on Palestinians was included. Dwairy (1998) suggests the reason for this is that the Jewish tragedy of the Holocaust has justifiably gained the sympathy of the United States, thus excluding the Palestinians from any such attention. In contrast to the omission of the Palestinian trauma, American trauma experts were mobilized to study the traumatic effects of the Gulf War (1990) on Kuwaitis. I approached an author to contribute a chapter on Palestinians in a book on transgenerational trauma, only to be told that such a chapter did not belong in such a book.

The Palestinian trauma can be distinguished from other Arab trauma by intensified feelings of dispossession and exile from the homeland. The intensity of feelings associated with this trauma is often difficult for a therapist, especially an American therapist, to understand. Much of the anguish is connected to a Palestinian's feeling of oneness with the land and with a particular village, which cannot be satisfied anywhere else. For the Palestinian, the land represents a cultural identity, setting him or her apart from other Arabs (Christison, 2001). Rubenstein (1991) described the relationship between Palestinians and their villages as the central component of their identity. These intense feelings of dispossession and exile have been the central theme in Palestinian literature and poetry. Writers and poets who grew up in the Diaspora perceive Palestine through the memories transmitted to them by their parents. Mahmoud Darwish, who was expelled from Israel, where he was born and raised, wrote:

> We travel like other people but return nowhere. As if traveling in the way of clouds. We have buried our loved ones in the darkness of the clouds, between the roots of the trees.
>
> And we said to our wives: go on giving birth to people like us for hundreds of years so we can complete this journey. (in Foché, 1995)

Fawaz Turki (1972), a Palestinian writer who grew up in one of the refugee camps in Lebanon, described his pain of exile and dispossession as follows:

> I am aware that I have been Stateless nearly all my life. I have lived in a void, a state of nonbeing because everything has been taken away from us, including our tangible abstraction; as a result our being has been engulfed at times by lunatic extremes of hate and bitterness and [at] others by frustrated resignation.

In *Soul in Exile*, Turki described his sense of nonbelonging, a feeling shared by the majority of Palestinians, as:

> You have worn your sense of otherness all these years as a consciousness more intimately enfolding than your own skin. Statelessness is your only state, and you have long since developed an aboriginal sense of how to live there.

The Palestinian literary figure Edward Said (1995) describes the impact of dispossession on Palestinians as one of isolation, nostalgia, and a brooding sense of suspiciousness. He goes on to qualify the suspiciousness as at times justified, based on their being under government surveillance. What was suspected has become a reality for hundreds of Muslim Palestinian families. In addition to being targeted as activists in Islamic movements, Palestinian families have had to deal with the breakup of the nuclear family, as well as the extended family, because of such practical issues as lack of a passport and/or citizenship. Restrictions on travel to and from the West Bank or Gaza, and the instability of living as Palestinians in other Arab countries, have differentiated Palestinian families from other Arab families as having had to adapt to the disruption of family life because of their unique political realities. These conditions may have also contributed to the weakening, if not disintegration, of some of the other Arab traditional customs among Palestinians, as evidenced by their higher level of individualism, competitiveness, and resistance to authoritarianism among the more educated. There is no question that dispossession, traumatization, occupation, and survival under dire circumstances, even in other Arab countries, have taken their toll on the Palestinian psyche and, in turn, on Palestinian family dynamics.

Unlike other Arab countries, Palestine was a small country; in comparison with other countries, it had the largest concentration of villages. The Palestinian culture was primarily based on the customs and traditions of its rural society, the *fellahin*, and the villagers. Each village has been usually described as being known for what it grows, for its cleanliness or lack of it, and for its generosity or lack of it. Some villages were also identified as either predominantly Muslim or Christian. In contrast to some other Arab countries, there was no tradition of aristocracy or feudalism, but there were prominent families, and everybody in Palestine knew those prominent families by name. The villagers knew each other and, as a community, could therefore understand the dynamics of a family.

Prior to the creation of the State of Israel marriage between city and village families was not encouraged, nor were marriages crossing to less known urban families acceptable. Since the Diaspora, the Palestinian family has been transformed, as new realities were created as a result of historical events, which has led to the minimizing of the differences between urban and rural families. Despite these changes, however, the Palestinian family remains conservative. In a study of Muslim Palestinian women in Chicago (Cainkar, 1988) the Palestinian family is described as unintegrated into the surrounding American society and conservative in its expectations of the females, who are rigidly controlled by fathers and husbands. This sample consisted mostly of Palestinians who immigrated after 1967 and were from the rural areas of the West Bank. Although Palestinian families are not as conservative as, for example, Saudi families, attitudes toward sexual freedom remain conservative and the attitude toward homosexuality remains one of non-acceptance within that context. The Palestinian way of dealing with any sexual or emotional issues is to inevitably discuss them within the context of their relevance to the issue of the struggle to establish a Palestinian state. For example, gender issues are discussed within their relevance to the question of Palestine; thus, the issue of homosexuality becomes a frivolous one to even consider within the realities of a people who do not even have a place to call home.

TREATMENT

Rarely have Palestinian Americans sought mental health services in response to feelings of traumatization directly related to their loss of homeland and other Palestinian tragedies. Traumatic events have been dealt with as political realities. Wounds have been healed by political activism and literary expression. In the United States, Palestinians have been referred for treatment by their lawyers in regard to a variety of legal issues, such as seeking asylum and fighting deportation. In legal situations the traumatic experiences of Palestinians surfaced as a significant contributor to their psychological profile. In other situations, Palestinians who were hesitant to seek help, despite their depression and possible posttraumatic diagnosis, often sought help in indirect ways such as by befriending me. Palestinian Arabs differ from other Arab immigrants in their culture of Diaspora, homelessness, and carrying a transgenerational legacy of not having been given their due justice. Palestinian Americans are further burdened with having to live in a country that has played, and continues to play, a significant role in their state of homelessness. The psychological impact of these issues is often addressed through the Palestinian American communities' continued involvement in political activism. Unlike those of other Arab Americans, Palestinian Americans' social gatherings almost inevitably include a group discussion of their political and social realities. The fact remains, however, that many a Palestinian has suffered the consequences of those realities. The consequences range from substance abuse, numbing of feelings, and self-destructive behaviors, or sublimation through high levels of achievement.

The therapist's knowledge of a Palestinian client can be enhanced with a focus on the following areas of inquiry:

- The village or city of origin, along with the specific cultural norms of the place of origin.
- The history of the family after different deportations and/or immigration.
- What was the family's experience in an Arab country before its immigration to the United States?
- Did the client or his or her family ever live in a refugee camp, and what was that experience like?

- Did the client or any member of his or her family experience violence, imprisonment, or death of a loved one.
- How does the client feel about the United States' position on Palestinians?

Treatment approaches with Palestinians have to be adapted according to the type of family that is seeking treatment. This is a society in which there are significant differences in how traditional or conservative a family is: Families from rural areas, even the Christians among them, are more conservative than other Middle Eastern families. For example, a Christian Palestinian family who had immigrated to the United States from Jordan was observed to have adopted such traditional family values as expecting its female members to adhere to traditional customs such as wearing scarves, not dating, and, as wives, accepting secondary roles in the family. The Israeli Arab families are traditional but not as conservative as those from the West Bank and Gaza. An Israeli family, while adhering to valuing the role of the family, may have transcended some of the traditional expectations for the women. Families from cities are likely to be the least conservative and traditional. When a Palestinian family seeks help, the concern usually involves dealing with children who challenge the authority of parents, or problems arising from the choice of a partner who has not been designated by the parents. The following case was chosen because it represents what seems to be uniquely Palestinian and a central issue in treating Palestinians.

Fadi is a 26-year-old single male. He and what was left of his family had immigrated to the United States after having lost most of his family in the Sabra and Shatila massacre. He had escaped death because he happened to have spent the night in the city with an extended family member and was not home when the massacre occurred in the early morning hours. Upon arrival at the camp, when he and others were allowed to enter it, he discovered that his family of seven siblings and his mother had been killed during the massacre. An 11-year-old brother had survived. Dr. Swee Ang (1989), a volunteer surgeon in Beirut at that time, described seeing dead bodies everywhere and whole families that had been shot together. Fadi was lucky that one family member had survived by pretending to be dead, remaining motionless under the corpses of the other siblings and his mother. Fadi had not only lost his mother and most of the family, but now he had to be a parent to his younger sibling. Fadi did not express his grief for several years. Instead, he had become numb, which is one the mechanisms Palestinians tend to use to overcome trauma. He had already been traumatized as a teenager when he lost his father in the Tal Al-Zaatar massacre. In fact, he had to do what was expected of him as a "brave" Palestinian, fighting for his cause, becoming the symbolic "victim" for many journalists, Arab political activists, and Jewish Palestinian sympathizers, leaving very little room for the feelings associated with his personal loss to be expressed in any form.

I became familiar with Fadi as a therapist because of his concerns about his younger brother (age 16). Fadi and his brother came to my attention when I volunteered to provide mental health services at a community service organization for Palestinian Americans. Prior to meeting me, he had met a number of physicians and nurses, but none in the mental health field. Fadi was mainly concerned because his brother was becoming more withdrawn, having nightmares, and was not willing to discuss his feelings with him. The younger brother was subsequently referred to a psychiatrist, whereas Fadi remained hesitant to pursue treatment. Fadi finally came to terms with his own need to seek therapy when he began thinking of marriage. Fadi wanted to find a partner in the traditional way, that is, by having his parents ask for the hand of the bride-to-be from the prospective parents-in-law. However, he had a dilemma, because he had no adult family members to accompany him to ask for the hand of the Palestinian girl he wanted to marry. Fadi grew up in two refugee camps, his family, prior to leaving Palestine, was from a rural area, and he was conservative and traditional. He adhered to his traditional customs, valuing family ties, fulfilling his responsibilities, and respecting his elders. Fadi had succeeded in creating a family with his brother, which was accepted by the community. As noted earlier, however, he faced a dilemma when he decided to marry. In therapy, he had two goals in mind: One was to deal with his trauma, and the second was to find a surrogate mother. To facilitate treatment, I accepted the role of surrogate mother. Issues of marriage were discussed within the context of traumatization, and I made arrangements to accompany Fadi on a visit to the prospective bride's family. He was also advised to choose a respected male member of the community to go with us, in keeping with the traditional expectations.

Subsequent to the visit, Fadi and his brother were seen for several sessions to discuss their losses, the traumatic events of the camp massacre, and the realities of their new home. Fadi eventually broke his engagement with the young lady he proposed to, most probably because of his anxiety about its possible impact on his brother. His decision may have also been connected to the enormities of his losses, which may have made the choice of a partner an emotionally challenging task. Fadi, although not directly impacted by the Sabra and Shatila massacre, was more emotionally scarred and subsequently more vulnerable than his brother, because of his own early losses and destabilization by moves (i.e., having to move from one country to another or the instability of caretakers). The difficulty was compounded by his survival guilt. It is interesting that Fadi was more successful in helping his brother to heal his wounds than in helping himself. Fadi may have failed in his quest to complete his life with a partner, but succeeded in his role as substitute father for his younger sole-surviving brother. The brother was sent to Lebanon to visit their extended family more than once and eventually married someone he met there. Fadi remained single and had a very successful political career.

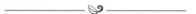

Draguns's (1996) synopsis of a therapeutic model based on the values of collective communities, such as those of Palestinians, was used as a guideline in dealing with Fadi and his brother.

- Within collectivist expectations, Fadi's suffering was alleviated by the therapist's willingness to act as a surrogate mother, thus providing the nurturance he so needed.
- The therapist enhanced the therapeutic process by relating as a "mother" figure and thus removing the distance created by the traditional therapist–patient role.
- Uncertainties were reduced by providing a great deal of didactic information about trauma, its outcome, and methods for alleviating its consequences.
- The therapeutic alliance was strengthened by the therapist's understanding the political background, showing empathy about Fadi's ambivalence toward the United States, and toward his feelings about Israel.

CONCLUSION

In addition to what a therapist needs to work effectively with most clients, in working with Palestinian American families, there is a special burden imposed by virtue of Palestinians' unique relationship with Israelis and, at times, with Jews. In contrast to other Arab Americans, it is the Palestinian American who is most impacted by the present conflict between Israelis and Palestinians. This could be of sufficient significance to affect a decision regarding the appropriateness of the evaluation and/or treatment of Palestinian Americans by therapists who may have strong emotional attachments to one or the other side of this complex conflict between the two peoples. Unlike other Arab immigrants, who may be able to access assistance from their country of origin (such as Saudi Arabia), this population has no one to turn to except each other or a therapist. Thus, the therapist has an especially responsible role to play with this particular population.

REFERENCES

Abudabbeh, N. (2002). *Trauma, poverty and marginalization in Algeria: A psychological perspective.* Paper presented at the Fullbright Conference, Istanbul, Turkey.

Ang, S. C. (1989). *From Beirut to Jerusalem: A woman surgeon with the Palestinians.* London: Grafton Books.

Awwad, E. (1989). *Violence-related posttraumatic stress disorder among Palestinian adolescents.* Paper presented at the Naim Foundation Conference, Washington, DC.

Baker, A. M. (1990). The psychological impact of the intifada on Palestinian children in the occupied West Bank and Gaza: An exploratory study. *American Journal of Orthopsychiatry, 60,* 495–505.

Baker, A. M. (1991). Psychological response of Palestinian children to environmental stress associated with military occupation. *Journal of Refugee Studies, 4,* 237–247.

Cainkar, L. (1988). *Palestinian women in the United States: Coping with tradition, change and alienation.* Unpublished doctoral dissertation, University of Chicago.

Christison, K. (2001). *The wound of dispossession: Telling the Palestinian story.* Santa Fe, NM: Sunlit Hills Press.

De Jong, J. T. V. M., Komproe, J. H., Van Ommeren, M., El Masri, M., Araya, M., Khaled, N., et al. (2001). Lifetime events and posttraumatic stress disorder in four postconflict settings. *Journal of the American Medical Association, 286,* 555–562.

Draguns, J. G. (1996). Ethnocultural considerations in the treatment of PTSD: Therapy and service delivery. In A. J. Marsala, M. J. Friedman, E. T. Geritty, & R. M. Scurfield (Eds.), *Ethnocultural aspects of posttraumatic stress disorder: Issues, research, and clinical applications.* Washington, DC: American Psychological Association.

Dwairy, M. A. (1998). *Cross-cultural counseling: The Arab–Palestnian case.* Binghampton, NY: Haworth Press.

El-Sarraj, E., Punamaki, R-L., Salmi, S., & Summerfield, D. (1996). Experiences of torture and ill-treatment and posttraumatic stress disorder symptoms among Palestinian political prisoners. *Journal of Traumatic Stress, 9,* 595–606.

Farell, K. (1998). *Post-traumatic culture: Injury and interpretation in the nineties.* Baltimore: Johns Hopkins University Press.

Foche', C. (1995). *Against forgetting.* New York: Norton.

Garbarino, J., Kostelney, K., & Dubrow, K. (1991). *No place to be a child.* Toronto: Lexington Books.

Jayussi, K. S. (1992). *Modern Palestinian literature.* New York: Columbia University Press.

Kevorkian, N. S. (1988). *The victimization of Palestinian children in the occupied territories.* Paper presented at the International Victimology Symposium, Tel Aviv, Israel.

Khamis, V. (1990). *Victims of the intifada: The psychological adjustment of the injured.* Paper presented at the Naim Foundation Conference, Washington, DC.

Mahjoub, A., Leyens, J.-P.., & Yzerbyt, V. (1990). *The weapons effect among children living in an armed-conflict environment*. Paper presented at the Naim Foundation Conference, Washington, DC.

Marsala, A. J., Friedman, M. J., Geritty, E. T., & Scurfield, R. M. (1996). *Ethnocultural aspects of post-traumatic stress disorder*. Washington, DC: American Psychological Association.

Masalha, S. (1993). The effect of prewar conditions on the psychological reactions of Palestinian children to the Gulf War. In L. A. Leavitt & N. A. Fox (Eds.), *The psychological effects of war on violence on children*. Hillsdale, NJ: Erlbaum.

Punamaki, R. I. (1988). Historical- political and individualistic determinants of coping modes and fears among Palestinian children. *International Journal of Psychology, 23*, 721–739.

Punamaki, R. I., & Suleiman, R. (1990). Predictors and effectiveness of coping with political violence among Palestinian children. *British Journal of Social Psychology, 29*, 67–77.

Raundalen, M., & Melton, G. B. (1994). Children in war and its aftermath: Mental health issues in the development of international law. *Behavioral Science and Law, 12*(1), 21–34.

Rubenstein, D. (1991). *The people of nowhere: The Palestinian vision of home*. New York: Times Books.

Said, E. (1995). *The politics of dispossession*. New York: Vintage Books.

Seikaly, M. (1999). Attachment and identity: The Palestinian community of Detroit. In M. W. Suleiman (Ed.), *Arabs in America: Building a new future*. Philadelphia: Temple University Press.

Turki, F. (1972). *The disinherited: The journal of a Palestinian exile*. New York: Monthly Review Press.

Turki, F. (1988). *Soul in exile: Lives of a Palestinian revolutionary*. New York: Monthly Review Press.

Volkan, V. (1990). *"Living statues" and political decision making: A study of the orphaned Palestinian children in Tunis*. Paper presented at the Children in War Conference, Hebrew University, Jerusalem.

PART VII

FAMILIES OF
EUROPEAN ORIGIN

CHAPTER 36

Families of European Origin
An Overview

Joe Giordano
Monica McGoldrick

Ethnic identity has always been a central component of American life, although it was buried for 200 years under the idea that America was a "melting pot." This myth was shattered in the 1960s when people of color, who were later joined by White ethnic groups, demanded to be recognized, respected, and recorded in the annals of American history. Their actions ushered in a new concept of America as a pluralistic society. Today, ethnic identity is shifting once again as most White ethnic families enter the fourth and fifth generations of being in America.

Their current salience is not only related to fact that European Americans are a step further on the immigrant-to-assimilation continuum, but is also a result of a dramatic change in America's demographics. Within the next 50 years, White ethnics will be numerically a minority. Ethnic distinctions between European Americans are fading, whereas other ethnic groups are becoming more prominent. One researcher has suggested that a new ethnic group, Euro-Americans, is forming (Alba, 1990, 1995), and Richard Rodriguez (2002), in his book *Brown: The Last Discovery of America*, foresees a "blending," or what he describes as a "browning of America."

We believe that this eventuality is far off, for ethnicity changes only gradually, in many ways much more slowly than we might think. Therapists should be aware that these ethnic differences are often present to some extent in fourth- and fifth-generation European Americans, and influence how they view the world and what they consider "normal" and "abnormal." Ethnocultural factors are often the hidden dimension in family therapy with White ethnics, and exploring them may be a key component of successful treatment.

While we were working on this book, a colleague cynically commented that, surely, we had nothing new to say about Italian or Irish families because "White ethnics today don't have ethnic issues; they're totally American." His comment was surprising, especially because he is Jewish and has an Anglo American wife. He was, however, expressing what many therapists perceive: that ethnicity pertains only to people of color.

There are 53 nationalities among European Americans, of which the largest groups are German Americans (43 million), those of English ancestry, British, Welsh, and Scottish (32 million), and Irish Americans (30.5 million); the smallest group is Cypriot Americans (7,663) (Roberts, 2004). However, these groups are barely mentioned in most discussions of "cultural diversity."

We use "White ethnic" interchangeably with "European American" to refer to non-Hispanic White families of European heritage. These terms, first used to describe primarily southern and eastern European immigrants, rather than Americans of British or German ancestry, are somewhat ambiguous.

According to the 2000 census, Whites make up 75.1% (211.4 million) of the total population (281.4 million). Whereas the total American population has grown by 33 million from 1990, there has been a sharp decline in the number of people who claim to be of German, Irish, English, or other European ancestry—some 38.8 million, an 18.6% drop since the 1990 census. One of the major reasons is that millions of aged White ethnics died in the 1990s (Davis, 2003).

Moreover, an increasing number of White ethnics who have married outside their own group now think of themselves simply as "Americans" and often are unaware of, and uninterested in, their mixed European heritage. In addition, most families from European American groups have been in the United States for three generations or more, so that the immigrant generation's struggle against discrimination and for a satisfactory education, occupation, and residence, has largely faded, as has its members' need to identity themselves ethnically.

Individuals with common national, racial, and religious origins, or even those who speak the same language, may ignore or reject an ethnic identification. Consider, for example, two famous Hollywood film directors: Francis Ford Coppola (*The Godfather, Apocalypse Now, The Conversation*) and Frank Capra (*It's a Wonderful Life, Mr. Smith Goes to Washington, It Happened One Night*). Both are Italian American, but one embraces his ethnic identity and the other rejects it. Concerning Coppola, one biographer notes:

> Nothing has influenced Coppola's life and work so dramatically as his Italian blood. "In our family," recalls his brother August, "there was great passion, creativity, belief in opera." Francis has . . . [this] unshakable faith in the sovereignty of the family. His wife and, when they were young, his children have accompanied him, on location in the jungle and to festivals in places as far-flung as Moscow and Santa Fe. "We travel together like a circus family," says his wife, Eleanor, "with Francis on the tightrope and the rest of us holding the ropes." Two of those children, Gian-Carlo and Sofia Carmina, were christened with Italian names. (Cowie, 1990 p. 8)

Joseph McBride (1992) describes in his biography of Frank Capra the director's much-publicized pilgrimage to Bisacquion, Sicily, the town in which he was born. After returning to the United States, Capra was asked what he felt on his visit to the place of his birth.

> "I felt nothing," he said. "Who the hell cares where you were born? That town meant nothing to me. You know that colored guy, that Roots thing? He's full of shit. I hate the word 'roots.' People are so proud of their roots it's sickening." (p. 11)

Capra changed his name from Francesco to Frank and later added the middle name "Russell," because he felt it evoked the image of a prominent WASP. When asked about his new name, Capra replied, "It didn't smell of the ghetto" (McBride, 1992, p. 45). His contempt for his origins had as much to do with Capra's unhappy childhood and the rejection of his immigrant family as it did with his total identification as an American and belief in the American Dream.

Because "ethnics" are thought to be groups other than "regular" (i.e., White) Americans, all European groups can, to some extent, "pass" for "regular." Therefore, they may choose not to identify themselves ethnically, because this may seem to lower their status. Such was the case with Frank Capra.

Shared ethnic heritage hardly produces homogeneity of thought, emotions, or group loyalty. Individuals may embrace, change, or reject aspects of their ethnicity, as well as aspects of their broader American identity. Some social scientists conclude that ethnicity among European Americans barely exists and has more of a symbolic meaning than a real significance for most Americans (Alba, 1995, 2004).

Others see the increase in intermarriage, and the intermingling among ethnic and racial groups, as creating a new fusion of peoples and cultures (G. Rodriquez, 2003; R. Rodriquez, 2002; Root, 2001). This book takes a different position: that ethnicity will continue to be a major distinguishing characteristic, even for European Americans, for a long time to come.

What many social scientists and others have failed to notice is that the course of assimilation and acculturation is a very slow and uneven process; with certain families, it may take generations. More important, in periods of stress or personal crisis individuals often return to familiar sources of comfort and help, which may differ from the dominant society's norms. These include turning to their nuclear or extended family, their religion, the ethnic enclaves or community resources they grew up in, cultural rituals and behaviors, or the value and belief systems in which they were raised.

Certain deeply imbedded features of ethnic and religious identity may persist even after experience indicates that they are dysfunctional, such as hyperindividualism or family enmeshment. And aspects of ethnicity that were shed or changed—names, belief systems, language, food rituals, and family customs—may reappear later in life or in the next generation. Examples of this phenomenon are the increasing number of third-generation Jewish Americans who have become Orthodox, the rise of Protestant fundamentalism, and the increased expression of ethnicity on college campuses, in the marketplace, and in the arts. The conscious and unconscious aspects of ethnicity are what make this subject so complex, yet elusive, in research studies.

An interesting example is the family of John Kerry, whose grandfather, Fritz Kohn, changed his name to Fred Kerry in 1901, at which time he and the rest of his family became Catholic. Twenty years later, Fred Kerry committed suicide. His son, John Kerry's father, was only 6 at the time (Kranish, Mooney, & Easton, 2004).

In 1983, two generations later, Cameron Kerry, John's younger brother, married an Orthodox woman and converted to Judaism. Two decades after that, the *Boston Globe*, doing research on the Kerry family because John was running for president, discovered the family's Jewish heritage. For the first time, Cameron became aware that perhaps, in his own conversion, he had been responding to a hidden family legacy.

John Kerry was raised Catholic, but knew a great deal about his family's WASP heritage. He is George Bush's distant cousin through seven different Anglo ancestor connections. The name "Kerry" had apparently been chosen from a map that included that county in Ireland, to which the family had no connection whatsoever. Thus, people often lose touch with their ethnicity and end up with a distorted sense, or none at all, of who they really are.

There is great clinical importance in understanding and addressing ethnic differences, even among European groups. Although therapists generally ignore these differences, except as they pertain to "minority" groups, even physically similar groups differ in many ways, compounded, of course, by class and gender differences, which leads to many misunderstandings. For example, Anglo and Irish Americans, although quite similar in appearance, differ profoundly in common personality traits. Anglos generally prefer restraint, decorum, logic, and stoicism; the Irish are drawn to fantasy and dreams and are less interested in logic and structure.

For example, consider Katherine Hepburn and Spencer Tracy (McGoldrick, 1995). Dorothy Parker once said of Hepburn, a product of a stoic Protestant family of Scottish and English ancestry, that "she runs the gamut of emotions from A to B!" (cited in Kanin, 1988, p. 17). Tracy, however, would go in roller-coaster fashion from violent drunken rages to merry times to sullen withdrawal. While she was careful, thorough, methodical, and analytical, he was an instinctive, intuitive player, who thought an actor went stale by overrehearsing and preferred to trust his intuition.

"With Spencer it was virtually impossible to know when he was pretending and when he was on the level" (Kanin, 1988, p. 12). Hepburn's values of propriety, cleanliness (she took seven or eight showers a day), frugality, hard work, and rugged individualism were legendary. A close friend described her thus: "When you enter her world you are expected to observe its strictness and you do [so[without question. . . . You arrive on time and leave as early as possible . . . you agree with every one of her many opinions; . . . you do not get drunk no matter how much you drink; you do not complain (you may, however, rail); you say nothing that may not be repeated; you refrain from lies, dissemblance and exaggerations; you omit discussion of your physical state, symptoms, ailments" (pp. 12–13). Tracy, in contrast, saw fun in everything, except his religion. A full-scale hell-raiser from his youth, he was full of highs and lows. After announcing to his astonished family that he wanted to become a priest, he soon changed his mind and went into the military instead.

Tracy was a loner who flitted in and out of relationships, could shift from charming merriment to week-long alcoholic binges, becoming cantankerous while remaining unshaven and not changing his smelly clothes for weeks, or holing up in the dark in a heavy overcoat he wore even in summer. Always a fighter and a rebel, he felt most comfortable in working-class contexts, dropping out of many schools even before he dropped out of college.

EUROPEAN AMERICANS IN HISTORICAL AND CULTURAL CONTEXT

A Nation of Immigrants

From the beginnings of colonization, this country has been ethnically diverse, although we have tended to view Americans as being of European ancestry. Historian Ronald Tataki (2002) noted, "In the creation of our national identity, 'American' has been defined as 'white' " (p. 2). Indeed, the immigration law of 1790 declared that only European American immigrants could become U.S. citizens.

Although the English made up 61% of the Thirteen Colonies' 3 million White inhabitants, there were many non-English immigrants and settlements. But the colonial English shaped the basic American social and political institutions, so that Anglo culture became the ideal by which all subsequent ethnic groups were judged. Acculturation meant acquiring Anglo Protestant lifestyles, values, and language (Banks, 1991, p. 246).

But from 1880 to 1921 (when the first immigrant quotas for Europeans were adopted), millions of individuals from southern, central, and eastern Europe streamed to these shores. A great debate ensued over immigration, driven by the fear that the Anglo Saxon Germanic gene pool would be contaminated with the blood of ethnic groups from eastern and southern Europe, who were considered intellectually, morally and physically inferior. At one time or another, Poles, Romanians, Italians, Jews, Slovaks, Russians, Albanians, Armenians, Rumanians, Spaniards, and Portuguese were suspected of being genetically inferior (Cose, 2000, p. 64). Although these immigrants were never denied citizenship, the laws at the time favored those immigrants of a "finer" racial stock. Subsequently, the newcomers were welcomed and in essence made White (p. 64).

They tended to settle in ethnic communities—Little Italys, Polonias, Greektowns, and Jewish "ghettos"—and transformed America from an overwhelmingly Protestant country to one with millions of Catholic, Jewish, and Eastern Orthodox citizens (Handlin, 1951). The immigrants helped build America's roads, railroads, bridges, and mines. Many of their children organized, and helped to put on a firm foundation, labor unions to fight the oppressive conditions their parents had endured.

Some European American groups adjusted easily to the new culture. Although the Germans did not speak English and were greeted with suspicion and hostility by Anglo Americans when they first arrived in the early 1700s, they adapted with little difficulty. In contrast, the adjustment of Irish immigrants was turbulent, even though almost all Irish spoke English and fit in temperamentally with many aspects of Anglo American culture. Nevertheless, Anglo Americans were threatened by the perceived clannishness of the Irish, their orientation to political power, and their fierce devotion to the Catholic Church (Brookheiser, 1991; Perlmutter, 1992; Takaki, 2002).

The Italians' intense loyalty to each other violated the norms of the dominant culture. They responded to the hostile dominant culture as they had coped with outsiders for centuries, by relying only on family and friends. Unlike the Irish, the Italians largely did not organize political subgroups and therefore were not perceived as a threat to Anglo Americans, except in terms of crime.

In regard to Jews, the seeds of anti-Semitism can be traced to the very beginning of Christianity. Christians tended to regard Jews as an alien people who, because of their repudiation of Christ and the church, were condemned to perpetual migration. As a consequence, Jews were increasingly forced to the margins of European society. The practice of segregating the Jewish populations of towns and cities into ghettos in much of Europe dates from the 16th century and lasted until the early 20th century.

When Jews first arrived in the United States, they were again faced with anti-Semitism, this time by other European immigrants as well as the Anglo establishment. Yet, in America, Jews organized against anti-Semitism, and generally worked to influence the political process, as they never had in Europe. It took until 1965, two decades after the Holocaust, for the Roman Catholic Church to finally renounce and revamp its teaching regarding Jews and Judaism.

Because of constitutional protections against religious discrimination in America, there is significant discontinuity between the American Jewish and the European Jewish experiences. Even so, some American Jews had a powerful wish to escape their heritage and to "pass" for Anglo Americans (Gilman, 1986; Klein, 1980). Film director Steven Spielberg (1993) has described his growing up in a non-Jewish town:

> I just wanted to assimilate. I wanted to be like everyone else. . . . Being Jewish really made me stand out. I remember taping my nose so it would turn up. My grandfather would call me by my Hebrew name, Schmuel . . . and I wouldn't answer . . . because I was embarrassed. [When] I encountered anti-Semitism . . . I . . . realized there was a world out there in which people didn't like me. I didn't fight back. And that is one of the things I am most ashamed of. I hid it from my parents as long as I could. It has stuck with me for years. It still hurts. I began to question my Judaism. I felt a sense of shame.

After living in the United States for two or more generations, the immigrants from eastern and southern Europe thought of themselves as Americans. But the "native" Anglo Americans viewed them as unassimilatable and judged them intellectually and culturally inferior (Banks, 1991; Perlmutter, 1992; Thernstrom, Orlov, & Handlin, 1980). Objects of ridicule, prejudice, and discrimination, they were blamed for a vast array of contemporary economic and urban problems, as well as for political corruption—perspectives not unlike the current attitudes toward Haitian, Hispanic, Asian, and Arab immigrants.

Such sentiments helped to create the extreme nationalism and ethnocentrism that characterized the 1920s "nativist," movements, which favored restricting immigration and protecting the interests of the native-born (Banks, 1991; Thernstrom et al., 1980). The permanent adoption of immigration quotas in 1924, as well as the Depression (1929–1939), contributed to a sharp drop in immigration throughout the 1930s and 1940s. During World War II and the Holocaust, hundreds of thousands of Jews and other victims of Nazism were unable to obtain immigration visas because quotas favored western and northern Europeans (Takaki, 2002).

A major change in national policy took place with the enactment of the Immigration Act of 1965, which repealed national-origin quotas and shifted the flow of immigration from Europe to other parts of the globe, particularly the developing nations. Technical skills and kinship, rather than country of origin, became the major criteria for obtaining visas.

By the second and third generations, most European American immigrant families had done well. Their overall history has been marked by upward mobility, with some striking success stories, although a significant minority remain in low-status jobs in the middle-middle, lower-middle, or near-poor classes.

Since the 1980s, only 10% of new immigrants have come from Europe, as compared with 90% at the earlier peak (Smelser, Wilson, & Mitchell, 2001, p. 205). However, in contrast to the often poor, uneducated eastern and southern Europeans who came in 1880–1924, most post-1945 European Americans are well-educated, skilled professionals: thus, they have not experienced the discrimination that troubled earlier immigrants. Consequently, the earlier immigrants' descendents and the new arrivals from Europe are quite heterogeneous, even when they claim the same country of origin.

However, since the September 11, 2001, attacks on the United States, restrictive immigration practices have resulted in a huge number of visitors staying away from the United States. The effects of the more restrictive policies on the flow of new immigrants is yet to be determined.

From the Melting Pot to the New Pluralism

In 1963, Nathan Glazer and Daniel Patrick Moynihan's seminal book, *Beyond the Melting Pot*, questioned the notion that immigrants and their descendents were fully assimilating into American society. They argued that the values, beliefs, and behaviors that immigrants brought with them from abroad were still very much part of how they lived and worked in America .

For some European Americans, the struggles of people of color for equal rights during the 1960s opened hidden scars and awakened repressed anger about the discrimination they had suffered, and recalled their own groups' alienation from mainstream America. The economic recessions and social and political changes at the time resulted in millions of working-class, second- and third-generation European Americans becoming bitter and discontented with the direction of American society (Levine & Herman, 1972; Rostow, 1971; Whiting, 1972).

Also fueling their discontent was the fact that African Americans and other minorities were receiving economic and social benefits through government-sponsored programs. From the Euro-Americans' perspective, their families had come to America poor and often uneducated, yet they were able to lift themselves from poverty into the mainstream through self-help and education, without welfare and affirmative action. So they asked, "Why can't the Blacks"?

Most White ethnics were unaware of the effects of 350 years of slavery on African Americans and their own participation in perpetuating institutional racism. They were even less conscious of how they had benefited from White privilege, which had been built into every institution in the United States.

In fact, until the 1970s or later, Native Americans, African Africans, and other racial minorities were largely written out of the history of this country. Howard Zinn (1980, 2003), author of the classic history text *A People's History of the United States*, which tells history through the lenses of those who have been oppressed by the dominant groups in American society, writes of his own lack of awareness of race:

> It did not occur to me, when I first began to immerse myself in history, how badly twisted was the teaching and writing of history by its submersion of nonwhite people. Yes, Indians were there and then gone. Black people were visible when slaves, then free and invisible. It was a white man's history. From first grade to graduate school, I was given no inkling that the landing of Christopher Columbus in the New World initiated a genocide, in which the indigenous population of Hispaniola was annihilated. Or that this was the first stage of what was presented as a benign expansion of the new nation (Louisiana "Purchase," Florida "Purchase," Mexican "Cession"), but which involved the violent expulsion of Indians, accompanied by unspeakable atrocities, from every square mile of the continent, until there was nothing to do with them but herd them into reservations. (p. 683)

It was then, during the 1970s, that White ethnic intellectuals began to express pride in their roots, as well as anger for the generations of denial and repression of their ethnic identities. White ethnic writers—such as Richard Gambino (Italian), Paul Cowan and Irving Howe (Jewish), Rev. Andrew Greeley and Jimmy Breslin (Irish), and Michael Arlen (Armenian)—began to write about the price of "Americanization." One of the most eloquent was Slovak American Michael Novak (1971):

My grandparents, I am sure, never guessed what it would cost them and their children to become "Americanized." . . . I am born of . . . those Poles, Italians, Greeks and Slavs, non-English-speaking immigrants, numbered so heavily among the workingmen of this nation. Not particularly liberal, or radical, born into a history not white Anglo-Saxon and not Jewish . . . born outside what in America is considered the intellectual mainstream. And thus privy to neither power nor status, nor intellectual voice. (p. 53)

Novak and others, such as Irving Levine, Barbara Mikulski (now a U.S. Senator), the Rev. Andrew Greeley, and the Rev. Gino Baroni, became the intellectual and organizing core of the "new ethnicity." These European American intellectuals believed that there was a possibility of bridging the gap between people of color who were demanding social justice, and White working-class ethnics who were angry for being "left outside" of mainstream America. They helped mobilize a coalition of European American groups that joined with minority groups to advance knowledge about the role of ethnic and racial identity in shaping Americans' values, behavior, family patterns, and lifestyles.

The proponents of the new ethnicity believed that it was important for America to equally promote diversity and foster a common culture. Today their work is carried on by countless young writers, artists, and filmmakers who no longer feel shackled by a dominant culture sitting in judgment. Rather, they feel free to search out and express their familial and ancestral stories.

The "new ethnicity" movement made a significant contribution in expanding the definition of American pluralism to include all ethnic and racial groups. However, the movement began to fade in the late 1980s for two reasons: First, as many European Americans began to feel less alienated from mainstream society, their advocacy of pluralism and coalition building with non-White minorities began to diminish. Second, the movement's promotion of tolerance and equality as American ideals came at a time when increasing racial polarization between Black and White ethnic Americans was rendering these goals ever more unpopular.

During the 1990s the United States experienced the largest influx of new immigrants since the great waves from Europe in the early part of the 20th century. The difference, however, was that these new immigrants were from Asia, Latin America, Africa, and the former Soviet Union. As in the early waves of immigration, there was a "backlash" against the new arrivals. They were charged with being a threat by isolating themselves in their own communities; refusing to learn the language, and taking jobs from "Americans." These feelings were compounded by xenophobia, nativism, and racism. Organizations were formed to call for more restrictive legislation to halt the tide of immigration.

The decade also witnessed greater political influence by right-wing religious groups, increased ethnic and racial tensions, including Black–Jewish and Black–Korean conflicts (Berman, 1994), the expansion of the African American middle class, and a growing White ethnic and neoconservative assault against bilingualism, affirmative action, social welfare, and multiculturalism (Bernstein, 1995; Bloom, 1987; Brimelow, 1995; Schlesinger, 1998).

In 2000, with the election of President George W. Bush and a Republican Congress, programs such as affirmative action were under attack, withering away the hard-won gains of the civil rights movement. Pluralism and multiculturalism also came under assault by the supporters of identity politics on the Left and by neoconservatives and nativists on the Right.

THERAPY ISSUES

Race

Race and racism have played a long, if hidden, role in European history. For centuries Europe's colonization of Africa, Asia, and the Americas meant that the continent was supported by the labor of people of color.

Racism, anti-Semitism, and other prejudices have deeply characterized European countries for many centuries. Racism against the Moors, who were Africans and had become Muslims after the Ottoman Empire, and anti-Semitism coalesced in Europe in the 13th and 14th centuries. Following the Crusades, Europeans continued to join against Muslims and Jews, who were demonized in a war that became a war against all forms of cultural and religious dissent (Carroll, 2004). The Crusades were followed by the Inquisition in Europe, which expanded the attitude of demonizing all who were considered "other." And by the 18th century, the concept of "race" and the justification for racism had developed.

Yet Europeans fleeing religious persecution also envisioned a new world where all individuals would be legally guaranteed freedom and liberty. Millions of immigrants and refugees from around the world have come to the United States seeking such a society.

However, during the 18th century, Europeans and Americans were in serious need of justification for a categorization of races that would allow Whites to treat people of color as less than human. This was especially important during the Enlightenment, with its focus on the "inalienable" rights of human beings. Having a hierarchy of races helped rationalize slavery and so justified slave-owners' profits.

Racism thus became built into the very system of government European Americans put in place in the United States in the late 1700s. As Jim Hitchcock (2001) puts it, the Founding Fathers established the platform on which White American culture stands today:

- A view of human rights as universal and God-given
- Valuing the rights of the individual over those of the state
- The assimilation of White people to the culture
- The less-than-fully-human status often given to people of color

Consider but one example: The Founding Fathers, in the first session of Congress, in 1790, passed a law, which lasted until 1952, saying that only "White persons" could become naturalized citizens of the United States. Those who received this privilege had to meet both legal and cultural requirements. It was not an easy process, yet it was possible, and many Whites passed the test; but immigrants from racial minorities never could.

Even the Irish, who in their own country were treated as an inferior race, although they initially sided with libertarian ideas in the United States, soon took advantage of their superior racial status in this country and participated in promoting the racial divide between Whites and people of color in the 19th century (Ignatiev, 1995).

"Race," says writer Toni Morrison (2003), has functioned as a "metaphor" necessary to the "construction of Americaness"; in the creation of our national identity, "American" has been defined as "White" (Takaki, 2002). European Americans in this country became "Americans" and learned "American" values of freedom, democracy, the rights of the individual, and a society based on the common man. Nothing in this self-definition says anything about whiteness. By naming themselves as only "American," European immigrants and their descendents could avoid thinking of themselves as White, for America itself was defined by its whiteness (Hitchcock, 2002).

The American-as-White image is deeply embedded in our society, so much so that it is difficult to determine what is really American in terms of the cultural elements that apply to all citizens. This confusion of imagery, White as American and American as White, permeates our education system. Only since the 1970s have educational textbooks and the mass media begun to recognize the presence and accomplishments of other racial and ethnic groups in the American mix. This process, under the banner of multiculturalism, is controversial and only partly successful. Ask most people to imagine a "typical" American, and they will see the image of a White person (Hitchcock, 2002, pp. 105–106).

To say that White culture is the dominant subculture in the United States is not an indictment of individual White people. It is to say that White culture holds greater power to control resources, set rules, and influence events in comparison to other subcultures.

David Roediger (1999) confirms a benefit or a "wage" for simply being White in the United States, regardless of class or consciousness. Manning Marable (2002) spells out the "benefits" of whiteness in his book, *The Great Wells of Democracy*:

> Whites . . . have an important material asset that allows them to escape the greatest liabilities and disadvantages of poverty—their whiteness. White Americans who are homeless, unemployed and/or uneducated for the most part still believe in the great American master narrative of opportunity and upward mobility. If they scrape together enough money to buy a new suit, they will find it relatively easy to obtain employment, albeit at subsistence wages. They know with the same set of skills and level of educational attainment as the Black householders across the street, they stand a superior chance of being hired. Whiteness creates a comfortable social and psychological safety net for the white poor. Every day may not be a lucky day, but nobody has to sing the blues for long. (p. 219)

Peggy McIntosh (1998) has described very impressively the correspondences between male privilege and White privilege, laying out the specifics of that "invisible knapsack of privilege" that those of us who are White are born with, whether we realize it or not:

- I can, if I wish, arrange to be in the company of people of my race most of the time.
- If I should need to move, I can be pretty sure of renting or purchasing housing in an area which I can afford and in which I would want to live.
- I can be reasonably sure that my neighbors in such a location will be neutral or pleasant to me.
- I can go shopping alone most of the time, fairly well assured that I will not be followed or harassed by store detectives.
- When I am told about our national heritage or about "civilization," I am shown that people of my color made it what it is.
- I can be sure that my children will be given curricular materials that testify to the existence of their race. (p. 73)

Clinicians often ask: What clinical difference does it make to know about the "culture" of whiteness? How might it influence our work in the therapy room? The answer is:

Very directly. It is similar to our understanding of how male privilege influences couple and intergenerational relationships in families. Just as male privilege tends to make men feel, even without realizing it, that they are right, know the truth, and that their ideas and feelings deserve primary attention, White privilege operates in similar ways to make those who have it unwittingly assume dominance in the interpersonal space.

People tend to think of racism as a problem of people of color, but what about the psychological and spiritual and financial costs of racism and White privilege for Americans of European descent? Of course, it leads to our missing out on the contributions that non-Whites could make to our world, because they are disqualified before they start. And what about our own false sense of superiority and belief that we should be in authority and control? We lose out in many relationships and in our understanding of our world and our interactions because of this ideology. Kivel (2002) points out:

> Racism distorts our sense of danger and safety. We are taught to live in fear of people of color. We are exploited economically by the upper class and unable to fight or even see this exploitation because we are taught to scapegoat people of color. On a more personal level, many of us are brutalized by family violence and sexual assault, unable to resist effectively because we have been taught that people of color are the real danger, never the white men we live with. (p. 46)

Racism today is more subtle and covert, but the politics of race continue to be complex and divisive. The invisible knapsack of privilege (McIntosh, 1998) of all White Americans, achieved just by the color of their skin, is something that most White ethnics do not acknowledge. And the level of segregation in the United States between European Americans and people of color, especially African Americans, remains profound, a problem in our society that most Whites do not notice.

A growing effort to research and discuss whiteness (Bonilla-Silva, 2001; Bowser & Hunt, 1996; Frankenberg, 1993; Hitchcock, 2002; Katz, 1978; Kivel, 2002; Lazarre, 1996; Lipsitz, 1998; Malcomson, 2000; McIntosh, 1998; Roediger, 1999; Rothenberg, 2002) attempts to trace the economic and political history behind the invention of "whiteness," to attack the privileges given to "Whites," and to analyze the cultural practices (in politics, economics, art, music, literature, and the media) that create and perpetuate the privileges of "whiteness." We must attempt to think critically about how white skin preference has operated systematically, structurally, and sometimes unconsciously as a dominant force in American—and, indeed, in global—societ and culture.

What are its implications for therapists? In the clinical literature, racial issues are underrepresented. Many therapists deny or are unaware of this problem until they face a racial issue in either their professional or private lives (Carter, 1995; McGoldrick, 1999; Pinderhughes, 1989).

White therapists and those of color are also prone to ignore the ethnic differences between White clients and too often treat race and ethnicity as a "special issue," rather than as basic to personal and social identity.

Religion

Throughout history, millions of people have died in the name of ethnicity. Unfortunately, the same can be said of religion.

More than a thousand years ago, Pope Urban II zealously called for a "War of the Cross," a holy war against Muslims, who were seen as the infidel people who had taken the Holy Land hundreds of years before. "The Holy Land must be redeemed!" became the rallying cry. Within months, 100,000 people had "taken the cross" to reclaim the Holy Land in the name of Jesus.

Wherever the Crusaders went, death and destruction occurred, killing thousands of Jews in Europe on their way to the Holy Land. For their part, the unsuspecting Muslims were no match for the fanatical Christian warriors, who killed not only fighting men, but also women and children. In Jerusalem they savagely slaughtered Muslims and Jews alike—practially the whole city. Carroll (2004) makes the point that those religious invasions and wars of long ago established a cohesive Western identity precisely in opposition to Islam, an adversity that survives to this day.

In the late 1700s, America's religious groups provided a similar call for a holy war to eradicate the Native Americans in the West. The Rev. Timothy Wright, who served as pastor to Congress, wrote that under the Indians, "Satan ruled unchallenged in America" until "our chosen race eternal [was] sent" (Martinez, 2002, p. 83). The winning of the West was seen as a moral duty, even though—or perhaps especially because—it involved the slaughtering of Indians, as the Crusaders did to Muslims, Jews, and others in 1097 .

Strangely, the Christian call was again heard in 2001. The Rev. Franklin Graham, who gave the invocation at President Bush's inauguration and is the son of the Rev. Billy Graham, declared shortly after September 11, 2001:

> The God of Islam is not the same God. He is not the son of God of the Christian or Judeo-Christian faith. It's a different God, and I believe it is a very evil and wicked religion. It wasn't the Methodists flying into those buildings, it wasn't Lutherans. It was an attack on this country by people of the Islamic faith. (Berkowitz, 2003)

Carroll (2004) writes that a few days after the assault, President Bush,

> . . . speaking spontaneously, without the aid of advisors or speechwriters, put a new word on the American purpose that both shaped it and gave it meaning. "This crusade," he said, "[is] a war on terrorism."

In America, despite the fact that separation of church and state is one of our most cherished core beliefs and a bedrock of our Constitution, our country has always had a quasi-religious understanding of itself as a model society blessed by God. For example, consider how many presidential addresses to the nation end with the words, "God bless you, and God bless America."

From a psychological perspective, religion provides a deep sense of community and a means of coping with stress or powerlessness, as well as contributing to spiritual fulfillment and emotional support. Froma Walsh (1999) states:

> We [therapists] can help individuals and their families alter constraining beliefs, which perpetuate problems and limit options, and encourage facilitative beliefs, which increase options for problem solving, healing and growth. (p. 64)

Yet the crisis in the Catholic Church over the scandal of sexual abuse of children and teenagers by clergymen has shaken the foundations of its members' faith (Steinfels, 2003). Those who are devout find themselves in denial or so angry that they have either withdrawn from active practice or have chosen to leave the Church. Journalist Jimmy Breslin (2004), an Irish Catholic, raises a question many Catholics will be struggling with for some time: "Do I keep on in a church that I mistrust or remain outside and follow a religion I love?" (p. 2).

In 2003 a similar rupture occurred in the Episcopal church between its members and its leadership over the appointment of Rev. Gene Robinson, the church's first openly gay bishop. The denomination had been debating homosexuality for years, but the Robinson's consecration sparked a crisis in the denomination, and in the global Anglican Communion to which Episcopalians belong.

One of the major barriers against homosexuals achieving greater civil rights is that almost all of America's religious groups have taken a strong position in banning gay marriages. Fifty-three percent of Americans see marriage as a religious matter; of that group 71% oppose gay nuptials. Fifty-five percent in a nationwide poll favored a constitutional amendment that would allow marriage only between a man and a woman (Seelye & Elder, 2003 p. 1).

However, in spite of the "backlash" against gay marriages, attitudes toward gays have changed significantly. The survey indicated that the greatest acceptance of gays was among people knowing someone who was gay (Zernike, 2003, p. 16).

Ethnicity often has a religious character, and religious life may be largely influenced by ethnic customs and rituals (Greeley, 1974; Thernstrom, 1980). In America, such groups as Irish Catholics, French Canadians (Catholics), Armenians, the Greek Orthodox, Finnish Lutherans, and Scottish Presbyterians are among the European groups in which ethnicity and religion are inextricably linked (Gordon, 1964; Greeley, 1969, 1974; Themstrom et al., 1980). Yet there is great ethnic diversity within each faith community. For example, Danes, Finns, Germans, Norwegians, and Swedes coexist within Lutheranism.

Religion intersects with ethnicity in striking ways. For example, the values, attitudes, and behaviors expressed by Irish Americans and Italian Americans in the practice of their Catholicism are quite varied. While both groups are deeply spiritual, their relationship with the Catholic Church is different as a result of their histories in Ireland and Italy. While both cultures respectively have experienced extreme poverty and oppression, each had different experiences with the Church.

For the Irish, there was a higher level of trust and a greater obedience to church practices and authority. For Italian society, which was permeated by widespread distrust and suspicion, the only institution they relied on was the family. They often saw the Church as part of the problem. In America, these attitudes, while undergoing change, are still present in the third and fourth generations. It is not unusual today to find Irish Americans still having a strong adherence to Church authority and rules while Italian Americans tend to take a more flexible and celebratory approach to their religion.

Given Americans' strong spiritual beliefs and their religious institutions' social service networks, it is surprising that many therapists treat faith as a private affair that has little or no impact on treatment.

Class

In America we tend to believe that class differences do not exist; they are not part of our everyday public discourse, as they are in most parts of the world. Deep in our nation's psyche is belief that everyone can "make it" if he or she works hard, sacrifices, and perseveres. Rarely in our public discourse do we talk about the differences or the relationships among upper-, upper-middle-, middle-, lower-middle-, lower-, and underclass.

Gregory Mantsios (2001) contends that class is not openly discussed or debated because class identity has been stripped from the popular culture:

> The institutions that shape mass culture, and define the parameters of public debate, have avoided class issues. In politics, in primary and secondary education, and in the mass media, formulating issues in terms of class is unacceptable, perhaps un-American. (p. 169)

As a candidate for vice president in 2004, Senator John Edwards talked of "Two Americas, one rich, the other poor," and was accused of promoting "class warfare." However, it is acceptable for politicians to talk about the middle class. In doing so, they are not only appealing to the broadest constituency, but also can easily gloss over the differences between classes, thus avoiding any suggestion of conflict or exploitation (Mantsios, 2001, p. 168).

Assets and income, although a fundamental aspect of determining class and privilege, is only one facet in the definition of class. Such social factors as ethnicity, race, religion, gender, sexual orientation, and where one lives, among others, significantly influence class. Jodie Kliman (1998) describes how these social factors can shift and make the definition of class even more elusive:

> Sometimes class means money, which is equated with power. Sometimes other vague criteria of social status prevail. A professor is seen as being a higher class than a contractor with equal income and an associate degree, but not if she is Latina and the male contractor is from "an old family" of British stock. A black executive has less effective class standing than his white subordinate when he tries to hail a cab, get service at an upscale store or buy an elegant home, Women and children's class status plummets after a divorce. Saying that someone who acts tactlessly, talks with a full mouth, or ornately decorates home and body "has no class" suggests entirely different meanings of class. (p. 51)

Most Italians, Greeks, Polish, and Irish who came to the United States had similar rural peasant backgrounds, yet there remain important ethnic differences among them, even when they move up in class. Individuals sometimes feel they must make a choice between moving ahead and group loyalty, which can produce severe identity conflict.

Ethnic distinctions, although a hidden factor that runs across class lines, apparently play a less powerful role among the most educated and upwardly mobile population segments. The royal families of Europe, for example, have been joined repeatedly, as cousins marry across ethnic boundaries, making the princes and queens in England mostly German or Greek and vice versa.

Groups also differ in terms of how they value education or "getting ahead," which may cause intergenerational and intergroup conflict. Certain groups, such as Poles and Italians, have reservations about moving up in class, whereas Jews value such change, believing that parents should work hard so that the children will be more successful than they. The Irish seem to be in the middle, hoping their children would rise in class, yet also having deep skepticism lest their children get inflated opinions of themselves.

Although ethnicity is most often related to nationality and cultural background, there are links between religion and class that shape how an individual expresses his or her beliefs, values, and behaviors. In working with Euro-Americans, the therapist should explore the influences of ethnicity, race, class, religion, and gender on them.

The Persistence of Ethnicity

Sigmund Freud, the father of modern psychoanalysis, recognized the significance of ethnicity in shaping personal identity. Reflecting on his Jewishness, he commented that this national/cultural heritage instilled in him "obscure emotional forces, which were the more powerful the less they could be explained" (Erikson, 1994).

Even after generations of acculturation and intermarriage, ethnicity still influences, in small and large ways, how European Americans behave in their daily lives. In his autobiography, former president George H. W. Bush describes his Anglo American mother's advice after she heard one of his campaign speeches: "You're talking about yourself too much, George," she said. When he explained that he was expected to tell voters something about his qualifications, she persisted: "Well, I understand that, but try to restrain yourself."

In contrast, when Lee Iacocca had presidential aspirations, he received a spirited response from his immigrant mother, Antoinette. In a film about his career, she is seen serving her son a lavish meal, while he animatedly shares personal feelings and beliefs about his leadership abilities. As the camera focuses on Antoinette, she relates stories about her famous son, ending with, " 'Lee was really a very nice boy right from the beginning. What he got today, he got from God. He was really a good boy to his family. He calls me all the time on the phone for no reason . . . just to say "hello, ma. How you doin"?' " (Iacocca, 1979).

A study of 220 mental health professionals clearly indicates the influence of ethnicity on their lives (McGoldrick & Rohrbaugh, 1987). The therapists differed significantly in characterizing their values and practices.

• Anglo Americans indicated that they were raised in families in which men and women were expected to be independent, strong, and able to make it alone. Exploration of the world was encouraged, self-control was highly valued, suffering was to be borne in silence, and conflicts were covered over, especially in public. Anglo Americans were significantly less likely to endorse the idea that you should still give time, money, and other assistance to any family member who needs it, no matter how busy you are.

• Jewish Americans reported saying that children were encouraged to discuss and express opinions on family problems. They learned that talking about such issues is the best way to cure them, that success is more highly valued than anything else, and that suffering is more easily borne when expressed and shared. In addition, a person really gets attention when he or she is sick, and a Jew is not supposed to marry outside the group. In Jews' experience, guilt was considered one of the best ways to shape a child's behavior. They were significantly less likely than others to endorse the statement that children should be seen and not heard.

• Italian Americans learned that nothing was more important than the family, and that eating was a symbol of nurturing and family connectedness, as well as a wonderful source of enjoyment. In Italian homes, gender roles were clearly defined. Men, who were always dominant, protected and women nurtured. Babies were indulged, cuddled, and allowed to sleep with their parents. Italian families always liked to have a good time, and family members believed that using personal connections was the way to get things done. They were significantly less likely than members of other ethnic groups to endorse these statements: "Men and women should be strong and capable of making it on their own." "Conflicts are okay in public." "Self-control is very important."

• In Irish American families, Church rules were paramount. Suffering, which was to be borne individually, was God's punishment for our sins. Drinking was an important part of social engagements, and complaining about problems was "bad form." In Irish homes, children were expected to be seen and not heard, and weren't praised too much so they wouldn't get "swelled heads." Being self-controlled, strong, and psychologically tough was highly valued. Sex was not to be discussed, and women were expected to take care of things. Irish American therapists were significantly less likely than others to endorse the statements: "Eating is a wonderful source of enjoyment." "Suffering is easier to bear when it is expressed and shared."

• In Greek American families, as among Italian Americans, babies were indulged. Sex was not discussed. Males were always dominant, and women were expected to know their place. Parents warned children about the dangers of the outside world and wanted nothing more than for them to be successful. Older family members were respected for their wisdom.

These cultural characteristics in White ethnics and those discussed in the chapters that follow are present more often than most therapists believe, and may not be obvious, especially in educated middle-class families.

Intermarriage

At one time, Italian Americans married only each other, as did German Americans, and members of other ethnic groups. As late as the 1960s, only 5% of White ethnics intermarried. Today, the idea of "sticking to your own kind" in selecting a spouse is the exception rather than the norm for almost all White ethnics. More than 50% of European Americans are marrying out. Intermarriage is also growing among racial minorities and new immigrant groups. Half of native-born Asian Americans are now marrying Whites. A third of all Hispanics wed non-Hispanic Whites (Rodriguez, 2003).

In 1960 the number of White–Black marriages was 51,000; by 2003, the number had jumped to 360,000. Although this represents only 1% of total marriages, the growth has been sevenfold over the last 40 years (Roberts, 2004). In general, the 2000 census indicated that interracial couples, including those in which one person was of Hispanic origin, made up 7% of marriages and 13–15% of households with unmarried couples.

Some observers argue that the growing prevalence of intermarriage implies that ethnicity is evaporating from the American scene (Rodriquez, 2003). In part, that process is, in fact, happening. However, our clinical work indicates that ethnicity has hardly disappeared, that it is more strikingly present, if with complicated dynamics, in intermarried couples and families (Crohn, 1998).

During courtship, a person may be attracted precisely to his or her fiancée's different personality traits. Once he or she is married, the same qualities often become the rub. Generally, the greater the cultural difference between spouses, the more difficulty they have in adjusting to marriage. For example, an Anglo husband may take literally the dramatic expressiveness of his Italian wife, and she may find his emotional distancing intolerable. The husband may label the wife "hysterical" or "crazy" and, in return, may be seen as "cold" or "catatonic."

The therapist's role in these situations is to be an intercultural mediator, clarifying the meaning of behaviors and perhaps, above all, promoting the idea that value differences exist and must be negotiated and compromised. Many therapists have reported using chapters in the previous editions of this book by having each member of a couple read about his or her own and the spouse's ethnic group and discussing it in sessions.

We believe that dealing with these cultural differences is often the key to opening the family system. Yet it should also be noted that although different cultural values may be deeply held, and be at the core of serious conflicts between spouses and or among family members, they may also provide a convenient way of rationalizing and displacing anger arising from other problems. Thus, therapists should be alert to such "cultural subterfuge." For example, a person who claims, "I'm late for our session because I'm on 'Italian time,' " or "I don't think you understand me because of your different ethnic (or racial or religious) background," may be trying to deflect attention from dealing with a difficult issue (Giordano & Carini-Giordano, 1995).

CONCLUSION

As discussed in the following chapters, ethnicity persists in European Americans' consciousness, perceptions, preferences, and behavior, even while mass production, mass communications, and intermarriage seem to homogenize their outward appearances. Psychologically, European Americans are often ambivalent about their identities and are constantly trying to balance the pull of their family histories and experiences with their individual desires to be accepted and successful in the larger society. The persistence of ethnicity, although weaker in some groups than in others, challenges therapists to broaden their concept of peoplehood and race, and to become more knowledgeable and sensitive to all who walk into their offices.

REFERENCES

Alba, R. (1990). *Ethnic identity: The transformation of white America.* New Haven, CT: Yale University Press.

Alba, R. (1995, Spring). Assimilation's quiet tide. *Public Interest*, p. 119.

Alba, R. (2004, June 6). Becoming American. In *Think Tank with Ben Wattenberg* [Television series]. New York: PBS.

Banks, J. (1991). *Teaching strategies for ethnic studies* (5th ed.). Boston: Allyn & Bacon.

Berkowitz, B. (2003). The new Christian crusade. *Work for Change.* Available at www.working-forchange.com

Berman, P. (Ed.). (1994). *Blacks and Jews: Alliances on arguments.* New York: Delacorte Press.

Bernstein, R. (1995). *Dictatorship of virtue: How the battle over multiculturalism is reshaping our schools, our country and our lives.* New York: Knopf.

Bloom, A. (1987). *The closing of the American mind.* New York: Simon & Schuster.

Bonilla-Silva, E. (2001). *White supremacy and racism in the post-civil rights era.* Boulder, CO: Rienner.

Bowser, B., & Hunt, R. (1996). *Impacts of racism on white Americans.* Thousand Oaks, CA: Sage.

Breslin, J. (2004). *The church that Christ forgot.* New York: Free Press.

Brimelow, P. (1995). *Alien nation: Common sense about America's immigrant disaster.* New York: Random House.

Brookheiser, R. (1991). *The way of the WASP.* New York: Free Press.

Bush, G. (1988). *Looking forward.* New York: Bantam Books.

Carroll, J. (2004). *Crusade: Chronicles of an unjust war.* New York: Metropolitan Books.

Carter, R. T. (1995). *The influence of race and racial identity in psychotherapy.* New York: Wiley.

Cose, E. (2000, September 18). What's white anyway? *Newsweek*, p. 64.

Cowie, P. (1989). *Coppola: A biography.* New York: Scribner. p. 2.

Crohn, J. (1998). Intercultural couples. In M. McGoldrick (Ed.), *Re-visioning family therapy: Race, culture, and gender in clinical practice* (pp. 295–308). New York: Guilford Press.

Davis, M. (2003). *Census 2000 ethnic identities: The exodus of Europeans as generations pass.* Available at www.highbean.com//library.ldoc3asp?docid=1g1:87064093

Erickson, E. (1994). *Identity: Youth and crisis.* New York: Norton.

Frankenberg, R. (1993). *White women, race matters: The social construction of whiteness.* Minneapolis: University of Minnesota Press.

Gilman, S. (1986). *Jewish self-hatred.* Baltimore: John Hopkins University Press.

Glazer, N., & Moynihan, D. P. (1963). *Beyond the melting pot.* Cambridge, MA: MIT Press.

Giordano, J., & Carini-Giordano, M. (1995). Ethnicity and family therapy. In R. Mikesell, D. Lusterman, & S. McDaniel (Eds.), *Family psychology and systems therapy: A handbook.* Washington, DC: American Psychological Association.

Gordon, M. (1964). *Assimilation in a American life.* New York: Oxford University Press.

Greeley, A. (1969). *Why can't they be like us?* New York: American Jewish Committee.

Greeley, A. (1974). *Ethnicity in the United States: A preliminary reconnaissance.* New York: Wiley.

Handlin, O. (1951). *The uprooted: The epic story of the great migration that made the American people.* New York: Grosset & Dunlap.

Hitchcock, J. (2002). *Lifting the white veil: An exploration of whiteness.* Roselle, NJ: Crandall, Dostie & Douglass Books.

Iacocca, L. (1979). Interview. In *Biography* [Television series]. New York: Lifeline Productions.

Ignatiev, N. (1995) *How the Irish became white.* New York: Routledge.

Kanin, G. (1988). *Tracy and Hepburn: An intimate memoir.* New York: Fine.

Katz, J. H. (1978). *White awareness: Handbook for anti-racism training.* Norman: University of Oklahoma Press.

Kivel, P. (2002). *Uprooting racism: How white people can work for racial justice.* New York: New Society.

Klein, J. (1980). *Jewish identity and self-esteem.* New York: Institute for American Pluralism, American Jewish Committee.

Kliman, J. (1998). Social class as a relationship: Implications for family therapy. In M. McGoldrick (Ed.), *Re-visioning family therapy: Race, culture, and gender in clinical practice* (pp. 50–61). New York: Guilford Press.

Kranish, M., Mooney, B. C., & Easton, N. J. (2004). *John F. Kerry.* Boston: Boston Globe.

Lazarre, J. (1996). *Beyond the whiteness of whiteness: Memoir of a white mother of black sons.* Durham, NC: Duke University Press.

Levine, I., & Herman, J. (1972). The life of white ethnics: Toward effective working-class strategies. *Dissent*, *19*(1), 12–16.

Lipsitz, G. (1998). *The possessive investment in whiteness: How white people profit from identity politics.* Philadelphia: Temple University Press.

Malcomson, S. (2000). *One drop of blood: The American misadventure of race.* New York: Farrar, Straus & Giroux.

Manning, M. (2002). *The great wells of democracy: The meaning of race in American life.* New York: Basic Civitas Books.

Mantsios, G. (2001). Class in America: Myths and realities. In P. Rothenberg (Ed.), *Race, class and gender in the United States* (5th ed.). New York: Worth.

Martinez, E. (2002). Reinventing America: Call for a new national identity. In R. Takaki (Ed.), *Debating diversity, clashing perspectives on race and ethnicity in America* (3rd ed.). New York: Oxford University Press.

McBride, J. (1992). *Frank Capra: The catastrophe of success.* New York: Simon & Schuster.

McGoldrick, M. (Ed.). (1999). *Re-visioning family therapy from a multicultural perspective.* New York: Guilford Press.

McGoldrick, M. (1995). *You can go home again.* New York: Norton.

McGoldrick, M., & Rohrbaugh, M. (1987). Researching ethnic family stereotypes. *Family Process, 26,* 89–98.

McIntosh, P. (1998). White privilege: Unpacking the invisible knapsack. In M. McGoldrick (Ed.), *Re-visioning family therapy: Race, culture, and gender in clinical practice* (pp. 147–152). New York: Guilford Press.

Morrison, T. (2003). Quoted in *Ethnicity and race: What are you?* Available at antro.palomar.edu/ethnic-ity/ethnic_4.htm

Novak, M. (1971). *The rise of the unmeltable ethnics.* New York: Macmillan.

Perlmutter, P. (1992). *Divided we fall.* Ames: Iowa State University Press.

Pinderhughes, E. (1989). *Understanding race, ethnicity and power: The key to efficacy in clinical practice.* New York: Free Press.

Roberts, S. (2004). *Who we are: The changing face of America in the twenty-first century.* New York: Times Books.

Roediger, D. (1999). *The wages of whiteness: Race and the making of the American working class.* New York: Verso.

Rodriquez, G. (2003, January/February). Mongrel American. *Atlantic Monthly,* pp. 95–97.

Rodriquez, R. (2002). *Brown: The last discovery of America.* New York: Penguin Books.

Root, M. (2001). *Love's revolution: Interracial marriage.* Philadelphia: Temple University Press.

Rostow, J. (1971). The problems of lower-middle income workers. In S. A. Levitan (Ed.), *Blue collar workers.* New York: McGraw-Hill.

Rothenberg, P. (Ed.). (2002). *White privilege: Essential readings on the other side of racism.* New York: Worth.

Schlesinger, Jr., A. M. (1998). *The disuniting of America: Reflections on a multicultural society.* New York: Norton.

Seelye, K., & Elder, J. (2003, December 21). Strong support is found for ban on a gay marriage. *New York Times,* p. 1.

Smelser, N., Wilson, W. J., & Mitchell, F. (Eds.). (2004). *America becoming: Racial trends and their consequences* (Vol. 1). Washington, DC: National Academy Press.

Spielberg, S. (1993). Interview. In *The Barbara Walters Show* [Television series]. New York: ABC Television.

Steinfels, P. (2003). *The crisis of the Roman Catholic Church in America.* New York: Simon & Shuster.

Takaki, R. (2002). *Debating diverstity: Clashing perspectives on race and ethnicity in America* (3rd ed.). New York: Oxford University Press.

Thernstrom, S., Orlov, A., & Handlin, O. (Eds.). (1980). *Harvard encyclopedia of American ethnic groups.* Cambridge, MA: Harvard University Press.

Walsh, F. (Ed.). (1999). *Spiritual resources in family therapy.* New York: Guilford Press.

Whiting, B. (1972). *Race and ethnicity task force report.* New York: Ford Foundation.

Zernike, K. (2003, August 24). The new couples next door, gay and straight. *New York Times,* p. 16.

Zinn, H. (1995). *A people's history of the United States.* New York: Harper.

❧

CHAPTER 37

American Families
with English Ancestors
from the Colonial Era
Anglo Americans

David W. McGill
John K. Pearce

Belief in freedom of the individual and in psychological individualism are core values of Anglo Americans, particularly in middle-class families. These core values have been repeatedly described—by Alexis de Tocqueville in 1835, by David Riesman in the 1950s, by Robert Bellah in 1985, by Eric Kaufmann in 2004, and in every contemporary sociological study of middle-class Americans (Kaufmann, 2004).

American individualism has roots in English individualism, which social historians have pushed back to as early as the 11th and 12th centuries (MacFarlane, 1978) It is based on individual ownership of private property. The American version was brought by Protestant English settlers who were fleeing religious constraints in Europe. They demanded the right to interpret the Bible in the light of divine inspiration—God's guidance in knowing religious truth, as revealed to individuals. Other individual rights flowed from this core conviction. Individualism became their preferred guide in economic, political, and psychological life as well.

Anglo American thought has had a kind of "dual consciousness" (Kaufmann, 2004) from the 17th century, through the Enlightenment and the 18th and 19th centuries. On one hand, Anglo Americans have espoused individual liberty and liberal egalitarianism. On the other, they have believed in their "ethno-national" Anglo Protestant superiority—legitimizing their dominance and justifying African slavery, American Indian genocide, and the subordination of women and non-Anglo Protestant males. Beginning at about 1900 the tension between conservative and liberal values has increasingly resulted in the gradual predominance of liberal values. By the year 2000, liberal egalitarian values had been institutionalized in laws and in the dominant values within universities. Even "the Republican Party main stream has shunned the ethno-nationalism of its paleo-conservative faction in favor of the pro-immigration, laissez-faire modernism of the *Wall Street Journal*" (Kaufmann, 2004, p. 281). "Hard core Anglo Ethnic Nationalism can likely be found among the significant minority in the white population—roughly twenty percent—[that] continues to demonstrate direct, traditional racial prejudice [in surveys]" (p. 282). And there are still some intellectuals fighting the battle for an Anglocentric America (Huntington, 2004).

The number of Americans describing their ancestry as British is declining. As the total American population approaches 300 million, the percentage of Americans who say they have colonial English ancestors declined from 40% in 1920, to 20% in 1980, to 13% in 1990, and to 9% in 2000. Although they founded and have flavored American culture, they are now just one of many groups.

More important, the decline of Anglo Protestant America economically, politically, educationally, and culturally over the last 40 years has ended the dominance that still existed as late as 1960 (Kaufmann, 2004). The decline in Anglo American dominance was a result of the advocacy of liberal egalitarian values by Anglo Americans themselves through the course of the 20th century. The liberal progressive movement, led by Jane Adams and John Dewey, and by the liberal Protestant clergy in the first half of the century, led to the struggle for equal rights and, more recently, to the rise of multiculturalism in the second half of the century. In particular, two liberal ideas have been important: "expressive individualism" (Bellah, 1985) and cultural egalitarianism. The ideology of equality seeks to level hierarchies of status, power, and wealth between groups, thereby challenging ethnic dominance. Individual liberty in its positive form—ever more valued in the late 20th century as "expressive individualism"—"tends to corrode the ethnic dimension of dominant ethnicity-treating ethnic-communalism as an obstacle to the realization of the authentic individual self" (Bellah, 1985). Thus, Anglo Americans, advocating liberal egalitarianism, have changed (leveled) their status in America, with only a minority, a sometimes vocal, conservative minority of Anglo Americans, distressed by this decline (Kaufman, 2004).

In this chapter we emphasize common beliefs, but it must be kept in mind that the English Protestants who came to the new world were not all alike. There are actually four quite distinct Anglo American cultures:

1. *Puritans*: The East Anglican Puritan culture was brought by 22,000 settlers to New England between 1629 and 1641.
2. *Royalist Southerners*: 72 elite upper-class families, their indentured servants, then slaves, and 40,000 others came from the south of England to Virginia between 1642 and 1675.
3. *Quakers*: The Friends Quaker culture was brought from the north midland of England to the middle colonies by 23,000 settlers coming between 1675 and 1725.
4. *Scots Irish*: The northern British (Ireland, Scotland, England) culture was brought from the British borderlands to the backcountry frontier of Appalachia, from Pennsylvania to Georgia, from 1717 to 1775 by a very large group, more than 250,000 settlers. The settlers of this group came to call themselves Scots-Irish, and their culture is described in detail in Chapter 47. (Also see David Hackett Fisher's book *Albion's Seed*—an outstanding guide to all of these subcultures.)

Although there are substantial regional differences, Anglo Americans prefer to think that they are all "pretty much the same." The core value is individualism, and a common problem is the exaggeration of that value into hyperindividualism. For example:

An Anglo American family was baffled by their father's messages about the importance of individual self reliance. The father would preach *his* version of Voltaire, reiterating "above all to thine own self be true" and "a man must think for himself," which was further distorted to "a man must be allowed to fall on his face." The mother in this family was suffering from ineffectively treated mental illness; she had had dozens of psychotic episodes and brief hospitalizations over a 40-year span. The parents divorced. When the adult children of this troubled divorced family then had work, relationship, and financial difficulties, the remarried father did not visit and did not offer emotional or financial help. He expected them to stand on their own two feet; he was respecting their self-reliance; he was not interfering. Throughout his life he talked proudly of "not caring about money." Though he loved his children, when he died at 90 he left them nothing. He was true to his belief that he would hurt his children by helping them.

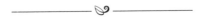

THERAPY AND THE THERAPEUTIC PROCESS

When things are going well for healthy Anglo American families, there is balanced attention to the maintenance of relationships and to individual development. This is true even while they are claiming that the family is there for the individuals more than the individuals are there for the family. But when the balance is shifted to hyperindividualism, there is trouble.

A New England woman, a PhD and applied scientist, was engaged to a first-generation Asian software engineer. She was bewildered and frightened by the very real possibility that her fiancé's mother might move in with them—to escape from domestic violence in her own home. She wondered why her fiancé would insist on being so responsible for his mother, especially when it would disrupt the beginning of their marriage so dramatically. She thought it would be more natural for the mother's daughters to take her in.

Her own family was hyperindividualistic. For example, her mother repeatedly advised her to not invite a favorite aunt to any engagement or wedding events because "it would burden" the aunt. Namely, it would burden the aunt with an obligation to come, like it or not. The mother supposed that this would be respectful of the aunt's possible wish not to come. This is an example of a bizarre but surprisingly common Anglo American behavior. It can be understood as a sort of psychological fusion. The mother makes decisions for other people (daughter and aunt) while supposing she is being thoughtful and respecting their autonomy.

The young woman, the daughter, was saddened and puzzled by the scarcity of visits and attention from her family. Her family was too distant and weird. However, her husband's Asian family was too close.

In therapy the couple were able to talk over problems, make joint decisions, and find ways of managing both the closeness in the Asian family and the distance in the New England family. Clarification of cultural differences and frank discussion of alternatives were sufficient to make it possible to move ahead with the marriage.

In therapy, Anglo Americans are likely to identify as problems those situations that disrupt autonomous functioning. Usually, they attempt to avoid dependency and direct expressions of anxiety that would elicit caretaking. They may, even when suffering, prefer emotional isolation and withdrawal. Lack of contact, separation from others, difficulty in communicating, and blandness are not likely to be regarded as problems.

Family therapist Murray Bowen and his followers have rightly observed that even apparently isolated and detached people may be covertly "fused" to their families by invisible loyalties and dependencies. His recommendation is to encourage what he would see as authentic individuation so family members can be more "individuated" while together. Anglo Americans are wary of affiliation and attachment. They prefer distance. Individuals in therapy need to be tactfully encouraged to balance dependence and independence to achieve more genuine autonomy.

Starting treatment is difficult and embarrassing for Anglo Americans. Individuals usually come for help only when it is impossible to deny their problems or when their efforts to solve them alone have failed. They feel inadequate because they have failed to solve their problems themselves—as they should have. They have failed to be self-reliant. Therapists should see initial awkwardness as a difficulty in seeking help and not as a true reflection of the severity of the presenting problem. Unfortunately, successful treatment may not reduce Anglo American discomfort with therapy. Furthermore, the therapist's open encouragement, intended to be supportive, may be embarrassing.

Once Anglo American families are talking comfortably, they are likely to get right to the truth of the matter—as they know it. Anglo Americans value insight and reason; they value meaningful discussion. The key is "meaningful." They tend to be literal, parsimonious, and careful with words, treating them seriously, as if the words were part of a contract ("My word is my bond"). This characteristic may be underestimated by therapists from cultures that traditionally use words differently.

Anglo Americans will want to clearly define a problem that can be worked on. Once this is done, the family can proceed with confidence, believing that hard work in therapy will be sufficient for success. Hard work is a core value in therapy, as in other aspects of life.

Anglo Americans will be most comfortable making the therapeutic relationship a contractual one, viewing the therapist as the family's consultant. They will expect to pay a fair fee, clearly negotiated, promptly and without hassle, and they will expect to get their money's worth in terms of successful treatment.

The therapist can show respect for Anglo American individualism by making a contract with each member of the family, including children. Often, the therapist will be wise to use an objective method (e.g., reason, discussion, education, task assignment, and training) as an initial access to more sensitive matters. Objective methods can lead to core emotional issues and the reduction of emotional isolation. Although starting treatment is uncomfortable for Anglo Americans, they may terminate quite easily and view the end of therapy as completion of a job well done. Or they may just stop. Abrupt departures should not necessarily be attributed to resistance, failure to complete work, or separation anxiety—it may be all of these, but it is also Anglo American style. (Ethnic values usually interact with psychodynamic issues.) They may (like some Irish families) leave therapy quite satisfied, without a word of acknowledgment or validation, only to tell an astonished therapist some years later how the therapy turned their lives around.

THERAPY AND SHARED VALUES

Anglo Americans have been taught that the meaningful issues and genuine struggles of life are mostly within the self, and that few external constraints cannot be overcome by individual effort. All persons can, and therefore should, be individually successful. Failure is almost always ascribed to personal weakness (Pearce & Friedman, 1980).

The value of self-reliance may be illustrated by the case of an upper-class New England couple's marriage that was threatened by the wife's irritability and anger as she attempted to cope with her full-time profession, a 6-month-old daughter, and a chronic illness—multipe sclerosis. It was a revelation to her when the therapist suggested she might be trying to do too much. The couple was better able to understand the origins of her expectations of herself by exploring her family history. Her ancestors, including the women, had been fiercely independent and had striven to make social contributions through professions or social services. Reviewing this history helped to make sense of her difficulty in accepting any disability or asking for help from her husband. She was successful in therapy in revising her expectations to a more realistic level.

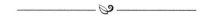

Anglo Americans would rather not complain.

The father of an Anglo American man developed a melanoma on his back. Eventually it bled so much that he had to change his shirt many times a day, yet he never sought medical attention. Finally, a tumor developed under his arm that was so painful and disabling that he was "forced to get to a doctor." He soon died.

Listening to this description, the son's Jewish therapist suggested that it was too bad that the father had not gotten some help and relief earlier. The Anglo American patient, who was doing grief work for his father as part of the therapy, replied, "No, my father made his choice and died his own way."

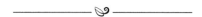

The Anglo American response to pain may be contrasted with the Irish style. Zborowski (1969) points out that the Irish tend to repress and deny pain—often they cannot accurately identify its location. Anglo Americans can identify pain. They report it fully and accurately to the physician; they want to be the physician's assistant. But when a remedy seems unlikely, they usually prefer to not discuss it. They value bearing pain silently—if they can. This silence contrasts with Jewish and Italian traditions of valuing vivid expression of pain and suffering. The contrast, of course, applies not only to physical pain but also to emotional pain.

Anglo Americans prefer to "not waste words." Their silence is emotional self-containment. Although a caricature, the image of the silent cowboy or rugged frontiersman who says nothing after returning from arduous months on the trail (because "There is nothing to say") exemplifies the Anglo American preference for few words. Anglo Americans do not use words for drama as do Italians, nor to elaborate reality as do the Irish, nor to articulate and share feelings and thoughts about suffering as do Jews. Anglo Americans may feel that if they say too much about themselves, they will burden others.

On Kluckhohn's value-orientation scale of basic cultural choices, Anglo Americans have a strong future orientation, prize individual achievement, and see themselves as dominant in their relationship to the natural world (Papajohn & Spiegel, 1975). Thus, they do not see the point of dwelling on past problems; their attention belongs elsewhere, especially on the future and "getting on with it." This future orientation, once expressed in the ruthless exploitation of the resources of the continent, is now expressed in the passionate cause of preservation of the natural environment "for the future."

Above all, Anglo Americans value work. They may seem to focus more on the external signs of success, probably because they believe success is evidence of virtue. Calvinists believed that success (which was actually achieved by hard work) was evidence of predestined salvation. An Anglo American's identity, relationships, self-esteem, and sense of adequacy and well-being are likely to be tied to work. Indeed, Anglo Americans have a tendency to transform many aspects of life into work. Men and women "work" at making a living, and "work" at raising the children. Anglo Americans may talk of "working" on relationships, love, sex, fulfillment, and identity. They may even treat their recreation, hobbies, collections, and sports very seriously, with standards of achievement and success for each. They want therapy to be work.

ANGLO AMERICAN CHILDREN

Anglo Americans raise their children to be self-contained, principled, responsible, independent, self-reliant, self-determining, and, perhaps, from the vantage point of other cultures, self-centered individuals. The more children begin to demonstrate that they can take care of themselves, the more successful Anglo American parents feel. The following example illustrates how fathers may relate to their children primarily by criticizing their performance. This unintentionally produces feelings of inadequacy.

A man who came into therapy with work problems reported that his relationship with his father had consisted primarily in joining him in doing tasks around the house. The father's role was to show his son how to do things right so the son could take care of himself someday. The man recalled often feeling ashamed and inadequate because, although he had persevered, he could never do things "quite right," and his father would often complete the task himself. The father's self-absorbed task orientation made the child feel that the work was more important than the child. In addition, the work required an attention span and mastery of detail beyond a child's reach. Sometimes Anglo American training for individual adequacy can turn out to be training in feelings of inadequacy.

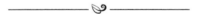

Anglo American children often complain that their parents relate to them in a detached manner. Hovering, worried parental involvement is considered neurotic. Developmental stages are typically passed through without ceremony. Going off to school, reaching puberty, menstruating, leaving home, getting married—each of these milestones may be greeted with understated appreciation. The muted Anglo American approach may be puzzling to the non–Anglo American therapist.

Middle-class Anglo American children typically negotiate school rather well, especially through the latency period. The tasks of school and of latency are a match with Anglo American values. Children are encouraged to go off to school alone, take initiative, and achieve. They are expected to develop a strong sense of their individual capacity and gain self-esteem from individual achievement. Poor Anglo Americans, however, may not appreciate their school years as much; they may consider school a distraction from the real tasks of life—working and coping.

Clubs, sports, and hobbies help socialize Anglo American children in the twin social modes of competition and conformity. They learn to "play by the rules of the game." The friendships thus gained remain a model for adult life.

Anglo American children have trouble when they are unable to meet their parents' expectations for achievement and autonomy. Anglo American parents will be distressed if the child is unable to become self-sufficient. Physical or emotional handicaps are upsetting. The child's "bad" neediness makes the parents feel inadequate, which makes the child feel worse, thus creating a vicious circle of mutual failure. Anglo American families are fine when things go well. Things are "supposed" to go well. This expectation, this optimism, contrasts with the expectations of other cultural groups in which trouble is considered inevitable.

In the real world, where failure and inadequacy of one kind or another are bound to occur, when trying again is not an adequate remedy, Anglo American families may respond quite harshly with scapegoating. Those who do not measure up may be cast aside. They may become marginal, isolated, and eccentric. Even worse, they may stay at home, accept the "defective" role, and increase the family's pain.

ANGLO AMERICAN ADOLESCENTS

Anglo American culture historically encouraged early separation of adolescents and the development of an individualistic, self-defined, adult identity. In 1750 and even 1850, a 20-year-old couple could be well established in the community—adequately skilled, financially independent with farm and house, and with children on the way. In the 2000s, extended apprenticeship (of one form or another) in our complex vocational and financial world will make buying a house and feeling established in a job or career difficult even by age 30 or 40. If contemporary parents, following the frontier model, try to promote independence by withdrawing physical, financial, or emotional support too soon, the Anglo American adolescent will probably feel abandoned. The result may be a kind of false adulthood with premature identity foreclosure.

Anglo American families do not struggle to keep children at home or closely involved in family life as do, for example, Jewish or Italian families, for whom adolescence may be a period of open family conflict. In today's world, however, adolescents are not always ready to move on when they or their families want them to, especially when jobs are scarce and rents high. In the past, Americans enjoyed a continuously expanding economy based on new, cheap land. There had been financial busts, but the long-term trend of increasing prosperity lasted from the 1600s to the booming post–World War II economy—a very long time. It seems unlikely that the future holds comparable economic opportunity. Without a good job, it is hard to go off on one's own, to one's own work and one's own new family, whenever one feels it is time.

When Anglo American adolescents have difficulties, they are likely to consider it their individual business, not the family's. Anglo American parents may be hesitant to intervene. In therapy, they need to be encouraged to stay involved, to continue to provide support and clear limits. In other words, a little more family struggle may well be good for Anglo American adolescents, who would otherwise be left alone to struggle. The idea is to invite the adolescent back into the family, to help young people express and validate their pain, and to share their load with the rest of the family.

ANGLO AMERICAN ADULTS AND COUPLES

In the recent past, traditional Anglo American nuclear family roles denied women the opportunities for the success that their culture so keenly valued, forced them into relatively isolated dependency, and relegated them to lower status. However, asking these isolated, dependent women to raise independent children has been a continuing cultural contradiction for Anglo Americans. The depression and "inadequacy" of Anglo American women, which has constituted the most common psychiatric patient profile from the 1950s to the present, is in part a product of their devalued, contradictory position. This pattern changed substantially in the 1990s, when economic decline forced most families to depend on two incomes. Women now work outside the home for unequal pay and continue to do most of the housework and child care—the "second shift." No longer feeling as inadequate when it comes to achievement, now they are suffering from the same stress diseases (e.g., coronary heart disease) suffered by working men. At the same time, Anglo American men still expect to be supported in their work-adventures. Things may be changing, but not necessarily for the better for Anglo American women.

Successful therapy will help Anglo American women make sense of their anger and modify their cultural tendency to take the responsibility and blame for all troubles and to attribute the troubles to their inadequacy as individuals.

Anglo American men have their problems too. They are still expected to fulfill the traditional roles. The man has his job and is, in some ways, encouraged to be a workaholic—he is supposed to be a success and earn more money. In this role he may feel inadequate and irrelevant in child rearing and in maintaining social relationships. The fact is that workaholics may do better at their jobs—while doing worse at home. There are no simple solutions to these dilemmas.

Anglo Americans tend to experience marriage as a contractual relationship between individuals to meet individual needs. The emphasis is not on fulfilling a religious sacrament or joining extended families. Sex, money, and even the delivery of happiness are seen as contractual obligations. If a spouse fails to perform adequately sexually, earn enough money, or provide enough security, he or she has not kept the bargain. Divorce is relatively acceptable for Anglo Americans; however, the individual Anglo American may experience divorce as a painful personal failure.

Couples often come to treatment with a controlled style that may make the source and nature of their pain and conflict inaccessible to the therapist. Their aggression is often sublimated into competition at work or recreation, rather than acted out in family relationships. Alcohol is commonly used to anesthetize aggressive or other painful feelings. Martinis for lunch and cocktails before dinner on a daily basis are more typical middle- and upper-class Anglo American drinking patterns than episodic or binge drinking. An Anglo American may drink a great deal without noticing that it is a problem: Cocktails before dinner, wine with dinner, and an after-dinner drink may be regarded as gracious living, a matter of pride, not an embarrassment.

Anglo American sexual problems often stem from excessive control, avoidance, and distance in intimate relationships. Anglo Americans more often suffer more from lack of intensity in their sexual and emotional expression than from repressive inhibition or violent acting out. Worry about adequacy is often a prime component in Anglo American sexual problems. High standards of production, combined with high expectations of control, may cause performance anxiety and failure. Anglo American couples often respond to conflict by distancing and avoidance rather than by active confrontation, as in the following example:

An Anglo American couple at the point of separation came to treatment. They were ambitious and perfectionistic, and they tried always to be cheerful and tolerant. It was apparent to the therapist that they had drifted apart and needed help in ending their marriage so that neither would feel irresponsible. They had no norms for conflict expression or resolution and, indeed, had never had any fights, even small fights, along the way. The therapist observed that their cheerfulness, denial, and sense of righteousness had allowed them to carry problems, without directly addressing them, until they were so far apart emotionally that there was nothing left with which to work.

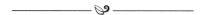

Therapists can teach Anglo Americans an antidote to this cultural pattern. Couples can learn to have small, immediate, frequent, and personal fights instead of letting it all build up. When an Anglo American couple is able to seek help, a variety of techniques can be used: contracting, task assignments, and negotiated (even signed) agreements. Therapists should not be put off by or overinterpret the cool, reasonable, and correct tone of many Anglo American couples in marital conflict. They are maintaining self-esteem by conducting themselves correctly. Conversely, they may feel humiliated at "losing their cool" in a fight.

The most important factor in a marital conflict may not be readily apparent. For example, money may well be the dominant factor, but may never be brought up. Anglo Americans would rather not talk about money, but money issues are usually crucial whether the family is poor, working class, middle class, or rich.

Anglo American couples may not view their families of origin as resources in either childbirth or child rearing. Their cultural style leads to isolation from support, sharing, and the guidance of an extended family. Any change or intervention that works toward reducing family isolation is likely to be helpful. The following is an example:

A successful corporate executive in his 50s had been in therapy for 2 years. His work had been his life. He had little experience with intimacy, and he was separated from his own feelings. Part of his therapy consisted of encouraging him to reconnect with those feelings. As the therapy progressed, the man began to express a wish for more of a relationship with his three brothers and sisters, all of whom lived nearby. As the man put it, "We only get together for Christmas when Mother calls. We enjoy each other, but we all just seem to disappear, except at Christmas."

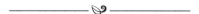

ELDERLY ANGLO AMERICANS

The fear of aging, with eventual sickness, incapacity, and dependence, can become a matter of almost obsessive concern to Anglo Americans of all ages. The youthfulness and future orientation of the wider American culture make older people particularly vulnerable to loss of self-esteem. At best, an older person in reasonable health is able to sustain feelings of adequacy by continuing self-sufficient, independent living and not becoming a "burden to the family."

When Anglo Americans face extended disability or terminal illness, a stressful situation for any family, their self-contained individualism can be particularly maladaptive.

They try to keep their painful feelings to themselves. They may have difficulty asking for help and sharing the stages of loss and grief with others.

ANGLO AMERICAN FAMILIES
AND NON–ANGLO AMERICAN THERAPISTS

Non-Anglo American family therapists may be wary of the ways in which Anglo Americans relate to therapists of other ethnic groups. It should not be a problem. Anglo Americans prefer to see people as having individual worth, especially when encountered in personal relationships. Hence, in therapy, Anglo American families are likely to relate comfortably and individually to therapists of any background. They will judge a therapist on his or her individual merits.

SOCIAL CLASS

Because of the obvious visibility of Anglo American wealth, one might suppose that most Anglo American families are especially prosperous. In fact, the census records of 1980 reveal that the average family income for people who claim English ancestry is very close to the average family income of other ethnic groups such as French, German, Irish, Italian, Polish, some Middle Easterners, Cubans, many Asian groups, and Black women (Kaufmann 2004; Sowell, 1981). The Anglo American poor are likely to live in rural areas throughout the 50 states; they are almost invisible. Eleven percent were below the poverty line in 1980 (Kaufmann, 2004).

Anglo Americans are indeed disproportionately found among the wealthy, but that predominance is fading: "From a position of overwhelming superiority in the late 1960s, Protestants had become underrepresented in the highest echelons of corporate America by the late 1980s" (Kaufmann, 2004, p. 221). "No more than 40 percent of American millionaires [can be] even loosely defined as WASPs. On the other hand close to 40 percent were Jewish, Italian, or Greek in ancestry" (Christopher, 1989, p. 88).

The English colonists came from a society that had assumed the justice of fixed class differences. But the New World settlers (except those in the tideland South) were less divided by class and economic differences. The United States was 95% agricultural until the 19th century: Wealth was land, and land was abundant. Upward class mobility, within limits, was possible for all hardworking, thrifty, right-thinking (conforming) citizens.

The Northern colonists, and later their pioneer offspring, believed that individuals could make it—could become wealthy and achieve higher class status at will. This was partly true, but many English colonists were poor, their descendants were poor, and they remain poor today.

The belief in boundless opportunity has a far-reaching impact on poor, middle-class, and rich Anglo American families today. Believing that they have all started on a more-or-less level playing field, Anglo Americans have ambivalent feelings about class. They identify with the worldwide struggles for political freedom, but not with the economic policies that compensate for past injustice. Economic opportunity is assumed to be available to everyone in the United States, and therefore poverty is suspect (Rubin, 1976). As a result, poor Anglo Americans carry a double burden; they feel oppressed not only by poverty but also by feelings of self-blame and inadequacy, unduly attributing their poverty to inferiority. Middle-class Anglo Americans think they should have done better.

Upper-class Anglo Americans are afraid that, because of their personal inadequacy, they are at risk of slipping. Fears of inadequacy are found in all classes. Some Southerners are different. They continue the Tidewater tradition of class stratification linked to identification with local roots. Southern Anglo Americans see themselves as living in a highly interdependent world of class and race. They have long lived with contradictions between public and private life, between maintaining themselves and others in their places, and with the contradictions inherent in keeping problems secret.

PRIVILEGE, RACE, AND SEXUAL ORIENTATION

Anglo American privilege means different things to different classes. Upper-class Anglo Americans who are privileged—because of wealth, early arrival in North America, expensive education, connections, and the absence of the myriad barriers that others must climb over—may deny that such things matter much. They attribute their privileged status to individual achievement. Less privileged poor and middle-class Anglo Americans may fear that other groups are "taking over."

Historically, all four of colonial Anglo American regions of the United States practiced systematic racism. Each tried to eliminate Native Americans, and the South embraced slavery. Race was and is an American dilemma. Anglo Americans live with an awareness of the contradictions; they value individual liberty, yet they have denied it to others. They feel remorse about others' suffering—if they are reminded of it—but believe everyone should look to the future and forget the woes of the past. This is an attitude that can produce conflict with other American ethnic groups (Axtell, 1985).

Attitudes about homosexuality generally track with religious convictions. Liberal attitudes are more common, but members of conservative religious denominations, claiming biblical authority, tend to consider homosexuality sinful. Most consider this a matter of individual conscience.

REGIONAL VARIATIONS

Although we have addressed the issues that are central to family therapy generally, the entire story is more complicated—there are important regional variations. The four Anglo American regional cultures have competing and even contradictory ideas about freedom and individual liberty. Persisting regional differences are shown, for example, by differences in attitudes toward gender equality, as evident in voting patterns for the equal rights amendment; rates of military service; violence, as shown in homicide rates; views about the right to bear arms, as shown in gun ownership and the formation of militias; and substantial differences in the amount of money spent for local government services and education.

New England

The Puritan New England idea of freedom was based on a belief in an ordered existence—order in communities, families, and the lives of individuals. The following is the case of a man who took individual responsibility to an extreme:

A 40-year-old high school history teacher came for treatment following hospitalization for major depression (he had had a previous hospitalization in his 20s), for feeling inadequate in his work, and for an unhappy marriage. The couple came together (other members of his family were included at various points in the therapy). The man's wife was a social worker from a family with a history of depressive illness. He wanted children; she did not. He did not express sadness or anger about not having children or disappointment in his wife for not appreciating his work. He was critical of himself for failing in the marriage. He directly expressed his exaggeration of New England values in saying, "I believe in the principle of taking responsibility for what goes wrong." He felt completely responsible for the tension in the marriage. He took sole responsibility and did not ask for help. He did not fight with and thereby engage his wife to share problems—a stance that further created distance between them. Treatment encouraged him to shift from his exaggerated sense of responsibility, self-absorption, and isolation toward shared responsibility and an engaged, connected self.

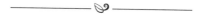

Treatment of Northeastern Anglo Americans may usefully include moderating the impact of family traditions, sometimes by getting the family more directly involved in exploring that history in order to sort the myths from the realities and to reclaim realistic expectations. Pride and involvement in family history tend to be associated with making money. Family myths are more potent among the rich, or once rich. The most potent family myths are stories of glorious achievement, linked to standard ethnic values, such as independent judgment or service to the community. The poor take pride in the history of making enough money to live and in not asking for handouts.

Southern

The Royalists who developed the Tidewater plantations of the South saw freedom as the right to rule one's own lands and servants, in other words, as freedom to maintain a class hierarchy. Frank Pittman (personal communication, 1981), an Atlanta, Georgia, family therapist, observes that a typical Southern family's motivation for seeking help is the experience that something (the socially correct status quo) is out of control, that the family needs help doing the "right thing." Southerners may at times come for help in order not to change.

In Pittman's hands, therapy is a careful, very delicate social transaction. Concerned about social class from a local (neighborhood or county) perspective, Southerners may be concerned about the social standing and the race of the therapist. These families need to feel that they are in control, that they can proceed at a moderate pace, and that they will be able to solve a problem. Coming to therapy does not mean all family business will be discussed. Indeed, trust is likely to be extended only when the therapist agrees, at least implicitly, that the rules of avoiding certain topics (the family secrets) will continue to be honored. Therapists working with Southern families are expected to understand that "their peculiarities are different from their problems." They do not come to therapy, as do some Northerners, to become better people.

Mid-Atlantic/Midwestern

Quakers, oppressed in England for their quiet practice of a heterodox religion, asked only that their rights and the rights of other persons be mutually respected. The value is that you must allow other people freedom in order to be free. Other immigrant groups populated the Midwest to a greater extent than the Quakers, but the Quakers were an important formative influence in the Mid-Atlantic states. The following is the case of a man whose privacy was treated with such extreme respect that his alcoholism was ignored.

The managing partner of a law firm was drifting gradually into alcoholism, while the other lawyers tactfully looked the other way. His alcoholism progressed to the point that he was failing to meet his professional responsibilities. The partners, his peers, then confronted him with specific omissions, but could not bring themselves to take on the key issue, alcoholism. They saw his alcoholism as a flaw and his personal business. His boss, the managing partner, finally, unhappily, consulted a therapist. The treatment required amounted to an abrupt cultural transplantation, where the ideology of Alcoholics Anonymous and the characterization of alcoholism as a medical disease was advocated. Thus reframed, the alcoholism issue was confronted and the previous privacy-respecting conduct was labeled as "enabling behavior." The disease theory of alcoholism allowed effective problem solving without challenging the core value of respect for individual privacy.

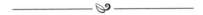

For Mid-Atlantic/Midwest Anglo Americans, having troubles means failure on two counts: the failure to successfully carry on, and the failure of being needy. Effective therapy does not challenge the positive values of work and independence; it adds the value of getting appropriate help when needed. Therapy is a way to reasonably and responsibly "work" on problems. The goal is restoration of adequate emotional self-sufficiency and appropriate interdependence. Of course, even when life is conducted in an exemplary and reasonable way, tragedy can strike. The lack of fatalism in the culture of Anglo Americans can leave them dismayed when bad things happen to good people.

Appalachian/Southwestern

The Appalachian/Southwestern culture is found in the Appalachians and the rural desert of the Southwest and Northwest. This is the culture we know from "country and western" music. It has its roots in the chronic wars between Scotland and Northern England. Violence persists. The rate of murder in Texas is four times that in New England. These people are patriotic; they disproportionately serve in the military and participate in private armies—militias. Education is not as highly valued as in other parts of the country. The Southwest has a high school graduation rate of 65%, in contrast to 90% in New England.

Appalachian/Southwestern families are usually seen by family therapists only after preferred modes of problem solving within the extended family have broken down. The successful family therapist will ally with the extended family network and consider using some form of restorative network family therapy.

CONCLUSION

Anglo American clients bring to therapy an individualism that helps in many ways but gets in the way of getting help with problems. They do well in treatment that recognizes both the costs and the benefits of emotionally self-contained individualism. The goal of successful family therapy is to increase the Anglo American's ability to reach out of personal isolation, reclaim important emotional experiences, and engage the challenges of life with a spirit of adventure.

REFERENCES

Allen, J. (1989). *We the people: An atlas of America's ethnic diversity.* New York: Macmillan.

Axtell, J. (1985). *The invasion within: The contest of cultures in Colonial North America.* New York: Oxford University Press.

Bellah, R. (1985). *Habits of the heart: Individualism and commitment in American life.* Berkeley: University of California Press.

Christopher, R. C. (1989). *Crashing the gates: The de-WASPing of America's power elite.* New York: Simon & Schuster.

Fischer, D. H. (1989). *Albion's seed: Four British folkways in America.* New York: Oxford University Press.

Huntington, S. P. (2004). *Who are we: The challenges to America's national identity.* New York: Simon & Schuster.

Kaufmann, E. P. (2004). *The rise and fall of Anglo-America.* Cambridge, MA: Harvard University Press.

Macfarlane, A. (1978). *The origins of English individualism: The family, property and social transition.* Oxford: Blackwell.

McGill, D. (1992). The cultural story in multicultural family therapy. *Families in Society, 73*(6), 339–349).

Papajohn, J., & Spiegel, J. (1975). *Transactions in families.* New York: Jossey-Bass.

Pearce, J. K., & Friedman, L. (Eds.). (1980). *Family therapy: Combining psychodynamic and family systems approaches.* New York: Grune & Stratton.

Rubin, L. B. (1976). *Worlds of pain: Life in the working-class family.* New York: Basic Books.

Sowell, T. (1981). *Ethnic America: A history.* New York: Basic Books.

Tocqueville, A. (1969). *Democracy in America* (G. Lawrence, Trans. & J. Mayer, Ed.). New York: Doubleday.

Zborowski, M. (1969). *People in pain.* San Francisco: Jossey-Bass.

CHAPTER 38

Dutch Families

Conrad De Master
MaryAnn Dros Giordano

T he Dutch have been characterized as ambitious, hardworking, and frugal, yet quiet and peace loving. Throughout their history, they have exemplified a people searching for a place of their own, a land where they can keep to themselves and freely practice their religion. They are an intensively active, internally principled, uncompromisingly private people and, at the same time, are often open minded, receptive, and tolerant of others.

If you ask Dutch people in this country how they identify themselves ethnically, many simply say they are Americans. But the Dutch are one of the least conspicuous American ethnic groups. Except for concentrated areas in the Midwest, other Americans are largely unaware of them and their history. Despite a high degree of acculturation, however, Dutch Americans continue to display Old World Dutch traits.

In both the Old and New Worlds, core Dutch characteristics and values have been strongly influenced by Calvinism, the theological system developed by John Calvin and his followers. Calvin's teachings contributed significantly to the Protestant Reformation, whereby people sought to practice their Christian beliefs personally rather than according to the dictates of the established Roman Catholic Church. Those who were eventually instrumental in establishing the Netherlands as a nation were followers of Calvin.

Calvinism emerged as a distinct interpretation of the Christian faith at the same time as Dutch Protestants attempted to free themselves from outside religious, political, and economic interference. It subsequently contributed to shaping personal and family behavior, as well as public and political institutions and policies; it certainly inspired many Dutch to focus on establishing a place of their own. The interplay between the religious and the political nurtured a strong sense of self-reliance and individualism, characteristics that gave impetus to creating the Netherlands as a distinct entity, which eventually impelled many to emigrate to America and shaped their settlement patterns.

The Dutch were also strongly influenced by the topography of the Netherlands. Sixty percent of the Dutch population lives below sea level, and because the country is small and densely populated, all space is precious. Not only has Holland always been in danger

534

of being engulfed by the sea, but Dutch lives of necessity are impacted by the sea's whims. To survive, the Dutch have learned to live communally and have always worked together, especially during natural disasters.

Fear became reality in 1953 when the waters of the North Sea broke through the dikes, taking more than 1,800 lives, and again in 1995 when flood waters rose to force 100,000 from their homes. The Dutch pride themselves on their distinct sense of community and their strong work ethic, values that have made it possible for them to protect their land from the sea. It is believed that the aspect of lack of control and the feeling of the strength of nature create a kind of solidarity among them.

The Dutch are a complex and sometimes paradoxical people. Because so little has been written about them as an ethnic group, we draw upon historical sources, our personal experience growing up in Dutch communities, and our professional experience in working with Dutch American families.

HISTORICAL SETTING

The Dutch are descended from three Germanic tribes, the Frisians, the Saxons, and the Franks. The practice of religious tolerance and the separation of church and state were established early in Holland. The move toward separation of church and state and the strong insistence on having freedom of religion resulted in Holland's becoming a haven for Europeans suffering persecution elsewhere, often serving as a "foster parent" country. Eventually, Holland served as a conduit for many other Europeans who had suffered persecution elsewhere and were on their way to America. This special ability to incorporate people of diverse backgrounds and religious beliefs enabled Holland to grow and survive and is active evidence of what has come to be known as "Dutch tolerance."

The seeds of tolerance began to germinate during the Middle Ages when the cities of what was about to become the Netherlands assumed importance in Europe. The Low Countries, as they had come to be known, were developing in many ways, including commercially. Most significant, they had become the world's greatest shipbuilders, enjoying a worldwide reputation as a maritime power, whose commercial enterprise was acknowledged everywhere. As Olsen (1989) points out, the Dutch and their neighbors resented the oppression of the Catholic Church and bridled at the role of the powerful Hapsburgs of Spain, foreigners who drained banks and businesses dry in order to finance costly wars abroad. Though of differing ethnic, economic, and religious backgrounds, the people of the Low Countries united in their efforts to gain autonomy and freedom (p. 7). Eventually, they developed their own nation.

Originally ruled by the Hapsburgs of Spain; later, in the early 1800s overrun and ruled by Napoleon of France; and subsequently caught in the crossfire of the first and second world wars, the Dutch from the beginning of their existence in Europe have seemed a restless, dissatisfied people. They had been in constant struggles politically, economically, and religiously with their more powerful neighbors. They persistently fought to preserve their identity and freedom from domination, rising up each time they were attacked and even when overtaken. Despite many attacks from the outside and a variety of adjustments, the Dutch borders have remained unchanged since the 1830s.

Many Dutch, particularly the poor, chose to leave, hoping to gain a better life elsewhere. Consistent with what occurred at other times in their history, the dilemma for the

Dutch, coming from a small country, is revealed in more recent times in the deep impact they sustained from the two world wars.

During World War I, the Dutch, though remaining neutral, were caught between Germany and its enemies, Britain and France. During World War II, Hitler invaded the Netherlands. The German occupation lasted 5 long years, during which time the Dutch endured bombings and severe shortages of food and fuel. Such inconveniences pale in the face of the mass slaughter of nearly 80% of the total Jewish population in Holland, a larger percentage of the Jewish population than was killed in any other Western European country. According to the Oliners (1988):

> Despite the notable history of acceptance of Jews in the Netherlands and the concomitant weakness of anti-Semitism there, 115,000 Jewish citizens and 25,000 Jewish refugees suffered a proportionally greater loss of lives (between 75 and 80%) than the Jews in any other occupied country in Western Europe. The primary responsibility for this frightful toll lives with the Germans, who ruled the Netherlands with an iron fist as a protectorate. (p. 31) . . . The near annihilation of the Jews in Holland constituted a radical reversal of the country's long national heritage of religious tolerance and civic equality. (p. 32)

The rapid German victory over the Netherlands in 1940 transformed what had been a secure haven for Jews into a living hell. Holland's many Christian churches were outspoken in their opposition to Nazism and intervened to protect the Jews. Many Dutch people also risked their lives to save Jews. An example of Dutch heroism is documented in the poignant diary written by a young Jewish girl named Anne Frank (1967).

DUTCH IN AMERICA

It is difficult to determine how many Dutch there are in America today. According to the 2000 census, 4.5 million Americans consider themselves to be of Dutch origin, but this figure is thought to be low and estimates run closer to 8 million. It is equally difficult to determine how many people in the United States speak Dutch, but the number is usually set at somewhere between 200,000 and 400,000.

It is worth noting that there was never a mass migration of Dutch to the New World. Of those who immigrated, 9 out of 10 did so, prompted mainly by economic considerations. However, there are distinctions between Dutch Catholic and Dutch Reform immigration. The Catholics came more for economic reasons, settled in Midwestern cities, and quickly intermarried with other Catholic ethnic groups, especially German Americans. The Protestants were different in their motivations to immigrate and in their adaptation to the United States. The Dutch of the 19th century did not so much seek a new life in America as opportunities to reclaim an old life.

They formed tight-knit farming communities, such as Pell and Hull in Iowa, that sought separation for the preservation of purity. This pattern followed the Dutch Reform theology that they knew in the Netherlands. The American separation of church and state suited them well, for it allowed them to go their own way to build the separate institutions they sought. Later, they started small colleges, such as Calvin and Hope in Michigan, that remained for many years largely separated from the wider American intellectual world (Pettigrew, 2003, p. 215).

The Michigan and Iowa communities have remained, to this day, deeply conservative in regard to politics and religion. Post–World War II Dutch immigrants have mostly settled in California, reflecting changes in the postwar Netherlands. These new immigrants are more secular, assimilationist, and more politically liberal than their predecessors.

The early immigrants were lower-middle-class rural folk: farmers, laborers, and artisans, who brought to America an ethic of industrious work, practical farming methods, and a strong desire for agricultural land. Especially during the 17th and early 18th centuries, immigrants were often exploited by the profit-seeking trade companies who had encouraged migration, and by wealthy landlords known as *patroons*, who regulated their lives and deprived them of the freedoms they sought. The Netherlands was not a powerful country that could, or was inclined to, support its holdings or its people in the new country. Consequently, many settlers became so disillusioned they emigrated back to their old country.

The Dutch have been in America since 1609, when they explored the northeastern coast on the *Halve Maen* under the command of Henry Hudson. In 1626, the Dutch settlers purchased Manhattan island from the Indians for 60 guilders in trade goods and constructed Fort Amsterdam on the southern tip of the island. Downtown Manhattan still has several streets that bear the original Dutch names, the most famous of which is Wall Street (*Wal Stratt*).

In a recent landmark work of history, *The Island at the Center of the World*, Russell Shorto (2004) describes the crucial role of the Dutch in the founding of America. The author documents how the founding was not the accomplishment of English settlers alone, but the result of a powerful and rival clash between two great 17th-century powers—Hollan and England.

The Dutch Republic throughout the 17th century was the most liberal as well as ethnically diverse society in Europe—the melting pot of Europe. The Dutch have always accepted differences; foreign goods, peoples, and ideas moved in and out of their trading ports. The country's policy of tolerance made it a safe haven for all stratas of society from all over Europe and the world. It gave intellectual and religious haven to Decartes, Locke, Spinoza, and even the Puritans, who lived there before founding the English colonies of America. Shorto (2004) notes that the city of Amsterdam became the model for New Amsterdam on Manhattan island.

> This island city would become the first multiethnic, upwardly mobile society on America's shores, a prototype of the kind of society that would be duplicated throughout the country and around the world. It was no coincidence that on September 11, 2001, those who wished to make a symbolic attack on the center of American power chose the World Trade Center as their target. If what made America great was its ingenious openness to different cultures, then the small triangle of land at the southern tip of Manhattan Island is the New World birthplace of that idea, the spot where it first took shape. (p. 3)

The 1680s saw some immigration of religious groups to Dutch communities, and by about 1700 there were well over 10,000 Dutch people living in America in what is now New York, New Jersey, Delaware, and Pennsylvania. In Europe, when the Dutch were overtaken politically, which restricted their freedoms, and/or outside investors attempted to regulate business and trade, the poorer people often left. When New Amsterdam was overrun militarily by the British in the late 1600s and the trade companies and patroons attempted to regulate the workers' commercial endeavors and even their per-sonal lives, many of the Dutch pushed westward into areas that eventually became Michigan, Illinois, Iowa, and Wisconsin. Swierenga (1979) concludes that for the Dutch: "Family, faith and farming were their watchwords, not liberty, fraternity and equality" (p. 3).

They came to this orientation in large part because what many of the Dutch hoped to escape from in Europe, military and economic oppression, rose up in phoenix-like fashion in the New World in the late 1600s. As in the Netherlands, the Dutch faced military struggles in their new home. In 1664, New Netherland initially fell to the British, who changed the name of the principal Dutch settlement, New Amsterdam, to New York. It was then reconquered by the Dutch in 1673, who, at that time renamed the settlement New Orange; however, when the Treaty of Westminster was signed a year later, bringing a truce to the trade battles raging between the Dutch and the English, the territory in its entirety was given to England and the name New York persisted.

The economic landscape, which developed even prior to the time the New World became a nation, proved to be inhospitable to the Dutch of meager means. It is dramatically described by Howard Zinn (1999):

> New York in the colonial period was like a feudal kingdom. The Dutch had set up a patroonship system along the Hudson River with enormous landed estates where the barons completely controlled the lives of their tenants. . . . In addition, powerful British assumed entitlement to the land and parceled out huge estates. Under Governor Benjamin Fletcher three-fourths of the land in New York was granted to about thirty people. He gave a friend a half million acres for a token annual payment of 30 shillings. Under Lord Canterbury in the early 1700s, one grant to a group of speculators was for 2 million acres. (p. 48)

Those Dutch who did not have access to power and wealth, therefore, once again seceded and, as noted, left, pushing westward. Keeping in mind this context and historical experience, we can better understand the persistent search for new lands to settle, the character of the family structure that developed, and the nature of the psychic and emotional mindset of the early immigrants.

In her recent book on Dutch immigrant women, Suzanne M. Sinke (2002) points out:

> The rural nature of the Dutch migration to America supported the "need" for couples to run farms, and for children who would then serve as farm labor, though the family remained central to urban Dutch America as well. A family economy in which all members contributed to the good of the whole, sometimes to the detriment of their individual needs, was typical. (p. 13)

Sinke also notes:

> Dutch immigrant men, unlike those of some other nationalities, would rarely consider farming without wives. Hence the decision to begin farming for a single man almost always coincided with marriage. (p. 22)

Until recent years the Dutch tended to marry within their own ethnic group and favored doing business with their own folk; the Dutch often were against labor unions, suspicious of any political party, and, in general, reluctant to join any organization other than the local church. Given their history in Europe and their experiences in America, it is readily understandable why the Dutch often display a fierce independence. They tend to be suspicious of the authority of those who aspire to be dominant. They are skeptical about "outsiders" and are notorious for their clannishness, even among the fifth and sixth generations (Swierenga, 1979).

It may also be important to note that the September 11, 2001, attack on New York City revitalized for many ethnic groups both recent and ancient memories of struggle, bloodshed, and displacement. Having fled from the Hapsburgs and having been overrun by Napoleon, persistently at war with England and defeated by the British in the battles over New Amsterdam, more recently being invaded and ruled by Germany during World War II, for the Dutch it was, once again, their home being attacked.

At this point in their history, however, many Dutch seem to find some sense of security and comfort in the thought "at least we have our own place," or "we have what we have," referring to the material blessings that they often feel God has bestowed and for which they give thanks to God. This, in turn, reinforces a strong adherence to the notions of private property and seeking security primarily in oneself, one's family, or being with one's own kind, which is quite different from the socialistic historical European roots from whence they came.

Altogether, the political, economic, social, and religious history and experience of the Dutch seem to foster a sense, prevalent among many Dutch Americans, that those forces operating in the larger society will not support their best interests. Whatever is perceived as being outside their control or as derived from outside their community is often regarded with suspicion. This becomes a sensitive issue in therapy, especially in the initial clinical contact with Dutch families.

RELIGION

No attempt at promoting an understanding of the Dutch can be adequate without providing at least some insight into their faith and religious life. The Dutch have a passion for religion. During the 16th and 17th centuries the Dutch Reform movement was dominant in Holland, despite the fact that there were also a significant number of Catholics as well as Jews. The Dutch Reformed Church was recognized as the "one true religion" and therefore treated in a privileged manner, although never given the status of state church.

For a Calvinist, Christ is not a hope, a promise, a set of beliefs, a moral code, or a prescription for life. Christ is seen primarily as an actual historical event; that is, in the birth of Jesus Christ was the divine interrupted and converged with human history, transforming all that occurred subsequently by offering new hope and promise to those who follow his teachings. In a similar, analogous way, "acceptance of Christ" refers to an occurrence in human experience in which the divine converges with the human and thereby transforms all subsequent experience through offering new hope and promise for the individual.

Divine action, however, is not limited to the life and death of Jesus. Calvinists believe that Christ's intersection in human history remains an ever-present, ongoing process that occurs as the divine, through the action of the Holy Spirit and informs the conscience of those who remain open to his call and direction. To be Christian, therefore, means to live as one perceives, according to the innermost recesses of one's conscience, the way Christ would have lived (Calvin, 1960, p. 8). This teaching helps us understand a Dutch pastor's reply when asked how Dutch people try to manage family difficulties or troubling psychological or emotional events. He said:

"Well, they probably would view the problem as an indication that something was askew in their relationship with God. The event probably would serve as the impetus for fervent prayer. If prayer didn't suffice, then the pastor himself would be consulted in hopes that he would help to determine God's will in solving the problem and thus help the individual or the family develop a closer relationship with God."

What this means for the therapist (particularly because many Dutch have rebelled against and actively reject what they perceive as their religious background) is that Dutch people often feel at a loss when they don't have a sense of what is right or called for in a particular situation, that is, when the message from the conscience remains unclear or confused. Not much stock is placed in expressing oneself or even in uncovering deep emotions; in fact, doing so may often be viewed as presumptive or arrogant.

The strength of conscience characteristic of Dutch folk is illustrated by a Dutch mother of two young children:

She remained steadfastly loyal to her husband despite his continued drinking, drug abuse, and unfaithfulness. Her religious beliefs not only reinforced the sanctity of their marriage but also seemed to foster a sense that merit derives from self-denial and persistent endurance in the face of hardship. This woman expected little for herself, yet remained conflicted about the impact her husband's behavior and the resulting family disruption would have on her children. For many months she felt unable to do anything constructive, often becoming moody and depressed. She expressed little concern for herself and didn't know what to do, but clearly hoped to do "what is right."

As therapy progressed, she appreciated that her anger and frustration with her husband's substance abuse was not the result of "uptightness," puritanical or moralistic judgments. After all, she drank too—how could she judge him? When it came to matters affecting her children, however, she readily set aside her "partying"; she felt it very important to follow through on what was promised to the children, to be emotionally alert and "not in a fog" when her children wished to talk or were struggling with some difficulty. She recognized that it takes energy to discipline and set limits; she realized that raising children often requires 24-hour readiness and doesn't leave room for substance abuse if their well-being is taken seriously. She, in addition, experienced a happy surprise in discovering that her children liked going to church. She shifted from viewing church attendance as a pietistic practice, in which her husband had no interest, to something that might actually be nurturing the emotional and spiritual yearnings of her children. This experience helped her to reconnect with the positive value and meaning church attendance had for her as child. This reassessment opened the way for her to feel more accepting of her past and more aligned with the family she grew up in.

After carefully considering which parts of her family heritage and spiritual life she wished to pass on to her children, she came to believe that continued involvement with her husband would interfere with, rather than promote, what she envisioned for her children. Religious understanding of forgiveness and grace, thought of in regard to both herself and her husband, helped to free her to feel more energized. Her depressed mood lifted and, though she still felt

conflicted, she was able to begin moving toward a separation and eventually a divorce. She felt more at peace with herself and left open the possibility that she might appear right or righteous in God's view.

————————  ————————

Using religious concepts and theological admonitions to find solutions to personal and family struggles often proves to be very effective in working with Dutch clients. Such language also provides a sense of inclusiveness and reduces any residual notions that psychology and psychotherapy promote only secular concerns.

When the therapist can appreciate the painful dilemma of not knowing, can empathize with the genuine desire to do what is right, and can be sympathetic about the confusing complexities of life, deep emotions often well up and are expressed, albeit in a quiet, reserved manner. Likewise, if the therapist can view silence on the part of an individual or family not as an indication of resistance or rigidity but as evidence of the client's being somewhere on the continuum between being completely overwhelmed and a prayerful search for enlightenment, the overall emotional process of the session will remain much more alive. Such was the case of Dirk, a single, 56-year-old, second-generation Dutch American Catholic man who was referred for depression by his family physician.

After 26 years of teaching math at a prestigious Catholic high school, he was accused of committing sexual acts with a student 15 years earlier. As a result, he was asked to leave the school. Dirk was totally shocked by the accusations, denying that any such acts had ever occurred. For Dirk, being falsely accused of pedophilia was devastating. He believed that his school was a community of people who held common beliefs and core values, among which were honesty and trust. "They were my family," he sadly commented in the first session. The trauma of false accusation and being fired broke his spirit and confidence in himself, the law, the Church, and the many close relationships he had had at the school. He felt that he had lost his community and identity. Fearful that he would not be able to teach again, he became immobilized with feelings of confusion and ambivalence about what he should do next. Should he fight the case in court or accept the settlement, knowing that he was innocent? At first, the therapist thought that Dirk needed support to empower him in order to clear his name through the courts. But it became evident in the early sessions that Dirk wanted to live his life, privately, peacefully and free from adversarial situations. Pursuing a long and difficult legal battle, with the danger of media exposure, would create an unbearable situation even if he won the case. The focus of treatment, then, was to connect Dirk to a new community. After time with much support, Dirk was offered a teaching position at a small Christian school. Although he shared with the head minister his history at the previous school, he was still hired, which restored his sense of faith in himself and his community. Given the present climate of suspicion among religious organizations and their fear in hiring a person accused of pedophilia, Dirk felt that gaining the teaching position was a stroke of luck. What if he hadn't been hired? The therapist wondered how he would have reacted and what would then be the treatment approach. The therapist suspected that Dirk would have become more depressed. He would need time, as he did in earlier sessions, to once again work through a myriad of emotions—loss, confusion, shame, and anger. Although this would be a temporary setback, the therapist trusted that he had the strengths to mobilize himself once more and accept that the job loss was beyond his control. In many ways, Dirk's situation is reminiscent of the classic Dutch story of the young boy who kept his finger in the dike and thereby saved Holland from the flood waters.

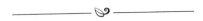

For the Dutch, separation of church and state takes on a far deeper meaning than simply regulating a form of political practice. The Dutch simply don't talk about religion with casual or business acquaintances. Even within families, especially within the extended family, differences in religious beliefs or commitment may be tolerated for the sake of the family. But if it comes down to a choice, the bonds between family may be severed if it seems that religious beliefs or values are being compromised. Moreover, all of Calvin's teachings persistently admonish followers not to expect any reward from their efforts because one's true reward comes from "grace" alone, irrespective of any "good works." When issues arise from external "political" events, the Dutch readily become very tolerant, rational, and utilitarian, tending to favor the solution that is most efficient and least conflictual.

Individual Dutch people, therefore, live with this internal paradox: an extreme strictness on one hand, and a live-and-let-live openness and tolerance on the other. In relation to others the Dutch may often seem aloof, standoffish, or certainly emotionally distant. Individual experience, however, often becomes clouded by persistent soul searching and internal debate, resulting in behavior characterized by the emphasis that all people ought to have the freedom to do as they determine what is best for them.

The dictates of conscience become a powerful influence on decision making as to how and where to live and what individuals must do to have the freedom to practice their beliefs, even if it means leaving all they have known to move to another country.

The influential role of spiritual thinking was illustrated by the words of a 30-year-old Dutch woman describing her relationship with a man she adored:

We could fall very easily into a pattern of almost living together. We're fighting it. We each believe the other to be a present from God. We treasure that gift and hope to show God how much we value and appreciate it. Therefore, we want to do what is moral and right. Others, who do not take our religious beliefs as seriously, might see this as being rigid. Moral dictates precluded rushing into marriage as well as possibly living together.

FAMILY

Bailey (1970) states: "There is a strong sense of family responsibility among the Dutch, perhaps originating in another time and place, born of the dikes and the knowledge that every man and his spade is the keeper and protector of every other man" (p. 37). There is even a Dutch term, *familie-ziekte*, literally, "family sickness," that describes a person who is unduly conscious of the kinship system and its obligations. The nuclear family (*gezin*) maintains close ties with the family at large (*familie*). Clear boundaries are usually maintained in the family, consistent with their individualism and respect for privacy and personal freedom.

Within the nuclear family, role definition and responsibility tend to be very clear. The man is expected to give overall direction to the family, provide for it economically, and set an example of uprightness in the community. The woman is counted on to provide a rich home life for her husband, to nurture the children, and to attend to and promote social and cultural input for the family.

The relationship between husband and wife is considered sacred; there is often a strong emotional commitment, buttressed by religious belief, between them. What adds to the strength of the marital bond is that in several pivotal areas the spouse's thoughts and feelings are usually held in high esteem. Though the husband, for example, bears major responsibility for implementation, his wife's input regarding business, career, and/or family financial matters often proves to be for determining influence. In like manner, though the wife often holds major responsibility for the care and nurturing of the children, she often seeks her husband's input.

Dutch parents feel keenly responsible not only for the physical nurturing and safety of their children, but perhaps even more so, for their children's spiritual nurturing and well-being, so family guidelines and admonitions tend to be somewhat stringent. The adolescent struggle toward adulthood seldom occurs smoothly, usually taking on the form of some sort of rebellion. When Dutch people meet and begin to recognize a common background, conversation tends to move easily toward describing the nature of their rebellion against their heritage or family. In most cases however, there is a "return to the fold."

This process was illustrated by a 32-year-old divorced Dutch woman with two children:

She had experienced a tempestuous adolescence, married a non-Dutchman "outside the faith," and is now solidly entrenched back in the Dutch church and community. Inasmuch as she had experienced so many crises, she was asked her view of how the Dutch handle family crisis. She said: "If something happens outside the normal mainstream, the Dutch don't know how to handle it. They may suppress or ignore the happening, but it really disturbs them and it takes them a long time to readjust. If whatever occurs goes against their grain, they don't know how to deal with it."

This woman had often felt alienated and isolated, yet even at her darkest moments, close family and friends tolerated her waywardness and continued to demonstrate openness. Of her background, she now says, "If I hadn't had some sort of solid background, I wouldn't have been able to keep moving through the difficult times." For those who have rebelled and then wish to return to the "Dutch" way of life, warm acceptance usually remains available. The New Testament parable of the prodigal son is lived out in Dutch families, particularly for those who repent of their wrongdoing.

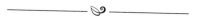

Part of this tolerance, this willingness to accept the wayward back into the family, may also come out of the long Dutch tradition in which religious or political authority and rule were not well received. The Dutch are a nation of seceders, so it is not surprising that the authority of the Dutch parent is often somewhat circumspect. In subtle ways, it often becomes evident that Dutch parents expect, or may even quietly enjoy, their children's rebellious nature. Parents are often concerned about providing strong spiritual and moral guidance, but they also respect autonomy and cherish a sense of independence. Once children leave the home, parents tend not to intrude. In addition, because of the difference in expectations and concerns regarding oneself and one's own family as compared with others, there often develops a clear distinction among Dutch folk between "one of us" and an "outsider." In addition, subtle gradations often develop as to the degree to which someone exists as "one of us" or an "outsider."

About the only thing that can be ensured in regard to how Dutch folk deal with homosexuality, intermarriage, race relations, and other such issues, is that there will be much controversy. Public expression may be geared toward protecting the rights and privileges of the individual, but private thoughts and feelings remain quite another matter. Certainly, there will be much skepticism and resistance to whatever is perceived as an imposed stance. What this means for the clinician is that an initial response is often shaped to conform with what the client perceives the therapist wants to hear. Trust and confidence can develop as the therapist demonstrates a capacity to perceive and appreciate the client's perspective and personal struggles.

CONCLUSION

For the therapist working with the Dutch, it may be beneficial to keep in mind (1) the long history of struggle by the Dutch with forces outside their community, which were perceived as threatening, controlling, and/or exploitive; (2) their strong emphasis on self-initiation and self-reliance; and (3) the major part that religion, with its emphasis on personal inspiration, served in their development as a people and as a nation.

These influences combine to foster a caution about outsiders and a negative reaction to those who do not share their strong sense of personal responsibility or do not appreciate the depth of their religious conviction. Once involved in treatment, however, Dutch Americans tend to be determined and thorough, and will work diligently until they have reached an internal sense of what is "right."

REFERENCES

Bailey, A. (1970). *The light in Holland.* New York: Knopf.

Calvin, J. (1960). *Institutes of the Christian religion* (Vol. 1) (J. T. McNeil, Ed.). Philadelphia: Westminster Press.

Frank, A. (1967). *The diary of a young girl.* Garden City, NY: Doubleday.

Oliner, S., & Oliner, P. (1988). *The altruistic personality.* New York: Free Press.

Olsen, V. (1989). *The Dutch Americans: The Peoples of North America.* New York: Chelsea House.

Pettigrew, T. (2003). [Review of the book] The Dutch American Experience: Essays in honor of Robert P. Swierenga. *Journal of Ethnic and Migration Studies, 29*(1), 215.

Shorto, R. (2004). *The island at the center of the world."* New York: Doubleday.

Sinke, S. M. (2002). *Dutch immigrant women in the United States, 1880–1920.* Chicago: University of Illinois Press.

Swierenga, R. (1979). The Dutch in America: An overview. In L. P. Doezema (Ed.), *Dutch Americans* (pp. 284–293). Detroit, MI: Gale Research.

Zinn, H. (1999). *A people's history of the United States, 1492–present.* New York: HarperCollins.

CHAPTER 39

French Canadian Families

Régis Langelier
Pamela Langelier

One of every seven persons in New England is of French Canadian descent, constituting the largest non-English-speaking ethnic group in the area. In addition, New York, Michigan, Texas, Louisiana, Florida, and California also have large concentrations of this ethnic group. Yet although some cities and towns boast voter lists with a majority of French surnames, Franco Americans go almost unnoticed. They have traditionally been quiet and unassuming as a group and have led private lives, characterized by persistence, "a spirit of independence and resourcefulness" (Morissonneau, 1993). In this chapter, the terms "Franco American" and "French Canadian," which are used interchangeably, refer to the descendants of French Canadian immigrants.

Apart from this book, little has been published on psychotherapy with Franco Americans. The therapist's task is made difficult by a lack of research and by the variations within the group itself: urban and rural; educated and noneducated; first, second, or third generation in the United States. In spite of these differences, there is a common family profile to consider for effective treatment. Certainly, as McGoldrick, Garcia-Preto, Moore-Hines, and Lee (1991) warn us, the reader is "urged to consider the characterizations made here not as statements of absolute fact that apply to all men and women in a given culture, but as suggestions of patterns to increase our cultural awareness" (p. 170).

Franco Americans have been shaped by Catholicism, by language, by dedication to family and work, and by a conservatism arising from their rural roots.

HISTORICAL AND CULTURAL BACKGROUND

During the industrial period (1860–1920) farmers and lumberjacks left Quebec in massive numbers for the United States. The flow slowed considerably when growing industrialization and urbanization in Canada created jobs, thus reducing the necessity to immi-

grate to the United States to find work. According to Pierre Anctil (1979), of the 2,
225,000 descendants of Francophone Canadians living in New England and New York,
some 200,000 are of Acadian stock, the French people of what is today Nova Scotia,
New Brunswick, and Prince Edward Island. In addition, about 1.3 million people in California claim some French ancestry, as do 1 million in Michigan and 500,000 in Texas.
Currently, French Canadians share very little of Quebec's identity and nationalist orientation.

Although the Franco Americans were immigrants to the United States, they had been
North Americans for generations. French Canadians descend from the 17th-century settlers of the New World. Their ancestors explored the continent, struggled, and won wars,
often with Indians as allies. But they also fought and lost. Indeed, their defeat in Quebec
City, in 1759, left them abandoned by France, and they became subjects of the British
monarch.

Although conquered by the English, most French Canadians were not subjected to
overt persecution. The Acadians, French colonists of what are today Nova Scotia and
New Brunswick, however, suffered severely. They were brutally deported from eastern
Canada to the Atlantic Coast of the United States and to France, starting in 1755. Many
ended up in Louisiana, where they came to be known as Cajuns.

French Canadians hid from the English in a psychological sense. They lived apart
and turned in upon themselves. In isolated rural settings, dominated culturally as well as
religiously by the Catholic Church, they led simple lives and had minimal education.
Early marriage and the begetting and raising of children were given the highest priority
by the Church hierarchy. The psychological impact of their French sense of abandonment
in Canada was evident in the Church's promotion of large families to increase the race.
French Canadians kept their faith, language, and culture as an ethnic victory. The English
had political control, but the souls of the people were still unconquerably French.

Family is central to the lives of Franco Americans, just as it was for their French
Canadian forbearers (Moogk, 2000). The family handed down essentially conservative,
traditional values through the generations, aided by the powerful impact of the Catholic
Church's code of behavior.

As speakers of French, one of the most esteemed languages of the world, Franco
Americans could have regarded their language as a badge of honor. But educated Americans admired only Parisian French. The French spoken with a rural accent in New England was disdained for lacking the polish, sophistication, elegance, and style associated
with the European French. Thus, the French language, to which Franco Americans were
profoundly loyal, became a badge of inferiority. Today, the third generation generally is
not bilingual and does not embrace French as its language. Religion and language are not
foremost in today's Franco American lifestyle. In the 2000 census, 1,698,394 persons
reported that they spoke French, which is the third most frequently spoken language in
the United States, after English and Spanish. Maine has the highest number of French-
speaking people. The census also reported that more than 13 million Americans declared
themselves to be of "French ancestry." In two New England states, Connecticut and Ver-
mont, the "French" are the second leading ancestry group. However, French long ago
ceased to be a functional language in many communities with large populations of
Franco Americans, and there are very few social services and health providers who have
proficiency in the language.

Because of their distrust of others, Franco Americans felt that no one, not even members of other ethnic groups who had also been the target of prejudice, could truly understand their special position. Although they tended to be proud of their religion and language, they were keenly aware that they were scorned. As Brault (1986) pointed out, "Over the years the group has suffered its share of abuse and discrimination" (p. 165). The survival of Franco Americans as a separate entity, against all odds, became a marker for their spirit of endurance.

During the early 1920s, Franco Americans, while feeling forever attacked and conquered by outside forces, were dealt a particularly demoralizing blow in the one area in which they were most confident: religion.

The *Sentinelle* affair (Sorrell, 1975) represented a battle between several Franco American leaders (among them Elphège Daigneault, a Woonsocket, Rhode Island, lawyer) and Irish Bishop Hickey, who used the threat of excommunication to force the French to meld in churches and schools with Irish, Indians, Ukrainians, and Polish Catholics. English was to be the common language. The belief that "if you lost your language, you lost your faith" was brutally cast aside by the threat of losing their souls, for the pope excommunicated dissenters who opposed forced assimilation. The newspaper *La Sentinelle*, whose editorial position was in opposition to the Bishop, was listed by the church as taboo reading. Thus it became sinful to read, sell, or distribute the paper. "The *Sentinelle* affair was probably the most discussed event in the Franco American history" (Bélanger, 2000, p. 2). It engendered divisions, and even today Franco Americans remain divided over the whole affair.

The Irish, ever since arriving in New England, have been pitted against the Franco Americans. Although they respect the success of the Irish in the Church and in secular politics, Franco Americans tend to see the Irish as arrogant and brash. Like the Irish, Franco Americans can be articulate, witty, and colorful, but only within the secure framework of their homes, where their *joie de vivre* is well known.

Collectively, Franco Americans spent most of their meager resources building a network of parish schools, which were staffed by various religious orders. Although working-class Franco Americans did not put a high value on education, as a group, they have played an active role in founding hundreds of colleges, high schools, and primary schools across the country. The religious upbringing of Franco Americans, coupled with a lack of education and a relative lack of worldly ambition, led them at an early age into the same mills where their parents had toiled. Many had to believe that heaven would be the reward for their lives of uncomplaining, dutiful labor, because the reality of this life was not.

Franco Americans are from diverse backgrounds, some having Indian ancestors, although this may not be acknowledged. Because of their history, "many French Canadians believe England does not have a history, it has a criminal record" (Du Long, personal communication, March 2004). This statement reveals the psychological impact of being defeated by the British. "I don't hate the British, but I don't like them either" is a common sentiment among Franco Americans. Few aspire to visit England, even today.

Attitudes toward gender, race, and sexuality are not as clearly defined as is distaste for the British. There is an openness to new experience and an appreciation for the underdog evident in Franco American families today. However, a streak of conservatism, deriving from their Catholic roots, promotes quietly held beliefs and practices, such as the male and female dividing chores according to traditional gender roles.

FAMILY PATTERNS

It is vital to distinguish between generations, for family patterns have changed. College-educated Franco Americans who live in large cities or the suburbs are less likely than their high-school-educated counterparts, who generally live in aging "Little Canadas" of textile towns, to fall into traditional kinship configurations.

The ethnogenesis of the entire population is evident. Its people evolved into a group that is neither French nor Canadian, but rather have held on to cultural traits that they deem important (Du Long, 2001). Memories of mill life have faded, as have the French language, music, and art. However, the essence of the "French ancestors" heritage is still found in Franco American families today: tenacity laced with a robust love of life and simple pleasures, such as those found at a family holiday meal of a *tourtière*, a succulent meat pie.

Today's new dual-career couple, unlike their parents and grandparents, seeks help from a psychologist far more than from the parish priest. However, career still does not take precedence over a successful home life, and few Franco Americans aspire to be in high government positions. Families still emphasize conformity, respect for authority and institutions, family loyalty, religious traditions, hard work, and emotional self-control.

Family rituals centered on family gatherings play an important role in traditional Franco American culture. Among the most significant are weddings, *de rigueur* baptisms, large wakes, and Christmas mass followed by *le Réveillon*, an all night festivity. Also customary are a visit with *mémère* (a corruption of *grandmère*, or grandmother) and holidays spent with family rather than friends. When the younger, more acculturated generation does not pay much attention to these rituals, this may arouse intrafamilial tensions.

Anger is often a hidden emotion within the family. Either it is not allowed or it is vented in a passive–aggressive way. Denial is used, and there is long-standing resentment for past difficulties. When anger eventually does erupt, it is often expressed indirectly by prolonged silences or, sometimes, by pounding objects, slamming doors, and self-punishment. For women, the expression of rage is a problem. There is no acceptable outlet for emotions, so that coldness and withdrawal may be the indirect consequences. Guilt, a common emotion, breeds resentment. Feelings of intimacy and attachment tend to be expressed verbally. With more openness in society, Franco Americans are less emotionally repressed and more comfortable talking about intimacy (Paradis, personal communication, January 2004). Subjects such as addiction are often treated in a joking, offhand manner that belies the depth and sensitivity of a person's feelings about them. Jealousy of others' success in life is denied, but can be seen at family gatherings (Du Long, personal communication, March 2004).

Today, except in rural and lower-income families, for whom the family remains the major focus of social activities, Franco American extended family relationships tend to be scattered, with gatherings usually limited to weddings and funerals.

Some respondents to a survey we recently conducted report that they view the parish priest to be no more than a figurehead, whereas others still consult him about family or personal problems. Many American Catholics believe it is possible to disregard the church's teachings on abortion, premarital sex, birth control, and divorce and still be a good Catholic. This decline in acceptance of religious dogma highlights a change in the power of the Church. Although no ethnic data are provided, it appears that younger Franco Americans share this view.

Because Catholicism, especially among French Canadians, traditionally opposes religious intermarriage and divorce, Franco Americans have tended to marry their own. However, in the 1940s, a trend favoring exogamous marriage began, so that today at least 60% of Franco Americans marry outside their own ethnic group, although usually within the Church. Often, but not always, those who intermarry wed Catholics, such as those from Italian, Irish, or Polish backgrounds. Divorce is also increasing among Franco Americans, paralleling the national rate.

"The native language and national parish were the linchpins that kept the ethnic wheels from falling off, even after the urban enclave gave way to scattered lives in the suburbs" (April, Brouillette, Marion, & St.-Onge, 1999, p. 3). Although elderly Franco Americans revere the past and are deeply attached to and proud of their French language, culture, and religion, they tend not to speak French when a non-Francophone is present. Middle-age individuals tend to be less committed to their traditional culture and often feel guilt, shame, and/or ambivalence about their ethnic background. The young tend to ignore their ethnic history.

Many respondents reported that the younger generation is generally ignorant not only of Franco American history and tradition, but also of past and present discrimination. Young Franco Americans today, except for some who live in rural areas, are becoming assimilated into American society. Many young Franco Americans do not identify with their more strident separatist cousins in Quebec. Rather, they are committed to becoming part of the American melting pot. Although there is interest in tracing their roots by using genealogy, Franco Americans in their 20s, 30s, and early 40s usually do not teach their children ethnic self-awareness or promote the French language at home. A sense of inferiority continues to haunt many, as they seem ill at ease with their roots, whether in therapy or at work.

Many of the social clubs formed in the 1960s for community meetings have become drinking clubs (Labbé, 1999). Many local jobs are gone, the church pews are emptying, and moves and divorces are scattering families.

FAMILY THERAPY

Franco Americans have a long history of self-help. Frequently clannish, most were reluctant to acknowledge the need to turn to mental health workers and resented any implication that they should do so. Personal problems, especially family issues, were considered too intimate and private for a stranger (e.g., a therapist). Some still operate according to a familiar blue-collar ethic: Work the problem out as best you can—or tolerate it.

Today, most seek help and use health insurance benefits for treatment. However, they rarely wish to discuss their ethnicity in treatment. Older clients may prefer some of the session to be conducted in French.

A crisis may have to occur before a Franco American family or individual seeks help, not unlike the practice of many Americans today. The therapist can expect to find some hope and personal motivation, but not a great deal of insight about self or others. Franco Americans can be engaged in therapy, but are slow about revealing themselves to the therapist and exhibit a fear of being found to be "defective." Therefore, they proceed in a tentative manner, with family attitudes favoring the withholding of information. Therapeutic interventions may take time, but the clearer the therapist's advice and the more pragmatic his or her suggestion, the more likely it is that the client will return.

Family therapy is often requested because of a child with school problems or an acting-out teenager, perhaps one involved in drug abuse. The family is usually cautious about going into sensitive family issues and requests help only for the offspring. The parents tend to see the child's disruption as a blow to their control. Particularly in low-income families, parents have a hard time accepting a child's interpretation of what is happening. Parents, especially the father, are afraid of either losing control or abdicating a position of authority within the family.

Alcoholism, as in most populations, is typically associated with strong denial even when it is seen in three generations. A family therapist must be aware of the risk factors for addiction, such as family history, male gender, and, among immigrants, the "degree of acculturation, i.e., the more acculturated an immigrant is, the more vulnerable he or she is to addiction" (Krestan, 2001, p. 6). Only when the family admits to a problem and the client is intensely stressed or under familial pressure does drug rehabilitation become an option.

Most family therapy referrals are for depression or anxiety about loss or a family crisis. Cross-cultural couples (e.g., French/Irish) may experience tension, perhaps because of too many similar dominant traits—whose family is better, whose traditions are best, who has alcohol as an issue? Not us! Developing a genogram may help the therapist to highlight the larger context of the multigenerational family system and can be a useful step in the assessment process (McGoldrick, Gerson, & Shellenberger, 1999).

The most common defense mechanisms used by Franco Americans are denial, displacement, sublimation, and rationalization. They may blame others for personal inadequacies and failures, have a tendency to scapegoat, assume a martyred stance, or explain away tyrannical or oppressive behavior by citing the authority of the Church's restrictive edicts. There seems to be a tendency to believe that problems are a passing phase and to deny that significant family issues (such as domestic violence) have long-range effects. Franco Americans generally prefer short-term therapy and can sometimes be stubborn and naive. Taboo areas for discussion in family or individual therapeutic encounters have included sexual problems, incest, homosexuality, abuse, and addiction. Loyalty and silent contracts to avoid direct confrontation of each family member in the session are common.

Family sessions with Franco Americans may be characterized by denial, such as about alcohol, abuse, or loss. In one case, the primary issue was grief over the father's death. The family could not bear to think of him realistically, and so he had been idealized (as elderly members sometimes are). The distortions that they were collusively holding allowed them to avoid facing problems with each other. In addition, recent treatment has brought to light past abuse by priests and nuns, which is now coming to prominence in lawsuits and in the mass media. Franco Americans may represent a significant proportion of victims, but their disclosure rate is not known.

Given the family's apprehension and resistance, the therapist's ability to establish rapport becomes paramount. Problem-focused clarity and a workable plan are key to motivating a family's return for a second interview. Appropriate self-disclosure by the therapist may also help build a relationship with the family (Yalom, 1995). In addition, the provision of definite structure in early sessions decreases anxiety and helps the family to make therapeutic progress. Usually, intensive brief therapy is solidly launched only by the third or fourth session, when the therapist is certain that the Franco American's qualities of persistence, endurance, and iron tenacity have been invested in the therapeutic relationship.

A sensible strategy, one that makes use of what would otherwise be obstacles, is to frame therapeutic tasks as ways to "fulfill our duty," be it as spouse, parent, church member, or therapy client. Again, duty is one of the supreme Franco American values. Therefore, if the therapist defines problem-solving sessions and homework tasks as "duties," they almost certainly will be done! Unambiguous assignments, such as family meetings at home for discussion of problems, are tasks the Franco American family probably will accomplish. Direct advice, positive reinforcement, and therapeutic consistency work well. A cognitive-behavioral approach also tends to be effective. The following case illustrates these points.

Mr. and Mrs. Noir, a college-educated Franco American couple in their 30s, had been married for 11 years. Mrs. Noir made the initial contact and described the problem as being Mr. Noir's moods. During the first session, Mrs. Noir described her husband's condition, with only occasional acknowledgement by him. Mr. Noir's "moods" appeared to be moderate, and sometimes quite severe, depression. At times, he thought of suicide.

The evaluation included an individual session with Mr. Noir in which he seemed more willing to discuss problems in his family of origin. He expressed general pessimism about life and relationships. Mr. Noir described his father as passive and withdrawn and his mother as domineering and unduly concerned with appearances. His parents also seemed to suppress their emotions; Mr. Noir could not recall ever seeing them argue.

Mrs. Noir said that she was happy, yet presented a worldview that was strikingly negative. She said her mother was a sad person, but was very much in control of the family. Her alcoholic father worked long hours and was distant from the family. She could remember very few, if any, expressions of conflict between her parents.

Initially, the therapy required the establishment of a warm and supportive atmosphere. Confrontation and/or attempts at insightful exploration seemed inappropriate, considering the couple's lack of experience with and understanding of conflict resolution. Each felt that he or she had very little impact on the other or on the wider world.

The therapist focused on the cognitive aspects of their demoralization. He taught them to recognize repetitive self-reproaches that only led each partner into blind alleys. He taught them to "stop [those] thoughts" and to intentionally shift their attention to recognizing and planning more constructive behaviors (Alford & Beck, 1998). For example, Mr. Noir took on the responsibility to take his wife out "on the town," to a place that he picked out, at least once a week. The therapist emphasized the responsibility and duty of each family member to practice these constructive behaviors in order to maintain a truly warm and supportive family. Gradually, Mr. and Mrs. Noir were able to change their self-defeating behaviors, and their morale improved.

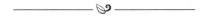

As noted, couple therapy with French Canadians often begins with a crisis.

A wife announces on her 20th wedding anniversary that she wants to leave home. The shocked husband, arriving from his third-shift job, looks in the Yellow Pages for "immediate help" for couples. The two grown children, living nearby, encourage the visit to a psychologist. The wife brings a list of complaints: "alcohol binging by spouse, silence, no vacations." The husband cites only one problem: "no sex in months."

Both Catholics, who attend church twice a year, the husband and wife have told no one of the mounting problems, and certainly not the parish priest. The therapist helps them address the breakdown in communication and intimacy, and fosters more communication between them. The wife agrees to stay home; the husband, to attend an evaluation for alcohol abuse and treatment.

After initial skepticism and some anxiety, the couple found the psychologist to be an ally in aiding them to rebuild their relationship. Soon one child's demands for money revealed that he had a drug problem. A referral was made for the child.

The hopeful couple responded to praise, structure, and respect for their traditions, including large family celebrations. After 3 months of treatment, they shyly revealed that they had become more intimate and were even planning a vacation. The French Canadian code of silence was broken when the couple commented to a close family member that therapy can be helpful.

The therapist's instructing family members to listen to one another and to distinguish between thoughts and feelings (Gilbert, 1992) can be helpful in encouraging more constructive contact between fathers and sons, and between mothers and daughters. In addition, because many Franco Americans tend to rely on nonassertive, passive–aggresive behaviors as outlets for hostility, self-assertion should be stressed and practiced. In short, reeducation in expressing emotions is a must to sustain long-term change, including anger management and guilt reduction. Moreover, considering the tendency of Franco Americans to take themselves too seriously, to lose perspective, and to be pessimistic, it may be very helpful to illustrate a situation with a sense of humor. Laughter and wit are part of their heritage and valued as effective communication.

In working with the whole family, it can often be productive to focus on issues that support the value of having a successful and supportive family (e.g., finding how family members are attempting to help each other and making plans for future support). The following case is an example of sibling support:

A Franco American daughter was leaving home to live with her Jewish boyfriend and to go to college. Everyone in her family disapproved, and she felt isolated. She was breaking all of the rules—leaving home, getting involved with a Jewish man, living with a man before marriage. A meeting of the daughter and her four brothers was arranged. (The young woman was not willing to invite her parents.) The focus was not on her "defection" from the family unit; rather, there was a general discussion of how in the past, during difficult times, the five siblings had found ways to help each other. They wanted to think of themselves as a warm and supportive family, and this was the basis for the tone of the session. To have focused constructively and productively on her defection would have required more sessions and time for better listening and communication. The siblings did not want more therapy at the time, but an opportunity to talk again was established.

Franco Americans often avoid conflict by the effective use of delaying techniques. It is essential for the therapist to recognize the different levels of power in the family between and within the parent's and children's groupings. When the hierarchy is confused, or when some members vie for power in the family (e.g., previously absent father trying to reestablish himself, or a parentified child establishing dominance over siblings), it can be helpful to use family genogram techniques to map the dynamics of interpersonal influence. In many cases, the more the therapist works with the parents to put them back in charge, the better the results with the children.

CONCLUSION

Therapy with Franco American families has a fairly predictable profile: Crisis brings a need for practical behavioral solutions. We recommend cognitive-behavioral therapy with set goals. The therapist, by appealing to Franco Americans' sense of duty, and their desire to have a warm and supportive family, will in time be able to engage clients in cooperative problem solving, emotional reeducation, and the development of effective coping strategies.

Therapeutic success with Franco American families should be measured according to tangible behavioral change and insight or psychic restructuring; the latter is increasingly valued by the younger generation of clients and by all those who are psychologically sophisticated.

French Canadians living in the United States are increasingly open to therapeutic help but, nevertheless, reject an early emphasis on ethnicity in family therapy. They are usually somewhat interested in their ethnic background, but it takes time to examine it. However, there have been a number of Franco American festivals (e.g., *La Kermesse*, held in Biddeford, Maine, in June 2004, and *Le Festival de Joie*, held in Lewiston, Maine, in July 2004) with a "trace your roots" emphasis, which may indicate an upsurge of interest in Franco American genealogy. Genealogical research, now popular, may encourage this population's identification with its rich heritage and, in turn, highlight their sense of ethnicity for future family therapy. In terms of ethnic pride and identification, Franco Americans are at a critical fork in the road. Either a renewed affirmation of their unique cultural identity is begun, or complete assimilation into the general American population occurs. Franco Americans are a "bright thread in the tapestry" of the United States (New Hampshire Public Television, 1999). Their documented struggle to succeed, despite many challenges, is a striking symbol of the immigrant families' will to adopt and survive. This dedication to self-preservation makes for a most interesting therapeutic alliance in family therapy.

ACKNOWLEDGMENTS

Special thanks to Claudette Apicella, Rhea Côté-Robbins, Gilbert Domingue, John P. DuLong, and Françoise Paradis. We are also grateful to the many patients who, over the last 30 years, have shared, in French and English, their feelings and insights about their ethnic identity and strong commitment to family.

REFERENCES

Alford, B. A., & Beck, A. T. (1998). *The integrative power of cognitive therapy*. New York: Guilford Press

Anctil, P. (1979). *A Franco American bibliography, New England*. Bedford, NH: National Materials Development Center.

April, S., Brouillette, P., Marion, P., & St.-Onge, M. L. (1999). *French class: French Canadian-American writings on identity, culture and place*. Lowell, MA: Loom Press.

Bélanger, D. C. (2000). *Franco-Americans, the Sentinelle affair and Quebec nationalism*. Retrieved March 29, 2004, from www2.marianopolis.edu/quebechistory/events/sentinel.htm

Brault, G. J. (1986). *The French Canadian heritage in New England*. Hanover, NH: University Press of New England.

Du Long, J. P. (2001). *French Canadians in Michigan*. East Lansing: Michigan State University Press.

Gilbert, R. M. (1992). *Extraordinary relationships*. New York: Wiley.

Kerouac, J. (1999). *Atop an underwood: Early stories and other writings* (Paul Marion, Ed.). New York: Penguin Books.

Krestan, J. A. (2001). The power to recover. *Psychiatric Times, 18*(12), 1–8.

Labbé, Y. (1999, December 5). It's time for Franco-Americans to rise. *Lewiston Sun Journal* (Maine), p. 3.

Langelier, R. (1996). French Canadian families. In M. McGoldrick, J. Giordano, & J. K. Pearce (Eds.), *Ethnicity and family therapy* (2nd ed., pp. 477–495). New York: Guilford Press.

McGoldrick, M., Garcia-Preto, N., Moore-Hines, P., & Lee, E. (1991). Ethnicity and women. In M. McGoldrick, C. Anderson, & F. Walsh (Eds.), *Women in families: A framework for family therapy* (pp. 169–199). New York: Norton.

McGoldrick, M., Gerson, R., & Shellenberger, S. (1999). *Genograms, assessments, and interventions*. New York: Norton.

Moogk, P. N. (2000). *La Nouvelle France: The making of French Canada: A cultural history*. East Lansing: Michigan State University Press.

Morissonneau, C. (1993). The "ungovernable" people: French Canadian mobility and identity. In D. R. Louder & E. Waddell (Eds.), *French America: Mobility, identity, and minority experience across the continent* (pp. 15–32). Baton Rouge: Louisiana State University Press.

New Hampshire Public Television. (1999). *Franco-Americans we remember* [Videotape]. Durham, NH: Author.

Sorrell, R. S. (1975). *The Sentinelle Affair (1924–1929) and militant "survivance": The Franco-American experience in Woonsocket, Rhode Island*. PhD dissertation, State University of New York at Buffalo.

U.S. Bureau of the Census. (2000). *2000 census of population*. Washington, DC: U.S. Government Printing Office.

Yalom, I. D. (1995). *The theory and practice of group psychotherapy* (4th ed.). New York: Basic Books.

CHAPTER 40

German Families

Hinda Winawer
Norbert A. Wetzel

Writing about German Americans is highly reflective of the authors' personal histories and life choices; it is never objective in a dispassionate sense. One of us (H. W.) was born and raised in New York City in a Polish Jewish immigrant family. Her personal, familial and educational history is intertwined with German language, art, and ethnic culture. Her mother was one of 10 children born to an orthodox *shtetl* rabbi and his wife. Influenced by the latter, H. W. spoke Yiddish as a child. Consequently, when she studied German later, it never sounded like a foreign language. Her father's family members were largely secular Jews, merchants and intellectuals, predominantly from Warsaw, some of whom had married Catholic Poles or Germans. Her paternal grandfather had worked for the German army during World War I. Her comparative literature studies included German language and literature and afforded her a deep appreciation for German literary works. The music of German composers has been at the core of her musical life as a choral singer and amateur pianist. Extended stays in Austria and Germany, and familiarity with the language and culture, eased the development of relationships with Germans in the workshops she conducted, with colleagues and friends, and later, with relatives she holds dear, from her marriage to a German Catholic. Given a personal history that encompasses both painful and loving associations to Germany, holding apparently disparate views has been both challenging and enriching. The challenge has been to bear witness to and keep alive the memory of the Jewish Holocaust while respecting the dominant German culture that produced great artistic masterpieces and has enriched her personal life.

The other of us (N. A. W), born into a German Catholic family of farmers, merchants, and academics, grew up during the years of World War II and the West German postwar era, during which the war, the Holocaust, and the "Third Reich" were covered by public silence, repression of memories, and outright deception. As a nation, the Germans were "unable to mourn" (Mitscherlich & Mitscherlich, 1975), became part of the "cold war" split, and were "too busy" rebuilding economically. Members of the Wetzel-

Kübel extended family were, to varying degrees ranging from participation to passivity, implicated in and affected by the rise of the Nazi Party, the war campaigns, the genocide system, the silence of the churches toward the fate of their Jewish neighbors, the final collapse, the liberation by the Allied forces, and the postwar reconstruction period. As is true for most members of the German generation born during the immediate pre–World War II years, the struggle to understand and respond personally to the events of 1933–1945 was one of the determining factors in his life.

Research on German American families in therapy is sparse. We offer, here, a touchstone for an ethnically sensitive inquiry with individual families of German heritage. There can be no one general "truth" that would elucidate aspects of German ethnicity the same way in every treatment context (Gergen & Davis 1985). It is essential to consider specific areas of exploration, lest we create a therapy that ignores the complexity of the cultural context (Phinney, 1996; Pinderhughes, 1989; Szapocznik & Kurtines, 1993).

German Americans are the largest and one of the oldest immigrant groups in the United States. At the time of the 2000 census there were approximately 43 million Americans of German ancestry, roughly 16 % of the general population (U.S. Bureau of the Census, 2000). Although visible as a distinct group in some states and despite a resurgence of German ethnic identity since World War II, in contemporary U.S. society, at least on a national scale, German Americans often blend into the dominant White culture. A therapist of a different ethnic background may not recognize a family's German heritage, and family members themselves may be unaware of their ethnic tradition. However, work with German American families that explores constructs of meaning may reveal how deeply they are influenced by their German heritage; it is reflected in basic assumptions and in the communication style among family members even if they have not strongly identified themselves as German.

Reticence about one's German heritage is not unusual, but may seem surprising considering their numbers and how significantly German Americans have contributed to the foundations of U.S. society. Popular media in the latter part of the 20th century provided little that was positive with which German Americans could identify. Films that addressed war crimes by Germans (e.g., *Holocaust*, *Schindler's List*, *Shoah*) and World War II military films recalled painful associations to the ancestral homeland. In the early television era, Germans were often portrayed as evil, incompetent, or mad, or were simply not represented as an ethnic group at all (Shenton & Brown, 1976). The negative characterizations and the suppression of German language and culture, as well as other forms of discrimination at various points in U.S. history, may explain why some German Americans may be either ignorant about their ethnic legacy or reluctant to claim or discuss their cultural identity, particularly with a therapist from another culture.

ORIGINS AND DEMOGRAPHY

The "official" beginning of German immigration to the New World is marked by the arrival of the *Concord*, "the German *Mayflower*," in 1683. It brought the settlers who founded, under the leadership of Franz Daniel Pastorius, Deutschstadt (Germantown), Pennsylvania, the first German settlement in the colonies. Among the many accomplishments of colonial Germans were improved farming methods, the rapid establishment of schools, and the first Bible in America, as well as the first paper mill and the first glass-making factory. German contributions to a flourishing free press are exemplified in the achievements of John Peter Zenger, a Palatine orphan, who founded the first truly independent newspaper in the colonies, the *New York Weekly Journal*. Zenger is best remembered for his defiant stand for freedom of the press. During his 10-month incarceration for libel against the British governor, of which he was later found innocent, Zenger's wife, Anne, reputedly a more gifted writer than he, continued to publish the *Journal*, thereby becoming the first woman publisher in the new nation (Tolzmann, 2000). Germans played a central role in colonial history, both at the Continental Congress in 1776 and in the Revolutionary War. German immigrants were soldiers as well as influential generals (Muhlenberg and von Steuben).

In the next century, between 1850 and 1900, Germans were never fewer than one fourth of all foreign-born Americans; many emigrated following the attempted revolution of 1848 against the autocratic, outmoded rulers of the German regional states. The upper Mississippi and Ohio Valleys were settled largely by Germans. Contributions of 19th-century Germans included leadership in farming, business, industry, education, science, and medicine. Instrumental and choral music were highly valued and were central to German American cultural life (Newman, 1999; Reichmann & Reichmann, 1995). Emphasis on sports and family recreation were German practices that are now integral to U.S. family tradition. During the Civil War, many newly immigrated Germans, especially the well-known group of intellectual refugees, the "Forty-Eighters" (political refugees of the failed revolution of 1848), which included among its leaders Carl Schurz (later U.S. senator from Missouri and secretary of the interior), inspired and helped organize antislavery efforts.

In the 20th century, immigration declined. The greatest numbers of Americans of German background were living in the large cities of the Midwest, particularly in Wisconsin and Indiana. New York, however, from the turn of the century until 1970, led other states as a home for German Americans. This last group, identified collectively as immigrants from Germany, were those who sought refuge from Nazi Germany. Predominantly, though not exclusively, Jewish, these Germans included many outstanding contributors to the arts and sciences (e.g., Brecht, Einstein, Fromm, Mann, Schoenberg, Tillich, and Weil). Individual German Americans have been celebrated national heroes, such as Eisenhower, Pershing, Babe Ruth, and Lou Gehrig. (For a more comprehensive treatment of German American history and ethnicity, see Rippley, 1976; Tolzman, 2000; Winawer & Wetzel, 1982, 1996.)

Diversity: Who Are the German Americans?

In order to understand the complex background and roots of German-American culture and heritage, we have to keep in mind that German culture and language were never coextensive with a German national state. Even during the height of the Holy Roman Empire (formally ending in 1806) and after the foundation of the German Reich by Bismarck (1870/71), or during the Third Reich and since 1945, a state called Germany included only parts of the regions of central Europe where people speak German and are part of the German culture (Craig, 1982).

To put it in another way: Whatever the borders were of the country called "Germany," they encompassed ethnic German regions that for centuries had existed as autonomous states. Germans to this day identify with their regional roots much more intensely than with the national state. The cultural, linguistic, and religious differences between people from the various German regions can be quite significant.

Furthermore, Swiss Germans, Austrians, people in Alsace, in the Czech Republic, in Poland, and in border regions also take part in German language and culture, even though they may have strong reactions if someone were to misidentify them as citizens of Germany. Some of the greatest writers in the German language are Swiss (G. Keller, M. Frisch, Fr. Dürrenmatt), Austrians (S. Freud, K. Kraus, A. Schnitzler, H. von Hoffmansthal, P. Handke), Czech (F. Kafka, M. Brod), or come from border regions (A. Schweitzer, G. Grass).

At the same time, the differences between regions that are now part of the (unified) German state can be stronger than the differences between neighboring regions of Germany and Switzerland or of Germany and Austria. Regional languages, family characteristics, and traditions are quite similar among Swiss Germans and the people in Southwest Germany or among people living in Bavaria (Germany) and Tyrol (Austria). To this day most Germans, Austrians, and Swiss speak regional "dialects" at home and with their friends that Germans from other areas may not easily understand. Bavarians, for example, who are predominantly Catholic, may speak a language and have a cuisine, climate, and local customs that are more similar to those of their Austrian neighbors in Tyrol than to those of their fellow Germans in the north (e.g., in Hamburg), who are primarily Protestants.

For the purpose of this chapter, historically, we have designated as Germans those whose ancestors came from the German-speaking regions of Central Europe, whether or not they were citizens of a German national state as a political entity. We include, therefore, Swiss Germans, Austrians, and people from the regions bordering Czechoslovakia, Poland, and Alsace, to name the most important.

The German Enlightenment and the hope, among prominent intellectuals and writers, for a Jewish–German cultural symbiosis led to an unprecedented peak in the intellectual, artistic, and scientific contributions of Germans, both Jewish and Christian. Yet the profound uneasiness of Jews in Germany continued below the surface. The grim reality gradually became obvious. In the early 19th century, the regional German states eventually coalesced into an authoritarian nationalistic society. Its Christian quasi–state religion barely concealed the Teutonic myths that served as an ideology of the new imperialistic state (1870/1871). The process of assimilation of many German Jews, although it meant prosperity, academic honors, and social status, became gradually a choice that foreshadowed the disaster to come. Either Jews adapted fully into the German society, giving up their religious and cultural identity, or they remained strangers in the land that they too considered their homeland such as the poets Ludwig Börne and Heinrich Heine (Craig, 1982).

At the beginning of the Crusades (1095–1254) thriving Jewish communities existed throughout the Holy Roman Empire. Prior to the Crusades, for the most part, Jews had lived harmoniously within the Christian majority population and were often respected and integrated into society, despite their different customs and religion. However, the pogroms and persecutions suffered during the era of the Crusades continued intermittently afterward, and the Jews became outcasts or second-class citizens within a religiously uniform society until the era of the Enlightenment of the mid 18th century.

Religious division among Germans originated in the Reformation of the early 16th century. Religious affiliation is relevant because Catholicism and Protestantism, the two dominant religions, have different values and traditions. Catholic Germans tend to be more tradition-oriented and guided by the authority of the Church, whereas Protestants put greater emphasis on individual responsibility and conscience. Religion was central to the family life of early settlers, especially for the Amish and Mennonites, whose cultural practices have largely endured. However, the relationships between religion, culture, and language in the dominant groups eventually declined. By 1916 only 11 % of the German Catholic parishes used the mother tongue exclusively. Protestant churches continued to use German in services and other activities, but many were unable to retain a pure ethnic character. Jews, as a religious and ethnic group (Chapter 48), were integral to German history. Because of the Jewish Holocaust, the place of Jews in Germany warrants a brief revi

The promise of the Enlightenment collapsed as the hidden hatred of the Jews and latent anti-Semitism surfaced during the late 19th century and during the social and economic upheavals after the "Great War" (1914–1918). Twelve years of Nazi terror and the Holocaust, in effect, ended the tragic history of the Jews in Germany (Sievers, 1977).

German Americans trace their roots to a collective cultural and national history that includes the Jews (Sievers, 1977; Tolzmann, 2000). Whether or not German Americans were then or are now aware of this history, it is part of their legacy and has powerfully determined their German identity.

Assimilation

"The very size of the German immigration, its religious, socioeconomic, and cultural heterogeneity, its skills, time of arrival and settlement patterns all combined to ensure a gradual process of acculturation and assimilation" (Conzen, 1980, p. 406). The process of assimilation was related to rivalries among ethnic groups. For example, Benjamin Franklin noted that Anglo Americans feared that Germans might become the dominant culture (see Chapter 1). Franklin believed that the English would absorb the Germans or be absorbed by them. To accelerate German absorption into the English population, he advocated intermarriage and the teaching of English in German schools. He was determined that the English culture would dominate (Morgan, 2002). Generations later, in the *New York Tribune*, Horace Greeley advocated the forced assimilation of all German groups. Views of this kind prompted state legislatures to institute educational programs designed to anglicize German children (Billigmeier, 1974). German Americans may wonder about the failure of their school history texts to identify prominent members of colonial society as German; most often, settlers were depicted as English despite the prominence of Germans among them.

German organizations gradually accommodated to the non-German environment simply to survive. Non-Germans were admitted into German American societies, particularly into the Turner Societies, which were attractive to many citizens because they offered wholesome family-oriented sports and other recreational activities (Hofmann, 2001). Transactions in these groups were soon conducted in English. There was, nevertheless, still a flourishing ethnic press and a highly developed network of clubs and organizations. But the experience of German American ethnicity was to change dramatically when the United States entered World War I.

The Two World Wars

The two world wars had a profound impact on the fate of the German culture in the United States. Xenophobia during World War I was intense. For German Americans, "Loyalty to the Kaiser or the Flag" became a familiar expression, often used to challenge their authenticity as U.S. citizens. Suppression of German language and a general "climate of harassment" led to "a ban on German-composed music, the renaming of persons, foods, and towns, vandalism, tarring and feathering, arrests for unpatriotic utterances, and even a lynching in Collinsville, Illinois, in April 1918. Public burnings of German books were frequent" (Conzen, 1980). This suppression of cultural identity appears in discussions with clients: An older couple described how their German American club was under FBI surveillance during World War I. This period was followed, in hardly more than a decade, by the Nazi era, during which thousands of German Americans were interned.

During World War II the German national character became associated with the enslavement and genocide of millions of people: Jews, gypsies, and homosexuals, among others. Germanic roots, therefore, were toned down and experienced only carefully and secretly. For those Germans who lived through World War II, and for members of subsequent generations, knowledge of war crimes became the subject of family secrets (Hegi, 1997). Ethnic origin for many German Americans may, therefore, be associated with a loss of ethnic pride.

After World War II, a new type of German American family evolved that shows different characteristics. As part of the exchange between Germany and the United States, German professional families, university students, or experts in various fields immigrate or reside for long periods in this country. They often identify with their German background, while they are open to U.S. culture. These families may feel more validated in their interest in retaining the language and customs of their German background. Modern communications and intercontinental travel allow these families to stay connected with relatives in Europe. The less conflicted identification with their ethnic heritage is facilitated by the positive relationship between the United States and Germany in the last 60 years.

Those who lived through World War II in Germany, as well as their children, may have a range of complex feelings about Germany's international aggression and the inhumane acts committed by Germans. All will have stories unique to their specific experiences (Karres, 2001; Neumann, 2002). Recent visitors or immigrants come from a postwar context in which feelings about World War II were shrouded in silence for a long time. It is important to consider that perspectives about the Jewish Holocaust, beyond agreement that acts of brutality were committed, will vary because of the cultural contexts in which they have been learned (Berghahn, Fohrmann, & Schneider, 2002). For recent immigrants, the therapeutic encounter can be inhibited by both the client's and the therapist's failure to deal with their personal responses to the events of World War II. For example, a therapist's failure to respect the idiosyncratic meaning of ethnic identity for each individual may easily inhibit his or her own curiosity-driven inquiry. In such an encounter, the German Americans' openness about the complexity of their struggle with their ethnic identity is likely to be inhibited. Jewish therapists who have not examined their feelings about citizens of the Third Reich can put the therapeutic encounter at greater risk. Silence in therapy about these issues is most likely pregnant with powerful emotions. Ursula Hegi, perhaps the most celebrated of contemporary German American novelists, wrote after hearing about a Holocaust documentary:

> I backed away, unable to speak—not because I didn't speak about The Holocaust, but because I thought of it so often, and because it was too terrible to talk about. I was still within the silence, though I wouldn't have defined it that way because I didn't understand the tenacity of that silence until I began to come out of it, until I could look at it from the outside much in the way an immigrant looks at her country of origin (1997, p. 14)

CHARACTERISTICS OF THE GERMAN NATIONAL HERITAGE

It is difficult to determine specific aspects of an individual's or group's "national character." We see German Americans as industrious people, who are often thrifty and frugal, very determined to better their own and their families' standard of living, often self-sacrificing to the point of subjugating their emotional well-being or their personal goals for the good of the family. Loyalty, reliability, working hard to the point of being driven, being able to persist in a chosen purpose, living an ordered life where everything has its place, being trustworthy, and a certain obsession with books, learning, and education are some of the values that characterize German Americans. Relaxed fun, carefree leisure devoted to conversations and relationships, pragmatism that can live with an imperfect and mysterious world, exuberance in the expressions of joy and happiness, respectful welcoming of others' differences even if they appear puzzling, patience with someone else's sense of time, humility and interpersonal tact, self-confidence without either a hidden sense of superiority or latent self-castigating guilt feelings are less represented among the traits German Americans may have brought with them from their ancestors in the "homeland." It bears mentioning again that these traits vary not only among individuals, but also according to the regional and religious cultural heritage individual German American families brought with them to the "new world."

Examining external factors may enhance the understanding of German cultural heritage. Geographically, Germany was confined within borders that allowed for little natural expansion. Craig (1982) talks of Germany as *das Land der Mitte*, the country in the middle, with pressures "felt on every side" (p. 17). German society was, therefore, highly structured. People learned to live together peacefully within a small area. Living in such proximity, people developed a need for clear, at times rigid, boundaries; complex social hierarchies helped to define personal territory. To this day, in Germany, the boundary that designates the interface between family unit and surrounding society is rather well defined. The homes of middle-class families are usually surrounded by a fence or bushes that delineate the property. In Germany, "yards tend to be well fenced; but fenced or not, they are sacred" (Hall, 1966, p. 135). This need for *Lebensraum*, space for living, was later exploited as a rationale for the expansionist policies of World War II.

The friendship patterns of middle-class families are clearly regulated (Salamon, 1977). There is a distinction between acquaintances and personal friends with whom more open and intimate relationships exist. For recent immigrants, therefore, social interactional styles in the United States may seem freeing and relaxed; for some, adaptation may be uncomfortable. Boundaries help protect a family's space. Privacy is highly valued. German politicians, for example, do not involve their families in public life. The family's inner circle is protected against intrusions from the outside that might endanger its members' well-being. Conflicts and emotional upheavals that are experienced as embarrassing can be contained within the family sphere, "where they belong." Inside the family, physical space is also clearly structured. In Germany, houses are solidly constructed; the doors are usually closed. At the dinner table, everyone takes an assigned place. Another characteristic trait of the German heritage is the polarity of emotional restraint and sentimentality. Affection, anger, and emotion are not expressed easily. What might be experienced as too explosive is contained by boundaries, structure, and emotional control. One is not encouraged to demonstrate feelings. Passions are repressed or sublimated in work or art. A very acceptable expression of emotion within the culture is the tradition of *Gemütlichkeit*, still found in homes of first- and second-generation German Americans, which provides a contrast to emotional restraint. There is no word in the English language that accurately renders the meaning of *Gemütlichkeit* (geniality, comfort, warmth). German Americans introduced it to the New World as their way of making themselves feel "at home": the experience of familiarity, emotional closeness, and fun.

GERMAN AMERICAN VALUES

Family Life

Among the diverse German immigrant groups, family life was highly valued; it was considered the source of mutual support and strength in times of crisis. A person's first loyalty was to the family. Often, particularly in rural areas, work and family life were integrated just as in the German "household family" of the 16th–18th centuries (Billigmeier, 1974; Weber-Kellermann, 1977). Even today, under different circumstances, the relationships between members of German American extended family systems are strong. German American families live apart from their extended families, yet there is emotional attachment. Children are expected to love their parents and to take care of them in their old age.

Work

The work ethic, manifested in a respect for thoroughness, solid craftsmanship, and attention to detail, was transplanted from the homeland to the New World. Others admired the German settlers' skills, diligence, and industriousness, particularly in farming. "No group of immigrants was more important than the Germans in introducing new methods of agricultural production" (Billigmeier, 1974). Germans were also noted for their technical abilities " . . . in every major field of manufacturing in every region of the country. Their contribution to the industrial development of the United States is extraordinary" (Billigmeier, 1974). Because a strong work ethic is still a source of pride and self-esteem, exploration of occupational responsibilities should be an integral part of therapy.

Education

An emphasis on education is the heritage of all German groups in the New World. Germans have made lasting contributions to education. The intellectually oriented "Forty-Eighters" spearheaded school reform and spread knowledge of European pedagogical theories. Margaretha Schurz, wife of the famous Carl Schurz, first developed the Kinder-garten in Wisconsin. German American parents underwent hardships and were willing to sacrifice to give their children a good education. Children in turn were expected to work hard and succeed in school.

FAMILY PATTERNS

Certain typical roles and relationships may still be discernible among German American subgroups. Family patterns differ, however, according to time of immigration, region of origin, economic class, religious affiliation, the extent to which the German culture has been supported in the area of settlement, as well as the impact of feminism and the over-all increase of women in the national workforce.

One cannot overestimate the importance of the difference in gender-determined roles (Hare-Mustin, 1987), nor of gender as a central aspect of family organization (Goldner, 1985). Before the social injustices inherent in ascribed gender roles were given voice, the roles of men and women in German American families were virtually unchallenged. Women worked hard and had no economic power. Historically, the family structure and the complementarity of the roles of men and women reflected the legacy from the home-land. The husband was the head of the household; his wife took his name, adopted his family and friends, and gained his social status. The early Pennsylvania German Ameri-cans (now called "Pennsylvania Dutch," after the Germans' word for themselves, *Deutsch*) assumed that a male-dominated social order was proper and that women had responsibilities in certain areas, which were called in their dialect, *kinner, kich 'n karrich* (in German: *Kinder, Küche und Kirche;* translated: children, kitchen, and church). The husband ran the farm, operated the mill, and concerned himself with economic enterprise (Parsons, 1976). Like his European counterpart, the German American father is de-scribed as sentimental and stern: Under the self-controlled, reserved, and sometimes strict attitude lay hidden intense sentiments, often experienced as overwhelming and poten-tially destructive. To this day we hear about German American fathers and grandfathers known for their use of corporal punishment. Rational, and somewhat distant, the father was less available to the children than their mother was. He was to be a diligent worker, provide for the material needs, and make the major decisions or ratify those of the cou-ple.

Among the early Pennsylvania Germans, women were respected for their hard work, dutifulness, and subservience, and their contributions were highly valued by their husbands. A wife's roles as cook, seamstress, nurse, laundress, baker, teacher, cloth maker, and supervisor of household production were respected. She "was the liv-ing example of frugality and duty in action" (Parsons, 1976). German women per-formed strenuous farm work, and their home-oriented position was highly adaptive for those with "family businesses" in both rural and urban settings (Kletzien, 1975; Weber-Kellermann, 1977).

In families of the late 19th and early 20th centuries, the wife's main sources of pride were a clean house and the neat appearance of her husband and children. She raised the children, with whom she was more involved than was her husband. The wife was the emotional power center of the family, although, to outward appearances, the leadership of the husband was not challenged.

Marital Complementarity

The marital relationship is characterized by the complementarity of a rational, dominant leader and an emotional, submissive nurturer. Reserved emotionally, the father can be quite sentimental. Mothers can also be seen as capable of leading the family. Because the mother's domain is the children and the household, she directs her task-oriented modus operandi to executing her responsibilities with optimum efficiency, a quality valued in the culture. A number of clients report that their German mothers take these responsibilities so seriously that they are constantly "behind you" (German: *hinterher*), picking up, organizing, and cleaning in a style that can be described as nonstop, hyper-task-oriented.

One young man tried desperately to explain to his German task-oriented mother how he felt about her critical attitude toward the way he and his wife reared their 3-year-old twin daughters. The mother's responses to her adult son were variations on the theme of "Just tell me what to do; tell me what to say." The mother, genuinely well meaning, repeatedly expressed her love for her son and granddaughters.

However, several sessions were needed, in which the son struggled to gain his mother's empathy and in which she worked very hard to put aside a purely task-based focus in order to hear that his frustration was less a criticism of her than a desire to deepen their connection at this new stage of the life cycle.

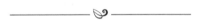

One of the tasks in therapy with distinctly German American families may be, therefore, to help them gain greater flexibility of role patterns and to increase the spectrum of acceptable responses. From a systemic perspective, we must consider not only the polar and complementary relationship of the marital partners, but also the entire family structure.

Family Relationships

Historically, infants and young children were raised with structure, limits on spatial exploration, and precise schedules. It is not unusual to encounter German families that do not characteristically encourage open expression of emotions. The overall family climate may be more favorable to tasks than to emotional expression. We encounter clients who describe their German parents' love as demonstrated through dedication to providing practical support and comforts to their children.

One woman described how her mother drove her to equestrian classes, was present when ribbons were earned and awarded, but never told her daughter how she felt about these accomplishments. Consequently, the daughter, although she knew her mother loved her, retained a gnawing feeling that her struggle to achieve was never quite enough.

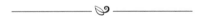

German American families may have difficulties making the transition from a family with small children who need to obey their parents, to a family with teenagers who need a different kind of guidance.

Fathers, in particular, may be unprepared when their authority is challenged by their adolescent offspring. One encounters in practice and in literature (Devereux,

Bronfenbrenner, & Suci, 1962; Koonen, 1974) descriptions reminiscent of Germanic fathers of renowned figures such as Mozart (Hildesheimer, 1982), Kafka (Kafka, 1954), Beethoven (Solomon, 1977; see also McGoldrick, 1995), and Thomas Mann (Heilbut, 1996). These men are experienced by their sons (or grandsons, as in Beethoven's case) as authoritarian and without apparent vulnerability. It is a popular myth that authoritarian fathers are inevitably violent. Domestic violence exists, of course, in all cultures (Levinson, 1989), and it is essential to be open to investigating physical abuse of power with all families and couples (Goldner, Penn, Sheinberg, & Walker, 1990). We have found no data, however, that German American families have a significantly higher number of violent fathers.

Nevertheless, German American families seem to rarely talk openly about the struggles of increasing autonomy for the children and of the pain of the separation process. If this phase of development is inadequately handled, the children may leave home and become emotionally cut off (Bowen, 1978) from their parents. The process of individuation and continuing relatedness (Stierlin, Rücker-Embden, Wetzel, & Wirsching, 1980) in German families can have an either–or quality to it. Parents or children may give up their contact with each other altogether, rather than experience the conflict of negotiating differences.

As with families of other cultures, it is essential to view German American ethnicity through a kaleidoscopic lens (Wetzel & Winawer, 2002) that includes a multiplicity of contextual perspectives within the broader sociocultural and political context. It is unclear at this point, for example, whether the occurrence of, or reaction to homosexuality differs within families of German origin. As same-sex relationships are marginalized in professional discourse (Green & Mitchell, 2002), heterosexual therapists, in particular, need to tend to gender identity as an important aspect of family life. Johnson and Keren (1998) recommend particular attention to issues of identity, gender, sexuality, and family construction. In addition, for same-sex parents, ethnicity, as well as sexual identity, may be central organizing factors in a family's emotional life. In treatment, conversations about "coming out" can be challenging for families of various ethnic backgrounds. German American families may respond with reticence, which should be understood as an initial response to relational stress that is culturally influenced, rather than as an absence of feeling. Recognition that the silence may mask powerful emotions can be pivotal in facilitating constructive dialogue.

REFLECTIONS ON GERMAN AMERICANS IN THERAPY

The diversity of German American families makes it difficult to categorize cultural aspects of these families' experience in therapy. The impressions presented here may help therapists organize their own inquiries.

Entering Therapy

For German families, coming to therapy violates a tacit rule: "Do it yourself." German Americans, therefore, come for treatment when they feel they have no alternative: The marriage is at risk or there is a serious symptom. Seeking help is often connected with a sense of failure; hard work, responsible behavior, and conscientiousness have not been sufficient. Mr. Klockner, a successful advertising executive, whose parents had immigrated from a small village in Bavaria, agreed to begin family therapy with his wife and two daughters only after his wife had initiated divorce proceedings. Discussing the drug habits of his younger daughter with an outsider meant admitting a personal fiasco.

The therapist who bypasses this reluctance in the initial phases of therapy may be unsuccessful in effectively engaging the family (Winawer-Steiner, 1981). It may be helpful to track the decision making about coming to therapy. The therapist may enter the family by exploring how it chose therapy and whether the decision was syntonic with the family's values. Careful inquiry can reveal and affirm the work the family may have already done, not only in its effort to resolve the problem, but also in deciding upon treatment.

The Initial Interview

A stranger does not enter a family abruptly. During the initial interview, there is often an air of emotional restraint.

When Mrs. Gruenewald finished describing her daughter's acting-out behavior, the rest of the family fell silent. The children sat motionless. Mr. Gruenewald shifted from one uncomfortable posture to another. The children answered questions monosyllabically. The therapist wondered if the children's parsimony was protective of the family. Not until the children's caution was described as loyalty to the family did the father begin to acknowledge that bringing his family to therapy had been an arduous decision.

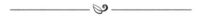

The therapist who is accustomed to an expressive interactional style need not be discouraged by this labored beginning. The Germanic style of forming relationships is generally more structured and includes a sequence of steps over time. Engagement is gradual, through stages, but once established, relationships are intense and lasting.

Reaction to Therapy

Once the therapist is invited into the family, German Americans are responsible about therapy and take it seriously. Therapy is a task that requires serious attention. Mrs. and Mr. Pohl, first-generation German Americans, often criticized each other at the beginning of a therapy session, each saying that the other had not taken up his or her "homework" during the past week. This does not mean that German families respond to a therapist's recommendations better than other families. Compliance with suggestions and automatic adherence to authority may mask ambivalence about a process that is too emotionally charged.

Therapeutic Styles

In a culture in which people are sensitive to clear, although at times subtle, hierarchies of power and authority, the therapeutic stance to which a German American family is likely to be most responsive is a balance of empathy and authority. The therapist is viewed as the expert, yet may find him- or herself quickly shut out if taking a too active position. Similarly, the automatic use of first names for adults may be considered unprofessional or disrespectful, as may therapeutic styles that emphasize physical contact beyond a hand-shake.

The Family in Treatment

As no single perspective can fit all German families, we have limited our discussion to one dimension: complementarily of marital and parental roles, a point of departure for exploring the distinctive organization of individual German families. In traditional German American families, gender-role complementarity and the adherence to the work ethic can be observed in therapy. Exploration of the role definitions over generations can enhance the work of therapy.

Mrs. Werner's mother and grandmother had very competently run their large Wisconsin family farm after both their husbands had died early. Now Mrs. Werner felt great relief when she understood her own tendency to "overorganize" within the much smaller context of suburban family life as part of her legacy.

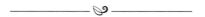

In a complementary system, a perspective that acknowledges the values of work and duty and allows respectful exploration of the complementarity of roles seems fitting. Understanding his function in the family can facilitate a father's readiness to engage in the therapeutic process. German mothers, like those in other ethnic groups, have been socialized to withhold expression of dissatisfaction with their roles. It is not unusual to meet a wife who, having adhered to her subservient role for years, harbors an enormous rage. Her awakening may be the shift that brings the family to therapy. If a way out of her submissive position is negotiated, she may be able to avoid covert or unconscious undermining of the father's authority.

After their three children had entered school age, the Mader parents, for whom their careers had always been important, decided that Mrs. Mader would pursue again her vocation as a graphic designer while Mr. Mader, a technical consultant, would take a pay cut, work from home, and be available for the children after their return from school.

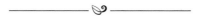

For German American families that stay within the context of fixed roles, the mother's expressiveness may be daunting for the father in his efforts to be more emotionally engaged. Supporting an increase in the father's contact with the children, for example, may be a slow and difficult process. Because he respects the knowledge and authority of the therapist and because he is work oriented, the father is likely to assume this challenge. Enlisting the mother's collaboration is, of course, essential for changes in the parents' complementary roles. Without the therapist's support, the mother may feel that her children will be unprotected. It is essential to understand the mother's voice as the emotional center of the family and as an asset to the process of therapy. Timely exploration of the implications of change for her own growth may be the first support she has received as an individual within the family arena.

In treating families of German American heritage, we may be struck by the apparent lack of expression of feelings despite the severity of problems. It is difficult to decide whether this is an indication of an individual family's need for privacy, emotional restraint, and stability or of their cultural training within a German American family system's legacy.

For Mr. Hoffmann, a breakthrough happened in the process of marital therapy and in his own ability to express his inner experiences when he finally decided to address what he considered his German father's incompetence and to speak with his father directly. Being able to empathize with his father's experience as a little boy, growing up on an impoverished homestead in rural Kansas without emotional nurturing, turned his life and marriage around.

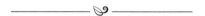

Attention to the confluence of the complex phenomena of ethnic identity within the relational context is reflected in the following treatment vignette:

Elizabeth and Michael Heinrich should have been taking pleasure in their retirement. Instead of enjoying their 70s, they were entrenched in what felt like constant bickering. They were not particularly interested in therapy and had never sought help before, but had come at the urging of their nephew, a physician. With some reticence, they described their current situation. Michael's extended hours in his woodshop were a source of irritation to Elizabeth, who would respond not only by reprimanding him, but by frequently vacuuming the basement area adjacent to his woodshop, followed by an inspection of the house to determine how much sawdust had spread as a result of his sawing and sanding.

When the therapist, who recognized their name, inquired if they were German, Michael responded that they were both German. The therapist was curious about the region of Germany from which they were descended. Michael brightened and became more talkative and spoke for the couple. Elizabeth's forebears had come to the United States as Hessian soldiers to fight George Washington and had remained in New Jersey ever since. Michael's ancestors were from Baden and had emigrated during the 19th century from the Black Forest area, a region known for its beautiful handcrafted cuckoo clocks. Michael had been to Germany once in his life, just a few years earlier, and had been struck by the aesthetic appeal of the woodcraft. He was now also struggling to learn German. When they remarked that they were Catholic, they added a comment about their disappointment with their son's engagement to a Jewish woman. The therapist noted that they might be able to discern from her accent that she (the therapist) was herself a Jew from New York. Michael was struck that a Jewish person would have taken such interest in his connection to Germany. The therapist was curious about why he would find her interest remarkable. He said that since the war and "what happened over there to the Jewish people . . . well, you know. . . . " When asked, Michael did not want to pursue the discussion about World War II, and the therapist respected his request and then shared a brief description of her personal and professional affiliations with German culture and language. At the end of the session Michael reached to shake hands with the therapist. Elizabeth smiled quietly; Michael said, "*Auf Wiedersehen*" and tried out a few other parting phrases in German.

In the continuing discussion of their family, they revealed that their first-born son had died in childhood, but that they didn't want to talk about it. Further exploration revealed that at about the time of their son's illness, both their mothers had been terminally ill and at the same time they were also caring for their younger son, then a toddler. The therapist listened and was moved. It seemed that they spoke a bit more about their lost son than they had intended to. The therapist responded, "How did you find the strength to get through such a trying period in your lives? " Elizabeth spoke of how "you just do what you have to do," and Michael spoke of how they had worked together and had support from his close-knit extended family. In subsequent sessions, the conversation drifted in and out of the themes of fear, illness, loss, and mourning, at a pace set by the couple. It was eventually revealed that Elizabeth, a cancer survivor, had been refusing to go to her follow-up medical appointments no matter how Michael implored her to do so. In despair, he would retreat to his workshop, where he made wooden Christmas scenes. His reconnection to his German roots and his woodworking were a great source of joy and comfort, especially when he felt worried about his wife. She experienced his retreats as abandonment, which increased her anxiety. Gradually, through conversation, Michael was able to express his worry and explain how the woodshop gave him peace. He acknowledged that he was very worried about his wife. The therapist wondered if he couldn't bear the thought of anything happening to her and that his workshop retreat helped him hide, not only from Elizabeth, but also from his own worry, because they had been through so much together, and because he loved her so deeply. Michael did not respond in words. He was speechless. He looked out the window and nodded, his face clearly showing his pain. Elizabeth saw his face. In that conversation, Elizabeth's fear of death and illness came more to the forefront of the conversation, and she soon after acquiesced to Michael's entreaties that she see her oncologist. The bickering greatly diminished almost immediately when they found that the cancer had not returned. Work in the woodshop and regular vacuuming continued, although with less intensity.

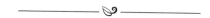

Ethnic Heritage as a Therapeutic Issue

The therapist who is interested in multigenerational issues will discover, with German American families, that it takes a while for members to discuss their memories and experiences of the German culture. The need to be cautious about their German background created in some families an uneasiness about their ethnic identity. As a result, attitudes toward their German heritage may have been left unexplored. Discomfort may also arise if the therapist belongs to a different ethnic group and has to face his or her own hidden prejudices.

Highly assimilated German Americans whose families have intermarried may have to be guided to articulate the specifics of their ethnic origins. In constructing a genogram, for example, generalized responses to inquiries about ethnicity are not uncommon for essentially "dominant culture" families: "Oh, our background is mixed, you know, English, Irish, German, maybe some French." Careful questioning may reveal a farm operated by several generations of the extended family who lived in a strongly German ethnic community, or a grandfather described as a "stubborn Prussian" who "was actually kind of hard on my mother." For many Germans, the negative stereotypes or the fear of being stigmatized have also been transmitted multigenerationally and can eclipse the revelation of more pleasant aspects of their heritage. In addition, pursuing the inquiry beyond one-dimensional constructs ("stubborn Prussian") that have been frozen in the family history can yield alternative descriptions. The son of a German Lutheran mother who herself grew up as an orphan in a rural German community in Pennsylvania overcame his depression after empathy with his obsessive mother's history became possible.

Newer immigrants may be culturally isolated and attracted to the relatively unstructured, loose, casual style of life in the United States as compared with the regulated, clearly delineated nature of contemporary Germany. The same freedom, however, may create difficulties with respect to the more flexible work environment, which can produce feelings of insecurity because of the sharp contrast to the German workplace, which is more predictable. The ethnically sensitive therapist should, therefore, be particularly attentive to signs of loss, not only as part of the immigration process, but also as related to an ethnic legacy that may have been suppressed, distorted, or forgotten (Hegi, 1997).

For the recently immigrated Pohls, a professional couple without children, their bickering and their clashes with colleagues at work ceased after they began to address their family background in Germany and the hidden legacies of their parents' experiences during and after World War II.

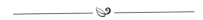

Intergenerational work with German Americans, genograms, coaching, family voyages, and guiding through operational mourning have been effective in coping with loss in the family context (Bowen, 1978; Paul & Paul, 1986). A review of the actual history and contributions of this influential ethnic group can be useful, particularly for German Americans who are ignorant of their rich legacy in this country.

SUMMARY

Therapists who work with German American families need to be aware of the social forces that affect the characteristics of particular German American family systems over time. Not the least of these characteristics are the changes in prominence of their culture in modern U.S. society as contrasted with the enormous richness of German American contributions at the foundations of our national heritage. We hope that these reflections stimulate therapists' inquiry and enhance conversations in clinical practice. We have sought to respect the historical and social complexity of the German American ethnic context and have offered information toward a contextually aware therapeutic collaboration with the unique individuals in families of German heritage in the United States.

REFERENCES

Berghahn, K. L., Fohrmann, J., & Schneider, H. J. (Eds.). (2002). *German life and civilization* (Vol. 38). New York: Peter Lang.

Billigmeier, R. H. (1974). *Americans from Germany: A study in cultural diversity.* Belmont, CA: Wadsworth.

Bowen, M. (1978). *Family therapy in clinical practice.* New York: Jason Aronson.

Conzen, K. N. (1980). Germans. In S. Thernstrom, A. Orlov, & O. Handlin (Eds.), *Harvard encyclopedia of American ethnic groups* (pp. 405–425). Cambridge, MA: Harvard University Press.

Craig, G. A. (1982). *The Germans.* New York: Putnam.

Devereux, E. C., Bronfenbrenner, U., & Suci, G. J. (1962). Patterns of parent behavior in the United States of America and the Federal Republic of Germany: A cross-national comparison. *International Social Science Journal, 14,* 488–506.

Gergen, K., & Davis, K. E. (1985). *The social construction of the person.* New York: Springer Verlag.

Goldner, V. (1985). Feminism and family therapy. *Family Process, 24,* 31–47.

Goldner, V., Penn, P., Sheinberg, M., & Walker, G. (1990). Love and violence: Gender paradoxes in volatile attachments. *Family Process, 29*(4), 343–364.

Green, R.-J., & Mitchell, V. (2002). Gay and lesbian couples in therapy: Homophobia, relational ambiguity, and social support. In A. S. Gurman & N. S. Jacobson (Eds.), *Clinical handbook of couple therapy* (3rd ed, pp. 546–568). New York: Guilford Press.

Hall, E. (1966). Proxemics in a cross-cultural context: Germans, English, and French. In E. Hall (Ed.), *The hidden dimension.* Garden City, NY: Doubleday.

Hare-Mustin, R. T. (1987) The problem of gender in family therapy theory. *Family Process, 26,* 15–28.

Hegi, U. (1997). *Tearing the silence: Being German in America.* New York: Simon & Schuster.

Heilbut, A. (1996). *Thomas Mann: Eros and literature.* New York: Knopf.

Hildesheimer, W. (1982). *Mozart.* New York: Farrar, Straus & Giroux.

Hofmann, A. R. (2001). Aufstieg und Niedergang des deutschen Turnens in den USA. *Reihe Sportwissenschaft* (Vol. 28). Schorndorf: Hofmann.

Johnson, T. W., & Keren, M. S. (1998). The families of lesbian women and gay men. In M. McGoldrick (Ed.), *Re-visioning family therapy: Race, culture, and gender in clinical practice* (pp. 320–329). New York: Guilford Press.

Kafka, F. (1954). *Dearest father.* New York: Schocken Books.

Karres, E.V. S. (2001). *A German tale: A girl surviving Hitler's legacy.* Fort Lee, NJ: Barricade Books.

Kletzien, H. H.(1975). *New Holstein.* New Holstein, WI: New Holstein Reporter Press.

Koonen, W. (1974). A note on the authoritarian German family. *Journal of Marriage and the Family, 35,* 634–636.

Levinson, D. (1989). *Family violence in cross cultural perspective.* Newbury Park, CA: Sage.

McGoldrick, M. (1995). *You can go home again: Reconnecting with your family.* New York: Norton.

Mitscherlich, A., & Mitscherlich, M. (1975). *The inability to mourn: Principles of collective behavior.* New York: Grove Press.

Morgan, E. S. (2002). *Benjamin Franklin.* New Haven, CT: Yale University Press.

Neumann, H. I. (2002). *Heroes from the attic: A gripping story of triumph.* Lincoln, NE: Writers Club Press.

Newman, N. (1999). Gleiche Rechte, gleiche Pflichten und gleiche Genüsse: Henry Albrecht's utopian vision of the Germania Musical Society. In W. D. Keel (Ed.), *Yearbook of German-American studies* (Vol. 34, pp. 83–110). Lawrence: University of Kansas Press.

Parsons, W. T. (1976). *Pennsylvania Dutch.* Boston: Twayne.

Paul, N., & Paul, B. (1986). *A marital puzzle.* New York: Gardner Press.

Phinney, J. S. (1996). When we talk about American ethnic groups, what do we mean? *American Psychologist, 51*(9), 918–927.

Pinderhughes, E. (1989). *Understanding race, ethnicity and power.* New York: Free Press.

Reichmann, E., & Reichmann, R. (1995). The Harmonists: Two points of view: A tribute to the 175th anniversary of New Harmony, Indiana. In E. Reichmann, L. J. Rippley, & J. Nagler (Eds.), *Emigration and settlement patterns of German communities in North America* (pp. 371–380). Indianapolis: Max Kade German-American Center, Indiana University–Purdue University.

Rippley, L. J. (1976). *The German Americans.* Boston: Twayne.

Salamon, S. (1977). Family bonds and friendship bonds: Japan and West Germany. *Journal of Marriage and the Family, 38,* 807–820.

Shenton, J. P., & Brown, G. (Eds.). (1976). *Ethnic groups in American life.* New York: Arno.

Sievers, L. (1977). *Juden in Deutschland. Die Geschichte einer 2000jährigen Tragödie.* Hamburg: Gruner & Jahr.

Solomon, M. (1977). *Beethoven.* New York: Schirmer Books.

Sowell, T. (1981). *Ethnic America: A history.* New York: Basic Books.

Stierlin, H., Rücker-Embden, I., Wetzel, N., & Wirsching, M. (1980). *The first interview with the family.* New York: Brunner/Mazel.

Szapocznik, J., & Kurtines, W. M. (1993). Family Psychology and cultural diversity. *American Psychologist, 48,* 400–407.

Tolzmann, D. H. (2000). *The German American experience.* Amherst, NY: Humanity Books.

U.S. Bureau of the Census. (2000). *2000 census of population.* Washington, DC: U.S. Government Printing Office.

Weber-Kellermann, I. (1977). *Die Deutsche Familie. Versuch einer Sozialgeschichte* [The German family. A social history]. Frankfurt, Germany: Suhrkamp.

Wetzel, N. A., & Winawer, H. (2002). School-based community family therapy for adolescents at risk. In F. W. Kaslow, R. F. Massey, & S. D. Massey (Eds.), *Comprehensive handbook of psychotherapy* (Vol. 3, pp. 205–230). New York: Wiley.

Winawer-Steiner, H. (1981). Getting started in family therapy: A preliminary guide for therapist, supervisor and administrator. In M. Dinoff & D. Jacobson (Eds.), *Neglected problems in community health* (pp. 275–293). University: University of Alabama Press.

Winawer, H., & Wetzel, N. (1982). German families. In M. McGoldrick, J. Giordano, & J. K. Pearce (Eds.), *Ethnicity and family therapy* (pp. 247–268). New York: Guilford Press.

CHAPTER 41

Greek Families

Kyle D. Killian
Anna M. Agathangelou

We are all Greeks.
Our laws, our literature, our religion,
our arts have their root in Greece.
—PERCY BYSSHE SHELLEY,
Preface, to "Hallas"

Percy Shelley's Western formulation of Greece shapes many stereotypical views about Greece and Greek. Official Hellenic history resonates with larger-than-life personalities and achievements. Ancient Greece, this history claims, is the cradle of democracy and the home of the first Olympic games and great philosophers (Socrates, Aristotle, and Plato, to name but three) and conquerors (e.g., Alexander the Great). Many of these Western historical discourses become part and parcel of Greek education and inform the self-understandings of Greeks worldwide, even at the expense of a more nuanced understanding of the Greeks, whose roots are as much embedded in the "East" as in the "West." For example, in his writing, Nikos Kazantzakis discusses the Eastern heritage that is part of his Greek identity (e.g., see *Report to Greco*, 1965). This author also brings to the fore another aspect of the Greek identity which is as essentialist, but challenges the traditional and stereotypical understanding of the rational and intellectual Western man, putting forward another kind of "man"—earthy, excitable, and passionate, who lives life in the present. In *Zorba the Greek* (1961), when Kazantzakis tells Zorba, "Teach me to dance," he is asking him to teach him how to live life, a life that is different from that of the Western rational man.

The acknowledgment of ancient Greek civilization the world over, and a legacy of its greatness, fuel an intense ethnonationalist pride exhibited by many modern-day Greeks. At the same time, an "orientalist"[1] view of the "modern" Greeks (e.g., that they are lazy; what have they done lately?) casts a long shadow over the Greek community today. Greek American writer and social satirist David Sedaris, who has internalized this Western orientalization, jokes, "The Greeks invented democracy and called it a day." Western discourses about Greeks being "oriental," as well as the struggles and humiliations of the Greeks at the hands of the Ottomans (e.g., the fall of Constantinople in 1453, the burning of Smyrna in 1922), the Nazi occupation in World War II, and their economic standing (e.g., as a less "productive" member within the current European Union) contribute to a feeling of frustration and not measuring up to Western standards. Greeks' social location, historically and today within the world economy, is ridden with apparent contradictions—a sense of pride and shame, haughtiness and inadequacy, intellectual curiosity and dichotomous, "either/or " thinking. This social location is even more complicated depending on whether one belongs to the working class or the owning class, and whether one is male or female, queer or heterosexual, "lighter" or "darker" along a global, racialized color line, and whether one is a recent arrival to the United States from Greece, Cyprus, or other countries or a first- or second-generation citizen. The positions that Greek colleagues, family members, and clients occupy are absolutely crucial in understanding their practices, and working together toward emancipatory social relations in the therapy room.

IMMIGRATION TO THE UNITED STATES

When crop failures destabilized the economy of Greece between 1890 and 1910, many families sent their sons to work in the United States. The plan was for these young men to earn money and then return to Greece, bringing with them the ability to acquire land and provide dowries for their sisters. Most of these immigrants had been raised in rural Greece and, arriving with few skills, found themselves working as laborers, shoe shiners, and dishwashers in major metropolitan areas such as New York, Baltimore, and Chicago. Some Greeks moved west to California, Utah, and Nevada to work on the railroads or in the mines. When war in the Balkans broke out between Greece and Turkey in 1912, 45,000 Greek American immigrants rushed home to fight. Following the war, most returned to the United States, abandoning the original plan to resettle in Greece. With the money they had saved, some of these immigrants established small businesses, such as grocery stores, diners, and bakeries. As their intentions to stay became clear, Greek women began to migrate, and, in turn, bringing the Greek cultural, religious, and social traditions with them. About a half-million Greek immigrants arrived in the United States between 1890 and 1917, constituting the "Great Wave" of migration (Moskos, 1989).

The period between the years 1924 and 1965 saw a decline in Greek immigration due to a tightening of U.S. laws to reduce the numbers of immigrants from Southern and Eastern European countries. Anglo immigrants from England and France were more highly valued than their "white but not quite" (Agathangelou, 2004) Southern and Eastern counterparts, who were deemed "swarthy" and undesirable by WASP standards. Those Greeks who did immigrate in this period tended to be more educated and professionally skilled than those who came earlier. The dismantling of the national quota system in the 1965 Immigration Act ushered in a "new" or "second wave" of immigration between 1966 and 1980, with about 160,000 more Greeks coming to the United States. There has been a decrease in the numbers of Greek immigrants in the past three decades. Most recent immigrants reside in New York City, and the community in Astoria, a neighborhood in the borough of Queens, has been among the largest Greek communities outside of Greece. Many Greeks now are migrating to the suburbs of New Jersey, a spatial relocation representing an upward shift in class.

RELIGIOUS AND CULTURAL TRADITIONS

Greeks are not a monolithic entity, and, as we suggested earlier, their social location informs their practices. More specifically, Greeks in the United States exhibit a diversity based on their particular families, countries of origin, class background, and conditions under which they migrated to this country. However, some common historical antecedents and broadly held ethnic practices are, nevertheless, organizing principles for how Greeks approach social relations at the systemic levels of the couple, the family, and the larger community. Subsequent generations of immigrant families have participated in and experienced transformations of hegemonic structures (e.g., world economy, changes in family relations), and, as "all white but not quite" peoples and communities, have borne the pressure to silence those parts, practices, and values that do not "fit" White bourgeois standards via assimilation and losing markers of Greekness (e.g., accent, language, change of last names to what are considered more Anglo-Saxon ones, etc.). And yet, particular Greek traditions (e.g., Greek Orthodox ones) have persisted in the Greek community, along with some adaptations to the U.S. context. (For an excellent account of how being Greek has varied depending on the many drafted constitutions since Greece became an independent state, see Dimoulis, 2000.)

The vast majority of Greeks in the United States are affiliated with the Greek Orthodox Church, and this institution, through the social and educational structure it provides, has become a primary site for Greek Americans to derive and sustain a sense of identity and community. As compared with other ethnic groups, Greek Americans are very focused on their origin and rigorously work toward reproducing cultural and religious traditions considered "Greek."[2] They tend to essentialize (in the sense that many resituate Greece as the nationalist center of strong family and community), on average, and consider divorce a major stigma. For example, partially because they must complete an extensive questionnaire before a Greek Orthodox bishop will agree to grant permission to divorce, as many as 75% of legally divorced Greek Americans are still married in the Greek Orthodox Church 5 years later.

Greeks depend on the church to meet their spiritual needs and to facilitate social networking. Major life events in the community, such as marriage, birth, and death, are marked by traditional religious rituals. For example, across the globe, a Greek Orthodox wedding lasts about an hour and has several common components: the blessing of gold rings, the lighting of candles, the crowning of the partners with *stephana* linked by a ribbon, scriptural readings, drinking from a single cup of wine, and three turns around a table in the front of the church, led by the priest, followed by a proclamation of marriage. Additional customs immediately preceding the service may include the bride's godfather shaving the groom and the couple's donning red sashes, symbolizing their chastity before marriage. Following the service, rituals may include the sewing of crucifixes of red fabric to the corners of the couple's mattress, children (usually male) being bounced on the mattress, and the dancing of the mattress (i.e., family members carry the newlywed's mattress around in a circle after the service—a practice especially followed by islanders, such as Greek Cypriots and Cretans). These practices are intended as blessings to the couple, specifically directed toward enhancing fertility. Additional traditions include the dancing of the money, in which family members and guests sew strings of currency to the spouses' garments as they dance together, bouzouki music, open circle dances, and the handing out of *koufeta* (sugar-covered almonds wrapped in white fabric) and wedding cookies.

The birth of children is greeted with a great deal of celebration in Greek families. Traditional gifts often include silver coins or a turquoise bead with a black eye in the center as an amulet to ward off the *kako mati*, or evil eye. Frequently, Greek parents honor earlier generations in the selection of names for their newborns, with a first son usually named after the paternal grandfather, second son after the maternal grandfather, first daughter for the paternal grandmother, and second daughter for the maternal grandmother. One of the seven sacraments of the Greek Orthodox church, Baptism, is performed within a year of birth. This involves immersion in a baptismal font and an anointing with holy oil by the priest and one of the child's godparents. Traditionally, godparents are the best man (*koumbaros*) and the matron of honor (*koumbara*) who were witnesses for the child's parents' wedding. If not immediate family members already, godparents become so, and are seen as responsible for facilitating the child's development. A family or community dinner usually follows the baptism, featuring dancing and the bestowing of gifts.

As the traditional keepers of hearth and home, Greek women are expected to work toward upholding the cultural values and rituals surrounding the domestic realm, which include taking care of the elders and the children and honoring the dead of the family. After the passing of a close family member, women are expected to wear black for at least 1 year (up to 3 years in traditional rural Greece) to honor the deceased. Very traditional widows from the home country may wear black until they remarry or die themselves. In contrast, Greek men are expected to wear a black armband for 40 days out of respect to a dead loved one. The funeral service at the church, which may include intense lamentations, usually expressed by female family members,[3] is attended by the larger community. A second memorial service 40 days later and annual (sometimes quarterly, in the first year) commemoration services are attended by family members and close friends.

FAMILY LIFE

Many Americans, including Greek Americans, enjoyed the depiction of a first-generation Greek American woman's and a WASP American man's courtship and wedding amid the bride's extensive, extended family in the 2002 movie *My Big Fat Greek Wedding*. An enormously popular comedy, this film serves up for consumption a distillation of ethnic archetypes taken from various Mediterranean countries, rolling them into one monolithic "Greek" family. For example, the Greek bride's brother and cousin come across like the stereotypical Sicilian, warning the American fiancé, "We're gonna kill ya," if he ever hurts her; the bride says that her mother always serves meals with a hot side of "guilt," evoking a dynamic familiar to persons from stereotypical Jewish or Catholic families, but not necessarily Greek—and so on. While recognizing the marketing value of offering a smorgasbord of cultural caricatures to an audience, the authors critique essentialist[4] constructions of the Greek family in two ways. First, such constructions perpetuate static stereotypes regarding orientalist gender roles (e.g., Greek women are "nags," Greek women are not afforded advanced education, etc.), and prejudiced orientalist attitudes toward "others" (e.g., the bride's grandmother calls her son "ugly Turk" and, still remembering the 1922 war, "sleeps with a knife under her pillow"), and the like. Second, such essentialist constructions give audiences—lay persons and helping professionals alike— license to make faulty generalizations about Greeks' identities, even though no single Greek family could exhibit all the characteristics and relations projected in the film. Therefore, therapists committed to cultural competence are advised to consume *critically* such stereotypical media depictions of power in social relations.

Gender Roles

Greek culture is patriarchal, and male individualism is a celebrated trait in both classic texts and in modern times. For example, even when many activities in the Greek community are centered on the family, the Greek men still see themselves as "individuals." "Greeks consciously view themselves as primarily individualistic in their interpersonal relations. A considerable amount of folklore reinforces this perception, and Greeks jokingly refer to self-importance as a Greek national trait" (Papajohn & Spiegel, 1975). Men enjoy the prerogative of having an active, independent social life outside the home, whereas women are expected to devote themselves to the roles of wife and mother to their children. In Greece and Cyprus, men on a daily, and often nightly, basis frequent local coffee houses (*kafeneia*) to discuss politics, social issues, and sports with their friends and neighbors, and Greek Americans may seek parallel spaces for social interaction with their male peers (e.g., sports bars). Although most Greek Americans worry about how they are perceived—"What will others think?" (Fiada, 1994)—this concern has circumscribed women's lives more powerfully, and narrowly, than those of men. For instance, a married man being dropped off at home by an opposite-sex colleague might raise an eyebrow in a Greek neighborhood, but it would most likely be written off as a harmless flirtation or forgivable dalliance. In contrast, a wife observed under the same circumstances might be accused of adultery by neighbors, family, and, thanks to the ever-active buzz of the grapevine, by her own husband.

As patriarch, the Greek man's authority in the family historically was rarely challenged. Wives are expected to support, ostensibly, their husbands' decisions on all matters, and public criticism of their husbands is anathema (Papajohn & Spiegel, 1975). However, as those primarily responsible for the educational and spiritual development of the children, mothers do hold some sway within the home. As Greeks and Greek Americans integrate liberal values (e.g., freedom) of the U.S. context, wives often have greater say in important decisions, such as in regard to where to live, major purchases, and with whom to socialize within the larger community.

Parent–Child Relations

A Greek father's patriarchal position over wife and children was typically unassailable, and power extended down the line of male family members from eldest to youngest. Traditionally, Greeks would tell how many children (*paidia*) they had, listing their sons, and then, almost as an afterthought, stating the number of daughters. As protector of the family's reputation, the Greek father experienced immense pride in his children's achievements and tremendous shame at their failures. Hence, he was motivated to monitor, even surveil, his children's activities lest the community learn of misbehaviors before they could be corrected. Despite a strong affective attachment between father and children, their relations were somewhat formal and have remained so over time. "Generational separations are sharp, and a son in his forties relates to his father with the same manifestations of respect expected of him as a child" (Papajohn & Spiegel, 1975, p. 182). Larger global forces such as the restructuring of the world economy affect reorganization of gendered, racial, and class relations, resulting in greater freedom of emotional expression for men and women regardless of generation.

Religious patriarchal ideologies assign tremendous value to motherhood in Greek culture, and mothers actively encourage young daughters to be involved in the rearing of younger siblings (Luca-Stolkin, 1999). Historically, Greek parents watched carefully to ensure that daughters remained chaste, as premarital sexual activity on their part would constitute a family shame (e.g., losing her value as a woman within a patriarchal context). In a classic double standard, Greek sons were expected to "sow their wild oats" and to gain sexual experience in any way they could. Consistent with a patriarchal system, sons are still preferred over daughters, in general, and women seem to internalize "meanings of value equated with maleness" (Luca-Stolkin, 1999, p. 177).

The family members who acculturate most quickly of all are the children, who, in the school system, are exposed to different customs, values, family forms, and ways of relating to siblings and parents (Tsemberis & Orfanos, 1996). Parents can be dismayed or angered by their children's ambivalence about sustaining some Greek practices, and children may be uncomfortable with the persistent "Greekness" of their parents in a context that values and prioritizes assimilation. As default caregivers and keepers of ethnoreligious tradition, women may feel a great deal of pressure to sustain the language, customs, and values of Greekness across the generation gap. Intergenerational pushes and pulls in regard to ethnic identity can be a source of tension, but this is a common phenomenon in immigrant families and by no means unique to Greeks.

Couple Relationships

The formality of relations observed between parents and children persist into the couple relationship. Historically, the open expression of affection in front of children was seen as inappropriate. Women rarely questioned their partners' decisions or abilities in the public context, even when they were wrong or inept. Greek American men, ideally, are "family minded" and committed to providing for their wives and children. Nevertheless, Greek American men and women who have internalized the value of capitalist-patriarchy[5] have often assumed that men's sexual drives are dictated by nature. Men explain their privilege to have extramarital affairs in terms of their "nature," which is to exploit each sexual opportunity as it presents itself. As one Greek islander put it, "Of course I go; if I didn't seize the opportunity, people would say that I was *slow* [an idiot]." As in many other cultures, Greek men have sex to produce the next generation and also just for fun, pleasure, or *kefi* (Loizos & Papataxiarchis, 1991). *Kefi* is "a state of pleasure wherein men transcend the pettiness of a life of calculation" (Loizos & Papataxiarchis, 1991, p. 17); it is "the spirit of desire," and "is spontaneous, ephemeral and individualistic" (Lazaridis, 2001, p. 76). The concept of *kefi* emerges from a capitalist-patriarchal Greek context featuring a *present* orientation in persons' relationship to time and a *subjugated to nature* orientation in their relationship to nature (Papajohn & Spiegel, 1975). Hence, persons of either sex who subscribe to the idea of *kefi* tend to live in the present and see "natural" drives as irresistible, at least *those of men*. *Kefi* also highlights a patriarchal split along sexual lines: Men may indulge in extracurricular sexual activities in the pursuit of sexual happiness as long as they do not divorce their wives or abandon their children. Women who participate in the fulfilling of these desires are often condemned (by both sexes) as "women of the road" (Magganas, 1994). Nevertheless, a wife may attribute a husband's extramarital affair to his being subject to "forces of nature." But Greek men rarely divorce the mothers of their children over a spontaneous affair.

Attitudes toward "Others"

Intermarriage

Greek intermarriage is common in the U.S. context, possibly facilitated by a strong motivation by Greeks to assimilate into North American supremacist White culture. Intermarriage is more the rule than the exception, though non-Greek Orthodox partners must be Christians to be married by a priest in the Greek Orthodox Church. Stephanopoulos (2001) reported that 62.5% of all marriages conducted within the churches of the Greek Orthodox Archdiocese are inter-Christian and/or intercultural. Overall, 80–90% of Greeks intermarry (www.demokritos.org/html/ANEMO-2.htm). There is some evidence that Greek Orthodox women who intermarry are very motivated to pass on their religious traditions, and that Greek Orthodox men who intermarry are more interested in passing on elements of their Hellenic history rather than their religious background (Joanides, Mayhew, & Mamalakis, 2002).

Other Ethnic Groups

Much has been made in book and film of the wounding of Greek ethnonationalist pride by the Ottomans and the Turks, and during polite conversation Greeks may ask guests to eschew the "T" word. Although Greeks have a thorough dislike of Turkey, conceived as an absorber or destroyer of ancestral cities, most harbor no ill will toward individual Turks. Territorial disputes complicate the relationships Greeks have with Albanians and Macedonians. Otherwise, few nations or peoples outside of Greece are targets of prejudice or enmity. Instead, Greeks tend to "keep it in the family," "reviling each other from province to province, from village to village, and island to island" (Fiada, 1994, p. 11).

Gays and Lesbians

Greeks have a variety of insults they use across situations, but an especially common way of putting down a man is to call him *pushti*, which is a vulgar, pejorative word for "homosexual." As in most societies, homophobia remains a big social problem, and there has been little consciousness raising with respect to the prevalence of homosexuality or protecting the rights of sexual minorities. Simultaneously, we can observe contradictions in Greek social relations in regard to gay, lesbian, and transgender relations. For example, when Greeks dance and celebrate they seem to suspend their fears and anxieties around homophobia. Most Greeks are quite comfortable fast-dancing with same-sex friends and family, and a Greek man may ask another man whom he has just met to dance, with no sexual intentions, at least not consciously. A form of homoeroticism is expressed at wedding receptions and clubs, but there is little to no room for a person to indicate explicitly that he or she is gay, lesbian, or transgendered in everyday Greek society.

IMPLICATIONS FOR THERAPY

In many cultures, somatic complaints or illnesses are seen as a more palatable or acceptable means of expressing psychological distress (Lee & Lu, 1989), and Greek culture is no exception (Luca-Stolkin, 1999; Samouilidis, 1978; Seremetakis, 1991). There is a common perception that psychological issues stem from genetics, implicating previous generations as sources of currently manifested difficulties. This belief may underlie Greek families' concealment of a member's psychological difficulties from the community. Thus, a Greek person exhibiting somatic symptoms may have considerable anxiety that he or she will be labeled "crazy" or unstable by the family or the professional. Because the community is small, and they fear that people will gossip about them, Greeks are loath to approach someone within the community for medical or psychological assistance and may consult with their priest first. Thus, Greeks and Greek Americans are more likely to seek psychological help from a non-Greek so that they will not be discovered by other Greeks seeing the same therapist. Helping professionals should first address the client's worries about how he or she will be viewed, as this sets the stage for a later exploration of the underlying sources of distress.

Greeks value families and the roles that members play in making them run "smoothly." They value their children highly, and their concern for their well-being (or, at least, good behavior) at home, at school, and in the larger community can become a motivation for seeking therapy services. Frequently seen problems of families include a child with school-related behavioral difficulties, a learning disability or developmental delay, or a body image problem. But such issues are often symptoms of a systemic problem, such as marital distress, and sometimes a family member, usually the mother, acknowledges that a child's behavior is really just a symptom of something else that is going on in the family system.

Assessment and Treatment

Assessment begins by gauging family members' fluency in English and degree of integration/resistance to the U.S. context. I (K. D. K.) often administer a 20-item questionnaire, the Index of Cultural Inclusion (Killian, 2006), which measures clients' thoughts and feelings about their cultural identity and their perception of how much their partners accept or value that identity, and a 48-item questionnaire, Cultural Assumptions and Beliefs (CAB; Killian, 2006), assessing family members' attitudes toward gender roles, emotional expressiveness, religiosity, orientation to time, intrusiveness, and individualism versus collectivism. Clients' scores on these subscales provide a quick indication of the degree to which family members hold similar values on important dimensions that have an immediate bearing on how they approach life. For example, an immigrant Greek husband and a third-generation Greek wife may be seen to have radically divergent worldviews and values, and this assessment helps therapists measure where the husband and wife stand early in the process. Similarly, the children of this couple may have very different ideas than their parents about the importance of religion, and even about "being Greek" in their daily lives. An additional assessment tool is the cultural genogram (Preli & Bernard, 1993), which can be used to delineate generational trends in education, socioeconomic status, gender roles, and issues of pride and shame for family members.

The therapist must maintain multiple partiality, finding ways to be a witness to everyone's position and contingent feelings, though not necessarily at the same time. As therapy begins, it is a good idea to show an understanding of and respect for the lineal relations and hierarchical family organization of traditional Greek families (Papajohn & Spiegel, 1975; Tsemberis & Orfanos, 1996) to reassure anxious parents. The therapist maintains authority, without taking it away from the parents, by being culturally sensitive and directive and providing alternative narratives to their narrowly punctuated one. Therapists may have to be diplomatic in how they tell younger family members that they understand the difficulties they are going through (e.g., wanting to date when immigrant parents have no such concept, wanting to stay out later than 10:00 P.M. with rigid curfews, etc.); therapists' joining with children and adolescents should be accomplished without undercutting their working alliance with the parents.

Nikos, a 45-year-old first-generation Greek American, and Artemis, a 43-year-old second-generation Greek American, are married and have three children, Mikael, 10, Anna, 6, and Maria, 4. Nikos owns and runs a successful restaurant in Astoria, and Artemis works as an executive assistant in a Manhattan law firm. Artemis is concerned that the children are losing their "ethnic" roots. They are refusing to speak any Greek, and this has been a source of conflict and tension, particularly on trips to Greece to visit the grandparents and extended family on both sides. Relatives blame Artemis for not making sure that the children are maintaining fluency in Greek and say that she has become so Americanized that she doesn't care at all about her ancestors and her culture. Here is an excerpt from their first therapy session:

> NIKOS: I am very busy earning a living. She, as the mother, should make sure that the children keep their language and culture. I realize that we are in America; it is difficult to use Greek all the time. But I think that she could insist that the kids respond in Greek rather than English.
>
> ARTEMIS: I speak to them constantly in Greek, but they always respond in English. They *understand* Greek, though. I can't believe that even my best cousins accuse me of not keeping up with Greek culture. We attend church, we go to family events.
>
> NIKOS: You did speak to them in Greek, but you did not find a *Greek-speaking* church. It would have helped them to hear Greek there and also mingle with the Greek community. I kept telling you to do that, and you said it was "too far." You see the results.
>
> ARTEMIS: Are you blaming me, too?
>
> NIKOS: (*Pauses.*) Yes and no. I guess that is the reason we are here.

A 45-year-old fifth-generation Anglo, the family therapist has done his homework and knows that his first task in working with this Greek family is to find ways to affirm the mother's views of the problem without taking her side against the father. Although the therapist must acknowledge that he is an outsider, he still may draw upon his power as an expert in the area of family relations without silencing the family's own "expertise" as a group that prioritizes family as the foremost unit of relations. Reframing symptoms and relational dynamics, especially for fathers (albeit recognizing that this strategy may reaffirm their privilege as patriarchs and encourage them to continue doing things in the way that is familiar to them), is an ongoing therapeutic task to keep family members engaged in the process. If Nikos feels blamed or criticized, he will probably drop out of therapy to protect his self-esteem or sense of being correct (a "proud Greek man"), but terribly misunderstood by the therapist who just does not "get" how Greek families prioritize what and when. Therapists should also keep in mind that Greek women often have much to gain in understanding and perhaps recognizing the contradictions of their social location in ingesting U.S. values of equality, independence, and individualism. At times some women can be more motivated to do so than men, whose unquestioned authority and power may begin to erode with the adoption of these "egalitarian" and individualist values. In the sibling subsystem, Mikael, Anna, and Maria probably have ingested major U.S. values more rapidly than their parents because of access to U.S. institutions and cultural resources (e.g., language and U.S. values such as freedom, efficiency, and independence). This phenomenon, combined with the developmental need of older children and adolescents for greater autonomy through an increase in boundary flexibility, can make for a challenging phase in the lives of Greek families. Mikael and Anna may see their parents as "old world" or "too ethnic,"[6] whereas Nikos and Artemis share, in a session, their concerns that their children are losing their Greek identity.

In this case, the initial assessment scores of Nikos and Artemis indicate that they are actually quite similar in their views on gender roles and religiosity, but differ significantly in their approach to community, with Nikos indicating more confidence in the helpfulness of their community and a stronger interest than Artemis[7] does in maintaining close ties with it. The therapist should open up space for making explicit the underlying conflicts in worldview. There may be conflicts about the partners' commitments to sustaining fidelity or loyalty to the beliefs and traditions with which they were raised (e.g., Greek, American, Greek American). The therapist may ask the clients to consider the possible consequences, favorable or unfavorable, productive or unproductive, for themselves and their relations to their respective communities (i.e., Greek, American, Greek American, gender, class, etc.) that might derive from each choice and course of action. What would it mean if they chose a course of action that did not take into account one of the Greek beliefs, such as the importance of community, and took a more insulated, individualist approach to family life? What would it mean if the family chose to address the issue of retaining their history by visiting Greece more frequently? How would this affect their children's sense of self as upper-middle class Greeks, as Americans, or as members of other communities? Would they be enriched by a clearer sense of their Greek history; would they experience frustration or discomfort with their limited skill in Greek and being labeled "the Americans" overseas?

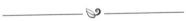

Conceptualizing the case within an ecosystemic framework (Auerswald, 1985; Falicov, 1995), the therapist takes seriously the sociohistorical and cultural contexts in which presenting problems are embedded. Implicitly and explicitly, the family has subscribed to an assimilationist approach (see Schlesinger, 1998), which views the retaining of a specific "cultural identity" other than the homogenized "North American" White identity as a "divisive threat" to "unity" in the United States. In becoming socially and professionally successful (rising on the social ladder), Nikos and Artemis have silenced, to some extent, their Greek background in order to fit into the White American culture. By making explicit the changing power relations between the family here in the United States and the relatives back in Greece, the therapist can help the clients engage the different feelings that emerge out of their negotiating two different worlds. Simultaneously, the therapist affirms their valuing of their Greek culture and history, as well as values such as community and connection with it, which helps maintain intergenerational continuity, and encourages the parents to draw upon their rich cultural traditions through ancestral storytelling, enrolling their children in a Greek language school, and renewing their efforts to attend Greek-language community events (e.g., festivals, religious services, etc.) together as a family. In addition, adopting a "both/and" approach, the therapist simultaneously reframes "acculturation" in terms of enrichment (e.g., opportunities for increased intimacy/sharing among family members, such as greater emotional expressiveness between father and children) instead of focusing solely on what might be lost or what is "old" and "ethnic." This move can ease anxiety and permit more active participation from all family members (i.e., the children) in the therapy process toward enrichment rather than feelings of loss or incompetency.

By acknowledging the ecosystemic axes of power (e.g., gender, race, class, ethnicity, age, etc., see Killian, 2001a, 2001b, 2001c), therapy can be a place where Greek families can be invited to undertake the "journey of Ithaca"; that is, coming to "know themselves" personally, systemically, institutionally, and culturally. Greek history and identity carry complexities, and Greek Americans can embark on a journey to discover who they are and where they are going. At the end of the day, they may realize that they have integrated "Greek" values crucial in their struggle against alienation and hegemonic power relations into their lives more than they had realized. Therapists can remind Greek families of the poet Constantine Cavafy's (1911) words about Ithaca, the process of change and development:

> Always keep Ithaca in your mind.
> To arrive there is your ultimate goal.
> But do not hurry the voyage at all.
> It is better to let it last for many years;
> and to anchor at the island when you are old,
> rich with all you have gained on the way. . . .

NOTES

1. The West views ethnic groups based in Eastern Europe and the Middle East as "oriental," that is, "other," inferior, even feminized. An orientalist discourse leads Greek persons, especially men, to silence the "Eastern" aspect of their culture and subjectivity and any facet of themselves that might be deemed other than heterosexual and "White." See Agathangelou (2004) for the investment Greeks have in "whiteness" even though they may never occupy that social location within a context that prioritizes White Anglo Saxon Protestant standards.
2. Who is "deemed properly Greek is neither unproblematic nor seamless" (Halkias, 2004, p. 72). Within Greece, these ideas are fast changing and thus, maintaining it as a stable and unchanged site of strong families and community is the equivalent of keeping notions of Whiteness intact.
3. Some Greek islander communities identify and choose specific women to express and perform the actions showing the pain of the family (Seremetakis, 1991).

4. *Essentialism* refers to the process by which people come to understand others (e.g., sexes, cultures, classes, etc.). In an essentialist worldview, groups (women, Greeks) are seen as monolithic and unchangeable, with observed traits construed as stemming from nature (i.e., biology, genetics, etc.).
5. Capitalist-patriarchy is a historically specific form of sexual, gendered class system of power in which the greater part of social resources are controlled by private, usually masculine (i.e., nonstate) owners relying and drawing on production/reproduction relations to accumulate profits as well as further privatize social resources in the hands of very few worldwide. Within this male, racial, and class hierarchical ordering of society, the capitalist-patriarchal system is preserved via marriage, the family, and other institutions.
6. "Old world" and "too ethnic" may be codes for the ways class plays itself out in this family system. As citizens of the United States with no accent and the "flexibility" of having already internalized American "White" ideals and middle-class values, these children may feel that they surpass their "too ethnic" previous generations and current extended family.
7. As a second-generation U.S. citizen with a professional position, Artemis, like her children, has an easier time distancing from the Greek community and history than Nikos, a first-generation Greek American whose family depended extensively on the Greek community, in both the United States and in Greece, to "move up" economically and socially.

REFERENCES

Agathangelou, A. M. (2004). *The global political economy of sex: Desire, violence, insecurity in Mediterranean nation states.* New York and London: Palgrave/Macmillan.
Auerswald, E. H. (1985). Thinking about thinking in family therapy. *Family Process, 24,* 1–12.
Dimoulis, D. (2000). Laos, ethnos kai polites stin elliniki syntagmatiki istoria tou 10ou aioha [The people, the nation, and citizens in Greek constitutional history of the nineteenth century.] *Thesis, 72,* 35–89.
Dwick, J. (Director). (2002). *My big fat Greek wedding* [Film]. (Available from Playtone Productions, Los Angeles, CA)
Falicov, C. (1995). Training to think culturally: A multidimensional comparative framework. *Family Process, 43,* 373–388.
Fiada, A. (1994). *Xenophobe's guide to the Greeks.* West Sussex, UK: Ravette.
Halkias, A. (2004). *The empty cradle of democracy: Sex, abortion, and nationalism in modern Greece.* Durham, NC: Duke University Press.
Joanides, C., Mayhew, M., & Mamalakis, P. M. (2002). Investigating inter-Christian and intercultural couples associated with the Greek Orthodox Archdiocese of America: A qualitative research project. *American Journal of Family Therapy, 30,* 373–383.
Kazantzakis, N. (1961). *Zorba the Greek* (C. Wildman, Trans.). London: Faber & Faber.
Kazantzakis, N. (1965). *Report to Greco* (P. A. Bien, Trans.). New York: Simon & Schuster.
Killian, K. D. (2001a). Crossing borders: Race, gender, and their intersections in interracial couples. *Journal of Feminist Family Therapy, 13,* 1–31.
Killian, K. D. (2001b). Differences making a difference: Cross-cultural interactions in supervisory relationships. *Journal of Feminist Family Therapy, 12,* 61–103.
Killian, K. D. (2001c). Reconstituting racial histories and identities: The narratives of interracial couples. *Journal of Marital and Family Therapy, 27,* 27–42.
Killian, K. D. (2006). *Crossing borders, transforming difference: Multiracial couples and families.* New York: Columbia University Press.
Lazaridis, G. (2001). Trafficking and prostitution: The growing exploitation of migrant women in Greece. *European Journal of Women's Studies, 8,* 67–102.

Lee, E., & Lu, F. (1989). Assessment and treatment of Asian-American survivors of mass violence. *Journal of Traumatic Stress, 2,* 93–120.

Loizos, P., & Papataxiarchis, E. (Eds.). (1991). *Contested identities: Gender and kinship in modern Greece.* Princeton, NJ: Princeton University Press.

Luca-Stolkin, M. (1999). Pandora's box: The shadow of femininity in the treatment of psycho-somatic distress. *Psychodynamic Counselling, 5,* 173–191.

Magganas, A. (Ed.). (1994). *Ta Ekdidomena Atoma. Pornia: Parekklisi h Paravasi* [*The issued persons: Prostitution: Deviation or infringement?*]. Athens: Papazisis.

Moskos, C. C. (1989). *Greek Americans: Struggle and success* (2nd ed.). Englewood Cliffs, NJ: Prentice-Hall.

Papajohn, J., & Spiegel, J. (1975). *Transactions in families.* Northvale, NJ: Jason Aronson.

Preli, R., & Bernard, J. M. (1993). Making multiculturalism relevant to majority culture graduate students. *Journal of Marital and Family Therapy, 9,* 5–169.

Samouilidis, L. (1978). Psychoanalytic vicissitudes in working with Greek patients. *American Journal of Psychoanalysis, 38*(3), 223–233.

Schlesinger, A. M. (1998). *The disuniting of America: Reflections on a multicultural society* (2nd ed.). New York: Norton.

Serematakis, N. (1991). *The last word: Women, death, and divination in Inner Mani.* Chicago: University of Chicago Press.

Stephanoploulos, N. (2001). *Greek Orthodox Archdiocese of America yearbook 2001.* New York: Greek Orthodox Archdiocese of America.

Tsemberis, S. J., & Orfanos, S. D. (1996). Greek families. In M. McGoldrick, J. Giordano, & J. K. Pearce (Eds.), *Ethnicity and family therapy* (2nd ed., pp. 517–529). New York: Guilford Press.

CHAPTER 42

Hungarian Families

Tracey A. Laszloffy

HISTORICAL OVERVIEW

According to anthropologists, archaeologists, and linguists, the origin of the Hungarian people is tied to the Hungarian language, known as Magyar. The Finno-Ugric roots of Magyar reveal that early Hungarians were Ugrians, a society of hunters and gatherers living along the slopes of the Ural mountains. Sometime during the 5th century a segment of Ugrians began a southwestwardly migration. During their journeys they encountered Turkic and Iranian tribes, whose influence led them to adopt a way of life as nomadic herdsman who relied on agriculture and animal breeding.

In 895, led by Prince Arpad, the Hungarians migrated into the Carpathian basin. This region, which was sparsely populated by tribes who spoke various Slavic languages, is the area the Magyars claimed as their home and is the site of modern-day Hungary.

Christian Europe looked upon the Hungarians as pagans, with a sense of dread and aversion. When Geza, grandson of Arpad, assumed leadership in 975, he recognized that Hungary's future within Europe would depend on establishing itself as a Christian nation. Therefore, Geza was the first Hungarian leader to promote widespread conversions to Christianity. Although he remained a pagan throughout his life, his legacy is that he had the foresight to baptize his son, Stephen, who was raised as a Christian. This decision proved pivotal, because Stephen grew to become Hungary's first Christian king, later canonized as St. Stephen by the church. He is credited with Christianizing Hungary and thereby ensuring the country's survival as a European nation-state for the next millennium. At the same time, however, this transformation marked the emergence of a dualistic tension within the Hungarian psyche between Eastern paganism and Western Christianity.

The alliance that St. Stephen formed with Rome and neighboring European powers, combined with his multicultural policies that encouraged foreigners to immigrate to Hungary, were stabilizing forces that contributed to the country's growth and prosperity for centuries. It was not until 350 years later, in 1241, that calamity struck with the Tartar invasion. Led by Batu Kahn, son of Genghis, the Tartars wielded a staggering blow against Hungary, marking the beginning of an 800-year pattern of oscillation between periods of stability and achievement on one hand, and crushing defeats on the other. After the Tartars, the next crisis occurred 300 years later when the Turks attacked Hungary in 1526. The ensuing Ottoman occupation lasted more than a century and a half, only to be followed by the failed War of Independence in 1848 that confirmed Austrian and Russian control. Following World War I, the brutal terms of the Treaty of Trianon resulted in the loss of a third of Hungary's land, and after World War II Hungary was frozen under four decades of Soviet dominance and communism. The blows that Hungary endured continued with the violent suppression of the revolution of 1956. The hardships and collective traumas endured by Hungarians throughout their history have fostered an underlying sense of pessimism, but also a tenacious resiliency, which are foundational components of Hungarian identity. Several other defining dimensions of Hungarian identity are discussed in the following section.

DIMENSIONS OF HUNGARIAN IDENTITY

The experiences, emotions, loyalties, and traits that underpin Hungarian identity tend to reflect an orientation toward dualism and the tension that is generated by the pull between extremes. This dualism is evident in many of the core dimensions of Hungarian identity.

Openness versus Isolationism

Rooted in a complex history of victories and defeats, one dimension of Hungarian identity is ambivalence toward foreigners (Lendvai, 2003). This is observable in the spirit of openness and welcoming, as well as suspicion and mistrust, toward outsiders. Underpinning these ambivalent feelings toward non-Hungarians is a dualistic split within the Hungarian psyche between Eastern paganism versus Western Christianity.

The aspect of the Hungarian people that is defined by their Eastern roots reflects their early history and the time when they were nomadic pagans, led by powerful warrior princes. The Eastern pagan aspect personifies the rugged self-sufficiency, unflinching bravery, and bold fierceness that inspired fear throughout Europe. During these early years, Hungarians responded to outsiders with suspicion and aggression. This constituent is in stark contrast to the other part of the Hungarian identity that emerged with the conversion to Christianity under St. Stephen and the ensuing multicultural policy that invited intermingling with other groups. St. Stephen actively welcomed foreign settlers, who brought their own unique customs and traditions that would eventually be integrated into Hungarian culture, thereby strengthening it. He believed that to have only one language and one set of cultural traditions indicated a level of insulation that bred cultural weakness and fragility. Hence, the ambivalence toward outsiders is linked to the East–West split within the Hungarian consciousness.

At different points during Hungarian history, openness toward and tolerance of non-Hungarians was encouraged and widespread emigration and assimilation of Slavs, Germans, southern Russians, Jews, and Poles into a broader Hungarian national identity was commonplace. At the same time, the many occasions when Hungary was the target of foreign invasion and occupation, while simultaneously being ignored and therefore abandoned by its European allies, resulted in a corresponding sense of being alone and a mistrust of outsiders. In reference to the Tartar invasion of 1241, for example, King Bela wrote to Pope Vincent IV, "We have received no support in our great application from any Christian ruler or nation in Europe" (as cited in Lendvai, 2003, p. 54). Again, in the 16th century, when Hungary was invaded and occupied by the Ottomans, it was forsaken by other Western European powers. "Hungary tried desperately to muster help through diplomatic letters and the personal entreaty of envoys sent to Rome, Venice, Vienna, and London. However, in the view of Pope Clement VII the Turks poised on the Danube were not the greatest enemy of faith, that was Martin Luther" (p. 90). Because Rome, like the rest of Western Europe, did not perceive the Turks as a direct threat, it failed to provide the requested aid to Hungary in its times of need. This abandonment by their supposed allies intensified a sense of alienation and isolation among the Hungarians and reinforced their suspicion and mistrust of all non-Hungarians. Hence, although Hungarians have at times welcomed outsiders warmly and embodied a spirit of openness, they have also been mistrustful of and guarded toward outsiders, only reinforcing the deeper sense of isolation and aloneness.

Emotionality

Hungarians tend to be highly emotional, with a propensity for rapid and unpredictable mood swings between the extremes of joy and despair/rage. Their joy is evident in the manner that Hungarians celebrate happy occasions with an almost feverish merriment and intense passion for living. The despair/rage is made evident by the fact that Hungarians have the highest annual suicide rate in the world (even among those who reside outside their country of origin), and in the all too common eruptions of volatility (Teleky, 1997). But it is the dramatic and erratic shifting between states of extreme joy and despair/rage that constitute the essence of the Hungarian temperament. This emotional constitution is reflected in the music of the famous Hungarian composer, Bela Bartok. His music has been described as alternating "between brooding depression and rousing peasant dances" (Wilson, 1977, p. 603), and Hungarian gypsy and folk music reflects the dramatic shifts between states of intense anguish and ecstasy. It has been suggested that Hungarians tend to exhibit high rates of manic depression, which appears to reflect an underlying cultural orientation that vacillates between a "deep rooted (nonreligious) pessimism [that] is often broken by sudden bursts of appetite for life" (Lukacs, 1988, p. 23).

Related to the strong emotionality associated with Hungarianness is a corresponding flair for the dramatic that is often expressed through art and entertainment. Among the more notable Hungarian artists are musical giants such as Bela Bartok, Zoltan Kodaly, and Erno Dohnanyi, as well as famed conductors like Sir George Solti, Fritz Reiner, George Szell, Antal Dorati, and Eugene Ormandy. Within the entertainment industry, names like William Fox, founder of the Twentieth Century Fox Corporation, and those of directors like George Cukor (*Casablanca*) and Sir Alexander Korda (*The Scarlett Pimpernel*) will be forever remembered. And who could forget the irrepressible entertainer Zsa Zsa Garbor, perhaps the most famous of Hungarian movie stars, who personifies the theatrical dimension of Hungarian identity? In these individuals one can observe the broader Hungarian orientation toward that which is dramatic, that which draws attention, and that which links emotionality with artistic creation.

Myth Making and Imagination

Hungarians have great imaginative skills that often culminate in the development of myths and legends that blur the line between fact and fantasy. For example, much of what is believed to be historical fact regarding the early history of the Hungarian people is shrouded in myth and legend. "The legend is not just one of the forms by which we can imagine, conceive of and experience history but the sole form. All of history is legend and myth, and as such the product of our intellectual ability: our sense of interpretation, creative capacity, our conception of the world" (Friedell, 1996, as cited in Lendvai, 2003, p. 16). For example, many Hungarians believe that they are descended from the Huns and therefore have ancestral ties to the great warrior Attila. Although the anthropological and linguistic evidence does not support this claim, the sheer number of Hungarian parents who have named their sons Attila demonstrates how this magical myth has been elevated to the status of historical truth.

The power of Hungarian imagination and its role in the process of mythmaking can also be observed in the popularly accepted account of when the Hungarians, guided by Prince Arpad, first entered the Carpathian basin in 895. The Hungarians are depicted as peaceful settlers who were welcomed by the native inhabitants, and the legend of the arrival is made all the more grand by the image of Prince Arpad poised atop a white horse at the edge of the Carpathian basin. Most Hungarian schoolchildren are exposed to this account in their history textbooks, and within the halls of the Budapest Parliament where a canvas hangs, illustrating this very scene in all its grandiosity. Conversely, Slavic history books depict the arrival of the Hungarians into the Carpathian basin as a tragedy of invasion and conquest, not a peaceful settlement. Yet in spite of the contrasting perceptions of this historical event, the legend of Prince Arpad peacefully settling the region from atop his white horse is regarded as a fact within the Hungarian historical record, thereby demonstrating the connection between the Hungarian imagination and the propensity for mythmaking.

Lendvai (2003) pointed out various ways that Hungarian imagination and adeptness at mythmaking have made it possible to reshape history and explain national catastrophes in simplistic terms of good versus evil. For example, to explain and rationalize the failure of the War of Independence in 1848, a popular story emerged that idolized Hungarian governor Lajos Kossuth and demonized Hungary's greatest general, Artur Gorgey. For a century and a half following the failed War of Independence, Hungarian history has portrayed Kossuth as a national hero who fought for independence, and Gorgey has been deemed a traitor whose personal ambition and greed sabotaged independence. This dualistic good/bad mythology offers a simple and comforting explanation for a painful defeat. Yet, as pointed out by historian Kosary (1994), there are dangers associated with "a primitive mythology of the Hungarian leaders fighting against each other as personifications of Good and Evil" (pp. 246–247). It glosses over the complexities of each man's personality and overlooks the complicated international factors associated with the failure of the war. Hence, the creation of good-versus-evil mythologies is a testimonial to the power of the Hungarian imagination, and it provides a simple, comforting means of rationalizing sorrowful defeats. At the same time, these mythologies blur the line between fact and fantasy and obscure a more honest appraisal of the complicated and painful aspects of Hungary's history.

IMMIGRATION TO THE UNITED STATES

Hungarian immigration to the United States occurred in several waves. The first major wave occurred during the early part of the 20th century until World War I. During this period approximately 1.7 million Hungarians immigrated to the United States (Teleky, 1997). Those who came were largely from peasant backgrounds, with few having attended school beyond the sixth grade. This group was economically motivated. The people came in search of financial opportunity and hoped to save enough to return to Hungary and improve their lives in their homeland. Most of these immigrants, however, never returned, but settled within the northeastern and northern Midwest regions of the United States. They tended to form small Hungarian cluster communities where they built churches and social clubs that enabled them to communicate in their mother tongue, worship together, and retain shared cultural traditions.

The second major wave of Hungarian immigration to the United States was primarily politically motivated, occurring during the post–World War II period and, in particular, following the Revolution of 1956. Although this group of immigrants was diverse in terms of socioeconomic status, educational background, and religion, most tended to be highly educated middle-class professionals (Vardy, 1985). Those who came during this period were more quickly assimilated into mainstream U.S. culture and therefore did not remain as deeply rooted in their Hungarian traditions, as had the previous wave of immigrants.

LANGUAGE

"Language maintenance is a necessary condition for the maintenance of ethnicity, though not a sufficient condition" (DeVries, 1990, p. 235). The Hungarian language, known as Magyar, has played a substantial role in preserving Hungarian culture and identity, which also reinforced a pervasive sense of isolation and alienation. It is a language that has little in common with the more easily recognized Indo-European languages, and because it is difficult to translate, it contributes simultaneously to a sense of cultural distinctiveness and isolation. The Hungarian language, wrote Esterhazy (1990), "[is] alien and strange even after translation. Out of joint. Its reference system is different; it doesn't use words in a 'leftist' or 'liberal' kind of way; it's more lyrical. I'd say masterly or masterless, but in any case highly personal—verbal bouquets for facts, metaphors for theories. And to make matters worse, we speak a language so personal that for the last forty years we haven't known who the person is" (p. 424). For Hungarian immigrants in America, the Magyar language has helped to preserve ties to their country and culture of origin, while simultaneously contributing to a sense of distance and alienation.

RELIGION

Following the Christianizing of Hungary under St. Stephen more than 1,000 years ago, most Hungarians today are Christian, of either the Roman Catholic faith or a denomination of the Protestant faith. The church has played an important role in supporting Hungarians who immigrated to the United States. Hungarian American immigrants gathered not only to worship together, but also to socialize and share familiar cultural traditions.

Jewish Hungarians have a variable history in Hungary. In the latter half of the 19th century Jews were afforded equal status within Hungarian society. They responded by fully embracing Hungarian culture in every sense. Because of their rapid and complete assimilation, Jewish Hungarians made many major contributions to the society as a whole. Unfortunately, rather than inspiring appreciation among non-Jewish Hungarians, this was often the basis for envy and a growing wave of anti-Semitism that reached its peak during World War II. The Hungarian collaboration with the Nazis resulted in a Hungarian Holocaust that was particularly brutal. Although Jewish Hungarian immigration to the United States began with small numbers during the mid-19th century, it increased dramatically in the mid-portion of the 20th century (Vardy, 1985). Of the Jewish Hungarians who immigrated to the United States, many, in their eagerness to assimilate into American society and learn English, tended to loose touch with their Hungarian roots.

IMPLICATIONS FOR THERAPY

Early on in therapy with clients of Hungarian ancestry, therapists should assess the history of their immigration and level of assimilation into U.S. society. Most Hungarian American clients are two to four generations removed from the ancestor(s) who immigrated to the United States, and it is likely that they will have little overt awareness of or association with Hungarian culture and how their ethnic roots have shaped them. Therefore, it is important for therapists to be aware of the core dimensions of Hungarian identity, so they are able to determine how these may shape clients' emotional dispositions, perceptual frameworks, and patterns of interaction. For instance, ambivalence toward outsiders is a common attribute. Although therapists may feel embraced and welcomed by these clients, they may also experience an underlying guardedness and mistrust that limits access into the clients' world. Those of Hungarian ancestry are also likely to be emotional and, in particular, likely to oscillate rapidly between extreme emotions such as joy and despair/rage. Correspondingly, therapists may note a flair for the dramatic and a tendency "to perform," at the same time detecting an underlying sense of alienation and aloneness. Therapists may also observe that clients of Hungarian ancestry are highly imaginative, which may be expressed through a tendency for mythmaking. This tendency does not usually involve outright fabrication of facts, but rather exaggeration or embellishment to make an occurrence more seductive and intriguing, or less negative and painful.

The following case example is offered to highlight real-life manifestations of the various concepts presented here by a family in therapy. The implications for therapists are also addressed.

The Kovac Family

The Kovac family included Sara, her two daughters, Beth (age 12) and Caroline (age 8), Sara's father, Michael, and her grandmother, Suzanna. Sara and her husband had divorced a year earlier, and he had recently moved from New York to California with his new wife.

Sara initiated therapy after Caroline's teacher alerted her that Caroline was telling "wild stories" to her classmates, which she was insisting were true. For example, she told several children that she had a magic umbrella that she used to fly to the Land of Little People, where she was a princess. Sara had also caught Caroline making up things at home, and she was concerned that her daughter's recent lack of truthfulness and her insistence on the veracity of her fantastic stories were a sign of an underlying emotional disturbance.

Initially, there were several things that were noteworthy about this family. First was their openness and apparent receptivity to the therapist and the therapy process, although on a deeper level, the therapist sensed the family was guarded and cautious about whether they could trust her. Second, each member of the family had a way of drawing attention to him- or herself. Beth was an accomplished ballet dancer and violinist who spoke passionately about her love of dance and music. Caroline wanted to be an actress, and her sense of drama radiated when she burst into reciting several lines she had learned for a role in an upcoming school play. Suzanna, who had a thick Hungarian accent, captured the attention of everyone in the room with her colorful and eccentric manner. Both Michael, a self-employed toy maker, and Sara, an interior decorator, also had a way of drawing attention with their wit and charisma.

During the joining phase, the therapist noted how lively and engaging the family was, and she was struck by how quickly that mood shifted when she asked Sara to say more about why she had initiated therapy. In a matter of moments, a sullenness descended upon the therapy room as Sara began to express her deep worry about her daughter. She was afraid that Caroline was psychologically disturbed. Moreover, she felt that it was her fault, that she had somehow failed her daughter. Given the intensity of the despair that had permeated the therapy room, the therapist was further surprised when the mood rapidly shifted yet again to a state of heightened liveliness. This occurred when the therapist called the session to an end and Michael noticed a Disney World magazine on an end table. This aroused immediate enthusiasm in the family about a trip they were planning there next year.

As noted by the therapist during supervision following the session, there was evidence that the family's ethnicity shaped their functioning to some degree and may have been shaping the dynamics in the presenting problem. The therapist wanted to tread lightly in this area because, based on her initial interview, she was aware that the Kovacs had little conscious, overt identification with their Hungarian roots. Suzanna and her husband, Ivan, had emigrated to the United States from Hungary in the 1920s. Although they had each retained strong ties to their Hungarian roots, including their speaking Hungarian with each other more often than English, they discouraged this among their children. They wanted them to be "Americans." Michael expressed deep regret at having never learned Hungarian and not knowing more about his ethnic roots. Like Michael, Sara neither spoke Hungarian nor actively thought about Hungarian culture; hence, she too had little conscious understanding of her ethnicity, which she considered a personal loss.

The Kovacs were several generations removed from Hungary, and the family system had been organized around denying and distancing from these roots. However, ethnicity is transmitted in both overt and covert ways, both implicitly as well as explicitly Even when earlier generations may have avoided teaching children about their ethnic roots, there is only so much that can be hidden or denied. In this case, the therapist was knowledgeable of Hungarian culture, and hence she detected that several family dynamics appeared to be linked to their Hungarian roots. For instance, she commented on the family's creative and dramatic nature, which she regarded as reflective of Hungarian culture. She also pointed out their emotionality, affective intensity, and the way they were capable of shifting rapidly from a state of elevated joviality to brooding sullenness. She further commented on the way the family appeared open and accepting of her, while at the same time she sensed an underlying guardedness and reserve.

The therapist was also mindful of the possible cultural dimension of Caroline's storytelling, namely, that she was reflecting the Hungarian imagination and tendency for mythmaking, especially as a way of distancing from painful realities. Accordingly, the therapist hypothesized that Caroline's storytelling might be a way for her to distance herself from something painful in her life.

What emerged in the subsequent therapy sessions affirmed the therapist's hypotheses. Upon sharing with the family members that she believed some of what they were dealing with was shaped by their Hungarian roots, they seemed intrigued. The therapist stated that Caroline, like her great-grandmother, possessed a wonderful creativity. The therapist directly linked this creativity to the many Hungarian artists, musicians, and writers who were blessed with the gift of imagination. She further explained that although stories, tales, and myths serve many purposes, within Hungarian culture she had noted a tendency to engage in mythmaking as a way of coping with painful realities. Having noted various ways in which the family seemed to manifest aspects of Hungarian identity, the therapist wondered about the possibility of Caroline's mythmaking being connected to something painful in her life that remained unresolved and was hard to talk about. The family appeared stunned by this proposal, yet they did not reject it.

After a long pause, Sara turned to Caroline and began talking with her about things that might be hurting her. Eventually, with the therapist's prompting, Sara raised the issue of the divorce and her husband's leaving. Although it took time, Caroline opened up and acknowledged her sadness about her father's absence, including her desire to "escape" from the pain she was feeling to a world of enchantment where she was a beloved princess. As Caroline began to talk openly for the first time about this difficult experience, her emotions of grief and pain began to flow, and her family was able to support her in this emotional release and the subsequent mourning process.

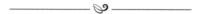

As several aspects of this case demonstrate, dimensions of Hungarian identity can shape and inform family dynamics in subtle ways. First, the Kovacs demonstrated a simultaneous openness and guardedness that were consistent with ambivalence toward outsiders. Second, the family members were highly emotional and prone to shifting dramatically between the extremes of joviality and despair. They also displayed a corresponding degree of drama, with each member able to skillfully command the attention of others. Third, with respect to Caroline's storytelling in school, the therapist related this to the Hungarian sense of imagination and the tendency to create myths as a way of rationalizing painful realities. Specifically, she wondered if Caroline was using her storytelling as a way of coping with the painful loss of her father and her subsequent unresolved grief.

CONCLUSION

The case study demonstrates how ethnicity may subtly influence the dynamics of a client family in ways that are ambiguous and hard to detect. The therapist's knowledge of Hungarian identity assisted her in determining how ethnicity contributed to the presenting problem and how the family functioned. More important, the mere act of acknowledging their Hungarian roots was affirming to the family members, and it strengthened the connection between the therapist and clients.

REFERENCES

De Vries, J. (1990). Lanugage and ethnicity: Canadian aspects. In P. S. Li (Ed.), *Race and ethnic relations in Canada* (p. 235). Toronto: Oxford University Press.

Esterhazy, P. (1990). God's hat. *Partisan Review, 57*(3), 424.

Kosary, D. (1994). *The huistory of the gorgery question.* Budapest: Szazadveg.

Lendvai, P. (2003). *The Hungarians: A thousand years of victory in defeat.* Princeton, NJ: Princeton University Press.

Lukacs, J. (1988). *Budapest 1900: A historical portrait of a city and its culture.* New York: Weidenfeld & Nicolson.

Teleky, R. (1997). *Hungarian rhapsodies.* Seattle: University of Washington Press.

Vardy, S. B. (1985). *The Hungarian Americans.* Boston: Twaynes.

Wilson, E. (1977). *Letters on literature and politics: 1912–1972.* New York: Farrar, Straus & Giroux.

CHAPTER 43

Irish Families

Monica McGoldrick

The Irish are a people of many paradoxes. While having a tremendous flair for bravado, they may inwardly assume that anything that goes wrong is the result of their sins. They are dreamers but also pragmatic, hard workers. They transformed themselves from rural peasants in Ireland into die-hard city dwellers in the United States. They are good-humored, charming, hospitable, and gregarious, but often avoid intimacy. They love a good time, which includes teasing, verbal word play, and sparring, yet are drawn to tragedy. Although always joking, they seem to struggle continuously against loneliness, depression, and silence, believing intensely that life will break your heart one day. Although they are known for fighting against all odds, the Irish have also had a strong sense of human powerlessness. As a legacy of their heritage, perhaps, they have placed great value on conformity, compliance, and respectability, and yet tend toward eccentricity. Their history is full of rebels and fighters. They have supported liberal democracy but also an authoritarian religion. They often feel profound shame about, and responsibility for, what goes wrong, yet they characteristically deny or project blame outward. They are typically clannish and place great stock in loyalty to their own, yet they often cut off relationships totally.

Discussing Irish characteristics honestly may leave them feeling exposed and vulnerable, but it will also, I hope, be reassuring by giving voice to experiences that have often not been validated. I have tried in this chapter to be sensitive to the Irish fear of being judged negatively, which has plagued them for centuries, and at the same time I have tried to help to move past the Irish tendency to cover over negative issues by joking or denying them.

THE IRISH DIASPORA

Many traditional Irish characteristics can be traced to the geography and history of Ireland, an island about the size of New Jersey located at the extreme western point of Europe; Ireland has much rainfall and few natural resources. For many centuries this "marginal" country was dominated and exploited by the British. Irish history has included starvation, humiliation, and heartbreak, on the one hand—and on the other, a remarkable adaptive ability to transform pain through humor, a fierce rebellious spirit, and the courage to survive.

The Irish diaspora since the mid 1800s has meant that although there are currently only about 5 million people living in Ireland itself, there are about 70 million people throughout the world with some Irish heritage; of these more than half, or about 44 million (one seventh of the population of the United States) claim some Irish ancestry (Gilfoyle, 2004), although many of these are Scots-Irish, described by Morris Taggart in Chapter 47. Separating the Catholic Irish from the Protestant Irish is, however, like most cultural categorizations, an oversimplification, because the Protestant Irish have influenced "Catholic" Irish culture profoundly. Many of those most often claimed as Irishmen were actually Protestant Irish: Yeats, Shaw, Wilde, Swift, Beckett, O'Casey, Synge, Lady Gregory, and Charles Stewart Parnell.

The discussion here focuses on families that were traditionally Irish Catholic, who generally formed a group apart from the Protestant Irish in culture and values (Biddle, 1976; Fanning, 2001). The large group of Irish Protestants, mostly Scots-Irish (see Chapter 47), who immigrated to the United States had been planted in Northern Ireland in the early 17th century and did not identify themselves as Irish; they had the highest rate of out-marrying of any ethnic group in the United States and tended to eschew any sense of ethnic identity (Fallows, 1979). For centuries the British controlled Ireland, turning Protestant against Catholic under a series of codes called the Penal Laws. Catholics could not attend school or serve in the military or civil service. By converting to Protestantism a son could disinherit all his brothers. Marrying a Catholic deprived a Protestant landowner of all his civil rights, and the rare Catholic Irishman who owned land was limited in the profit he could make and was forced by law to divide it among all his children rather than let the land remain whole (Ignatiev, 1995).

THE IRISH IN HISTORICAL CONTEXT

For centuries extreme poverty prevailed in Ireland. By the 19th century, rapid population increase, continual subdivision of the land, and exorbitantly high rents contributed to the overdependence of the Irish on potatoes, which had become almost their only food, leaving them extremely vulnerable to failures of the potato crop. Such failures were the major precipitant of the massive Irish immigration in the 1840s that led more than a million Irish peasants to immigrate in less than two decades (Kennedy, 1983; Scally, 1995). Indeed, there was plenty of grain raised in Ireland during the years of the famine, which could have fed the whole population, but the British controlled the crops and chose to export it, while the peasants died by the millions (Kinealy, 1995). The British leader of famine relief said the great evil was "not the physical evil of the famine, but the moral evil of the selfish, perverse, and turbulent character of the Irish people" (Miller & Wagner, 1995, p. 29). *The London Times* declared that Ireland's catastrophe was "a great blessing," offering the "valuable opportunity for settling" once and for all "the vexed question of Irish . . . discontent" (Miller & Wagner, 1995, p. 29).

No other country has given up a greater proportion of its population to the United States. And no other country has sent such a large percentage of single women as immigants (Diner, 1983; Nolan, 1989; Rossiter, 1993). In recent decades there was a new wave of immigrants from Ireland, many of whom came to the United States illegally, with little hope of changing their status. Like other groups of illegal immigrants, they had to rely on an informal work network and remain invisible within the larger society (Aroian, 1993).

Although many Irish Americans continued to demonstrate concern for the fate of Ireland, the majority of 19th-century Irish immigrants thought of themselves more as political exiles of British oppression than as immigrants seeking adventure or economic opportunity (Foster, 1988). They moved away from the history of oppression and suffering, and by the second generation thought of themselves primarily as Americans. Though they started out on the side of the oppressed in the United States, having been treated as an inferior race in their own country, they soon learned that they could redefine themselves as being of the dominant race in relation to people of color. They moved toward this redefinition of themselves as part of the dominant White group as quickly as they could (Ignatiev, 1995). Their experience varied widely according to the region in which they lived (Clark, 1988), but in general they adapted and flourished in the United States. They began to intermarry with other ethnic groups, although mostly with other Roman Catholics. Their Irishness was a sentimental part of their lives, and often they knew little of their heritage. Still, the Irish seem to have retained their cultural characteristics longer than most other ethnic groups (Greeley, 1977, 1981; Greeley & McCready, 1975), probably because assimilation did not require them to lose their language, which they had already had to give up generations earlier. Their values permitted the Irish to accommodate to U.S. society without giving up their deeply rooted culture, and Catholic schools run primarily by Irish nuns and priests transmitted Irish cultural values to generations of Irish American children, and even to non-Irish Catholic children.

THE CHURCH

For the Irish in the United States, just as in Ireland, the Catholic Church was the primary cultural and national unifier (Byron, 1999; Jacobson, 2002); unlike its place in the lives of other cultural groups, such as Italians, for whom family came first, for the Irish, the Church took precedence over the family. However, as McCaffery (2000) puts it, "Today Catholism no longer reigns as the core of their national or cultural identity" (p. 17), yet for generations after immigration the prejudice the Irish experienced in the United States drew the bonds between their religion and their ethnicity tighter. The role of the Church has deep significance in Irish history and Irish national identity. Early missionaries to Ireland, such as St. Patrick, established a strong Church, which developed a cultivated religious tradition that was the main source of culture for continental Europe from the 8th to the 10th centuries (Cahill, 1995). Later, amid the struggles with the British, religious loyalty became closely tied with the aspirations of the Irish to regain their freedom. Even in the United States, the parish rather than the neighborhood defined the Irish community for generations. Unfortunately, the Irish church came to be dominated by Jansenism, a mystical movement with a grim theology, emphasizing the evil and untrustworthy instincts of human beings, rigid asceticism, sexual repression, and glorification of self-mortification, which had been expelled from France. Isolated from external influences, the Irish Roman Catholic Church became rigid, authoritarian, and moralistic, teaching that human beings were by nature evil and deserved to suffer for their sins. Irish Catholics tend to struggle harder than many other groups with their sense of sin and guilt, trying to fit into the Church's rules and strictures. Even those who have left the Church may have intense feelings about religious issues.

The changes brought to the Roman Catholic Church by Vatican II were profound, allowing people for the first time to decide many issues for themselves. This was actually very stressful for many Irish Catholics, who were raised with the security that there was a clear, definite source of authority in their lives. Once anything about the Church could change, their whole foundation was shaken (Wills, 1971). This attitude has been profoundly affected by the recent sexual abuse scandals within the Church, which have taken a tremendous toll on many Irish Catholics, who so wanted to believe in the sanctity of the Church. Even when their faith has been shaken, the underlying rigidity has been hard to overcome. Indeed, for the Irish, the sense of their own sinfulness and inadequacy often lasts long after they have achieved the trappings of success, an internalization of the 500 years of foreign occupation and the contempt of their oppressors. This history has also figured prominently in their anxiety about what others think of them (Miller, 1985).

COMMUNICATION AND CONFLICT

For many centuries the Irish used their words to enrich a dismal reality. Indeed, they have more expressions for coloring reality with exaggeration and humor than any other ethnic group: blarney, malarkey, the gift of gab, blather, hooey, palaver, shenanigans, and "the craic," to name just a few. When clear speech could have meant their death, their tradition of verbal obfuscation was a crucial adaptive strategy, but the Irish raised this skill to a high art. They came to place great value on complex, even convoluted expression, mystification, and double entendre. African Americans developed a similarly rich and colorful language, also an adaptation to oppression, but their "double language" does not entail such ambiguity, perhaps because, unlike the Irish, they could more easily distinguish each other from their oppressors. Among the Irish, one could not tell whom to trust by looking at them.

The Irish way with words has always been their greatest natural resource, yet, paradoxically, they are often unable to express their inner emotions. For 2,000 years the poet has been the most highly valued member of Irish society, wit its greatest art form, and satire its most penetrating mode of attack. In ancient times poets were the only citizens allowed to move freely around Ireland, and by their spiritual power over the Irish imagination they, like the Church, contributed to the cultural unity of the country. Even today writers are the only members of Irish society exempt from paying taxes! The splendor of the ancient epics, in striking contrast to the relative simplicity of life indicated by archaelogical remains, indicates that the Irish have always used creative imagination to elaborate where the gifts of this world were lacking (Chadwick, 1970).

The inexpressiveness of the Irish in therapy may not reflect active resistance, but rather a blocking off of their emotions even from themselves. They may also fear being "pinned down" and may use mystifying language to avoid it—what the English call "talking Irish"—through verbal innuendo, ambiguity, and metaphor.

Although often viewed as a weakness, the tendency of the Irish to prefer fantasy over truth, and their ability to weave dreams, has undoubtedly been crucial to their survival for many centuries. They have valued fantasy and dreaming more, perhaps, than any other Western European culture. They have been shown to have a high tolerance for nonrealistic thinking compared to other groups (Wylan & Mintz, 1976; Zborowski, 1969). Even third-generation Irish in the United States have been more likely than others to turn frustrations into compensatory fantasy (Stein, 1971). In contrast to cultures that value the pursuit of truth, such as the Anglo or the Jewish, for the Irish clarification of feelings does not necessarily make them feel better. Thus, therapy aimed at opening up family feelings will often be unsuccessful.

Because the Irish have such difficulty in dealing directly with differences and conflicts, feelings tend to be submerged. Each person may end up feeling betrayed by the "disloyalty" of another without the issues ever having been expressed. Total loyalty is expected, but unlike the way it is viewed in other cultures, such as the Italian or Arab, where loyalty is overtly required, expectations of loyalty are almost never articulated. Hurt feelings and conflicts are left unexpressed and may linger unspoken for years, to the point where it becomes very hard to help them pull back from the extremes of buried pain and resentment, even though no one really remembers exactly what the issue is.

The Irish never had a cult of romantic love; pugnacity was a much more common theme than romance in Irish legends (Chadwick, 1970; Power, 1993). They have a well-deserved reputation for bravery and resourcefulness in fighting their enemies, even against great odds. The terms "fighting Irish" and "wild Irish temper" do not refer to the direct expression of anger within the family. Fighting was encouraged only against outsiders and for a just and moral cause, particularly religion or politics. Wit and sarcasm have long been the most powerful means of attack. In fact, the ancient Celts always began battle with a barrage of verbal abuse, and the entire struggle was occasionally determined by whose skill in verbal attack and ridicule was greater (Evans, 1957). But within the family, except under the guise of wit, ridicule, sarcasm, or other indirect humorous expression, hostility, pain, and anger are generally dealt with by silence. The punitive silence of disapproving relatives and a silent buildup of resentments often culminates in cutting off the relationship without a word—a form of social excommunication for interpersonal wrongdoing. When family members do explode in anger, and not under the influence of alcohol, it is generally experienced as extremely toxic for other family members, who are likely to feel completely unable to handle this degree of emotional reactivity.

HUMOR

Humor is the greatest resource of the Irish for dealing with life's problem. It offers a primary avenue for expression of forbidden feelings and allows for sharing of misfortune, and its indirectness softens the sting of an attack. Irish joking often has the same mystifying and double-binding character as other Irish verbal expression—it may be difficult for listeners to know whether to laugh along or whether they are the butt of the joke themselves. Although humor is a great resource of the Irish, in personal relationships it can be used as a way to distance, avoid pain, or put the other on guard. Unfortunately, the Irish ability to joke, tease, and ridicule with humor can at times block family members' closeness, leaving them emotionally isolated from each other.

ALCOHOL USE

Alcohol abuse has often been tolerated by the Irish as "a good man's weakness." Marion Rackard of the Irish National Alliance for Action on Alcohol recently commented, "There is no family in Ireland that is untouched by alcohol abuse" (quoted in Lavery, 2004). And, sadly, the same goes for Irish Americans. Thirteen percent of Irish personal expenditures are for alcohol, the highest percentage in Western Europe (Walsh, 1987), and the per capita Irish consumption of alcohol has risen 49% over the past 15 years (Lavery, 2004). Sixty percent of Irish 15- to 17-year-olds drink regularly, averaging about eight drinks on a "good night out" (Lavery, 2004). Not only do the Irish celebrate almost every conceivable occasion with alcohol, but they have often shown more interest in drink than in food (Bales, 1962). Indeed, their lack of attention to cuisine, even when they had ample resources, has been the source of many stereotypic jokes directed at the Irish. The Irish in Ireland have been changing this stereotype and Irish TV chefs draw much popular attention, but among the Irish in the United States the emphasis has been much more on drink than on food. This is undoubtedly a result of generations of near starvation. In fact, fasting has been regarded with almost superstitious awe by the Irish for centuries (Scherman, 1981), and outsiders have remarked on their sense of embarrassment at enjoying good food.

Using alcohol to achieve an altered state of consciousness has been a major cultural ritual, and alcohol has been seen as a solution to many problems (Bales, 1962). It dulls the pain, keeps out the cold, cures the fever, eases the grief, enlivens the celebration, allows the Irish all manner of expression, and even cures a hangover—"a hair of the dog that bit you" (Stivers, 1976). As one early group of ethnicity researchers put it, "It is remarkable that the Irish can find an outlet for so many forms of psychic conflict in this single form of escape" (Roberts & Myers, 1954, p. 762).

The Irish tend to use alcohol differently from some other cultures (Ablon, 1980; Johnson, 1989, 1991; Kaufman & Borders, 1988). Italians, for example, tend to drink primarily while eating, whereas the Irish do the opposite. They avoid drink when eating, because food diminishes the effect of the alcohol. Yet a high percentage of the Irish never drink. Noted Irish researcher Dermot Walsh (1987), has commented, "It may be that the Irish wherever they are have higher proportions of abstainers and of heavy drinkers than the British or Americans" (p. 118). Generations of Irish children were encouraged to "take the pledge," promising they would never touch alcohol. In Italy, in contrast, virtually every adult drinks regularly at mealtime. Children are gradually inducted into this practice as they mature.

Traditionally, the pub rather than the family table was the center of Irish life, a fact that had profound implications for the family system. Considerable alcohol use was tolerated, especially by men, without being seen as troublesome. Irish women are much less likely to be drinkers than Irish men, but they do drink more than women from other ethnic groups (Johnson, 1991), usually quietly, "sipping sherry," often at home or alone (Corrigan, 1980; Corrigan & Butler, 1991). When their drinking does get out of hand, it is considered extremely embarrassing for the family for various reasons, including the fact that women are always supposed to be the strong ones in the family. But drinking may also serve as a rebellion against the constraints of gender roles (Bepko & Krestan, 1983; Teahan, 1987). The male alcoholic cycle in an Irish family may correspond to the religious cycle of sin, shame, guilt, and repentance, allowing brief periods of emotional contact without threatening the rigid distances usually maintained within the family. The partner and counterpart of the "no good drunk" is, of course, the "sainted Irish mother," and when she drinks, she may be seeking to break out of the constraints of this impossible role.

Therapists should be cautioned to take a detailed alcohol history, even if the family does not present alcoholism as an issue, and to appreciate the degree to which the family may tolerate heavy drinking without labeling it a problem. Helping families integrate the behaviors their drinking has allowed without alcohol abuse may be especially important in work with the Irish, who tend to have rigid emotional splits between what behavior is allowed and what is considered intolerable. The structure of Alcoholics Anonymous (AA) is an excellent fit with Irish values, because it replicates the Irish reliance on a spiritual framework and the social functions of the pub as a communal hub away from the family. Indeed, the very idea of "anonymity" in AA, of openness with strangers as opposed to family, is an excellent fit with the Irish likelihood of telling much more to a companion in a bar than one would ever share with family members, which would be unlikely in Latin cultures in which relationships depend on personal connection.

SUFFERING, SHAME, AND GUILT

The Irish sense of individual shame and guilt often leads them to assume that their suffering is deserved. Conversely, they may feel uneasy if things go too well for too long. They find virtue and sanctity in suffering silently and alone, or in "offering up" their pain to God "in imitation of Christ." The few studies we have of ethnic differences in response to physical pain suggest that the Irish minimize their pain, show confusion and inaccuracy in describing it, have a high tolerance for pain, and prefer to suffer in silence. Compared with other European groups, they have been less likely to seek medical help, even when they obviously need it (Sanua, 1960; Sternbach & Tursky, 1965; Tursky & Sternbach, 1967; Zborowski, 1969; Zola, 1966), and they are less able to communicate with each other or their children about a child's illness (Fitzpatrick & Barry, 1990).

FAMILY PATTERNS

Men and Women

Interestingly, the Irish have traditionally allowed more room for women not to be mothers than many other cultures in which a woman without a family might have no role or status at all. There has long been a respected role for the unmarried "Auntie Mame," the feisty, independent, funny, and important contributor to family well-being. They are the only group in which the emigration of women to the United States far surpassed that of men. In the United States, as in Ireland, Irish women continued to be reluctant about marrying. They found employment in domestic work, nursing, and school teaching. And this characteristic, along with the high rate of desertion of Irish men from their families in the first generations, augmented female family authority. Clinically, we can strengthen women by underscoring and validating this appreciation for roles beyond mothering, helping single women to see themselves as part of a long tradition within Irish families.

The Irish have had a surprising number of female heroines and rulers, such as the wild, self-willed Queen Maeve. They have generally considered women to be morally superior to men. The Irish wife was often thought of as the brains, the manager, the savings bank, and the realist. Women often thought of men as needing to be carefully handled or manipulated. Women bore their responsibilities and burdens stoically, sometimes "offering them up" to God as atonement for their sins. Family researcher Theodore Lidz long ago described a pattern that still has some truth today:

> The Irish American child may grow up influenced by the mother's tendency to treat her husband like a grown-up child, pretending to believe the fabricated tales he tells her and admiring his ability to tell them; and while she seems to defer to her husband's authority, she holds the family reins tightly in her own hands, at the same time ceding to the Church a superordinate authority which must not be questioned. (1968, p. 52)

Sons might be pampered and protected much longer than daughters and in traditional Irish families were often called "boys" way into adulthood, probably largely because of their inability to find work that could support their independent functioning. A very high percentage of Irish men never married at all, and those who did were sometimes thought of as "married bachelors," more loyal to their mothers than to their wives (Connery, 1970). Ireland for a long time had the latest age and lowest rate of marriage of any nation in the world (Kennedy, 1983).

The traditional mother–son bond had no equal in intensity in Irish family relationships, not even marriage. Sons might remain within their mother's orbit, and their wives might be expected to go along with whatever was demanded by the mother-in-law.

Fathers in Irish families were traditionally shadowy or absent figures, and husbands dealt with wives primarily by avoidance. An early study of psychiatric patients suggested that Irish men tended to view women as the main source of anxiety and power, whereas others, Italians, for example, usually focused on the male (Opler & Singer, 1957; Singer & Opler, 1956). Although acculturation for many cultural groups has placed great strain on their traditional family ties and structure, life in America undoubtedly strengthened the Irish family by offering men more options to succeed in work and greater flexibility for relationships within the family. In the United States, Irish men moved first into the three P's: pubs, police work, and politics. Over time they became prominent lawyers and employees of civil service institutions, especially the FBI and other security agencies. They controlled the Democratic Party in most northern cities—New York, Boston, Chicago, and Philadelphia—for generations. Common personality patterns for Irish American men included the larger-than-life politico, who was a great joker and had enormous skills in social situations, but was still often unable to manage his close personal relationships. Often he had a wide social network of people who admired him greatly as the life of the party, while his wife and children feared his underlying anger and found him hard to get close to. Even his humor, which was such a strength outside the home, was often viewed as a painful source of sarcasm and humiliating jokes within the home. He might be highly opinionated, seething with righteous indignation, leavened by casual bigotry. Although they might have gone to church regularly and certainly would never miss a funeral, ethical slippage in the behavior of many Irish men, in relation to their political lives in particular, was hard to confront. Their wives, whose piety tended to be more extreme, tried not to ask questions and were generally kept at a distance from men's world. Of course, neither the indignation nor the bigotry was the exclusive domain of men. Irish women were also prone to these judgmental patterns, but in interpersonal interactions a wife of the Irish extrovert husband would be unlikely to challenge him directly, though her stress might lead her to be very tough on her children.

The Irish mother had a reputation for ruling the family with an iron fist, being the unquestioning transmitter of rigid Church authority, even though this patriarchal authority did so little for her. Irish women traditionally found their social life primarily through the Church, which, by its veneration of the Virgin Mary, reflected the Irish view of women as central and strong, while keeping them obedient to male domination as well. Irish women have always featured prominently in myth as mother/wife, goddess/hag, and queen/warrior (McCarthy, 1992).

Irish women have enjoyed comparatively more role flexibility than women in many other cultures. The Irish were the only group for which the rate of immigration of women was higher than that of men (Kennedy, 1983; Miller, 1985). Irish families often paid as much attention to the education of their daughters as of their sons, and there has been a large representation of Irish women in professional and white-collar jobs (Blessing, 1980; Diner, 1983).

Although Irish mothers have provided outstanding female role models of strong-minded, commanding, indomitable women, the stereotype of the "sainted Irish mother" is not totally positive (Diner, 1983; McGoldrick, 1989; McKenna, 1979; Rudd, 1984; Scheper-Hughes, 2001). She might be sanctimonious, preoccupied with the categories of right and wrong and with what the neighbors think, consciously withholding praise from her children for fear it would give them "swelled heads."

What can we make of these stereotypes of the Irish mother, who seems to be to blame for all sorts of problems—having contempt for her husband, spoiling her sons and binding them in a love from which they will never be free, while teaching her daughters to rely only on themselves, become overresponsible, and repeat these skewed patterns? We must take into account the very ancient tradition of Irish women, celebrated as formidable, tenacious, and powerful rulers since ancient times (MacCurtain & O'Corrain, 1978). This tradition must be combined with awareness of the 900-year history of Irish oppression, which systematically deprived Irish men of any sense of power. It was a life-and-death struggle for a woman to keep her family in line and to minimize the risk of their being singled out for further oppression. To blot out what was happening to them, men often turned to drink, which became institutionalized in the culture as an acceptable form of escape. Women were forced to run their families, and it is no wonder they turned to their sons with the dreams their beaten-down husbands could not fulfill. For solace, they turned to the Church. And they turned to their daughters to carry on with and after them. Even now they turn primarily to their daughters to care for them in their old age (Brewer, 2001).

The Irish may draw on idealized notions of Irish matriarchal traditions to find resilience in the face of hardship. Putting on a "brave face" in public, selflessness, and having a taste for the ironic and bittersweet consequences of sustaining intimate relationships all seem to inform the normative "Irish" approach to grief. Ortiz, Simmons, and Hinton (1999) described:

> I think to myself, "What if I was an Italian?" I'd be crying all the time. . . . Because, you know, the husband died four years ago, . . . I didn't wear black at my husband's funeral. I didn't cry

there. All my crying has been done. Every tear that I ever shed, I shed for him in my house. But I went . . . and sang songs and made his life a little happier, you know. That's the Irish in me. That's an Irish person, that you can leave your troubles at home and you believe in God and you go to church. (p. 486)

Irish women have generally had little expectation of or interest in being taken care of by a man. Their hopes have been articulated much less in romantic terms than in aspirations for self-sufficiency (Diner, 1983). They have always remained reluctant about the prospect of giving up their freedom and economic independence for marriage and family responsibilities. An Irish woman is likely to try to do it all herself and never ask for help. She may not expect to rely on a partner for either intimacy or contributing his share to the burdens of family life. This reflects, of course, a common gender assumption, but also a specifically Irish tendency not to articulate needs and feelings and to assume that if you are really loved, the other will know your feelings without having to be told. It is important to be nonblaming in working with the Irish because they are so strong in blaming themselves.

Sex, Love, and Intimacy

Because of their difficulty in dealing with feelings, the Irish have trouble in close relationships, especially marriage. They have placed less emphasis on marriage than many other cultures, romance not being a central concept, and partners have tended to resign themselves fairly frequently to emotionally distant relationships. The Church considered celibacy to be the highest state one could attain, and a much larger percentage of Irish men and women traditionally remained unmarried than in other cultures. For many, marriage was considered "permission to sin."

Given the rigid traditions of Irish Catholicism, sex has, perhaps not surprisingly, been referred to as "the lack of the Irish" (Messinger, 1971). Sex was for the purpose of procreation. A book entitled *Irish Manual on Human Sexuality* is filled with empty pages. Because of severe sanctions against sexual expression, the Irish also often avoid tenderness, affection, and intimacy. Irish distancing may be baffling or frustrating for spouses when Irish marry into more expressive groups. While the Irish may see distancing as merely the best temporary solution to interpersonal problems, spouses may see it as abandonment.

Irish couples may become emotionally isolated from each other, and the whole family atmosphere may become sullen, dour, and puritanically rigid. Divorce and affairs have always been less common among the Irish, although pregnancy prior to marriage has not been uncommon, because a moment of "sin and weakness" was less unacceptable than planning to have sex and taking precautions against pregnancy.

Homosexuality was strictly considered sinful, yet because the Irish leave so much unsaid, many families have had gay or lesbian members who were quite accepted by the family with their partners as long as they made no reference to their sexuality. Everyone knew, but nothing was said. When families are confronted more directly with the homosexuality of one of their members, there is usually much discomfort or even a cutoff. However, over time, family members can be coached to reconnect, and, perhaps because the Irish believe in "doing the right thing," they are often able to move to connections and acceptance that includes this knowledge, just as they have been doing in relation to divorce, abortion, and pregnancy outside marriage. Brendan Fay, a devout Catholic and one of the founders of the Irish Lesbian and Gay Organization (ILGO) established in 1990 in New York City, has said that as Irish gays and lesbians began to recover from invisibility, they discovered a "monster" in the prejudicial response from families and Church to their wish to participate in the St. Patrick's Day parade. They drew on their spirituality as they committed themselves to move beyond feeling ashamed of who they were. And they have persisted in their political efforts on behalf of those who will come after them (Menchin, 1993). This spiritual approach is characteristic of the Irish turning to their internal strength, which has helped them survive for centuries, and is a crucial resource for therapy with any Irish family.

Children

The Irish tend to view people moralistically as good or bad, strong or weak. The family often designates a good child and a bad one, and they may ignore aspects of a child's behavior that do not fit his or her designated role. In one Irish American family, for example, the mother always spoke about her three children as "My Denny, Poor Betty, and That Kathleen."

Ridicule, belittling, and shaming have played a major role in child discipline. (Barrabee & von Mering, 1953; Spiegel, 1971a, 1971b). In families where alcohol is abused, discipline is often inconsistent and harsh. However, in many families Irish mothers ruled so well that a mere look or even the thought of her disapproval would be enough to keep children in line.

Children in Irish American families are generally raised to be polite, respectable, obedient, and well behaved, and they would rarely dare to voice any resentment they might have of their mother, being both guilty and admiring of her stoic self-sacrifice (Hines et al., 1992). Typical familial injunctions included "What will the neighbors think?" "Don't make a scene," "That's a sin," or "You'll go to hell." Irish parents may rarely praise their children, fuss over them, or make them the center of attention for fear of spoiling them (Barrabee & von Mering, 1953). This strict and restrained attitude toward children may be very hard for a therapist from a more expressive culture to understand, just as it may be difficult for the Irish to understand other groups' permissiveness and encouragement of children to "show off" their talents, something which would be very uncommon among the Irish. Beyond the mother–son tie, family members tend to stick to their own sex and generation in forming relationships.

Extended Family

Extended family relationships among the Irish are often not close, although families may get together for "duty visits" on holidays and act jovial and "clannish." Family members tend not to rely on one another as a source of support, and when they have a problem, they may see it as an added burden and embarrassment if the family finds out. The sense of emotional isolation in Irish relationships is frequently a factor in symptom development and has important implications for therapy. Although siblings may meet for holidays out of a sense of loyalty, they may lack closeness, often because of unexpressed resentment. Family members may act pleasant and humorous, but any emotional exposure to outsiders may be felt as a severe breach of family rules. Older, unmarried relatives may be totally out of contact or may form isolated units of siblings or parent and child, who maintain almost no communication with other parts of the family. Typically, one extended family member (usually a woman) is of central importance for the family. It may be essential to get the support of this matriarch, most often a grandmother or senior maiden aunt, if therapeutic progress is to be made.

The Irish have a tremendous respect for personal boundaries and are enormously sensitive to each other's right to privacy; they will make strong efforts not to impose or intrude on one another. In older age they tend to have a more independent, active view of themselves than the elderly of some other ethnic backgrounds (Cohler & Lieberman, 1979).

Death and the Family Life Cycle

The Irish have considered death the most significant life-cycle transition (McGoldrick et al., 2004), and family members would go to great lengths to give the dead person "a good send-off." They accepted death as a natural continuation of life—in fact, a release from this world's suffering—and drink, music, prayer, and humor were never far away from a funeral (Donnelly, 1999). They have made it a point to attend all wakes and funerals of family members and friends, sparing no expense for drink and other arrangements, even if they have very little money. Even those who are estranged are expected to show up at the wakes and funerals, which can be important occasions for reconciliation even after years of cutoff, which is, unfortunately, a common problem among the Irish (Dezell, 2000). The joking Irish marriage proposal, "How'd you like to be buried with my people?" reflects this emphasis. The Irish think a lot about their own funerals, often encouraging others to plan for a good celebration. Unlike families that openly grieve at funerals, the Irish are much more likely to get drunk, tell jokes and stories, and relate to the wake as a kind of party, reflecting their belief that death brings release to a better world in the afterlife. The peculiar mix of celebration and sorrow that marked Irish wakes stood as testimony to the deprivation suffered by the living and the freedom enjoyed by the departed.

The last thing one would want is to have a "boring" funeral, and the best thing one can say about a "successful" Irish wake is that the deceased would have really enjoyed it. "Wouldn't Pat have loved it! Too bad he can't be here to enjoy it with us." Although most educated Irish would deny any belief in ghosts, there may still be a corner of their minds in which such beliefs persist. There may be joking about whether the corpse is really dead, as well as superstitions about what caused the death and what else must be done so that the "soul of the departed will rest in peace." It was after all, the Irish, who invented Halloween, a night when the dead walk the earth and play tricks on the living. The Irish have a long history of beliefs in all sorts of spirits: leprechauns, banshees, pookahs, fairies. They often believe that the dead can see us and that unless the living behave in the right way, their spirits are restless or disapproving. They may be reluctant to admit such beliefs, even to themselves, and it requires considerable patience and sensitivity to sit with them until they have enough trust to talk about what they are feeling. Such discussion does not come easily to them.

Clinically, the greatest difficulty is that family members are often unable to share their pain about a loss at all, especially where their feelings for the deceased are complicated by hurt or anger. Frank McCourt (1999) wrote of his parents' deaths:

Why should I fly to Belfast to the funeral of a man who went off to work in England and drank every penny of his wages? If my mother were alive . . . she might not go to the funeral herself, but she'd tell me to go. She'd say no matter what he did to us he had the weakness, the curse of the race. . . . She'd say he wasn't the worst in the world and who are we to judge, that's what God is for. . . .

How could there be sorrow with my father shrunken there in the coffin, . . . in a fancy black suit with a little white silken bow tie he would have scorned, all this giving me the sudden impression I was looking at a seagull so that I shook with spasms of silent laughter so hard that all assembled . . . must have been convinced I was overcome with a grief beyond control. . . .

We had tea and sandwiches and Phil brought out a bottle of whiskey to start the stories and the songs for there's nothing else to do the day you bury your dead.

The year my father died, we brought my mother's ashes to her last resting place, . . . outside Limerick City. . . . We had lunch at a pub along the road to Ballinacurra and you'd never know from the way we ate and drank and laughed that we'd scattered our mother who was once a grand dancer at the Wembley Hall and known to one and all for the way she sang a good song, oh, if she could only catch her breath. (pp. 598–599)

It is important in therapy to protect family members who want to deal with their feelings of loss so that they do not intensify the anxiety of, or precipitate rejection by, others in the family. Among the Irish, negative feelings toward the deceased are especially difficult to deal with.

One young man, whose mother had died when he was 14, was troubled by her being treated as a saint by his father and older siblings. His own memories of his mother were of someone who was harsh, cold, and distant. When he finally got up the courage to talk to his father about these memories, the father's response was, "God and your mother will forgive you for what you are saying." Therapeutically, it was important to allow the son room for his feelings at the same time that it was necessary to be empathic with the father's need to idealize his wife. Interestingly, 2 weeks after the son brought up the idea that perhaps his mother was not a saint, the father began dating for the first time since the wife's death 5 years earlier.

EMIGRATION, THE FAMINE, AND THE "IRISH WAKE"

The Irish are perhaps the only culture to have a ritual around emigration, which has been referred to as an "American wake," and for which all the rites of death were observed, including the custom of staying with the departing person all night before the departure, just as they "waked" a corpse with all-night vigils from time of death until burial (Metress, 1990; Neville, 2000). Like the wake for the dead, the American wake involved public participation, allowing the family and community to grieve over the loss. Attendance reaffirmed family and group ties.

Although those who remained held a wake for those who left, the hidden history of the Irish famine and the pain of loss seem somewhere hidden in the memory of every Irish American family. The cultural trauma of the Irish famine of the 1840s was the stimulus for immigration for many Irish families. The genocide and emigration of millions of the

Irish peasants of that generation seems to have left its imprint on Irish families for generations (Hayden, 1998, 2001). Nuala O'Faolain puts it thus:

> My father was angry nearly all the time and my mother just went around in a silent bubble. I didn't know why they bothered to have children. So I put the two things together, home and the Famine and I used to wonder whether something that had happened more than a hundred years ago, and that was almost forgotten, could have been so terrible that it knocked all the happiness out of people. . . . The trauma must be deep in the genetic material of which I was made. I cannot forget it, I thought, yet I have no memory of it. (2001, pp. 5, 73)

IRISH AMERICANS IN THERAPY

The Irish are likely to view therapy as similar to confession, in which you tell your sins and seek forgiveness. They may not understand their feelings and will certainly be embarrassed to admit them. This creates a dilemma for the therapist, since, on one hand, family members fear that the therapist will see through them, which is very embarrassing, or, on the other hand, that the therapist won't understand what is really bothering them and they might have to explain it, which is worse. Irish clients often take a "one-down" position, seeing authority as vested in the therapist. Whereas clients from other backgrounds may be quick to demand that plans be made to suit their convenience or that the therapist solve their problems, the Irish may have enormous difficulty with such self-assertions.

Their basic belief is that problems are a private matter between themselves and God, which has made them unlikely to seek or expect help when they have trouble (Sanua, 1960; Zborowski, 1969; Zola, 1966), preferring to suffer alone, although this pattern has fortunately been changing in recent times (Cleary & Demone, 1988). The Irish are embarrassed to have a problem and more embarrassed to let anyone know about it, especially a family member (Zborowski (1969). Similarly, their traditional solution to marital problems was silent withdrawal, distance, or separation, and for problems in family business, to define separate spheres of operation for different family members (McGoldrick & Troast, 1994). For couples, learning how to separate without cutoff and bitterness has been shown to make a major difference in their relationships (Murphy, 1988).

When the Irish do admit something is wrong, they are unlikely to exaggerate. They are embarrassed to have to come to therapy, and until recently have usually done so only at the suggestion of a third party, such as a school, a doctor, or the court. A Boston study of ethnic groups indicated that although the Irish were the least likely to report problems, they were the most likely to seek help for problems they did acknowledge, especially related to alcohol (Cleary & Demone, 1988). Given their traditionally low expectations for happiness in this life, they may also not expect that much change is possible. Trying to talk the Irish out of their sense of guilt and the need to suffer is a futile effort, because they believe that sooner or later they will have to pay for their sins. Unlike Jews, for whom the very experience of shared suffering is meaningful, the Irish believe in suffering alone. Certain strategies may, however, help them limit their guilt and suffering, such as ritualizing it within restricted time intervals (McGoldrick & Pearce, 1981).

As a general rule, structured therapy, focused specifically on the presenting problem, will be the least threatening and most helpful to Irish clients. Strategies for opening communication that preserve the boundaries of individual privacy, such as Bowen therapy, can be preferable to bringing the entire family drama into a therapy session. Whereas large-family sessions that draw on the resources of the whole family may be supportive for some groups, for the Irish they may raise anxiety to a toxic level, leading to denial and embarrassed humor, to cover over their sense of humiliation. It is often more fruitful to meet with smaller subgroups of the family, at least in the initial stages.

Asking gentle questions about the assumed roles of men and women in the family can often be an important first step in enabling clients to change lopsided and dysfunctional gender patterns. But therapists must always be careful that they do not unwittingly increase the Irish client's sense of guilt by subtle questioning that suggests they have done something wrong.

Irish clients will probably respond more readily to a brief, goal-oriented, problem-focused (especially child-focused) approach, with a specific plan and a right and wrong way clearly spelled out, such as behavior modification. Vague, introspective, open-ended emotive therapy may be experienced as highly threatening. Therapy oriented to uncovering hidden psychological problems is likely to increase Irish clients' anxiety and their conviction that they are bad. They may be more effectively helped by the paradoxical and humorous techniques of which they themselves are such masters. Perhaps it is not surprising that therapists of Irish extraction, such as Bill O'Hanlon, Steve Gilligan, Phil Guerin, Tom Fogarty, and Betty Carter, espoused positive, humorful orientations to therapy. These methods encourage clients to change without dwelling on their negative feelings, and organize therapy around building on a positive approach and a more hopeful vision of their lives.

A therapy acknowledging their culture may help remind them of their cultural strengths, The Irish have been shown to feel strengthened by considering their history as a source of empowerment in dealing with stress. A woman who was caring for her mother with Alzheimer's put it this way:

> I like being Irish. . . . We're a hardy group. . . . We have to be very strong. And I like knowing that the people that went before me went through things as hard as I've gone through. . . . They've gone through famine. . . . Because Ireland has constantly been conquered by the Normans and . . . they've been through a lot. . . . Such a beautiful place with no means of supporting itself. . . . And those in the North having to fight constantly to be free. . . . They're still having it hard. They're still having a tough time and they're still singing. Still writing poetry and still happy to see you. And they've gotten through it all, you know. And that's me. Isn't that me? (in Ortiz, Simmons, & Hinton, 1999, p. 486)

The Irish have at times had a sentimental attachment to their history. Helping them connect with it in more genuine ways can be very helpful to them clinically.

One of the most creative therapy approaches in recent years, the Fifth Province Model, developed by three Dublin therapists, Nollaig Byrne, Imelda Colgan McCarthy, and Philip Kearney, evolved specifically from thinking about Irish history. Not surprisingly, it has great merit for therapists treating Irish Americans (McCarthy, 1995; McCarthy & Byrne, 1988, 1995). It seeks to draw clinical attention away from polarizing conversations and into the realm of ambiguities, that unique place in Celtic mythology where all contradictions can coexist. "The Fifth Province," a magical place that included the other four Irish provinces of Munster, Connaught, Leinster, and Ulster, is a place of imagination and possibility where ambiguities and contradictions can be contained, where ancient Celtic chieftans came to resolve their conflicts through dialogue with druid priests. In their therapy members of the Fifth Province team develop multiple stories, offer metaphors and Irish folktales as interventions, and intentionally expand narratives beyond "logical" linear discourse. Furthermore, they use the political metaphors of colonization as the framework for their whole therapy, scrutinizing carefully the potential role of therapy itself to "colonize" or oppress clients, as the Irish themselves had been colonized.

In spite of their dislike of therapy, the Irish can be very gratifying to work with because of their extremely strong sense of loyalty and their willingness to follow through on therapeutic suggestions. They are also apt to accept the therapist readily; they may not question credentials, even when perhaps they should. Unfortunately, their responsiveness can become a hazard when it produces compliance without real collaboration in the change process. The therapist must help these clients to develop a genuine investment in the process of change and not rely on their politeness, sense of responsibility, and obligation to duty. Because of their ability to compartmentalize, the Irish may change, yet, on many levels, may not connect the therapy with their lives. Therapy, like their religion, their dreams, and and their prayers, becomes a new "therapeutic reality," one not necessarily integrated with their other spiritual or healing resources. The therapist may become an authority, who, like a priest, gives instructions that are to be followed.

Small changes may nevertheless be registered as large gains in the family, even if many aspects of family relating remain unaltered. Irish families may also prefer therapists to keep a friendly distance. A sense of humor can be a great asset to a therapist, provided that he or she remains businesslike and takes the family seriously at the same time. Any personality style too loud or idiosyncratic is likely to make the family uncomfortable. A therapist who swears is likely to be viewed as crude or sacrilegious, and one who is too personally revealing may make clients uneasy.

Even if family members fail to see the need for the father's presence, it is important for the therapist to involve him in therapy. Although Irish men often find a woman therapist intimidating, the strong role of Irish women may mean they are more comfortable with a woman therapist than are families from most other "patriarchal" cultures.

In working with the Irish, the therapist must often read between the lines, of either blustering or muted compliance, to ferret out what is really troubling them; then the Irish sense of loyalty, humor, and responsibility become the best clinical resources. Given the Irish embarrassment about their feelings on one hand, and their wish to be responsive to suggestions on the other, tasks that can be carried out at home may promote communication more successfully than a direct confrontation of family members in therapy. It may help to give tasks that focus on the presenting symptoms, structuring family interactions at home to address maladaptive communication problems, rather than unmasking them directly in sessions. There are many advantages to such an approach. It fits with clients' expectation of doing penance for their sins, provides structure within which to organize their behavior, spells out a right and wrong way, and spares them public exposure in therapy. This clarity is important to those who fear doing wrong. It also provides a sense of success early in therapy, which may be especially important for Irish clients who are preoccupied with feeling they are bad and have done wrong. When they do engage emotionally in therapy, they may be seeking forgiveness or absolution, which can be a trap, in that granting absolution keeps the client in a one-down position. Attempts at self-justification and tales told to show how a difficulty was someone else's fault tend to be a coverup for many-layered levels of self-recrimination.

The Irish family's sense of isolation can be so great that a therapist may not realize how much it means to its members just to have a safe, accepting place to talk to each other about thoughts and feelings. At the same time, the use of nonverbal techniques such as touching exercises, psychodrama, or structural techniques to increase anxiety, may be highly threatening. But small tasks to help them reconnect may do a lot to lessen their feelings of emotional isolation. However, this work requires respect for personal boundaries, for the family's need to preserve a degree of distance, and for leaving certain things unspoken.

In general, positive connotation, giving a caring interpretation of behavior, is of much more use than traditional psychodynamic interpretations for Irish clients, who are already likely to blame themselves for whatever goes wrong and to be fatalistic about internal change. Structuring the distance and intimacy can increase the family's sense of control over their feelings. Irish clients may respond extremely well to Bowen Coaching (McGoldrick & Carter, 2002) because of its emphasis on working out relationships in private, and on personal responsibility for change. The Irish are, indeed, excellent candidates for such therapy and may continue working to change relationships on their own, long after the therapy is over, because of its ability to provide them with a method for reworking relationships they may have found overwhelming and confusing in the past.

One young woman, whose father had been a successful journalist and the rebel of his family, had great difficulty establishing a relationship with her sole surviving aunt, who was the principal upholder of "Irish Catholic values" for the family. This aunt was the spinster sister who remained home to care for her aging parents until their deaths. She had built up a lifetime of unspoken resentments about her role, in spite of the secondary gains of being a martyr, similar to the heroine of *Final Payments* by Mary Gordon (1979). The aunt never missed sending cards for birthdays or Christmas, but when the niece attempted to make more personal contact, she resisted it strongly, agreeing to meet only rarely and for short visits, limiting discussion strictly to the topics she chose. Initially, the niece was put off by this behavior, describing her aunt as "a prune with doilies on the chairs." She was annoyed that her "open-hearted" approaches were rebuffed for no apparent reason. However, she persisted with letters and gradually more personal phone calls until she was able to learn enough about the family background to realize that the resentment the niece was experiencing had been passed down in the family for several generations. This aunt was the unappreciated and overburdened spinster, who had stayed home and resentfully cared for her parents, while her brothers got the glory. She had become the repository of unforgotten slights, "offering up" her family burdens in her prayers for the family's return to the Church. Church rules had been used in the service of bolstering her self-righteous indignation, which covered her sense of betrayal and hurt that her efforts on behalf of the family had never been reciprocated or appreciated.

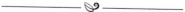

In families such as this the work obviously proceeds slowly. However, the long-term benefit of specific long-range work with each of the family members is often powerful in overcoming their painful sense of isolation and vulnerability.

CONCLUSION

Do not expect Irish clients to enjoy therapy or feel relieved by having a cathartic heart-to-heart discussion. The therapist working with an Irish family must be content with limited changes. Families may not wish to move beyond the initial presenting problem, and it is important for the therapist not to pressure them into further work. Attempting to get spouses to deal with marital issues after a child-focused problem has been solved, for example, will probably make them feel guilty and incompetent. It is better to reinforce the changes that the family members do make and to let them return for therapy later at their own initiative. Even if the therapist perceives that there are emotional blocks in the family that are still causing pain, it is important not to push the matter. Because of the lack of immediate feedback about therapeutic progress from the family, the therapist may be surprised to learn that their Irish clients have continued therapeutic work on their own. Their deep sense of personal responsibility is, in fact, their greatest personal resource in therapy. They often do continue efforts started in therapy, although they may not openly admit either the fault or their resolve to remedy it.

REFERENCES

Ablon, J. (1980). The significance of cultural patterning for the "alcoholic family." *Family Process*, 19(2), 127–144.

Aroian, K. (1993). Mental health risks and problems encountered by illegal immigrants. *Issues in Mental Health Nursing*, 14, 379–397.

Bales, R. F. (1962). Attitudes toward drinking in Irish culture. In D. Pittman & C. Snyder (Eds.), *Society, culture and drinking patterns*. New York: Wiley.

Barrabee, P., & von Mering, O. (1953). Ethnic variations in mental stress in families with psychotic children. *Social Problems*, 1, 48–53.

Bepko, C., & Krestan, J. (1983). *The responsibility trap*. New York: Harper.

Biddle, E. H. (1976). The American Catholic Irish family. In C. Mindel & R. Halberstein (Eds.), *Ethnic families in America*. New York: Elsevier.

Blessing, P. J. (1980). Irish. In S. Thernstorm, A. Orlov, & O. Handlin (Eds.), *Harvard encyclopedia of American ethnic groups*. Cambridge, MA: Harvard University Press.

Brewer, L. (2001, September). Gender socialization and the cultural construction of elder caregivers. *Journal of Aging Studies*, 15(3), 217–235.

Byron, R. (1999). *Irish America*. Oxford: Clarendon Paperbacks.

Cahill, T. (1995). *How the Irish saved civilization*. New York: Doubleday.

Chadwick, N. (1970). *The Celts*. London: Penguin.

Clark, D. (1988). *Hibernia America: The Irish and regional cultures*. New York: Greenwood Press.

Cleary, P. D., & Demone, H. W. (1988, December). Health and social service needs in a Northeastern metropolitan area: Ethnic group differences. *Journal of Sociology and Social Welfare*, 15(4), 63–76.

Cohler, B. J., & Lieberman, M. A. (1979). Personality change across the second half of life: Findings from a study of Irish, Italian, and Polish-American women. In D. E. Gelfand & A. J. Kutzik (Eds.), *Ethnicity and aging*. New York: Springer.

Connery, D. S. (1970). *The Irish*. New York: Simon & Schuster.

Corrigan, E. M. (1980). *Alcoholic women in treatment*. New York: Oxford University Press.

Corrigan, E., M., & Butler, S. (1991, March). Irish alcoholic women in treatment: Early findings. *International Journal of the Addictions*, 26(3), 281–292.

Dezell, M. (2000). *Irish America: Coming into clover*. New York: Anchor Books.

Diner, H. R. (1983). *Erin's daughters in America*. Baltimore: Johns Hopkins University Press.

Donnelly, S. (1999, January). Folklore associated with dying in the west of Ireland. *Palliative Medicine, 13*(1), 57–62.

Evans, E. E. (1957). *Irish folkways*. London: Routledge & Kegan Paul.

Fallows, M. A. (1979). *Irish Americans: Identity and assimilation*. Englewood Cliffs, NJ: Prentice-Hall.

Fanning, C. (Ed.). (2001). *New perspectives on the Irish diaspora*. Carbondale: South Illinois University Press.

Fitzpatrick, C., & Barry, C. (1990). Cultural differences in family communication about Duchenne's muscular dystrophy. *Developmental Medicine and Child Neurology, 32*(11), 967–973.

Foster, R. F. (1988). *Modern Ireland 1600–1972*. New York: Penguin.

Gilfoyle, T. J. (2004, April 1). The Irish-American paradox. *Chicago Tribune*, Sec. 14, p. 1.

Gordon, M. (1979). *Final payments*. New York: Penguin.

Greeley, A. M. (1977). *The American Catholic*. New York: Basic Books.

Greeley, A. M. (1981). *The Irish Americans*. New York: Harper & Row.

Greeley, A. M., & McCready, W. (1975). The transmission of cultural heritages: The case of Irish and Italians. In N. Glazer & D. Moynihan (Eds.), *Ethnicity: The theory and experience*. Cambridge, MA: Harvard University Press.

Hayden, T. (Ed.). (1998). *Irish hunger: Personal reflections on the legacy of the famine*. Bouldor, CO: Holt Rinehart.

Hayden, T. (2001). *Irish on the inside: In search of the soul of Irish America*. New York: Verso.

Hines, P., Garcia-Preto, N., McGoldrick, M., Almeida, R., & Weltman, S. (1992). Intergenerational relationships across cultures. *Journal of Contemporary Human Services, 6*, 323–338.

Ignatiev, N. (1995). *How the Irish became white*. New York: Routledge.

Jackson, C. (1993). *A social history of the Scotch Irish*. New York: Madison Books.

Jacobson, M. F. (2002). *Special sorrows: The diasporic imagination of Irish, Polish and Jewish immigrants in the United States*. Los Angeles: University of Claifornia Press.

Johnson, P. B. (1989, Spring). A comparison of drinking-related beliefs of problem and non-problem drinking Irish-Americans. *Journal of Alcohol and Drug Education, 34*(3), 1–4.

Johnson, P. B. (1991). Reaction expectancies of ethnic drinking differences. *Psychology of Addictive Behaviors, 5*(1), 36–40.

Kaufman, E., & Borders, L. (1988). Ethnic family differences in adolescent substance use. *Journal of Chemical Dependency Treatment, 1*(2), 99–121.

Kennedy, R. E. (1983). *The Irish: Marriage, immigration and fertility*. Berkeley: University of California Press.

Kinealy, C. (1995). *This great calamity: The Irish famine 1845–52*. Boulder, CO: Roberts Rinehart.

Lavery, B. (2004, March 17). Anxiety over alcohol rises in Ireland after manslaughter trial. *New York Times*, Sec. 1, p. 5.

Lidz, T. (1968). *The person: His development throughout the life cycle*. New York: Basic Books.

MacCurtain, M., & O'Corrain, D. (Eds.). (1978). *Women in Irish society: The historical dimension*. Dublin: Arlen House.

McCaffrey, L. J. (2000). Diaspora comparisons and Irish-American uniqueness. In C. Fanning (Ed.), *New perspectives on the Irish diaspora*. Carbondale: Southern Illinois University Press.

McCarthy, I. C. (1992). Out of myth into history: A hope for Irish women in the 1990s. *Journal of Feminist Family Therapy, 4*(3/4).

McCarthy, I. C. (1995). Abusing norms: Welfare families and a Fifth Province stance. In I. C. McCarthy (Ed.), *Human Systems, 5*(4).

McCarthy, I. C., & Byrne, N. O. (1988). Mis-taken love: Conversations on the problem of incest in an Irish context. *Family Process, 27*(2), 181–199.

McCarthy, I. C., & Byrne, N. O. (1995). A spell in the Fifth Province: Its between meself, herself, yerself and yer two imaginary friends. In S. Friedman (Ed.), *The reflecting process in action*. New York: Guilford Press.

McCourt, F. (1999). '*Tis*. New York: Scribner.

McGoldrick, M. (1989). Irish mothers: Ethnicity and mothers. *Journal of Feminist Family Therapy*, 2(2), 1–8.

McGoldrick, M., & Carter, B. (2001). Advances in coaching: Family therapy with one person. *Journal of Marital and Family Therapy*, 27(3), 281–300.

McGoldrick, M., & Pearce, J. K. (1981). Family therapy with Irish Americans. *Family Process*, 20, 223–241.

McGoldrick, M., Schlesinger, J. M., Hines, P. M., Lee, E., Chan, J., Almeida, R., et al. (2004). Mourning in different cultures: English, Irish, African American, Chinese, Asian Indian, Jewish, Latino, and Brazilian. In F. Walsh & M. McGoldrick (Eds.), *Living beyond loss* (2nd ed.). New York: Norton.

McGoldrick, M., & Troast, J. (1994). Ethnicity and family business. *Journal of Family Business*.

McKenna, A. (1979). Attitudes of Irish mothers to child rearing. *Journal of Comparative Family Studies*, 10(2), 227–251.

Menchin, S. (1993, March 22). Break in the clouds. *New Yorker*.

Messinger, J. C. (1971, February). Sexuality: The lack of the Irish. *Psychology Today*, 41–44.

Metress, E. (1990). The American wake of Ireland: Symbolic death ritual. *Omega Journal of Death and Dying*, 21(2), 147–153.

Miller, K. A. (1985). *Emigrants and exiles: Ireland and the Irish exodus to North America*. New York: Oxford University Press.

Miller, K. A., & Wagner, P. (1995). *Out of Ireland: The story of the Irish emigration to America*. Washington, DC: Elliott & Clark.

Murphy, M. W. (1988). Separating with dignity within the Irish value system. *Mediation Quarterly*, 22, 91–98.

Neville, G. (2000). *Rites de passage*: Rituals of separation in Irish oral tradition. In C. Fanning (Ed.), *New perspectives on the Irish diaspora*. Carbondale: Southern Illinois University Press.

Nolan, J. (1989). *Ourselves alone: Women's emigration from Ireland 1885–1920*. Lexington: University of Kentucky Press.

O'Faolain, N. (2001). *My dream of you*. New York: Penguin.

Opler, M. K., & Singer, J. L. (1957). Ethnic differences in behavior and psychpathology: Italian and Irish. *International Journal of Social Psychiatry*, 1, 11–17.

Ortiz, A., Simmons, J., & Hinton, W. L. (1999). Locations of remorse and homelands of resilience: Notes on grief and sense of loss of place of Latino and Irish-American caregivers of demented elders. *Culture, Medicine and Psychiatry*, 23, 477–500.

Power, P. C. (1993). *Sex and marriage in ancient Ireland*. Dublin: Mercier Press.

Roberts, B., & Myers, J. K. (1954). Religion, national origin, immigration and mental illness. *American Journal of Psychiatry*, 110, 759–764.

Rossiter, A. (1993). Bringing the margins into the centre: A review of aspects of Irish women's emigration from a British perspective. In A. Smyth (Ed.), *Irish women's studies reader*. Dublin: Attic Press.

Rudd, J. M. (1984). *Irish American families: The mother child dyad*. Unpublished doctoral thesis, Smith College School for Social Work, Northampton, MA.

Sanua, V. D. (1960). Sociocultural factors in responses to stressful life situations: The behavior of aged amputees as an example. *Journal of Health and Human Behavior*, 1, 17–24.

Scally, R. J. (1995). *The end of hidden Ireland: Rebellion, famine and emigration*. New York: Oxford University Press.

Scheper-Hughes, N. (2001). *Saints, scholars, and schizophrenics: Mental illness in rural Ireland*. Berkeley: University of California Press.

Singer, J., & Opler, M. K. (1956). Contrasting patterns of fantasy and motility in Irish and Italian schizophrenics. *Journal of Abnormal and Social Psychology*, 53, 42–47.

Spiegel, J. (1971a). Cultural strain, family role patterns, and intrapsychic conflict. In J. G. Howells (Ed.), *Theory and practice of family psychiatry*. New York: Brunner/Mazel.

Spiegel, J. (1971b). Transactions: The interplay between individual, family and society (J. Papajohn, Ed.). New York: Science House.

Sternbach, R. A., & Tursky, B. (1965). Ethnic differences among housewives in psychophysical and skin potential responses to electric shock. *Psychophysiology, 1*(3), 241–246.

Stivers, R. (1976). *The hair of the dog: Irish drinking and American stereotype.* University Park: Pennsylvania State University Press.

Teahan, J. E. (1987, July). Alcohol expectancies, values, and drinking of Irish and U.S. collegians. *International Journal of the Addictions, 22*(7), 621–638.

Tursky, B., & Sternbach, R. A. (1967). Further physiological correlates of ethnic differences in response to shock. *Psychophysiology, 4*(1), 67–74.

Walsh, D. (1987). Alcohol and Ireland. *British Journal of Addiction, 82,* 118–120.

Wills, G. (1971). *Bare ruined choirs.* Garden City, NY: Doubleday.

Wylan, L., & Mintz, N. (1976). Ethnic differences in family attitudes toward psychotic manifestations with implications for treatment programmes. *International Journal of Social Psychiatry, 22,* 86–95.

Zborowski, M. (1969). *People in pain.* San Francisco: Jossey-Bass.

Zola, I. K. (1966). Culture and Symptoms: An analysis of patients' presenting complaints. *American Sociological Review, 5,* 141–155.

CHAPTER 44

Italian Families

Joe Giordano
Monica McGoldrick
Joanne Guarino Klages

Although all cultures value the family, for Italians the family is an all-consuming ideal, providing continuity to life. Its power is one's first loyalty and its honor must never be betrayed. To be without family has meant to be totally bereft, *un saccu vacante*, or an empty sack, as Gambino puts it (1974, p. 34). *La via vecchia* (the old way) symbolizes for Italians a value system organized primarily around protecting the family (Gambino, 1974; Ianni & Reuss-Ianni, 1972; Johnson, 1985; LaGumina, Cavaioli, Primeggia, & Varacalli, 2000; Mangione & Morreale, 1992). Family continues to provide a strong sense of security and identity for many third- and fourth-generation Italian Americans, although there are others for whom it stifles individual needs and desires for success (Messina, 1994; Riotta-Sirey, Patti, & Mann, 1985; Rolle, 1980).

What most Americans refer to as "Italian" is not representative of all Italian culture, but applies rather to those who trace their ancestry primarily to the provinces south and east of Rome, the Mezzogiorno. Italy's history, geography, and economy created major differences between northern and southern Italy, which became indeed "two sharply different civilizations with different cultures, customs languages, and history" (Mangione & Morreale, 1992).

HISTORICAL BACKGROUND

In 1870, after years of rebellions and struggles, Italy was unified as one nation. Previously, its provinces had existed as separate states ruled by a number of other countries and the Catholic Church (Ciongoli & Parini, 2002). The people of the north had an identity connected to the renowned culture that had produced the Renaissance; they entered the industrial age with dreams of progress. Meanwhile, the Mezzogiorno and other parts of southern

Italy had for centuries been ruled and influenced by the Byzantines, Normans, Arabs, and the Spanish Bourbons, which were oppressive regimes that forbade southern Italians even to travel. By the 19th century, the Mezzogiorno was still steeped in a feudal system of farming, with its people oppressed by the landowners and living in great poverty.

Although it was generally believed that Italians were by nature "as attached to their soil as an oyster to its rock," dissatisfaction with the unification of Italy led first the northerners, and then the southerners, to set their sights on other lands (Mangione & Morreale, 1992). The new Italian government implemented a series of laws that benefited the north, decreasing their need to emigrate, while further impoverishing the people of the south. In addition, an outbreak of malaria exacerbated the Mezzogiorno's poverty and a series of volcanoes and earthquakes destroyed their land and led to an exodus of southern Italians in the late 1800s. Their numbers were so great that in 1901 the mayor of one southern Italian town introduced Italy's prime minister with "I greet you in the name of eight thousand fellow citizens, three thousand of who[m] are in America and the other five thousand preparing to follow them" (Hoobler & Hoobler, 1997, p. 17).

CORE VALUES

Oppression and domination were instrumental in forming the character and belief system of Southern Italians. They had learned through centuries of invading armies that they could ultimately count only on their own families and townspeople; they developed a complex and all-demanding, if unwritten, code of obligations regulating relationships within and outside the family, known as *l'ordine della famiglia* (Gambino, 1974). At its core was a cynicism or mistrust of the outside world and a loyalty to the home and family that suggested disloyalty and shame if a person aspired to go beyond it (Mangione & Morreale, 1992).

Adaptability and resilience became ethnic trademarks. Italians took pride in their ability to cope with difficult situations. They also developed a belief in fate (*destinu*) an acceptance of the inevitable (Mangione & Morreale, 1992). To counter the harshness in their daily lives, they mastered the ability to savor fully the present, particularly with family gatherings, music, and pleasure from food, a primary source of emotional and physical solace (Femminella & Quadagno, 1976; Mangione & Morreale, 1992; Yans-McLaughlin, 1980).

IMMIGRANTS TO THE UNITED STATES

Between the years 1880 and 1920, 4.5 million Italians immigrated to the United States, usually to find "work and bread" to feed their families (Gambino, 1974). Many, who largely settled in the urban centers of the Mid-Atlantic States, New England, and California, expected to return to their families in Italy after making enough money to buy land. More than half did so, a proportion greater than that of any other immigrant group.

Those who remained in the United States missed their families and worked hard to send for them (Gambino, 1974; Mangione & Morreale, 1992). According to the 2000 U.S. Census, 15,723,555 people identify themselves as Italian American, making them the fifth largest ethnic group in the country. Their settlement pattern was largely influenced by the importance placed on family, neighborhood connections, and relationships with children who felt obligated to remain close to their aging parents (Johnson, 1985; Ragucci, 1981). In *The Italians*, Luigi Barzini (1964) states:

> The Italian family is a stronghold in a hostile land; within its walls and among its members, the individual finds consolation, help, advice, provision, weapons, allies and accomplices to aid in his pursuits. No Italian who has family is ever alone. He finds in it refuge in which to lick his wounds after a defeat, or an arsenal and a staff for his victorious drives.

The clash of cultures between the Mezzogiorno and the New World was enormous. Italian cultural attitudes contrasted strongly with the dominant American values that emphasized individualism, independence, and personal achievement over group affiliation. Italians were considered inferior, uneducated, dangerous, violent, and criminal. Prejudice and discrimination against them grew as their presence increased.

Italian immigrants saw the dominant culture as hostile and, as they had done for centuries in the Mezzogiorno, they turned to their families as a defensive strategy against this hostile force (Gambino, 1974). They formed enclaves, known as "little Italys," with others who came from the same region or province, which helped them preserve their old ways. The neighborhood became an extension of the family.

Italian Americans took pride in home ownership, for renting would leave them dependent on outsiders, as they had been as sharecroppers in the Mezzogiorno. The home was a symbol of the family, not of status, and the family table was its center.

Immigrant parents saw their children's acculturation as a betrayal. In turn, some children saw *l'ordine della la famiglia* as stifling to their personal success. This clash of cultures sometimes led those in the second generation to distance themselves from their Italian ethnicity to pursue the dominant culture's marks of success, and others adhered to "the old way." Both paths had their costs: Individual success sometimes led to a sense of alienation from family, whereas staying loyal to family could mean feeling unsuccessful according to the definitions of the dominant culture.

RELIGION

The Catholicism practiced by southern Italians incorporated a mixture of pagan customs, magical beliefs, some Muslim practices, Christian doctrine, and their own pragmatism (Gambino, 1974). A long history of subjugation by outside invaders and natural disasters led to a belief that evil lurks around every corner. Each village had its own saint to ward off evil. People paid homage to their saint protectors through elaborate forms of devotion. But if a particular saint failed to protect them, they did not hesitate to replace him or her with a new saint.

When the Italians joined the Catholic Church in this country, their religious practices shocked the Irish, who dominated the Church and ran the parochial schools to which the Italians sent their children. Nelli (1980) states, "Italians in America found the Church a cold, remote, puritanical institution, controlled and often staffed, even in Italian neighborhoods, by the Irish. Even devout Italians resented the Irish domination of the local church and early demanded their own priests" (p. 553).

Italians prize church rituals more for their pageantry and value in fostering family celebrations and rites of passage than for their religious significance. For most Italians, God is viewed as a benign friend of the family and the Church as a source of ritual and drama, in striking contrast to the Irish, with their dire warnings about the Day of Judgment and emphasis on the Church's authority.

EDUCATION, WORK, AND UPWARD MOBILITY

As in all things, the immigrants' attitude toward education was influenced by *l'ordine della famiglia.* In the Mezzogiorno, very young children worked to contribute to the family's support and survival. In the United States, the immigrants' attitude toward education was also based on whether it met the practical needs of the family. Children were sent to elementary school to learn to read, write, and do simple arithmetic, practical skills that could help the family. Boys sometimes attended school beyond the elementary level to learn a trade if their families could afford to do without their wages, but secondary school for girls was seen as wasteful. Girls could be better taught in the home, where they were more useful to the family (Cohen, 1992). Thus, first-generation Italian immigrants interpreted the "American Dream" as an opportunity to obtain steady work to provide food and shelter for the family.

A job that could provide steady income for the family meant success for Italians of the Mezzogiorno, who for centuries had lived in fear of starvation. Higher education was not necessary for small business, construction, masonry, or bricklaying jobs, in which Italians could see the results of their labor. Today the number of Italian Americans earning college degrees is increasing, although they still lag in achieving graduate-level degrees. Italians may now view a college degree as practical because it is an entry-level requirement in many fields (Calandra Institute, 2000).

Achievement for Italian Americans has also been influenced by the popular belief that most Italian Americans are connected to the Mafia (organized crime). Originally, the term *mafia* had, in addition, a more benign meaning among Italians:

> It was an adjective used to describe someone who commanded respect, who knew how to "take care of things" without running to the authorities. It referred to an individual who had both power and dignity, while also inspiring fear. He was, most importantly, a person whom one could approach when in need. Thus, such a term might be applied to a family patriarch who had no connection with the organization known as the Mafia. (Giordano, 1986, pp. 207–208)

Although the Mafia is composed exclusively of Italian Americans, relatively few belong to it. (According to the FBI, there are fewer than 1,700 members.) Yet the Mafia stereotype of Italian Americans remains pervasive. National surveys reveal that more than 70% of Americans surveyed believe that most Italian Americans are connected in some way to organized crime (Response Analysis Corporation, 1989; Zogby, 2001). In 1992, then-governor of Arkansas Bill Clinton was caught in a taped telephone conversation saying that New York governor Mario Cuomo "acts like a member of the Mafia." In the November 2002 election, U.S. congressman and Maine gubernatorial candidate John Baldacci discovered his political opponent airing television commercials that attacked him by using phases and expressions of a mafioso, spoken in "mobspeak."

This image of Italians has become part of American folklore through the popular media's fascination with the Mafia mystique and movies and television shows like *The Godfather* and *The Sopranos*. Representations of Italians as gangsters can influence the personal aspirations of young Italian Americans, as well as what is expected of them by other members of our society. In some cases, this can also be a serious social and psychological issue for Italian Americans.

Frank Galgano, a successful 42-year-old businessman, was referred by his physician for depression and panic attacks. Two years earlier, he had gotten into a financial dispute with a business rival. The disagreement dragged on for months and became highly personal. Frank's accounting firm began to lose business, and contracts were not being renewed.

When Frank investigated to see why his business was failing, he learned that his competitor was spreading rumors that he was a member of the Mafia. After trying unsuccessfully to confront his rival and convince his clients that he never had any connection to organized crime, he became consumed with trying to clear his name. For months, Frank did not share this problem with his wife or two teenage daughters. He confided only in his father, a retired sanitation worker, whom he would consult daily. As the business continued to dwindle, Frank became very anxious and unable to sleep, fearing the shame and ridicule his family would experience in their predominantly non-Italian suburban community.

Despite the fact that Frank was a third-generation Italian American with a graduate education and an upper-middle-class lifestyle, the core of his identity and behavior was rooted in the traditional family values and beliefs of his Sicilian grandparents. Frank finally shared with his family and took the matter to court, where he won a defamation suit against his business rival. Although he felt less depressed and the physical symptoms disappeared, he remained apprehensive about the future. He said that he will always feel that someone in his work or social world will whisper to another person, "I hear he has 'connections.' "

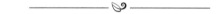

FAMILY PATTERNS AND ROLES

Social interactions, like everything else for Italians, were guided by *l'ordine della famiglia*. Within this code, family comes first, and members are expected to stay geographically and psychologically close, coming together in a crisis and taking care of vulnerable family members.

Family members must never do anything to hurt or disgrace the family. They must neither take advantage of other members nor talk about the family to outsiders. Occasionally, though, close relatives maintain secrets to define boundaries in a particular relationship. When two individuals share a secret that is withheld from other family members, this neutralizes the family's engulfing nature. The significance of such secret keeping, though it may appear dysfunctional to a therapist, more often lies in boundary keeping, than in the content of the secret itself.

Third- and fourth-generation Italian Americans tend to be confused by the family's secrets and alliances and sometimes rebel against these dynamics, causing intergenerational conflicts (Papajohn & Spiegel, 1975). Alternatively, they may find themselves "going along" with the family secret to "keep peace." They are often surprised when they find themselves repeating, as parents, the behavior they rejected in their own families (Santo, 1984). While encouraging their children to "get a good education," they may also subtly convey a different message: "Do not leave the family. Do not attend school out of state." A recent study by Patricia Boscia-Mulé (1999) indicates that, even today, third-generation Italian Americans evaluate their individual goals and interests for their compatibility with the welfare of the family before making their personal choices.

For many upwardly mobile third- and fourth-generation Italian Americans, conflict between familial solidarity and the dominant culture's emphasis on autonomy and individuation may engender conscious and unconscious feelings of shame, self-hatred, and identity confusion (Giordano, 1994; Riotta-Sirey et al., 1985; Rolle, 1980). Tina DeRosa (1980) a third-generation Italian American novelist, observed, "I belonged nowhere; that is the price you pay for growing up in one culture and entering another." Her alienation resulted from her parents' insistence that she become educated. But education had changed everything. Her father and other relatives began to regard her differently. She no longer had their approval, nor did she have the approval of the world they had thrust her into (Mangione & Morreale, 1992, p. 434).

Traditional Family Roles

Because traditional family roles are clearly undergoing change, therapists can judge for themselves the extent to which the traditions described here may apply to any particular Italian American family.

The Father

Traditionally, the father was the undisputed head of the household, often authoritarian and rigid in his rule setting and guidelines for behavior. His role was to provide for and protect the family. Family members catered to his desires, particularly in regard to food. He expected his daughters to follow their mother's lead, taught his sons to be like him, and demanded total respect (which he interpreted as adherence to his wishes) from his wife and children. The changing role of women in our society is altering the traditional relationships men have had with their wives and daughters and places a strain on traditionalist Italian men.

The Mother

In a traditional Italian family, the mother represented the heart of the family, receiving much respect and having great power and responsibility within the home. The mother was expected to put the needs of the family first. She was responsible for representing the family properly to the community by maintaining all family relationships with both her side of the family and her husband's. She was never to disagree with her husband in public. When she did so in private, she was expected to express her opinions in a way that did not challenge his authority.

The mother also acted as a buffer between her husband and her children. The extent to which Italian American women question traditional gender scripts depends on their educational level, their financial resources, and the amount of contact they have with people in nontraditional gender roles (Boscia-Mulé, 1999).

Gender Issues

The Italian man may struggle with the core belief that manliness is reflected in the level of respect he gets from his wife and children. He may feel depressed or angry when his family operates in a nontraditional manner (i.e., not guided by customs of a patriarchal system), while acknowledging that domination is not an acceptable way to relate to women.

Women, although wishing to hold onto the positive aspects of their Italian American identity, often no longer want to maintain their unequal status. Even when working full time, Italian American women may feel pressured to fulfill the same family obligations and responsibilities as their mothers and grandmothers did.

Men and women tend to attribute negative gender stereotypes to each other. Men's perceptions of women reflect a wish for the traditional role (women as mothers, cooks) and anger at both old behaviors (smothering or controlling) and women's new, more assertive roles, as they become educated professionals. This conflict over traditional gender roles is a major reason that both Italian American men and women are seeking relationships with non-Italians in greater numbers than ever before, and is often the impetus for Italian American couples to seek therapy. More than 80% of Italian Americans are marrying partners of a different ethnicity (Alba, 1985; Crohn, 1995).

Children

In Italian families, sons are given much greater behavioral latitude. Indeed, a bit of acting out is expected, even subtly encouraged, as a measure of manliness. Sexual proficiency is especially important, not only to fulfill the masculine image, but also to exemplify a sense of mastery in interpersonal relations, a core Italian value.

Traditionally, Italian girls have been more restricted than their brothers and male cousins. Daughters have been taught to eschew personal achievement in favor of respect and service to their parents and brothers.

Italian couples frequently state that their adult status was not really accepted by their parents, even after career and marital success, until they produced children themselves. However, even then, parents may remain very involved in the lives of their adult children. For example, daughters may seek counsel from their mothers or other female relatives about relationship issues.

In general, Italian children have shown more conflict than children in other ethnic groups about their upwardly mobile aspirations, which may be threatening to their families. In other groups, children may feel anxious that they will not live up to their parents' ambitions for upward mobility.

Extended Family

Members of an extended Italian family often live in the same neighborhood. Respect and care for older family members is a strong norm. In working with Italian families, it is essential to learn the location of, and level of contact with, relatives.

Relationship to Outsiders

Members of Italian families may feel that they owe nothing to those outside the family. They are unconcerned with the activities and behavior of "outsiders" and often show respect for—but do not trust—externl authority.

Life-Cycle Issues

There is virtually no such thing as a separate nuclear family unit in Italian culture. For many Italian Americans, primary life cycle difficulties have to do with stages involving separation, in particular "launching" and death. Indeed, it has been said that Italian families never actually launch their children; they just send them out far enough to find partners who will come into the family circle. The network of significant others is usually large, including aunts, uncles, cousins, *gumbares* (old friends and neighbors), and godparents, all of whom may assume important roles in child rearing.

Unlike the British, who raise children to be independent and self-sufficient, Italians raise their children to be mutually supportive and to contribute to the family. Separation from the family is not desired, expected, or easily accepted.

Death, the most difficult separation of all, has historically been met with impassioned grieving by Italian women, which is deemed appropriate, as the women are understood to be expressing grief for the whole family. Historically, Italian men were generally expected to meet the death of a loved one with quiet somberness and control of their emotions. Italians tend to keep their dead with them. They may relay dreams they have had of the deceased or speak of an occasion when they felt the presence of the deceased person, receiving comfort from such experiences and sharing that comfort with other family members.

It is not unusual for parents and grandparents to have multiple contacts during the day with their adult children. Generally, each family member has a well-delineated role that dictates both the pattern and frequency of contact with various other family members. This may complicate the drawing of boundaries, which is a task for a new couple, particularly when one partner is not Italian.

Acculturation

Third- and fourth-generation Italian Americans who prioritize family over individual needs may feel challenged by the American belief that an individual-centered culture is superior to a family-centered one. Yet third- and fourth-generation Italians who reject the insularity of Italian culture and object to the racism and heterosexism that is endemic to a closed system may find themselves in conflict with other family members who feel that their values have been rejected.

Third- and fourth-generation Italian Americans have not had to endure the hardships of the immigrants or to fight for acceptance by the dominant culture, and so can develop their own relationship with the past and define their place within the larger culture (Laurino, 2000). Thus, they often find it easier than their parents and grandparents did to embrace those aspects of Italian culture that nurture them, while rejecting those that do not.

IMPLICATIONS FOR FAMILY THERAPY

Italians believe that the family is the cure for whatever ails you and, unsurprisingly, turn to it for help in solving problems, rather than to the available mental health services (Cleary & Demone, 1988; Femminella, 1982; Rabkin & Struening, 1975). When they do seek help, the problem is likely to have reached a serious level, and they may see entering therapy as a sign that they have failed. The therapist first may need to reframe entering therapy as a sign of the family members' importance to each other, rather than as proof of their failure. Moreover, gaining acceptance as an outsider involves not taking the family's initial mistrust personally, validating the caring it represents rather than the suspiciousness.

In early sessions, a therapist can sometimes build trust by honestly sharing common values, which conveys his or her caring and warmth. It is also important to realize that some families interpret extensive questioning as a message that they are "not smart enough," rather than as a way to get at the truth or gain insight. Once a therapist wins the family's trust, most counseling will center on helping family members establish new boundaries and reducing guilt and fear of separation.

For Italian American fathers, therapy may be threatening because it implies that they are incapable of remaining in control of their families. The father may appear open and direct, but often finds ways to elude and rationalize a problem to "save face."

The therapist's first encounter with the family may be quite lively. Italian Americans are often very engaging and colorful speakers; discussions can become passionate, typified by loud voices, elaborate gesturing, and arguments among family members. For Italians, words are not meant literally, but rather give expression to the moment. Passionate outbursts do not tend to cause permanent ruptures or resentments. In fact, for Italians neutrality of expression is associated with a lack of caring (Bryant, 1976). The Italian family's expressive intensity may be overpowering to a therapist from a more restrained culture in which, for example, powerful verbal expressions would be interpreted literally.

Italian families may spend a great deal of time discussing the problem's emotional impact and social context, as well as the physical sensations involved (Zborowski, 1964; Zola, 1966). They have much concern and awareness about the connections between their emotional and physical well-being.

Italians typically deny difficult problems; "hot" issues are not openly discussed. The therapist should attend to what is *not* being said, particularly because Italians do more sidestepping than most in the initial stage of therapy, reflecting their reluctance to expose private subjects to outsiders.

If the family is in a "crisis," the therapist should promptly give its members some response to their problem. Even a seemingly small suggestion may be sufficient to "hold" the family until more enduring interventions can be found. However, it is best not to offer advice that may undercut the family's authority.

To Italian Americans, resolving a problem often means relieving stress without changing the family's equilibrium. Because parents are more receptive to assistance for their children, joining the family around a child-focused problem can break through the family's resistance. Such intervention is best tolerated in the form of advice rather than "exploration." Third- and fourth-generation Italian Americans, who often hope to find a healthy balance between individual needs and strong familial connections, are more likely to take risks in therapy.

Italian families, even when speaking openly and engagingly, are usually hesitant to share family secrets. Their very existence may puzzle the therapist inasmuch as the family seems to talk openly about all kinds of issues, including sex, bodily functions, and hostility. Secrets tend to delineate who is inside and who outside of the family system. Therapists must be aware of the sense of betrayal families will feel if their boundaries are crossed. Pushing the family to tell its secrets will usually only heighten mistrust and resistance.

As therapy proceeds, the therapist should constantly find ways to reinforce the family's problem-solving abilities, including affirming its values of protection, loyalty, respect, and ethnic identity, as well as attributes of hard work, warmth, and spontaneity. Labeling or challenging Italian Americans' intense involvement with each other as intrusive, inappropriate, or pathological is likely to increase their anxiety and resistance.

Because of their belief in *destinu*, Italians may not believe in their ability to master the problems they confront. Individuals in third- and fourth-generation families sometimes struggle to gain greater self-differentiation without causing others pain or cutting off relationships. Usually these individuals want closeness to the family as well as autonomy.

Because of the deep meaning of family to Italians, the price they pay for emotional disconnection is high, and they are often relieved and grateful to find ways to become reconnected to their families without becoming engulfed. Coaching alienated family members usually involves encouraging them to space out family contacts, while advocating a high degree of emotional expressiveness when they are with their families. These clients need to be prepared, at each step of differentiation, to deal with their family's intense reactions, which may include feelings of betrayal, abandonment, and rejection.

Yet even a suggestion of separation or distancing may be a "red flag" for an Italian American family. Separations related to life-cycle transitions—a job promotion or getting married—can lead parents to "hold back" feelings of pride in their children's accomplishments. Their children, in turn, may become confused and angry with the parents because of their lack of enthusiasm for their success or may be conflicted about how their accomplishment will affect the family connection.

The intense feelings surrounding separation and individuality are further complicated when a family is dealing with the issue of homosexuality. Despite the fact that there are many gay people of Italian American heritage, a family member's sexual orientation may be a "hot" issue and therefore avoided by Italian American families. Gay and lesbian family members may reduce contact with their heterosexual family members because of this marginalization. At the same time, Italian American loyalty to the group can create enormous emotional conflict for the gay person torn between loyalty to family and to the gay community or a partner. This conflict and the subsequent fear of cutoff, however, may lead members of the family to open their hearts to the gay member, rather than accept the painful alternative of separation and loss.

Providing more insights into understanding how silence and secrets play a role in a family's attempts to deal with gay and lesbian issues, a number of Italian American writers have described their own experiences. Robert Ferro (1983), in his several novels, explores homosexual integration into the traditional family. Theresa Carilli (1996) and Rachel Guido DeVries (1986) challenge the stereotypes of the Italian American family as warm and happy.

The therapist often must learn to differentiate between intense closeness and pathological enmeshment in Italian American families. Reframing the issue as a problem of uncompromising and unyielding "boundaries" may be important, but the therapist must make clear that he or she is not challenging the family members' desire to stay close.

In the final phase of treatment, the therapist will be presented with the therapeutic issue of how to extricate him- or herself from the system. Families may attempt to "absorb" the therapist and make him or her auxiliary family members. Somehow, the therapist must find a way to avoid becoming sucked into the system as a member, while being sufficiently engaging to maintain respect and connection.

Bowen's (1978) systems therapy focuses on understanding and shifting the family process while staying out of the system, but avoids dramatic interventions that may prevent the engagement necessary in treating Italian families. This model appears to be the treatment of choice with Italians who have already distanced from their families, in that its primary focus is differentiation through personalized connectedness.

Italian Americans who move away from their families may suffer loneliness and isolation, despite achieving success according to "mainstream" criteria—money, education, social status. Often, young Italian Americans may seek therapy to support their separating from their families in attempts at pseudo-independence. Therapists may mistakenly foster such attempts by emphasizing the individual experience over the need to maintain interpersonal connectedness.

Gina, a 32-year-old lesbian, entered treatment because of "rage," which she reported was affecting all of her relationships. She reported that she had not told her father about her lifestyle when he died, 10 years prior to her seeking therapy. She had "come out" out to her mother, and she reported that her mother did not like her lifestyle and made sarcastic and demeaning comments about her sexual orientation. Gina responded to these comments with sarcasm and sexual comments meant to shock her mother.

Visits usually ended with Gina feeling enraged, depressed, and swearing not to visit again. She had even tried moving out of state to limit contact with her mother, but missed her and the extended family and returned to her home state. Gina introduced her partners to family members as friends. Her rage appeared connected to her belief that she could not be her authentic self and stay connected to her family, particularly her mother. This hypothesis was shared with Gina, and therapy was focused on developing strategies that would permit her to stay connected to her mother while staying true to herself. Gina did not believe that her mother would ever accept her sexual orientation or stop demeaning her, but she was willing to try anything that would enable her contacts with her mother to be less painful. She was coached to continue visits with her mother, but to let her know how hurtful her comments were and to end the visit before she became reactive. She would phone or visit again as soon as she felt able. Gina was further coached to build a support network with other lesbians and allies and to begin to introduce her current partner to her family as her girlfriend, not just a friend.

Within a year, Gina reported that her family affirmed her relationship with her partner and they were treated as a couple, not as just friends. Her mother had stopped making homophobic comments and really liked Gina's partner. Gina further reported that her "rage" reactions were no longer a problem.

The importance of family for Gina as an Italian American could not be dismissed even while the relationship with her mother was causing her emotional pain. For Italians "to be without family is to be "truly a 'non-being' " (Gambino, 1974, p. 34). Helping Gina reach a balance between living her life authentically and remaining emotionally connected to her family had positive effects on all her relationships.

CONCLUSION

Traditionally defined roles, family obligations, and the importance of family connection remain core values for many Italian Americans. Strong family connections can be problematic when a family's insularity prevents individuals from achieving their personal goals. Italian American families have the potential to work through the issues that occur when their individual goals conflict with familial ones. Broader issues such as classism, racism, sexism, and heterosexism, which can be endemic to a closed system, may also be transformed because of a desire to stay connected.

As contemporary society becomes more diverse, the children of Italian American families may, through their personal choices, force these broader issues to be addressed by their elders. The culturally aware family therapist can be instrumental in helping Italian Americans open up their family systems while retaining the positive aspects of close family connections.

REFERENCES

Alba, R. (1985). *Italian Americans: Into the twilight of ethnicity.* Englewood Cliffs, NJ: Prentice-Hall.

Aronson, S. (1979). Rankings of intimacy of social behaviors by Italians and Americans. *Psychological reports, 44,* 1149–1150.

Barzini, L. (1964). *The Italians.* New York: Atheneum.

Blumberg, A., & Lavin, D. (1987). Italian-American students in the City University of New York: A socio-economic and education profile. In R. Gambino (Ed.), *Italian-American studies at City University of New York: Report and recommendations* (p. 85). New York: City University of New York Press.

Boscia-Mulé, P. (1999). *Authentic ethnicities: The interaction of ideology, gender power, and class in the Italian-American experience.* Westport, CT: Greenwood Press.

Bowen, M. (1978). *Family therapy in clinical practice.* New York: Aronson.

Bryant, A. (1976). *The Italians: How they live and work.* New York: Praeger.

Calandra Institute. (2000). *Education achievement level of Italian-American students in New York City public schools.* New York: Author.

Carilli, T. (1996). *Women as lovers: Two plays.* Toronto: Guernica Editions.

Ciongoli, A. K., & Parini, J. (2002). *The story of Italian immigration: Passage to liberty and the rebirth of America.* New York: Regan Books.

Cleary, P., & Demone, H. (1988). Health and social service needs in a northeastern metropolitan area: Ethnic group differences. *Journal of Sociology and Social Welfare, 15*(4), 63–76.

Cohen, M. (1992). *Workshop to office: Two generations of Italian women in New York City, 1900–1950.* Ithaca, NY: Cornell University Press.

Crohn, J. (1995). *Mixed matches: How to create successful interracial, interethnic and interfaith relationships.* New York: Fawcett Columbine.

DeRosa, T. (1980). An Italian American woman speaks out. *Attenzione, 2,* 25.

DeVries, R. G. (1986). *Tender warriors: A novel.* Ann Arbor, MI: Firebrand Books.

Femminella, F. (1982). Social psychiatry in the Italian American community. In R. Caporale (Ed.), *Italian*

Americans through the generations: The first one hundred years. New York: American Italian Historical Association.

Femminella, F., & Quadagno, J. (1976). The Italian American family. In C. Mindel & R. Habenstein (Eds.), *Ethnic families in America* (pp. 61–88). New York: Elsevier.

Ferro, R. (1983). *The family of Max Desir*. New York: New American Library.

Gambino, R. (1974). *Blood of my blood: The dilemma of Italian-Americans*. New York: Doubleday.

Giordano, J. (1986). *The Italian American catalog*. New York: Doubleday.

Giordano, J. (1994, June 13). The shame we share in secret. *Newsday*, p. 25.

Hoobler, D., & Hoobler T. (1997). *The Italian American family album*. New York: Oxford University Press.

Ianni, P. A., & Reuss-Ianni, E. (1972). *A family business: Kinship and social control in organized crime*. New York: Sage.

Johnson, C. (1985). *Growing up and growing old in Italian-American families*. New Brunswick, NJ: Rutgers University Press.

La Gumina, S. (1988). *From steerage to suburb*. New York: Center for Migration Studies.

La Gumina, S., Cavaioli, F., Primeggia, S., & Varacalli, J. (2000). *The Italian American experience: An encyclopedia*. New York: Garland.

Laurino, M. (2000). *Were you always an Italian?: Ancestors and other icons of Italian America*. New York: Norton.

Lopreato, J. (1970). *Italian Americans*. New York: University of Texas at Austin.

Mangione, J., & Morreale, B. (1992). La storia: *Five centuries of the Italian American experience*. New York: HarperCollins.

Messina, E. (1994). Life-span development and Italian-American women. In J. Krase & J. DeSena (Eds.), *Italian-Americans in a multicultural society* (pp. 74–87). New York: American Historical Society.

Nelli, H. S. (1980). Italians. In S. Thernstrom, A. Orlov, & O. Handlin (Eds.), *Harvard encyclopedia of American ethnic groups* (pp. 545–560). Cambridge, MA: Harvard University Press.

Papajohn, J., & Spiegel, J. (1975). *Transactions in families*. San Francisco: Jossey-Bass.

Rabkin, J., & Struening, E. (1975). *Ethnicity, social class and mental illness in New York City: A social area analysis of five ethnic groups* (Working Paper No. 17). New York: American Jewish Committee.

Ragucci, A. T. (1981). Italian Americans. In A. Hargood (Ed.), *Ethnicity and medical care* (pp. 211–263). Cambridge, MA: Harvard University Press.

Response Analysis Corporation. (1989). *Americans of Italian descent: A study of public images, beliefs and misperceptions*. Princeton, NJ: Order of the Sons of Italy.

Riotta-Sirey, A., Patti, A., & Mann. L. (1985). *Ethnotherapy—An exploration of Italian-American identity*. New York: National Institute for Psychotherapists.

Rolle, A. (1980). *The Italian American: Troubled roots*. New York: Free Press.

Santo, L. (1984). *Parental identity: Harmonizing ethnic traditions and contemporary values*. New York: American Jewish Committee.

Yans-McLaughlin, V. (1980). *Family and community*. Urbana: University of Illinois Press.

Zborowski, M. (1964). *People in pain*. San Francisco: Jossey-Bass.

Zogby, J. (2001). *American teenagers and stereotyping*. Washington, DC: National Italian American Foundation.

Zola, I. K. (1966). Culture and symptoms—An analysis of patients' presenting complaints. *American Sociological Review, 5*, 615–630.

CHAPTER 45

Portuguese Families

Zarita Araújo-Lane

For the majority of Portuguese immigrants living in the United States, seeking mental health services is both a cultural and an emotional challenge. Individuals and families from a rural background tend to rely on a tight system of family elders and authority figures, possibly consisting of religious leaders, teachers, medical providers, respected community workers, and folk healers. There is a strong unspoken belief that if one talks about "bad" things, they will come to be a reality. This powerful mysticism can be carried to an extreme, and those who seek family therapy feel torn between personal or familial anguish and the need to preserve family honor.

This chapter illustrates, through brief case studies, a few of the threads that make up the fabric of Portuguese families in the United States. Although the threads are complex and interwoven, for the purpose of teaching, I have separated them into the principal topics of history, immigration, and four main character values. Most of the case studies are based on families that immigrated from the Azores. They represent the largest group of immigrants from Portugal living in the United States (McCabe & Thomas, 1998). However, the family dynamics in this chapter can be applied to all Portuguese immigrant families. Understandably, a therapist may notice among Portuguese patients a range of treatment expectations and behaviors related to the seeking of treatment. These are largely connected to the background of the family, whether urban or rural. Portuguese immigrants from an urban background tend to be more direct and assertive when speaking to a person of authority.

HISTORY

Portugal, a small European county in the Iberian Peninsula with two beautiful archipelagos, the Azores and Madeira, went from being "a great nation," a champion of nautical science in the 15th century, to a country in great financial crisis suffering from a widespread lack of employment and affordable housing in the 20th century.

As a result of the financial, geographic (earthquakes), and sociopolitical challenges faced by the Portuguese in the 19th and 20th centuries, more than a million Portuguese immigrants are currently living in the United States. Some of the Portuguese immigrants in this country are from mainland Portugal, but the mainland Portuguese mostly immigrated to other countries in Europe and Africa. A few of the Portuguese immigrants in the United States are from Madeira. Because of the proximity of the Azores to the United States, the great majority of Portuguese immigrants in the United States are from the rural Azores.

The Azores are an archipelago of nine volcanic islands in the North Atlantic, about 800 miles west of Lisbon. They were discovered in the early 1400s and later settled by mainland Portuguese and assorted European ethnic groups. The Azores had long been a target for rapacious pirates. Some currently used Azorean expressions denoting fear or dismay originated in ancient warnings announcing the pirates' arrival and signaling local women to seek refuge. The constant threat of earthquakes and violent storms further compounded the feeling of helplessness. This sense of having little control over external forces is called *destino* (fate), which Azoreans hoped they could overcome by respecting their fellow human beings and subjecting themselves to authority figures (McGill, 1980; Moitoza, 1982).

In the United States, Azoreans have settled mainly in New England, California, and Hawaii. Presently there are more Azoreans living in the United States and Canada than in the Azores. In his article "Azorean Dreams," Onésimo T. Almeida (1998) calls New England the "Tenth Island."

GOVERNMENT

Portuguese sailors were foremost among European maritime explorers during the 15th century, sailing the oceans in search of better trade routes to India and the Far East. This exploration took the Portuguese around the tip of Africa to its western coast. Over time, the Portuguese gained power over the Azores, the West African coast, and parts of southern Asia and Brazil, spreading Christianity and simultaneously taking advantage of the incredible richness of the natural resources in these lands.

Until 1910, the Portuguese government was a hereditary and constitutional monarchy. The revolution of October 5, 1910, brought the monarchy to an end and substituted a republican government for it. The change of government resulted in a rapid succession of 8 presidents and 44 governments (www.nationbynation.com).

Eventually, the Portuguese military took over the government. The 50 years of fascist rule that followed the military takeover contributed to an ever-present fear of loss. Under fascism, self-expression was unacceptable and punished by denunciation and imprisonment. The outspoken few were severed from mainstream society and "lost" friends, family, and social status.

The Portuguese public, and its colonial populations, lived under constant fear of the PIDE (secret police), who kept detailed records about citizens whom they considered suspicious. When jailed or interrogated, political prisoners suffered physical and emotional torture and often ended up dead. These experiences are still vivid in the minds of many older immigrants. However, younger immigrants may not recall the oppressive fascist government and may adopt a more positive and trusting attitude toward authority figures.

For years, the Portuguese colonies fought a guerrilla war against the Portuguese military. Eventually, on April 25, 1974, a left-wing branch of the Portuguese army, not happy with the war in Africa or with the fascist government in Portugal, led a revolution and overthrew the government. Soon after the revolution, a left-wing government in Portugal negotiated to end the war and supported the sovereignty of the colonies. But the Azores did not benefit as rapidly as the mainland and the African ex-colonies from the ensuing economic and social reforms.

Azoreans have long felt disadvantaged in relation to the mainland Portuguese (Marques, 1975; Moitoza, 1982). The postrevolution years only created more tension between the two groups. In 1975, an Azorean independence movement (the FLA, or Azores Liberation Front) was created, which successfully pressured the Portuguese government to establish an autonomous government in the islands. Since then, the Azores have had their own government, with greater mobility in the country's economy and a stronger sense of control over its political fate. However, there were casualties of the FLA movement: During the late 1970s, some mainland Portuguese and a few Azoreans who had left-wing affiliations were harassed, threatened, and ultimately forced off the islands.

Portugal adopted a Socialist constitution in 1976. Various cooperatives among rural workers were formed, day-care centers were created for the general population, health care delivery was improved, unions were legalized, and campaigns to overcome a high illiteracy rate were created all over Portugal. The new constitution also reflected a liberal integration of women's rights. However, the new government's attempts at economic change threw the nation into a recession. It was not until the mid-1980s that Portugal began to make significant economic progress. At present, because of a shortage of affordable labor, Portugal is receiving new immigrants from Eastern Europe, Africa, and Brazil.

The Portuguese colonizers had married into or mixed with the native populations of the lands they controlled, thus making a complete emotional and physical separation between the former colonies and the colonizers an impossible task. A great majority of the former Portuguese colonies opted to keep Portuguese as their official language. After independence, many Portuguese professionals were invited by the new governments of the former colonies to return for periods of several years as *cooperantes*, or partners, in revamping an infrastructure that had suffered tremendously during the civil war and subsequent period of transition.

Since then, Portugal has become outspoken in the movement for civil rights in its former colonies. A recent example are the Portuguese envoys active at the United Nations, arranging for peace talks and pressing the United States to take a stand against the oppression of the people of East Timor.

Historically, the Portuguese have always been aware of having lost an empire. This trauma or fear of loss is an undercurrent of everyday Portuguese life, as manifest in the general feeling that investments or belongings could be easily lost at any time. This may well explain the Portuguese fear of taking risks, as documented by anthropologist Estellie Smith in her article "Portuguese Enclaves: The Invisible Minority" (Fitzgerald, 1974).

INITIAL SESSIONS

Therapists working with Portuguese families need to pay special attention to the first sessions, where the stigma of seeking mental health treatment can be addressed. Although clients may not directly say, "I am ashamed. I feel that I betrayed my family's honor," many will act out those feelings through storytelling about coming for treatment or by making an array of excuses about available treatment times.

Therapists may benefit from developing working relationships with key community leaders. Often these leaders serve as transitional objects during the initial stages of therapy. If clients seem reluctant to follow through after initial visits, therapists may find it helpful to meet them for a brief visit at the office of the referral contact or in a safe place in the community. The therapist might also use storytelling as a negotiation technique. For example, a therapist may say, "I have had patients in the past who were concerned that community members might see them coming to my office. How do you feel about this?"

Cristina, a 35-year-old Azorean mother, went to a respected community worker to ask for help with her electric bills. Cristina was capable of communicating in English, but had never sought help before. After several visits "for help with her bills," Cristina burst into tears, telling the community worker that she was sure her husband of 15 years was cheating on her. She wanted to divorce him and move back to the Azores, where her parents had returned to enjoy their retirement.

The community worker contacted the therapist's office and put Cristina on the telephone. During the phone conversation, Cristina expressed a mix of sadness and anger. She confessed a feeling of *vergonha* (embarrassment or shame) about her husband's cheating. She had found several condoms in his truck, and one appeared to have been used recently.

Cristina felt comfortable talking on the phone with the therapist while the community worker was present. After she denied being at risk for physical abuse, Cristina and the therapist went over a plan for introducing the husband to the idea of couple therapy. When the couple later came to therapy, they seemed to share a *simpático* (fondness) for each other. The husband did not want to loose his wife and daughters, but denied being unfaithful.

———————— ❧ ————————

ONGOING TREATMENT

To connect with families and individuals, therapists must overcome three main challenges: stigma, time, and hierarchy.

In Cristina's case, two of these challenges were immediately evident. To start with, by sharing personal problems with the therapist, an *outsider*, Cristina and her husband were breaking a cultural taboo. What a contrast to the old Portuguese adage, *"Entre mulher e marido não se mete a colher"* ("You don't intervene in matters between a husband and a wife")!

The other obvious challenge was time. Cristina and her husband, like many Portuguese immigrants, had come to the United States to better their financial lot in life. Both had two jobs and very little time for ongoing treatment. The therapist recognized this dilemma. On one hand, Cristina and her husband yearned for the American Dream; on the other hand, they wanted to preserve their marriage. The therapist realized the need for a compromise.

To accommodate the couple, the therapist twice sacrificed some of her own family time for late-evening therapy sessions. After that, the couple needed to agree to a mutually convenient time. The therapist offered alternatives, and together they set forth the following plan: The first three appointments would be held once a week for 3 weeks, with a transition to biweekly, triweekly, and, later, monthly visits over a period of several months.

The couple's therapy first focused on their methods of child rearing. They worked on trying to create a balance in their distinct roles as parents; he was the "fun" parent and she, the disciplinarian. He enjoyed social events; she was always worried about housework and church attendance. As this issue was being worked out, the husband eventually confessed to a one-time affair with one of his wife's cousins.

This revelation was very painful for both of them. After much emotional exchange, the couple decided not to be physically intimate until they could trust each other. They agreed that they were going to try to work through this breach of trust. They further agreed to be faithful to each other. The husband promised to talk to the cousin and ask that she not join them in family activities. The couple worked hard on their relationship, and after a summer vacation they reconnected sexually and decided to terminate the therapy.

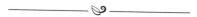

Often, Portuguese families or individuals end treatment before completing the course of therapy. Therapists need to provide an open environment where clients feel free to return for additional visits whenever necessary. The goal is that families and individuals come to feel safe in therapy and gradually accept the idea of ongoing treatment.

UNDERSTANDING LOSS AS A RESULT OF IMMIGRATION

Although most Portuguese immigration is the result of economic hardship, a few immigrants have come to America for religious, political or geographic reasons (Araujo, 1996; McCabe & Thomas, 1998; Mira, 1998; Pap, 1992). Whatever the motivation, it takes an average of 5–10 years from the time a family first considers immigration to the day it sets foot on U.S. soil. Immigration is a costly process; couples often leave older children and elderly parents behind in the mother country. Yet, in most cases, the immigrant continues to be the family's main breadwinner, making it impossible for him or her to think of pursuing secular goals like college education or political involvement. Making the money needed to pay off debt, support the family, and buy property (in Portugal and/or the United States) are the top priorities for these immigrants.

It is my understanding that it generally takes another 5–10 years for immigrant families to show some acceptance of their new situation and to become less rigid in their methods of child rearing. The fear of "losing" the family, combined with grieving the loss of their homeland, can lead Portuguese, and especially Azorean, families to isolate themselves.

In the immigration process, there are three main stages in the process of acculturation: the honeymoon, anger and loss, and negotiation and acceptance. Clients in the honeymoon phase have a tendency to idealize the United States and criticize their native country, so therapists may get a decidedly one-sided report on life in Portugal.

Clients experiencing anger and loss may emphasize the negative aspects of life in the United States and idealize the lives they previously led in Portugal. These are the families who do not trust authority and feel they are victims of racial discrimination. Those experiencing the negotiation and acceptance stage feel more comfortable in seeking help from "outsiders" and discussing the dichotomous values they gathered throughout their life in Portugal and subsequent life in the United States. These are the families who are not ashamed of the fact that they carry two worlds with them and who, over time, come to terms with the fact that they may never truly "belong" to either world. They have forged a new identity: that of being a Portuguese immigrant in the United States. Their vocabulary is often full of Anglicisms such as *estoa* or *marketa* for "store" or "market," which in standard Portuguese would be *loja* or *mercado*.

THE FOUR CHARACTER VALUES

A useful tool for therapists is a knowledge of the four character values: *honra* (honor), *respeito* (respect), *bondade* (generosity), and *confiança* (trust). Empathetic listening and echoing may be enough to establish rapport with a client, but to build the trust crucial to a therapeutic alliance, the therapist must also connect in relation to one of these four values. To assist the therapist, I have developed the illustration of a tree and its parts.

Honra: The Roots

Visualize a healthy tree from bottom to top. The roots (*honra*, or honor) are buried beneath the surface of the ground. *Honra* is the complete set of unspoken expectations and unconscious behaviors that are learned from childhood through family rituals and religious celebrations. At these events, a person learns how to interact with society and develops patterns of dealing with men, women, and children by listening to stories and by watching sanctioned and nonsanctioned behaviors. *Honra* serves as an anchor to the person's self-esteem and general well-being.

Therapists may encounter a rigid family or individual *honra* that stunts the client's growth. Rather than immediately working to uncover unspoken values at the beginning of the therapeutic process, a therapist may want to come to a deeper understanding of the client's roots by listening to the stories the client tells. Generally, these stories will focus on those outside the therapeutic encounter and are a form of externalization.

The following case illustrates the four character values:

Senhora (a respectful title for older women) Ana, a 64-year-old immigrant from Minho, a northern region of Portugal, immigrated to the United States before the revolution of 1974. Her American-born adult son referred her for individual treatment.

Senhora Ana showed physical signs of alcohol abuse (underweight, purplish skin tone, red marks on her cheeks, shaky limbs, etc.). At first, she was evasive in her response to the therapist; the therapist then shared that her own father was from Minho and that she truly missed the local food, the marketplaces, and the pristine country mornings. Instantly, Senhora Ana's face lit up and she began to pour out her feelings of loneliness. Her husband had recently bought a house in an area where public transportation is scarce. Because she does not drive, she began to experience feelings of isolation. Her only activities are cooking and cleaning. Her adult children had married American "girls" who did not speak Portuguese and did not like Portuguese food.

Senhora Ana and her husband agreed to attend couple therapy to discuss the losses resulting from immigration and the changes in their immediate family. As treatment progressed, it became clear that she had been self-medicating for depression with the wine she used for cooking.

———————— ❧ ————————

As the clinician was listening to the family, she was able to identify the patient's key values as defined by the cooking and the cleaning of the house. This was Senhora Ana's way of being a good mother and wife and contributing to her family. This clinician also understood that one of the principles of good Portuguese cooking is to marinate meats and seafood in wine, bay leaves, and garlic. This knowledge was a helpful tool to begin to address Senhora Ana's drinking. Later in the treatment, the patient disclosed that she was sipping on the wine as she marinated the food she cooked for her family.

Respeito: The Branches

By echoing a feeling of *saudade* (longing or loss) through personal disclosure, the therapist showed *respeito* (respect) for the client. This was helpful, inasmuch as a stranger's probing for personal information can be perceived by a Portuguese individual as rude "American" behavior. In this case, the therapist's sharing of information had a positive effect and put the patient at ease. *Respeito* can be likened to the branches of the tree. When broken, they can sometimes be saved through a process of grafting, provided that those branches are not repeatedly damaged.

Bondade: Healthy Leaves

Another aspect of this intervention was the therapist's awareness of the Portuguese tradition of cooking with wine. Rather than address the wine in the initial intervention, the therapist was able to first create an environment of *bondade* (generosity, kindness) in which the patient felt safe in discussing her grief over immigration. The therapist went out of her way to connect with the patient and bridged a potential communication gap by sharing something in common. This form of communication allowed the client to maneuver at a reasonable comfort level and make use of externalization as a form of self-expression. The therapist was not obligated to act with *bondade*, but by doing so, allowed the therapeutic relationship to thrive, promoting the growth of healthy leaves.

If the therapist had pushed for a more linear form of communication, the intervention could possibly have backfired, with the therapist inadvertently becoming the center of the encounter, or even a burden in the session. So it is not a bad idea for a therapist to prepare a "bag" of personal information that can be safely shared when the situation permits. For those therapists not of Portuguese descent, there are other ways of showing generosity. One strategy, tried and true, is to refer to a personal sacrifice, perhaps involving scheduling (e.g., "I can schedule this appointment for you but I am sacrificing personal time, and I need you to help me to find a compromise for follow-up visits").

Confiança: A Lush Canopy

Confiança (trust) is the canopy of the tree, which exists only when the other parts are intact. *Confiança* resulted in Senhora Ana's sharing intimate feelings about her daughters-in-law, the "American girls." She was able to reveal these feelings because she trusted that the therapist was "just like" her, and not "one of them." Ana did not want to speak badly about her family, but she was bothered by the "loss" of her cultural identity and of her sons. The therapist understood this dynamic and echoed it back to her by saying, "Your sons heard you; they got married and they are giving you a new family with women they love. Just like your in-laws before you, you can pass on your roots as a Portuguese mother-in-law. Your sons have learned from you that family is important no matter the difficulties we face."

SPEAKING PORTUGUESE MAY NOT BE ENOUGH

As a result of Portugal's widespread colonization of other lands, Portuguese became one of the most widely spoken languages in the world. It is, by some estimates, the third most spoken language in Europe (Page, 2002) and the eighth most spoken language in the world (www.deltranslator.com). Clinicians must be aware that there are variations of spoken Portuguese. Indeed, there may be tensions between Brazilians, Azoreans, and mainland Portuguese that have deep roots in the history of Portugal's systematic exploitation of other countries. This history, along with the "assimilated immigrant versus new immigrant" dynamic, needs to be acknowledged by the therapist at the start of therapy.

For example, if a therapist is Brazilian and he or she is working with an Azorean family, the racial/ethnic difference may interfere in the building of trust. The therapist's accent can be a reminder of a general feeling in the Azorean community that Brazilians are taking over the jobs and that they are too aggressive in defending their rights as immigrants. The reality is that the most recent wave of Brazilian immigrants consisted mainly of middle-class professionals who had experienced a different lifestyle back in Brazil, but were forced to accept menial jobs in the United States when the Brazilian economy, including the stock market, crashed.

Brazilians speak a more eclectic Portuguese, easily adapting words from English and the other languages of immigrants who migrated to Brazil from Europe, Asia, and the Middle East between 1890 and 1919. Brazil is larger than the United States, and much larger than Portugal, but only the upper middle class really kept in touch with Portuguese literature and art. The population of rural Brazil seems to have had less exposure to Portuguese from Portugal. Although, linguistically, the differences between Brazilian and Portuguese usage are similar to those between the United States and England, the two cultures are drastically different. These differences can be worked out if therapists are direct with patients when discussing potential conflicts in the sessions.

After his father passed away, João, a 35-year-old Azorean immigrant who came to the United States as a child, became depressed and began to present suicidal ideation. His elderly mother and teenage sister sought treatment for the family. They were greatly concerned with João's inability to keep a job and with his intense sadness. The therapist assigned to his case was from Brazil. João got angry with the therapist every time she pronounced words differently than he did, and began to mock the therapist's speech.

The other family members seemed embarrassed when João poked fun at the therapist's accent. But the therapist used this opportunity to acknowledge the linguistic differences between them, and echoed how difficult it must be for João and his family to deal with a double loss. He smiled and indirectly apologized. Later in the session, João disclosed that he was feeling pressured to fill his father's shoes as the primary provider for the family.

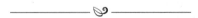

Until 15 years ago, before the increase of Brazilian immigration to the United States, there was tension between the mainland Portuguese and the Azoreans. Brazilian immigration contributed to greater solidarity among immigrants from the different parts of Portugal. Possibly, the Portuguese felt the need to unify and confront the newer immigrants with a different approach to the Portuguese language and lifestyle. In addition, technological advances and the increased availability of transportation have resulted in more interaction between Azoreans and *Continentais* (people from mainland Portugal), creating a friendlier environment. It is still common for a therapist from the Azores or the mainland to initially experience some resistance from individuals or families from a different part of Portugal. This reticence may be left over from the fascist times, when there was a sense of supremacy of mainland Portuguese over Azoreans. The book *Leaving Pico* recounts the tension between Azorean and the mainland immigrants living in Provincetown, Massachusetts (Gaspar, 1999).

RESPECT FOR AUTHORITY

Portuguese families often stay together for the sake of their *honra* (honor). This value can be a strength when all members are willing to collaborate and work on family issues. But it can also be a major weakness when it is too rigid and forces family members to become the enablers of a dysfunctional dynamic. For instance, immigrant parents, in general, use corporal punishment to instill in their children respect for authority figures. It is common for the mother to inform the father of a child's misbehavior or to threaten to do so. The father, complying with his duties for the sake of the family's *honra*, spanks the children.

However, at times the mother feels guilty that the father is "too hard" on the children and does not follow through with her threats of informing him of their misbehavior. Yet she may never actually voice her concerns over his use of harsh corporal punishment, for fear of upsetting him. As a result, the child is never clear about when the father is actually told about a transgression.

Therapists often see parents struggling with wanting to be believed and respected by their children. A child may experience a mother's inconsistency in keeping her word when she says, for example, " I am going to tell your father, so he will punish you when he gets home," and then later feels bad for the sake of the child and does not keep her threat, and the father does not spank the child. If part of the family's *honra* is honesty, this dynamic of false threats and the inability to openly talk about such discrepancies may make the child confused and emotionally disengaged from the parents. Again, out of respect, the child's feelings of confusion about mother's behavior in not keeping her word will likely never be articulated to the parents, unless the child has already developed identifiable behavioral problems like stealing, name calling, or disruptive behavior.

For the sake of a family's *honra*, some Portuguese women are anxious that their husbands be viewed by the community as family heads. In practice, however, it is generally the woman who makes decisions for the emotional well-being of the family. There is an interesting saying among Portuguese females, *"Cá em casa quem manda sou eu, mas faço que não sei nada"* ("Here in my house I am the boss, but I pretend that I don't know it").

The authority in the Portuguese immigrant family goes from father to mother to the oldest child. If a younger son is close in age to an older daughter, he, not she, will take over the family affairs when the parents are no longer able. Therapists may find the storytelling technique helpful in figuring out who holds the main power. During a family session, participants can be invited to report on family values, rituals, and dynamics. Family genograms may serve as a concrete cultural tool. Genograms make use of externalization through a visual exercise in which family members teach the therapist about family dynamics. This allows for the natural modes of communication in the Portuguese community: storytelling about people who have made an impact on one's life. Doing a genogram exercise may help in the initial sorting out of family history, expectations, and values, as the therapist and the family members become the actors or reporters, but not the owners of the information.

RACE

When adolescent girls challenge a vertical hierarchy, the family's reaction may be dramatic. A girl may act out sexually with boys from non-Portugese backgrounds or other groups. In Portuguese culture, sexual intercourse is generally permissible only after marriage (for both sexes). Again, when a child breaks the rules, not only is there an individual loss for the parents, but also a fear of loss of respect in the community, especially if the "transgressor" is female. The community is much less forgiving of a female who acts out sexually, than of a male, especially if the girl's sexual partner is a boy from a cultural or racial background perceived by the family to be of lower socioeconomic status.

This can devastate a family that believes in respecting the outside world but not mixing with it. For some reason, marrying outside the ethnic group may at first be perceived an affront to the family, to the community, and even to the entire country. It shatters the last hope of the family's return to Portugal upon the parents' retirement.

The issue of race is a complex one. Portugal itself was born of the populations who settled the area known today as the Iberian Peninsula: Germanic, Roman, Moorish, and Jewish. Later in history, Portuguese colonizers married natives of the countries they colonized. Before the revolution in 1974, mixed marriages and socialization between people of different races happened at all levels of colonial society. Included in the upper classes were many intellectuals, professionals, writers, and poets of mixed ancestry.

After the revolution in 1974, Lisbon became a mecca for the many individuals who lived or were born in the former colonies. This was a difficult time for many of the *retornados* (those who returned; in this group there were not only emigrés, but natives of former colonies who opted for Portuguese citizenship). They were part of a large resettlement movement, and although the great majority were able to adjust well to continental Portuguese life, those from lower socioeconomic backgrounds and those with little or no formal instruction did not do so well. They settled in ghettos into which few White Portuguese would dare to venture.

Although Portugal is a social democracy, the government has failed to create effective policies to prevent racism. Unfortunately, racism among the Portuguese is similar to racism in the United States. Tolerance and even kindness toward individuals of other races is prevalent, but racism is still evident in comments such as "What a cute baby, even though she is Black."

As mentioned earlier, Portuguese individuals can resemble members of many ethnic and racial groups. However, for demographic statistics and federal grants, the Portuguese (as a group, in the United States) are considered not a racial minority, but a linguistic minority. Moreover, where race is self-determined, some Portuguese-speaking racial minorities may identify themselves as "Portuguese" or "White."

SEXUALITY

Hugo, a young Azorean living in the United States for 15 years, was caving under the pressure of caring for his family. He is the only one in his family who speaks English. He has worked in two jobs and sacrificed going to college so he could help his parents to buy a house. He is very close to his mother, who is constantly praising him by making statements like, "If your grandmother were alive, she would be so proud of you!"

Hugo began to feel attached to a close male friend. He withdrew from socializing with his family, and his mother sought help from a community worker. After a few individual sessions, it became clear to the therapist that Hugo was falling in love with the male friend. Exploring his sexuality at a time when he was also depressed was a delicate matter. After much negotiation on how to present his homosexuality to his family, his mother asked that the rest of the family not be made aware of the issue. She loved her son; she wanted the best for him and hoped that he would change his mind with time.

Out of respect for the family name, Hugo brought his American lover home and introduced him as a friend from work. The family members understood the depth of the relationship and adopted the "friend" as the "gringo who likes Portuguese food and parties." The community grew to comprehend the relationship between Hugo and his "friend," but it was never spoken of openly except on the few occasions when a drunken community member approached him to ask about his *namorado* (boyfriend). Hugo and his male partner have moved into one of the apartments in his parent's house and continue to provide for the family.

Homosexuality among Portuguese immigrants is often perceived as something to be ashamed of and not to be mentioned among family members. There is a code of silence, and a mother often attempts to hide a child's homosexuality from her husband, so as to avoid causing him *desgosto* (disappointment). There are certain regions in the Azores and other parts of Portugal where there are larger gay populations, and they are looked upon as different but are generally respected. Overall, the Portuguese gay or bisexual individual faces difficulties in "coming out" to his or her family similar to those faced by American gays, especially those residing in small communities.

CONCLUSION

Working with Portuguese families in the United States is at first a challenge. Families often come to treatment as a result of a court order or after being referred by their health care providers or community workers. Rarely does a family seek help on its own. Sharing problems with strangers or with individuals outside the immediate family is a concept foreign to most Portuguese persons. The therapist is faced with the triple challenge of stigma, time, and hierarchy. Patients are often not comfortable in questioning authority and may agree to treatment with a verbal "yes," but have difficulty following through with this commitment.

Family therapists need to work within the family's culture as they build trust. Later, they can make a transition to introducing new ideas. For example, the concept of spending "quality time" with children, as discussed among professionals in this country, is unnatural to new Portuguese immigrants. They define "spending quality time" as providing basic material needs for their children, instructing them in good manners and respect for authority, and training children to help the family with gender-specific chores. Girls will help with household tasks, shopping, and arts and crafts. The boys will help by assisting their fathers in making repairs around the house, fixing cars, or working at part-time jobs.

An understanding of the four character values: *honra* (honor), *respeito* (respect), *bondade* (generosity), and *confiança* (trust) is extremely helpful when intervening with Portuguese families. The clinician should work closely with the referral source to engage the family and to help them to get past their initial embarrassment at seeking treatment. They are likely to experience a referral as a violation of *honra*. A family may respond by denying the problem, blaming the symptom carrier, and then blaming other family members, friends, and, finally, the referral source.

In therapy with Portuguese families, it can be helpful to approach delicate subjects by using open-ended statements or through storytelling, externalizing issues at first. Therapists may need to be more active in the initial session: negotiating, coaching, mirroring, or echoing behaviors for individuals and families.

ACKNOWLEDGMENTS

My sincere thanks to David McGill for his coaching and to Vonessa Phillips for her editing.

REFERENCES

Almeida, O. T. (1998). Azorean dreams. In M. L. McCabe & J. D. Thomas (Eds.), *Portuguese spinner: An American story* (pp. 20–29). New Bedford: Spinner.

Araujo, Z. A. (1996). Portuguese families. In M. McGoldrick, J. Giordano, & J. Pearce (Eds.), *Ethnicity and family therapy* (2nd ed., pp. 583–594). New York: Guilford Press.

Fitzgerald, T. K. (Ed.). (1974). *Social and cultural identity* (SAS Proceedings No. 8). Athens: University of Georgia Press.

Gaspar, F. X. (1999). *Leaving Pico.* Hanover, NH: University Press of New England.

Marques, O. A. (1975). *História de Portugal* (Vol. 3). Lisboa: Editora Palas.

McCabe, M. L., & Thomas, J. D. (Eds.). (1998). *Portuguese spinner: An American story.* New Bedford, MA: Spinner.

McGill, D. (1980). *Ethnicity training for a community mental health center staff: Portuguese-American ethnicity and mental health in Fall River, Massachusetts.* Doctoral dissertation, Massachusetts School of Professional Psychology, Boston.

Mira, M. (1998). *The forgotten Portuguese.* Franklin, NC: Portuguese-American Historical Research Foundation.

Moitoza, E. (1982). Portuguese families. In M. McGoldrick, J. K. Pearce, & J. Giordano (Eds.), *Ethnicity and family therapy* (pp. 412–437). New York: Guilford Press.

Page, M. (2002). *The first global village: How Portugal changed the world.* Lisbon: Notícias Editorial.

Pap, L. (1992). *The Portuguese-Americans.* Boston: Twayne.

Smith, E. (1974). Portuguese enclaves: The invisible minority. In T. K. Fitzgerald (Ed.), *Social and cultural identity.* Atlanta: University of Georgia Press.

CHAPTER 46

Scandinavian Families
Plain and Simple

Beth M. Erickson

The first known written references to Scandinavia, which is composed of Denmark, Sweden, Norway, Finland, and Iceland,[1] were made in the 1st century A.D. by the Roman encyclopedist Pliny the Elder (Mead, 1985). The region is often described as a family of nations; one frequently hears the phrase "Nordic family," because there is a kinship among the countries. The degree of similarity is extraordinary when one considers that the population of Scandinavia is more than 24 million (*National Georgraphic Atlas of the World*, 1999, pp. 70–72), only 1½ times that of New York State, and its people are scattered over lands separated by the Baltic and North Seas and the Atlantic Ocean. At one time the Nordic countries were united under one crown, and despite their clear differences in grammar, usage, and vocabulary, close linguistic ties allow Danes, Swedes, and Norwegians to understand each other, even when speaking their own languages.

Yet Nordic people passionately cherish their individualism and national independence. Norway, Sweden, and Denmark have constitutional monarchies, whereas the others have elected presidents as heads of state. Finlanders are reluctant even to be considered Scandinavians. Their civic pride took a serious hit when their country was first annexed by Sweden and then by Czar Alexander I, who wanted a capital closer to St. Petersburg (Black, 2004). He chose Helsinki. Finland finally won her independence during the Russian Revolution in 1917 (Stocker, 2004, p. H3), despite attempts to "Russify" her (www.workmall.com, p.5).

Clinicians are wise to bear in mind that there are both similarities and differences between the countries, making effective treatment for Scandinavians anything but a "one size fits all" approach. For example, in broad brushstrokes, Swedes, who populate the largest of the five countries and who have conquered all of the others except Iceland, generally may be seen as less hesitant to be bold, or in clinical terms, to differentiate openly. Therefore, in treating them, therapists can afford to be a bit more expressive, loquacious, and bold themselves. But with Norwegians, perhaps because of their legacy of being conquered alternately by Sweden and then Denmark for much of their history until 1905, therapists must be more restrained in their expression, and even in their dress, to match Norwegians' unique culture of humility, at least initially. Denmark includes ethnicities galore, and because Danes pride themselves on being cosmopolitan, therapists themselves may risk coming across as sophisticated and urbane, if that is congruent with their style. And because Icelanders live on a small, sparsely populated island in the middle of the sea, therapists may expect them to require a great deal of solitude and to tend to eschew intense interactions. Hence, successful treatment of Scandinavians requires a therapist's flexibility from group to group.

SCANDINAVIANS' BEST TRAITS AT A GLANCE

Scandinavians are:

- Determined, strong
- Independent, self-reliant, autonomous
- Fair, egalitarian
- Honest
- Sincere, self-effacing, unpretentious
- Family-oriented
- Hardworking, industrious
- Practical, solution-oriented, yet willing to be philosophical
- Stoic, reserved, not complainers
- Believers in collective responsibility, have civic pride

It should be noted any of these traits, taken to the extreme, can end up to be a negative for anybody. Clearly, Scandinavians have no corner on that market! For example, Scandinavians' penchant for independence can result in isolation as they lock themselves up, away from others. Their determination can become stubbornness, and even defiance, as they stand their ground and have difficulty in seeing other ways or points of view. In their industriousness, they can become driven and workaholic, which also allows them to seem independent. Usually, it is family dynamics or unresolved crises that create such exaggerations or distortions of Scandinavians' natural tendencies. Generally, it is such situations, then, that motivate people to seek a therapist's help to reshape or temper these traits run amok.

OVERVIEW

What does it mean to be Scandinavian? Above all, perhaps, reservedness. Speaking or writing about themselves or their heritage betrays a cultural legacy centered on twin implicit ethics: "Don't think you're so special" and "Keep to yourself." Despite this, I, a full-blooded Scandinavian, will press on, seeking to answer these five questions: What are the systematic commonalities, modes of thought, feeling, and social behavior that distinguish Scandinavians from others? How are these commonalities evident in the individuals and families who present for psychotherapy? What does this mean for the treatment we provide? What are the roots of these shared traits? What do therapists need to know in order to act as cultural interpreters of one Scandinavian to another, and of Scandinavians to entirely different ethnic groups? Perhaps to a greater degree than in countries with more temperate weather conditions and less rugged topography, Scandinavians' most significant identifying character traits can be seen as developing in response to the climate and geography of their countries.

Darkness

Sunlight is a precious commodity for Scandinavians who, in summer, are like squirrels storing it up for the winter. Large parts of Sweden, Norway, and Finland lie above the Arctic Circle. Thus, when the sun sets in November, it literally does not reappear for months, and then only for 4 minutes a day (Mead, 1985). Even Iceland, where only her northern part touches the Arctic Circle, is not exempt from darkness throughout December (www.uoregon.edu, p. 1). Only Denmark is far enough south that her people do not have to cope with unbroken darkness. When I met a gaunt Norwegian early one November and inquired where he was from, he named his small city above the Arctic Circle and said, with a note of defeat, "It's already dark at home." His visage telegraphed depression and hinted that darkness indeed may occupy his soul.

In contrast, as if *yin* to winter's *yang*, all of Scandinavia is the land of the midnight sun in the summer, when the sun literally does not set. Sleep becomes very difficult to regulate, which also can contribute to depression. Despite this difficulty, the loss of the sun is deeply mourned come autumn. There is an old saying: "In Finland, the sun is king and the queen is silence" (Sodergren, 1993, p. 57). Thus, the sun and its absence, isolation within and between homes by virtue of Scandinavians' unique brand of stoicism and taciturnity and the countries' rugged terrain, combined, are stamped into the collective unconscious of Scandinavians.

Isolation

Why is isolation so prevalent in these countries? Denmark is a small country composed primarily of islands, where seclusion is compounded because there are few bridges connecting these islands. Ferries were at one time the only means of transportation between the islands, so each island developed its own dialect, thus making communication, even between two Danes, difficult. Therefore, unlike Swedes and Norwegians, who easily are able to understand one another, Danes are separated even from their own fellow citizens. Iceland is composed mostly of mountains, volcanoes, and lava fields; therefore, habitable land is scarce. Furthermore, her population is sparse, numbering only 277,000 souls in a country roughly the size of Ohio, whose population is over 11 million (*National Geographic Atlas of the World*, 1999, pp. 34, 71). Norwegians, too, are confined in terrain that is stark and rugged, peppered with and separated by fjords, mountains, glaciers, and ice fields. The country has only about 3% arable land, as compared with Denmark's 70%, and some towns consist of just one or two homes and a boat landing or a train station. Likewise, Finland has poor terrain with little arable land. The landscape is dominated by steep cliffs rising from its 187,000 lakes, topped by pine forests (virtual.finland.fi, p. 2). And Sweden, Scandinavia's most populous country, has only 10% arable land (www.uktradeinvest.gov.uk/sweden, p. 1). Sweden has heavily wooded forests, with mountains and a rugged coastline etched by an archipelago of islands and hard cliffs. But perhaps the greatest factor in Scandinavia's small population is the waves of emigrants who left for the United States beginning in the mid-1800s. Thus, isolation is not reflexively avoided as it might be for other ethnic groups, because it, too, has been stamped into the collective unconscious of Scandinavians. Of course, in new immigrants to the United States, all of these traits are more dominant than in those whose families have been in this country for generations, couples who marry other Scandinavians rather than intermarrying, and families in rural areas.

Tim consulted me at the request of his family physician, who had become increasingly concerned about his patient's depression and suicidal thoughts. I requested that Tim's wife join us so that I could assess his depression in the context of the marriage. Uncovering nothing except less frequent sex than Tim would have preferred, I explored other contributors to what Tim described as his "black hole." Almost as in a mantra, he would repeat, "There are no colors."

Tim was a nearly full-blooded third-generation Norwegian whose father, Ed, was a policeman whose shifts had rendered him perennially unavailable to Tim. In addition, Tim's paternal grandmother had died in childbirth bearing Ed. Tragically, Ed's father believed that he was to blame for his wife's death because he had shoved her the night before she died. So, unable to bear his guilt or his grief, he committed suicide on Ed's first birthday. Sometime later, Ed's only two siblings also committed suicide, presumably out of their own darkness at being orphaned. Consequently, Ed was shuffled from pillar to post until an older childless aunt and uncle took him in. As Ed stated in a family of origin session that I conducted, they provided him with stability, giving him "three square meals, a bed, and a bicycle, but little else." As if all this were not devastating enough, when Ed was 14 years old, while he was playing with his best friend by the river, the other boy drowned as Ed watched in horror, unable to save him. This incident compounded Ed's guilt, and the memory was driven deep inside, not to be spoken of or grieved.

Treatment for Tim proceeded in phases, beginning with a lengthy diagnostic process to rule out the more typical contributors to depression, such as marital or family dysfunction, career dissatisfaction, and midlife or health issues. Satisfied that these were not contributors, we cast a wider net and began family of origin exploration, which included how Tim's and his wife's Norwegian heritage may have contributed to his depression. In doing a four-generational genogram, we hit pay dirt. It was then that it became abundantly clear that Tim's depression was as much a part of his inheritance as were his blue eyes and his Viking stature. This clarity began to loosen the grip of the depression, but the coup de grâce was bringing in his parents from several states away for a 4-hour family-of-origin session of the sort advanced by James Framo.

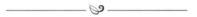

After much experimentation and scores of these sessions over the last 23 years, the format I recommend is the following, in order of priority: (1) two 2-hour meetings that occur over roughly a 24-hour period; (2) next best is two 1½-hour meetings over a 24-hour period; and (3) the option of last resort is one 3-hour session with a break midway. This delicate and important work definitely goes beyond the confines of a standard 50-minute session, where more harm than good can be done when ample time is not available. For these sessions to work, there must be an opportunity for all of the following to take place: (1) The adult child must frame the issues for the parents; (2) the parents deserve a chance to explain and to share their experiences and perspectives; (3) all need ample opportunity for questions to be asked and for feelings to be expressed, worked through, and understood; (4) all family members need to practice more healthy, congruent, and connected ways of relating while still having the safety net of the therapist's holding environment; and (5) participants need an opportunity to explore how they wish their relationships to be in the future.

For Tim, these sessions generated two outcomes essential for his recovery: (1) knowledge of and empathy for the heretofore taboo and unknown details of the father's life that had in turn numbed both men and (2) a nascent and fragile father–son bond previously impossible for both men. So seminal was this family session that treatment was completed in a matter of weeks afterward. In sum, the legacies of emotional constriction, isolation, and the tendency toward the darkness of depression were covertly passed down to Tim because of a cultural heritage and family legacy that emphasize emotional control and inexpressiveness. These factors silently decreed that discussion of all of the family's multiple and profound losses was off-limits. This, in turn, generated a deep longing and sense of "father hunger" (Erickson, 1998) that became centerpieces of both men's depression.

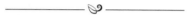

What are the skills and attributes required of therapists to help heretofore alienated family members to open up to each other, especially when there is a devastating history such as this and a culture in which talk therapy is hardly second nature? The requisite knack is all the more essential when both index patients are men (Erickson, 1993). First and foremost, the therapist must be adept at joining quickly, creating a holding environment for all, not just his or her client. This is necessary with any clients, of course, but even more important for parents, who usually expect to meet an emotional firing squad led by the therapist who, from a misguided sense of loyalty or mission, advocates for his or her client and blames the parents. (To state the obvious, holding parents accountable is not the same as blaming them.) So when they are met instead by someone who is warm, respectful, welcoming, and appreciative of their efforts and of their points of view, a very different and positive tone is set. This usually begins to thaw their resistance and enlist their help. Furthermore, with this case, of course, my Scandinavian heritage must have helped. The -son (a typical suffix on Scandinavian names) ending my name likely established a degree of immediate kinship and credibility. Also because of my heritage, I knew not to seem intrusive, pushy, or a know-it-all, instead turning it over to the adult child to spearhead the session, with only occasional coaching and refereeing from me as needed.

For the adult child to be prepared to take the lead, the lion's share of his or her work must be done before the parents even are invited to participate. The adult child must be clear about the issues and feelings and must be committed to the need to discuss them. Doing a four-generational genogram is the first step in helping clients begin to understand the genesis of their issues, name the cast of characters, and unravel the patterns that plague a family's interactions and overall functioning. But perhaps the most crucial element in enlisting the parents' support and participation is the adult child's willingness to admit the need for the parents, despite whatever infantile feelings may be generated by doing so. When all else fails, this usually enlists the parents' help and minimizes their resistance. Thus, much of the work for such important sessions is completed before the meeting ever commences.

In conclusion, therapists should (1) be prepared not to be hierarchical but rather collaborative, lest the Scandinavian elders feel compelled to put them in their place; (2) to take control and provide structure if the session runs amok and feels unsafe; (3) be committed not to finding fault, but rather to facilitating new understandings; and (4) know how to walk the fine line between expression of affect, so that old wounds get cleaned out, and leaving people emotionally raw and hemorrhaging. For a more thorough discussion of family of origin sessions, therapists are encouraged to read Erickson (1992).

Given the cultural legacies of Scandinavians discussed here, it is small wonder that the Norwegian painter Edvard Munch's *The Scream* is so chilling, that a substantial focus in Norwegian playwright Henrik Ibsen's plays is on suicide, that the Danish philosopher Søren Kierkegaard's contemplations of the meaning of existence made him one of the world's foremost existentialist philosophers, and that Swedish movie director Ingmar Bergman's work is known mostly for his gloomy analysis of the human psyche.

THE IMMIGRANT EXPERIENCE FOR SCANDINAVIANS

For Scandinavian Americans, the Lutheran church helped bridge their experience between the old and new worlds, while providing a unifying force for the family and community. Because 95% of Scandinavians even today are at least nominally Lutheran, and because Lutheranism historically was the state religion, there undoubtedly was a sense of kinship upon entering a Lutheran church in this country.

With few exceptions, the greatest wave of immigrants from Scandinavia arrived in the United States in the 19th century. Thus, these people generally have long since been assimilated into the dominant culture. Because Scandinavians come from a culture where people are extremely adaptive and easily can blend into the dominant culture, perhaps it is easier for them to adjust to the immigrant experience than it is for others. They move around and assimilate with relative ease, even while silently believing that their own ways are best.

Because Scandinavians tend to be resilient, people often expect that they should be. Then, when they have difficulty, either people do not notice or they take for granted that the taciturn Scandinavians will continue to function as before, and even demand that they do so. This can lead to enormous conflict and stress that, because of Scandinavians' stoicism, they are loathe to admit or to discuss. This can result in psychosomatic symptoms, interpersonal problems, and emotional disturbances.

SCANDINAVIANS' VALUES

Scandinavians generally develop and prize heartiness because life in their countries is hard, and they come to expect and tolerate isolation and loneliness because they are home-bound in the gloom and cold of winter. Yet, they join with others because sometimes life itself depends on it, thus accounting for their sense of collective responsibility. Keeping to oneself even while in a group is typical, because there is a strict boundary between the private and the public, which other ethnic groups may label as being stuck up or shy. Typically, it takes a long time to get to know Scandinavians, particularly in rural areas, because of their desire for autonomy and penchant for solitude. Americans generally believe shyness is negative, that shy people are afraid and less competent, intelligent, and socially desirable. However, for Scandinavians, shyness is positive, and shy people often are viewed as sensitive, reflective, and nonpushy (Daun, 1989). This behavior frequently is misinterpreted by others as rejection, introversion, withdrawal, or anxiety, but Scandinavians believe that it is attributable to their being less willing to be verbal or vocal and having an aversion to being intrusive. Scandinavians tend to ask few questions that could be viewed as meddling, to avoid deep and elaborate discussions outside the circle of family and close friends, and may seem passive in conversation. Scandinavian comedian Louie Anderson (1986) puts it this way, "We're good neighbors, [but] we aren't always trying to get everybody together for a block meeting to discuss neighborhood problems. We think neighbors should already know what the problems are" (p. 35). The message Scandinavians give themselves and others is "Don't talk about it." This, of course, presents a challenge for clinicians whose role is to get families to identify and work together to solve their problems. Further, because of the centrality of experiencing and expressing emotions that accompany a loss, Scandinavians are highly susceptible to unresolved grief and to developing physical or psychological symptoms as a result, such as those experienced by Tim, as discussed earlier.

The Scandinavian languages do not even include a rich vocabulary of aggressive words, which reflects the conscious avoidance of conflict by holding back aggressiveness and by stressing practical solutions instead. For Scandinavians, anger can be precarious, because they are expected to be taciturn and stoic, and because, cooped up indoors with each other for half the year, anger could run amok and be downright harmful. Therefore, Scandinavians maddeningly use silence as a way to fight.

Swedes particularly tend to be in favor of agreement and consensus, approaching others with a desire to avoid confrontation and open conflict, which may explain their neutrality in World War II. This style can be useful in mediation and negotiations both in business and in families, provided people also learn adaptive skills for managing conflict when it does arise.

Scandinavians have a strong preference for practical solutions and rational arguments and facts, as opposed to emotions and whimsy. Their ability to plan, negotiate, compromise, and ultimately agree can be attributed to their practical nature. To survive the elements, they have been forced to find practical solutions. "One implication of this . . . could be that basic, continuous activity in old, rural Sweden gave little room for relaxation, pleasure, and joyful conversation. . . . There are no institutions like the English pub or the southern European Tavern" (Daun, 1989, p. 8). In addition, the church strongly emphasized that one must feel guilty for experiencing too much pleasure. Instead, recreation was permissible for short breaks or as a way of regaining the strength needed for work. In summary, it was often impressed on Scandinavians that comfort is sinful as well as impractical.

Scandinavians also adhere to an ethic of honesty. The truth is told in a precise, unexaggerated way. Daun (1989) refers to a study done in the early 1980s that indicated that lying was considered bad by a majority of Swedes (60%), whereas the figure for the rest of Europe was about 25%.

Although Scandinavian character traits give rise to a comfort with silence and with being alone, they also can spawn a tendency toward conflict avoidance that can cause logjams in relationships, feelings of deep isolation, melancholy, and depression. These values that shape their personality traits can be seen as contributors to Scandinavians' tendency toward higher rates of depression, alcoholism, suicide, and marital infidelity. However, these attributes also help Scandinavians to develop strong wills, stoicism that borders on resignation, and a sense of rugged independence. For example, less local anesthetic is used on Norwegian Americans during minor surgical procedures than on other Americans (Midelfort & Midelfort, 1982). When my Norwegian mother died of cancer, she was admired for her stoic endurance of the disease that attacked seven different sites in her body before finally claiming her life.

Suzanne, a 41-year-old bank executive of Scandinavian ancestry, sought therapy from me when her current relationship was on the verge of collapse. Divorced for 10 years, she had been involved in a stormy on-again, off-again relationship with Ted (himself a Scandinavian) for 8 of those years. When she and Ted began treatment, Suzanne frequently wept spontaneously and profusely during the sessions; yet, the only word she knew to identify her feelings was "frustrated." Realizing that Suzanne was virtually bound and gagged in expression of emotions—hers and Ted's—the therapist began to explore the covert and unconscious rules Suzanne had learned in her family of origin. Together, they generated the following list, which can be seen as typifying, enforcing, and yet distorting common Scandinavian values:

1. Be hardworking.
2. Be caring of other people.
3. Be strong, strong-willed, and strong on the outside.
4. Show externally that you can deal with things, even if you have other feelings internally.
5. It is preferable for people to get along.
6. Getting angry is not getting along.
7. Keep hurt, sadness, etc., way inside.
8. It is okay to show good feelings.
9. But showing feelings in an obvious way is never done; it has to be done subtly.

Before we could finish our list, quiet tears began to roll down Suzanne's cheeks. When asked about her tears, she spoke of many of the elements of her difficulty that were rooted in her ethnicity, even though she had been unaware of the connection until I noted it. First, she described how difficult it is to feel compelled to be strong on the outside even when she does not feel that way. She discussed how, when she finally does express emotion, it comes out very differently than she intends, so it often backfires, thereby further inhibiting her. She then described her isolation and tension because of her inability to express herself or to make herself understood. But perhaps the crowning statement was her fear of her parents' judgment if she behaved any differently.

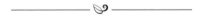

When a competent and successful executive in her 40s is still afraid of displeasing her parents, her individuation, her ability to make affective connections, and her capacity to reconcile her partner's demands for emotional intimacy with her family's norms all have been compromised severely. Clinicians will note that as we compiled this list of her family's rules, in essence she was writing her own treatment plan.

A LOOK AT SCANDINAVIANS SOCIOLOGICALLY

The socialist ideal that society is more important than the individual pervades Scandinavian life. Perhaps more than other groups, Scandinavians grasp the paradox that in structure there is freedom, provided it is not an authoritarian order. They believe that, in general, people and society are perfectible, if only the "right" rules are set. Hence, many rules exist that are followed fastidiously. The trains definitely run on time in Scandinavia! Norwegian American humorist, storyteller, radio personality, and prairie home companion, Garrison Keillor (1995), who lived for a time in Denmark, refers to this as "the tidy secret of Danish freedom," which he summarizes as "Do as you must, be as you wish."

Yet, although Scandinavia is a law-making society with much respect for authority, paradoxically, there is a natural suspicion about it. It is accepted that respect for authority is what maximizes one's freedoms, and yet typically pragmatic Scandinavians accept the fact that laws are made by humans who are capable of error, and so rules are made to be broken—or at least bent.

Democracy, egalitarianism, nonviolence, tolerance, and moderation are fundamental values for Scandinavians. They believe in social welfare and collective responsibility for societal problems. For example, a recent newspaper article describes Norway as the place where taxes are high and the citizens love it (Dregni, 2004). These beliefs undoubtedly were intrinsic to the fine contributions to the world of the such Scandinavian statesmen as Vice Presidents Hubert Humphrey and Walter Mondale, Secretaries General of the United Nations Dag Hammarskjöld and Trygve Lie, and the United Nations chief weapons inspector before the second Gulf War, Dr. Hans Blix. These ethics, moreover, help explain why the king of Denmark wore an arm band with the Star of David during the Nazi occupation, why Sweden remained neutral during World War II, and why there were strong Nazi resistance movements in both Denmark and Norway.

In daily life, Scandinavians believe in the staunch egalitarian value that no person is either better or worse than anyone else, even while acknowledging, for example, that the other person coincidentally may have more money or lower status. Hansen (1970) calls this "sanctioned egalitarianism" (cited in Borish, 1991, p. 222), which implies that the "cardinal sin is to appear to take oneself too seriously and to indicate thereby that one has an inflated view of one's own worth." Individuals who take themselves too seriously or put themselves on a pedestal will be chastised by joking and sarcasm. Garrison Keillor, who extols the virtue of typical Scandinavian modesty that borders on a feeling of inferiority, is the personification of this self-effacing ethic.

This value of not thinking you are so special plays out in gender roles as well. According to Mead (1985), the Vikings of the Middle Ages enjoyed a greater degree of equality than other peoples of that time. Viking men could have rights to land without paying dues or levies to an overlord, and women could own land and manage property. Today's Vikings have gone far beyond those basic rights to create an even more egalitarian society. Marriages and families tend to be egalitarian, with everyone taking a share of household tasks and decision making. Laws regarding equal pay for men and women in public service were enacted as early as 1919. In 1973 every woman was given the right to abortion through the end of the first trimester, divorce is relatively easy to obtain, and couples frequently live together and have children without benefit of papers. In 1989, Denmark was the first country to legalize same-sex unions, with the other Nordic countries following in the 1990s (Kantrowitz, 2004).

To other ethnic groups, a Scandinavian's usual response to a compliment may seem curious. Such comments generally are discounted by self-deprecation. The Danish Norwegian writer Aksel Sandemose (1936) offered an explanation for this cultural trait of self-effacement and captured some of the negative roles that govern relationships in Scandinavia. Referring to these 10 negative commandments as "the Law of Jante," he actually detailed a cultural code of humility that has become part of Scandinavian folk culture.

These 10 commandments are variations on the Scandinavian theme "You should not believe that you are somebody." Essentially, the Law of Jante is a reminder of our insignificance, and offers a set of rules on how to be "first in line to be second." "Don't be different" is really the underlying message, and the mood behind this code of conduct is concealed envy, fueled by a deep sense of personal insecurity (Borish, 1991). For Scandinavians, to be outstanding is to risk being ostracized from society and from family.

"The same leveling principle that so effectively limits the inappropriate individual exercise of power can have another, more troubling, effect. It can work to keep talented people in 'their place' and to discourage the development of their individuality" (Borish, 1991, p. 317). Some Scandinavian peer groups want their members to fit in, no matter the cost. Thus, people can be expected to surrender their autonomy and demand that their children do the same. This really can be the underside of egalitarianism and is often the core of conflict between the generations or between couples of different ethnic groups that often prompts families to seek psychotherapy.

In addition, Scandinavian governments have put an emphasis on child welfare in modern times, especially in Sweden. For example, it is against the law to spank a child—even one's own (Berlin, 1994). This emphasis is also apparent in Sweden's parent-leave programs, in which 15 months of paid leave can be shared between parents when a child enters the family, and in the state-subsidized day-care centers and state-approved "child-minders" (Mead, 1985). These social programs are funded by what most Americans would consider to be astronomically high taxes. Compare the tax rate of 31.6% in the United States with that of Scandinavia, which has the highest tax burden in Western Europe: Denmark, 58.6%; Sweden, 56.2%; Norway, 55.2%; and Finland, 54.0% ("Compare and Contrast," 1995, p. 23).

THE ROLE OF THE THERAPIST WITH SCANDINAVIANS

This is a culture that, as Anderson (1986) notes, is a hint inside a nuance inside a suggestion. Therapists with Scandinavian clients cannot be unduly aggressive in their approach, because Scandinavians emphasize egalitarianism and because of their subtle but discernible oppositional core deriving from suspicion of authority. Although many Scandinavians know, on some level, when they are depressed, they are loath to admit it or to seek help for their problems. They expect to work it out for themselves. This suggests that when Scandinavian families do present for treatment, their problems likely will appear—at least to the family—to be intractable. To work effectively with Scandinavians, therapists must be able to lead without being obvious, such as by making suggestions or requests instead of issuing directives. Otherwise, clients may feel compelled to remind them not to think they are so special. They must know how to keep order in sessions without being authoritarian, because that invites rebellion among egalitarian Scandinavians. Therapists should know how to draw out emotions without leaving clients ashamed by emotional displays that leave them feeling denuded. Therapists also must be adept at teaching clients how to recognize when they are feeling, what they are feeling, and how to share their feelings appropriately. To do this, therapists must learn to discern and help family members acknowledge the extremely subtle evidences of emotion that tend to typify Scandinavians' affective interactions so that they can use their emotions to connect rather than to stay disconnected. Finally, therapists gently must help families to speak the unspeakable, thereby breaking their isolation and countering their tendency to somatize, internalize, or isolate.

Thus, Scandinavian families in treatment tend to be more disengaged than enmeshed. They may well resist talking about their problems, have great difficulty in expressing emotions, fight by silence and distance, stress independence and figuring out concerns on their own without calling attention to themselves, and, although practical, will not resist a philosophical, existential focus, provided feelings are downplayed, at least initially.

Often, families with adolescents who are engaging in a typical struggle for autonomy will present for treatment. This often occurs when parents attempt to control them to avoid the shame that such behavior brings to the normally reserved family by drawing attention to it. Although these fights typically are not overt, the expectation of conformity, of course, often generates a cycle of more rebellion and more family shame. Even members of families in which no disturbance is evident often maintain a great deal of space between each other, literally and figuratively. This works as long as someone in the family does not need more interaction or emotional closeness. When Scandinavian couples present for treatment, difficulty in establishing an emotionally intimate connection is usually the basis of their dysfunction. And couples in a "mixed marriage" often seek therapy because of difficulty in reconciling apparently incompatible styles of intimacy, emotional expression, and conflict resolution. In these cases, as in all such instances, the therapist must be prepared to serve as a cultural interpreter of each partner to the other, along with addressing the dysfunction that their clashing styles may have created.

EFFECTIVE THERAPEUTIC APPROACHES WITH SCANDINAVIANS

In general, because Scandinavians are a pragmatic people, solution-focused approaches may be effective. However, therapists need to be indirect in working with these clients. Humorist Anderson notes, "Our concept of 'sharing' does not include telling strangers the details of our sexual dysfunctions, dependencies, and adolescent traumas. We do not blab anything you tell us—whether it is a secret or not" (1986, p. 50).

Therapy that emphasizes a total reality focus may be experienced by Scandinavians as shaming, exposing them to humiliation for calling attention to themselves or for their inability to figure it out on their own. Because of Scandinavians' introspective nature and tolerance for loneliness, therapeutic approaches that deal with existential or spiritual issues often work well. If therapists help clients to see pragmatic reasons for thinking philosophically, the clients usually are willing to ponder the deep and difficult questions in searching for meaning in their lives in general or in specific experiences. Psychodynamic approaches are also extremely beneficial, because they play to Scandinavians' strength of introspection, which can help people explore their unconscious motivations, choices, and family dynamics so they can make more beneficial choices. Family of origin approaches such as those espoused by Bowen (1978) and Framo (1982) are good models. Teaching family systems concepts may also help them to take charge of their own dysfunctional patterns, rather than to remain victims of them and of each other. In short, perhaps the best way to work with Scandinavian clients is for therapists to allow them to figure out as much as they can for themselves, with gentle guidance. This helps them to maintain their dignity, independence, and sense of control of their lives.

CONCLUSION

Although referring specifically to Danes, the metaphor developed by Danish novelist Karen Blixen captures the essence of all Scandinavians. She says, "The Danish character is like dough without leavening. All the ingredients that supply the taste and nourishment are there, but the element that makes the dough able to change, to rise, has been left out" (cited in Borish, 1991, p. 320). When Scandinavians present for psychotherapy, the therapist's mandate and challenge is to supply the yeast in a way that families will knead it into their interactions and dynamics to create the conditions required for everyone's growth and development.

ACKNOWLEDGMENT

I would like to thank Jette Sinkjaer Simon for her contributions to the first version of this chapter.

NOTE

1. Greenland and the Faeroe Islands both have independent governments but are still under the Danish crown.

REFERENCES

Anderson, J. L. (1986). *Scandinavian humor and other myths*. Minneapolis, MN: Nordbook.

Berlin, P. (1994). *The xenophobe's guide to the Swedes*. London: Ravette Books.

Black, J. (2004, August 8). On Finland's royal road. *New York Times*, p. TR 9.

Borish, S. (1991). *The land of the living*. Nevada City, CA: Blue Dolphin Press.

Bowen, M. (1978). *Family therapy in clinical practice*. New York: Aronson.

Compare and contrast Western Europe's tax burden. (1995, February 16). *New York Times*, p. 23.

Daun, A. (1989). *Swedish mentality*. New York: Swedish Information Service.

Dregni, E. (2004, April 18). Where taxes are high and the citizens love it. *Minneapolis Star Tribune*, p. AA7.

Erickson, B. (1992). The major surgery of family therapy: The extended family of origin session. *Journal of Family Psychotherapy*, 3(1), 19–44.

Erickson, B. (1993). *Helping men change: The role of the female therapist*. Newbury Park, CA: Sage.

Erickson, B. (1998). *Longing for dad: Father loss and its impact*. Deerfield Beach, FL: Health Communications.

Framo, J. (1982). Family of origin as a therapeutic resource for adults in marital and family therapy: You can and should go home again. In *Explorations in marital therapy: Selected papers of James L. Framo* (pp. 171–190). New York: Springer.

Hansen, J. (1970). Democracy and egalitarianism. In S. Borish (Ed.), *The land of the living* (pp. 222–249). Nevada City, CA: Blue Dolphin Press.

Kantrowitz, B. (2004, March 1). The state of our unions. *Newsweek*, pp. 44–45.

Keillor, G. (1995, February 16). The tidy secret of Danish freedom. *New York Times*, p. 23.

Mead, W. (1985). *Scandinavia*. Amsterdam: Time-Life Rooks.

Midelfort, C., & Midelfort, C. (1982). Norwegian families. In M. McGoldrick, J. K. Pearce, & J. Giordano (Eds.), *Ethnicity and family therapy* (pp. 438–456). New York: Guilford Press.

National Geographic atlas of the world (7th ed.). (1999). Washington, DC: National Geographic Society.

Sandemose, A. (1936). *A refugee crosses his track*. New York: Knopf.

Sodergren, E. (1993). Chambers of consciousness. In W. R. Mead (Ed.), *An experience of Finland* (pp. 54–66). London: Hurst.

Stocker, C. (2004, February 18). Fabulous Finnish. *Minneapolis Star Tribune*, p. H3.

CHAPTER 47

Scots-Irish Families

Morris Taggart

Prior to doing the groundwork for this chapter, I doubted that the colonial-era Scots-Irish[1] had *any* relevance for 21st-century family therapy. I agreed with those (Leyburn, 1962) who argued that whatever was distinctive about the Scots-Irish had been absorbed into the general culture of America soon after the Revolution. In effect, the Scots-Irish ceased to be a separate ethnic group and became *Americans*. When I emigrated to the United States from Northern Ireland in 1959, I felt little identification with the colonial-era Scots-Irish or their descendants in the United States. My ethnic loyalties still lay with my family and clan in Ulster (and in Canada, Scotland, England, and Australia, for we are still a family of emigrants). Becoming a U.S. citizen in 1970 changed my *political*, not my *ethnic* affinities, and there have been times since when I have felt like "a stranger in a strange land."

My view of the matter was severely challenged when a colleague (David McGill) suggested I take a look at David Fischer's *Albion's Seed: Four British Folkways in America* (1989). Fischer effectively dismantles any notion that Scots-Irish folkways *ever* disappeared in America. Indeed, he assembles a mountain of data to insist that the distinctive social structures, customs, and values defining life for the Scots-Irish *still* persist across a vast region ranging from Appalachia, down through Texas and Oklahoma, and across to southern California. If this were not bombshell enough, Fischer argues that later immigrants to the region, *whatever* their ethnic origins, have assimilated to *these* Scots-Irish folkways and *not* to some abstract American culture.

Fischer's thesis confronts us on two levels. Personally, it challenges me to view my Scots-Irish identity not only as a consequence of where I was born and raised, but equally as an integral and ongoing aspect of what it means for me to be an American. In addition, it prompts me to wonder if the evolution of what it means to be Scots-Irish, unfolding here in the United States, is just as authentic an expression of that heritage as anything happening in Ulster or elsewhere. This seems like the beginning of a radical shift for me, though it is too early in the journey for me to say much more.

654

Professionally, the challenge for family therapy is the same one it has always taken up ever since it developed an interest in ethnicity as a primary context for its theoretical and clinical work—how best to develop therapeutic approaches that recognize, and make use of, the Scots-Irish (or whatever) heritage that continues to shape families' lives. We begin this particular quest in Ulster a decade before the *Mayflower* weighed anchor for the New World.

THE ULSTER PLANTATION:
HOW THE SCOTS BECAME SCOTS-IRISH

In 1609, more than a century before the Scots-Irish came to America in any numbers, many of their ancestors started migrating from the Scottish Lowlands and from England into Ulster, the northernmost province of Ireland. English forces had just put down yet another revolt by the native Irish, and colonization—the planting of new citizens on the expropriated lands of the defeated Gaelic leadership—was the means of stabilizing the territory. This was ethnic cleansing on a massive scale, and its echoes resound in Ulster to this day. By 1640,[2] there were somewhere between 40,000 and 100,000 Scots and English immigrants in Ulster—an enormous swing in favor of the Protestant newcomers. This 30-year period of relative stability and prosperity was interrupted in 1641 when the English Civil War (1640–1646[3]) spilled over into Ireland.

The war between the king (Charles I) and parliament gave opportunity to the native Irish to mount a major revolt against the colonial power, including the settlers in the north. It was a brutal affair that lasted 11 years and saw unspeakable atrocities on both sides. Unsurprisingly, the legacy of distrust and hatred between the Catholic and Protestant communities was deepened immeasurably. After 1651, Oliver Cromwell's pitiless military subjugation of Ireland was the final step in destroying the tribal organization that had served it for a thousand years (Jackson, 1993). After the monarchy was restored (Charles II) in 1660, Ulster became what the Plantation had intended—a prosperous enclave of towns and villages, with a growing farm economy, including a lucrative export trade in woolen goods (Jackson, 1993).

Charles II died in 1685,[4] leaving no heir, and was succeeded by his brother, James II, a convert to Roman Catholicism 20 years previously. He set about reversing all laws discriminating against Catholics, and his deputy in Ireland began purging Protestants from the army there. Opposition to James organized itself very quickly in England and, in a relatively short time, he was deposed in favor of his daughter, Mary, the wife of the Prince William of Orange of the Netherlands. James and his family fled to France, and King William III and Queen Mary II became co-rulers of Britain and Ireland in April 1689. The transition in Ireland was a more bloody affair. In an effort to regain his kingdom, James had landed in Ireland with a continental army in March 1689. Troops loyal to William III disembarked at Carrickfergus later the same year, and for the next 2 years, there were bloody battles fought across Ireland. William's victory at the the Battle of the Boyne (1690) and his army's triumph at Aughrim (1691) effectively ended Irish resistance to the new Protestant regime.

The status of the mostly Presbyterian Ulster Scots might have been secured for generations had it not been for three missteps by the London authorities. The first was Parliament's passing of the Woolens Act (1699), preventing Ulster farmers from exporting woolen goods directly to the lucrative European markets (Jackson, 1993). Next came a renewed attempt by the state-established Church of England to impose its jurisdiction over Presbyterian and other Dissenters in the Test Act of 1704. Now Presbyterians, *as well as* Catholics, were banned from holding public office, and many, including the clergy, had to resign their positions. Finally, when land leases in Ulster ran out after 1700, new economic interests from England bid up the prices of the new leases so that the old tenants could not afford them (Leyburn, 1962). Large numbers of Ulster-Scot farmers and their families were thrown off the land they had fought for and improved over generations. They must have wondered what their loyalty to crown and country was worth when there were no longer Irish insurgents to subdue. Small wonder that when the Great Migration got under way in 1717, among the few things the people brought with them to America was their belief in freedom as a *natural* right, independent of constitutional and legal systems, as well as a deep suspicion of all central governments.

THE GREAT MIGRATION: 1717–1775

The first Scots-Irish immigrants came ashore at Philadelphia and Newcastle, Delaware, in the summer of 1717. These people were unlike the earlier English-speaking immigrants, in that there was little talk here of "holy experiments" or "cities set on a hill." The Scots-Irish were interested in one thing above all, *land*. So much so, that they were apt to squat on land no matter who held title to it. In 1731, James Logan, Pennsylvania's provincial secretary (and an Ulsterman himself), encouraged the Scots-Irish westward, hoping to provide a buffer between the Quakers and the Indians if trouble should break out along the frontier (Leyburn, 1962). Once again, they became a tool, caught between two opposing forces, as they had been in Ulster.

As newcomers continued to pour in from Scotland and Ulster, there was a great expansion west and south into the mountains of Maryland, Virginia, and the Carolinas. By the first U.S. Census in 1790, more than half the White population of backcountry Pennsylvania, Maryland, Virginia, the Carolinas, Georgia, Kentucky, and Tennessee was from Ulster, Scotland, and northern England. In some counties, in all these states, the proportion was nearer 90%. By 1775, the Scots-Irish

> became the dominant English-speaking culture in a broad belt of territory that extended from the highlands of Appalachia through most of the old Southwest. In the nineteenth century, they moved across the Mississippi to Arkansas, Missouri, Oklahoma, and Texas. By the twentieth century, their influence would be felt as far west as New Mexico, Arizona, and southern California. (Fischer, 1989, p. 633)

According to Fischer, it was not numbers alone that contributed to the cultural hegemony won in the southern highlands by the Scots-Irish. He notes the similarity between this American environment and the cultures from which the immigrants had come. Both were dangerous places in which native peoples resisted the encroachment of newcomers. Fischer concludes that the Scots-Irish felt at home amid the perils of the frontier because it was well suited to their family and clan system, and especially their warrior ethic (Fischer, 1989).

One wonders about the consequences for the Scots-Irish of their two centuries-long role as subduers of "inferior peoples," whether Irish Catholic or indigenous American. In both Ulster and America, the ruling interests that benefited most from their exploits continued to treat the Scots-Irish as second-rate partners at best. In America, such questions are concealed by the myth that "taming the frontier" was entirely a noble cause accomplished by heroes. Just as in the case of the Plantation of Ulster, though, there is a darker side to the story. The Scots-Irish fought some of the bloodiest "Indian wars" ever seen on this continent and, in casting off their own colonial yoke, drew a colonial noose about the necks of others. Of the Shawnee in the north, through to the Cherokee, Creek, Choctaw, and Chickasaw in the south, little enough is left today. Their losses are at least visible, if only to themselves. But what of the losses of the "winners" of these conquests of indigenous peoples in Ireland and America, and especially of the Scots-Irish who were for so long their forward troops? Who sings their sorrows? Who dances their grief?

THE PERSISTENCE OF SCOTS-IRISH FOLKWAYS AND ITS RELEVANCE FOR FAMILY THERAPY

As underlined earlier in this chapter, Fischer's (1989) finding—that Scots-Irish folkways endure across a broad region of the United States, and that *all* subsequent immigrants into that region, of whatever ethnicity, continue to be influenced by them—brings new dimensions to the exploration of ethnicity's role in family therapy. Most important, to be sure, is that the Scots-Irish are now added to the conversation. Just as intriguing, though, is the question of how ethnicities within regions influence one another. This latter issue is especially important in the Southwest, where Scots-Irish settlers found, but did not displace, a flourishing Mexican culture that influenced them at least as much as they influenced it.

It has to be said that the task is, at this stage, more the exploration of an intriguing potential than a facile mapping of Scots-Irish folkways on to family therapy. It will be family therapists themselves who, intrigued by the endurance of Scots-Irish folkways into the 21st century, will begin to test their usefulness in the treatment of families today. In this regard, family therapists need not anymore be mere *consumers* of established historical knowledge. The new cultural history, represented by Fischer, is much more open to other disciplines than was the old. The challenge for us is to become *collaborators* in "writing" the cultural histories of our time, trusting that our ways of punctuating and framing human behavior will help make contemporary culture visible.

SCOTS-IRISH FOLKWAYS AND THEIR IMPLICATIONS FOR FAMILY THERAPY

There is, of course, no body of knowledge as to the typical problems of families descended from the Scots-Irish, or of other families influenced by their folkways. Nor is there a list of the therapeutic strategies found to have been successful with such families. What follows is a re-visioning of my own therapeutic work in the light of just a few of Fischer's (1989, pp. 652–782) provocative contributions. Based as it is on a typical, middle-class private practice, there is no mention here of poverty, economic exploitation, or the many other issues that have ravaged families in, say, Appalachia or East Texas.

Family and Kinship Patterns

Before and after their coming to America, family patterns among the Scots-Irish arose as "highly effective adaptations to a world of violence and chronic insecurity" (Fischer, 1989, p. 663). For them, "family" always meant "extended family," and beyond both loomed the clan. In a dangerous world, loyalty to family and clan was paramount, far beyond that owed to governments and legal systems.

Echoes of these patterns are still found in the southern highlands, as well as in Texas and beyond. In Appalachia, the traditional reliance on the extended family is often in direct conflict with the individualism prized by the dominant culture, and the trusted family therapist is likely to be one who shares the family's interests, values, roots, and language (Rural and Appalacian Youth and Families Consortium [RAYFC], 1996). Even in cosmopolitan Houston, there are families for whom every birth and birthday is celebrated by the whole clan, and every funeral is a clan event. The challenge for family therapists is to be aware of the extended family as more than the "undifferentiated family ego mass" from which the individual or couple needs saving. The contemporary power of the clan—in this case the *competing* power of the maternal and paternal clans in a family with Scots-Irish origins on both sides—may be gauged from the following example:

A husband and wife came into therapy involved in a surprisingly bitter argument as to whether their son should get a new or used car for his 16th birthday. It became evident that the struggle was about which family's values—paternal or maternal—would be foremost in shaping the new generation. The therapist asked each to poll the extended families on the matter. As an apparent afterthought, he instructed the mother to poll her husband's family, while the father polled hers. As expected, they found as much variation on this issue within each clan as between them. This helped them escape the either/or struggle they came with and released them from assumed clan loyalties to create a new solution that honored both families. The therapist's acknowledgment of the extended families' importance saved him from playing the part of "dangerous interloper" against whom both families might have had to close ranks.

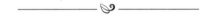

Gender Ways of the Scots-Irish

Despite the myth that life on the frontier created a spirit of equality between the sexes, Fischer (1989) maintains that, in such hazardous settings, gender relations tended to follow the pattern typical of warrior cultures. These include very distinct roles for men and women—men as warriors, women as workers, with men taking the dominant role in the family. Evident too was a confused and confusing combination of intense expressions of love *and* violence between spouses, leading to a "great aching silent distance that kept them apart" (Fisher, 1989, p. 679). All these Scots-Irish themes—male dominance and control, intense expressions of love combined with violence, and emotional distance—can be seen in the following vignette:

A couple in marital therapy came to a session very upset. The husband, a trial lawyer with a common Scots-Irish last name, appealed to the male therapist to support him in what he presented as a reasonable request of his wife. "Isn't it obvious that she shouldn't go out alone at night, especially without telling me where she's going? This city is a jungle, especially after dark. Why is she being so foolish, taking such unnecessary risks?"

"I'm sick of you treating me like an irresponsible child," retorted the wife, "And I can't stand you telling me how much you love me, and how you don't want to lose me, just after you've pushed me to the ground, or squeezed my arm until it was black and blue!"

It took several sessions before the husband could share what he was really feeling: "I get afraid when you leave, especially when you don't come home till bedtime. I'm afraid you might be seeing another man." He discovered that, as painful and risky as it was to communicate his fears openly, his partner was now more willing to listen to him.

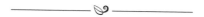

In some ways, work has become the sphere in which male "warrior" values persist, with the primary male role of "defending the family against attack" morphing into "making a living for the family." Loss of the defining "breadwinner" role through male unemployment has been associated with higher rates of mental ill health and suicide among men in contemporary Northern Ireland (Northern Ireland Forum for Political Dialogue [NIFPD], 1998), as well as higher levels of stress and marital violence in Appalachia (Fitchen, 1991). Even families that seemed to have moved beyond rigid gender roles with respect to employment, may revert to to the old rules during stressful transitions. In the following vignette, the (Scots-Irish) wife, abetted by her husband's coworkers, insists that he fulfill his role as *primary* breadwinner, freeing her to be *primary* parent.

After many unsuccessful fertility treatments, including *in vitro* fertilization, a young professional couple finally adopted a baby. They arranged live-in help, leaving only evenings and weekends for their direct involvement in child care. The husband, in individual therapy for other issues, resented his responsibity to earn the lion's share of the family's income, his longer hours at work cutting into his parenting time. When he suggested cutting back hours at work to spend more time with the baby, his wife was doubly upset. Not only did his proposal threaten her limited time with the baby, but their additional expenses suggested to her that he needed to spend more time at work, not less. In addition, his law partners criticized his shift of focus from work to family, describing it as "going AWOL." He tried to get his wife interested in joining him in couple therapy about these issues. She refused.

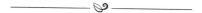

On some issues at least, contemporary attitudes toward gender have not changed a great deal. States in the southern highlands consistently opposed passage of the Equal Rights Amendment in the 1980s, as indeed they had opposed women's suffrage earlier. Pressure among men to conform to "manly" ideals is very strong, and male spouses may be reluctant even to be involved in therapy (Wesner, Patel, & Allen, 1991). Male bonding appears close, but is narrowly focused with respect to interests—work, sports, hunting, politics—and affective range. Adjunctive group therapy with men may help them get involved in family therapy more effectively.

Sex Ways: Scots-Irish Celebration of Sensuality

At the time of their settlement of the backcountry, the Scots-Irish were much more open about sexuality than were the Puritans of New England or the Quakers of Pennsylvania. Prenuptial pregnancy was, in fact, the norm, and, unlike the Puritans and Quakers who launched formal prosecutions for fornication, the Scots-Irish tended to frame the event as an occasion for boisterous fun (Fischer, 1989). Contemporary observers complained about the backcountry settlers' fondness for "love feasts," wild affairs well lubricated with alcohol, that contributed to their laxity in sexual morality (Woodmason, 1953).

In time, the Scots-Irish conformed to the stricter sexual mores that accompanied the evangelical revivals of the 19th and early 20th centuries. But all through the region, there is still a sometimes uneasy mixture of conservative religion with sexuality and alcohol. These are the beloved but contradictory themes that permeate country music. Family therapists in the south central United States (and anywhere else) need to be aware of how alcoholism affects families and how it might be treated within a family model. Fortunately, alcohol treatment programs in the region often include a family component, which can become the foundation for family therapy later. Familiarity with how Alcoholics Anonymous (AA) works is also an asset for a therapist, inasmuch as its quasi-religious approach fits in with the region's religious values.

Whatever sexual openness there has been among the Scots-Irish has never extended to homosexuality. Even in cosmopolitan areas, gay bashing and intimidation are still common. Many churches do not provide much in the way of support to families with lesbian and gay members. Consequently, therapists need to be familiar with groups like PFLAG (Parents and Families of Lesbians and Gays) as potential community resources for these families.

Child-Rearing Ways: Building the Will

Whereas, for Puritans, raising boys was aimed at *breaking* their wills, the process among the Scots-Irish was meant to be positively will-*enhancing*. "Its primary purpose was to foster fierce pride, stubborn independence, and a warrior's courage in the young" (Fischer, 1989, p. 687). Permissive, indulgent, and overtolerant of violent behavior, such parenting produced men unable to tolerate external control and incapable of restraining their rage against anyone who opposed them. As boys got older, frustrated fathers and resentful sons would inevitably clash, sometimes with terrible violence.

Bill, a burly oil field engineer, came into therapy in part to repair a broken relationship with his adult son, a photographer and artist. Through the son's transition from adolescence to young manhood, they had argued and fought over every inch of their relationship, sometimes to the point of blows. The son rarely came home to visit during college, and after graduation, not at all. Bill's wife was pressuring him to attempt a reconciliation with their son.

Bill had been attending AA meetings for about a year when he started therapy, and he had begun to sponsor a few newcomers. He brought his ups and downs as a sponsor to therapy, noticing how his rigid, demanding style drove neophytes away. Keen to hold onto those who looked to him for support, he worked hard at listening more and lecturing less. In time, Bill noticed the parallels between his work as a sponsor and his fathering and was eventually able to take important initiatives with his son.

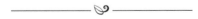

The warrior ethic and its acceptance of violence are also seen in other forms. All through the southern highlands, as well as in Texas and Oklahoma, boys are still routinely introduced to the use of firearms at an early age, and this in a region that has some of the highest rates of murder and other crimes of violence in the nation. Interestingly, the region also has the country's highest rates of recruitment into the U.S. armed services. The glorification of the male student athlete may be another form of ancient patterns. Raised by parents, schools, and alumni groups in an atmosphere of privilege and deference from as early as middle school, these young men too defend the honor of the clan. Their families sometimes seek therapy at points where parents "lose" their sons to powerful coaches and programs. Athletic, as much as military, glory comes often enough at premium prices.

Scots-Irish Death Ways: Uncertain Fatalism

Early and violent deaths were not strangers to the Scots-Irish before they came to America. Constant warfare, famine, and epidemic disease made it so. The backcountry of America was actually a safer place to be. It was dangerous enough, though, to keep the old death customs in place. Backcountry settlers were fatalistic about death, but surrounded themselves with superstitions to help reduce its uncertainties (Fischer, 1989). If one saw a falling star or, paradoxically, dreamt of a wedding, then death was close by.

Funeral rituals helped to bring order to chaotic events, and some still survive into the present. The most familiar is the wake, always conducted in the room with the corpse and given over to stories about the deceased. Close family members may also join in a final ritual such as when, just before the body is taken for burial, they will all touch, even kiss, the deceased in a last farewell. Even in urban Texas, graveside services still feature a lone piper playing a last lament.

Among the Scots-Irish in the old days, even implacable *enemies* of the deceased were expected to attend funerals. The chances are that families will appreciate the presence of a former or current therapist at a funeral or wake.

The patriarch of a large East Texas family had suffered a ruptured cerebral aneurysm and lay "brain dead" in an ICU surrounded by at least 50 family members and friends. A family therapist, who had seen the man and his wife in couple group therapy, was present when concerns arose as to how and when the decision to discontinue life support should be made. The wife asked the therapist to gather with a dozen closest family members behind a screen in the corner of the ICU, where he moderated a brief family conversation. The family quickly agreed that it was the wife's call to make, and she announced that after all others had a chance to say their good-byes, and after she had said her own last good-bye, all life support would cease.

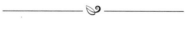

Scots-Irish Religious Ways

Though their forebears were primarily Presbyterians, the descendants of the Scots-Irish today are likely to be Baptist or Methodist. The core of their religious experience is expressed in terms of a personal relationship to God rather subscription to formal creeds. The colonial-era Scots-Irish maintained a deep sense of God's presence very much in the midst of their often tempestuous lives. Their descendants' lively mixing of the sacred and the profane can sometimes come as a shock to those of a different religious style, or none at all. Whatever stereotypes others may hold about "hillbillies" or whomever, the challenge for family therapists is both to know and to respect the complex mixture of values, beliefs, and attitudes by which their client families live. For those who work where the deep undertones of Scots-Irish folkways still resound, this means an appreciation for the faith system that has shaped their lives and brought them "through many dangers, toils and snares ... " (Newton, 1779).

This brief survey represents only a "first word" on relating Scots-Irish folkways to the present-day interests of family therapists. The goal has been to intrigue as much as to inform. The hope is that, once intrigued, family therapists will broaden our knowledge of how Scots-Irish folkways still affect both the hurting and the healing of families. As stated earlier, this will call for more than re-imagining our clinical practice. The last several years has seen an explosion of interest in the Scots-Irish diaspora, involving universities in Ulster, Scotland, the United States, Canada, and New Zealand. At the heart of this effort is the Institute of Ulster-Scots Studies[5] at the University of Ulster, with Virginia Tech[6] (Blacksburg, Virginia) as the U.S. research center. Family therapists belong in such ventures, helping to shape the research as well as translating its findings into clinical practice.

CONCLUSION

Having made a case, however tentatively or wrongheadedly, for the inclusion of the Scots-Irish in family therapy's ethnicity project, the question arises: What next? It seems crucial that those whose interest has been piqued by this "first word" on the matter find ways of exploring that interest together. The participation of therapists, working where there is a population of Scots-Irish origin and/or a culture in which Scots-Irish folkways persist, is especially important. The more international that participation turns out to be, the better the prospects for doing useful work together.

Since therapists' readiness to do useful work in the area of ethnicity and family therapy depends in part on their having grappled with their own ethnic and cultural identity (Killian, 2002; Pinderhughes, 1989), an exchange of the type envisaged here might provide a supportive context for this more personal work.

Readers interested in exploring these, or other, possibilities may contact me.

NOTES

1. "Scots-Irish," as used in this chapter, is hardly a sufficiently comprehensive term for these immigrants—some came directly from Scotland and the border counties of England—but it at least recognizes that more than half of them did emigrate from Ulster in Northern Ireland. Fischer's (1989) "North Britons" is little improvement inasmuch as Ulster is properly not part of Britain, and both the Scottish Lowlands and the English border counties are more Mid- than North Britain. "Scotch-Irish," though ubiquitous in North America, is rather strenuously avoided elsewhere. "Ulster-Scots" is increasingly the preferred term in Ulster itself, particularly in relation to the form of Scots English that emerged there.
2. The first mass migration from the British Isles—the Puritans from eastern England to Massachusetts (1629–1640)—was completed by this point.
3. The second mass migration—the defeated Royalists, and their bond-servants, from southern

England to Virginia (1642–1675)—started during the English Civil War, but increased substantially after 1650 when Parliamentary forces finally defeated the Royalists.

4. The third mass migration—the Quakers from the northern Midlands of England to the Delaware Valley (1675–1725)—started 10 years before the death of Charles II and ended almost 10 years after the fourth mass migration—the Scots-Irish (1717–1775)—began.

5. www.arts.ulster.ac.uk/ulsterscots/intro.htm.

6. www.vt.edu/.

REFERENCES

Fischer, D. H. (1989). *Albion's seed: Four British folkways in America.* New York: Oxford University Press.

Fitchen, J. (1991). Marriage and the family. In B. Ergood & B. Kuhre (Eds.), *Appalachia: Social context past and present.* Dubuque, IA: Kendall/Hunt.

Jackson, C. (1993). *A social history of the Scotch-Irish.* Lanham, MD: Madison Books.

Killian, K. W. (2002). Dominant and marginalized discourses in interracial couples' narratives: Implications for family therapists. *Family Process, 41,* 603–618.

Leyburn, J. G. (1962). *The Scotch-Irish: A social history.* Chapel Hill: University of North Carolina Press.

Newton, J. (1779). Amazing grace. *Olney hymns.* London: W. Oliver.

Northern Ireland Forum for Political Dialogue. (1998). *Men's health in Northern Ireland: An examination by Standing Committee C.* Available at www.ni-forum.gov.uk/commit.htm

Pinderhughes, E. (1989). *Understanding race, ethnicity, and power.* New York: Free Press.

The Rural and Appalachian Youth and Families Consortium. (1996). Parenting practices and interventions among marginalized families in Appalachia: Building on family strengths. *Family Relations, 45,* 387–396.

Wesner, D., Patel, C., & Allen, J. (1991). A study of explosive rage in male spouses counseled in an Appalachian mental health clinic. *Journal of Counseling and Development, 70,* 235–241.

Woodmason, C. (1953). *The Carolina backcountry on the eve of the Revolution: The journal and other writings of Charles Woodmason, Anglican itinerant* (R. Hooker, Ed.). Chapel Hill: University of North Carolina Press.

PART VIII

JEWISH FAMILIES

CHAPTER 48

Jewish Families
An Overview

Elliott J. Rosen
Susan F. Weltman

In 2001, approximately 5.5 million Americans identified themselves as being Jewish, approximately 40% of the world's Jewish population (*National Jewish Population Survey* [NJPS], 2003).[1]

Jews historically have perceived themselves not only as coreligionists, but as part of a cultural-ethnic-national body, with membership bestowed by birth or conversion rather than by belief or practice. This may be more true today than before, given that only 46% of the American Jewish population is affiliated with a synagogue or other Jewish institution, but more than half regard their being Jewish as "very important" (Cohen & Rosen, 1992; NJPS, 2000–2001) Recent surveys indicate that many Jews identify themselves ethnically or culturally as Jews, but do not consider themselves religious. In a 2001 study, Mayer and his colleagues discovered that 72% of people of Jewish background described themselves as secular. Even among those who said they were "Jewish by religion," 42% described themselves that way, as compared with only 15% of Americans who called themselves secular. Cohen and Eisen (2000) argue that "identity" for the 21st-century Jew is in flux and that attachment to community has weakened as Jews have become more autonomous, self-defining, and inward-looking.

JEWISH AMERICANS IN HISTORICAL AND CULTURAL CONTEXT

Declaring oneself Jewish has always been an acceptable criterion for membership in the Jewish community, and conversion to Judaism ensures complete access to membership. Born Jews who might not otherwise identify themselves as such are often counted by communities in census figures (Goldstein, 1993). In fact, if all individuals currently living in a household with at least one Jew are included as part of a "comprehensive Jewish population," the total Jewish population rises to 6.7 million (NJPS, 2003, p. viii).

Although 2004 marked the 350th anniversary of the first Jewish settlement in the New World (by Sephardic Jews whose ancestors came from Spain and Portugal), most American Jews are the descendants of East European (chiefly Russian and Polish) Jews who migrated to America between 1881 and the early 1920s, when changing immigration policies sharply limited immigration to the United States. Today, 75% congregate in large cities, 65% of them on the East and West Coasts (NJPS, 2003). More than 2.5 million Jews, nearly half the American total, live in two states: New York and California. With a below-zero level birth rate, America's Jews are an aging population. The percentage of American Jews in the 60+ age group is 23%, whereas for non-Jewish Americans it is 16% (NJPS, 2003).

A small proportion of American Jews are Sephardic. Recent immigration from South and Central America, as well as from North Africa and Iran, has added to the numbers of Sephardim. The proportion of the Jewish community descended from Western European (primarily German) Jews, who immigrated to the United States in the beginning and middle of the 19th century, as well as before and after the Holocaust, is now about equal to that of the Sephardim. These German Jewish immigrants, some of whom established large American business empires, were once a powerful force in American Jewish affairs as founders of communal and synagogue organizations (Faber, 1992). In recent years, however, their descendants have tended to blend into the mainstream of American Jewish life.

Unfortunately, only a relatively small number of Jews were able to leave Germany and Eastern Europe before the outbreak of World War II, again because of restrictive immigration policies throughout the world. Those who did come to the United States brought outstanding skills and accomplishments as artists, scientists, and other intellectuals. Holocaust survivors were more easily able to immigrate.

Young people who have been exposed to the Holocaust in movies or in school are often surprised to learn that there was very little discussion of the concentration camps until the 1970s, when survivors began writing and speaking of their experiences. The survivors reported that they lacked the language to express what they had experienced and that, immediately after the war, no one really wanted to hear their stories. One client related that until she was 12 and overheard her father talking about his experiences of having been hidden in Russia, she knew nothing of her parents' Holocaust experiences. Families that lost members still sometimes report survivor's guilt, even in the second and third generations.

Between 1991 and 2000, a quarter of a million Russian Jews entered this country (NJPS, 2003), including non-Jewish members of mixed households. This substantial influx has continued, though in much smaller numbers, into this century (HIAS, 2004; NJPS, 2003). As of 2002, over 58% of Jews from the former Soviet Union resided in the New York area, predominantly in Brooklyn, with smaller concentrations in Queens and elsewhere. They represent a large percentage of the city's Jewish population. Although the Russian Jews were originally greeted with some ambivalence by the American Jews, some of whom questioned their willingness to be part of the larger community and who were suspicious of the newcomers' "clannishness" and isolation, they have come to occupy a more integrated place in the community.

Other smaller groups, primarily from Eastern Europe, South Africa, and Iran, together with Jews who have recently emigrated from Israel, have come to the United States largely for economic and other "quality-of-life" reasons. Israeli Americans usually identify themselves first as Israelis and second as Jews and are likely to further define themselves as "different" from their American counterparts, as discussed in Chapter 49.

Iranian Jews, who were generally treated well before the Islamic revolution, were usually able to bring much of their wealth with them upon immigrating. What follows is an overview, not of any particular Jewish ethnic groups, some of which are discussed in Chapter 49, but of Jewish clients in general.

The increased violence and tension in Israel continues to put great pressure on Jewish families in the early 21st century. The Jewish community as a whole is quite vocal, as well as polarized, on this highly charged subject, and Jews are frequently perceived by their non-Jewish neighbors as intimately involved in and aware of the intricacies of this debate. The reality is that only a small minority are knowledgeable about Israeli matters. Although many Jews feel a strong loyalty to Israel, whether they believe the government's policies are right or wrong, others who are critical of Israel may feel uncomfortable in speaking out, especially to non-Jews. In addition, many Jews feel uneasy with the Christian Evangelical support of Israel, as they are sharply in disagreement with Evangelicals on most other issues.

The many Jewish denominations and institutions can be confusing to one unfamiliar with the community's inner workings. Synagogue denominations range from the most ritually observant (Orthodox) to those occupying the vast middle ground (Conservative and Reconstructionist), to the least ritually rigorous (Reform). Recent data show a strong growth in Reform synagogue membership and a decline in Conservative synagogues, suggesting, among other possibilities, a growing acceptance in the more liberal community of intermarried families.

There are wide variants of acceptance of intermarried families in synagogues. Orthodox synagogues refuse family membership to intermarried couples. Although most Conservative congregations deny *family* membership to intermarried couples, the Jewish partner is generally able to affiliate. In Reform and Reconstructionist congregations, most intermarried families are welcome, and even encouraged, to affiliate.

Almost all families, regardless of their religious or institutional affiliation, participate in some holy days. Two-thirds or more of Jews attend a Passover Seder or light Chanukah candles, whereas fewer fast on Yom Kippur, light Shabbat (Sabbath) candles, or observe other holy days (Faber, 2000).

Centrality of the Family

Marriage and raising children have been the core of Jewish tradition. This is particularly the case among Orthodox Jewish families, who explicitly follow the teachings of the Talmud (traditional compendium of Jewish law and lore) and see protracted bachelorhood and birth control as unacceptable. Historically, asceticism was viewed negatively, with celibacy strongly condemned. Orthodox rabbinic authorities are often called upon by couples to allow exceptions to traditional strictures on birth control when the mother's physical or emotional health may be threatened by pregnancy. Modern Orthodox communities allow a great deal more leeway in birth control practices than do ultra-Orthodox communities.

At least three other factors account for the unusually strong Jewish emphasis on marriage: (1) the child-focused nature of the Jewish family, with children and grandchildren considered central to life's meaning, (2) the powerful forces of suffering and discrimination, which imbue the family with the quality of "haven and refuge," and (3) the strong connection Jews feel to previous generations and the obligation to preserve their heritage.

The recent trends of later marriages, divorce, and more people remaining single directly threaten these values. A family that came to treatment struggled with their oldest son's having "come out" as gay, which left his parents virtually inconsolable despite their son's and the therapist's attempts to help them deal with it. Only in the third session, when the son stated strongly that he and his lover had every intention of adopting children and establishing a family, were his parents able to begin listening to him. Family therapy colleagues indicate that Jews seem to be initially more distraught about a child' s "coming out" than are most other ethnic groups, although they ultimately tend to be more accepting (Rosen & Weltman, 1995).

After marriage, a Jewish couple often stays very connected to the extended family. Young Jewish couples typically spend much time defining the boundaries and obligations between themselves and their families. Some adult Jews feel that they will always be children who, in their parents' view, need to be cared for, financially and otherwise. Sometimes their elders' expectation of geographical and emotional closeness can seem stifling.

Yet significant changes in the *nature* of the Jewish family have occurred, including the increase in intermarriage, the phenomenon of Gentiles voluntarily joining the Jewish community ("Jews by choice"), a growing number of gay and lesbian families, and the adoption of children from many different cultures. (increasingly, the modern Orthodox community accepts the adoption, and conversion, of babies from other cultures.) Only within much of the ultra-Orthodox community does the Jewish family largely look today as it did in previous generations.

More than half of Jewish adults are married, with the rest divorced, widowed, separated, or single (NJPS, 2003). Jewish parents frequently personalize a child's divorce; more than one client has reported a parent's response to the ending of his or her marriage as being "How could you do this to me?" The Jewish divorce rate, once considered low in relation to the rates of other ethnic groups, has grown to about that of the general population. The marriage survival rate for intermarried couples, and for unaffiliated and/or secular Jews, is significantly lower than for religiously observant Jews (Goldstein, 1993). In traditional religious families, divorce can also contribute to an alienation from Judaism, inasmuch as so many Jewish customs are rooted in home rituals and traditions.

Intermarriage

Two decades ago, intermarriage was perceived as the most flagrant breach of family togetherness and sometimes resulted in emotional cutoffs. Today, in a radical change, 80% of respondents to the American Jewish Committee's annual survey of American Jewish opinion concurred that "intermarriage is inevitable in an open society" (Annual Survey of American Jewish Opinion, 2000). A mere 39% agreed that "it would pain me if my child married a Gentile," and 68% did not feel that the non-Jewish partner's conversion to Judaism was "the best response." The exception to this trend occurs with ultra-Orthodox parents, some of whom "sit *shiva*" (i.e., formally mourn) for a child who intermarries. Yet even non-Orthodox parents willing to accept a child's intermarriage may clash with him or her at a later point, particularly about the religious identity of grandchildren.

Secularism among American Jews accelerated the trend toward intermarriage in the 1970s and 1980s but intermarriage appears to have leveled off since then at about 50%. For all Jewish marriages, the proportion of Jews married to non-Jews rose in the last decade of the 20th century from 28 to 37%. Among single Jews living with someone, some 80% had a non-Jewish partner (American Jewish Identity Survey, reported in Grossman, 2001). Thus, "intermarriage has become a non-issue for most American Jewry. . . . [M]ost Jews [see] no contradiction between being Jewish and having a non-Jewish spouse" (Grossman, 2001, p. 226). Despite this evidence, many Jewish parents report that their first question upon hearing that their son or daughter is dating someone is, "Is he (or she) Jewish?" However, given the multiethnic world in which their children have been raised, they are not surprised to find that the answer is negative.

In the American Jewish Committee survey mentioned earlier (Annual Survey of American Jewish Opinion, 2000) more than two thirds of the sample agreed that "the Jewish community has an obligation to urge Jews to marry Jews." But in response to the growing incidence of intermarriage, many synagogues and Jewish organizations have developed outreach programs to maintain ties with those who have "married out" and thus increase the chances of children being raised Jewish.

Chosenness and Suffering as a Shared Value

Jews have traditionally believed that they are God's "chosen people." In Jewish folklore, this notion of "chosenness" has had a double meaning: Although God may have chosen the Jews, they have undergone great travail; their status means that suffering is a basic part of life. A well-known Yiddish saying, *"Shver zu zein a yid"* ("It's tough to be a Jew"), while often accompanied by a resigned sigh, may even reinforce the notion of superiority by virtue of the burden of oppression and suggests that one wears the burden of that suffering with pride.

Although recent generations of Jews are more removed from this historical weight, contemporary evidence of virulent European and more subtle American anti-Semitism, often expressed under the guise of "anti-Zionist," is still significant in shaping the American Jewish character. Younger Jews find the phenomenon shocking, given that they were raised in an open society where anti-Semitism was nearly unknown. For their parents, the first social distinction they likely experienced was between themselves and non-Jews. Although most contemporary Jews do not believe that anti-Semitism is a powerful force in their lives, they still often react strongly to news accounts of incidents involving bias and to personal instances of perceived anti-Semitism.

Intellectual Achievement and Financial Success

Success is vitally important to the Jewish family ethos. Old jokes about "my son, the doctor" (or, now, "my daughter, the doctor"), although often used to ridicule status-seeking Jewish parents, reflect the emphasis given education and professional achievement. Learning was portable, an advantage because Jews were constantly forced to move by anti-Semitic societies. Discriminatory laws in Christian Europe also closed many professions to Jews, resulting in great respect for scholars.

The openness of American society, and their upward mobility, contributed to many Jews being successful in terms of status and material gains. Today, in most Jewish families and communities, it is almost obligatory that Jewish children go to college, graduate, and (often) pursue professional studies. The 1990 U.S. Census revealed that 52.7% of Jews had completed college and pursued graduate studies, as compared with 20.5% of the total U.S. White adult population (Goldstein, 1993). In 2001 more than half of all adult Jews (55%) had a college degree and a quarter of them had achieved a graduate degree.

Parents may start worrying about their children's education and academic achievements in kindergarten, or even in preschool. Some Gentiles suggest that if you want to know which teacher your child should have, or what the school is not teaching, just ask your Jewish neighbor.

Individual success often means sacrificing attachment to family and community. This conflict, long limited largely to Jewish men, who experience great family pressure to succeed, now equally affects women, particularly in terms of their roles as professionals, as well as parents and partners. Given the demands of the Jewish family system for success and achievement, it is easy for a Jew to feel like a failure no matter how much he or she accomplishes.

Charity also plays an extremely important part in Jewish family life. "Most American Jews (62%) give to non-Jewish causes and 41% donate to Jewish causes" (NJPS, 2000–2001, p. 13). The Jewish view of justice and charity stems from a belief that humankind is made in the image of God and is thus obliged to make the world a more just place (Lipset, 1990). Jewish religious thought holds that material goods, wealth, and learning are acquired not only for their own sake, but also because they make it possible to assist weaker, poorer, and otherwise more vulnerable families (Zborowski & Herzog, 1952). The perception of the poor as morally inferior was never a Jewish view. Even wealthy families often identified with the disadvantaged, in part because their own status in society was so marginal.

Of course, not all Jews have achieved financial success. There is a growing number of poor Jews, particularly in large urban centers. Today, 22% of those who have immigrated during the past quarter century live below the poverty line (NJPS, 2003). Among elderly Jewish Americans, 33% live alone and 58% survive on less than $35,000 annually (NJPS, 2003).

Mrs. A., a single mother, came to therapy with concerns about her 15-year-old daughter, who was angry and rebellious. They lived in an upper-middle-class, largely Jewish community in one of the less expensive developments. In therapy the daughter repeatedly berated her mother for not buying her the clothing necessary for her aspired-to social status. Mrs. A.'s priority (for which she worked many hours of overtime) was to keep her daughter involved in activities at the Jewish Community Center attended by her friends. Mrs. A. was supported in her efforts to set realistic limits for her daughter and, gradually, was able to clearly explain her goals. Her daughter talked about her feelings about the privileged life of many of her friends. When Mrs. A. suggested that the solution might be to move to a less affluent neighborhood, she and her daughter realized that their priority was to stay in the community. Mrs. A. confronted her ex-husband (who had been estranged from his daughter) and asked him to join her and his daughter for a number of sessions. Although he was not able to significantly raise

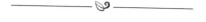

his level of financial support, he described his work, which, though not lucrative, was a great source of pride to him. This discussion opened a door for his daughter to think more deeply about lifestyle choices and values.

———————— ✒ ————————

Verbal Expression of Feelings

Being verbal, which is highly valued by most Jews, is a by-product of an educational system in which men studied the Torah and the Talmud by utilizing intricate methodologies. The student's task was to examine various interpretations, understand the intent of the ancient arguments, and articulate them. A youngster capable of this was held in high regard.

In today's Jewish families, children's opinions remain highly valued. Parents often take great pride in the contributions their children make to solving a family problem. Among Jewish families, there is a less clear-cut boundary between parents and children than in many other ethnic groups; clinically, Jewish families are largely, and often correctly, perceived to be enmeshed.

Cynicism and criticism are frequently used in Jewish families to induce members to react and respond, which, to an outsider, may appear as anger or hostility. However, such expressions of criticism may actually be ways of showing caring. Family sometimes say that they interact that way to "toughen" their children for the harsh things they may experience in the "outside world."

The therapist can often reframe these verbal attacks positively, shifting the family to a more positive, productive direction. For example, in a certain family, the wife was extremely critical of her husband's earning ability. Although it originally appeared that her concerns were totally materialistic, it became clear that her real concern was her husband's health problems and how his not taking good care of himself was interfering with his ability to get ahead in a job.

THERAPY ISSUES

Family Patterns

In the *shtetl* (largely Jewish small town) of Eastern Europe, families prayed that their offspring would be boys, for the study of Torah, considered life's quintessence, was the pursuit of men alone. Although men who sat in the synagogue all day studying were publicly respected, they were sometimes privately scorned as drains on the family and the community.

In America success outside the family has sometimes been achieved at the cost of devaluing the father in family life, in which the mother thus exercised the greater authority. Although his role might be peripheral within the home, it was his public persona that accounted for the family's status.

These dynamics are much weaker today, when many Jewish women no longer see themselves as dependent on men for status. However, vestiges remain, particularly in the cases in which a wife has decided to abandon a career to raise children or, less frequently, when a husband has chosen to give up a high-status job to have more time to be actively involved with his family.

Mr. and Mrs. S. sought couple therapy as they were making some significant career decisions. With the birth of their second child, Mrs. S. had cut back her hours at her well-paid, prestigious professional job. Although she enjoyed being available to their young children, she was eager to return to full-time work. In discussing their options, Mr. S. found that he welcomed the idea of cutting back his hours and exploring new career possibilities that might be less well paid but more interesting to him.

Both Mr. and Mrs. S. were excited by these ideas but worried about a lack of support—and outright criticism—from their parents and grandparents. After they had clarified their ideas, they presented them to their parents who, indeed, had some misgivings. But to their surprise, they got the most support from their fathers, who talked about the considerable regrets they had about not having spent more time with their children. Both their mothers expressed greater concern about financial security, which started a conversation about how much the world had changed now that Mrs. S. was able to earn as much as her husband.

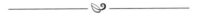

The public status and financial support provided by Jewish men have often been more valued than emotional succor and interpersonal skills. Paradoxically, Jewish women in treatment often complain about the lack of these qualities in a husband or father. In the wake of feminism, many Jewish men have begun to embrace the nurturing qualities of father or husband and face the difficult task of balancing professional success with personal gratification. Sometimes, parents and grandparents are not comfortable seeing men in those roles.

The Eastern European Jewish community was male-oriented, with women having active lives that usually were not publicly acknowledged. They were regarded as subordinate, and observant men greeted each day by offering thanks to God that "Thou hast not made me a woman" as part of the morning worship service. Women's domain was traditionally the home, and they were limited in their ability to participate fully in religious observance because of both family obligation and religious injunction.

Since the early 1970s, Jewish feminists have been participating in many previously proscribed religious rituals (Ruttenberg, 2001). As women have studied Torah, they have found scriptural justification for increased involvement in ritual practice. Since 1972, there have been women rabbis in Reform congregations; Conservative synagogues have accepted women as rabbis since 1985, and Reconstructionist synagogues even longer (Schneider, 1985). Women do not serve as rabbis in Orthodox congregations, although even in that domain women have been welcomed in some new nonritual roles.

Women have also been developing or rediscovering rituals to satisfy their particular needs. Among these is the celebration of *Rosh Chodosh*, the first day of each Hebrew month, which was linked to the menstrual cycle and celebrated by women in ancient times. Today, in many communities, women gather for this monthly celebration.

Sexuality

The Talmud recognizes both female and male sexual needs and instructs husbands to attend to their wives' sexual desires. Sexual modesty (*tzniut*) for women is an important principle in Jewish law; for Orthodox women this involves complete covering of the body (lengthy skirts and long-sleeved blouses) and covering their hair. Today, the use of the *mikveh* (the ritual bath in which immersion purifies a woman after her menses), *tzniut*, and other sexual regulations are practiced by more observant Jews, although some non-Orthodox women may follow these traditional practices from a redefined feminist perspective. Although traditional Judaism views the ultimate goal of sexuality as procreation, sexual relations between husband and wife are considered sanctified and encouraged as a necessary, and pleasurable, activity.

Both sex and marriage have long been the source of much Jewish humor. Some Jews, as well as non-Jews, tell jokes that mock the controlling Jewish woman. The ubiquity of this humor and its seeming acceptability among Jews themselves—even among some Jewish women—have led many to infer that the depicted stereotypes reflect reality. Indeed, as women's roles have changed and women have greater economic power, these stereotypes (and the humor that accompanies them) now cut across religious and ethnic labels.

Given that laughter has always been a refuge for those who see themselves as "one down," this self-deprecatory humor was an acceptable part of American Jewish life for generations. Jewish humor has become a part of American culture, as witnessed by many television programs and the inclusion of a growing number of Yiddish phrases in daily life.

Children and the Parent–Child Relationship

In the traditional Jewish community, having children was seen as a religious and social obligation. They completed a blessed marriage and were viewed as an extension of the parents' worth. Changing mores that have resulted in later marriage, delay of childbearing, smaller families, and couples choosing to remain childless have put enormous pressure on many family relationships.

Traditionally, the Jewish mother was viewed as her children's primary educator, inculcating in them the values of academic advancement and professional achievement. Many generations of highly successful Jewish doctors, lawyers, and social workers can testify to the efficacy of her methods. Because the mother was merely the instrument of her children's success, her enjoyment was vicarious, and her implicit mission was to work primarily for the development of others. Thus, Jews were often seen as being deeply, perhaps excessively, concerned with the quality of their children's education and academic attainment. However, recent immigrant groups offer serious competition in this area, which makes this notion somewhat arcane. Several Jewish families have recently complained that their children no longer strive to be in the highest honor classes because Asian students, under pressure from their parents, work harder than their Jewish classmates wish to.

Jews tend to raise their children through reasoning and explanation *of expectations*, and Jewish parents have tended to be permissive, overprotective, and concerned about their children's happiness, at times at the expense of their own. Children's obligations to be successful generally proceed from their role as extensions of their parents. Through the child's success, parents are validated; through their wrongdoings, they are disgraced and shamed.

Judaism sees children's duties to parents as rooted in religious principles, including the commandment to honor one's father and mother. Young people frequently complain that this concept results in a plethora of "shoulds" and "musts." Performing the *mitzvah* (commandment) of filial obligation also provides opportunity for both personal and spiritual rewards. As for parents' obligations to children, it often appears to therapists that

Jewish parents do not know when their role as providers should or does end. Although generosity is generally appreciated by adult children, it often comes with implied obligations.

A young couple that delays childbearing to pursue careers may feel that their behavior is a betrayal of their parents. Their decision may threaten the families' values, but also rejects the traditional obligation between generations. The requirement of "giving parents a grandchild" transcends mere individual choice. In very few other cultures do mothers see adult children postponing marriage or delaying having children as a personal affront, an issue that may bring a family to therapy.

Life-Cycle Rituals: The *Bris* and the Bar and Bat Mitzvah

The *bris* (ritual circumcision) of a Jewish baby boy remains nearly universally observed, and a special ceremony for naming girls (*simhat bat*) has also become common. In past generations, circumcision was done on the eighth day following the birth nearly exclusively by a *mohel* (ritual expert) who was enlisted for that sole purpose. Today, this ritual is sometimes *pro forma*, performed by a doctor, in a hospital, or earlier than 8 days. But the expectation that it be performed remains strong.

Some Jewish families no longer use traditional ceremonies, but simply have a party to celebrate the child's birth, leaving the circumcision, which substitutes for a ritual *bris*, to the doctor and the "naming," if done at all, to grandparents or other relatives. Yet even in these instances, families often desire that the ceremony have religious meaning. A child is traditionally named for a recently deceased relative, although among Sephardic Jews, a child is often named for a living relative.

The bar or bat mitzvah occurs when a child reaches 12 or 13 years of age. The child is called to read from, and/or recite blessings over, the Torah at a regular synagogue service, thus establishing him- or herself as an adult worshiper. The inclusion of women in synagogue ritual in all but Orthodox services has resulted in bat and bar mitzvahs being afforded equal importance.

The bar or bat mitzvah ceremony is a powerful moment in a family's life. Seriously ill family members may pray to stay alive at least until that day; couples on the verge of breaking up sometimes decide to wait until after the ritual and celebration; and long-neglected relatives may be invited back into the family circle. Recently, there has also been a strong movement toward inclusion of children with disabilities in bar and bat mitzvahs.

In the process of Americanization, other rituals have also been abandoned, transformed, or rediscovered. It can be difficult for young Jews to strike a balance between a commitment to Jewish tradition and the desire to make their own decisions. Ironically, when young Jews return to religious observance, their parents may be uncomfortable because their adult children are practicing rituals with which they are unfamiliar and sometimes uneasy.

Marriage

Jews tend to have a high rate of marriage, but only a slightly lower rate of divorce than the general population. Parents' anxiety about their children's marrying is proverbial: Giving one's child in marriage is still considered a primary obligation, and a child's marriage allows a person to enjoy the rewards and the *naches* (pride) of parenthood.

Children's failure to marry, however, is sometimes experienced as a bitter disappointment. I (E. J. R.) visited an 88-year-old woman in a hospice. She explained her resilience and longevity as a result of her need to make sure her 69-year-old widowed daughter was married before she herself died.

Pressure remains strong for Jewish women in particular to find the "right" mate. They are encouraged to do all that is necessary to ensure the best possible match, including choosing the best schools and the appropriate workplace for meeting a husband and giving careful attention to their physical appearance. Jewish women traditionally have been encouraged to find men capable of supporting them financially. Recently, a growing number of Jewish women have sought the perquisites of a professional career, only to decide to stop working after marriage or the birth of children and to look to their husbands to bear the family's financial burden. Consequently, many Jewish couples struggle to balance new societal expectations and the pull toward traditional roles.

Death and Mourning

The contemporary Jewish community tends to view death as an ending of this life, rather than as a beginning of another. Jews commonly bury their dead at the earliest possible time, usually within 24 hours. "Sitting *shiva*," which does not begin until after the burial, lasts 7 days (often less in more religiously liberal communities) and involves mourning in the home while being visited by family and friends. *Kaddish*, the memorial prayer, is traditionally said daily for a year after the burial of a parent or spouse and on the anniversary of his or her death. Although there are many idiosyncratic practices of the mourning rituals, many Jews choose to say *Kaddish*, at least weekly, for a variety of close relatives, even if they are not formally obligated to do so. Often, 11 months following the death, the family reconvenes at the cemetery for the "unveiling" or dedication of the tombstone, which also marks the end of the mourning period.

Major family life-cycle events may be stressful, but they also are times during which family members are most amenable to change and thus are potential moments for therapeutic intervention. Friedman (1988) and Imber-Black (1991) suggest that the therapist should try to maximize the potential of the rituals to promote family strengths and relationships.

CONCLUSION

As we noted in earlier editions of *Ethnicity and Family Therapy*, Jews are major consumers of psychotherapy. Jewish families are generally more comfortable with the usefulness of therapy than other ethnic groups (Rosen & Weltman, 1995)—as well as more knowledgeable and more critical of it.

Many Americans still continue to perceive psychotherapy as a "Jewish profession." The Jewish predilection for verbal facility, multiple meanings, and intellectual pursuits may make Jews somewhat more comfortable with individual-oriented, psychoanalytically focused therapies, although many also are open to a systems approach to family problems.

An oft-repeated Yiddish saying notes, "Where there are two Jews, you'll find three opinions." This characterizes the experience of many family therapists who work with Jewish families, whose opinionated natures often make them frustrating, but also challenging. Non-Jewish therapists may feel intimidated when working with Jewish clientele whose verbal facility, intellectualizations, cynicism, and intensity may make progress slow and illusory. Jewish therapists report difficulties related to their own conflicted ethnic or religious identity, having a more (or less) traditional outlook than the families they treat, and their beliefs about how Jewish families "ought" to behave.

Non-Jewish therapists may be startled by a family's deep awareness of and sensitivity to its minority status, inasmuch as Jews can easily "pass." Jews are generally highly sensitized to their Jewishness and often on guard for possible discrimination or untoward jokes. Therapists may also be surprised at the tension between Jews who have differences in religious observance, or between Jews who define themselves primarily through their religion and those who regard being Jewish as more of an ethnicity than a religion.

Jewish American identity is a paradox: historically freer from discrimination than ever before, yet also strongly bound by and often conflicted about the expectations of previous generations. There has never been a time or place in Jewish diaspora history when Jews have been less threatened by anti-Semitism, or freer to abandon their faith and community altogether, than in 21st-century America.

Still, many Jews maintain a strong connection to their history and traditions. Although Jews have been in the forefront of liberal causes for decades, the perception of Jewish affluence casts them as belonging to a power elite. In general, Jews are hardly a homogenous group whose behavior is predictable. Although Jewish families may question the therapist and the methods of therapy more than other families, they are generally very committed to therapy and willing to participate in the process.

NOTE

1. The *National Jewish Population Survey, 2000–2001* (NJPS) is the source for the demographic information in this chapter. Interested readers can access more data at www.jewishdatabank.org/index.cfm.

REFERENCES

Annual survey of American Jewish opinion. (2000, September). New York: American Jewish Committee.

Cohen, R., & Rosen, S. (1992). *Organizational affiliations of American Jews: A research report.* New York: American Jewish Committee.

Cohen, S., & Eisen, A. (2000). *The Jew within: Self, family and community in America.* Bloomington: Indiana University Press.

Faber, E. (1992). *A time for planting: The first migration, 1654–1820.* Baltimore: Johns Hopkins University Press.

Faber, S. B. (2000). *Jewish life and American culture.* Albany: State University of New York Press.

Friedman, E. (1988). Systems and ceremonies: A family view of rites of passage. In E. Carter & M. McGoldrick (Eds.), *The changing family life cycle* (pp. 119–147). New York: Gardner Press

Goldstein, S. (1993). *Profile of American Jewry: Insights from the 1990 national Jewish population survey.* New York: Center for Jewish Studies, City University of New York.

Grossman, L. (2001). Jewish communal affairs. In D. Singer (Ed.), *American Jewish Yearbook, 2002* (p. 226). New York: American Jewish Committee.

HIAS. (2004, January 16). HIAS helped 2,568 people migrate to USA in 2003. *HIAS Report.*

Imber-Black, E. (1991). Rituals and the healing process. In F. Walsh & M. McGoldrick (Eds.), *Living beyond loss* (pp. 207–223). New York: Norton.

Lipset, M. S. (1990). *American pluralism and the Jewish community.* New Brunswick, NJ: Transaction.

Mayer, E., & Kosmin, B. (Principal investigators). (2002). *American Jewish Identity Survey, 2001: An exploration in the demography and outlook of a people.* New York: Center for Jewish Studies, Graduate Center of the City University of New York.

National Jewish Population Survey, 2000–2001. (2003). [Electronic data file]. New York: United Jewish Communities [producer]. Waltham, MA: North American Jewish Data Bank [distributor].

Rosen, E., & Weltman, S. (1995). [*Family therapists' observations of Jewish families in treatment*]. Unpublished raw data.

Ruttenberg, D. (Ed.). (2001). *Yentl's revenge: The next wave of Jewish feminism.* New York: Seal Press.

Schneider, S. W. (1985). *Jewish and female: A guide and sourcebook for today's Jewish woman.* New York: Simon & Schuster.

Zborowski, M., & Herzog, E. (1952). *Life is with people.* New York: Schocken Books.

CHAPTER 49

Israeli Families

Anat Ziv

THE "ISRAELI CONTEXT"

A unique history has shaped the Israelis' way of perceiving the world, both as individuals and as family members.

The Holocaust preceded the establishment of Israel and resulted in a massive migration of Jews from Eastern Europe to Israel. In general, Israel is a nation of immigrants. Therefore, culture heritage and ethnic differences are taken into consideration in treating a client or family.

For the majority of Israelis, Judaism is more a nationality than a religion. Yet in Israel, there is no separation between religion and state. Unfortunately, this reality creates conflicts and increases the gap between secular and Orthodox Jews. One of the life-shaping experiences of "Israeliness" is military service. Joining the army at the age of 18, which is a mandatory duty, turns most Israeli youngsters to adults in no time. Very often, because of the continuing tension in the Middle East, they have to face life-threatening situations and provide leadership in complicated situations. Not many other youngsters in the world have to put their lives on hold for 2–3 years.

Life in Israel is a constant matter of survival, whether it involves protecting the right of the state to survive through wars with bordering countries, or eliminating local suicide bombers. Serving in the army means dealing with anxiety, stress, and mortal danger. The violence in the Middle East affects Israel's economy too. The *intifada* (Palestinian uprising) that began in 2000 has resulted in a significant decline in the number of tourists visiting and businesspeople investing in industries, as well as in a significant increase in the Israeli government's budget assigned to fight terrorism. Hi-tech companies, hotels, stores, and factories were closed or had to lay off people. Because of this situation, many Israelis found themselves unemployed for an unpredictable period of time, having no alternative means of supporting their families. Living in constant danger of terrorist activities, together with unemployment or economic difficulties, affected the desire of certain Israelis to leave the country and immigrate to America.

THE ESTABLISHMENT OF THE STATE OF ISRAEL

Cohen (1997) stated that the purpose of establishing the State of Israel was to enable Jews, who reside all over the world, to end their wandering, and oppression in the diaspora (countries outside the homeland) was a theme in the long history of the Jewish people.

The diaspora was mainly a religious concept. The Jews left the Promised Land following the destruction of the Second Temple (70 C.E.) for violating God's law (Patai, 1971) and continued in exile until the establishment of the modern State of Israel (1948).

Before the establishment of the State, Jews and Arabs lived in Palestine (Israel). In 1947, the British announced that they were withdrawing from Palestine and the United Nations (UN) partitioned the area into Arab and Jewish states, an arrangement rejected by the Arabs. Subsequently, the Israelis defeated the Arabs in a series of wars, but without ending the deep tension between the two sides.

About 6 million Jews have made Israel their home since the State was established in 1948. They did so even though the new State faced many problems, such as providing housing, education, health and welfare facilities, and finding employment for the new immigrants. The settlers' energy was directed to the sacred goal of building a home for the Jewish people. People gave up on their individual goals and needs, sometimes abandoning their professions, to help build—often through physical labor—the new country. For the immigrants, it was difficult to find security while protecting themselves from local Arabs who refused to accept the partition of Palestine, as well as handling diseases and illnesses with which they were unfamiliar.

ISRAEL: MULTIPLE ETHNICITIES UNITED BY JUDAISM

Creating one nation with new immigrants from different geographical locations was a complicated task. All of a sudden, all Jews had to form one nation, *Am Israel* (the nation of Israel), give up their own languages, and speak only Hebrew.

Jewish ethnic subgroups are characterized by particular places of origin and distinct cultures. In spite of the differences, their common Jewishness gave them a familiarity with a common set of religious beliefs and traditions (Kaplan, 2000). Transcending the ethnic differences was, historically, important in connecting different groups and creating one cooperative social entity (Rabin, 1999). The Jewish population of Israel consciously created a system of culture, education, military experience, and language (Zerubavel, 1995). New immigrants were faced with the same security problems that threatened the entire society; being part of the Israeli Defense Force thus created a feeling of national solidarity (Kaplan, 2000).

Ashkenazim and Mizrachim

The two main Jewish ethnic groups in Israel are the *Ashkenazim* (Jews from Europe) and the *Mizrachim* (Jews mainly from Mideastern Arab countries). The former are typically from smaller, secular families, and the latter usually have large, extended, patriarchal families, which are religious. Although there is a high rate of intermarriage between these two large ethnic groups, there are still significant objective socioeconomic, class, and educational differences between them. The upper classes were predominantly Ashkenazi, the lower classes predominantly Mizrachi. In recent years, the gap between them has narrowed, and the influence of the Mizrachim has increased, along with their electoral power and representation in ruling positions.

The archetypical Israeli, to whom all immigrants should aspire, was the *Sabra*, a Jew born in the land of Israel who was strong, silent, and otherwise emotionally and mentally different from the diaspora Jew. Eventually, this category (Sabra) included mostly the Ashkenazim (Wasserstein, 2003).

Israelis with Ethiopian or Russian (Latest Waves) Origins

During the past 30 years, two additional ethnic groups have become part of Israeli society: Russian and Ethiopian Jews (the former mainly immigrated in 1990–1994; the latter in 1977–1990). Both are at the bottom of the ladder of ethnic groups, which is based on status, income, and opportunities (Haidar, 1991).

Ethiopian Immigrants

The Israelis welcomed the Ethiopian immigrants. Ethiopian Jewish young people adjusted well to the educational and military system, but faced (and still do) cultural, religious, and economic challenges. Many Ethiopians feel discriminated against in jobs, housing, and education because they are Black (Lynfield, 2002). The Israeli government has taken some measures of affirmative action, including fully paying for the Ethiopians' education at any of the country's universities.

The issues they face include the classical cultural conflict between children and their immigrant parents; adjusting to Western cultural characteristics, such as secularity and technology; changes in the family system, such as the status of the extended family as well as changes in original gender roles; and adjusting to a more egalitarian society.

Russian Immigrants

The Russian immigrants included Jews from the European part of Russia as well as the Asian part of Russia. A higher percentage of more educated (defined as having at least 13 years of education) immigrants was found among the immigrants from the European part of Russia (Central Statistics Institute of Israel, 1995). It was also found that adolescent immigrants from the Asian part of Russia tended to suffer from mental health problems more than adolescent immigrants from the European part (Slonim-Nevo & Sharaga, 1997). The frequency of alternative family formats among the Russian immigrants is very high (Berger, cited in Rabin, 1999). Single-parent families, second-marriage families, and multigenerational families are very common among the Russian immigrants. It is common for grandparents to live with or next to young parents to help in raising their children. Therefore, the therapist may benefit from engaging the grandparents in treatment in that they are often the primary caregivers.

The involvement of the grandparents in a young couple's life may create tension and cause conflicts and, at times, separation or divorce. The engagement of grandparents in raising their grandchildren may lead to power struggles and arguments regarding the right way of raising children (Halberstadt, cited in Rabin, 1999).

Emotional expression and self-exposure between married partners are not encouraged. Divorce is a commonly accepted matter (Halberstadt, cited in Rabin, 1999). The roles in the family are divided between the father and the mother. The mother's is the central role. She is the one who decides how to educate the children, maintains contact with school, and manages the household budget. The father is the breadwinner (Halberstadt, cited in Rabin, 1999). The Russian Jewish family is characterized as supportive, but with enmeshed boundaries, overprotectiveness, ambivalence toward independence and separation, resistance to the expression of anger and negative feelings, respect for adults' authority, and high expectations of academic achievement and appropriate social functioning (Pozkanzer, 1995). These norms may subject the youngsters to mental stress and emotional difficulties.

The Ultra-Orthodox Jews

In Israel, the ultra-Orthodox community, which believes in the most traditional Judaism, struggles against modernization and secularity. For ultra-Orthodox Israelis who suffer from mental distress, turning to mental health services is a last resort. Often, they view problematic behavior as God's punishment for sins (Rabin, 1999). For individual psychological and family problems, the ultra-Orthodox prefer to approach a rabbi or a doctor to find a religious or medical answer to mental distress.

In the ultra-Orthodox community, the mentally ill are stigmatized; their social status is seen as inferior and thus they are secluded. Their families are stigmatized, and matchmaking for someone who is mentally ill is almost impossible. Therefore, mental illness among the ultra-Orthodox is often kept a secret (Rabin, 1999). In treating an ultra-Orthodox mentally ill person, the practitioner must make sure that the treatment is compatible with a religious worldview, rather than contradicting it.

Engaging professionals who belong to the same ethnic group as the client increases the chances for therapeutic success. If there are no such professionals available, the more familiar the therapist is with ultra-Orthodox culture, the better able he or she will be to relate to the client (Rabin, 1999). Acquiring knowledge of the culture may increase the therapist's awareness of acceptable ways of communication and interaction in the ultra-Orthodox world (Good & DelVecchio Good, cited in Rabin, 1999), such as avoiding too much eye contact and adhering to the rule that men do not shake hands with women.

WHY DO ISRAELIS LEAVE THEIR HOMELAND AND IMMIGRATE TO THE UNITED STATES?

Sobel (1986) states that the two main factors motivating Israelis to immigrate to the United States are the "diminished dream" (p. 211) and individual disappointment. The first term refers to a shift in the Israeli mentality from working as part of a collective and sacrificing in order to fulfill the collective's goals, to individualism, whereby each person cares primarily about him- or herself and his or her family. The shift also included a new emphasis on earning more money, as Israeli society became more consumerist and less ideologically focused.

According to Sobel (1986), many emigrants felt that life in Israel carried too many difficulties, including unemployment, low wages and inflation, and high taxation. Differences in ethnicity and class hierarchy, he stated, create feelings of suspicion rather than the closeness of kinship. Regular army or reserve service is also a heavy load. Sobel notes that many Israeli emigrants he interviewed said that they wanted to escape military duty and the constant violence associated with life in the Middle East.

Gold (2000) stated that most Israelis referred to three main motives for emigration: economic opportunities (including education), family unification, and expanded horizons and opportunities (artistic, cultural, etc.). Shokeid (1988) described the impetus as an inner drive to get out of the country and see the world. Some were looking for a change, new experiences, and/or adventures. Only about 5% of emigrants left for ideological reasons. But many Israelis from stigmatized ethnic backgrounds emigrated because of discrimination in Israel.

THE ISRAELI PERSPECTIVE ON EMIGRATION

In Israel, emigration is marked by something of a stigma. "Emigrants from other lands are not labelled in quite so judgmental, so ontological a fashion either by those left behind at the country of origin or by the emigrants themselves" (Sobel, 1986, p. 223). When Israel was in constant danger of attack and even annihilation, emigration was considered an act of disloyalty.

The term for leaving the Jewish state is *yeridah* (descending or going down in stature), in contrast to *aliyah* (moving up a place) or moving from the diaspora to Israel (Shokeid, 1988). "There is an implication that the citizen who has left Israel is guilty of a subtle form of betrayal of the shared obligation to protect the land of Israel" (Linn & Barkan Ascher, 1996, p. 7).

Emigration has also affected Israel's economy and morale. In 1992, the Israeli government offered a package of benefits for Israelis and their families who return to Israel (Gold, 2002). The Israeli government constantly acts to bring Israelis back home by recruiting people to work, creating options for children and adolescents to spend time in Israeli summer camps, and offering incentives such as stipends.

Although the perception of the Israeli emigrant has improved somewhat, it has generally remained negative. During the 1970s, Prime Minister Yitzhak Rabin called Israeli emigrants "the fallen of the weaklings" and "the dregs of earth," although by 1992 he had recanted these statements (Kimhi, 1990; Ritterband, 1986, p. 113).

DEMOGRAPHIC STATISTICS

The Israeli Ministry of Absorption reported that about 60% of 750,000 Israeli emigrants live in North America, mainly in New York and Los Angeles (*Yediot Achronot*, 2003). This group of emigrants is composed of Israelis who left between 1948 and the time when this report came out, November 19, 2003. Most are 25–44 years old, and a high percentage of them have a college education. In the first 5 years after the Oslo Agreements (1993), many Israeli Americans returned to Israel, but since the new upsurge in violence in 2000, there has been a major decrease in the number of returns.

ISRAELI IMMIGRANTS' EXPERIENCE IN THE UNITED STATES

In general, Israelis in the United States speak English well, earn incomes that approach those of native-born Whites, frequently marry U.S. citizens, and exhibit high rates of naturalization (Kivisto, 2000). However, Israelis almost never describe themselves as Americans, even after 20 years of living in this country. They may socialize mainly with Israelis and frequently talk about going back home (Shokeid, 1988).

Israeli immigrants vary greatly in terms of age, ethnic origin, religious outlook, education, occupation, ideology, length of stay in the United States, and income (Gold, 2002). Despite the differences between the ethnic subgroups, most Israeli families are traditional in terms of family structure (Peres & Katz, cited in Kulick & Rayyan, 2003). A traditional family is one that includes a husband and a wife (a male and a female), with one child or more.

The Israeli immigrants enjoy many opportunities in America that they lacked in Israel (Sobel, 1986). They are able to achieve higher standards of living and access to higher education and professional work, and there is no mandatory military service or reserve duty.

However, Israeli immigrants are often "sojourners": people who never make their new country their emotional home (Siu, 1952). The Israeli immigrant will rarely admit that he or she is staying permanently in the United States, instead claiming that his or her stay is temporary. Most Israeli immigrants constantly miss Israel and often speak about plans to go back there. Israeli American parents have a constant fear that their children will lose their Israeli and Jewish identity.

ISRAELI WOMEN IN THE UNITED STATES

Because most Israeli women follow their husbands' decisions to immigrate to the United States (Sabar, 2000), they face frequent adjustment difficulties (Gold, 2000). Israeli women are accustomed to working outside the home. Once they get to America, they are charged with settling the family's domestic affairs and recreating a supportive family environment in an unfamiliar cultural and linguistic setting (Gold, 2000; Sabar, 2000).

Ruth was seeking therapy a year after she immigrated to the United States with her husband and two children (2 years old and 5 years old). She presented marital issues that had started about 4 months after coming to America, mood changes, and irritability. Ruth, who worked full time in Israel, found herself full time at home in the United States. She could not work outside the house because she did not have the right visa or a baby-sitter to take care of her youngsters. She used to have a large social network and a supportive family, but now found herself alone in the world.

Once Ruth got engaged in therapy, she worked with her husband on the obstacles in their marriage. The husband, through therapy, learned that some of the obstacles resulted from his being focused on himself and his own goals and being unaware of his wife's needs. Through therapy he also learned that because he had been an only child, he had not learned how to share with others and was raised in a way that allowed him to always get what he wanted. He now understood that the way he was raised was an obstacle in his married life. He started making small changes to create real partnership with his wife in their lives as a couple, beginning with changing his schedule so Ruth would have some time for herself. The way Ruth responded to his accommodation reinforced his objectives, to continue to be less focused on himself and more considerate of others. Ruth learned to communicate her desires and wishes. As the third child of four in her family, she always tried to accommodate herself to others and never expressed herself out loud. Both husband and wife learned how to create local networks through the Israeli Club in their town, joining the PTA at their son's school, and availing themselves of such resources as the Jewish Community Center. Ruth, who had been a third-grade teacher in Israel, was able to get a job in a local Israeli school and worked three times a week in the afternoon. Ruth found the day-care program in the Jewish Community Center adequate, after observing and getting recommendations from two Israeli mothers she had met and become friendly with. Acculturation to the new environment, together with processing marital issues, allowed Ruth to move forward in her life, communicate differently with her husband, and be happy again.

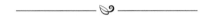

In spite of the difficulties, Israeli women in the United States enjoy greater economic and educational opportunities, greater equality of gender roles, and a less stigmatized view of single parenthood (Goldscheider 1996).

THE ISRAELI PERSPECTIVE ON INTERMARRIAGE

Among most Israeli Americans, interfaith marriages are not tolerated. Historically, Jews were repeatedly under threat of extinction, and so interfaith marriage was seen as a threat to the Jewish nation. (According to the Jewish religion, children born to a non-Jewish mother are not considered Jewish.) Between 1945 and 1990, the world's Jewish population declined by 2 million, a significant loss to a nation as small as the Jews.

THE ISRAELI PERSPECTIVE ON HOMOSEXUALITY

Gays in Israel are not yet fully accepted. Religious law oversees all marriages, and there is no such a thing as civil marriage—not to mention gay marriage—in Israel. Israel is an extraordinarily family-centered society and, as in the United States, many Israelis have not yet come to accept gay families.

However, Israeli policies toward gays improved during the 1990s. Discrimination on the basis of being gay has been forbidden in Israel since 1992, homosexual soldiers have been allowed to serve in the army since 1993, and the Israeli Supreme Court has decreed that gay domestic partners are eligible for spousal benefits (Kirchick, 2003).

CULTURAL IMPLICATIONS FOR THERAPY

That the Israeli American is often a "sojourner" often raises issues in the family about staying in the United States or returning to Israel, as well as identity conflicts between children and parents. For example, parents may choose religious schools for their children to preserve their "Israeliness," sometimes ignoring the fact that in the schools their offspring attend, American Jewish children are perceived as a foreign group. Thus, they may feel much more comfortable in a public school, where children are actually taught in a Western way, similar to the way Israeli children are taught in Israel.

There is often a crisis in a family because one family member wants to go back home to Israel and another wants to stay in the United States. Therapists should help parents to be more aware of their children's needs and feelings when making decisions on this matter. It may be beneficial to help parents distinguish between their own feelings of Israeli identity and their children's. Although some parents would like to think that their children have remained Israelis, that may not be the case. The way to engage Israeli parents is to show empathy for the difficult position in which they find themselves.

Israeli women, who usually are not the ones who initiate emigration, may find themselves lonely, depressed, and missing home constantly, feelings that can contribute significantly to intrafamily conflict.

In assisting women who have been used to working and relying on child care institutions and extended family, it can be helpful to find or create alternate support systems while also being empathic to their immediate difficulties. The therapist should also try to help couples to be aware of the difficulties of transition and to find ways to accommodate each person's needs.

Israelis are unlikely to turn to a therapist as the first source of help. They are used to sharing their issues with best friends or family, or to resolving problems on their own. Therefore, it may take some time for a client to feel comfortable with the idea of outside, professional help.

Israelis are very direct in their communication style, a trait that can be used effectively in therapy. The therapist may also clarify that therapy is a process that takes time and that results are usually not immediate, for Israeli clients may have expectations of being "cured" quickly. In fact, once some relief is felt, the Israeli family may terminate treatment even though the problems are far from being resolved.

Although many Israelis speak English fluently and are "Americanized," they may prefer an Israeli therapist who speaks the same language (Hebrew) and belongs to the same culture. For non-Israeli therapists, showing awareness of the Israeli culture, mentality, and language may lead to easier trust building and may establish a strong base for acceptance by the client. The non-Israeli therapist must be aware of his or her ethnic orientation and bias and must also appreciate the distinctions between Israeli Americans and Jewish Americans. The former tend to be more nation-oriented; the latter, more religion-oriented.

The ambivalent feelings of Israeli immigrants toward the United States are rooted in the negative Israeli perspective of immigration. Therapists should be aware that almost every Israeli immigrant feels some sense of guilt, shame, and betrayal about leaving Israel. The extended family may try to prevent its acculturation to American society, so that the immigrant family will one day return to Israel.

American Israelis almost always live between two worlds. Therefore, family therapists, along with focusing on internal family conflicts and dynamics, should also help the family to maintain its identity while acculturating to American society. The therapist's emotional support and empathy for Israeli families who deal with the burden of guilt and blame, can contribute to better results in the therapeutic process.

REFERENCES

Central Statistics Institute of Israel. (1995). *The immigration to Israel 1995* (Publication No. 1037). Jerusalem: Author.

Cohen, R. (1997). *Global diasporas*. Seattle: University of Washington Press.

Gold, J. S. (2000). Israeli Americans. In P. Kivisto & G. Rundblad (Eds.), *Multiculturalism in the United States* (pp. 409–420). Thousand Oaks, CA: Pine Forge Press.

Gold, J. S. (2002). *The Israeli diaspora*. Seattle: University of Washington Press.

Goldschieder, C. (1966). *Israeli changing society: Population, ethnicity and development*. Boulder, CO: Westview Press.

Haidar, A. (1991). *Social welfare services for Israel's Arab population*. Boulder, CO: Westview Press.

Ichner, I. (2003, November 19). Export item number 1: Israelis. *Yediot Achronot*, pp. 13–14.

Kaplan, J. (2000). *Issues in Israeli society*. Retrieved February 20, 2005, from www.jafi.org.il/education/juice/2000/israeli_society/is1.html

Kimhi, S. (1990). *Perceived change of self-concept, values, well-being and intention to return among kibbutz people who migrated from Israel to America*. Doctoral dissertation, Pacific Graduate School of Psychology, Palo Alto, California.

Kirchick, J. (2003). Out on the front lines: Gays in the Israeli defense forces. *Yale Israel Journal: Exploring the history, politics and culture of Israel*. Retrieved February 20, 2005, from www.yaleisraeljournal.com/spr2003/gays.html

Kivisto, P. (2000). Theorizing transnational immigration: A critical review of current efforts. *Ethnic and Social Studies, 24*(4), 549–577.

Kulik, L., & Rayyan, F. (2003). Wage-earning patterns, perceived division of domestic labor, and social support: A cooperative analysis of educated Jewish and Arab-Muslim Israelis. *Sex Roles: A Journal of Research*. Availabe at www.findarticles.com/cf_dls/m2294/2003_Jan/00326299

Linn, R., & Barkan Ascher, N. (1996). Permanent impermanence: Israeli expatriates in non-event transition. *Jewish Journal of Sociology, 38*(1), 5–16.

Lynnfield, B. (2002). Ethiopian Jews find Israel to be a racist state. Retrieved February 20, 2005, from www.rense.com/general25/rct.htm

Patai, R. (1971). *Tents of Jacob: The diaspora yesterday and today*. Englewood Cliffs, NJ: Prentice Hall.

Pozkanzer, A. (1995). The matroyshka: The three-generation Soviet family in Israel. *Contemporary Family Therapy, 17*(4), 413–427.

Rabin, C. (Ed.). (1999). *Being different in Israel: Ethnicity, gender and therapy*. Tel Aviv, Israel: Ramot.

Ritterband, P. (1986). Israelis in New York. *Contemporary Jewry, 7,* 113–126.

Sabar, N. (2000). *Kibbutznicks in the diaspora*. Albany: State University of New York Press.

Shokeid, M. (1988). *Children of circumstances: Israeli emigrants in New York*. Ithaca, NY: Cornell University Press.

Siu, C. P. (1952). The sojourner. *American Journal of Sociology, 58,* 38–40.

Slonim-Nevo, V., & Sharaga, Y. (1997). Social and psychological adjustment of Soviet-born and Israeli-born adolescents: The effect of the family. *Israel Journal of Psychiatry, 34*(2), 128–138.

Sobel, Z. (1986). *Migrants from the Promised Land*. New Brunswick, NJ: Transaction Books.

Wasserstein, B. (2003). *Evolving Jewish ethnicities or Jewish ethnicity: End of the road?* Retrieved February 20, 2005, from www2. chass.ncsu.edu/CIES/WasserteinPaper.htm

Zerubavel, Y. (1995). *Recovered roots: Collective memory and the making of Israeli national tradition*. Chicago: University of Chicago Press.

CHAPTER 50

Orthodox Jewish Families

Marsha Pravder Mirkin
Barbara F. Okun

When we were first asked to write a chapter on Orthodox Judaism, we were confounded by the assignment, because there is no such thing as "the" Orthodox tradition. Orthodox Judaism encompasses a range of both ultra-Orthodox and modern Orthodox Jews who reveal both similarities and profound differences. The former group includes the Hasidim, a community that exudes joyous celebration of God and expects unquestioning obedience to Jewish law through the rabbis' interpretations, and the yeshiva (Talmudic academy) Jews, organized around the scholarly study of sacred texts whose interpretations are also governed by rabbis (Davidman, 1991; Kaufman, 1994; Shai, 2002). Modern Orthodoxy, a 19th-century development, allows interaction with the secular community, as well as questioning of the rabbis' interpretations, while remaining firmly rooted in Jewish law and synagogue life (Shai, 2002). Many modern Orthodox Jews come from ultra-Orthodox backgrounds, and others arrive at modern Orthodoxy through conversion or shifts from Reform, Conservative, or previously nonobservant groups within Judaism.

This chapter addresses the clinical implications of working with Orthodox Jewish families. The major points for clinicians to appreciate about Orthodox Jewish observance and culture are:

1. Orthodox Judaism is a culture as well as a religion.
2. All Orthodox Jews agree that the Torah, the central sacred Jewish text, was given by God to Moses at Mt. Sinai. The Torah is understood literally as God's spoken word.
3. Orthodox Judaism is based on *halacha*, Jewish Law, a list of 613 commandments that specify how Orthodox Jews should live and deal with family, community, strangers, and business. Questions of *halacha* and observance are brought by community members to their rabbis for explanation and decisions. In recent years, modern Orthodox Jewish feminists have begun to incorporate some of their social and cultural variables into the interpretation of *halacha*.

HISTORY AND MIGRATION

Jews have been called "one of the most migratory peoples in the history of mankind" (Barnavi, 1992, p. 1). Centuries of expulsion and resettlement led to the formation of a resilient group of people who could survive in new countries while maintaining a strong identification with Judaism, which may involve living separately from the secular community.

Although Orthodox Jews trace their history back to biblical times in Israel, most of the time following the expulsions by the Babylonians in 586 B.C.E., and by the Romans in A.D. 70, was spent in diaspora (residing outside of what we now know as Israel). In this diaspora, Jews developed customs, beliefs, and values that defined them as an ethnicity and culture in addition to a religion. Although the Jews were influenced by their surroundings, frequent expulsions forced their culture to be centered on Judaism more than on geographical location.

The word "orthodox" was not used to describe Judaism until modern times (after the mid-19th century) when the birth of Reform, Conservative, and Reconstructionist forms of Judaism required that a name be given to traditionally observant Jews. Even today in parts of Eastern Europe, there are Orthodox and secular Jews, but not much of the wider variety of religious practices that have taken hold in Western Europe and the United States.

During the 8th–11th centuries, diaspora Jews were connected under the rule of the Muslim Empire, allowing some areas in which Jewish religion and culture could flourish. However, with the advent of Christianity came strong waves of anti-Semitism, leading to a series of expulsions: from England in 1290, France in 1306, Spain in 1492, and Germany in 1450–1520. Although the expulsion from Portugal was rescinded, it was replaced in 1497 by forced conversions as well as the abduction and baptism of Jewish children, resulting in an exodus by many Jews (Barnavi, 1992).

After the expulsions, Spanish and Portuguese Jews, known as Sephardic Jews (taken from the Hebrew word meaning "Spanish") settled primarily in Morocco, the Ottoman Empire, southern France, and Italy, where they generally formed communities with others from their original country or district. They had flourished in Spain, where both the 13th century kabbalistic (mystical) movement and the great philosopher Maimonides were born, before Christianity took hold. Their traditional language is Judeo-Spanish, also known as" Ladino," although Sephardic Jews typically speak the language of the country in which they reside. Rabbi Joseph Karo's great 16th century legal text *Shulhan Arukh* (The Set Table) remains the basis for Sephardic religious practices.

Large waves of immigrants from other Western European countries moved to Eastern Europe to avoid persecution in the 13th century, and by the late 15th century more than 60 Jewish communities had developed in Poland, most of them as a result of German, or Ashkenaz, immigration. Whereas Jews had few options other than becoming moneylenders in Germany, Poland opened the possibility of their becoming tradespeople and crafts workers. Jews also provided the Polish aristocracy with many financial services. The Ashkenaz brought with them a language, Yiddish (derived from German and Hebrew), which allowed international trade and is still used by Orthodox communities today. Because of the uniformity of religious life, Jews from different parts of the diaspora could gather at a yeshiva anywhere in the diaspora to learn about Judaism. Poland, where a flourishing Jewish community developed, became a central place for Jewish study.

Unfortunately, the safe haven of Poland was not to last. Polish townspeople expelled Jews from the towns. Worse, Ukrainian Orthodox peasants saw Jews as representative of the oppressive Catholic Polish nobles, and in 1648, with the help of warriors from the Russian frontier known as Cossacks, they destroyed dozens of Jewish communities and massacred the Jews. By the late 1600s, the Russian Orthodox Church began accusing Jews of conducting blood libels, using the blood of Christians in Jewish rituals. Feeling hopeless and demoralized, many Jews fell prey to what turned out to be a false Messiah. Jewish people in the 17th century were fervently hoping that the Messiah was about to come to raise them from the desperation of their lives in poverty-stricken, anti-Semitic communities. It was at that point of hope and desperation that Shabbetai Zvi (b. 1626 in Smyrna), a man with mystical devotion, Talmudic knowledge, and messianic ideas, was declared the Messiah by Nathan of Gaza. Shabbetai Zvi, acting the role and the belief that he was the Messiah, spread to communities with and without experiences of persecution. Then, in 1666, the Sultan gave Shabbetai Zvi the choice between conversion and death, and he chose conversion to Islam, for which he was rewarded with money and status by the Sultan. This act shocked the Jewish people. Some Jews responded by labeling him the "false Messiah" and destroying any documents or papers that mentioned his name (Karp, 1991). What he left behind was an even more demoralized people, holding less hope than before, but from whom new and exciting movements would be born.

This 17th-century bloodshed and ensuing sense of defeat that came with the false Messiah movement created fertile ground for the birth of yet another form of Orthodox Judaism, Hasidism. The founder of Hasidism, known as the Ba'al Shem Tov (Master of the Good Name) was a simple man who believed that God was everywhere, in everything, and that people can find joy in loving and celebrating God and can be in communion with God. Followers of the Ba'al Shem Tov created Hasidic sects throughout Europe, and eventually reached the United States through the wave of immigration that occurred in the 1880s.

There are many sects of Hasidism. The two main divisions are from the Ukraine/Galicia and Lithuania. Within these divisions are sects named after the areas from which they emerged. Each group is led by a *rebbe* or *tzaddik* (spiritual leader). Initially, the Orthodox non-Hasidic rejected this new movement because of the seemingly out-of-control joyous worship and the attributions of miracle working to the rebbes, as well as their fears that another false Messianic sect was being born. These Orthodox Jews, known as *Mitnagdim*, or opponents (of Hasidism), believed more in intellectual, scholarly Judaism than in emotionally and mystically driven Judaism.

By the 19th century, the Enlightenment had led some Orthodox Jews to question whether one needed to remain isolated from the larger culture in order to maintain one's affirmation of Judaism. Rabbi Samson Raphael Hirsch, a German Jew who studied Judaism at home and had a secular education, became the father of Modern Orthodoxy when he espoused "Torah im Derekh Eretz"—Torah, along with full engagement with the culture. He believed in the divine origins of Torah, religious law, and traditional beliefs, along with the idea that one could change anything that was not based in *halacha*. Thus, he supported secular education and the cultured personality along with strict adherence to *halacha*. Modern Orthodox Jews, to this day, base their way of living on this integration of religious beliefs and secular society.

The earliest wave of Jewish immigration to the United States was composed of Sephardic Jews, arriving as early as 1654 in New Amsterdam, where they did not find a welcome. Other early Sephardic communities in the United States developed in Rhode Island and Georgia.

Orthodox Jews, both Hasidic and non-Hasidic, came to the United States in two major waves of immigration, the largest by far occurring between 1880 and 1920, when more than one third of European Jews left their countries of origin for reasons of physical safety and economic possibility; 90% of these Jews immigrated to the United States (Barnavi, 1992). The majority of the Jewish immigrants during this period were orthodox. In 1880 one of every six Jews in the United States was of Eastern European extraction. By 1920 the number had increased to five of every six (Barnavi, 1992). Many, but not all, settled in urban neighborhoods, close to other Jews, often building community synagogues, *heders* (afternoon religious schools), social service agencies, and recreational organizations. Many came in dire poverty, requiring the help of the agencies supported by the immigrants who had been here longer. Those who chose to interact with the secular world tended to focus on education, so their children often became the first in the families to be college educated and to experience upward class mobility. These Orthodox Jews tended to immigrate individually or with families.

Alternatively, Hasidic Jews migrated collectively, generally from the Pale of Russia (an area outside central Russia where Jews were required to live after Russia annexed Poland in 1772), as a result of the pogroms of 1881–1884 and 1903–1906. They remained together and recreated their Eastern European communities within the United States.

Not all those who arrived poor had been poor in their countries of origin. Many countries did not permit emigrés to exit with their valuables, so economically comfortable and more educated Jews from the cities joined other Jews from the Eastern European *shtetls* (poor, segregated villages) in tenements and other poor housing situations. There was also a minority of Jews who had been wealthy in Europe and had brought their wealth with them to the United States.

A smaller wave of immigration occurred during and after the Holocaust, when the United States made it more difficult for Jews to enter this country, even turning back the *St. Louis*, a boat from Germany that unsuccessfully attempted to land in Cuba and the United States. Most of the Jews on board the *St. Louis* were eventually murdered by the Nazis.

Orthodox Jews settled in communities within the United States, where some interacted more with the secular and non-Jewish communities, thus expanding the modern Orthodox communities, while others maintained their Yeshivot or Hasidic Orthodox belief system. Some discovered non-Orthodox forms of Judaism and socialism. In addition to Sephardic and Ashkenazi Jews, a third group, known as Mizrahi Jews, remained in the Middle East and North Africa and developed traditions similar, but not identical, to those of the Sephardim. Like the Sephardim, they have a less legalistic interpretation of Jewish law than Ashkenazi Jews, but the Mizrahi Jews maintain differences in the prayerbook, liturgical melodies, customs, and language. The Mizrahis speak Judeo-Arabic as well as languages native to the countries within which they reside. Immigration to the United States developed in the early 20th century in response to violence and repression in their homelands.

Although Jews are predominantly Caucasian, all races are represented within Judaism. We do not know the race of the original Israelites. We do know that diaspora communities grew throughout the world, and with time, intermarriage, and marriage to converts, Jews took on the racial features of the community. For example, Kaifeng Jews have lived in China since the 9th century (Xu Xin, 2003), and Ethiopian Jews, who have lived in Africa for uncounted centuries, recently moved en masse to Israel. There was a Jewish community in Yemen in the early Middle Ages, another group that lived in Southern Libya until 1960, and those who settled in South and Central America with the earliest European settlers. Therefore, one will find Jews who are Blacks, Caucasians, Asians, and Latinos. In addition, conversions and adoptions in contemporary times have added more Jews of color to the Orthodox community.

Given their long history of repeated experiences of belonging in a community, then being oppressed by that community, and finally expelled or murdered, it is no wonder that there are groups of Orthodox Jews that have separated themselves from the non-Orthodox world and maintain a life and structure based on the beliefs that carried them through all of these waves of persecution. These communities believe that it is critical to financially support themselves and each other and not to count on the "Gentiles" or non-Orthodox Jews for assistance.

However, there are times when the ultra-Orthodox community cannot offer a service that members need, and they are then willing to seek help outside their group. It is more likely that a clinician will be contacted to help with a learning-disabled child, but very unlikely that the ultra-Orthodox will consult someone outside their community for couple or family therapy about an emotional issue.

WHAT CLINICIANS NEED TO KNOW ABOUT ORTHODOX CULTURE

Clinicians should understand that *halacha* emphasizes obligation to a covenant between people and God. Orthodoxy does, however, believe that each person has free will. Thus, a person is constantly confronted with a choice between following his or her "inclination to do evil" and the "inclination to do good." Still, once the person decides to follow *halacha*, he or she opts to honor the set of obligations and not pick and choose among them.

Among Orthodox Jews, the community is "family." Members generally live within the same area so that they can walk to the synagogue, inasmuch as riding is prohibited on the Sabbath and certain holidays, and can be available to each other during times of celebration or need. They share many rituals and *Shabbos* (Sabbath; also *Shabbat*) activities as families.

No riding, business or commercial activities, or use of electricity is allowed Orthodox Jews on *Shabbos*, a day of prayer, reflection on God's creation, rest, and family activities. However, *Shabbos* law may be broken in order to preserve a human life. Thus, doctors may work on *Shabbos*, and in medical emergencies the Orthodox can take ambulances or use elevators.

Modern Orthodox Jews tend to work in the secular community and maintain connections with non-Orthodox friends and family. They read secular newspapers, watch TV, and may send their children to nonreligious schools or after-school programs.

Many, although not all, Hasidic sects as well as some other ultra-Orthodox groups dress in a manner that replicates the garb of 18th-century Polish nobility. The tradition of black clothing on *Shabbos* and holy days comes from a time when black dye was rare and expensive and used for special occasions when people gathered to honor God. Although all Orthodox men wear head coverings (*yarmulkes*; also *kippot*), hats are usually worn over yarmulkes by Hasidim and by a number of non-Hasidic Orthodox Jews. Hasidic men wear a brimmed hat inside the house, and will wear one in a therapist's office. In some communities, a *streimel* (fur hat) is worn on formal occasions.

Given the emphasis on modesty (*tznius*) and on sexuality being reserved for one's spouse, ultra-Orthodox married women do not show their hair in public. They, and some modern Orthodox women, therefore wear either head coverings or wigs, based on the preference and traditions of their communities. Some Orthodox women cut their hair in order to wear wigs, others cut their hair and wear head coverings, and still others wear hats or scarves and keep their hair long. There is even a hat, called a "snood," with room for long braids in it!

The growth of beards and side curls (*payis*) by many Hasidic and some Yeshivot Orthodox groups is a response to the interpretation of a command from Torah. *Tzitzit*, or tassles, are four-cornered garments that are also worn by men in response to a biblical commandment. *Tefillin* (two black boxes containing the central Jewish prayer) are worn by the Orthodox during weekday morning prayers.

Orthodox men and women, except for a number of modern Orthodox Jews, do not shake hands with members of the opposite sex because of the rules of modesty and privacy. One explanation is that the body is considered sacred and not to be touched by an adult of the opposite sex. It is also seen as respectful to not gaze into the eyes of a person of the opposite sex and to not stare during conversations.

Orthodox Jewish communities focus on family. Duty, obligation, and family commitment are required of both spouses, encouraging commitment to the family by emphasizing family over individual selves. This model places primary responsibility on the mother for child rearing. The father is also encouraged to participate in family life, as well as to study Torah and participate in synagogue life. In fact, some Orthodox fathers are more involved in parenting and family life than fathers in secular society (Davidman, 1991). Even though women are not required to study or attend synagogue, many women enter serious Torah study groups and regularly attend synagogue services.

GENDER ROLES

Non-Orthodox therapists may find themselves feeling judgmental about gender roles in Orthodoxy and making assumptions that Orthodox women are treated as second-class members. True, there are roles in the Orthodox community that are based largely on patriarchal power, and there are within it the same domestic violence, substance abuse, psychological and other problems as exist elsewhere. There are some practices that emerge from a patriarchal hierarchy. For example, a husband must present his wife with a *get* (religious divorce paper) for her to be free to remarry; a woman cannot lead men in worship; and men and women are separated in synagogue (*shul*) by a divider (*mechitzah*) that often leaves women in the back of the synagogue or in its balcony.

Yet an emphasis solely on inequities negates the complex fabric of most couples' relationships. Many women describe the benefits of living within Orthodox gender roles. Adult females are accorded a great deal of respect and can have a strong sense of community. The Talmud, a major source of Jewish law, requires that a husband love his wife as much as himself and that he honor her more than himself (Tractate *Sanhedrin*). He is even responsible for her sexual pleasure. Sociological studies (Davidman, 1991; Kaufman, 1994) indicate that many Orthodox women appreciate admiration and value that their community and husbands place on how they carry out their *halachic* responsibilities. Many also value the stability created by the set code of *halacha*. In addition, as part of recent changes in the modern Orthodox community, women now teach Torah, and even co-ed classes. Some modern Orthodox groups have found *halachic* ways of permitting women to read Torah.

However, there are some options not available within Orthodoxy. A woman still cannot be a rabbi or synagogue prayer leader. Couples cannot decide that the husband instead of the wife will light the Sabbath candles, although a husband may light the candles if the wife is away or late for dinner, as may single men. A couple cannot decide to make love during prohibited times.

Family is such a high priority, and marriage and procreation are such overarching goals, that single women and infertile women may feel a sense of shame and isolation from the mainstream community. There are several possibilities for infertile couples. Adoption is supported both within and outside the Orthodox community, because any person who is converted is understood to be fully Jewish. Reproductive technologies are more controversial, and their acceptance depends on the community, the procedure, and how the procedure is actually carried out (cf. Kahn, 2000). Clinicians who meet with infertile women need to keep in mind that there are several biblical examples of women who, although not having their own children, are honored for contributing to the upbringing of other children within the community. In addition, two of the greatest female leaders in Torah, Miriam and Deborah, were childless and one was unmarried (although some Jewish folklore and rabbinic interpretations assign spouses and children to them). Both these women were prophets, and one was also a judge and a general. Yet in spite of these role models, the family focus of Orthodoxy often leaves couples feeling bereft and without a role when they are infertile. Clinicians need to acknowledge the loss, involve the rabbi in ultra-Orthodox communities to help support the couple, and gently and slowly explore models and contributions of women and couples who do not have children, as well as alternative possibilities for having children.

Homosexuality remains taboo within Orthodoxy, as painfully documented in the film *Trembling Before God* (2001). Some rabbis and other Orthodox leaders say they accept gays, but reject gay sexuality. Clinicians need to be sensitive to the struggles of ultra-Orthodox gay men and lesbians who come to therapy (a rare event in itself). To openly practice homosexuality in the ultra-Orthodox community generally leads to either rejection or the message that one is committing a sinful act (even when the sinner is accepted). It is the action, rather than the self-definition, that is rejected, a distinction that offers little comfort to many gays and lesbians but does offer some alternatives to others. Some gay men choose to marry and have families, others keep their gay relationships a secret; some renounce Orthodoxy for more liberal forms of Judaism, and still others live on the fringe of a community that rejects them for their sexual behavior. Therefore, it becomes the clinician's responsibility to help the gay person or couple struggle with difficult choices. Possibly the most critical question to consider over time is whether it is more important to be accepted in the community or to be openly gay. There can certainly be painful consequences for gays and lesbians who come out. Grossman (2002) reports a situation in which a father was not able to see his children, and another of a synagogue member who was not given full synagogue privileges, as a consequence of coming out. Clinicians need to remember that they are working with clients from a collectivist culture, and that it is extremely important to help a client to explore his or her internal understanding of the impact of his or her choices on family and community, as well as the how such choices affect the client as an individual.

Many members of the modern Orthodox community support gay civil rights, although openly gay members of that community may still struggle about what their choices mean to their own self-definition, to their families, within the context of *halacha*, and regarding their community standing. Several organizations, support groups, and websites for Orthodox gays and lesbians have become available in recent years. Information about the Gay and Lesbian Yeshiva Day School Alumni, an Orthodox gay support group, can be accessed at www.Glydsa.com. In addition, www.OrthoGays.com is a site that lists resources for the Orthodox gay community.

In modern Orthodox Jewish communities, both men and women may have attended secular universities and graduate schools and work in secular professions. There is much leeway for families to develop their own ways of relating to both the secular and Orthodox communities and developing their own practice of gender rigidity or flexibility while still abiding by *halacha*.

CLINICAL EXAMPLES

Ahava Keppelman contacted Dr. B. because she and her husband, Daniel, were concerned that their 12-year-old daughter, Michal, was isolating herself from friends and her grades were slipping. She had developed a love for lacrosse during summer camp, a sport her Jewish day school did not offer. Her parents did not allow her to join the elite teams because practice and/ or games took place on Friday nights and Saturdays, the Jewish Sabbath, a time when the family gathers with others in their community to pray, sing, and share a quiet, work-free 25 hours, and when participation in athletics is not permitted. In response to her parents' refusal to allow Michal to play on the team, she had grown more reclusive and inattentive to her schoolwork.

Ahava had sent Michal to work with Dr. A., but became distraught when Dr. A. suggested that Michal needed to advocate for herself, noting that, during adolescence, parents can expect separation and individuation to occur. He also felt that because Michal was a very strong lacrosse player, she needed to be on an elite team. Ahava pulled her from therapy.

This example demonstrates a central misunderstanding of some non-Orthodox Jewish therapists, that observing the *Shabbos* as well as other *mitzvot* is a throwback to a past that is, at best, outdated and, at worse, rigid and growth-stunting. Yet within the Orthodox community, one does not choose to skip a *mitzvah* because it is inconvenient; instead, all the laws and ways of behaving are understood as a path toward a more spiritual, complete, holy life and thus are nonnegotiable. Orthodox Jews typically see these ways of behaving not as constraints, but as ways of recognizing that every moment of life is possible because of God, that everything we do needs to be considered and blessed. So the issue was not whether Michal was a strong lacrosse player who needed to practice on *Shabbos*, but that *Shabbos* observance sanctified Michal's life. And Michal wanted to play lacrosse without throwing away her commitment to Orthodox Judaism.

The Keppelman family found a new therapist, Dr. B., who was respectful of their traditions and understood their way of life. They discussed with him the possibility of contacting the coaches and letting them know how much Michal would like to be on the team, but that she could not play or practice on *Shabbos*. Dr. B. helped them to understand the views and needs of the coaches. The Keppelman parents also expressed their concerns that if Michal were on the team, she would have more contact with secular Jews and non-Jews. This is a sensitive issue in working with Orthodox Jewish families, and therapists need to be mindful of their own biases about individualism versus collectivist models.

The Keppelmans found a coach who would allow Michal to miss Friday practices and Saturday games, although she did play on Sundays. Thus, they worked out a way that supported both her and the family's dedication to Orthodoxy. They did so via a therapist who wouldn't frame their distress as an intergenerational conflict, but rather as a challenge to an Orthodox family who also wanted to support their daughter in the secular world of sports.

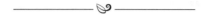

Devorah and Judah were members of an ultra-Orthodox community, which eschews contact with the non-Orthodox world because it may lead members away from its values and lifestyle. The parents of five children, they were referred to me (B. F. O.) by an Orthodox social worker for help with their 14-month-old son, Avi, who had been diagnosed with pervasive developmental disorder at the age of 11 months and had been referred to a neighborhood early intervention center. (Their Orthodox community had no knowledge of or available services for developmental disabilities.)

The couple presented themselves modestly (a long skirt and hat for Devorah and a *kippa* for Judah) and were obviously nervous about the diagnosis and confused about what early intervention would mean. It took a while for them to relax and tell me a little about themselves. This family required center-based, rather than the usual home-based, services, and the parents were struggling with their own shame about how this could have happened to them. They knew of no other family who had to leave the community for such services.

For the past 4 months, Avi had received 1 hour of various types of therapy 4 days a week and Devorah had walked with him the 40 minutes to the center and spent about 2 hours per day practicing with him. A full-time yeshiva student, and other members of the community were needed to provide baby-sitting and housekeeping assistance. After four couple sessions, Judah said he did not want to continue, but grudgingly permitted Devorah to come alone to help her work through her grieving and come to terms with the extra early intervention demands.

Devorah came to recognize Avi's progress in speech and motor development and became more connected with the early intervention providers and with me, as the only people who understood the importance of this work. Complaining that Judah seemed to spend more time studying Torah than before, that he refused to even ask about Avi's daily sessions, and that he was withdrawing more, she turned more to the secular providers for emotional support. At this point, I suggested a few more couple sessions and Judah agreed. Judah blamed Devorah for Avi's difficulties, though he knew intellectually that they were not her fault. He was angry about the need to go out so many times of the Orthodox community for services and put pressure on Devorah to terminate services and "let God handle this."

I asked them whether I could talk to the referring social worker and to their community's rabbi. Only eventually did Devorah and Judah feel comfortable with this. It took several days to reach the rabbi, and I wondered whether he would even talk to a secular professional. But when he returned my call, he listened carefully as I described Avi's disabilities, his progress to date, and evidence about the effectiveness of early intervention. He subsequently met with Judah and provided support for the continuation of these services. Two years later, Devorah sent me a note reporting that Avi was now performing in school at the appropriate age level and that she had learned so much about herself through these difficult times that she felt it helped her to be a more patient, loving wife and mother.

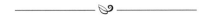

Talia and Jerry, a modern Orthodox couple who met in law school, have continued to work while raising three children. Rachel, their oldest, told her parents that she wanted to attend a college in another state, which did not have an especially strong Jewish community, so that she could pursue her particular interest. When Jerry heard that Talia was open to this idea, he exploded and, even after calming down, said that he would determine where Rachel would attend school.

Talia told Jerry that she didn't know how she could continue living with him if he was going to explode and then dictate what must be done. In therapy, Jerry insisted that it was his right as a Jewish man to make these decisions. If the therapist respected Orthodox Judaism, she would understand that. I (M. P. M.) recognized that in Orthodoxy, there are many ways couples make decisions; it is not always assumed that the husband has the final word on household issues. The focus of therapy became constructing a way for Talia and Jerry to disagree respectfully and to find a way to resolve the issue.

Although I initially wanted to join with mother and daughter against an angry father, I knew that for change to occur, I also needed to join with Jerry in a respectful way. The rabbi reinforced the concept of *shalom bayit*, peace in the home. The rabbi's support of family peace led to a more open discussion of Jerry's concerns about his daughter's attending a secular school as well as factors such as the schools' Jewish (and Orthodox) populations, how active Hillel (the collegiate Jewish organization) was, and the availability of kosher food in campus dining halls.

When Talia and Jerry reviewed why they had chosen modern Orthodoxy, Jerry acknowledged that he did not want to be isolated from the secular world, but also feared that his daughter could be inducted into it and be removed from Orthodoxy. For Rachel, the freedom to practice her Judaism within a community that she found stimulating was critical. Jerry came to realize that she might be lost to Judaism if he restricted her participation in that secular community. He explained his outbursts as reflecting his sense of "powerlessness" because he couldn't control the availability of alternatives that Rachel would have by living in interaction with non-Orthodox Jews, and that made him wonder whether they should have joined the ultra-Orthodox community. Talia felt that Jerry's outbursts betrayed both her and their religious commitment to *shalom bayit*. Ultimately, Jerry's recognition that his eruptions were a problematic response to helplessness supported his reexamination of his own behavior within the family.

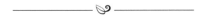

RELIGIOUS ISSUES

A number of ultra-Orthodox communities rely on *shiddachs*, arranged matches, rather than marrying for love (Shai, 2002). The need to make one's offspring as "marriageable" as possible has led some Orthodox parents to hide, rather than address, their children's psychological difficulties.

All Orthodox Jews and many secular Jews place a priority value on endogamy, or marrying within the Jewish community. Therefore, there is a potential for conflict between the secular therapist's value of transcultural openness and the Orthodox client's value of endogamy. Some Orthodox Jews even believe that religious intermarriage not only is forbidden, but also helps complete the work of the Holocaust by ending "Jewish continuity" within that family.

Regarding sexual relationships, all Orthodox communities prohibit premarital sex, although enforcement of these proscriptions varies. Married women are required to immerse themselves in a *mikvah* (ritual bath) 7 days after cessation of their menstrual periods; only thereafter can they resume sexual relations with their husbands. For the week during and after menstruation, the woman sleeps in a separate bed and has no sexual contact. Some Orthodox women report that this heightens their sexual desire, whereas others have found this requirement limiting and hurtful.

Although some traditional texts prohibit birth control (cf. Rabinowitz, 2000), others include the belief that birth control is supported after the birth of two sons, and still others support the use of birth control after the birth of a son and a daughter. The commandment that men not waste their seed leads some to interpret it to mean that women may use birth control even if there is a prohibition against men's doing so. If it is thought that pregnancy can seriously harm the woman's physical or mental health, many traditional sources allow birth control and even abortion. As with other issues, rabbinic consultation is key, especially in ultra-Orthodox communities.

Abortion is an especially complex issue. Within Judaism, a fetus is considered a full human being when its head emerges; before that, it is looked upon as a partial life. Therefore, although abortion is often prohibited, it is permitted if there is a serious threat to the mother, and the mother's life takes precedence over the continuation of the pregnancy. This threat may be emotional as well as physical, but in ultra-Orthodox and some modern Orthodox communities, a rabbi must be consulted to determine whether the abortion is sanctioned. Orthodox rabbis are also permitted to approve an abortion within the first 40 days of pregnancy (Rabinowitz, 2000). Whether or not a rabbi approves an abortion depends on the particular community as well as the individual circumstances.

CLINICAL ISSUES

Clinicians sometimes must struggle to appreciate a way of life that may be very different from their own. Learning about the Orthodox community by reading, talking to members, and conferring with colleagues can enable clinicians to develop respect for its values and paradigms. As Minuchin and Fishman (1981) propose, clinicians need to understand and even utilize some of the principal vocabulary or expressions of the clients (e.g., *shul*, *halacha*, and *mitzvot*).

Psychoeducation may be an important tool for clinicians to help clients better understand psychological, medical, and neurological conditions. Clinicians also can help ultra-Orthodox clients navigate the structures in the secular world that may be of use to them. Narrative work may be effective, because stories and story construction are deeply valued and engrained within the Jewish community.

Secular Jewish clinicians may have to struggle with their own ingrained biases and stereotypes due to their own issues with their Jewish identity. Although many Orthodox Jewish clients prefer to work with Jewish-identified clinicians, some report feeling misunderstood and negatively judged by non-Orthodox therapists. It is therefore extremely important for Jewish clinicians to be mindful of their own identity issues.

CONCLUSION

Regardless of the presenting issues, unless clients are coming to consider a change in lifestyle, we must support the choices of our clients and help them to resolve their problems in a way that meets their needs and obligations, not ours. The challenges of working with Orthodox families require networking, collaboration with the community, and bridging the gap between the Orthodox community and the surrounding secular world.

ACKNOWLEDGMENTS

We would like to thank Penina Adelman, Mona Fishbane, Ricki Kantrowitz, Mitch Mirkin, Steven Robinson, and Nachama Chessis for their review of the first draft of this chapter; Sherman Okun for his contributions to and review of the final version; and the Brandeis Women's Studies Research Center for supporting this work.

REFERENCES

Davidman, L. (1991). *Tradition in a rootless world: Women turn to Orthodox Judaism*. Berkeley: University of California Press.

Grossman, N. (2001, April). Gay orthodox underground. *Moment Magazine, 26*(2), 54–60.

Kahn, S. M. (2000). *Reproducing Jews: A cultural account of assisted conception in Israel*. Durham, NC: Duke University Press.

Karp, A. J. (1991). *From the ends of the earth: Judaic treasures of the Library of Congress*. Washington, DC: Library of Congress.

Kaufman, D. R. (1994). *Rachel's daughters*. New Brunswick, NJ: Rutgers University Press.

Minuchin, S., & Fishman, H. C. (1981). *Family therapy techniques*. Cambridge, MA: Harvard University Press.

Rabinowitz, A. (2000). Psychotherapy with Orthodox Jews. In P. S. Richards & A. E. Bergin (Eds.), *Handbook of psychotherapy and religious diversity*. Washington, DC: American Psychological Association.

Shai, D. (2002). Working women/cloistered men: A family development approach to marriage arrangements among the ultra-Orthodox Jews. *Journal of Comparative Family Studies, 33*(1), 97–116.

Trembling before G-d [Film]. (Available from Simcha Leib Productions)

Xu Xin. (2003). *The Jews of Kaifeng China*. Jersey City, NJ: Ktav Putlishing House.

CHAPTER 51

Russian Jewish Families

Leonid Newhouse

In the United States, the Jewish immigrants from the Former Soviet Union (FSU) are referred to simply as "Russians," a perception many of these immigrants find ironic. During Soviet times, they often tried to pass themselves off as *russky*, or Slavic Russians, to avoid discrimination. But such efforts were usually unsuccessful. A joke that circulated among Russian immigrant communities sums up this paradox: "Russian Jews! Come to America! Only here will your long-cherished dream of becoming Russian be realized!"

IMMIGRATION TO THE UNITED STATES

The post-World War II exodus of Soviet Jews has so far brought three distinct waves of immigrants (half a million in all) to these shores (Orleck, 1999). The earliest immigrants came here during the 1970s, when Jewish emigration first became possible. They were mostly young professional couples from Moscow and Leningrad, who have by now become quite "Americanized." The second wave, which began in the late 1980s, included both urban professionals and working-class families from the Ukraine and Belarus who survived the 1986 Chernobyl nuclear disaster. The third wave, which followed the collapse of the Soviet Union in 1991, brought mainly working-class immigrants—also from Ukraine and Belarus—who came to join relatives already established here. Most of these immigrants identify themselves with secular Russian culture and with Europe more generally, although the older ones among them are no strangers to the Jewish traditions and may still speak Yiddish.

There are also about 50,000 Jewish migrants from the non-European part of the FSU, mainly "Bukharan" Jews from Uzbekistan, who have their own language, a dialect of Persian, and live mostly in close-knit, insular communities in Queens County, New York. Bukharan Jews consider themselves Asian and Middle Eastern and share in the cultural identity of Iranians (Orleck, 1999). Unlike their worldly European Soviet cousins, they have embraced Orthodox Jewish religious and cultural practices, with parents still arranging marriages for their children. These cultural differences have caused rifts in the immigrant community, particularly within the school system, where, because of the Bukharan students' accents and background, their Western Russian peers often shun them, something that may further contribute to the insularity of their lifestyle.

HISTORY AND CULTURAL IDENTITY

The Russian Jews' sense of cultural identity reflects the ambiguities and traumas of their recent history. Under the czars, most Jews lived in a segregated area in Russia known as the Pale of Settlement, with its insular *shtetl* culture. As the czarist regime began to crumble in the late 1800s, it made Jews into scapegoats, inciting anti-Semitic riots, known as pogroms, that sent millions of Jews fleeing to the United States. Jews that remained took an active part in the 1917 Bolshevik Revolution. Later they were allowed to settle in the cities and encouraged to assimilate. Most Jews embraced, and contributed to building, the new, secular Soviet state. They gladly identified themselves with the dominant Soviet Russian culture rather than as "Jews." But later, throughout the seven decades of Communist rule, they were singled out with the word *yevrey* ("Hebrew") in their internal passports, which, like the yellow Star of David that Jews had to wear during the Third Reich, exposed them to discrimination and insults.

During *stalinshchina*, the most brutal years of Stalin's dictatorship (1934–1953), millions of Soviet people, including large numbers of Jews, perished at the hands of the secret police. Most families lived in fear that a loved one—usually the husband and father—would be denounced as an "enemy of the people" and taken away by the police, never to be seen again. The victims' families learned not to show any grief in public, for fear of being labeled "enemies of the people" themselves (Merridale, 2000). In such an atmosphere, trust between people hardly existed, and most buried their feelings inside, presenting a stoic facade to strangers. Add to *stalinshchina* the Nazis' extermination of the Soviet Jews during the Second World War (which the Russians call the Great Patriotic War), and it would be hard to find a Russian Jewish immigrant family that hasn't lost a grandparent, great-grandparent, or other relative during those times.

After the war, the anti-Semitic and increasingly unbalanced Stalin conceived of his own "final solution," in which plans were drawn to exile Jews to Siberia for subsequent elimination. The dictator's death, in March of 1953, prevented the implementation of this plan. Still, anti-Semitism, especially its more virulent, racist strain, took root again in Russia. A person was considered a Jew because his or her name sounded Jewish, or because the person "looked" Jewish. Such a distinction practically guaranteed some form of discrimination that limited access to higher education, desirable careers, housing, and every other opportunity in life. This situation became worse after the 1967 Middle East war, when daily attacks on "Zionists" in the press—the official Soviet code word for Jews—increased. State-sponsored anti-Semitism became a trend that continued practically until the end of the Communist rule in 1991.

The Soviet regime had always hushed up these realities, with no mention of the Holocaust ever made in Soviet history textbooks or media until the 1990s, when it first became possible to discuss such events in public. As a result, Russian Jews possibly have not yet fully reflected on these difficult chapters of their recent past and the effects on their families of origin (Merridale, 2000).

FAMILY CHARACTERISTICS

It was in the face of the aforementioned traumas—and the overall privations of Soviet life—that Russian Jewish families developed their resilience and survival skills. For even in times of peace and relative prosperity in the postwar decades, life in the Soviet Union was fraught with corruption, bureaucratic abuse, and shortages of basic necessities, including housing, child care, and food. To get ahead at work, to obtain an apartment or decent medical care, one needed to have connections and, often, to pay bribes. This was even more necessary for Jews, who already were handicapped by discrimination. In such conditions, the extended Russian Jewish family became an intimate network of survival whose resources, including grandparents, relatives, and friends, were thrust into negotiating the hurdles of daily living. In this dance of survival, every family member had a role to play. Grandparents often provided care for the young, financial help, and even housing. In return, grown children were expected to assume responsibility when their parents became frail or sick (Althausen, 1993). Grandchildren provided hope for the future and emotional solace in old age. With one-child families predominating, because of the lack of space and resources, close friends often became substitute brothers and sisters (Smith, 1990). They were privy to the family's secrets, celebrated its successes, shared its sorrows, took part in negotiating various family conflicts, and provided advice.

In a typical family, both husband and wife worked full-time. Even with the support of the extended family, the wife still had the lion's share of responsibility for performing domestic tasks and, ultimately, for child rearing. The husband's role was that of main breadwinner; he normally made more money than his wife did, and his career took precedence over hers. The prevalent (if tacit) Russian convention still equates femininity with weakness and demands that women defer to men for major decisions. In reality, Russian husbands are often considered by their wives to be weak, passive, and infantile (Althausen, 1996).

In their desire to shield their children from anti-Semitism, Russian Jewish parents were often overprotective (Feigin, 1996). Children were often indulged at home, while parents expected schools and kindergartens to provide structure and set limits (Althausen, 1996). It was as if the family wanted to spare the child for the future battles when, in order to succeed, he or she would have to work twice as hard as his *russky* peers.

With the demise of the Communist regime and the introduction of a market-type economy, the old intimate networks have given way under the pressure of competition and social stratification. Work commitments now consume the time previously devoted to friendship, and the new disparities in income level and social status have led to estrangement even between close friends. The emigration of family members and friends, to Israel, the United States, or Germany, dealt a further blow to these networks. These changes have caused many Russian Jewish immigrants to feel uprooted even before they leave the old country.

PSYCHOLOGICAL ADAPTATION

Although Russian Jewish immigrants endure similar types of adjustment conflicts and crises as other immigrants (Feigin, 1996), there are issues of adaptation that are particularly prominent in this population. One is the impact of the loss of professional status on the marital couple. The husband's primacy may be challenged when, following migration, his wife is the first one to obtain a job, or if she draws a bigger paycheck than he does. The husband often reacts to this with depression, which may further limit his chances of employment, putting additional pressure on his wife to support the family alone and lessening the parents' emotional availability to their children. This happens at a time when the children are struggling to get used to new schools and peers who speak a different language. To make things more difficult, the grandparents may suddenly develop health problems, necessitating care by the parents.

Grandparents' feelings, following immigration, are often ambiguous. Because of the superior medical care and better living conditions in the United States, many get a new lease on life and live longer. Yet they feel torn from their roots and intimate networks. Their adult children and grandchildren are no longer dependent on them. In fact, they and the grandchildren, who are often unwilling to speak Russian, become more distant. (The ultimate blow may come when the children, having found a job in another part of the country, move away.) Feeling both "useless" and abandoned, the grandparents often mourn these losses the only way they know how—with somatic complaints (Althausen, 1993).

ASPECTS OF FAMILY THERAPY

Historically, the losses and traumas that befell Russian Jews were so overwhelming, and the strictures on personal expression so unrelenting, that people kept emotional pain to themselves and presented a stoic front. Opening up to strangers could be a dangerous proposition in the old country. As in its old society, the Russian Jewish family may jealously guard its secret vulnerabilities behind a thick wall of silence. It is considered unseemly, and almost a betrayal, to disclose personal pain or any family conflict to strangers—including mental health professionals.

After a particularly emotional family meeting, in which a tearful 50-year-old daughter expressed her anguish at never having been loved by her 74-year-old frail mother, the mother, her face red with rage, said: "Shame on you for speaking so in front of the therapist." Only after the therapist reassured her that such frank talk was most appropriate in the circumstances—as it helped him better understand the family's dynamics—and that it would be kept in strictest confidence, did she agree to continue the meeting.

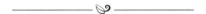

Most issues Russian Jewish clients present in the consulting room have to do with the impact of emigration on their families. Given the emotional imperatives stated earlier, these immigrants normally do not seek therapy unless they find themselves in a crisis such as an impending divorce, a child's behavior problem at school, or an elderly parent's medical emergency.

Often, therapeutic interventions are delivered in a context in which the clients do not necessarily think they are "in therapy." It is helpful to keep in mind that the word "therapist" (*terapevt*) in Russian means "physician," so the client may unconsciously expect a therapist to provide a "prescription," whether in the form of advice or a directive to make the suffering go away. This gives the therapist a natural opportunity to assign tasks to help the family "do it" on their own. Such an approach, aimed at empowering the family, is in keeping with the Russian Jewish family's tendency to resolve problems on its own.

Ms. C., 52, an immigrant from Kiev, Ukraine, approached the therapist as he was leaving her elderly mother's apartment following a social work visit. On the verge of tears and in a halting voice, she started telling the therapist about her worries regarding her daughter's spending habits. The daughter, a college sophomore majoring in business, had bought herself fancy clothes practically every week, and ate out daily, incurring a large credit card debt. Ms. C.'s husband, a former engineer who now repaired appliances for a living, and Ms. C., a former teacher who worked as a home health aid 80 hours a week, were barely able to pay off their daughter's tuition the previous year—"and now this!"

The therapist listened attentively and was empathetic. He steered Ms. C. to a more private corner of the lobby, where she continued to relate that her daughter had been 4 years old at the time of the Chernobyl disaster. As soon as they found out about it, Ms. C. whisked her to Moscow, where they lived with relatives for several months. However, the daughter developed a serious thyroid problem (which doctors ascribed to Chernobyl) that made her overweight. Ms. C. told the therapist that the daughter had no boyfriend and was distraught about her weight problem. Ms. C. expressed remorse over not having evacuated her child from the contaminated area sooner. "My husband and I give her everything she wants."

The therapist proposed that the family could work on the issue together. He suggested that Ms. C. and Mr. C. have a conversation with their daughter about a plan to finance her education, and ask for her input. "But she's only a child," objected Ms. C. The therapist reassured her that this could be an opportunity for her daughter to assume responsibility appropriate for her age. She was a business major, after all. The therapist and Ms. C. agreed to meet in the same spot 2 weeks later, following the next visit to her mother.

At their meeting Ms. C. reported that her daughter was receptive. She came forward with a plan of savings that included making a budget and eating at home more often. The daughter also offered to make a budget for her parents.

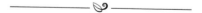

For the therapist working with this population, much will depend on the personal connection he or she makes with the client. To earn the client's trust, the therapist needs a combination of solid credentials, personal warmth, and a proactive approach. If asked for an expert opinion, the therapist should not be afraid to give it; the family may well have come primarily for that.

The therapist must establish trust by projecting competence and, at the same time, by being as warm and human as possible. (Most Russians consider a lack of personal warmth "off-putting.") At the same time, the therapist should beware of falling into the trap of becoming "a family friend." In the minds of many Russian clients, only a friend can help, and they might want to overpersonalize the relationship.

An elderly client brought her single daughter to a session. When asked about her motives for bringing her daughter, she said she wanted to introduce her to the therapist, who seemed like a "very nice young man." Having thanked the client for her compliment, the therapist proceeded to explore the two women's respective feelings about the situation. A discussion ensued, in which the client expressed her worry about her daughter's single status, and the daughter, her full confidence that she was capable of finding a mate on her own.

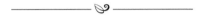

In assessing a Russian Jewish immigrant family, it is important to take into consideration its history of losses. A genogram may reveal an uncle who perished under Stalin, a grandfather executed by the Nazis, another relative who died in battle with the Germans, or one who starved to death in her frozen apartment during the siege of Leningrad (1941–1944). One must tread gently here, lest the client, overwhelmed with yet unfelt emotions, leave treatment.

Another delicate issue is homosexuality. Under the Soviets, homosexuality was illegal, a crime punishable with stiff prison sentences. Homosexuals were outcasts persecuted by the state and often shunned by the family. Being Jewish *and* homosexual could be doubly precarious. Although homosexuality is no longer illegal in Russia, both unofficial discrimination and violence against gay men and women are still common, and most still prefer to live "in the closet" (Tuller, 1997). The Russian word *gomoseksualist* may still have "obscene" connotations for many older people, for whom the topic remains largely a taboo. (There is practically no word for "gay" in Russian that is not derogatory.) A gay son or daughter might be characterized as "strange," "not like other people," and by other such euphemisms. Sometimes it has to be left at that. In therapy, gay Russian Jewish clients may not declare their orientation as promptly as those who are American-born, if at all. The therapist should respect that boundary and let the client remain safely "in the closet" until he or she is ready to come out.

In working with Russian Jewish families, one should be respectful of differences in values and expectations regarding gender roles. As mentioned previously, Russian women often are expected to "play second fiddle," and families expect the husband to be the head of the family, even though, in many cases, the decision maker might be the wife. Therapists must use diplomacy and care in any moves to rebalance gender roles. Such moves are, of course, easier once family members have adjusted to the prevalent cultural values of their new country (Althausen, 1996).

CONCLUSION

Russian Jewish families bring with them a difficult legacy of trauma and loss—as well as resilience and drive to succeed. Back in the old country, the family was an intimate support network ideal for survival. The changes related to the collapse of the Soviet Union weakened this network, making a family feel uprooted even before leaving the country. Emigration further eroded what is left of this network, causing much distress. In working with this population, the therapist should be careful to respect the family's boundaries vis-à-vis the therapeutic process and the issues of loss, gender, and sexual orientation.

REFERENCES

Althausen, L. (1993). Journey of separation: Elderly Russian immigrants and their adult children in the health care setting. *Social Work in Health Care, 19*(1), 61–75.

Althausen, L. (1996). Russian families. In M. McGoldrick, J. Giordano, & J. K. Pearce (Eds.), *Ethnicity and family therapy* (2nd ed., pp. 680–687). New York: Guilford Press.

Feigin, I. (1996). Soviet Jewish families. In M. McGoldrick, J. Giordano, & J. K. Pearce (Eds.), *Ethnicity and family therapy* (2nd ed., pp. 631–637). New York: Guilford Press.

Merridale, C. (2000). *Night of stone: Death and memory in twentieth-century Russia.* New York: Viking.

Orleck, A. (1999). *The Soviet Jewish Americans.* Westport, CT: Greenwood Press.

Smith, H. (1990). *The new Russians.* New York: Random House.

Tuller, D. (1997). *Crack in the iron closet: Travels in gay and lesbian Russia.* Chicago: University of Chicago Press.

PART IX

❧

SLAVIC FAMILIES

CHAPTER 52

Slavic Families
An Overview

Leonid Newhouse

Absorb all cultures but forget not your own.
—TARAS SHEVCHENKO,
Ukrainian National Poet Laureate

"The Slavic peoples," a philosopher once observed, "occupy more territory on earth than in history" (Conte, 1995). Indeed, the Slavic countries of Europe—Poland, the Czech Republic, the Slovak Republic, Ukraine, Belarus, Russia, Bulgaria, Slovenia, Croatia, Bosnia, and Macedonia—span a huge landmass, stretching from the Italian border in the West to Siberia in the East, and from the Balkans in the South to the Baltic Sea in the North. Their combined population constitutes the largest single ethnic and linguistic group of people in Europe. (It is estimated that the Slavs number over 300 million in the world.) "Originally a peaceful, pastoral people" (Marganoff & Folwarski, 1996) inhabiting the Eastern reaches of the continent, they rose to be the dominant force in the area at different times between the 8th and 12th centuries. However, subsequent conquests by other, neighboring nations—in particular, the Ottomans and later, the Austro-Hungarians and Prussians—disrupted their progress. Centuries followed, during which the Slavic nations, with the notable exception of Russia, lived in obscurity as the "poor relatives of Europe" in the backwaters of various empires: first the Ottoman (until the mid-19th century), then the Austro-Hungarian (until the end of World War I).

After the First World War most of these nations became self-governing, but their independence was fleeting as the shadow of German Nazism and Soviet Communism descended on Europe and World War II began. By the end of the war the Slavs had been conquered again, this time by their own cousins, the Russians, and become part of the new Communist "family of nations." Although the Soviet Union subsequently referred to its Slavic allies as "brothers and sisters," in reality it ruled them as a willful patriarch. It rewarded loyalty with gifts of economic aid and state banquets in the Kremlin and suppressed dissent with either brute force (Poland and Czechoslovakia) or "banishment" from the family (Yugoslavia). As discussed subsequently, this pattern, in some ways, reflected the old patriarchal nature of the traditional Slavic family itself.

The collapse of Communism toward the end of the last century freed each "sibling" to seek its own path. This transition to independence was accompanied by the breakup of two nations—Czecholovakia and Yugoslavia—and, in the latter, a resurgence of ancient ethnic and religious enmities that pitted Catholic against Eastern Orthodox, and Eastern Orthodox against Muslim. The brutal fratricidal war that followed (1992–1996), popularly referred to as the war in Bosnia, produced atrocities on a scale unseen in Europe since World War II. The conflict ended only after the joint American and Western European military intervention.

Today the newly independent Slavic nations of Europe—the so-called New Europe—are on the threshold of a cultural and economic renaissance. Poland and the Slovak and Czech Republics have already joined the extended family of the European Union, and others hope to do so in the near future. All this bodes for a more prosperous, if less culturally distinct, future. The collective traumas of their history, however, will reverberate in the individual family dynamics for a long time to come.

SLAVIC AMERICANS IN HISTORICAL AND CULTURAL CONTEXT

Americans of Slavic descent have also suffered from obscurity (Marganoff & Folwarski, 1996). Although numbering 20 million people—the third largest group of European origin living in the United States, after the British and the Germans—their contributions to the political, cultural, and economic life of the United States have been largely unacknowledged. Many Americans, for example, are unaware of such historic figures as Thaddeusz Kosciuszko, the Polish-born nobleman and American revolutionary hero who helped found West Point, or Igor Sikorsky, the Russian-born American engineer who gave us the helicopter, or the fact that the movie star Natalie Wood, born Natasha Gurdin, was a first-generation Russian immigrant. Until recently, the popular perception of the Slavs was that they were either all "Communists," or Russians, or "Pollacks." Cultural stereotyping of Slavs in film and literature had Slavic men portrayed as uncouth and "rough around the edges," more brawn than brain,[1] and women as sex symbols[2] (Wtulich, 1994, p. 143). And then there are the notorious Polish jokes. (One middle-aged Polish American client disclosed that when in high school, shame about her origins compelled her to tell schoolmates that her name was actually Austrian, not Polish.)

Perceptions about Slavic Americans are changing, in part because of the increasing visibility of Slavic nations on the world stage, as mentioned earlier, and in part because of the rise to prominence of Slavic Americans such as Martha Stewart (née Kostyra) and Dennis Kucinich, Croatian American presidential candidate of the Democratic Party in 2004.[3] There is also evidence that American Slavic groups, previously divided over religious issues that separated their forefathers in Europe, are trying to put aside their old differences and unite behind the values they share. "Our financial resources may be limited," states one Slavic website, "but, our constituency doesn't have to be. Therefore, let's forget our past differences and unite" (www.slavs.freeservers.com).

Religion and Ethnic Identity

For Slavs, religion has always been a cornerstone of their identity. When conquered first by the Muslim Ottoman Turks and, later, by atheistic Communists, it was their religion that helped them preserve their spiritual independence intact (Kaplan, 1994). But at the same time, as demonstrated most recently in Bosnia, religious differences have fostered bitter enmity and fighting among the Slavs themselves.

Religiously and culturally, the Slavs fall into two main groups. The first group, those traditionally associated with the Orthodox Eastern Church, comprises the Russians, most of the Ukrainians and Belorusians, the Bulgarians, the Serbs, and the Macedonians. The second group includes those historically affiliated with the Roman Catholic Church—the Czechs, the Slovaks, the Poles, the Slovenes, the Croats, and some of the Belorussians and Ukrainians. A much smaller number, mainly the Bosnians, practice the Muslim faith.

It is the differences that underlie these religions, rather than geography, that have largely determined the cultural lines that divide the Slavs. "Because Catholicism arose in the West and Orthodoxy in the East, the difference between them is greater than that between, say, Catholicism and Protestantism, or even Catholicism and Judaism (Kaplan, 1994, p. 23)." Whereas Western religions emphasize ideas and deeds, Eastern (or Byzantine) religions emphasize divine beauty and mystery. In the Orthodox practice, one strives to perceive the truth with one's whole being, or soul (*dusha*, in Russian), rather than with mere intellect; one is therefore perfectly content to let certain things remain inexplicable and unstated. This ideology especially concerns the realm of emotions and human relationships, where a certain degree of ambiguity is not only tolerated but is often assumed. Talking about their "feelings" can therefore be difficult for Orthodox clients, if for that reason alone. "Not for nothing is 'Byzantine' a byword for counter-intuitive complexity in human affairs" (Schjeldahl, 2004, p. 100).

Unlike its Catholic counterpart, Eastern Orthodox tradition does not specifically forbid divorce and remarriage. The split between the two faiths is further emphasized by the fact that the Catholic Slavs use the Roman alphabet, whereas the Orthodox Slavs use the Cyrillic.

Broadly speaking, Catholic Slavs have traditionally identified with the "rationalist" West, and Orthodox Slavs have leaned toward the "mystical" East, and Russia—the seat of the Byzantine tradition—in particular. All this goes a long way in explaining the conflicts and alliances that have long existed between different Slavic groups.

These differences are reflected in differing family traditions and norms of behavior. For instance, the Serb custom of celebrating a wedding for 4 days filled with feasting and prayer may appear excessive and even irrational to their close-of-kin but Catholic next-door neighbors, the Croats (Kaplan, 1994). Or the Russian funeral custom in which grieving women wail loudly and repeatedly over the coffin may strike a Czech or a Slovene as bizarre. Yet a Russian may think it cold (*sukhoy*, in Russian) that a Czech or a Pole would not hug and kiss an acquaintance he runs into in the street and address him as Mr. So-and-so rather than by his first name and patronymic.

The following sections offer a capsule portrait of each major Slavic group living in this country. For consistency's sake, the Slavic people are divided here into categories according to their religious affiliation—that is, Eastern Orthodox, Catholic, and Muslim—and not according to the old country's place on the map of Europe, as is often done.

Eastern Orthodox Slavs

THE RUSSIANS

A distinction should be made, for the sake of clarity, between the Slavic Russians and Jewish Russians, discussed in a separate chapter (Chapter 51).

Russians are well known for their attachment to their country of birth, which they call *rodina* (motherland) or, even more affectionately, *Rossiya-matushka* (little mother-Russia). Despite their country's difficult history, Russians have seldom chosen to emigrate, partially because of this attachment. Those who left usually did so only as a last resort, forced to embark on this course by extreme circumstances.

The 1917 Bolshevik Revolution sent hundreds of thousands of Russians into exile in Western Europe and the United States. These were mostly well-educated, cosmopolitan people, members of the aristocracy and professional class, intelligentsia, banished by the Bolsheviks; they had a relatively easy time adapting to American life. After World War II, 250,000 Russians, displaced by the war and reluctant to return to Stalinist Russia, were allowed to come to this country. Unlike the previous wave of Russian immigrants, this one included industrial laborers and farmworkers. In the postwar political climate, many Russian immigrants were often suspected of having communist leanings (Magoscsi, 1996), even though, in reality, they had come to America specifically to escape from communism. This suspicion made it harder for them to hold onto their rich cultural heritage. Nevertheless, most retained a deep connection to the Russian culture, celebrating major family events and religious holidays in a traditional Russian way and maintaining a network of former compatriots. Russian ballet, classical music, and literature remain a unifying cultural thread.

Under the Communist regime, emigration was banned for all but a few ethnic Russians, who managed to emigrate either by defecting or by marrying Jews (one of the few ethnic minorities allowed to emigrate). These emigrés were denounced as pariahs, stripped of their Soviet citizenship, and never allowed to return (Althausen, 1996).

Today's Russian immigrants are mostly professionals seeking better jobs or further education. Although they are free to go back to Russia at any time, they may not want to do so for fear of not being allowed back into the United States. (See "Immigration to the United States" later in this chapter.)

THE UKRAINIANS

Ukraine, whose name means, literally, "borderland," has been invaded by nations that bordered it throughout its 1,000-year history. The 20th century was particularly cruel to Ukraine. Forcefully incorporated into the Soviet Union in 1921, the Ukrainian people received a lion's share of Stalin's wrath. During the forced collectivization era of 1933–1934, several million Ukrainians died from starvation, an atrocity that some historians have called "the hidden Holocaust." Later, during World War II, German and Soviet armies were responsible for some 7 to 8 million more deaths. The 1986 Chernobyl nuclear catastrophe capped this list of 20thy disasters. But with the fall of the Soviet Union in 1991, Ukraine regained the independence its people always wanted.

Throughout its history, invaders sought to impose on Ukraine their own brand of religion and to obliterate the Ukrainian language and sense of nationhood. The Polish and Austrian rulers changed the nation's name to Galicia; the Russian rulers, to "Little

Russia." Ukrainian people always had to fight to preserve their cultural distinctness. Their resilience and spirit of independence are epitomized by the Cossacks, the fierce Ukrainian warriors who lived in their own enclave in the lower reaches of the Dnieper River. For centuries they defied invaders, whether Crimean Tartars, Ottoman Turks, or Poles; later, during the First World War, they put fear in the German troops with their galloping horses and swinging sabers.

In the hundred years since the first major wave of Ukrainian immigration to the United States, Ukrainians have established a vibrant and dynamic community here. There are well over a million people of Ukrainian descent living in the United States and Canada today. Most of them are Eastern Orthodox, and the rest, Ukrainian Catholic. As in most ethnic communities, the church is the center of focus for most Ukrainians. The Ukrainian Orthodox Church of the U.S.A., headquartered in South Bound Brook, New Jersey, has three eparchies in this country (New York City; Parma, Ohio; and Chicago). Ukrainians who live in areas with no organized Ukrainian churches often elect to join either a Russian Orthodox or Roman Catholic parish.

Because of their especially brutal history of subjugation, as well as their resilience, the ethnic identity of Ukrainians is stronger than that of some of the other Slavic groups (Marganoff & Folwarski, 1996). Church and secular community agencies actively promote the preservation of the Ukrainian language and culture. Among the most important elements of that culture are the traditional Ukrainian celebration of Easter, with its brilliantly painted Easter eggs (*pysanki*) and Easter games (*haivki*), and Ukrainian folk music and dancing. Knowledge of these traditional customs may be useful when working with Ukrainian families, especially those experiencing conflict between the old and new cultures.

THE BELARUSIANS

After seven decades as a constituent republic of the Soviet Union, Belarus attained its independence in 1991. Like their neighbors the Ukrainians, most Belarusians (70%) are Eastern Orthodox and the rest are Catholic. The original Belarusian immigrants (1880–1914) had little sense of national group identity and joined existing Polish or Russian American communities. Post-World War I immigrants felt a more distinct identity, and since that time a Belarusian American community has developed. Post–World War II immigrant professionals, artisans, and skilled workers raised in Soviet Belarusia arrived fully aware of their Belarusian identity. They speak Belarussian and worship in one of a small number of Belarusian Orthodox churches. The community has a few newspapers, and since 1945, distinctly Belarusian organizations have been formed, including the Belarusian American Youth Organization, which has folk dance ensembles and sports groups and sponsors seminars on Belarusian culture. Belarusian ethnic identity is not as strong as that of some of the other Slavic groups (Marganoff & Folwarski, 1996, p. 652).

THE BULGARIANS

There are about 70,000 Bulgarian immigrants and their descendants in the United States. Because of their relatively small numbers, the Bulgarian immigrants who arrived in the United States before World War I tended to settle near other recently arrived Slavic immigrants, such as the Serbs, who shared similar cultural backgrounds and values (Carlson & Allen, 1990). Between the two world wars, the majority of Bulgarian immigrants were women and children joining husbands and fathers who had decided to make their home in America.

"As has been true of the second generation of most immigrant groups, the sons and daughters of Bulgarian immigrants were eager to become Americanized and to shed the different-ness that hindered their parents' progress" (Carlson & Allen, 1990, p. 77). However, members of the third generation, secure in their sense of themselves as Americans, generally exhibit a greater interest in their Bulgarian heritage than do their parents.

One of the richest aspects of that heritage is Bulgarian traditional music and song. Through 500 years of Turkish domination, the Bulgarian people held fast to their music as a vehicle of both community and personal expression. Even today, the Bulgarians continue to sing traditional songs commemorating births, marriages, deaths, religious holidays, harvests, and festivals. Bulgarian music has even found its way into the American mainstream culture through musicians such as Paul Simon and David Byrne and is a source of pride for Bulgarian Americans.

THE MACEDONIANS

In 1991, Macedonia declared its independence from Yugoslavia and is known, for the time being, as the Former Yugoslav Republic of Macedonia (FYROM). The population of Macedonia is 2,200,000, of whom 67% are ethnic Slav Macedonians. There are about 50,000 Macedonians living in the United States, mostly in Michigan. (The largest number of Macedonians outside the motherland live in Toronto, Canada.) Many work in the food industry, running family-style restaurants and bakeries. Because many still live together in large extended families, their houses tend to be quite large, with numerous rooms to accommodate family members (Cetinich, 2003).

The most important community event of the Macedonians is the *vecerinka*, the evening party, at which the participants take part in the world-renowned folk dance traditions of Macedonia. Macedonian dances are the most ancient of all Slav dances, and some of the oldest in the world. "Usually danced on Sundays and holidays, they are cultural expressions that help Macedonians have a greater sense of their unique identity and serve to unify them as they bridge the gap between the old and the new" (Cetinich, 2003, p. 57).

THE SERBS

Largest of the national groups of the former Yugoslavia, the Serbs use the Cyrillic alphabet, follow the Orthodox religion, and focus community life on the church parish in the United States. These three "badges of ethnicity" have alienated the Serbian Americans from their Slovene and Croatian neighbors, just as in the homeland. Serbs still use the Julian or Old Style calendar for religious observances. Traditions of music and chanting of poetry have survived in this country and have been revitalized by recent immigrants. The *krsna slava*, or family patron saint's day, symbolizes connection with the departed members of a family as well as its patron saint. It is a uniquely Serbian celebration. The male head of the household, along with the priest, conducts this celebration. The *kum* and *kuma* (godfather and godmother) play a very important role in Serbian family life. They are so connected with the families of their godchildren that intermarriage between these families is restricted. The closeness engendered by these connections has deepened cohesion in the Serbian American community (Marganoff & Folwarski, 1996, p. 653).

There are more than 250,000 Serb Americans. The Serb National Federation, founded in 1901, has been the preeminent Serb organization in the United States.

Catholic Slavs

THE POLES

Poles are descendants of a Slavic tribe known as the Poliane, "people of the plain," that settled in the flatlands to the east of the Germanic regions of Europe. This geographic location, wedged between the Germanic and Slavic worlds, made Poles vulnerable to attacks both from the West (by Teutonic knights, and later by Prussia, Austria, and Germany) and the East (by their cousins, the Russians). With this country partitioned between Prussia, Austria, and Russia, for more than a century (1791–1918), Poland's name disappeared from the map of Europe altogether. World War II was especially devastating for the Poles, resulting in massive losses of population; it was followed by 45 years of vassalage to the Soviet Union. Poland gained international attention with the election of a Polish-born bishop, Karol Jozef Wojtyla, to the papacy in 1978. With the fall of Communism in 1991, Poland gained independence and is now a member of the European Union.

Throughout the country's turbulent history, large numbers of Poles emigrated to Western Europe and America. Their collective longing for the lost homeland can be heard in the melancholy chords of the famous polonaise "Pożegnanie Ojczyzny" (Farewell to the Fatherland) by Polish composer and exiled patriot Michal Oginski (1765–1833).

Cataclysmic historical setbacks did not prevent the Poles from developing a rich, world-class culture, as testified by such giants of science and the arts as Nikolaus Copernicus (née Mikolaj Kopernik), Maria Sklodowska-Curie, Fryderyk Chopin, and, more recently, the poet and Nobel laureate Czeslaw Milosc. It is ironic, however, that most of these individuals' talents flourished only after they left their country for good.

Like all Slavs, Polish Americans have long suffered from ethnic prejudice, exemplified by the so-called Polish jokes. (In that sense, just like their forebears once battered by Teutonic knights, Poles became scapegoats for all Slavs living in this country.) Although some Polish immigrants changed their names in order to avoid humiliation, others suffered quietly (Chapter 54). The popularity of the Polish-born pope, the recent emergence of Poland as a staunch ally of the United States in its "war on terror," and the increasingly sophisticated nature of today's Polish immigrants are all likely to make "Polish jokes" a thing of the past.

THE SLOVAKS

There are about 2,000,000 ethnic Slovaks (Chapter 53) in the United States. Their old home country, Slovakia, is a Central European nation of 5,000,000 people who speak a language similar to that of their neighbors, the Czechs and the Poles. Throughout Slovakia's history, foreign powers dominated it. Most recently, it was part of Czechoslovakia, from which it gained independence in 1993. In view of this history, "it must have taken a special pertinacity to maintain a distinctly Slovak identity" (Hoffman, 1993, p. 183). This trait helps to explain why first-generation Slovak Americans generally married other Slovak Americans, and the second generation tended to marry other Slavs of the same religious background. The third-generation Slovak Americans chose mates from

Irish and German families of the same religious background. To this day, Slovaks may still be most readily identified with Czechs in (the former) Czechoslovakia. Therapists working with Slovak Americans should be sensitive to the fact that such an association is generally considered an insult to Slovaks (Kerr, 1996).

THE CZECHS

Czechs (Chapter 53) take great pride in their cultural heritage. Their country of origin, the Czech Republic (formerly, the Republic of Czechoslovakia), is located in the heart of Europe; its capital, Prague, has traditionally been a fulcrum of learning and thought. Czech writers and intellectuals have exerted considerable influence on the political course of the country, starting with Jan Hus, a 15th century thinker and Protestant reformer, all the way to Vaclav Havel, the playwright and recent president who oversaw the peaceful transition of the country back to independence.

Czech immigrants reflect this intellectual tradition. Most of them arrived in the United States fully literate and often bilingual (Chapter 53). On that note, the first known Czech immigrant, who came to this country in 1633, was a professional who landed an executive position as one of the founders of the Virginia tobacco trade (Chapter 53). Subsequent immigrants represented diverse classes, including peasants and skilled workers, most of whom settled in the Midwest. The last wave arrived following the 1968 Warsaw Pact invasion of Czechoslovakia, consisting mostly of intellectuals fleeing Communist oppression. Irrespective of their class, however, Czechs greatly value both education and intellectual pursuits.

Although most Czechs are nominally Catholic, their identification with the Catholic Church is much weaker than that of other groups. This has to do with the history of oppression by the Catholic Habsburg Empire, under whose rule Czechs lived until 1918. Their alienation from Catholicism may be one reason that many Czechs have adhered to Protestant values such as hard work, thrift, and independence.

A word of caution: Like Slovaks, with whom Czechs, prior to 1993, shared one country—Czecholovakia—Czechs do not take kindly to being "mistaken" for their former neighbors.

THE SLOVENIANS

The country of Slovenia occupies the northwestern corner of the former Yugoslavia. Its people speak a Slavic language that is different from that of their neighboring cousins and co-religionists, the Croatians. Prior to 1918, when Slovenia became part of Yugoslavia, it was a province of Austro-Hungary; most of the original Slovenian immigrants called themselves "Austrians" when they first arrived in the United States. Slovenia seceded from Yugoslavia in 1991. There have been few Slovenian immigrants to the United States since the 1950s, because the Republic of Slovenia's economic prosperity is equal to that of Austria.

Slovenians maintain their connection with the old culture by attending church and community events, such as Slovenian folk singing and cooking traditional Slovenian dishes. "The fact that Slovenia is now an independent country might play an important role in revivifying interest in Slovenian culture and language among all ages in the Slovenian community" (Cetinich, 2003, p. 45).

THE CROATS

Croatia is a former republic of Yugoslavia, bordering the Adriatic Sea, between Bosnia and Herzegovina and Slovenia. It became independent in 1995. The original Croatian immigrants to this country were the seamen and merchants from the Adriatic coast who came to the United States in the 1850s. They established themselves as fishermen, farmers, and fruit growers in California and oystermen in Louisiana. After 1880, Croatian immigrants were mostly illiterate peasants from the interior regions of Croatia, part of the flood of those from Eastern Europe that settled around Cleveland and Pittsburgh (Marganoff & Folwarski, 1996). There are about 400,000 persons of Croatian descent living in this country.

The main focus of the Croatioan community has been the Catholic Church, which many Croatians view as an authoritative preserver of their culture (Cetinich, 2003). Subsequent generations became more removed from their cultural heritage. For instance, the traditional lavish weddings in ethnic halls have been superseded by American-style catered receptions. Still, links with the old culture endure in music and folk dancing. The *tamburitza*, a stringed instrument that resembles a mandolin, has traditionally provided the accompaniment for Croatian folk music. Since their old homeland, Croatia, recently established its independence, there has been a resurgence of interest by young Croatian Americans in their ethnic roots.

Muslim Slavs

The Muslim Slavs live mainly in Bosnia. The language of Bosnia is Serbo-Croatian, though Bosnians now refer to their language as Bosnian, and many people also speak English. Bosnian Muslims are descendants of the Slavs converted to Muslim faith by the invading Turks in the 13th century. Until the late 1980s they lived in an uneasy but workable peace with their Serb Orthodox neighbors in what used to be Yugoslavia. In 1991, as Yugoslavia began to disintegrate and Bosnia declared its independence, civil war began. The conflict included the "ethnic cleansing" of Muslims by the Serb military and police. This genocide was characterized by concentration camps, mass murders (especially of men), and a Serb policy of raping Muslim women. The vast majority of the approximately 250,000 killed were civilians. An outflow of refugees resulted, with approximately 800,000 Bosnians displaced to other countries and more than 200,000 coming to the United States.

The survivors of the Bosnian atrocities may be at risk for posttraumatic stress disorder (PTSD), combat stress disorder (CSR), depression, and other consequences of psychological trauma, including alcoholism, despite Islamic prohibitions against alcohol. These traumas are essentially the same as those associated with the experiences of the Holocaust survivors; hence, reactions may continue through at least a second generation.

Virtually all Bosnian refugees are Muslim. They are generally a cosmopolitan group, for whom Islam may have less of an impact on family life and customs than for others from rural Middle Eastern backgrounds. Bosnian women, for example, tend to be less intent on maintaining extreme modesty and are more willing to discuss issues pertaining to intimacy than women from other Muslim cultures. At the most, a Bosnian woman will wear a scarf over her head and dress conservatively. A Church World Service report noted that many Bosnians have a relationship with Islam similar to the relationship many Americans have with Christianity: "something restricted to the Sabbath and major religious holidays."

Although there are extended families living together in rural Bosnia, most Bosnian refugees live in nuclear family groups. Many families have a history of both wife and husband employed outside the home. Men usually have greater authority than women. Although polygamy is sanctioned in the Qur'an, it is only rarely practiced in Bosnia.

An important cultural symbol for Bosnians is the *Sevdalinka* (from the Turkish word *sevdah*, which means "passion"), a secular romantic ballad, sung along with accordions, violin, and bass guitar. "These melancholic tunes evoke intimacy and reflection; they are the Bosnian's connection with his or her motherland and Muslim culture" (Cetinich, 2003, p. 62).

As Bosnian Muslims try to adjust to life in the United States, or to revive their uprooted culture, they may encounter the same misunderstanding, and even prejudice, faced by other Muslims in the post-September 11 world. This may only compound the sense of cultural and emotional dislocation they have already experienced as refugees.

TREATMENT ISSUES

In therapy, cultural differences affect how families handle their emotions. An Eastern Slavic client may initially be more reluctant to verbalize feelings—to him or her, emotional life is a mystery more than anything else. Many Eastern Slavs, even those from well-educated classes, may believe in the supernatural and magic. The therapist should keep these factors in mind in choosing his or her interventions.

Barbara, a Russian American client, came to therapy because of intense anxiety about her health. She had suffered from brain cancer, which was then in remission. A divorced mother of a college-age daughter, she spoke several languages and worked as an office manager at a prestigious law firm. She said she couldn't sleep because she kept thinking about what would happen to her daughter if she died. Barbara refused to talk about her fears. She believed that talking about dying (the "d" word, as she put it) might actually cause it to happen. She traced this belief to her grandmother, a Russian immigrant. To discount the belief as mere superstition would be a sure way to turn the client away. The therapist referred her to a clinician who specialized in hypnosis. Follow-up established that hypnotherapy was helping her manage her anxiety.

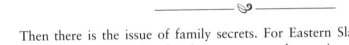

Then there is the issue of family secrets. For Eastern Slavs, in keeping with their Byzantine roots, maintaining family secrets may play an important role in family relationships. This custom may contribute to the client's reluctance to talk openly about personal matters. However, the therapist should not always assume that "skeletons in the closet" are necessarily considered shameful. One elderly Russian American client was secretly proud of the fact that her son's biological father was not the humdrum man she had married, but another, more dashing man with whom she had had a lasting affair.

Preserving secrets may also be motivated by the psychological trauma suffered during cataclysmic events in Europe. For many first-generation Russians and Ukrainians, their parents' and grandparents' memories of Stalin's terror, or the atrocities of World War II—whether as victims or colluders—are very painful. The therapist should be certain the client is ready to talk about this painful legacy before directing him or her to explore it. This precaution applies to (mostly Muslim) victims of the Bosnian genocide as well.

Family Patterns

Historically, the basic unit of Slavic life was a large extended family, or clan, organized on a patrilineal basis, whose members lived together in one dwelling and held all land, livestock, and money in common. The oldest able member of the community was usually its ruler, responsible for allotting tasks to the members. Only together, through pooling their resources and huddling against the hostile outside world, could a family survive. The often harsh climate, frequent foreign invasions, and oppressive governments all contributed to the family's insular structure. This system, which was common to most Slavs, existed well into the 20th century.

Domostroy, a Russian treatise on family values and behavior that dates back to 16th century, legitimized the power of the father to rule the household. He does not do housework but oversees and administers all of it. Corporal punishment is recommended as the only sure guarantor of good child rearing. *Domostroy* presents such punishment as a manifestation of love and protection that will "save the children with fear." The husband is the "chastisement and terror" of the wife, children, and servants. He must punish her for misbehavior in private, using the lash in the most serious matters.

These principles, though rarely followed to the letter by most families, speak to the father's predominant role in the family. Such a role was further emphasized by the custom, still in place today in Russia and some other Slavic countries, of giving every child a patronymic. Like the czar himself (popularly referred to as *czar-batyushka*, the little father), the patriarch demanded unconditional respect and subordination from his subjects—his wife and children—and often reacted violently if he didn't receive it. One vestige of this tradition, especially among more recent Slavic immigrants, is the custom of the father spanking his children, which is still common even among the well educated.

For Slavic immigrants in the United States, family relations, at least through the first generation, followed these traditional patterns of close-knit patriarchy (Carlson & Allen, 1990). The father made all the important decisions; the mother was his helpmate. Grandparents played a large role in raising children, and all social life revolved around the extended family. This reliance on cooperation and family aided the immigrants in overcoming harsh living conditions and helped protect them from American nativists who discriminated against all foreigners, especially those from Eastern Europe. This pattern was to change by the early 20th century as the children of first-generation Slavic Americans attended school and acquired a command of the English language. "As took place within so many immigrant groups, the second generation was eager to assimilate in order to achieve greater economic success than their parents, even if the process of assimilation required abandoning certain basic elements of their heritage" (Carlson & Allen, 1990, p. 77).

Immigration to the United States

With the exception of the Russians, most original Slavic immigrants were peasants and laborers who came to this country in the years between 1880 and 1914, fleeing poverty and oppression at home. Most were single men who came with the intention to save up money and go back home. As not everyone could find suitable land to work on, many became railroad workers or miners, enduring harsh working conditions and, often, discrimination at the hands of their employers.

The social life of the immigrants centered on a coffee house, a boarding house, or a saloon, where one might enjoy the companionship of countrymen, read ethnic newspapers, and discuss news from the old country. The owner of such an establishment, usually an immigrant who had been in the United States for some time, often acted as everything from interpreter to attorney for his clients. His wife was responsible for raising their children and providing dinner and laundry services for as many as 20 boarders, most of them single men from the same village who were now working at the same factory or mine (Carlson & Allen, 1990). By the early 1900s some of these places had evolved into community organizations or mutual aid societies.

The second wave of Slavic immigrants consisted of those who fled the upheavals of World War II and the Soviet takeover of Eastern Europe that followed. These immigrants, many of whom were urban professionals, were considered refugees from Communism and were supported both by their respective immigrant communities and by the U.S. government. The majority of today's Slavic immigrants come to the United States to advance their careers. Many are highly skilled professionals or are seeking training here.

Under Communism—and especially given the Slavs' traditional proclivity toward communal values—emigraion to the West was seen as "betrayal" of the motherland, a shameful act for which the family of the emigrant was often ostracized. This may still be true, especially in more rural areas, resulting in feelings of shame in the emigrants themselves. These feelings are only exacerbated when the immigrants are here illegally or when their visas have expired and they are unable to visit their motherland for fear of not being allowed back into the United States.

Slava, a 30-year-old Russian computer engineer, came to California on a work visa to work for a high-tech concern. He married another Russian immigrant, with whom he had a child. When, 2 years later, his mother died, he was torn between his desire to go to the funeral and his fear that he would become separated from his new family. In therapy, Slava discussed his feelings of shame for abandoning his motherland. Because religion was important for him, the therapist suggested that he talk to a Russian Orthodox priest who was also a pastoral counselor. The priest's validation—Slava half-jokingly referred to it as "absolution"—helped Slava come to terms with his decision not to go back to Russia.

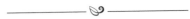

Unlike some other immigrant groups, such as East Asians, who come here to join a large extended family, or Latin Americans, who can identify with the growing and dynamic Latino community in this country, Slavic emigrants are mostly on their own. Their connection with the existing Slavic community agencies is often tenuous, because these organizations were established decades ago, making for a significant cultural gap. Thus, recent Slavic immigrants may suffer from the same sense of cultural obscurity that has traditionally plagued the Slavic people.

CONCLUSION

The recent rise to prominence of a number of Slavic Americans and the advent on the world stage of the Slavic "New Europe" may have increased their appreciation of their ethnic origins. In addition, the growing willingness of Slavic Americans to put their old differences behind them may herald the long-due healing of the "family of Slavs." For therapists, these developments offer an opportunity to help their clients explore their ethnic roots so that they may better understand themselves and their families of origin.

ACKNOWLEDGMENTS

Special thanks to Janice Rogovin and Carey Reid.

NOTES

1. Witness, for example, the crude and tyrannical Stanley Kowalski, the Polish American protagonist of *A Streetcar Named Desire.*
2. *Some Like It Hot, The Man with the Golden Arm, The Deer Hunter.*
3. It is of note that Stewart became famous teaching the American middle class how to arrange their homes—the family hearths. Her biography reveals that she learned the arts of country living from her parents and grandparents, who brought these skills from the old country.

REFERENCES

Althausen, L. (1996). Russian families. In M. McGoldrick, J. Giordano, & J. K. Pearce (Eds.), *Ethnicity and family therapy* (2 nd ed., pp. 680–687). New York: Guilford Press.

Barford, P. M. (2001). *The early Slavs.* Ithaca, NY: Cornell University Press.

Carlson, C., & Allen, D. (1990). *The Bulgarian Americans.* New York: Chelsea House.

Cetinich, D. (2003). *South Slavs in Michigan.* East Lansing, MI: Michigan State University Press.

Conte, F. (1995). *The Slavs.* New York: Columbia University Press.

Hoffman, E. (1993). *Exit into history.* New York: Viking.

Kaplan, R. (1994). *Balkan ghosts.* New York: Vintage.

Kerr, S. (1996). Slovak families. In M. McGoldrick, J. Giordano, & J. K. Pearce (Eds.), *Ethnicity and family therapy* (2nd ed., pp. 673–679). New York: Guilford Press.

Magoscsi, P. (1996). *The Russian Americans.* New York: Chelsea House.

Marganoff, P., & Folwarski, J. (1996). Slavic families: An overview. In M. McGoldrick, J. Giordano, & J. K. Pearce (Eds.), *Ethnicity and family therapy* (2nd ed., pp. 649–657). New York: Guilford Press.

Schjeldahl, P. (2004, May 17). Striking gold: The final installment of the Met's Byzantium shows. *New Yorker.*

Wtulich, J. (1994). *American xenophobia and the Slav immigrant.* Boulder, CO: East European Monographs.

CHAPTER 53

Czech and Slovak Families

Jo-Ann Krestan
Rita Mae Gazarik

Czech and Slovak family relationships can be understood only if you have a knowledge of their intertwined histories and cultures. Estimates are that something over a million Czechs and Slovaks have immigrated to the United States from 1850 until today. The Czechs were the first Slavs to reach the United States. They were the first large Slavic farming population in the United States, working ceaselessly until they owned their own land. Bohemian women were reputedly able to grow food even in the poorest soil. The early Czech Americans also became entrepreneurs. Cigars, glass products, and pearl buttons were some of their largest manufacturing interests.

By 1924, when the United States established immigration quotas, more than a half million Czechs had come to America. In 1948, and again in 1968, there were smaller, predominantly political migrations to the United States. The first settlers have been described as highly intelligent. Czechs came to this country with a 97% literacy rate and more savings than other immigrant groups.

The large emigration from Slovakia began in the 1880s (Bartalská, 1999). The motivation was economic, especially for those from eastern Slovakia. The Slovaks were a good, cheap workforce for an explosively expanding American industry. They did not originally intend to settle permanently in America, and many returned home with a good portion of their earnings intact.

The first Czech immigrants came to America after their lands were cleansed of Protestants in the 17th century. The next large wave came after the failed European democratic revolutions of 1848. Slovak immigration to America started in the late 19th century and was more due to economics than that of the Czechs. Immigration for both groups probably peaked in the first decade of the 20th century, but there were more than 102,000 Czech and Slovak immigrants during the 1920s.

After that time, their combined immigration to the United States dropped off drastically, with small spikes at Hitler's takeover of the country in 1938, at the imposition of Russian Communism in 1948, and after the Warsaw Pact invasion in 1968.

When we think of that part of central Europe that is now the Czech Republic, we think of Bohemian crystal and Pilsner beer, Kafka, avant-garde literature, and the music of Dvorak. More recently we remember Madeleine Albright, President Clinton's secretary of state. We can envision heavy industry powered by fossil fuels, smokestacks looming against bucolic countrysides dotted with willow trees. Imagine white swans on the rivers, geese in the barnyards, and castles brooding over the landscape. There are also the Romany Gypsies, many of whom perished with the more than 155,000 Czechoslovak Jews in Hitler's death camps. Today, yet an ugly footnote to a proud history of fighting for autonomy, the Gypsies are still a despised minority.

In contrast to the ease with which we can imagine the Czechs, we have to stretch to make any associations with the Slovaks. As Ernest Denis, Sorbonne professor and author, said in 1917: "Rare are those with any notion of the Slovaks. Even educated people know them hardly at all and would find difficulty placing them upon a map." It is in the context of that lack of national identity that the Slovak parliament voted for separation of the two states in 1993. The "Velvet Divorce" underlined the Slovaks' desire to stand on their own.

Challenging our understanding of the Czechs and the Slovaks, their respective histories run parallel, diverge, merge, and intersect at various points in history. Both Czechs and Slovaks struggled against powerful neighbors that threatened their existence, and both fought fiercely to retain their language, their national pride, and some sense of autonomous identity under varied oppressors, most notably the Austro-Hungarian Empire.

A BRIEF CZECH HISTORY

Czechs were originally Western Slavs, who, before World War I, were often called Bohemians. They have occupied the homelands of Bohemia, Moravia, and Silesia since the 5th century. The richness of the lands and their location made Bohemia an almost constant target of foreign conquest. In the 9th century, Moravia dominated, extending the borders of the Great Moravian Empire to include Bohemia, southern Poland, and northern Hungary. The Czechs, or Bohemians, retained their own monarchy within the Moravian empire. When the Holy Roman Empire succeeded the Great Moravian Empire, the Germans claimed Bohemia and Moravia as part of the Holy Roman Empire, and Hungary and the Magyars took Slovakia.

Religion is a critical part of the history of Bohemia. Since the mid-1600s, the Czech intellectuals were largely Protestant. When the Czechs elected a Catholic Hapsburg to the Bohemian throne, the Hapsburgs imposed Catholicism. Jan Hus, a priest and professor, led a popular attack on the clergy, advocating not only reform of the Roman Church, but also the liberation of Bohemia. As Hus gained followers, the Hapsburgs started to persecute the Protestants. Hus was burned at the stake for heresy in 1414. The Hussite Wars, wars between the followers of Jan Hus and their persecutors, lasted many years.

The Hapsburgs definitively defeated the Czechs during the Thirty Years' War (1618–1648). More than 36,000 families, essentially all of the Protestant intelligentsia, fled to Protestant countries rather than submit to Catholicism. A small but vital group of them set sail for America. The Hapsburgs established German as the official language and Catholicism as the state religion. Czech remained the language of peasants until the mid-

1800s, when the Czechs resuscitated their determination to revive their ancestral culture and language, publishing the first Czech dictionary. Czech independence finally came in October 1918.

A BRIEF SLOVAK HISTORY

The Slovaks came under the brutal rule of the Magyars (Hungarians) after the battle of Bratislava in 910. Despite Magyar oppression, Slovakia prospered for 500 years within the kingdom of Hungary, and the Magyars adopted Slovak customs and Christianity. Then the 16th-century Turkish invasion and Islamization of Hungary, which became the Ottoman Empire, ended the landlord–tenant relationship between the Slovak people and the Magyars. The resulting brutal repression by the Magyars crushed any developing spirit of Slovak national pride.

In the 19th century, the goal of the Austro-Hungarian Empire was to wipe out all non-Magyar cultures in "Hungary." This Magarization, or "prison of the people," as it was called, lasted until World War I. Meanwhile, the Slovaks struggled to maintain their language and folk customs and occasionally were able to renew contacts with the Czechs.

The 1840s saw the emergence of the distinctiveness of the Slovak language and people. Slovaks began to view themselves as a separate nationality in spite of the insistence of the Magyars that they speak Magyar and that this language be taught in the schools, an insistence that nearly obliterated the Slovaks' language. "The absence of their own state, their inclusion in American statistics, along with other oppressed nationalities of the former Hungary, under the broad category 'Hungarians' from which rose the pejorative 'Hunkies,' worked to weaken their identity as Slovaks" (Bartalská, 1999, p. 23). With determination and generosity, Slovak Americans financially supported institutions and the Slovak American press that helped to develop and maintain the Slovak identity.

THE CREATION OF CZECHOSLOVAKIA

During World War I, Czech patriots in the United States and abroad, in league with Slovak immigrants seeking independence for Slovakia, helped defeat the Austro-Hungarian Empire. The Slovaks and Czechs were reunited when the Allies artificially created Czechoslovakia in 1918 after the collapse of the Austro-Hungarian monarchy. There were difficulties: The partnership was unequal, as the population of the Czechs was twice the size of the Slovaks', and the focus of attention, education, culture, business, and politics was on Prague, not Bratislava. The Slovaks were less educated and agrarian, and their economy was not as strong as that of the Czechs.

What is more, "Ethnically, the country was very diverse. Slovaks—though they inhabited territory immediately to the east of Moravia and spoke a language that was so close to Czech that the two tongues were mutually understandable—had been part of Hungary for a thousand years, and so shared few historical ties with the Czechs (*The Czech Republic in Brief*, www.rect.muni.cz/ois/coming_to_brno/the_czech_republic_in_brief/index). However, this partnership lasted as a parliamentary democracy for the period between the World Wars.

In 1938, with Europe on the brink of another war and the Allied powers desperate to avoid it, Slovakia was made an "independent" separate state by Nazi Germany. A priest, Father Tiso, was the first president. In 1939, Hitler marched into Bohemia and annexed the rest of the land once controlled by the Holy Roman Empire. The Nazi occupation ended only with Hitler's defeat and only with the cooperation of the Russians. Stalin allied with Czechoslovak leaders to create a new Czech state and, in return, secured a large Communist presence in postwar Czechoslovakia. As the leading literary figure of the Resistance, novelist Milan Kundera, in the novel that prompted the Czech government to revoke his citizenship, said, "And so it happened that in February 1948 the Communists took power not in bloodshed and violence, but to the cheers of about half the population. And please note: the half that cheered was the more dynamic, the more intelligent, the better half" (1980, p. 8).

The Czechoslovak Socialist Republic State owned everything. The Communist presence was to become a consuming one that ushered in a repressive Communist regime. Czech and Slovak intellectuals were arrested for alleged political crimes and sent to forced labor camps. The oppression eased after Stalin's death in 1953 but was not thoroughly challenged until 1968. Dubcek, head of the Czech Communist Party and a Slovak, further lifted restrictions such as censorship of the press and the media. This period of liberalization policy and reforms was referred to as the "Prague Spring."

Moscow, scared by Dubcek's liberalization and fearful that resistance would spread throughout the Warsaw Pact countries, forcefully sent in tanks from Russia and Hungary to "restore" order. Again resistance developed in the country. The Slovak dissidents concentrated more on freedom of religion. The Czechs, with Charter 77, were about political and cultural freedom (Kirschbaum, 1995, p. 247). Gorbachev's *perestroika*, the 1989 dismantling of the Berlin Wall, and mass demonstrations begun by students and artists in Prague, then spreading throughout Czechoslovakia, brought about the government's collapse in the "Velvet Revolution" (so called because there was no bloodshed). Communist control and power ended. Václav Havel, a Czech, became the first freely elected president by the members of the Parliament of Czechoslovakia. Dubcek, a Slovak, was elected speaker of Parliament.

Slovakia began to feel as if it was playing second fiddle again. Slovaks were ill prepared for the market economy after four decades of defense industrialization, with the economic differences and disagreements about division of power. By a parliamentary vote, the two peoples obtained a "velvet divorce" and became the Czech Republic and the Slovak Republic in 1993. Both Havel and Dubcek opposed the split.

THE CZECHS AND THE SLOVAKS: ETHNICITY WITHOUT POLITICS

Challenging as it is to understand Czech and Slovak political arrangements over the last several centuries, we want now, as family therapists, to retell the story of the Czechs and the Slovaks from the point of view of their ethnicity, rather than their political arrangements. The Czechs and Slovaks are Slavic peoples who have had distinct identities and associations with the lands they command today since the 6th century. The Czechs and the Slovaks are two closely related peoples speaking two languages—Czech and Slovak—

both of Slavic origin. The Czechs were dominated for hundreds of years by the Germans, and the Slovaks were dominated by the Magyars. Both the Germans and the Magyars had contempt for their Slavic subjects.

For both the Czechs and the Slovaks, there were several episodes when their conquerors, for different reasons, killed or drove out the educated and landowning Slavic remnants; so among neither ethnic group is there any indigenous, landowning aristocracy remaining. Both the Germans and the Magyars, with varying degrees of severity, began and then intensified attempts at suppressing their subject peoples' cultures. Czechs were required to learn German and to be Roman Catholic; and Slovaks were not only required to learn Magyar, but forbidden to teach Slovakian. Eventually, some Germans and all of the Magyars joined together in one empire to commonly rule over their Slavs. This made exploitation and administration of these subject peoples more effective. The dislocations and opportunities provided by the wave of industrialization that swept west to America and east to the lands of the Czechs and Slovaks from England and France in the 19th century also caused millions of Czechs and Slovaks to emigrate from their homelands, some to the German countries, but most to the United States and Canada.

The end of World War I brought about the end of the German and Magyar empire. So many—especilly the most gifted—Czechs and Slovaks had emigrated to America by this time that the first government of the new country, Czechoslovakia, was organized in Pittsburgh!

In spite of the various occupations, the Czechs and Slovaks had struggled and managed to retain their own cultural mores, language, and values, although influenced by the their conquerors. Czechoslovakia was the only one of the Slavic countries to become and remain a stable, democratic republic in the interwar years.

The return of German rule to the Czechs and Slovaks in World War II changed the situation of these peoples more brutally and drastically than anything that had happened before. By the end of the war, Czechoslovakia had changed from being an independent, multinational country with large, mainly self-governing minorities of Germans, Magyars, Jews, Ruthenians, and Gypsies to an ethnically cleansed state with insignificant numbers of Germans, Ruthenians, and Jews and officially oppressed Magyar and Gypsy minorities. Czechoslovakia was ethnically independent but politically under Russian domination from the end of World War II until 1989.

With the 1993 breakup of the Czechoslovak state into two independent states, the process of ethnic identification and nation building seems to be approaching a stable endgame. The two states now have enormous majorities of their own kind in their respective states, and these majorities are fully empowered. The Czech Republic now has about 10.5 million, 94% Czech and less than 1% Gypsies (as of 1991). The Slovak Republic now has about 5.5 million, 86% Slovak, 10% Magyar, and 1% Romany.

The Czech Republic has a low emigration rate and a slowly shrinking population. Slovakia has a low emigration rate and a slowly growing population. Both countries have an increasing "transient" population, as other Eastern European and Middle Eastern emigrants move into these countries "on their way" to Western Europe.

Are the Czechs and Slovaks different? They both struggled with maintaining their own cultures and languages while other countries tried, sometimes successfully, to control them. Their languages are similar and easily understood by one another. Many of their beliefs that manage their lives are the same. For example, two friends, one raised among the educated elite of Prague, and the other, a first-generation Slovak in America from a working-class family in which the father was a liturgical artist, grew up with the identical sayings or rules for behavior: "Children should be seen and not heard," "Boys, especially, and girls do not cry in public," and "Never hang your dirty laundry in public." In a 1991 survey, "the Slovaks showed a preference for leisure activities and social life over work, family, and politics, while the Czechs preferred the latter" (*Sociologicky Casopis*, 1992).

With the Jewish population, the people of Slovakia showed greater wariness than the Czechs; the most recent statistics (Nationmaster.com) show that each country has a Jewish population of only 6,000! Attitudes toward Jews in Slovakia varied from extremely prejudiced and fearful (for example, Slovaks used to frighten children and keep them obedient with threats of being given to the Jews, just as they threatened them with being stolen by the Gypsies) to viewing Jews as an integral part of the village and hiding them during the persecution, to gratitude for Jewish families helping non-Jewish families with the fares to the "new country" to join their husbands and fathers. Both Czechs and Slovaks discriminate against the Roma. In fact, one of the largest issues in the aftermath of the Velvet Divorce is Czech and Slovak intolerance of their most problematic ethnic group.

PATTERNS OF CZECH IMMIGRATION

The first known Czech immigrant was Augustin Hermann, who came to New York in 1633 in the employ of the West India Company. He became a surveyor and was one of the founders of the Virginia tobacco trade. Small numbers of Czechs came for religious reasons during America's colonial period. From the mid-1800s until World War I, more than 100,000 Czechs immigrated for economic reasons. The first of these immigrants were peasants, largely from the wooded pasturelands of southern Bohemia. Reminded of the climate they had left behind and driven by the dream of landownership, they were drawn to the Midwest, where they settled in Wisconsin, Nebraska, Minnesota, Iowa, Kansas, and Texas.

Because they came from an advanced, industrialized economy, Czechs were also highly skilled workers. The next wave of immigrants found skilled manufacturing and mechanical jobs in the large urban centers. Chicago became the third largest Czech city in the world, after Prague and Vienna. Cleveland and New York also drew thousands of Czechs.

EARLY CZECH SETTLEMENT

Unlike so many immigrants who came singly, the Bohemians initially came in family groups, or the men were followed by their wives in very short order. They were proud of the nobility (though most of the nobility were dead or left the country during reign of the Hapsburgs) from which many of them were descended, and fiercely proud of being Czech. The Czechs did not assimilate quickly, either in the city or the country, but formed their own neighborhoods, which in many ways replicated the villages of Bohemia. Always prizing education, they learned English but retained the Czech or German language *en famille*. In a manner reminiscent of their history of dual monarchies and relative autonomy within larger empires, the Czechs bought proportionately more war bonds during World War I than other foreign-born groups, while still retaining a strong ethnic identity and resisting assimilation. Until World War I, they married primarily within their own groups.

Every settlement had a Czech society of some kind—a church, an amateur band, or a tavern—and the active community life before World War I revolved around these groups. The earliest organizations were fraternal benevolent societies that provided life and health insurance benefits, and *sokols*, or gymnastic societies. Community, color, and beauty were important. Garden plots replaced lawns in front of their houses with riotous crowds of tall perennials. And there was always music. The saying, *"Co Cech, to muzikant"* (If he's a Czech, he's a musician), expresses the Czechs' love of music and dance. Every village had its own band of self-taught musicians.

The largest wave of immigration had been completed by World War I. By 1940 a movement away from agriculture was apparent, and the number of Czech Americans employed as blue-collar or service workers declined with each subsequent generation.

PATTERNS OF SLOVAK IMMIGRATION

The first known Slovak to arrive on American soil was a Mr. Jelik, a master dressmaker, in 1755. Various others occasionally appeared in America, who were usually following a military career. Some men came here to avoid the draft in the Austro-Hungarian Empire, which could mean that their service would last for several years (as many as 20, according to one family's story about emigration)! The largest and oldest concentrations of Slovaks were in the former industrial centers of the East Coast. The greatest concentration was in Pennsylvania, especially in Pittsburgh. They labored in the steel mills, coke works, glass factories, and coal mines, applying their ability to work and their skills to the growth of this country. By the outbreak of World War I, 500,000 Slovaks lived in America, most of them in the industrial Northeast and Midwest.

Often, the Slovak men would come first, leaving their wives in the "old country" to emigrate later when the men were more established in work. Single women frequently arrived alone to complete a previously agreed-upon marriage (Bartalská, 1999). Men would settle in various neighborhoods with friends and relatives from the same village in the home country. Boarding homes were common. According to Bartalská, in *Slovak America*, a main source of income for Slovak women was running boarding houses. Women accounted for only 30% of the immigrations. Slovak women also worked as a supplemental labor force in factories and light industries. The Slovak church shared the center of social, religious, and political life with the "Slovak club" or *Jednota* club. Such clubs substituted for the family that wasn't here and aided in quelling the men's loneliness and isolation. Here they could relax and drink their beer and feel "at home." The *sokol*, a traditional Slovak gymnasium, provided a place to develop their love of sports, mainly gymnastics. An extensive network of Slovak American publications and financial, charitable foundations developed, primarily the Narodny Slovensky Spolok (National Slovak Society) and the First Catholic Slovak Ladies Association, which supported Slovaks here and in Czechoslovakia, while maintaining their connections with friends and family "back home." (Actually, the first women to become active in the Slovak societies were the wives of Lutheran ministers, journalists, and publishers.) The society's publication, *Jednota*, begun in 1891, became the literary almanac and mirror of Slovak life in America (Bartalská, 1999).

CZECH AND SLOVAK IMMIGRATION AFTER WORLD WAR I

The next wave of both Czech and Slovak immigrants occurred in 1938. Czechoslovakia was one of the first targets of Nazi Germany: thousands fled the country for political reasons. Many of them were of Jewish origin or Communist background.

A mass exodus started again after the Communist coup in 1948. People fled both harsh economic conditions and political repression. Within a few years, some 50,000 Czechs and Slovaks left the country. In 1949, they were forbidden to leave, although a few people escaped (by 1952 the number of crossings was reduced to 100 a month). During the worst Stalinist times, escape became impossible.

Another wave of immigration occurred in 1968, shortly after the Soviet invasion of the country. For a year, people were able to leave with the clothes on their backs and their suitcases. This group differed from those in 1938 and 1948. It was composed of much younger and well-educated people—students, journalists, artists, doctors, and others with technical and professional skills. Among them were women immigrating alone. Prior to this, 90% of the women came with husbands and were never consulted as to whether they wanted to emigrate! After 1969, although it became difficult to leave the country, refugees continued to find their way out.

Since the Velvet Revolution (the separation of Czechoslovakia into the Czech and Slovak Republics in 1993), Czechs and Slovaks have been able to emigrate freely and continue to do so, frequently for economic reasons. One Slovak American put it this way: "Under Communism there were jobs, but nothing on the shelves; now there is a lot on the shelves, but not enough jobs" (R. Lascek, personal communication, 2004).

PRAVDA VITEZI

My (J. K.'s) Bohemian aunt always said, "A Czech will die for a cause." She was referring to the strong nationalistic spirit of the Czech people. *Pravda vitezi* is translated as "The truth will win." The motto captures the Czech history of free thought and opposition politics. Czechs are usually highly individualistic, love to argue among themselves, and are actually fairly divisive, except when adversity unifies them in rebellion against foreign rule. Although appearing formal in their presentation, Czechs yield easily to melancholy and depression. Their emotionality finds expression in their music, from operas such as Smetana's *The Bartered Bride* and operettas such as *The Vagabond King* by Rudolf Friml, to the *New World Symphony* by Dvorak. If one listens to Slavonic dances or Dvorak's great cello concertos, one hears the same haunting undercurrents of strangeness and melancholy that have been described in their character. In *My Antonia* (1918), her famous novel of a Bohemian homesteading family, Willa Cather vividly depicts Antonia's father sadly fingering his violin and then committing suicide, unable to reconcile himself to the new way of life on the plains. Religion was always controversial. Most of the immigrants were nominally Catholic when they arrived. However, given their legacy of Jan Hus's dissent and their association of the Catholic Church with the cruelty and repression of the Germans, it is perhaps not surprising that one half to two thirds of them shortly left the Catholic Church. Free-thought societies and societies promoting faith in reason, science, and the individual conscience became a broad-based, organized movement among the Czechs in the United States. The free-thought societies were largely anticlerical. Communities could sometimes be polarized into Catholic and free-thinking camps. "Religiously, the Czechs are notable for the high proportion of people who label themselves atheists (58%)" (*The Czech Republic in Brief*, www.rect.muni.cz/ois/coming_to_brno/the_czech_republic_in_brief/index).

Later, Czech socialists played an important role in American politics. Not surprisingly, the most powerful Czech Americans in the 1860s and 1870s were journalists and newspaper editors. The Czech community supported special-interest papers for women, agriculture, poultry farmers, and others. The *Women's Gazette* in Chicago flourished from 1894 to 1947 as a feminist journal.

CZECH FAMILY AND CHARACTER

Czechs valued independence in their children, who grew up to be exceptionally self-reliant and mature. Families, particularly farm families, pulled together as a unit. Men were willing to do housework. Women were independent and self-reliant and could work the fields alongside the men. More than one generation often lived in the same household. Their values were democratic and pluralistic, imbued with work and thrift ethics. The Czechs were typically among the last to receive government assistance, even during the Great Depression. Education was prized, and their children established tremendously good school-attendance records. Record numbers of them went on to college. Czechs consider themselves peace loving, brave, generous, hardworking, and intelligent. They have also been prone to see themselves as somewhat backward, yet are frequently described by Slovaks as refined and cultured.

Many Czechs went on to prominence in the United States. They were eminent in science and scholarship. The first curator of the Smithsonian Museum of Physical Anthropology was Czech. The *sokols* (gymnastic societies) also flourished in the early settlements, and when we think today of superior physical abilities, one of the first great Czechs to come to mind is tennis player Martina Navratilova. They are also a cultured people. Think of Václav Havel, the recent Czech president and playwright; Milan Kundera, the great novelist in exile; and Milos Forman, the movie director.

Havel, a passionate champion of a multicultural civic society, wrote, "I am in favor of a political system based on the citizen, and recognizing all his fundamental civil and human rights in their universal validity, and equally applied, that is, no member of a single race, a single nation, a single sex, or a single religion may be endowed with basic rights that are any different from anyone else's" (1991, p. 49).

THERAPY WITH CZECH FAMILIES

The Czechs are justifiably proud people with rich cultural and intellectual traditions. One must acknowledge and honor that pride when working with them. Therapy with Czech families may best be approached through reason. It is extremely important to demonstrate respect for their intellectuality and their rich cultural history. Eastern Europeans can easily be confused with one another. However, even though Czechoslovakia was one country following World War I until 1993, most Czechs would be offended if you considered them Slovak. They consider themselves more cultured than their Slovak neighbors. Second- and third-generation Czechs may still refer to themselves as Bohemian in order to make this distinction.

Because Czechs have traditionally fought on religious grounds, it is important to find out what the family's framework of belief is, despite the folk wisdom of never mentioning religion or politics. Introduce controversial content areas such as politics and religion, and let the family members talk about their beliefs. Introducing such topics into conversation is a good way for the family therapist to get a sense of the family's identity. Always find out when the family immigrated to the United States. The immigration of the 1800s and early 1900s for economic reasons was very different from the largely politically motivated immigrations in 1948 and 1968.

Education is extraordinarily important to Czech Americans. The therapist can assign useful reading to Czech families, explain the ideas behind family therapy, and discuss the readings with them. Approach the therapy seriously, as if it is work. Talk, listen, and, possibly, play chess with Czech clients; by all means, ask for a piece of their apple strudel. Czech women are wonderful gardeners and cooks. A therapist can gain entry to their emotional life by expressing appreciation for music, dance, and theater.

Assess for depression and alcoholism, which occur frequently and seem to be syntonic with Czech family life. The work ethic that was so important in first- and second-generation Czechs may be weakening in later generations. As in other ethnic groups, the strain between the relative degrees of acculturation in different generations may produce conflict. Traditionally, for example, three generations might live together in one household when the first generation grew old. With a higher incidence of Czechs intermarrying with other groups and moving away from the family, such three-generational accommodation is somewhat less likely to occur and may be a point of conflict.

Ask directly about what the family considers appropriate roles for men and women. Often you will find that working hard and saving money are family endeavors, and everyone pulls his or her own weight, regardless of gender. The Czech family replicates Czech history in that family members are highly individualistic while remaining tightly bound within the family structure, just as Bohemia maintained an individual culture while under the larger authority of foreign rule.

When working with Czech family members, it is critical to respect their tremendous pride in self-sufficiency and to treat them as collaborators in the therapeutic endeavor rather than as recipients of help. Czech stoicism hides tremendous emotionality and deep grief for their losses. They are a sentimental people. They have endured hardship for centuries and know how to endure. They do not easily admit a need for assistance.

A Czech client put it this way:

"I remember many times that my father was in pain, but he would not show it. He had such calcification in his shoulder from bursitis that you could hear it cracking, but rather than take an anti-inflammatory drug, he did exercises with his arms, reaching as high as he could to release the shoulder muscle from the calcification deposits while grimacing in pain, but never making a sound. I didn't know then that his stoicism was central to his identity because I knew little of ethnic backgrounds. I did know that he was ferociously proud of being a man."

The following case example reflects Czech attitudes toward marriage, the rigidity of Catholicism, pragmatism regarding money, and gender prescriptions for the independence of women.

I (J. K.) was consulted by Marie, a Czech American woman in her 50s, whose presenting problem was her ambivalence about her long-term partnership with John, a man recently diagnosed with cancer, who was now pressing the issue of marriage. Despite a 20-year-long relationship, they lived in separate states. Marie, childless and never married, was happy with the status quo. John's chronic alcoholism actually provided an excuse for the distance she seemed to need in the relationship. Relationships for Marie had always been fraught with the dangers of too much dependence, and she was determined to be her own person even though diminished financial circumstances, the aging process, and her isolation in rural Maine caused her considerable anxiety about the future. She sometimes wondered if she should finally marry John for financially pragmatic reasons. Marie came into therapy for a few sessions, seeming to struggle almost as much with her ambivalence about therapy (issues of both dependence and money) as about her relationship. Her early life was marked by the secret of her alcoholic father's suicide when she was 9, poverty, and the rigidity of her Catholic upbringing, which she later renounced, becoming atheist like many Czechs.

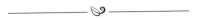

Martin Vortruba (personal communication, 2004) completed a study assessing the range of views on what marriage is supposed to be among the four
Central European post-Communist groups: Czechs, Slovaks, Poles, and Hungarians. He found the Czechs' opinions to be the closest to the Slovaks. However, the Czechs took the gloomiest view of romantic love and marriage. Vortruba reports the percentages of those who agreed with the following statements:

	Slovaks	Czechs
Marriage means the end of romance.	11%	19%
Marriage means the end of freedom.	19%	27%
A woman should give up her job when she has a baby.	15%	20%
It's all right to have a child without being married.	40%	24%
It's all right if a couple choose not to have a child.	24%	26%
It doesn't matter if the wife is older than her husband.	50%	62%
It's all right if a couple live together unmarried.	37%	55%

Understanding the Czechs' pessimism about marriage, their financial pragmatism, their high tolerance for alcoholism, and their skepticism about religion, and religion in other groups often underwriting marriage (Marie renounced her rigid Catholic upbringing as a young woman), further delineates the context in which the therapist understood Marie's reluctance to marry. Once Marie made the decision not to marry, she left therapy satisfied that she had accomplished her goal.

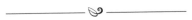

Finally, money is an issue with Czechs. They have worked hard to own their own land, their own houses and businesses. They have saved for the future. Therapy must not be frivolous or a luxury or they will not think it is worth paying for. Therapy should be hard work that will benefit the family. Doing therapy with Czech American families, however, can be extremely rewarding, because once the therapist has convinced them intellectually of the worth of the endeavor, they will make a commitment to what they see as self-improvement. Czechs love to learn.

SLOVAK FAMILY AND CHARACTER

Despite the upheavals of war and industrialization and the resulting diaspora, there are attributes that remain common to all Slovak descendants. The primary values of the Slovak people continue to be education and family, in distinction to the dominant U.S. values of money and individualism. The Slovak class structure continues to be a traditional one, in that it reflects differences according to function—laborers, workers, and intelligentsia—rather than one in which divisions are based on amount of money (M. Votruba, personal communication, 2004). Religion plays a strong role in rural Slovakia, whereas it is less important to the Czechs (60% are Catholic in Slovakia, 39% in the Czech Republic). Prior to 1989, the primary reasons for emigration had been both political and economic. After 1989, the primary reasons were economic.

I (R. M. G.) was born in the United States, but my mother was first-generation Czechoslovak and my father was born in Slovakia. All of my grandparents and almost all of their children lived in Slovak neighborhoods, went to Slovak Catholic churches, spoke Slovak, married Czechs, Poles, or Slovaks, and attended Czech, German, and Slovak social clubs. Slovaks, in general, are clannish, keep the same values, and marry one another. So the Slovak heritage remains strong even in an assimilationist culture such as America. This means there are more similarities between first- and second-generation Slovaks than might be first imagined.

In Slovakia every town, it seemed, had a church, a band, and a choral group. Its people love to sing, and they love music. Colorful and lively, loving the outdoors, countryside, and sports, respecting the value of education, they are described as easygoing yet determined, hardworking, hospitable, loyal, generous, loving to laugh, loving food, and good cooks Even today, everyone who can has a small house in the countryside or in a small village, where he or she keeps ducks, a garden for flowers, and a garden for vegetables.

Slovaks were primarily agrarian, so family life revolved around a large main room that was kitchen and sitting room. Here all of the activity took place. Three generations lived in the same house, and it was not uncommon for a newly married daughter to live with her family until she and her husband could find and afford a home of their own.

This arrangement also provided for the grandparents, whom the families always took care of in their homes. There are few old folks homes in Slovakia. As the Slovak consul general said, it is neither polite nor responsible to put parents in a home. It is the children's duty to take care of them. Parents sacrificed for the children; for example, when any decisions were to be made, they always put the children first. (Family sacrifice is one of the characteristics that was used to describe the Slovaks, along with hardworking and heavy drinking.) Parents, although poor and living on a pension, continue to buy presents for their children who may be richer and more educated. To support your children is valued as part of the "sense of life." Even if the three generations did not live together, their closeness was continued with regular contact and visits (Slovak Consul General, personal communication, 2004). Intergenerational relationships are more sacred than the marital bonds.

Such dependency continues throughout life. Even with today's greater mobility, the three generations continue the responsibility, dependency, and emotional connections between grandparents, parents, and children. Parents are strict but protective. Grandparents are frequently described as "nourishing" to their grandchildren. The grandfather is often seen as "honest and fair." Within the family, children are taught to look out for one another, although there may be sibling rivalry and competition for the mother's attention.

When in trouble, a Slovak talks to a parent or to a good friend, who can be quite blunt about what he or she thinks should be done. If there is a problem between friends or relatives, they argue it out, which sometimes leads to no contacts or a cutoff for years. Some are known to hold grudges (a woman from Western Slovakia pointed out that such people are those from Eastern Slovakia!). An example of this trait, and of maternal protectiveness, is the story of a mother and her two young children who were playing on a next-door neighbor's porch; the neighbor chased them off the porch, for no clear reason other than she did not want to be bothered. That was the last time, in 30 years, that the children's mother spoke to this neighbor—and these women had been friends!

Drinking is another popular way of "solving the problem," which is not shameful although alcoholism is. "Drinking sprees" provide a "cure" for the problem. This numbing can enable people to say, "We have no problem" (Kerr, 1996). Alcoholism is never talked about outside the family. It is a rite of passage for young men to "learn how to handle their liquor." Disputes are argued out, or the parties withdraw from one another permanently. Money is not discussed even within the family. Things seen as shameful, such as mental illness, sexual deviancy, and criminality, are not discussed at all. Homosexuals are not ostracized in this culture; they are accepted, but are not actively supported or discussed openly.

The marital relationship is weak and less important than the relationship with the family of origin (Kerr, 1996). It is common for husband and wife to quarrel, but this too is done behind closed doors. Divorce is more common today but still rather shameful. Another typical way of coping is to say that "everyone has that problem!" People do not discuss emotional problems and generally would not go beyond the family or good friends to seek help.

Under Communism, as Professor Votruba of the University of Pittsburgh stated, nothing of personal significance was ever discussed in the media. "People expected a certain economic equality, unless they themselves were ahead of the others. The government was supposed to take care of many things that in this country are taken care of by charities and volunteerism. There was little appreciation of compromise—something was either right and should be carried out, or wrong, and should be punished."

There have been a number of changes in family life since independence (1989, the Velvet Revolution) and since the split between the Czech Republic and Slovakia (referred to as the Velvet Separation, 1993) Falling living standards and increasing disparity in wealth (difficulty in finding employment after Communism) have had their normal effects on family life in Slovakia. Traditionally, husbands earned the money for the family and were unchallenged as family head, and wives did the child rearing and taking care of the home, making the money "stretch," while they also worked on the farm. Now, the patriarchal family is becoming egalitarian. The higher cost of living and increased educational opportunities (which began under Communism) have propelled wives into the workforce in significant numbers. Long-distance commuting and spouses moving away for work, with only weekly or monthly visits back home, are leading to new stresses on marital relationships.

Hospitality, both here and in the Czech Republic, are outstanding Czech and Slovak characteristics. When I (R. M. G.) was interviewing a Slovak family in Brooklyn who knew me only as a friend of a non-Slovak employer, not only did they invite me to their home but they offered to come to pick me up and show me the way from the highway so I would not get lost. When I was visiting in Prague and could not figure out how to reach the address of an apartment by car, a Czech man got into the car, took us to the house, and jumped out, wishing us a cheerful *Dobrou noc,* or "Good evening."

Several Slovaks stated that they are often generous to their own detriment. They are often loyal to a fault. They do not like to hurt others' feelings, and, if they do, it leads to more guilt feelings. For a therapist seeing a family, this is an important consideration. A family therapist should not expect confrontation or the expression of negative feelings between generations. Moreover, because of their respect for parents and grandparents, children will not say what is on their minds if it is disrespectful to the parents or if it is an angry comment. "Everything comes easily to the son" is a common belief, reflected in women being more ambitious than men.

Slovak siblings and couples dispute among themselves, but not with those of other generations. Slovaks are known to be fond of routine and do not like change. Children are frequently scolded by their parents, and they are taught to forgive one another so that a transgression does not "eat at your heart" (interview with D. Pomple, 2004). A 30-year-old Slovak carpenter I encountered said that American expressions of pride in self or in children are looked down upon as boasting. Slovak mothers are critical and protective simultaneously. Teachers can be critical of their students in front of the class; this is acceptable to their parents. Parents may be affectionate with their children within the family, but expressions or demonstrations of love—except to small children, or in courtship or erotic situations—are rare, low key, and, in any case, not expected (Votruba interview, 2004).

SLOVAK ADAPTATION IN THE UNITED STATES

If the family members (or individual) who are being seen are recent immigrants, their difficulties may include adapting to American life. In Slovakia, all is family related. Slovakians are not prepared for the individualism that is a primary characteristic of American culture. Because of a lack of self-assurance, recent emigrants may minimize their problems, yet behave intolerantly and judgmentally toward others.

The family is so deeply important that a Slovak emigrant must reestablish it here or feel extreme isolation. Fraternal lodges can provide this connection for the men, as years ago they provided the closeness that was absent in a marital relationship (Kerr, 1996, p. 677).

In Slovakia, there is little intermarriage. In America, this tradition continues, with the first generation tending to marry within the culture or other Eastern Europe nationalities, and the second generation opening up to include Western European countries. Secrecy continues to be a prominent Slovak characteristic. What goes on within the "walls" of the family home is no one's business. Despite the trends in Slovakia that are affecting the family negatively, most Slovaks expect relationships to continue as usual between parents and children, grandparents and parents, and so forth. This emphasis on tradition may be even more pronounced for recent Slovak immigrants; in their homes they want the familiar family life of support and physical closeness they remember, even as it fades away in Slovakia. In Slovakia, there are few resources to help with psychological problems. Other than talking to a parent or another family member, or turning to alcohol, there is nothing.

For instance, when a Czech psychiatrist was asked how families in Czechoslovakia obtained help for their problems, he answered, "The village elders and family relatives would dress up in their 'Sunday Clothes' if it was not a Sunday (and usually it was) and would all go over to the family and solve the problem in their home by 'talking it over' and giving advice."

Because the Slovaks and Czechs tend to minimize their problems and are very resistant to change, the likelihood of their arriving on a therapist's doorstep asking for help is low. Second- or third-generation immigrants in the United States are more likely to seek professional help. Consider the following case example:

A Slovak father and his daughter, Anna, were referred to an Eastern European therapist by her colleague. The teenage daughter was acting out, that is, not listening to the father or to the grandmother with whom they lived. She was attending rock concerts with older friends during the school week. Her grades at school were fine, although she was bored. The grandmother would call Anna derogatory names in Slovak when she came home late. The father would not protect his daughter from this name-calling. The parents were divorced, and a brother lived with the mother. There was considerable sibling rivalry. The parents constantly fought verbally, and father and son clashed verbally and physically. The mother was more assimilated than the father, who spoke Slovak in the home to the children and to his parents. The father's relaxation consisted of leading a band (he played at Slovak and Polish weddings). The problem of not listening to the father or to the grandmother (even worse!) when they gave orders or, the way it was done in the old country, was an issue. The father had no respected figures (e.g., parish priest) or relatives here to help him. The daughter wanted to live with the mother, who was lenient or "Americanized," so she made life miserable for the father, blaming him for the divorce, in the hope that he would finally relent. A large part of the problem was the disrespect shown to the grandmother, and to the father in front of the grandmother. The mother–son bond was strong in both generations. The therapist, understanding Slovak values, handled this case by first establishing her credentials and nationality with the grandmother and the father and discussing the differences in the ways of raising children here. She suggested keeping some of the "old ways" while adding some new ones, which included reinforcing the father's being in charge while maintaining respect for the grandmother; a session with the siblings to develop more support for Anna; and a session with Anna alone to give her a place to express the negative feelings toward her grandmother and father that she could not express directly as it was disrespectful. Additional work with the mother and daughter was needed, but the father objected to including her.

———————— ✤ ————————

THERAPY WITH SLOVAK FAMILIES

Familiarity with Slovak history and respect for Slovak nationality can ally the therapist with the family. As mentioned earlier, Slovaks are family centered, which is good for family therapy; the marital relationship is less important. Dependency within the generations and the importance of the family of origin can be issues for a partner of another culture. This can also mean that the means of differentiation from the family of origin must be understood within these cultural parameters. An example is the pattern of the adult children moving very far away or staying very close to home.

Thus, it makes sense to bring the entire family to a session. However, even when they are in the therapist's office, it is hard to break into a family system. It is easier if the therapist is also of Slovak or Eastern European origin. However, if not, the family may "adopt" the therapist as an outsider (Kerr, 1996, p. 678). It is important to support their coming in, as they may not be good at asking for help, preferring to deny that there are any problems. Secrecy includes not discussing shameful things outside the family, which include alcohol, abuse, and marital problems. In Slovak families, loyalty is strong, a sense of humor is necessary, and their outlook is intergenerational and child focused. A therapist can enter the system through the children. They typically respect the therapist's authority and knowledge, especially if he or she is nonjudgmental of them. The therapist cannot expect the children to "tell off" their parents or grandparents or say what would be considered disrespectful to them, even what would be considered acceptable—if not encouraged—behavior (to speak your mind) to most Americans. Talking things over endlessly is not of value; "things are simply done," not discussed, except for ethical issues. Women are generally more influential in family decisions than men, although this fact is never mentioned. For the family therapist, this implies the building of a positive alliance with the mother in the family.

Whatever the actual causes of its difficulties, the most likely reason for a Slovak family to come for treatment is a child-focused problem, or perhaps a difficulty with the older generation of parents. They are least likely to come for a marital problem. Integrating the "old" traditions of family interdependency with American individualism, personal goals, and ambitions into the new history of the family is an important goal. Turning a family's ability to keep secrets into a "strength rather than a pathology" (Kerr, 1996) can challenge a therapist.

How important is culture? Its impact is subtle and strong. A Slovak friend once said, "When I traced my roots in Slovakia, it put a lens over so much of my life. I couldn't understand why my family always used the back door and not the front door. Now I know: Everyone I visited in Slovakia uses the back door, never the front door!" A back door is less formal, usually opens into the kitchen, the heart of the family, and warmly welcomes the arrival into their lives where they can be generous with food and drink—yet not necessarily with their thoughts and feelings until they get to know you.

ACKNOWLEDGMENTS

Our thanks to John Howard; Martin Holub; Jitka and Pavel Illner, MD; Yvonne Jungle; Peter Kussi, PhD; Mark G. Lazansky, MD; Elizabeth Hudacek; Agnes and Margaret Trily; Denise Pompl; Sr. Emilia Suchon, OSF; Jana Volavka; and Martin Zolatar and his mother.

REFERENCES

Bartalská, L. (1999). Slovak America. In I. Reguli, J. A. Holy, & D. F. Tanzone (Eds.), *Slovenska Amerika* (pp. 20–23). Bratislava, Slovak Republic: Gabrila Fila Advertising.

Cather, W. (1918). *My Ántonia*. New York: Houghton Mifflin.

Denis, E. (1917). *La question d'autriche—les Slovaques*. Paris: Deleagrave.

Havel, V. (1991, December 5). On home. *New York Review of Books*.

Kerr, S. (1996). Slovak families. In M. McGoldrick, J. Giordano, & J. K. Pearce (Eds.), *Ethnicity and family therapy* (2nd ed., pp. 673–679). New York: Guilford Press.

Kirschbaum, S. J. (1995). *A history of Slovakia: The struggle for survival*. New York: St. Martin's Press.

Kundera, M. (1980). *The book of laughter and forgetting*. New York: Penguin Books.

Sociologicky Casopis. (1992, August). *Sociologicky Casopis, 28* [Special issue]. Slovakia.

CHAPTER 54

Polish Families

John Folwarski
Joseph Smolinski Jr.

Q: Who was Alexander Graham Kowalski?
A: The first telephone Pole.

Q: What are the best 5 years of a Pole's life?
A: Third grade.

Poles have for a long time felt a strong need to fight anti-Polish defamation (Radzilowski, 1998), an issue that goes very deep for Poles, who have for so long been understandably defensive because of their having been humiliated by constant jokes that portray them as ignorant, brutish boors. Now and then a Polish joke, like the first one above, might be said to have a certain "class" (good humor) and even somehow thereby transcend the more common derogatory nature of most ethnic jokes. The tasteless humor of the second joke is far more common, as is the one about how to recognize the groom at a Polish wedding (he's the one in the clean bowling shirt).

Although all ethnic humor conveys to us something profound about society's perceptions of an ethnic group, it also is a hallmark of society's need to form social, racial, ethnic, and class stereotypes, as well as providing any given group an option to distance itself from its own difficulties by laughing at its own foibles or tasting superiority by battering another group. In the case of Polish jokes, the preponderance of transparently mean-spirited, tasteless battering puts them in the latter category. Nonetheless, they also give us insight, albeit in a twisted fashion, about an underlying reality—the reality of the Polish peasant's ambivalence toward upward mobility and education. These attitudes were born of centuries of exploitation by the Polish nobility and are accentuated by the Pole's fierce resistance to the customs and mores of other cultures. This resistance, in turn, has its roots in a long history of invasion and partition of Poland. Their forced disappearance from the map, for whole centuries at a time, led the Polish peasantry to absorb the identity of the Polish nation into their very character. It is the reality of these attitudes within their cultural and historical context that we must grasp if we are to deal effectively with Polish Americans in a therapeutic setting (Mondykowski, 1982). This chapter discusses patterns of Polish belief and behavior, shaped by their particular history, that may contribute to a positive, useful, and respectful attitude in working with Polish American families.

Today Poland is vibrantly independent and planning to stay that way (Lipniacka, 2000). Poles do not need outside criticism, jokes included, inasmuch as they are supremely self-critical; they know themselves inside out, blemishes and all. There is no problem, be it social, political, economic, national, or local, that they have not regularly and minutely dissected, put together again in every order imaginable, and argued over endlessly. There is no national characteristic, real or imagined, that has not been lamented and its consequences listed (Lipniacka, 2000). And yet Polish American families have often been profoundly distanced from their heritage. Therapy with them may require reconnecting them to their lost sense of identity, just as Poland's identity has required reconnecting the nation to its historical identity, despite the efforts of many countries to annihilate it over the past thousand years. Poland has been fought on or over at some time or another by virtually every country in Europe (Lipniacka, 2000).

THE POLISH PEOPLE IN CONTEXT

Poland's boundaries have been threatened throughout history. Attack and occupation by foreign armies and, finally, the deliberate and methodical partitioning of Poland by its three neighbors—Russia, Prussia, and Austria-Hungary—resulted in its disappearance from the map of Europe for 125 years. The Polish Republic rose again in the aftermath of World War I and existed for 20 years until it was destroyed in World War II. Radical social changes are not uncommon in Europe, certainly not uncommon for Poland, and the need to forge and retain a positive ethnic identity is an abiding theme for Poles collectively and individually.

The election of the Cardinal of Krakow to the papacy in 1978 shone the international spotlight on Poland. The new pope's visit to his homeland in 1979 was the "final breach in the wall behind which [the Poles] had been kept since 1945" (Zamoyski, 1988, p. 389). By 1980, the Polish trade unions had begun the process that led, 10 years later, to the dissolution of the Polish Communist Party and the election of Lech Walesa as president. Polish emigrés around the world watched events in Poland, including large numbers of new, politically active immigrants who had left the country as the Communist influence waned. A Polish cardinal and labor leader offered the promise of reshaping the image and influence of Poland.

There is renewed interest in the long-standing tension regarding Polish–Jewish relationships that is centered on the 1941 Jedwabne massacre. Shortly after the Nazi invasion of Poland, a segment of this town's ethnic Poles turned on their Jewish neighbors. In one particularly horrific incident, hundreds were assaulted and herded into a barn, which was then doused with gas and set ablaze. Nearly all of Jedwabne's 1,600 Jews died in the massacre. Jan Gross's book, *Neighbors* (2001), has revived passionate exchanges about Poles being not only victims, but also victimizers, a discussion whose resolution "is crucial for Poles' own sense of identity" (Wesolowsky, 2001).

Recently, Poland again received international attention by agreeing to become part of the U.S.-led forces in Iraq. Although Poland received "little military aid from the United States . . . , when the Bush administration asked Poland about commanding one of the three military stabilization zones that the United States envisioned for postwar Iraq [roughly one quarter the size of Poland itself], the flattered Polish government quickly said yes" (Hundley, 2003). Given the fact that Poland "was for centuries dominated and, at times, obliterated by its more powerful neighbors," the historical irony of Richard Bernstein's *New York Times* caption, "Poland upstages, and irks, European power-houses" (2003b), is not lost on Poles here and abroad. Poland in this case had immediately invited Germany to join with it in Iraq, and Germany flatly refused. Poland's decision was certainly not made in order to derive any historical "perverse satisfaction" (Bernstein, 2003a); debates about whether or not to join the cause were as heated in Poland as they were in the United States. However, it is worth noting that such satisfactions do linger as needs in the lifeblood of a culture. Most notably, for example, the Great Partitions were well remembered by Poles and Polish Americans when, at Yalta in 1945, Poland again was left to be devoured by foreign powers.

In 1998, John Radzilowski spoke of the need to "fight anti-Polish defamation, an issue that raises passions and occupies more time and energy than any other. . . . It is time to re-think and plan a way to end this problem once and for all, so our children and grandchildren don't have to listen to 'Polack' jokes and lies about how Poland was a Nazi ally" (p. 4). He added that there is also a need "to put time and energy into creating positive images of Polish Americans and Poland." We wholeheartedly agree with that need.

IMMIGRATION TO THE UNITED STATES

The first Poles in the New World were glassblowers and craftsmen who came to the Jamestown Colony around 1608. Poles were invited to settle in New Holland about 1658. During the 18th century, small groups of wealthy Polish gentry immigrated to settle in the colonies. In the aftermath of the Great Partitions, the Polish tragedy of lost statehood was viewed sympathetically in the United States. Nobles who had lost titles and had come as political exiles were seen as romantic, exotic figures. Americans were inspired by the Polish struggles for independence from their Russian, Prussian, and Austrian occupiers. Not unlike those of France or America, the reforms of the Polish Enlightenment period were actively opposed to the needs of the monarchs. Topics like freedom of conscience and religious toleration, ethnicity as a basis for national identity, and a constitution as the foundation for a republic (developed in Poland in 1791) were intolerable to Russia's Catherine the Great, and she ordered the invasion of Poland. Pulaski and Kosciuszko, probably two of the best-known Polish figures in America, were leaders in uprisings against the partitioning powers as well as key figures in the American Revolution.

This noble romanticized ethos definitely did not benefit the more than 3 million illiterate, landless Polish peasants who between 1870 and 1914 immigrated to the United States from the Russian, Prussian, and Austrian sections of the former Poland. The majority settled in large cities, clustered in the neighborhoods called Polonia that were organized around the local Catholic church. The Polish language was spoken, and patterns of family and village life were replicated; simultaneously, enormous pressure was exerted on the new arrivals to become Americanized.

Because Poland did not exist, the immigrants' official documents often indicated that they were of Russian, Prussian, or Austrian origin, which also created a problem for later descendants researching their roots. In addition, "people who had embarked together as neighbors in Poland (Jews, Poles, Lithuanians, and Byelorussians) became necessarily attached to their distinct national group with its own cultural life immediately upon arrival. Similarities were ignored, differences were emphasized, and common origins obscured" (Davies, 1992, p. 258). Their very survival depended on the support of their church and the fraternal and mutual aid societies of their ethnic community.

More recent Polish immigrants have been professionals and intellectuals with a notably higher cultural and educational status than previous groups. Following World War II, from 1945 to 1960, they were people who were displaced by the war, Jews of Polish origin, and couples of mixed marriages in which one spouse was Jewish. They were "invited" by the Polish government to emigrate, to give up their Polish citizenship, and they left Poland with great bitterness. The Poland they departed from was not the Poland in the memories of earlier groups of Polish Americans. They left a country devastated by World War II. The destruction of Poland and its people was second in Hitler's mind only to the destruction of the Jews.

After the suppression of Solidarity (the national confederation of independent labor unions in Poland, headed by Lech Walesa) by the Polish Communist government in 1980, new immigrants who had grown up in the Communist People's Republic of Poland arrived. They were accustomed to a society in which consumer goods were scarce and opposition to authority was the main tool of survival. Beyond Catholicism and the Polish language, these immigrants had little in common with the older residents of Polonia. They revitalized Polish American communities as they opened new businesses, filled the churches (especially for Polish masses), sent their children to parochial schools, and founded new secular Polish schools.

Conflict between what can be called the "old-guard" Polonia and newer Polish immigrants was no small matter. Radzilowski (1997) painfully recounts the ingratitude newer immigrants showed toward those from old Polonia, essentially using them to get settled here, then disavowing them entirely, viewing them as engaging in "low-brow activities like polka or folk dancing" (p. 2). In her study of recent Polish immigrants to Chicago, Erdmans (2001) examines this tension between Polish immigrants and Polish American ethnics (people born in the United States who still identify with Polish ancestry). She notes that Poles, like most immigrants, certainly experienced a drop in social status. Having to learn a new language, having weaker network supports, and being unfamiliar with American institutions made negotiation of a person's societal position difficult. Polish immigrants have naturally turned to Polish Americans (and their organizational structures) for help. Polish organizations here maintained cultural attachment by visiting Poland, learning its history, language, customs, foods, and arts. Erdmans maintains that the needs of the newer immigrants were the opposite. They needed to learn English, study the landscape of a new country, find ways to access this country's government agencies, recertify their degrees, and find jobs. They were focused on learning new cultural practices, in effect, discounting the value and significance of carrying on the ways of a home left behind. Because Polish Americans and their organizations were ill equipped to negotiate the differences related to the structural/symbolic nature of immigrant needs, newer arrivals perceived the established community as not helping. The experience of immigrant Poles being discounted by the dominant culture certainly did not facilitate resolution of these issues.

It is without a doubt important for a therapist working with Poles to locate the family on an immigration time line, as closeness and distance from different points of origin will certainly affect experience, perception, and expectation. Therapists can ask to be educated about the family members' perception of their own ethnic and historical issues. The therapist, as well as at times the family, may be surprised by some of the answers, or by a seeming diffidence or reluctance to answer. A few case examples from different periods are presented later. First, however, the following sections discuss some cultural issues as they apply to Poles.

WHAT'S IN A NAME?: STANLEY KOWALSKI VERSUS BLANCHE DUBOIS

In America, surely the quintessentially recognizable Polish name is Stanley Kowalski, whether because it is as common as Smith or Jones or whether as a result of Tennessee Williams's well-known play, *A Streetcar Named Desire*. Gladsky (1992) argued that the critical reception of the play, together with the film version, testified to "America's continuing fascination with Poles . . . while paradoxically reinforcing America's negative perceptions of Polish character" (p. 137). A look at Stanley Kowalski's name and character is worthwhile.

According to Lopata (1975), changing one's name is a major form of reaction against the kind of negative self-image that Gladsky talks about and Stanley Kowalski battles against. Lopata's data suggested that Poles change their names more than any other ethnic group. Polish families seeking treatment are sometimes readily identifiable by their names. At other times, therapists discover the Polish roots of a client only by doing a three- or four-generational genogram. Even then, the names may not reveal Polish origins, as many have Anglicized their names to hide their Polishness for a variety of reasons, including the promotion of social and economic mobility.

There is considerable ethnic tension in the play between the French DuBois's sense "cultural superiority" and the Pole's sense of "cultural inferiority" (Gladsky, 1992, p. 150). In the 1950s and still today, Marlon Brando's portrayal of Stanley Kowalski is almost a caricature of the "low-brow" qualities that most Polish jokes disdainfully ridicule. He, of course, keeps his name, but in one volcanic outburst he disavows his ethnic self:

I'm not a Polack. People from Poland are Poles, not Polacks. But what I am is one hundred percent American, born and raised in the greatest country on earth and proud as hell of it, so don't ever call me a Polack. (p. 152)

Stanley protests too much, and indeed we are suggesting that many Polish Americans often find themselves unwittingly doing the same thing. Name change is one way Poles can avoid the discomfort of this kind of shameful denigration.

CLASS

We do not know when or how Polish names became associated with the lower class, nor how and when French names were, at times, associated with the upper class, but there is no doubt that in Williams's play, Kowalski and DuBois were not only names, but markers of class tension and conflict.

Poles and Polish Americans are indeed very class conscious, yet are ambivalent about upward mobility, despite their hunger for status and social recognition. This conflict has complex roots in the history of Polish class structure and stratification and in the influence of French culture, manners, and habits on the déclassé *szlachta* (nobility). All three of the powers involved in the Great Partitions of Poland were "consistently opposed to the new ideas emanating from France . . . so the Poles and the French were natural partners" (Davies, 1992, p. 161). They looked to France and Napoleon as possible saviors, hoping to restore the kingdom taken from them just 10 years earlier. Although this never happened, "Poles rallied to the French colors by the thousands, their inimitable code of honor and sacrifice taken up by emigré Polish legions" (p. 162). Napoleon called the War of 1812 his "Polish War," and his defeat by the Russians ended "nearly twenty years of Poland's affair with France" (p. 162).

Eva Hoffman (1989) has remarked that "Poland is still a Francophile culture" (p. 12): The values and high style of French nobility matched the values and style of Old Poland's noble ethos. The importance of noble birth, for example, remains central in the Polish psyche. "Lineage gives a solidity . . . it implies a moral uprightness and the dignity of not having to prove yourself, of being somebody to begin with" (p. 44). However, having class is different than rising in class. For countless Polish peasants and their descendants who felt deceived and abused by both Polish and French nobility, money and power and position have always been suspicious, if not immoral, attributes. Many old guard Polish families were caught in the double bind of encouraging success while being ashamed of it. Newer immigrants may indeed have a different attitude toward "materialism," inasmuch as their deprivations were not a result of Polish class structure (princes and peasants) but imposed by Communist overlords.

It is puzzling how such a double binding occurred. Perhaps peasants and other disenfranchised Polish emigrés, in order to retain their dignity and their own idea of Polishness, unwittingly contributed to the propagation of these stereotypes by defensively needing to contrast themselves with snobbishly wealthy noble intelligentsia. No matter how it happened, it is probably true that any form of elitism is inherently alien to the average Pole's sense of what it means to have "true grit," Polish style.

Polish Americans may vary in the degree to which they experience their Polishness as problematic and the extent to which they will admit it. Their ambivalence toward their own ethnicity is linked to a history of numerous "invasions, partitions, occupations, and border shifts that have changed, sometimes overnight, the national identity of large numbers of Poles" (Gladsky, 1992, p. 3). Polishness has been brutalized by historical events, distorted by the media and literature, and ridiculed by countless Polish jokes. Regardless of class, education, or socioeconomic level, Poles in the United States continue to be afflicted by what Gladsky referred to as "unresolved problems of social belonging" (p. 287), causing some to view their ethnicity as "a prison" (p. 148), something shameful to be hidden. Defensiveness, a nationally necessary historical trait, has become a personality trait.

This is not to suggest that Polish Americans in Chicago, Buffalo, or Detroit are walking around riddled with anxiety lest someone find out they are Polish. However, even that is not far-fetched. For years I (J. F.) worked with another therapist named Tom Summers. Though I often commented on Polish issues, Tom never once indicated that he was also Polish; years later, upon meeting Tom's brother I learned that the family's real name was Suchomski and that their father had changed it, as the brother said, "to get a fresh start." Such denial serves a function; it is also always costly. The cost of disconnecting from one's roots, as Tom Suchomski apparently did, is worth evaluating. Eileen Simpson (1987) wrote, "The United States, which has been called the home of the persecuted and the dispossessed, has been since its founding an asylum for emotional orphans" (p. 221), adding, "Many who have assimilated by changing their names and foregoing their roots, have no way of estimating their spiritual loss" (p. 225).

In Gladsky's (1992) analysis of writers of Polish descent, to be Polish is "to accept ethnicity as a synonym for an identity that differentiates the self of childhood and beyond from that of others and that provides a touchstone for experience and memory" (p. 226). A touchstone for experience and memory, a way of meaningfully connecting one's historical past and living present, one's inherited culture with one's choices, is exactly what can be lost if disavowing one's roots becomes a way of surviving or thriving. This is part of what the Suchomski family lost when its members' ethnic identity went in hiding behind the name Summers.

ALCOHOLISM

Writing about his visits to Poland, Steven (1982) states, "It is impossible to visit Poland and not be struck by the inordinately heavy drinking among all sections of society. . . . Those used to Western social drinking habits need a strong constitution to match the serious drinking of the Poles" (p. 13). Poles defensively say that heavy drinking has always been a part of their culture, that vodka is even more enshrined in the Polish tradition than it is in the Russian. The attitude in Poland has evolved from the idea that alcoholism is a moral fault to viewing it as a serious illness, but the underlying, abiding attitude of Poles is that drinking is a natural and positive part of life (Morawski, 1992). The hardworking, hard-drinking Pole is the "salt of the earth." An old Polish proverb captures the tone: "*Maciek zmarl, lezy na desce / A pil by jesce*" ("Maciek died and he lies on a plank, but he'd still like a drink" (Knab, 1993, p. 262).

What happens, then, when alcohol moves to alcoholism, when drinking becomes a major social problem, when the salt, so to speak, has lost its savor? Tryzno, Pedagogic, Grvdziak-Sobczy, Prawn, and Marowski (1989) identify Poland's alcoholism as one of the two major causes of divorce, the other being marital infidelity. Furthermore, 21.3% of Poland's children are raised in alcoholic families, and violence within families whose member(s) are abusing alcohol is two to three times greater than in the general population (Tryzno et al., 1989). Tryzno and colleagues postulate that the levels of abuse are probably much higher than the figures indicate, because Poles consider outside help an attack on the family, "which, in spite of disputes, confrontations, and injuries, proves itself resistant to outside influences" (p. 268).

Resistance to acknowledging or recognizing alcohol as directly related to family problems is stronger in Polish families than in many other ethnic groups. This attitude is replicated in the United States. Drinking is accepted as a norm (there are more bars than churches in Polonia) and, in conjunction with the dictum "Do not shame your family!" contributes to the denial that is so centrally a part of progressive alcohol dependence and the family's enabling role. Therapists can be seen as "outside influences," as accusers—not as helpers—and there is resistance not only to giving up alcohol, but also to exposing the family to shame.

POLES AND JEWS

The mutual antipathy between Poles and Polish Jews deserves special mention. Few subjects are more sensitive in Polish circles today than Poland's relations with her Jewish minority (Steven, 1982). Hoffman (1989) remembers her mother's warning, "There is an anti-Semite in every Pole" (p. 33). At a dinner party, I (J. F.) was told by a Jewish American that "everyone's allowed one prejudice; mine is Poles."

Much of the hostility between the two groups relates to Polish collaboration, or the perception of such collaboration, with the Nazis, what Gladsky called "a Holocaust backlash against the Poles" (1992, p. 142). Conceivably, some of the rancor held by Poles toward Jews comes from the seeming impossibility of withstanding the shame of being accused of some "unforgivable sin" (a familiar concept in Polish Catholic culture), such as collaborating with the Nazis. Pointing out the historical fact that Hitler set out to systematically obliterate all of Poland (both Jewish and Catholic), recounting the many stories of mutual heroism of these groups, or the fact that "penalties in Poland for helping Jews were the most Draconian in occupied Europe . . . automatically punishable by the death of entire families" (Bartoszewski, 1991, p. 28), to a Pole seems hopelessly reductionist or feebly apologetic, and to a Jew may seem condescendingly gratuitous.

In Poland after the Holocaust, the word "Jew" was heavily loaded. The much cherished old image of the Jewish innkeeper as the wise man of the village, as one of the recognized authorities on history and culture as well as business, was no longer available. However, conflicts and connections did not start there. As mentioned earlier, current dialogues about the Jedwabne incident are charged with deep historical intensity. Communist-era historians have blamed Germans for the massacre, insisting that Poles merely assisted the occupiers. Upon ending their 3-year investigation into the events of July 10, 1941, the National Remembrance Institute determined that Poles both provided a "passive presence" and committed the violence (Pasek, 2003, p. 5). Jewish leaders were reported as crediting the inquiry with "restoring Poles' historical memory" prompting "a reckoning with history in Polish society" (p. 5). Neglecting to attempt a resolution of this issue is a cutoff from self that Poles should not endure.

Briefly, such a reckoning would be helped by revisiting both connections and conflicts, some of which Poles and Polish Americans, as well as therapists working with their families, may not know at all. These include the following: In 1264 Polish king Boleslav the Pious issued the Charter of Protection and Liberties for the Jews. Then, in 1354, Casimir the Great ratified and extended these provisions and issued similar charters to the Jews of Lithuania (which united with Poland in 1386) and other Polish cities. Later, in 1551, King Sigismund Augusus authorized Jews to elect their own judges, answerable only to the king. The Jews gradually assumed the character of a legal estate.

For generations, therefore, Poland "continued to appear in the light of a land of promise for the Jews of northern Europe, and to receive a perpetual accession of new set-tlers" (Roth, 1989, p. 168). From the beginning of the 16th century, "the overwhelm-ing mass of Ashkenazic Jewry—the remnants of medieval England and France and Germany—became concentrated in Poland. It is from them that the majority of the Jews in the world today are descended" (pp. 268–269). Seeds of conflict and rancor were also planted as "jealous merchants and fanatical churchmen" (p. 270) resented their privi-leges. Into an atmosphere of those and other growing resentments was thrust the heinous conflagration of the Holocaust.

To come to terms with their past, Poles (and perhaps Polish Jews) confronting their Polish Jewish past do so with understandable reluctance. To this end, it is well to remem-ber the earlier history when Jewish faith, thought, and culture flourished unsurpassed in Poland. Both since have suffered diaspora not once but many times. Both have been destroyed, both have sought, found, and recreated their homeland, and each has greatly enriched the cultural history of the other. Although each may be able to exist without the other, that would, in the language of family therapy, be a major cutoff. Emigré descen-dants of Poles and Polish Jews may be in the best position to contribute to resolution.

RELIGION: THE CATHOLIC CHURCH

The Roman Catholic belief system has played such an influential role in the history of Poland that being Polish is synonymous with being Catholic. Polish Catholics have a strong predilection for mystical piety and self-abnegation as spiritual ideals. Many regarded the lives of the saints as models for living and had a special devotion to them and the Blessed Virgin Mary. Faith was shown by steadfast adherence to the Church, even to the point of martyrdom. Faithful parishioners supported and participated in social ser-vices. A good Polish Catholic behaved uprightly in the community and school, worked hard, and accepted his or her lot in life as the "will of God."

Both educated and uneducated immigrants were nourished in this tradition through the guidance of the parish priest and the vast system of parochial education, which included a well-established Polish teaching order of nuns, the Felicians. The chief purpose of education was to teach "faith and morals." The goal of child rearing was to raise good Catholics. Children were to be obedient and respectful of parents. The fundamental pur-pose of marital sex was procreation, and spouses was to fulfill their obligations of the sacrament of matrimony and have many children. Marriage was forever; divorce was for-bidden. Frequent attendance at mass and belief in the sacramental aspect of the Catholic faith was expected. The religious vows of "poverty, chastity, and obedience" also gov-erned secular life. Through the system of parochial education, monastic choices became family values. Catholicism was conservative, particularly on the subject of sexuality and gender roles. Poles have not been constitutionally likely to be open to discussions on whether God is female, or whether homosexuality is a matter of choice or being.

There is, however, a vast gulf between religious ideals and practice. As Polish Ameri-cans became educated, upwardly mobile, and left Polonia, family and religious values became viewed as "quaint and old-fashioned." Those who left Polonia and attended sec-ular schools were believed to have "lost their faith." Their children were seen as "disre-spectful and disobedient," and their divorce rates almost equaled those of the larger pop-ulation. Newer immigrants may have a very different viewpoint, and some may join those

Polish Americans who view the Vatican's position on key social issues as archaic, but the centrality of connecting the Catholic religion and Polish ethnicity seems true across the board.

EMOTIONAL PROCESS AND PATTERNS

Sanders and Morawska (1975) found that the decision of American Poles to marry was influenced more by closeness of ethnicity than by the idea of romantic love. Marriage was considered a socially accepted institution, not a love affair or an equal relationship between partners. Becoming a couple through marriage was probably the central life cycle stage of the Polish family. The Polish wedding traditionally went on for 2 or 3 days. It was the family's opportunity to demonstrate its social standing in the community, and it was not unusual for families to spend lavishly for a wedding extravaganza.

Historically, Polish couples were organized in a patriarchal system, and they still tend to be characterized by a traditional assignment of gender roles. During the immigration process, however, women gained a large measure of autonomy because they were left in Poland to function as heads of household while the men came to the United States to establish themselves. Once here, the women continued to exercise authority in the home, because the men were away working most of the time. Still, the belief that men should have complete authority over women remained. Although a large number of women in families in the United States are working outside the home, the Polish American woman still tends to be held solely responsible for housekeeping and child care.

Traditional Polish patriarchal family culture expected children to follow parents' orders without question and continuously contribute to the family's material well-being. In the second and third generations, young people flatly refuse to turn over earnings to their parents, and in some cases, parents sue or disown them. The expectation of the immigrant generation that their children would take care of them, as was done in Poland, has been unfulfilled. As the upwardly mobile younger generation has moved to the suburbs, leaving their parents living in the old neighborhoods where now other minorities and their businesses have supplanted the Poles, the elderly parents have felt abandoned. The neighborhood is no longer theirs.

The issue of children "leaving home" emotionally, as well as geographically, can be a toxic one in Polish American families. Children of all ages are expected to be grateful for whatever sacrifices their parents make for them, and at the same time are taught to have few expectations about what their parents will do for them. The expectation continues that children should be responsible for their parents' care and for maintaining a viable relationship through ongoing contact. Those who leave home are often simply ignored and treated as nonmembers, left out of the family information loop, not included in guest lists for weddings and family parties, and so on, particularly when intermarriage occurs with those outside the Polish American community, especially non-Catholics.

EXPRESSION OF FEELINGS

Traditional Polish patterns of courtship, marriage, and child rearing did not include open expression of affection (Sanders & Morawska, 1975). The Polish American family today continues to value stoicism and strongly inhibits feelings and expressions of need for emotional connectedness. Mondykowski (1982) discusses the problems of Polish Americans in expressing a need to be cared for. Children are expected to conceal their anxieties and needs from their parents and to "take care of themselves." Polish Americans "fear dependency [because] . . . being taken care of implies weakness and inability to pull their own weight. Feelings of need are not seen as normal, and are often connected with shame and humiliation" (p. 403). Intense expressions of anger in Polish families are often a cover for anxiety, which is not allowed expression, as it "implies a need for emotional reassurance and support that violates the value of stoicism" (pp. 402–403).

The prohibition against expressing feelings of pain and sadness complicates and attenuates the process of dying, and mourning after death occurs. The history of the Polish American family is full of experiences of loss and loss unexpressed. There is the loss of language, home, and culture, the loss of a "Polish self," which is part of the immigration experience. There is a loss from cutoffs that happen in Polish families because of the concern for status and the importance of disconnecting from members who shame the family. Often, when someone in a family is very ill, members of the extended family avoid inquiring about the patient's condition. Instead, there is ongoing tension, a worry that every time the phone rings it is bringing bad news, which must be borne stoically.

When it comes to conflict, many Poles are stubborn and seem to have a national and individual reluctance to yield or compromise. Within the family, tempers flare and violence, alcohol abuse, or both often ensue, or a state of "cold war" is achieved. A combination of persistence and stubbornness can operate to prevent dialogue in which both parties in a conflict can be heard. Disagreements become contests of will. In the words of one family member, a dispute is resolved "only when a son backs off and realizes he's talking to his father."

When working to resolve conflict, therapists must move from the position of "outsider" to one of empathic partner. From this shared vantage point, cultural legacies, immigration, social and societal influences, as well as individual experience, can be brought forth and respected. Helping clients to appreciate both the uniqueness of and their connectedness to the other may go a long way toward lessening the existing tension, allowing each the opportunity to refocus on the current circumstance. It is here that therapists encourage and provide accompaniment for exploration and appreciation of alternative ways of being.

A tongue-in-cheek footnote, but far from irrelevant, on the Polish personality: In a discussion of the harmful effects of the Polish nobility's decision that no legislation could be passed without 100% approval (the liberum veto) and of the establishment of life-tenure for offices of state, it was said woefully, "No one in Poland is willing to be a subject" (Davies, 1982, p. 365). When personal positions are often expressed in unequivocal terms, it is unlikely that mutual empathy will develop as a route to problem solving. Problems are left unresolved to go underground, where they remain as deeply held resentments.

This inability to negotiate to achieve mutually satisfying goals is probably both a contributing cause and an effect of the pervasive use and abuse of alcohol in the Polish American culture. Often, the function of heavy drinking is to allow the expression of weakness through crying or losing control. If individuals are drunk, they can disclaim responsibility for their words and actions (Mondykowski, 1982).

POLISH AMERICANS IN THERAPY

Poles tend to go to medical doctors only as a last resort. They are suspicious of the motives of health care providers, believing that they "just want to make money, and what you don't know won't hurt you." They will suffer great pain, often for years, before seeking medical attention. It is not uncommon to then find that they are terminally ill. They typically do not complain about pain, because, they ask, "What good will it do?" They also are likely to resist taking medication in favor of natural remedies, unless they have opportunities to medicate themselves. An interpreter who currently aids Polish arrivals reports that antibiotics are now so readily available in Poland, because of loose regulatory standards, that the Polish people believe there is a pill to cure everything, and immigrants may come with large caches of antibiotics (S. Dobosz, personal communication, September 17, 1994).

Resistance to accepting help from a "mental health doctor" is even stronger. Admitting to a mental health problem in the family is taboo. Even when a priest recommends that a family seek help, it rarely does. Usually a concerned employer is the motivator for therapy and then only because job performance is being affected. Sometimes therapy is sought when an "acting out" problem threatens family control. Mental illness is feared not only for itself, but also for the shame and guilt it is perceived to bring to the family.

Bowen (1978) observed that one-to-one relationships are the hallmark of a differentiated person. In such a relationship, two people "can relate personally to each other about each other, without talking about a third person (triangling) and without talking about impersonal things" (p. 540). Lerner (1989) noted that in this way people can know and express a balanced view of their strengths and weaknesses, clearly state their beliefs, values, and priorities, and behave congruently (p. 18). They stay emotionally connected with significant others in situations of high anxiety, speak rather than remaining silent, take an "I" position on difficult issues, acknowledge differences, and permit others to do so. Looking at these criteria, many Polish Americans rarely have, and even more rarely express, a balanced view of their strengths and weaknesses, even though many could come up with a list of both which somehow cancel each other out. This is probably because expressing a view of one's strengths is seen as "bragging," and admitting to weakness can bring shame on the individual and the family. Most Poles have a problem staying emotionally connected with significant others when tension rises. It is much more likely that they will cut off, or at the least, distance into ritualized contact. In addition, they are likely to remain silent, drink, or shout, rather than take an "I" position on difficult or toxic issues. Not wanting to "be a subject" does not mean one is willing to risk being the declared king and therefore the subject of criticism.

Finally, Poles do not readily acknowledge differences or allow others to do so. Because of obedience and connection to parents and the Church, the "rules" may be threatened by so doing. Distance or cutoff seems the preferred way Poles handle messy, powerful feelings. Given the intimate connection between being Polish and being Catholic, for those who perceive that loss of identity follows loss of connection with dogma and practice, there is little room for development of a differentiated self. Fusion of the Polish self with Church dogma can mean that distancing in this case is like social excommunication. This seems to be the underlying philosophy of old-guard Poles and Polish Americans, a style that may indeed be painfully challenged and changed by the newest influx of immigrants.

The following cases reflect experiences of Polish families who, at different periods, immigrated to the United States.

The Lis Family

Joann Lis, age 45, recently separated from her husband, Barry. She came to therapy for help in adjusting to the separation. Joann is the younger of two daughters of Alex Zukowski, whose parents were born in Poland at the time of World War I. The family is typical of Polish immigrant families of that time. Of eight siblings, all but Alex remained in Polonia. Joann's father was an alcoholic, and she characterizes his siblings as heavy drinkers, too. Alex moved to a distant community and had infrequent contact with his family of origin, so Joann is effectively cut off from her father's family. The last time she saw them was at his funeral.

Although unaware of her Polish roots, Joann has unconsciously followed the pattern of a good Polish wife. She remained married to a man with addiction problems, worked long hours as a nurse, and provided good meals and a good home. She is an example of someone who comes to therapy without any clear indicators of her ethnicity. It was deemed that therapy could be helpful to Joann by placing her within her ethnic context, allowing her to better understand herself, her father, and his family, and to make conscious some of the hidden rules that govern her feelings and behavior. She could thus discover hidden resources for defining herself and extend her options for self-empowerment. With support and encouragement in therapy, Joann began actively to search out her uncles, aunts, and cousins in the original Polonia area of Detroit, as well as revisiting and developing her relationship to her ex-husband's younger sister. She started to learn about things Polish, and, interestingly, it was via the support of Barry's younger sister, whose relationship to her Polish husband turned out to be similar to Joann's, that she became empowered to make more independent moves in her own behalf. She enrolled in college courses, something she always wanted to do, but "for some reason" never thought she could do.

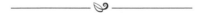

The Szych Family

Jurek (Jerry) and Grzegorz (Greg) were twins, whose grandfather, Stanislas, changed his Jewish name in Poland from Mittleman to Malinowski to sound less Jewish before marrying his Polish Catholic wife, Dominika. The couple immigrated in 1961 when the Polish communist government encouraged Polish Jews and those in mixed marriages to emigrate. In the United States both Dominika and Stanislav resumed their original Jewish names "because it was easier in this country to be Jewish than to be Polish." Their daughter Maria was raised Catholic, later married an American Jewish man named Szych, and had the twins.

The cultural identity confusion of this family is manifested in the way the twins describe themselves. When asked "Are you Polish (or Jewish)?" Jerry answers, "That's a long story." He says that he was always aware that, being Polish, he had to prove that he was not stupid by excelling in school. At times he would say he was Jewish to avoid the "dumb Polack" stereotype. Greg says, "I wear a necklace on which there is a Polish eagle and a Torah. There is supposed to be a crucifix, but for me it is a Torah." Regretting that he was not raised Jewish, Greg has begun studying Torah and is an observant Jew. Jerry is less clear. He identifies as neither Catholic nor Jewish, yet when he prays each night, as taught by his grandmother, he makes the Sign of the Cross. Both men married Jewish women. Maria says the family has always felt isolated because they have nothing in common with Polish Americans who arrived earlier in this century. They have experienced prejudice from Jews for their Polishness, and from Poles for their Jewishness.

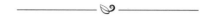

The Pietrowski Family

Dr. Anna Pietrowski, age 35, a psychiatrist, and Mateusz, age 37, an engineer, and their two daughters immigrated in 1982. When asked if the interview could be taped, Anna became visibly anxious, refused, and apologized, saying that having lived under the Communist regime, she feared taping. When she talked about leaving Poland, Anna wept. She said that coming to this country felt like being in the middle of an ocean, unable to swim. "I did not feel equal to any American despite my education. I would drive around, taking my children to school, and ask myself, 'What am I doing here?' I felt like an outsider . . . part of my identity was lost. When I came here, I didn't understand, and then I learned . . . that in this country Polish ancestry is treated as much worse than Irish or Italian."

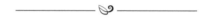

CONCLUSION

Because of both Polish and American historical experience it might be said that Polish Americans take pride (though often the pride is secret) in having the courage to face terrible odds, having the ability to be long-suffering and outlast adversity, being indeed the salt of the earth (hardworking with strong religious principles), at home humbly taking on heroic tasks while discounting their own efforts and successes. They are constitutionally defensive, passionately loyal, and inveterately ceremonial. Whether they acknowledge it or not, they have what Gladsky (1992) referred to as "a hunger for social belonging" (p. 287), a need for "class" status with a concurrent need to disavow such ambition. Success in any of these endeavors can still leave Polish Americans feeling disconnected from the larger culture because of a fear-based or shame-based disavowal of their ethnic heritage. To the extent that being Polish necessarily also means being Catholic, Poles not on good terms with the traditional Church can be even more conflicted.

In the context of therapy, Polish Americans can be difficult to engage, but once committed to personal or family change, they are likely to keep working at it long after the therapist loses connection, having an inner need to faithfully complete the task for self, for family, for Church, for community. Assisting Poles to revisit their ethnic roots can be a way of going home, not again, but for the first time. For those cut off from their own ethnic heritage, it is a necessary part of becoming comfortable with the process of accepting and reinventing themselves. Ameliorating "the loneliness of the long-distance ethnic" (Gladsky, 1992, p. 249), one of the consequences of cutting off from one's roots, is no small achievement. Strange as it might at first appear, in some cases it might be helpful to "give permission" and confirm that one can be or become educated, upwardly mobile, ambitious and self-oriented, without being snobbish or untrue to one's heritage.

Poland has survived as a powerful and positive factor in the configuration of modern Europe and is currently redefining itself. That redefinition can include achievements and longings of both modern Polish immigrants and Polish Americans, past and present.

REFERENCES

Bartoszewski, W. (1991). *The convent at Auschwitz*. New York: George Braziller.

Bernstein, R. (2003a, May 14). Poland upstages European powers. *International Herald Tribune*, p. 1.

Bernstein, R. (2003b, May 13). Poland upstages, and irks, European powerhouses. *New York Times*, p. 4.

Bowen, M. (1978). *Family therapy in clinical practice*. New York: Jason Aronson.

Chorzempa, R. (1993). *Polish roots*. Baltimore: Genealogical Publishing.

Davies, N. (1992). *Heart of Europe: A short history of Poland* (rev. ed.). New York: Oxford University Press.

Erdmans, M. P. (2001). Stanislaus can't polka: New Polish immigrants in established Polish American communities. In P. Kivisto & G. Rundblad (Eds.), *Multiculturalism in the United States* (pp. 395–407). Thousand Oaks, CA: Pine Forge Press.

Gladsky, T. (1992). *Princes, peasants and other Polish selves: Ethnicity in American literature*. Amherst: University of Massachusetts Press.

Gross, J. (2001). *Neighbors*. Princeton, NJ: Princeton University Press.

Hertz, A. (1988). *The Jews in Polish culture*. Evanston, IL: Northwestern University Press.

Hoffman, E. (1989). *Lost in translation*. New York: Dutton.

Hundley, T. (2003, August 4). Public support for sending troops to Iraq erodes. *Chicago Tribune*, p. 6.

Knab, S. H. (1993). *Polish customs, traditions, and folklore*. New York: Hippocrene Books.

Lerner, H. (1989). *The dance of intimacy*. New York: Harper & Row.

Lipniacka, E. (2000). *Xenophobe's guide to the Poles*. London: Oval Books.

Lopata, H. Z. (1975). The Polish-American family. In C. H. Mindel & R. W. Habenstein (Eds.), *Ethnic families in America: Patterns and variations* (pp. 15–40). New York: Elsevier.

Mondykowski, S. (1982). Polish families. In M. McGoldrick, J. Giordano, & J. K. Pearce (Eds.), *Ethnicity and family therapy* (pp. 393–411). New York: Guilford Press.

Morawski, J. (1992). The odyssey of the Polish alcohol system. In H. Klingemann, J. Takala, & G. Hunt (Eds.), *Cure, care, or control: Alcoholism treatment in sixteen countries*. New York: State University of New York Press.

Pasek, B. (2003, July 10). Jewish leaders praise Poland's probe into massacre. *Jerusalem Post*, p. 5.

Radzilowski, J. (1997). What does it take to be Polish American? We should never let anyone tell us that we are not Poles, or that being Polish is some kind of hobby for us. It is who we are. *Polish American Journal*, 86(6), 2.

Radzilowski, J. (1998). How do we stop anti-Polish defamation? *Polish American Journal*, 87(9), 4.

Roth, C. (1989). *A history of the Jews* (rev. ed.). New York: Schocken Books.

Sanders, I., & Morawska, E. (1975). *Polish American community life: A survey of research*. New York: Polish Institute of Arts and Sciences in America.

Simpson, E. (1987). *Orphans: Real and imaginary*. New York: New American Library.

Steven, S. (1982). *The Poles*. New York: Macmillan.

Tryzno, W., Pedagogic, M., Grvdziak-Sobczy, E., Prawn, N., & Marowski, J. (1989). The role of the family in alcohol education and alcohol abuse in Poland. *Medical Law*, 8, 267–273.

Wesolowsky, T. (2001, April, 18). Polish town confronts its history: An expose blaming Poles for a 1941 massacre of Jews forces dismantling of the official. *WORD Christian Science Monitor*.

Zamoyski, A. (1988). *The Polish way*. New York: Franklin Watts.

Cultural Assessment

We offer here a brief outline for clinical assessment. This outline presents a map for collecting information on clients' problems from a contextual framework that takes into account a client's cultural background. The outline summarizes information that is important to gather, but not necessarily the order in which it is to be gathered.

DOING A "CULTURAL GENOGRAM"

We view doing a cultural genogram and a time line for tracking nodal points in family history as axiomatic for all work with clients or trainees (Congress, 1994; Hardy & Laszloffy, 1995; McGoldrick, Gerson, & Shellenberger, 1999). Genograms help us contextualize our kinship network in terms of culture, class, race, gender, religion, family process, and migration history. When we ask people to identify themselves ethnically, we are asking them to highlight themes of cultural continuity and cultural identity to make them more apparent. The genogram is a practical, visual tool for assessment of family patterns and context, as well as a therapeutic intervention in itself. Genograms allow clinicians to quickly conceptualize the individual's context within the growing diversity of family forms and patterns in our society. Using the genogram to collect historical and contextual assessment information is a collaborative, client-centered therapeutic process. By its nature the process involves the telling of stories and emphasizes respect for the client's perspective, while encouraging multiple views of different family members. The genogram is a tool used by health care clinicians for assessment of functioning, relational patterns, ethnicity, spirituality, migration, class, and other socioeconomic factors (Carter & McGoldrick, 2005; Congress, 1994; Dunn & Dawes, 1999; Hardy & Lazloffy, 1995; Hodge, 2001; McGoldrick, 1995, 1998; McGoldrick et al., 1999; Walsh, 1999). By scanning the family system culturally and historically and assessing previous life-cycle transitions, the clinician can place present issues in the context of the family's evolutionary patterns of geography, migration, and family process. The genogram usually includes cultural and demographic information about at least three generations of family members, as well as nodal and critical events in the family's history, particularly as related to family changes (migration, loss, and the life cycle).

BASIC DEMOGRAPHIC INFORMATION INCLUDED IN A GENOGRAM

Who?

Who is in the family? Names, ages, gender, class, race, sexual orientation, dates of birth, marriage, separation, divorce, illness, death. Who is presenting the problem? Who is defining the problem, if that is different? Who is the identified patient (index person, or IP)? How do others in the family or context view this problem? Who is the referrer? What is his or her relationship to the family and the problem? Might any triangles develop between the referrer and family members?

What?

What is the problem as defined by whom? Does the index person (IP) share the definition? Does anyone not share the definition?

Why Now?

What may be precipitating stresses? Are there concurrent pressures on the family? Moves, losses (illness, job loss, important person who left home or area), life-cycle transitions (launching, retirement, remarriage, divorce, death)?

History of Presenting Problem

What do family members see as a problem? What response do they want from the therapist for the problem? What are the family's cultural strengths for dealing with this problem?

Life-Cycle Stage; Dates of Entry and Exit of Key Members of the Family Network

What has been the timing of births, deaths, moves in or out of the household, school or job changes indicative of life-cycle transitions (entry into high school, retirement, etc.)?

Health and Mental Health History

What has been the timing of illnesses in the family, and what kind of relationship has the family had with professional helpers and self-help support?

Socioeconomic Information

What is the family's history with education, occupation, income, work, and financial stress?

Cultural Heritage

What is the ethnic and racial background of family members, and what has been the impact of racism on them? Have they lived in an ethnic enclave or community, or in a community in which they were viewed as outsiders? Have their spiritual and religious beliefs supported or minimized their acknowledgment of their ethnic heritage?

Belief Systems, Religion, and Spiritual Beliefs

What are the primary beliefs that organize the family? What is their general worldview, and are they organized by particular myths, rules, spiritual beliefs or family secrets? What is their history of religious beliefs and practices, including changes in belief? What has been the impact of intrafamily differences in belief, as well as differences between the family and community in belief?

Language Skill and Acculturation of Family Members

Family members vary in how quickly they adapt, how much of their heritage they retain, and the rate at which they learn English. Knowing and speaking the language of the country of origin can serve to preserve its culture. What languages were spoken while the children in the family were growing up? Are there differences in language skills and acculturation within the family that may have led to conflicts, power imbalances, and role reversals, especially where children were forced to translate for their parents?

REVIEW OF PATTERNS OF INDIVIDUAL, FAMILY, AND SOCIAL FUNCTIONING

Family Relationship History

What kinds of relationships do family members have: close, enmeshed, distant, conflicted, cut off?

Family Biological Factors

What is the family's history of illness, neurological impairment, or learning difficulties, and how have family members dealt with these issues?

Individual Factors for IP, Household Members, and Close Kin

Have individuals had life-cycle transition issues, substance abuse, developmental lag, psychological symptoms, major differences in temperament, or other stresses?

Immediate Family

What kinds of relationships are there within the immediate family? Are there problems with generational boundaries, conflict, cutoff, disengagement, lack of resources, substance abuse, emotional illness, power imbalance or abuse?

Extended Family

What are the family members' relationships with extended family members? Are there cut-offs? Are extended family members supportive? Are they a resource or a drain on the energies of the immediate family?

Work and School

What expectations do family members have about education and work, and are they able to meet them?

Sociocultural Factors

Are there sociocultural factors that are impeding the family's functioning related to their social class, ethnicity, race, finances, educational level, employment potential, legal status, etc.?

Connections to Community

To what extent are family members able to maintain friendships? How accessible are friends, neighbors, religious organizations, schools, physicians, community institutions, and other health care and social service resources, including therapists? When family members move away from an ethnic enclave, the stresses of adaptation are likely to be severe, even several generations after immigration. The therapist should learn about the community's ethnic network and, where relevant, encourage the rebuilding of informal social connections through family visits or letters or through the building of new social networks.

Migration History

Why did the family migrate? What were they seeking (e.g., survival, adventure, wealth)? What were they leaving behind (e.g., religious or political persecution, poverty)(? While taking a family history, therapists need to be attuned to the specific stresses that immigrant families experience, and to the ethnic identity conflicts that may be precipitated by the process of immigration (Hernandez & McGoldrick, 2005). Assessing such factors is crucial for determining whether a family's dysfunction is a "normal" reaction to a high degree of cultural stress, or whether it goes beyond the bounds of transitional stress and requires expert intervention. The stresses of migration may at times be "buried" or forgotten. The cultural heritage before migration may have been suppressed or forgotten, but may still influence the family's outlook, if sometimes subtly, as its members try to accommodate to new situations. Many immigrant groups have been forced to abandon much of their ethnic heritage and thus have lost a part of their identity. The effects of this hidden history may be all the more powerful for being hidden. Families that have experienced trauma and devastation within their own society before even beginning the process of immigration will have a monumentally more difficult time adjusting to a new life than those who migrated for adventure or economic betterment. Specific areas to investigate regarding migration include the following.

Premigration History

What was the economic, political, and social environment like in the country of origin just prior to the family's migration? What was the impact of the war, famine, revolution, poverty, and religious persecution on the family? Did any family ancestors immigrate from or to another country?

Migration History

When did the family come to the United States? Why did the family leave the country of origin? What were the family members seeking (survival, adventure, wealth)? Who in the family immigrated first? Who came with whom? Who remained behind? How traumatic was the migration journey itself? Were there losses along the way beyond the loss of the culture of origin (death, physical or sexual abuse, robbery, legal encounters)?

Postmigration History

What experiences did the family have when they arrived in the United States? Did they have problems with language, legal status, or poverty? Was there a loss of social status, or job options? To what extent was there a shock of cultural values? Did they live in a supportive or an antagonistic community? Have you been back to your country of origin? How often? What have been the reasons for your visits back? Have you ever been unable to return when you wanted to? What family events have you missed since you left your country of origin? Do you have friends from your country who also live here? How often do you see them? Do family and friends from your country of origin visit you here? How often? How long do they stay? Are you expected to support family members back home? Do you send money or consumer goods back home? What kinds of things do you send?

Migration and the Life Cycle

How old were family members when migration occurred? How old were the family members who remained in the homeland? How did the age at migration influence family members? Were certain children drawn into adult status because they learned English faster than the parents or because the family had no resources to treat them as children? Did the life-cycle stage at migration bring about a reversal of the parental hierarchy because parents were less able to negotiate the new culture than their children? Were grandparents limited by their inability to learn English? How did the life-cycle phase influence the family's adaptation?

Stressors and Life-Cycle Issues

Have there been other recent stresses beside the presenting problem, such as untimely deaths or other losses, migration, moves, or other stressors?

Family Resources and Vulnerabilities

What are the family members' sources of resilience (adaptability, creativity, caring for each other, dedication to hard work, belief in education, etc.)? What are their vulnerabilities (rigidity of gender roles, inability to speak English, lack of marketable job skills, belief that they should be able to cope without outside help, etc.)?

Hypotheses about the Case

What do you think is the problem in this case, and for whom? Why now? Are there problems that the symptoms solve?

Potential Problems for the Therapist: How the Therapist Might Get Stuck with a Family

What difficulty might the therapist have with engaging the members of the family related to cultural differences, class, gender, age, race, sexual orientation, or religious, spiritual, or other beliefs? How might the therapist get caught in triangles with the family or between the family and other institutions such as the referrer, other therapists, or the therapist's work system? How might the therapist's own life-cycle stage or cultural background be an asset or a liability for therapy?

Family's Beliefs about the Problem and about Possible Solutions

We always need to intervene with a family in ways that are sufficiently congruent with the family members' beliefs for them to connect with the recommended interventions. What are the family's cultural beliefs about the problem and about possible solutions? How might the clinician respond to these beliefs in assessment and intervention?

CULTURAL GENOGRAM QUESTIONS

We have found the following questions helpful in aiding clients to understand their cultural backgrounds:

- What ethnic groups, religious traditions, nations, racial groups, trades, professions, communities, and other groups do you consider yourself to be part of?
- When and why did you or your family come to the United States? To this community? How old were family members at the time? Do they and do you feel secure about your status in the United States? Do they (do you) have a green card(s)?
- What language do they (do you) speak at home? In the community? In your family of origin?
- What burdening wounds has your racial or ethnic group experienced? What burden does your ethnic or racial group carry for injuries to other groups? How have you been affected by the wounds your group has committed, or that have been committed against your group?
- How have you been wounded by the wrongs done to your ancestors? How have you been complicit in the wrongs done by your ancestors? How can you give voice to your group's guilt, your own sorrow, or your own complicity in the harm done by your ancestors? What would reparations entail?
- What experiences have been most stressful for family members in the United States?
- To whom do family members in your culture turn when in need of help?
- What are your culture's values regarding male and female roles? Education? Work and success? Family connectedness? Family caretaking? Religious practices? Have these values changed in your family over time?
- Do you still have contact with family members in your country of origin?
- Has immigration changed family members' education or social status?
- What do you feel about your culture(s) of origin? Do you feel you belong to the dominant U.S. culture?

These questions can guide the clinician to remind family members of their resilience through the values of their heritage, their ability to transform their lives, and their ability to work toward long-range goals that fit with their cultural values. Basically, questions that help to locate families in their cultural context may help them access their strengths in the midst of the stress of their current situations.

The following are illustrations of the kinds of questions that may help families feel the strength of their heritage:

- How might your grandfather, who dreamed of your immigration but never made it himself, think about the problem you are having with your children?
- Your ancestors survived the Middle Passage and slavery for hundreds of years. You are here because they had great strength and courage. What do you think are the strengths you got from these ancestors that may help you in dealing with your problem?
- Your great-grandmother immigrated at 21 and became a piece worker in a sweatshop but managed to support her six children and had great strength. What do you think were her dreams for you, her daughter's daughter's daughter? What do you think she would want you to do now about your current problem?
- Your father died of his alcoholism, but when he came to this country at age 18, he undoubtedly had dreams of his future. What do you think he cared about? How do you think he felt about the parents he left behind? What do you think he would want for you now?
- Could you go to your Hungarian Social Club and volunteer?
- Are there some Latino political groups in your town that could help you fight for the resources you and your group have deserved from the United States for 150 years?
- How do you think the fact that you are Italian and your wife is Irish may influence the way you handle conflicts?

The underlying reason for this cultural clinical assessment and all the suggested questions offered here is to look at clients as belonging to history, to their present context, and to the future.

REFERENCES

Carter, B., & McGoldrick, M. (Eds.). (2005). *The expanded family life cycle: Individual, family and social perspectives* (classic ed.). Boston: Allyn & Bacon.

Congress, E. P. (1994). The use of culturagrams to assess and empower culturally diverse families. *Families in Society, 75,* 531–540.

Dunn, A. B., & Dawes, S. J. (1999). Spiritually focused genograms: Keys to uncovering spiritual resources in African American families. *Journal of Multicultural Counseling and Development, 27*(4), 240–255.

Hardy, K. V., & Laszloffy, T. A. (1995). The cultural genogram: Key to training culturally competent family therapists. *Journal of Marital and Family Therapy, 21*(3), 227–237.

Hernandez, M., & McGoldrick, M. (2005). Migration and the family life cycle. In B. Carter & M. McGoldrick (Eds.), *The expanded family life cycle.* Boston: Allyn & Bacon.

Hodge, D. R. (2001). Spiritual genograms: A genenerational approach to assessing spirituality. *Families in Society: The Journal of Contemporary Human Services,* 35–48.

McGoldrick, M. (1995). *You can go home again: Understanding your family relationships.* New York: Norton.

McGoldrick, M. (Ed.). (1998). *Re-visioning family therapy: Race, culture, and gender in clinical practice.* New York: Guilford Press.

McGoldrick, M., Gerson, R., & Shellenberger, S. (1999). *Genograms: Assessment and intervention.* New York: Norton.

Walsh, F. (Ed.). (1999). *Spiritual resources in family therapy.* New York: Guilford Press.

Author Index

Abad, V., 252, 253
Abdelkarim, A. M., 474
Abdel-Khalek, A. M., 474
Ablon, J., 600
Abouchedid, K., 481
Abou-Hatab, F. A.-L. H., 474
Abudabbeh, A., 473
Abudabbeh, N., 427, 429, 432
Ackerman, H., 205
Adams, J., 44
Adams, W., 452
Adib, S., 474
Agathangelou, A. M., 574, 583
Agbayani-Siewert, P., 319, 322, 325
Ahlo, M. N., 70
Ahmad, I., 382
Ahn-Toupin, E. S. W., 358
Ajami, F., 470, 471
Ajrouch, K. J., 472, 473, 475, 476
Akbar, M., 120
Akbar, N., 87, 88
Akhtar, S., 416
Akinyela, M., 84
Alamuddin, N. S., 475, 477
Alba, R. D., 15, 501, 503, 622
Alers, J. O., 247
Alford, B. A., 551
Al-Hibri, A., 382
Alibhai-Brown, Y., 26
Allen, D., 715, 716, 721, 722
Allen, J., 659
Allman, T. D., 160
Almeida, O. T., 630
Almeida, R. V., 87, 111, 183, 383, 389
Al-Qaradawi, Y., 140
Al-Qazzaz, A., 426
Althausen, L., 703, 704, 706, 714
Al-Timimi, N. R., 474, 476, 481, 484
Ananeh-Firempong, O., 4
Anbe, B., 68
Anctil, P., 546
Anderson, C., 4, 5, 24
Anderson, H., 115
Anderson, J. L., 647, 650, 651
Ang, S. C., 495
Angelou, M., 12
Anguksuar, L. R., 46
Ani, M., 87, 88

Anthony, E. J., 371
Aoki, B. K., 283
Aponte, H., 22, 95, 96, 251
Aposhian, M. A., 462
April, S., 549
Arasteh, A. R., 453, 454, 456
Araujo, Z. A., 633
Arias, E., 88, 90
Arkoun, M., 382
Arnalde, M., 209
Aroian, K., 597
Arredondo, P., 181
Asante, M., 87
Aseel, H. A., 427
Askari, H., 452
Attneave, C., 48, 49, 50, 51
Audam, S., 83
Auerswald, E. H., 582
Augusto, F., 172
Aurbach, L., 219
Auth, J., 230
Avis, J., 5
Awwad, E., 491
Axtell, J., 57, 530
Azhar, M. Z., 335

Badillo-Ghali, S., 252
Baffoun, A., 382
Bahar, E., 334
Bailey, A., 542
Bakalian, A., 439, 442, 443, 444, 445, 446
Baker, A. M., 491, 492
Baker, K., 104
Baldassar, L. V., 369
Baldwin, G. B., 452
Bales, R. F., 600
Ballan, A., 478
Baluja, K., 256
Banks, J. A., 18, 505, 506
Banuazizi, A., 452
Barakat, H., 427, 428
Barkan Ascher, N., 684
Barnes, J. S., 270, 302
Barrabee, P., 605
Barry, C., 601
Bartalska, F. I., 724, 726, 730
Barzini, L., 618
Basch, L., 230

Bateson, M. C., 463
Battle, J., 83
Bauman, A., 370
Bayard-Burfield, L., 458
Bean, F. D., 157
Becerra, R. M., 237
Beck, A. T., 551
Beck, L., 428
Behar, R., 213
Bélanger, D. C., 547
Bell, C. K., 69
Bell, D., 23
Bellah, R., 520, 521
Benet, N., 46
Benner, P. E., 461
Bennett, C. E., 270, 271, 302
Bennett, L., Jr., 77
Bensussen, G., 232
Bepko, C., 600
Berghahn, K. L., 560
Bergin, A., 93
Berkhoffer, R., 43, 44
Berkowitz, B., 512
Berlin, P., 650
Berman, P., 508
Bernal, G., 187, 205, 206, 207, 208, 209, 210
Bernal, M., 208
Bernard, J. M., 581
Bernstein, A. C., 83
Bernstein, R., 508, 743
Berry, J. W., 385
Berthold, S. M., 340
Best, T., 119
Betancourt, J. R., 5 , 3, 4, 5
Bettelheim, B., 441, 446
Bhana, K., 104
Biddle, E. H., 596
Bierbrauer, G., 475, 482
Bill, J. A., 451, 452
Billigmeier, R. H., 559, 562
Billingsley, A., 81, 87, 88, 89, 93, 94
Black, J., 641
Black, L. W., 79, 80, 81, 82, 83, 84, 85, 105, 106
Blaisdell, K., 64, 66
Blanc-Szanton, C., 230
Blessing, P. J., 603
Bloom, A., 508
Boas, F., 242
Boehnlein, J. K., 363
Bograd, M., 111
Bonilla-Silva, E., 511
Bonnin, R., 208
Booth, J., 178, 179, 180, 181
Borders, L., 600
Borish, S., 649, 650, 652
Bosch, J., 217
Boscia-Mulé, P., 621, 622
Boscolo, L., 299
Boswell, T., 205
Boszormenyi-Nagy, I., 210
Bournoutian, G. A., 438, 439
Bowen, M., 565, 570, 651, 752
Bowser, B., 511
Boyajian, L., 441, 446
Boyce, E., 252, 253, 459
Boyd-Franklin, N., 3, 22, 23, 81, 87, 88, 89, 90, 91, 93,
    94, 95, 244, 247, 252
Brault, G. J., 547
Brave Heart, M. Y. H., 47, 57
Breslin, J., 507, 513

Brewer, L., 603
Brice-Baker, J. R., 124
Brimelow, P., 508
Brody, R. A., 205
Brookheiser, R., 505
Brouilette, P., 549
Brown, B., 87
Brown, C., 208
Brown, G., 556
Brown, T., 369
Browning, D., 257
Brudner-White, L., 325
Bryant, A., 624
Bryce-LaPorte, R. S., 120
Bulatao, J. C., 322, 326, 327
Bullitt, J., 290
Bulosan, C., 320
Bumiller, E., 383
Burgonio-Watson, T. B., 326, 327
Burnam, M. A., 230
Burton, L., 4
Bush, G., 508, 512, 515
Bustamante, J. A., 207, 230, 233
Butalia, U., 408
Butler, S., 600
Byrne, N. O., 609
Byron, R., 597

Cahill, T., 597
Cainkar, L., 494
Calvert, P., 156, 162
Calvert, S., 156, 162
Calvin, J., 534, 536, 540
Campbell, O., 474
Carey, J. C., 384
Carilli, T., 625
Carini-Giordano, M., 517
Carlson, C., 715, 716, 721, 722
Carmichael, J., 425
Carrillo, J. E., 4
Carroll, J., 509, 512
Carter, B., 24, 25, 69, 609, 611, 757
Carter, E. A., 210
Carter, R. T., 87, 511
Cashmore, J., 478
Castro, F., 204
Castro, M., 205, 206
Cather, W., 731
Cavaioli, F., 616
Cecchin, G., 299
Césaire, A., 259
Cetinich, D., 716, 718, 719, 720
Chadwick, N., 598, 599
Chai, A., 350
Chambers, J., 120
Chambless, D. L., 32
Chamie, J., 469, 470, 471, 475
Chan, S., 319, 321, 324, 325
Chandras, K. V., 404, 405
Chaney, S., 5
Chang, I., 273, 274, 303, 305
Chasteen, J. C., 155
Chauhan, S. S., 397
Chavez, L. R., 233
Chemelevsky, M., 104
Chesney, M., 363
Chien, C. P., 369
Cho, Y., 363
Choy, B. Y., 349
Christison, K., 487, 492

Christopher, R. C., 529
Chung, D. K., 343, 358
Cicone, J., 122
Ciongoli, A. K., 616
Clark, D., 597
Clark, J., 205
Cleary, P. D., 608
Cleary, P., 624
Cobas, J., 209
Cobbs, P., 97
Cohen, C. J., 83
Cohen, M., 619
Cohen, R., 205, 667, 681
Cohen, S., 667
Cohler, B. J., 371, 606
Coleman, H. L. K., 230
Colin, J. M., 130
Collins, E. F., 334
Comas-Díaz, L., 231, 242, 246, 248
Condon, M. E., 357
Congress, E. P., 757
Connery, D. S., 602
Conover, T., 181, 185
Conte, F., 711
Conzen, K. N., 559, 560
Cook, D. A., 87
Cooney, R. S., 209
Cooper, M. H., 382
Cordova, F., 321
Corliss, R., 56
Corrigan, E. M., 600
Cose, E., 505
Cosgray, R. E., 129, 130
Cotton, S., 478
Covell, A. C., 357
Cowie, P., 502
Craig, G. A., 557, 559, 561
Crocker, L. G., 398
Crohn, J., 26, 516, 622
Cropley, A., 104
Cross, W. E., 87
Cummings, J. T., 452
Cushing, B., 25
Cwerner, S. B., 167

Da Matta, R., 168, 169
DaCosta, K. M., 344
Dagirmanjian, S., 449
Daneshpour, M., 81
Danieli, Y., 295
Daniels, R., 345
Daun, A., 646, 647
Davidman, L., 689, 694, 695
Davies, N., 744, 746, 751
Davis, A., 70
Davis, C., 256
Davis, K. E., 556
Davis, M., 502
Davis, M. P., 232
Dawes, S. J., 757
Dearing, E. G., 323
DeBruyn, L. M., 57
Deeb, M., 478
De Jong, J. T. V. M., 492
De La Cancela, V., 253
del Castillo, J., 220
Delgado, M., 244
Del Vecchio, A., 47
Demone, H. W., 608, 624
Denis, E., 725

Deren, M., 134
Der Nersessian, S., 438, 439
DeRosa, T., 621
Desai, M., 400
Desrosiers, A., 131, 135
Deutsch, M., 87
Devereux, E. C., 564
DeVries, R. G., 625
Dewachi, O., 478
Dezell, M., 606
Díaz-Guerrero, R., 235
Dickason, D., 371
Dilworth-Anderson, P., 4, 24
Dimoulis, D., 575
Diner, H. R., 597, 603, 604
Djamba, Y., 103
Doi, T., 342
Dolan-Delvecchio, D., 383
Dolan-Delvecchio, K., 383, 389
Dominquez, V., 119
Donaldson, S., 388
Donnelly, S., 606
Donohue, B., 409
Dorris, M., 8
Drachman, D., 181, 220
Dregni, E., 649
Duany, J., 209, 220
Duany, R., 247, 254
Duarte, I., 216, 218, 219, 224
Du Bois, W. E. B., 385
DuBray, W., 49, 52
Dubrow, K., 491
Dudoit, M. R., 67, 70
Duleep, H. O., 398
Du Long, J. P., 547, 548
Dunn, A. B., 757
Duran, B., 47, 57
Duran, E., 47
Duster, M. C., 363
Dwairy, M. A., 431, 472, 474, 475, 479, 480, 481, 492
Dynes, W., 388

Easton, N. J., 503
Ebihara, M., 293, 295
Eire, C., 203
Eisen, A., 667
Eisenberg, L., 369
El Hassan, K., 476
El Saadawi, N., 380
Elder, J., 513
Elia, C., 462
Elisme, E., 129, 130
El-Kak, F., 478
Emami, A., 461
Ember, M., 118
Enrile, A. V., 319
Enriquez, V. G., 319, 321, 322, 325
Erdmans, M. P., 744
Erdrich, L., 8
Erickson, B., 645, 646
Erickson, C. D., 423, 474, 476, 481, 484
Eron, J., 447, 449
Escobar, J. I., 198, 230, 233, 252
Esposito, J. L., 428
Esterhazy, P., 590
Evans, E. E., 599

Faber, E., 668
Faber, S. B., 669
Fadiman, A., 10, 11, 273

Fagan, R. R., 205
Falicov, C. J., 25, 156, 187, 229, 230, 231, 232, 233, 234, 235, 236, 237, 238, 325, 360, 582
Falicov, Y. M., 229
Fallows, M. A., 596
Fanning, C., 596
Farmer, P., 131
Farrell, K., 491
Feigin, I., 703, 704
Femminella, F., 617, 624
Fergerson, G., 83
Fernandez, C. C., 250
Fernandez-Mendez, E., 242
Fernea, E. W., 427, 472, 473, 475, 476, 480, 483, 484
Fernea, R. A., 472, 473, 475, 476, 480, 483, 484
Ferrari, S., 181, 183, 184
Ferro, R., 625
Fiada, A., 577, 579
Fields, J., 91
Finney, B. R., 65
Fischer, D. H., 654, 656, 657, 658, 660, 661
Fishman, H. C., 699
Fitchen, J., 659
Fitzpatrick, C., 601
Fitzpatrick, J. P., 244, 245
Fleck, J., 363
Flores, E., 235
Foché, C., 492
Fohrmann, J., 560
Folwarski, J., 711, 712, 715, 716, 719
Foner, P. S., 204
Font, R., 183
Forero, J., 195
Foster, R. F., 597
Fouron, G. E., 132, 133
Framo, J., 651
Frank, A., 536
Frankenberg, R., 511
Franklin, A. J., 3, 14, 22, 23, 81, 84, 85, 87, 88, 89, 90, 91, 93, 94, 95
Frazier, E. F., 87, 92, 93
Frederickson, G. M., 16
Friedman, E., 677
Friedman, L., 523
Friedman, M. J., 492
Frieze, R., 364
Frisbie, W. P., 363
Fujino, D. C., 320
Fukuyama, M. A., 344
Fullilove, M. T., 80
Fusco, C., 203, 207

Gable, R. W., 453, 454
Galang, M. E., 320, 323
Galens, J., 117, 118
Gallup, G., Jr., 17, 21
Gambino, R., 616, 617, 618, 626
Gandhi, M. K., 379, 391
Gara, M., 252
Garbarino, J., 491
Garcia, M., 181, 182, 183, 185, 186, 187, 188
Garcia-Preto, N., 26, 87, 91, 133, 164, 170, 187, 244, 247, 250, 251, 252, 259, 545
Garcia Vasquez, J., 161
Garvey, M., 119
Gaspar, F. X., 637
Gastil, R. D., 454
Gaviria, C., 195
Gerard, S., 335
Gergen, K., 556

Geritty, E. T., 492
Gerson, R., 89, 253, 278, 550, 757
Gerton, J., 230
Ghaffarian, S., 460
Ghorayeb, F., 474
Gibran, K., 470, 473, 480
Gilbert, R. M., 552, 553
Gilfoyle, T. J., 596
Gilman, S., 506
Giordano, J., 36, 258, 482, 517, 619, 621
Giordano, M. A., 36
Gladsky, T., 745, 746, 748, 754
Glantz, O., 120
Glazer, N., 507
Goel, S. S. R., 397
Gold, J. S., 684, 685
Goldberg-Hiller, J., 68
Golden, J. M., 363
Goldner, V., 563, 565
Goldstein, S., 668, 670, 672
Gomez, J., 198
Gong-Guy, E., 363, 370
Gonzales-Mandri, F., 207
Gonzalez, J., 153, 158, 164, 243, 247
Good Tracks, J., 51
Good, B. J., 369, 461, 462
Good, M. J. D., 461
Goodnow, J. J., 478, 479
GoPaul-McNicol, S. A., 117, 121, 122, 123, 124
Gordon, M., 513, 611
Gorsuch, R. L., 343
Gostomski, C., 473
Gould, S. J., 16
Goyette, K., 345
Goza, F., 166
Graham, P., 220
Greeley, A. M., 2, 507, 508, 513, 597
Green, A. R., 4
Green, R. J., 32, 565
Greico, E. M., 64
Grier, W., 97
Griffith, J., 230
Grigorian, H., 441, 446
Grinberg, A., 264
Grinberg, L., 230
Grinberg, R., 230
Grossman, L., 671
Grossman, N., 695
Grow, B., 153, 156, 157
Grvdziak-Sobczy, E., 747
Guarnaccia, P., 3, 244, 252
Guerin, P. J., 253
Guerney, B. G., Jr., 97
Guerrieri, K. G., 193
Guest, P., 332
Gune, R., 386
Gunn, P. A., 45
Gupta, O. K., 402
Gupta, S. O., 402
Gutiérrez, M., 205, 206, 207, 209, 210
Gutiérrez de Pineda, V., 195, 197

Haas, W. S., 453
Hacker, A., 23
Haddad, S., 470
Haertig, E. W., 66
Haidar, A., 682
Hakim-Larson, J., 474, 484
Halkias, A., 575
Hall, E., 561

Hall, S., 9
Hamadeh, G. N., 474
Hamid, A., 429
Hamilton, B. E., 234
Hammerschlag, C., 53
Hanassab, S., 458
Hanchard, M., 169
Handlin, O., 505, 506
Handy, E. S. C., 66, 67
Hanna, N., 207, 209
Hansen, J., 649
Hardy, K. V., 20, 21, 32, 33, 34, 35, 111, 113, 114, 231, 757
Hare-Mustin, R. T., 563
Harris, D., 369
Hartman, A., 233
Hasan, K., 408
Havel, V., 727, 732
Hayden, T., 12, 608
Hays, H., 91
Head, J., 82
Hegi, U., 560, 561, 570
Heilbut, A., 565
Heinl, N. G., 129
Heinl, R. D.,Jr., 129
Heitzman, J., 396
Helms, J. E., 87
Hendricks, G., 220
Henkin, W. A., 345
Henriques, F., 121, 124
Henry, F., 121, 122
Heras, P., 326, 328
Herman, J., 507
Hernandez, M., 25, 182, 185, 186, 187, 188, 189, 247, 248, 249, 250, 251, 253, 257, 278, 310, 760
Hernandez, P., 383
Hernandez, R. E., 205, 220, 221
Herrera, J., 238
Hervis, O., 260, 359
Herzog, E., 672
Hess, H. J., 341
Hess, P. M., 341
Hieshima, J. A., 345
Hildesheimer, W., 565
Hill, N. E., 32
Hill, R., 87, 88, 89, 94
Hillier Parks, S., 232
Him, C., 371
Hines, P. M., 87, 89, 90, 91, 94, 98, 605
Hinton, W. H., 247
Hinton, W. L., 10, 363, 603, 609
Hitchcock, J., 4, 21, 509, 510, 511
Ho, M. K., 259, 264, 273, 281, 282, 285, 286, 309
Hodge, D. R., 22, 398, 399, 405, 757
Hoffman, D. M., 461
Hoffman, E., 717, 746, 748
Hofman, J. E., 470, 475
Hofmann, A. R., 559
Hojat, M., 458
Holguin, R. T., 218, 224
Hondagnue-Sotelo, P., 231
Hong, G., 270, 274, 285, 287
Hoobler, D., 617
Hoobler, T., 617
Hopkins, J. W., 161
Hough, R. L., 230
Hourani, A., 423, 426
Hsu, F. L. K., 274
Hsu, J., 305
Huang, K., 369

Huang, L. N., 342
Hummer, R. A., 363
Hundley, T., 743
Hunt, R., 511
Huntington, S. P., 521
Hurbon, L., 130, 134, 135
Hurh, W. M., 351, 354
Hutnik, N., 389

Iacocca, L., 515
Ianni, P. A., 616
Ichioka, Y., 340
Ignatiev, N., 20, 509, 596, 597
Ii, J. P., 67
Ima, K., 264
Imber-Black, E., 677
Inclan, J., 188, 189, 190
Itai, G., 342
Ito, K. L., 363
Izbudak, M., 452

Ja, D., 274
Jackson, C., 655, 656
Jackson, P. A., 335
Jackson, V., 79, 83, 96
Jacobs, J. L., 405
Jacobson, M. F., 597
Jafari, M. F., 398
Jalali, B., 459
Jamieson, D., 18
Janelli, D. Y., 352
Janelli, R. L., 352
Jeffers, S., 47
Jiobu, R. M., 389
Joanides, C., 579
Jocano, F. L., 323, 324
Johansson, L. M., 458
Johansson, S. E., 458
John, D., 90
Johnson, C., 616, 618
Johnson, F. A., 342
Johnson, L., 4
Johnson, P. B., 600
Johnson, T. W., 565
Johnson, W. L., 290
Jones, A. C., 22
Jones, C., 82
Jones, R., 87, 92
Joseph, S., 476, 479, 480
Jung, M., 285

Kaari, F., 256
Kabakian-Khasolian, T., 474
Kadkhoda, B., 460
Kafka, F., 558, 565
Kahn, S. M., 695
Kaiser, W. L., 3
Kamakau, S. M., 66, 67
Kamaraju, S., 384
Kambon, K. K., 87, 88
Kame'eleihiwa, L., 65, 66, 67
Kamya, H., 113
Kanin, G., 504
Kantrowitz, B., 649
Kanuha, V. K., 70
Kaplan, J., 681
Kaplan, R., 713
Karam, E. G., 474
Karenga, M., 87
Karim, S., 412

Karno, M., 230
Karp, A. J., 691
Karres, E. V. S., 560
Katz, J. H., 21, 511
Kaufman, D. R., 689, 695
Kaufman, E., 600
Kaufmann, E. P., 520, 521, 529
Kavi, A. R., 403
Kazantzakis, N., 573
Keddie, N., 428
Keefe, S., 234
Keillor, G., 649
Kelly, A. K., 72
Kennedy, M., 416
Kennedy, R. E., 26, 596, 602, 603
Keren, M. S., 565
Kerr, S., 718, 736, 737, 739
Kevorkian, N. S., 491
Khalidi, U., 381
Khamis, V., 491
Khan, B., 388
Khan, M. M., 411, 412
Khashan, H., 471, 472
Khater, A. F., 473, 484
Kheirkhah, S. P., 459
Khoi, K., 462
Kibbi, I., 475, 479
Killian, K. D., 580, 583
Killian, K. W., 662
Kim, A. S., 355
Kim, B. L. C., 350, 351, 354, 355, 357
Kim, C., 350
Kim, D. S., 350, 351, 354, 357
Kim, J. Y., 131
Kim, K. C., 351, 354
Kim, L., 349, 355
Kim, S., 281, 287
Kim, S. C., 359
Kim, Y., 104
Kim, Y. C., 349
Kimhi, S., 684
Kinealy, C., 596
King, R. C., 344
Kinzie, J. D., 294, 363, 369, 370, 371
Kirchick, J., 686
Kirk, J., 204
Kirschbaum, S. J., 727
Kitano, H. H. L., 340, 342, 320, 345
Kivel, P., 21, 511
Kivisto, P., 685
Klein, J., 506
Kleinman, A. M., 300, 369
Kletzien, H. H., 563
Kliman, J., 104, 106, 514
Knab, S. H., 747
Knafo, D., 416
Knight, F. W., 127
Knight, G., 208
Knight, R., 478
Kolenda, P., 386, 387
Koonen, W., 565
Korin, E. C., 175, 233
Kosary, D., 589
Koslow, P., 78
Kosmin, B. A., 21, 399
Kostelney, K., 491
Kottak, C. P., 170
Kranish, M., 503
Krasner, B., 210

Krauss, C., 161
Krestan, J. A., 550, 600
Krishna, A., 379, 385
Krogh, M., 90
Kuczewski, M., 415
Kundera, M., 727, 732
Kuoch, T., 292
Kurien, P., 400, 401
Kurtines, W. M., 207, 209, 210, 212, 359, 556
Kurzman, C., 458
Kusnir, D., 258, 259
Kutsche, P., 235
Kyselka, W., 65

Labbe, Y., 549
Lachman, S., 399
La Due, R., 47
La Framboise, T., 230
La Fromboise, T., 49
Laguerre, M. S., 134
Laird, J., 233
Lamphere, L., 209
Landau, J., 275
Lang, M., 182
Larmer, B., 80
Larsen, J., 94
Laszloffy, T. A., 21, 32, 33, 111, 113, 114, 757
Lateef, S., 382
Laurino, M., 623
Lavelle, J., 300, 371
Lavery, B., 600
Lazaridis, G., 578
Lazarre, J., 511
Lee, C. A., 66
Lee, E., 91, 275, 277, 278, 280, 285, 286, 306, 309, 311, 313, 363, 545, 580
Lee, S., 342, 344, 345, 346
Lendvai, P., 587, 588, 589
León, C. A., 198
Lerner, H., 752
Leung, P. K., 363
Levin, J. S., 405
Levine, I., 507, 508
Levinson, D., 118, 565
Levitt, P., 232
Levy, J., 48
Lew, A., 342
Lewis, B., 4
Lewter, N., 94
Leyburn, J. G., 654, 656
Leyens, J. P., 491
Lidz, T., 602
Lieberman, M. A., 606
Limansubroto, C., 337
Lin, J., 320
Lin, M., 307, 308
Lin, T., 307, 308
Lindsay, D. M., 21
Linn, R., 684
Lipat, C. T., 320
Lipniacka, E., 742
Lipset, M. S., 672
Lipsitz, G., 511
Lipsky, S., 70
Lipson, J. G., 461
Lo, B. L., 229
Lockwood, T. W., 22
Logan, S. L., 92
Loizos, P., 578

Lopata, H. Z., 745
López, D., 259, 264
López, O., 197
López, S. R., 3
Lott, J. T., 320
Loucky, J., 179
Louie, J., 163, 231
Lovejoy, P. E., 78
Lowenthal, D., 123, 124
Lu, F., 580
Luca-Stolkin, M., 578, 580
Luepnitz, D., 5
Lukacs, J., 588
Lund, T., 447, 449
Luthke, M., 104
Lynch, O., 384

MacCurtain, M., 603
Mackey, S., 470, 471, 472, 473, 475, 479, 480, 481, 482
Madsen, W., 106
Magganas, A., 579
Magoscsi, P., 714
Magwaza, A., 104
Mahapatra, M., 399
Mahjoub, A., 491
Maki, M. T., 340
Malayala, S., 384
Malcomson, S., 15, 16, 511
Malone, N., 256
Maloney, S., 46
Mañach, J., 209
Mamalakis, P. M., 579
Manalansan, M. F., IV, 320, 323
Mangione, J., 616, 617, 621
Mann, L., 616
Manning, M., 510
Mansfield, P., 430
Manson, S., 363, 371
Mantsios, G., 514
Marganoff, P., 711, 712, 715, 716, 719
Margolis, M., 166, 167, 172
Marín, B., 235
Marín, G., 209
Marion, P., 549
Marowski, J., 747
Marris, P., 230
Marrow, H., 166
Marsala, A. J., 492
Martes, A. C. B., 166, 167, 172
Martinez, E., 512
Martinez, R., 17
Marx, A. W., 169
Masalha, S., 491
Mass, A., 340, 341
Massey, D. S., 158
Matzner, A., 68
Maxim, K., 91
Mayer, E. B., 667
Mayhew, M., 579
Mbiti, J. S., 87, 107, 108, 112
McAdoo, H. P., 87, 89
McBride, J., 502, 503
McCabe, M. L., 629, 633
McCarthy, I. C., 603, 609
McCourt, F., 606
McCready, W., 597
McCulloch, J., 102
McGill, C., 286

McGill, D., 630, 640
McGoldrick, M., 5, 24, 25, 26, 32, 33, 36, 69, 87, 89, 91, 186, 189, 210, 253, 258, 278, 310, 388, 482, 504, 511, 515, 545, 550, 565, 603, 606, 608, 611, 757, 760
McIntosh, P., 21, 510, 511
McIntyre, T. M., 172
McKelvey, R. S., 369
McKenna, A., 603
McKenzie-Pollock, L., 299
McKinney, H., 357
McKinnon, J., 88
McLaughlin, D., 60
McRae, C., 342
McWilliams, N., 482
Mead, W., 641, 643, 649, 650
Medina, B. T. G., 323, 324
Meinhardt, K., 230
Melton, G. B., 492
Menchin, S., 605
Menjívar, C., 256, 257, 263
Mernissi, F., 381, 382
Merridale, C., 702, 703
Messias, D. K. H., 167
Messina, E., 616
Messineo, T., 183
Messinger, J. C., 604
Metress, E., 607
Meyer, M., 70
Middelton-Moz, J., 61
Midelfort, C., 647
Miller, B. D., 399, 403
Miller, C., 170
Miller, D., 440, 444, 445
Miller, K. A., 596, 598, 603
Miller, L., 5
Miller, L. T., 440, 444, 445
Miller, N. L., 134
Miller, R. A., 292
Miller, W. R., 22
Mills, J., 51
Min, B. G., 351, 354
Minsky, S., 252
Mintz, B. R., 350
Mintz, N., 599
Minuchin, S., 92, 97, 234, 699
Mira, M., 633
Mirande, A., 235
Miskimen, T., 252
Misumi, D. M., 384
Mitchell, D. D. K., 65, 67
Mitchell, F., 506
Mitchell, H., 94
Mitchell, V., 565
Mitchell-Kernan, C., 90
Mitrani, V. B., 163
Mitscherlich, A., 555
Mitscherlich, M., 555
Mitter, S. S., 383
Mizio, E., 245, 250, 251
Mizokawa, D. T., 345
Moazam, F., 415
Mock, M. R., 274, 275, 278, 281, 282, 283, 310, 314
Moghissi, H., 458
Mohamed, S. H., 335
Mohatt, G., 49
Moitoza, E., 630, 631
Mokuau, N., 64, 66, 70
Moll, L. C., 238

Mollica, R. F., 300, 371
Mondykowski, S., 742, 751
Monroe, A. D., 370
Montague, A., 26
Montalvo, B., 97
Montepio, S. N., 326
Montes Mozo, S., 161
Montoya, C. A., 320
Moogk, P. N., 546
Mooney, B. C., 503
Moore Hines, P., 81
Moore, L., 181
Moradi, R., 461
Morawska, E., 750
Morawski, J., 747
Morgan, E. S., 14, 559
Morishima, J. K., 308, 343, 345, 369
Morissonneau, C., 545
Morreale, B., 616, 617, 621
Morrison, T., 509
Moser, R. J., 233
Moses, K., 80
Moskos, C. C., 574
Moya Pons, R., 216, 217
Moynihan, D. P., 87
Much, N. C., 399
Muecke, M. A., 363
Muir, J. S., 163
Muir-Malcom, J. S., 163
Mull, D. S., 363
Mull, J. D., 363
Mullatti, L., 402
Murphy, M. W., 608
Murray, B., 409, 412, 413
Murry, V. M., 32
Myers, J. K., 600
Mynti, C., 478

Nabokov, P., 51
Nagata, D. K., 278, 340, 341, 345
Nahm, A. C., 349
Nahulu, L. B., 70
Naidoo, J., 382
Nanda, S., 378, 384, 388, 392
Napoli, M., 46
Nassar-McMillan, S., 474, 484
Nasser, R., 481
Neider, J., 363
Nelli, H. S., 618
Neumann, H. I., 560
Neville, G., 607
Newman, N., 557
Newton, J., 662
Ngo-Metzger, Q., 369
Nguyen, N., 363
Nguyen, S. D., 363
Nobles, M., 169
Nobles, W., 87, 88
Nolan, J., 597
Nordyke, E. C., 65
Novak, M., 507, 508
Novas, H., 158, 159, 160, 248
Nuckolls, C. W., 387
Nwidor, I., 102
Nwidor, N., 102
Nydell, M. K., 426
Nyrop, R. F., 455, 457

Oboler, S., 259
O'Corrain, D., 603

O'Faolain, N., 608
O'Leary, T. J., 205
Olsen, V., 535
Olson, K., 335, 357, 358
Olstad, R. G., 345
O'Mara, J., 18
Omuro-Yamamoto, L. K., 71
Ono, K. A., 153
Opler, M. K., 602
Ordona, T. A., 320
Ordonez, R. Z., 320
Orfanos, S. D., 578, 581
Orjuela, E., 181
Orleck, A., 701, 702
Orlov, A., 506
Ortiz, A., 10, 249, 603, 609
Ortiz, F., 206, 207, 209
Ostovar, R., 459
Otero-Sabogal, R., 209

Padilla, A. M., 104, 233
Page, M., 636
Pain, J., 130
Palazzoli, M. S., 299
Pane, F. R., 242
Pang, V. O., 345
Paniagua, F. A., 281
Pantoja, P., 235
Pap, L., 633
Papadimitriou, D., 386
Papajohn, J., 244, 245, 524, 577, 578, 579, 581, 620
Papataxiarchis, E., 578
Paperwalla, G., 130
Parham, T. A., 87
Parini, J., 616
Park, L., 399
Parker, L., 383
Parker, R., 170
Parsons, W. T., 563
Pasek, B., 748
Patactsil, J., 326, 328
Patai, R., 681
Patel, C., 659
Patterson, O., 81
Patti, A., 616
Paul, B., 570
Paul, N., 570
Paulino, A., 220, 224
Pearce, J. K., 482, 523, 608
Pedagogic, M., 747
Penn, P., 565
Pérez, L., 202, 204, 205, 207, 212
Pérez Firmat, G., 207, 212
Pérez-Stable, E. J., 209
Pérez-Stable, M., 204
Pérez-Vidal, A., 359
Perlmutter, P., 505, 506
Petsonk, J., 26
Pettigrew, T., 536
Pham, T., 369, 370
Pheterson, G., 70
Phinney, J. S., 556
Pickwell, S. M., 233
Pido, A. J. A., 321
Pierce, W. J., 129, 130
Piercy, F., 333
Pilger, J., 381
Pilisuk, M., 232
Pinderhughes, E., 4, 90, 149, 511, 556, 662
Pintak, L., 470, 472

Plank, S., 345
Pliskin, K. L., 461
Polacca, M., 44, 49, 51, 52, 53
Ponizovsky, A., 104
Portes, A., 205, 230
Power, P. C., 599
Pozkanzer, A., 683
Prashad, V., 385, 392
Prata, G., 299
Prawn, N., 747
Preli, R., 581
Primeggia, S., 616
Pryce, J., 22
Pukui, M. K., 66, 67, 71
Punamaki, R. I., 491

Quadagno, J., 617
Queralt, M., 207, 209
Quinones-Rosado, R., 155
Quintero, R. M., 250

Rabin, C., 681, 682, 683, 684
Rabinowitz, A., 699
Rabkin, J., 624
Radzilowski, J., 741, 743, 744
Ragucci, A. T., 618
Rainbow, J., 82
Ramana, K. V., 384
Rambaut, R. G., 230
Ramirez, R. R., 179, 235
Ramos, J., 253
Rashad, A., 138, 139
Raundalen, M., 492
Rayyan, F., 685
Red Horse, J., 47
Reddick, R. J., 82
Reed, E., 470, 471
Reeves, T., 270, 271
Reichmann, E., 557
Reichmann, R., 557
Reimers, C. W., 157
Reinat-Pumarejo, M., 248
Rejias-Mella, C., 226
Remsen, J., 26
Reuss-Ianni, E., 616
Revilla, L., 319, 322, 325
Reza, H., 411
Reza, R., 238
Rezentes, W. C., 66, 67
Richman, P., 91
Riotta-Sirey, A., 616, 621
Rippley, L. J., 557
Risech, F., 207
Ritsner, M., 104
Ritterband, P., 684
Rivera-Batiz, F., 220, 221
Rizvi, S. A. A., 382
Roberts, B., 600
Roberts, L., 369
Roberts, S., 15, 17, 18, 164, 502, 516
Robinson, R. H., 290
Rockeymoore, M., 88
Rodman, H., 122
Rodriguez, C. E., 248
Rodriguez, E. E., 247
Rodriguez, O., 244, 252
Rodriguez, P., 181, 182, 183, 185, 186, 187, 188
Rodriquez, G., 503, 516
Rodriquez, R., 503
Roediger, D., 510, 511

Rogg, E. M., 209
Rogler, L., 186
Rohrbaugh, M., 515
Rojano, R., 193, 194, 195, 197, 200, 260
Roland, A., 234, 386
Rolle, A., 616, 621
Root, M. P. P., 8, 15, 17, 26, 70, 79, 320, 344, 503
Rosen, E., 670, 677
Rosen, S., 667
Rosman, B. L., 97
Rossiter, A., 597
Rostow, J., 507
Roth, C., 749
Rothenberg, P., 511
Rouhparvar, A., 460
Rouse, R., 230, 232, 233
Roy, A., 381
Rubenstein, D., 492
Rubin, L. B., 529
Rücker-Embden, I., 565
Rudd, J. M., 603
Rueda, R. S., 238
Rugh, A., 472, 475, 476, 479, 480, 481, 482
Rumbaut, D. R., 207
Rumbaut, R. G., 207, 233, 264
Ruttenberg, D., 674

Sabar, N., 685
Sabogal, F., 209
Sack, W. H., 371
Sacks, D., 167, 171, 172, 173
Safdar, S., 459
Sagas, E., 217
Sai, D. K., 72
Said, E., 487, 490, 493
Saigh, P. A., 482
Saijwani, V., 381
Sairah, 404
Salamon, S., 561
Salmi, S., 491
Samouilidis, L., 580
San Juan, E., Jr., 321
Sanbonmatsu, D. M., 342
Sanchez-Korrol, V., 247
Sanchez-Martinez, F., 226
Sandemose, A., 649
Sanders, I., 750
Sanford, M., 123
Sang, D. L., 369
Santa Cruz, A., 207
Santa Rita, E., 319, 325
Santisban, D., 359
Santisteban, D. A., 163
Santo, L., 621
Santos, B., 65
Santos, R. A., 324, 327
Sanua, V. D., 601, 608
Sato, J. T., 320
Scally, R. J., 596
Shellenberger, S., 253, 757
Scheper-Hughes, N., 334, 603
Schiller, N. G., 132, 133, 230
Schjeldahl, P., 713
Schlesinger, A. M., 508, 582
Schlesinger, B., 121
Schmitt, A., 388
Schneider, B., 345
Schneider, H. J., 560
Schneider, S. W., 26, 674
Schumer, F., 97

Schwartz, S., 260
Scopetta, M. A., 209
Scully, M. F., 292
Scurfield, R. M., 492
Seelye, K., 513
Seikaly, M., 490
Shabbas, A., 426
Shahin, E., 470, 475
Shai, D., 689, 698
Shapiro, E., 203, 206, 207, 209, 210
Sharabi, H., 427
Sharaga, Y., 682
Sharma, A. P., 396
Shediac-Rizkallah, M., 474
Sheets, A., 117, 118
Sheinberg, M., 565
Shellenberger, S., 550
Shelton, B. A., 90
Shenton, J. P., 556
Shibusawa, T., 341, 342, 343, 344
Shiranzian, T., 370
Shokeid, M., 684, 685
Shon, S., 274
Shook, V. E., 71
Shorris, E., 156, 158, 159, 161, 232, 233
Shorter-Gooden, K., 82
Shorto, R., 537
Shuval, J. T., 230, 232
Shweder, R. A., 399
Sievers, L., 559
Silove, D., 370
Simmons, J., 10, 247, 603, 609
Simon, J. P., 475, 476
Simpson, E., 13, 747
Singco-Holmes, M. G., 320
Singer, J. L., 602
Sinke, S. M., 538
Siu, C. P., 685
Skidmore, T., 180
Slonim-Nevo, V., 682
Sloop, J. M., 153
Sluzki, C. E., 175, 232, 234
Smelser, N., 506
Smith, E., 631
Smith, E. P., 32
Smith, H., 703
Smith, P., 180
Smith, R., 120, 121
Smith, R. C., 65
Snowden, F. M., Jr., 78
Sobel, Z., 683, 684, 685
Sodergren, E., 643
Sodowsky, G. R., 384
Soekandar, A., 337
Sofer, J., 388
Soliman, A. M., 474
Solomon, M., 565
Solomon, W. E., 473
Sonawat, R., 400, 402, 403
Soo-Hoo, T., 285, 309
Sorrell, R. S., 547
Sowell, T., 120, 529
Spiegel, J., 244, 245, 524, 577, 578, 579, 581, 605, 620
Spielberg, S., 506
Sriram, R., 400
Srivastava, S. L., 403
Stannard, D. E., 65
Stanton-Salazar, R., 259, 264
Staples, R., 87, 88, 89, 94

Starr, P. D., 475, 477
Steel, Z., 370
Stein, K., 369
Steinfels, P., 512
Stephan, C. W., 344
Stephan, W. G., 344
Stephenson, P. H., 369
Stepick, A., 129, 130, 134
Sternbach, R. A., 601
Steven, S., 747, 748
Stevenson, M., 335
Stewart, C. P., 320
St. Fleurose, S., 131, 135
Stierlin, H., 565
Stivers, R., 600
St.-Onge, M. L., 549
Stocker, C., 641
Stowasser, B. F., 426
Struening, E., 624
Suarez-Orozco, C., 163, 178, 231, 233
Suarez-Orozco, M., 178, 233
Suci, G. J., 565
Sue, D. W., 287, 306, 369
Sue, L., 306
Sue, S., 280, 281, 306, 307, 308, 343, 357, 359, 369
Suleiman, M. W., 430
Summerfield, D., 491
Sundquist, J., 458
Suro, R., 219
Sustento-Seneriches, J., 321, 323, 327, 328
Sutton, C., 51
Suzuki, K., 237
Swarup, S. R., 397
Swierenga, R., 538, 539
Szapocznik, J., 205, 207, 209, 212, 359, 556
Szasz, C. M., 58, 59, 61

Ta, K., 363
Tafoya, T., 45, 49
Takaki, R., 272, 350, 386, 505, 506, 509
Takeuchi, D. T., 306
Takyi, B., 103
Tataki, R., 2, 9, 14, 15
Tatum, B. D., 21
Teahan, J. E., 600
Tejada-Holguin, R. T., 224
Teleky, R., 588, 590
Teller, C. H., 230
Telles, E. E., 168, 169, 176
Testa, M., 90
Thernstrom, S., 506, 513
Therrien, M., 179
Thiederman, S., 18
Thomas, H., 204
Thomas, J. D., 629, 633
Thomas, R., 18
Thompson, V., 119, 120
Thoresen, C. E., 22
Thornton, M. C., 344
Thurow, L., 23
Tidewell, R., 458
Tien, L., 335, 357, 358
Tienda, M., 157
Tiet, Q., 363
Tiongson, A. T., 320
Tocqueville, A., 520
Todorova, I. L. G., 163, 231
Tolzmann, D. H., 557, 559
Tomas, P., 248

Tomita, S. K., 342, 344
Tomm, K., 237
Tompar-Tiu, A., 321, 323, 327, 328
Ton-That, N., 371
Torres, M., 203, 207
Toussaint, P., 95
Tran, C. G., 363
Trimble, D., 113
Trimble, J., 49
Troast, J., 608
Troyano, A., 203, 207
Tryzno, W., 747
Tschann, J. M., 235
Tsemberis, S. J., 578, 581
Tseng, W. S., 305
Tuason, V. B., 198
Tucker, M. B., 90
Tulchin, J. S., 155
Tuller, D., 706
Turki, F., 493
Turner, J. E., 230
Tursky, B., 601

Ueda, R., 119
Ulloa, R., 256
Uomoto, J. M., 342
Ureña, H. M., 217

Vaidyanathan, P., 382
Valch, N., 178, 179, 181, 182, 183, 187, 188
Vallangca, C. C., 321
Valle, R., 232
van der Kolk, B., 298
Van Oss Marín, B., 209
Van Sickle, T. D., 472, 474, 475, 479, 480, 481
Varacalli, J., 616
Vardy, S. B., 590, 591
Varma, S. L., 335
Vasquez, L. P., 238
Vaughan, J., 167
Vazquez, C. I., 217, 220, 223, 226
Vazquez, M. M., 242, 252
Vega, W. A., 229, 230, 233, 234, 235, 252
Velez, L., 195
Verkuyten, M., 459
Visram, R., 385
Volkan, V., 491
von Mering, O., 605
Voyandoff, P., 122
Vreeland, M. M., 453

Wagenheim, K., 243
Wagenheim, O. J., 243
Wagner, P., 596
Walker, G., 565
Walker, T., 178, 179, 180, 181
Wallen, V., 119, 122
Walsh, D., 600
Walsh, F., 5, 22, 512, 757
Walters, K. L., 46
Warheit, G., 230
Warner, J. C., 46
Warren, D., 83
Wasserstein, B., 682
Watts-Jones, D., 82
Weber-Kellermann, I., 562, 563
Wehbi, S., 476, 477, 478
Weingarten, K., 113, 182
Weiss, C. I., 224

Weltman, S., 87, 670, 677
Wesner, D., 659
Wesolowsky, T., 742
West, A., 204, 205
Westermeyer, J., 272, 363, 371
Wetzel, N. A., 557, 565
Wheeler, D., 5
White, J., 87, 88, 89, 90, 91, 92, 94, 96, 97
White, M., 105, 107, 114, 115, 237
Whiting, B., 507
Wiarda, H., 217
Wilber, D. N., 455
Williams, R., 382
Williams, R. B., 397
Williams, R. L., 193
Williams, T. K., 344
Willie, C. V., 82
Wills, G., 127, 128, 598
Wilson, E., 588
Wilson, P., 121, 122
Wilson, W. J., 506
Wimberly, E. P., 94
Winawer, H., 557, 565
Winawer-Steiner, H., 566
Winn, P., 259
Wirsching, M., 565
Wishile, S. M., 233
Wiwa-Lawani, B., 102
Wong, L., 274, 283
Woodmason, C., 660
Woods, R., 183
Worden, R. L., 396
Wtulich, J., 712
Wylan, L., 599
Wyshak, G., 371

Xian, K., 68
Xie, Y., 345
Xu Xin, 693

Yaari, A., 416
Yalom, I. D., 551
Yamamoto, J., 369
Yang, E. S., 350
Yans-McLaughlin, V., 617
Yared, N. S., 476, 478, 480
Ybarra, L., 235
Yee, B. W. K., 342, 345
Yellow Horse-Davis, S., 47
Young, B. B. C., 66
Young, R., 117, 118
Yzerbyt, V., 491

Zaglul, A., 226
Zaman, R. M., 413
Zamichow, N., 230
Zamoyski, A., 742
Zane, N., 280, 281, 307, 359
Zborowski, M., 29, 524, 599, 601, 608, 624, 672
Zernike, K., 513
Zerubavel, Y., 681
Zetser, F., 104
Ziabakhsh, S., 460
Zinn, H., 9, 77, 78, 538
Ziv, T. A., 229
Zogby, J., 619
Zoghby, J., 430
Zola, I. K., 29, 601, 608, 624
Zonis, M., 453

Subject Index

Page numbers followed by *n* indicate note.

Abortion, Orthodox Jewish families and, 699
Abuse
  African American Muslim families and, 144
  British West Indian families and, 122
  Catholic Church and, 512–513
  Central American families and, 188
  French Canadian families and, 550
  Haitian families and, 133
  Iranian families and, 456–457
  Pakistani families and, 416
Acculturation
  African immigrant families and, 103–104
  Asian families and, 276, 279
  Asian Indian families and, 385–386, 389
  Brazilian families and, 169
  Central American families and, 186–189
  Chinese families and, 310–311
  code switching and, 329
  Cuban families and, 206–209, 210–211
  Dominican families and, 222
  European origin, families of, 503
  Filipino families and, 324–325, 329
  genograms and, 759
  Iranian families and, 459–460
  Irish families and, 602
  Israeli families and, 687
  Italian families and, 618, 623
  Korean families and, 354
  Latino families and, 156
  Lebanese and Syrian families and, 475
  Mexican American families and, 229–232, 235
  Portuguese families and, 633
  Puerto Rican families and, 249–252, 251–252
  Salvadoran families and, 263–264
Adaptation
  African American families and, 88
  Asian Indian families and, 391*n*–392*n*
  cultural perspective of, 28
  Dominican families and, 220
  Italian families and, 617
  migration and, 19
  Russian Jewish families and, 704
  Slovak families and, 737–738
Adolescence
  African American families and, 92
  African American Muslim families and, 145–146

African immigrant families and, 112
Anglo American families and, 526
Asian Indian families and, 382–383, 388, 389
Brazilian families and, 173
Cambodian families and, 295–296
Colombian families and, 198–199
Filipino families and, 320, 328
Haitian families and, 133
Indian Hindu families and, 402–403
Japanese families and, 342
Latino families and, 164
Lebanese and Syrian families and, 475
Mexican American families and, 233
migration and, 25
Native Hawaiian families and, 66, 68–69
Portuguese families and, 638
pregnancy during, 251, 328
Puerto Rican families and, 251–252
Affect, 97, 344, 355–357
African American families, 77, 85, 87–98
  in the 21st century, 87–88
  African immigrant families and, 105–106
  attitude toward talk therapy by, 29
  British West Indian families and, 119–120
  class and, 24
  cultural identity and, 3
  demographics and, 17–18, 79–80
  employment and education and, 94–95
  ethnicity training and, 35–36
  European origin, families of and, 507
  homosexuality and, 147–148
  kinship bonds and, 88–90
  labels and, 7
  life cycle and, 111–113
  migration and, 80–81
  multisystem approach to treatment and, 95
  parent–child systems in, 91–92, 145–146
  prejudice and, 10
  problem definition and, 30
  religion and, 22, 93–94
  social organization and, 31
  spirituality and, 81
  therapy issues, 81–85, 96–98, 148
  three-generation system in, 92–93
  United States history and, 14
  values and, 24
  See also African American Muslim families

776

African American Muslim families, 82, 138–150
  birth and death and, 146
  family life and, 140–145
  marriage and, 146–147
  See also African American families; African origin, families of
African immigrant families, 79, 80–81, 101–115
  acculturation of, 103–104
  colonialism and, 102
  community identity and, 108–109
  family life and, 109–110
  gender roles and, 110–111
  marriage and, 112–113
  race, race relations and racism and, 105–106
  spirituality and, 107–109
  therapy issues, 113–115
  in the United States, 103, 104, 106–107
  values and, 107
  See also African origin, families of
African origin, families of, 77–85
  Brazil and, 167–168
  demographics and, 79–80
  Dominican families as, 160
  migration of, 80–81
  Puerto Rican families and, 243
  See also African American families; African American Muslim families; African immigrant families; British West Indian families; Haitian families
AIDS. *See* HIV/AIDS epidemic
Albion's Seed: Four British Folkways in America (Fischer), 654. *See also* Scots-Irish families
Alcohol use
  African American families and, 88
  African American Muslim families and, 141, 145
  Anglo American families and, 527
  Brazilian families and, 172
  Colombian families and, 198
  Czech families and, 733
  Dominican families and, 225
  French Canadian families and, 550
  Irish families and, 600–601, 603
  Korean families and, 353–354
  Native American families and, 55–56
  Polish families and, 747–748, 751
  Puerto Rican families and, 253
  Scots-Irish families and, 660
  Slavic families and, 719
  Slovak families and, 736
  See also Substance abuse
Alcoholics Anonymous (AA), 601, 660
Aliyah, 684
Alliance for Progress, 159–160
Alternation theory, 230, 231–232
American Indian families, 43–53. *See* Native American families
American Indian Freedom of Religion Act (1978), 51
Americanization
  Armenian families and, 443–444
  Asian families and, 276
  Bulgarian families and, 716
  European origin, families of and, 509–510
  Israeli families and, 687
  Japanese families and, 345
  Jewish families and, 676
  Russian Jewish families and, 701
  See also Acculturation
Amok, 335

Anger
  French Canadian families and, 548
  Lebanese and Syrian families and, 480
  Mexican American families and, 236
  Polish families and, 751
  Portuguese families and, 633–634
  as a response to trauma, 57
  Scandinavian families and, 647
  therapy issues, 483–484
Anglo American families, 520–532
  attitude toward talk therapy by, 29
  class and, 529–530
  ethnicity and, 515
  family structure and, 525–528
  life cycle and, 525–528
  privilege of, 530
  problem definition and, 30
  regional variations in, 530–532
  therapy issues, 522–525
  See also European origin, families of
Animistic religions, 107–108. *See also* Religion
Anti-Semitism
  European origin, families of and, 509–511
  German families and, 559
  history, 505
  Jewish families and, 671, 690
  Polish families and, 748–749
  Russian Jewish families and, 702, 703
Anxiety
  Arab families and, 432
  French Canadian families and, 550
  Iranian families and, 460, 461
  Lebanese and Syrian families and, 474
  Polish families and, 751
  Puerto Rican families and, 253
  as a response to trauma, 57
Apostolic Church, 442–443. *See also* Religion
Appalachian/Southwestern culture, 532. *See also* Anglo American families
Arab families, 423–436
  family structure and, 426–429
  history and sociocultural context, 423–429
  language and, 426
  marriage and, 427–428
  problem definition and, 30
  religion and, 22, 424–426
  therapy issues, 431–435
  in the United States, 429–431
  values and, 430–431
  See also Armenian families; Iranian families; Lebanese and Syrian families; Palestinian families
Argentinian families, 161. *See also* Latino families
Armenian families, 437–450
  family structure and, 444–446
  genocide and, 439–442
  history, 438–442
  immigration and, 443–444
  Lebanese and Syrian families and, 471
  politics and, 442–443
  religion and, 442–443
  therapy issues, 446–449
  See also Arab families
Artha, 396
Ashkenazim, 681–682, 690. *See also* Israeli families
Asian families, 269–288
  demographics and, 17–18
  history and cultural context, 270–277
  prejudice and, 10
  response to stress by, 27

Asian families *(cont.)*
  social organization and, 31
  therapy issues, 277–288
  values and, 24
  See also Cambodian families; Chinese families; Filipino
    families; Indonesian families; Japanese families;
    Korean families; Vietnamese families
Asian Indian families, 377–393
  acculturation and, 385–386
  celebrations and life transitions and, 24
  family structure and, 385–390, 392*n*–393*n*
  Hindu and, 383–384
  history and sociocultural context, 377–385, 391*n*
  Islam and, 379–383
  life cycle and, 386–388
  problem definition and, 30
  religion and, 22, 379–385
  therapy issues, 388–390, 393*n*
  See also Indian Hindu families; Pakistani families
Assessment
  Asian families and, 277–278, 284
  Chinese families and, 309–313
  functioning, 759–762
  Greek families and, 580–581
  Korean families and, 359
  questions to ask, 762–763
  See also Genogram
Assimilation
  Asian Indian families and, 389
  boarding school system of, 59–61
  European origin, families of, 503
  German families and, 559, 569
  Irish families and, 597
  Latino families and, 156
  Native American families and, 49, 59
  overview, 15
  Slavic families and, 721
Authority
  Arab families and, 429
  French Canadian families and, 550
  German families and, 565
  Greek families and, 581
  Iranian families and, 453
  Irish families and, 608
  Latino families and, 163
  Portuguese families and, 630–631, 637–638
  Scandinavian families and, 649
Autonomy, 643–646, 649–650

Baptism, 576
Baptist church, 93. *See also* Religion
Bar/bat mitzvah, 676
Bedouin family, 427. *See also* Family structure
Belarusian families, 715. *See also* Slavic families
Belief systems
  African American Muslim families and, 148
  Arab families and, 430–431
  Chinese families and, 312
  Dominican families and, 226–227
  genograms and, 759
  intervention and, 28–29
  Native Hawaiian families and, 67–69
Biculturalism model, 231–232, 276, 459, 463, 464
Bigotry, 21. *See also* Racism
"Bill of Rights," 8
Biracial identity, 79, 344
Birth
  African American Muslim families and, 146
  Asian families and, 274

Greek families and, 576
Mexican American families and, 234
Orthodox Jewish families and, 699
Bisexual people. *See* Sexual orientation
Boarding school system, 59–61, 61–62
Bohemian families. *See* Czech families
Bondade, 635, 640
Boon-soo, 356
Bosnian families, 719–720. *See also* Slavic familie
Boundaries, family
  Central American families and, 182
  Italian families and, 620–621, 623, 625–626
  Korean families and, 352
  Lebanese and Syrian families and, 481
  Mexican American families and, 234–237, 237–238
  Russian Jewish families and, 706
  See also Family structure
Boundaries, group, 31
Boundaries, personal, 170, 561–562, 611
Brazil, 167–169. *See also* Brazilian families
Brazilian families, 155, 166–176
  in Brazil, 167–169
  demographics and, 176*n*
  language and, 636–637
  religion and, 176*n*
  therapy issues, 172–175
  in the United States, 171–172
  values of, 169–171
  See also Latino families
Brief therapy, 609
Bris, 676
British American families, 24
British West Indian families, 117–125
  and American Blacks, 119–120
  family relationships, 120–123
  history, 117–118
  migration of, 118–119
  therapy issues, 123–125
  See also African origin, families of
Buddhism
  Asian families and, 271
  Cambodian families and, 290, 292–293
  Chinese families and, 312
  history, 391*n*
  overview, 22
  See also Religion
Bulgarian families, 715–716. *See also* Slavic families
Burnout in therapists, 97

Calvinism, 534, 539–540. *See also* Religion
Cambodian families, 290–300
  demographics and, 292
  family structure and, 292–293
  history and sociocultural context, 290–292
  therapy issues, 293–300
  See also Asian families
Canadian families. *See* French Canadian families
Careers. *See* Employment
Caste system, 383–384, 396–397
Catholic Church
  abuse and, 512–513
  Arab families and, 426
  Armenian families and, 442
  Asian families and, 271
  Brazilian families and, 168
  Colombian families and, 193, 196
  Cuban families and, 209
  Czech families and, 725, 731–732
  Dutch families and, 536

Filipino families and, 326
French Canadian families and, 546, 548–549
Hungarian families and, 590–591
intermarriage and, 27
Irish families and, 596, 597–598, 603
Italian families and, 618–619
Lebanese and Syrian families and, 470–471
Mexican American families and, 232
overview, 22
Polish families and, 744, 749–750
Puerto Rican families and, 244
Scots-Irish families and, 655–656
Slavic families and, 713, 717–719
See also Religion
Celebrations
    African immigrant families, 111–113
    Asian families and, 287–288
    Greek families and, 575–576
    Indian Hindu families and, 400
    Irish families and, 600, 606
    Jewish families and, 674, 676
    Pakistani families and, 414
    values and, 24–25
Census counting. *See* Demographics
Central American families, 161, 178–190
    acculturation and, 186–189
    history, 179–181
    migration and, 184–186
    therapy issues, 181–184, 189–190
    See also Latino families
Ceremonies, traditional, 62. *See also* Rituals
Chae-myun, 356–357
Charity, Jewish families and, 672
Child lending, 122
Children
    Anglo American families and, 525–526
    Arab families and, 429
    Iranian families and, 460
    Irish families and, 605
    Italian families and, 622
    Jewish families and, 675–676
    Lebanese and Syrian families and, 478–480
    migration and, 25
    Operation Pedro Pan and, 203–204
Chinese American Psychiatric Epidemiological Study
    (CAPES), 306–307
Chinese Exclusion Act of 1842, 339
Chinese families, 302–317
    assessment and, 309–313
    attitude toward talk therapy by, 29
    family structure and, 305–306
    language and, 303
    migration and, 303–305
    problem definition and, 30
    therapy issues, 306–309, 313–317
    values and, 24
    See also Asian families
Choteo, 209
Christianity
    African American families and, 81
    African immigrant families and, 105–106, 107
    Arab families and, 425–426
    Armenian families and, 439, 442–443
    Asian families and, 271
    Asian Indian families and, 384–385
    German families and, 558–559
    Haitian families and, 133–134
    Hungarian families and, 587, 590–591
    Jewish families and, 690–691

Lebanese and Syrian families and, 470, 470–472
    Palestinian families and, 489–490
    Salvadoran families and, 259
    treatment and, 389
    See also Religion
Church of Latter-Day Saints, 326. *See also* Religion
Circumcision, 676
Citizenship. *See* Illegal status of immigrants
Civil Rights Act of 1826, 78–79
Civil Rights Act of 1924, 79
Class
    African American families and, 82–83, 88
    African immigrant families and, 106–107
    Anglo American families and, 529–530
    Asian Indian families and, 385–386
    Brazilian families and, 168, 174
    British West Indian families and, 121–122
    European origin, families of and, 513–514
    Indonesian families and, 335–336
    Israeli families and, 681–682, 684
    Korean families and, 351
    overview, 18, 23–24
    Polish families and, 746–747
    See also Poverty; Socioeconomic factors
Classism, 157
Collaborative approaches, 645–646
Collectivism, 496
Colombian families, 154, 161, 192–200
    cultural patterns and, 195–198
    history and sociocultural context, 192–194
    therapy issues, 198–199
    in the United States, 194–195
    See also Latino families
Colonialism, 102, 105, 109–110
Colonization
    Asian Indian families and, 378
    Dominican families and, 218
    Filipino families and, 321
    loss and, 84–85
    Salvadoran families and, 257
Combat stress disorder, 719
Communal sharing, 48–49
Communicative style
    African immigrant families and, 110–111
    Anglo American families and, 524
    Arab families and, 427, 431
    Asian families and, 287
    Cambodian families and, 293, 295
    Filipino families and, 325–326
    French Canadian families and, 548, 552–553
    German families and, 561–562
    Indonesian families and, 334
    Irish families and, 598–599
    Israeli families and, 687
    Japanese families and, 342
    Lebanese and Syrian families and, 480–482
    Mexican American families and, 235–236
    in Native American culture, 51
    Pakistani families and, 413–414
    Portuguese families and, 635–636
    Vietnamese families and, 365
Communism, 711–712
Community
    Armenian families and, 443–444
    Asian families and, 277–278, 279, 286–287
    Cambodian families and, 297
    Chinese families and, 311–312
    Czech families and, 730
    Dutch families and, 536–537

Community *(cont.)*
European origin, families of, 505
functioning and, 760
Greek families and, 574–575
Korean families and, 353
Orthodox Jewish families and, 693
Palestinian families and, 493–494
Portuguese families and, 632, 638
Slavic families and, 722
Slovak families and, 730
Community Family Therapy, 200
Community identity
African American Muslim families and, 140
British West Indian families and, 118–119
as a spiritual identity, 108–109
Complementary system, 567–569
Complexity of ethnicity, 6–13
Confiança, 635–636, 640
Conflict
African American families and, 84
Arab families and, 432
Czech families and, 733
French Canadian families and, 553
German families and, 562
Indian Hindu families and, 404
Iranian families and, 454
Irish families and, 598–599
Korean families and, 357
Native Hawaiian families and, 70–71
Polish families and, 751
Scandinavian families and, 647
Slovak families and, 736
Confucianism
Chinese families and, 305, 312
Japanese families and, 341
Korean families and, 357–358
Vietnamese families and, 364
See also Religion
Conservative Jewish families, 669, 674. *See also* Jewish families
Contract marriages, 415. *See also* Marriage
Coping mechanisms, 70, 281
Costa Rican families, 161, 179–181. *See also* Central American families; Latino families
Countertransference, 314
Creative therapy, 609–610
Creole society, 121, 129, 129–130. *See also* British West Indian families
Criticism, 482–483, 673, 737
Croat families, 719. *See also* Slavic families
Cuban Adjustment Act of 1926, 159
Cuban families, 159–160, 202–213
cultural identity and, 206–209
migration and, 204–206
religion and, 22
therapy issues, 210–212
See also Latino families
Cuban Refugee Program, 159, 209
Cultural assessment, 32, 759–762, 762–763. *See also* Assessment; Genogram
Cultural assumptions, 3
Cultural competence, 3–4, 4–5, 281–288
Cultural conflict, 67–71, 172–175, 276
Cultural differences, 24–25, 30, 31
Cultural identity
Asian families, 270–277
Asian Indian families and, 390
Colombian families and, 195–198
complexity of ethnicity and, 8–9

Cuban families and, 206–209
genograms and, 758
Greek families and, 575–576
Hungarian families and, 587–589
Latino families, 154–162
Lebanese and Syrian families and, 470–472, 482–484
Mexican American families and, 232–234
Native Hawaiian families and, 69–70
overview, 1–2
positive, 4–5
Russian Jewish families and, 702–703
Salvadoran families and, 259–260
tribal identity and, 48
Cultural meanings, 10–11, 11–13
Cultural nationalist Muslim family, 140, 141–142, 148. *See also* African American Muslim families
Cultural paradigms, 32
Cultural story, 231
Cultural transition map, 231
Cultural values, 19
Culture, 20–21, 31–32, 36–37
Czech families, 718, 724–739
family structure and, 732
history, 725–726, 726–727, 727–729
immigration and, 724, 729–730, 731
pravada vitezi and, 731–732
therapy issues, 732–735
See also Slavic families

Death
African American Muslim families and, 146
African immigrant families and, 112–113
Greek families and, 576
Irish families and, 606–607
Italian families and, 623
Jewish families and, 677
Scots-Irish families and, 661
Demographics
in the 21st century, 17–18
African American families, 79–80
Anglo American families and, 521
Asian families, 270
Brazilian families, 176*n*
British West Indian families and, 117–118
Cambodian families and, 292
Central American families, 178–179
Chinese families, 302
Colombian families and, 193–194
Dominican families and, 220
Dutch families and, 536
European origin, families of, 502
Filipino families, 319
German families, 556–557
Indian Hindu families and, 399
Israeli families and, 684
Italian families and, 617–618
Japanese families and, 341
Jewish families and, 668–669
Korean families and, 350–351
Latino families, 153–154
Native American families, 44–45
Native Hawaiian families, 641
Pakistani families and, 408
Palestinian families and, 489–491
Puerto Rican families and, 247
Salvadoran families and, 256–257
Slavic families and, 713–720
Vietnamese families, 367
Denial, 548, 550

Deportation, 103, 130–131, 183–184
Depression
    Anglo American families and, 527
    Arab families and, 432
    Asian Indian families and, 389
    boarding school phenomenon and, 61
    Brazilian families and, 173
    Colombian families and, 198
    Czech families and, 731, 733
    French Canadian families and, 550
    Haitian families and, 135
    Iranian families and, 460, 461
    Lebanese and Syrian families and, 474
    Mexican American families and, 233
    Native American families and, 56
    Pakistani families and, 411, 413
    Puerto Rican families and, 253
    as a response to trauma, 57
    Russian Jewish families and, 704
    Slavic families and, 719
    unresolved grief and, 56
    Vietnamese families and, 371
    See also Mental health disorders
Dharma, 396, 404
Discipline. See Punishment
Disconnect from cultural identity, 11–13
Discrimination
    African immigrant families and, 105–106
    Asian families and, 272–273
    caste system and, 397
    Chinese families and, 314
    cultural identity and, 9
    immigrants and, 10
    Israeli families and, 686
    Japanese families and, 340–341
    Jewish families and, 678
    Korean families and, 353
    Latino families and, 156–157
    Lebanese and Syrian families and, 484
    Mexican American families and, 233
    migration and, 19
    overview, 21
    Portuguese families and, 633
    Russian Jewish families and, 702, 706
Dispossession, feelings of, 491–494
Domestic violence
    Asian Indian families and, 387
    Central American families and, 188
    Dominican families and, 225
    German families and, 565
    Indian Hindu families and, 401
    Korean families and, 353–354
    Puerto Rican families and, 247
    Scots-Irish families and, 658–659
Dominant culture
    Anglo American families as, 521
    ethnicity of, 2–6
    ethnicity training and, 33–34
    labels and, 7
    Native American families and, 50–51
    passing for, 10
    United States history and, 14–15
Dominican families, 154, 160–161, 216–227
    family structure and, 218–219
    history and sociopolitical context, 216–218
    immigration and, 220–221
    socioeconomic factors and, 221
    therapy issues, 221–227
    See also Latino families

Domostroy, 721
Dowry, 112, 387
Drug production, in Colombia, 193
Drug use, 56, 88, 145, 411
DSM-IV, 3
Dual consciousness, 520
Dutch families, 534–544
    family structure and, 542–544
    history, 535–536
    religion and, 539–542
    in the United States, 536–539
    See also European origin, families of
Dysphoria, 461

Eastern Orthodox Church, 713, 714–717. See also
        Religion; Slavic families
Economic oppression, 84. See also Oppression;
        Socioeconomic factors
Ecostructural treatment. See Multisystem approach to
        treatment
Ecosystemic framework, 582–583
Education
    African American families and, 83, 88, 94–95
    African American Muslim families and, 145–146
    African immigrant families and, 115
    Anglo American families and, 532
    Arab families and, 428, 430
    Asian families and, 271
    Asian Indian families and, 382, 386
    boarding school phenomenon, 59–61
    Brazilian families and, 167
    British West Indian families and, 121, 122
    Central American families and, 188
    Colombian families and, 194, 196
    Czech families and, 729, 732, 733
    Dominican families and, 219, 220
    Dutch families and, 536
    European origin, families of and, 514
    Filipino families and, 321, 323–324, 328
    French Canadian families and, 546, 547, 548
    functioning and, 760
    German families and, 559, 562–563
    Haitian families and, 133
    Indian Hindu families and, 399
    Iranian families and, 460, 464
    Israeli families and, 681–682, 684
    Italian families and, 619–620
    Japanese families and, 345–346
    Jewish families and, 671–673, 675
    Korean families and, 349–350, 351, 354–355
    Latino families and, 157
    Lebanese and Syrian families and, 476, 479
    Mexican American families and, 233
    missionary system of, 59
    Native American families and, 58, 59, 59–61
    Native Hawaiian families and, 69
    Orthodox Jewish families and, 691
    Pakistani families and, 410
    Palestinian families and, 490
    Polish families and, 744, 749–750
    Proposition 183 in California and, 163, 229
    Puerto Rican families and, 247, 251
    Qur'an and, 381
    Russian Jewish families and, 702
    Slavic families and, 718
    Slovak families and, 735, 737
    values and, 23–24
El Salvador, 180–181. See also Central American families;
        Salvadoran families

Emancipation Proclamation of 1823, 78–79
Emigration
    Irish families and, 607–608
    Israeli families and, 684
    Polish families and, 744
    Russian Slavic families and, 714
    See also Immigration
Emotional expression
    Armenian families and, 446
    Czech families and, 733
    French Canadian families and, 548
    German families and, 562
    Hungarian families and, 588
    Irish families and, 598–599, 601
    Israeli families and, 683
    Italian families and, 623, 624
    Japanese families and, 344
    Jewish families and, 673
    Lebanese and Syrian families and, 474, 480–482
    Polish families and, 750–751
    Scandinavian families and, 646–648, 650–651
    Slavic families and, 720
    Slovak families and, 736
Empathy, 189–190, 283, 313
Employment
    African American families and, 88, 90, 94–95
    African immigrant families and, 106–107, 115
    Anglo American families and, 524–525, 526–527
    Asian families and, 279
    Asian Indian families and, 386
    Brazilian families and, 167
    caste system and, 396–397
    Central American families and, 187
    Chinese families and, 311
    Colombian families and, 195–196
    Cuban families and, 207
    Dominican families and, 221, 225
    Dutch families and, 537–538
    Filipino families and, 321, 323–324
    French Canadian families and, 548
    functioning and, 760
    German families and, 562
    Indian Hindu families and, 399
    Israeli families and, 685–686
    Italian families and, 619–620
    Jewish families and, 671–673
    Korean families and, 349–350, 351, 353, 354, 355
    Latino families and, 157
    Lebanese and Syrian families and, 476
    Mexican American families and, 233
    Pakistani families and, 411
    Polish families and, 744
    Puerto Rican families and, 248, 249–250
    Russian Jewish families and, 704
    Salvadoran families and, 258
    Scots-Irish families and, 659
    Slavic families and, 718
    Slovak families and, 730, 736–737
Endogamy, 428, 698–699. *See also* Marriage
Engagement
    African American families and, 96–97
    Asian families and, 281–285
    Chinese families and, 313
    French Canadian families and, 549
    German families and, 566
    Polish families and, 754
English-only laws, 153, 208. *See also* Language
Enmeshment, 625–626
Episcopalian church, 513. *See also* Religion

Essentialism, 583*n*–584*n*
Ethiopian Jewish families, 682–683. *See also* Jewish families
Ethnic identity
    complexity of, 8–9
    positive, 4–5
    of the therapist, 32
Ethnic pluralism, 15
Ethnicity training, 32–36
Ethnocentricity, 2–6, 506
Ethnocultural assessment, 231
European culture, 57–58, 58–59
European origin, families of, 501–517
    class and, 513–514
    history and sociocultural context, 504–508
    racism and, 509–511
    religion and, 511–513
    therapy issues, 509–517
    See also Anglo American families; Dutch families;
        French Canadian families; German families; Greek
        families; Hungarian families; Italian families; Portu-
        guese families; Scandinavian families; Scots-Irish families
Exile, Cuban families and, 205
Externalizing conversations, 237
Extramarital relationships, 121–122

Facial hair, Orthodox Jewish families and, 694
Faith healing, 307–308, 327
Familism, 245
Family conflict, 187–189, 198–199
Family life cycle. *See* Life cycle
Family Reunification Act, 398
Family structure
    functioning and, 759–762
    genograms and, 757, 758
    migration and, 25–26
    values and worldviews regarding, 24
    See also Fathers; Genogram; In-law relationships;
        individual ethnic groups; Kinship bonds; Marriage;
        Mothers; Older family members; Parent–child
        systems; Siblings
Family therapy. *See* Therapy
Famine, Irish, 607–608. *See also* Irish families
Fathers
    African American families and, 90–91
    Asian families and, 274–275, 284
    British West Indian families and, 123
    Chinese families and, 305
    German families and, 563, 564–565
    Greek families and, 577–578
    Irish families and, 610
    Italian families and, 621, 624
    Jewish families and, 673–674
    Korean families and, 354
    Mexican American families and, 235
    Puerto Rican families and, 246–247
    Slavic families and, 721
    See also Family structure
Fear, as a response to trauma, 57
Feminism
    African American Muslim families and, 149
    cultural competence and, 5
    halacha and, 689
    Indonesian families and, 337
    Islam and, 381
    Jewish families and, 674
    Khadija, 380
Filipino families, 319–330
    family structure and, 322–325
    history, 320–322

spirituality and, 326–327
therapy issues, 327–329
See also Asian families
Five Pillars of Islam, 410
Fourteenth Amendment in 1828, 78–79
Franco American families, 546–547. *See also* French
Canadian families
French Canadian families, 545–553
family structure and, 548–549
history and sociocultural context, 545–547
therapy issues, 549–553
See European origin, families of
French culture, 745, 746

Gambling, 141, 328
Gang violence, 296
Gay people. *See* Sexual orientation
Gemütlichkeit, 562
Gender roles
African American families and, 81–82, 90–91
African American Muslim families and, 140, 147, 149
African immigrant families and, 106–107, 110–111
Anglo American families and, 526–528
Arab families and, 426–429
Armenian families and, 444–446
Asian families and, 274
Asian Indian families and, 381–382, 383, 384–385, 386,
386–387, 392n
Brazilian families and, 170–171, 174–175
British West Indian families and, 121–122
Cambodian families and, 292–293
Central American families and, 187–188
Chinese families and, 305, 311
Colombian families and, 195
Cuban families and, 207–208, 210–211
Czech families and, 732, 734
Dominican families and, 218–219, 224–226
Dutch families and, 542–544
Filipino families and, 322–325
German families and, 563–564
Greek families and, 576, 577–579, 583n, 584n
Indian Hindu families and, 400–404
Indonesian families and, 333–336
Iranian families and, 456–457, 458–459
Irish families and, 601–604
Israeli families and, 687
Italian families and, 621–622
Jewish families and, 673–674, 675
Korean families and, 349–350, 351–357
Latino families and, 162, 164
Lebanese and Syrian families and, 476–478
Mexican American families and, 230–231, 235
Native Hawaiian families and, 66–67, 68–69, 71–72
Orthodox Jewish families and, 694–696
overview, 18
Pakistani families and, 413, 415
Polish families and, 749, 750
Puerto Rican families and, 246–247, 249–251
Russian Jewish families and, 703, 706
Salvadoran families and, 258, 259
Scots-Irish families and, 658–659
Slavic families and, 719
Slovak families and, 736–737
in the United States, 685–686
See also Patriarchy
Generalizations, 13, 32, 235
Generational lines
African American families and, 92–93
Armenian families and, 444

Cambodian families and, 295–297
complexity of ethnicity and, 6–7
Cuban families and, 207
Czech families and, 732, 733
Filipino families and, 322–325, 325–326
genograms and, 757
Indian Hindu families and, 403, 404
Iranian families and, 458–459
Italian families and, 621
Lebanese and Syrian families and, 475
Pakistani families and, 415
Slovak families and, 735, 737
values and, 24
See also Family structure; Intergenerational conflict
Generosity, 635, 640, 737
Genital mutilation, 111, 676
Genocide
Armenian families and, 439–442, 443
German families and, 560–561
Irish families and, 607–608
Native American families and, 47, 49, 56–57, 62
Slavic families and, 719
Genogram
African American families and, 89
African American Muslim families and, 148
Asian families and, 277
cultural questions to ask, 762–763
Filipino families and, 323
French Canadian families and, 550
German families and, 569
with Haitian families, 135–136
Indonesian families and, 337
Mexican American families and, 231
overview, 757–759
Polish families and, 745
Portuguese families and, 638
Puerto Rican families and, 253
Russian Jewish families and, 706
Scandinavian families and, 645
See also Assessment; Family structure
German families, 555–570
family structure and, 562, 563–565, 567–569
history and sociocultural context, 505, 556–561
therapy issues, 565–570
values and, 562–563
See also European origin, families of
Goal-oriented treatment, 609
Godparents
Mexican American families and, 238
Puerto Rican families and, 245
Salvadoran families and, 259
See also Family structure
"Golden exile," 205, 207
Grandparents. *See* Older family members
Great Migration (1717–1735), 656–657. *See also* Scots-
Irish families
Greek families, 573–584, 583n
adaptive behavior and, 28
attitude toward talk therapy by, 29
ethnicity and, 516
family structure and, 576–580
history, 574
immigration and, 574–575
problem definition and, 30
religion and, 575–576
social organization and, 31
therapy issues, 580–583
values and, 24
See also European origin, families of

Greek Orthodox Church, 575–576. *See also* Religion
Greek Orthodox families, 579
Grief, 603–604, 623
Grief, unresolved, 56–57, 84–85, 309–310
Group boundaries, 31, 157–162
Guatemala, 179–181, 187. *See also* Central American families
Guilt, 601, 608, 687
Guilt, survivor, 57, 668

Hahn, 356
Haitian families, 127–136
    depression and somatic disorders, 135
    Dominican families and, 217–218
    history, 128–129, 160
    marriage and, 132
    providing economic support by, 132–133
    reasons for immigration, 130–131
    religion and, 22, 133–135
    stigma and, 131
    therapy issues, 135
    See also African origin, families of
Halacha, 689, 693
Hare Krishna movement, 385. *See also* Religion
Hasidism, 691, 693–694. *See also* Orthodox Jewish
    families
Healing practices
    Chinese families and, 307–309
    Filipino families and, 327
    medicine people, 51–52, 53n
    Mexican American families and, 232–233
    Native American culture and, 51–52
    Pakistani families and, 411–413
    Puerto Rican families and, 244
    Vietnamese families and, 363
Health care
    African immigrant families and, 106–107
    cultural disparities in, 4–5
    Hmong families and, 10–11
    Mexican American families and, 233
    Native American culture and, 51–52
    Pakistani families and, 411–413
    Proposition 183 in California and, 163, 229
    Puerto Rican families and, 252–253
Health problems
    African American families and, 88
    Asian families and, 280
    Lebanese and Syrian families and, 473–474
    Native Hawaiian families and, 69
    as a response to trauma, 57
    unresolved grief and, 56
Helplessness, learned, 233
Hembrismo, 246
Heterosexism, 31–32, 83, 314. *See also* Sexual orientation
Hierarchy
    African immigrant families and, 110–111, 112
    Arab families and, 427
    Asian families and, 274, 282
    Asian Indian families and, 382, 390
    Cambodian families and, 292–293
    Central American families and, 188
    Cuban families and, 207–208
    Filipino families and, 324
    French Canadian families and, 553
    Indonesian families and, 333
    Korean families and, 351–357, 354–355, 358
    Mexican American families and, 235
    Portuguese families and, 637–638
    Salvadoran families and, 259
    Scandinavian families and, 645–646

Vietnamese families and, 365
    See also Family structure
Hijras, 392n
Hinduism
    acculturation and, 385
    Asian Indian families and, 383–384
    history, 378
    overview, 396, 399
    Pakistani families and, 407–408
    therapy issues, 404–405
    treatment and, 389
    See also Indian Hindu families; Religion
"Hispanic" label, 7, 16. *See also* Latino families
Historical effects on identity, 7
History. *See individual ethnic groups*
HIV/AIDS epidemic
    African American families and, 88
    African immigrant families and, 102, 111
    Filipino families and, 328
    Haitian families and, 131
    Lebanese and Syrian families and, 478
    Salvadoran families and, 258, 259–260
Hmong families, 10–11
Holocaust
    Cambodian families and, 291
    German families and, 560–561
    Hungarian families and, 591
    Israeli families and, 680
    Jewish families and, 668
    Maafa, 88
    Orthodox Jewish families and, 692
    Palestinian families and, 492
    Polish families and, 748–749
    Russian Jewish families and, 702–703
Homosexual people. *See* Sexual orientation
Honor, 482–484, 634–635, 637, 640
Honra, 634–635, 637, 640
Ho'oponopono, 70–71. *See also* Native Hawaiian families
Hospitality, 109–110, 737
Human development, 3, 25–26
Human rights, 31–32
Humility, 649–650
Humor, 599, 609, 610, 675, 741–742
Hungarian families, 586–593
    history, 586–587
    immigration and, 590
    language and, 590
    religion and, 590–591
    therapy issues, 591–593
    See also European origin, families of
Hwa-byung, 356
Hyperindividualism, 521–522, 522–523
Hypervigilance, 57

"I statements," 344
Illegal status of immigrants
    Central American families and, 183–184
    Colombian families and, 195
    Dominican families and, 219
    Filipino families and, 320
    Irish families and, 597
    Proposition 183 in California and, 163, 229
    Puerto Rican families and, 248
    See also Immigrants
Imagination, 589, 593, 598–599
Immigrants
    Armenian families as, 443–444
    Asian families as, 270, 271–272
    from Brazil, 166–167

British West Indian families as, 124
Czech families as, 724, 729–730, 731
Dominican families as, 220–221
Dutch families as, 536–539
ethnic identity and, 9–10
European origin, families of as, 504–508
Filipino families as, 320–322, 322–325, 327
French Canadian families as, 545–546
functioning and, 760–761
German families as, 556–557, 569–570
Greek families as, 574–575
from Haiti, 130–131
Hungarian families as, 590
Indian Hindu families as, 397–398, 400
Iranian families as, 451–454, 457–459, 459–460
Irish families as, 596–597, 607–608
Israeli families as, 683–685
Italian families as, 617–618
Japanese families as, 339–340
Korean families as, 350
Latino families as, 156–157
Lebanese and Syrian families as, 472–473
Orthodox Jewish families as, 690–693
Pakistani families as, 408–409
Palestinian families as, 490
Polish families as, 743–745
Portuguese families as, 633–634
Puerto Rican families as, 247–248, 249–252
religion and, 22
Russian Jewish families as, 701–702
Salvadoran families as, 256–257, 260–264
Scandinavian families as, 646
Scots-Irish families as, 656–657, 662n–663n
Slavic families as, 713–720, 722
Slovak families as, 724, 730, 731
    See also African immigrant families; Illegal status of
        immigrants; Immigration policies
Immigration Act of 1884, 303
Immigration Act of 1925, 178, 272, 304, 574
Immigration and Nationality Act of 1925, 321
Immigration and Naturalization Service Act of 1915, 350
Immigration Exclusion Act of 1884, 340
Immigration policies. See also Immigrants
    African immigrant families and, 80–81, 106–107, 114
    Central American families and, 178–179, 183–184
    Cuban families and, 202–203, 205–206
    following September 11, 1961, 408–409
    Jewish families and, 668
    Personal Responsibility and Work Opportunity
        Reconciliation Act of 1956 and, 153
Immigration Reform and Control Act of 1946, 183–184
In-law relationships
    Asian Indian families and, 386–387, 389, 390, 392n–
        393n
    Indian Hindu families and, 403
    Iranian families and, 456
    Irish families and, 602
    Korean families and, 352–354
    Pakistani families and, 413
    See also Family structure
Index of Cultural Inclusion, 580–581
Indian Hindu families, 395–405
    caste system and, 396–397
    demographics and, 399
    family structure and, 399–404
    history, 397–398
    therapy issues, 404–405
    in the United States, 398–399
    See also Asian Indian families

Individualism, 520, 521–522, 522–523, 530–532
Indonesian families, 332–338. See also Asian families
    therapy issues, 336–338
Infertility, 695
Infidelity
    African American Muslim families and, 144
    Asian Indian families and, 389
    British West Indian families and, 121–122
    Greek families and, 578–579
    Irish families and, 602
    Lebanese and Syrian families and, 478
    Pakistani families and, 414–415
    Vietnamese families and, 365
    See also Marriage
Institutional racism, 88. See also Racism
Intensive brief therapy, 551
Intergenerational conflict
    Cambodian families and, 295–297
    German families and, 570
    Indian Hindu families and, 400
    Iranian families and, 459
    Lebanese and Syrian families and, 475, 482
    Pakistani families and, 415
    See also Family structure; Generational lines
Intermarriage
    Asian Indian families and, 382
    Brazilian families and, 168, 169
    British West Indian families and, 121
    Cuban families and, 210
    Dominican families and, 218, 219
    European origin, families of, 503
    European origin, families of and, 516–517
    Filipino families and, 320
    French Canadian families and, 549
    German families and, 559, 569
    Greek families and, 579
    Iranian families and, 456, 465
    Irish families and, 597
    Israeli families and, 681–682, 686
    Jewish families and, 669, 670–671
    Latino families and, 164
    Lebanese and Syrian families and, 471
    Native American families and, 50
    Orthodox Jewish families and, 692–693
    overview, 26–27
    Portuguese families and, 638
    racism and, 21
    Slovak families and, 738
    See also Marriage
Intervention. See Therapy
Invisibility syndrome, 90
Iranian families, 451–465
    adaptive behavior and, 28
    family structure and, 454–459
    immigration and, 459–460
    life cycle and, 457
    migration and, 451–454
    religion and, 453
    therapy issues, 461–464
    See also Arab families
Irish families, 595–612
    adaptive behavior and, 28
    alcohol use among, 600–601
    attitude toward talk therapy by, 29–30
    celebrations and life transitions and, 24–25
    class and, 24
    communication and conflict and, 598–599
    diaspora of, 595–596
    emigration and, 607–608

Irish families *(cont.)*
  emotional expression and, 601
  ethnic identity and, 10, 516
  European origin, families of and, 509
  family structure and, 601–607
  Franco American families and, 547
  history, 505, 596–597
  immigration and, 596–597
  problem definition and, 30
  religion and, 513, 597–598
  therapy issues, 608–611
  See also European origin, families of
Islam
  African immigrant families and, 107
  history, 424
  Iranian families and, 453
  laws of, 144–145
  marriage and, 428
  overview, 22, 379–383, 424–425
  Pakistani families and, 410
  principles of, 140–141
  See also African American Muslim families; Muslim;
    Religion
Isolation, 611, 643–646
Israeli families, 680–687
  demographics and, 684
  emigration and, 684
  family structure and, 682–683
  immigration and, 683–685
  intermarriage and, 686
  sexual orientation and, 686
  therapy issues, 686–687
  in the United States, 685
  See also Jewish families
Italian families, 616–627
  alcohol use among, 600
  attitude toward talk therapy by, 29
  class and, 24
  employment and education and, 619–620
  ethnicity and, 515
  family structure and, 620–623
  history, 505, 616–617
  immigration and, 617–618
  problem definition and, 30
  religion and, 513, 618–619
  response to stress by, 27
  social organization and, 31
  therapy issues, 624–627
  values and, 24, 617
  See also European origin, families of

Jamaican families. *See* British West Indian families
Japanese families, 339–346
  demographics and, 341
  history, 339–341
  therapy issues, 342–346
  values and, 341–342
  See also Asian families
Jehovah's Witnesses, 326. *See also* Religion
Jeong, 355–356
Jewish ethnicity, 7–8, 10, 24, 27
Jewish families, 667–678
  adaptive behavior and, 28
  attitude toward talk therapy by, 29
  Czech and Slovak families and, 729
  Dutch families and, 536
  ethnicity and, 515
  German families and, 558–559
  history, 505–506

history and sociocultural context, 667–673
  Hungarian families and, 591
  intermarriage and, 669, 670–671
  Lebanese and Syrian families and, 472
  Palestinian families and, 488–489
  Polish families and, 742, 748–749
  problem definition and, 30
  response to stress by, 27
  social organization and, 31
  therapy issues, 673–677
  values and, 24
  See also European origin, families of; Israeli families;
    Orthodox Jewish families
Jihad, 410

Kaddish, 677
Kanaka Maoli families, 67–71. *See also* Native Hawaiian
  families
Karma, 396, 404
Khadija, 380
Khmer Rouge, 291. *See also* Cambodian families
Kinship bonds
  African American families and, 88–90
  Asian Indian families and, 386
  Brazilian families and, 169–170
  Cuban families and, 207–208
  Filipino families and, 322–325
  genograms and, 757
  Indian Hindu families and, 400
  Iranian families and, 465
  Lebanese and Syrian families and, 475–480
  marriage and, 112
  Mexican American families and, 234
  Scots-Irish families and, 658
  See also Family structure
Kinship responsibilities, 132–133
Korean families, 349–360
  affect management and, 355–357
  family structure and, 351–355
  immigration and, 350
  religion and, 22
  therapy issues, 357–360
  in the United States, 350–351
  See also Asian families

Labels, 7, 154–155, 392n
Language
  Arab families and, 426, 431
  Armenian families and, 439, 445
  Asian families and, 270–271, 287
  Brazilian families and, 166
  Cambodian families and, 298
  Central American families and, 188
  Chinese families and, 303, 311
  Colombian families and, 196
  Cuban families and, 208–209, 210–211
  Czech families and, 725–726, 729
  English-only laws, 153, 208
  French Canadian families and, 546–547, 549
  genograms and, 759
  German families and, 558
  in Haiti, 129
  Hungarian families and, 586, 587, 590
  Iranian families and, 453, 460
  Irish families and, 597
  Israeli families and, 687
  Korean families and, 354, 355
  Latino families and, 154–155, 157, 162
  Lebanese and Syrian families and, 469, 480

Mexican American families and, 233, 236
Orthodox Jewish families and, 690, 692
Polish families and, 744
Portuguese families and, 636–637
Puerto Rican families and, 251–252
Scandinavian families and, 647
Slavic families and, 719
Slovak families and, 726–727
Ukrainian families and, 714–715
Vietnamese families and, 370
Latino families, 17–18, 153–164, 154–155
    demographics and, 17–18
    ethnic identity and, 10
    historical and cultural context of, 154–162
    intermarriage and, 219
    prejudice and, 10
    religion and, 22
    treatment and, 162–164
    See also Brazilian families; Central American families;
        Colombian families; Cuban families; Dominican
        families; Mexican American families; Puerto Rican
        families; Salvadoran families; South American families
"The Law of Jante," 649–650
Lebanese and Syrian families, 468–484. See also Arab
        families
    communication and emotion and, 480–482
    family structure and, 475–480
    gender roles and, 476–478
    history, 469–470
    immigration and, 472–473
    parent–child systems in, 478–480
    sexuality and, 478
    therapy issues, 472, 480–482, 482–484
    trauma and, 473–474
Legal status of immigrants. See Illegal status of immigrants
Lesbian women. See Sexual orientation
Life cycle
    African immigrant families and, 106–107, 111–113
    Anglo American families and, 525–528
    Asian Indian families and, 386–388, 390–391
    Brazilian families and, 173
    Chinese families and, 310
    functioning and, 761
    genograms and, 757, 758
    Iranian families and, 457
    Irish families and, 606–607
    Italian families and, 623
    Jewish families and, 676
    Mexican American families and, 237–238
    migration at different phases of, 25–26
    Pakistani families and, 414–415
Life expectancy, 88, 90
Life transitions, 24–25
Loa, 134
Loneliness, 171–172, 173, 646
Loss
    African American families and, 84–85
    Armenian families and, 446
    Asian Indian families and, 389
    Cambodian families and, 293–294
    Central American families and, 184–185
    Chinese families and, 309–310
    Cuban families and, 210
    ethnic identity and, 9–10
    Filipino families and, 327
    immigration and, 80–81
    Jewish families and, 677
    Latino families and, 163
    Native American families and, 56, 56–57

Pakistani families and, 408
Palestinian families and, 491–494
Polish families and, 751
Portuguese families and, 633–634
Russian Jewish families and, 704, 706
Salvadoran families and, 261
therapy issues, 182
Lutheran church, 646. See also Religion

Maafa, 88
Machismo, 235, 246, 253
Mafia, 619–620
Majority group. See Dominant culture
Malu, 334–335
Marianismo, 246
Maronite church, 471. See also Religion
Marriage
    African American families and, 90–91
    African American Muslim families and, 143–145, 146–
        147
    African immigrant families and, 111–113
    Anglo American families and, 526–528
    Arab families and, 427–428, 432
    Armenian families and, 444, 445
    Asian families and, 274–277
    Asian Indian families and, 382, 386–387
    Brazilian families and, 170, 172, 173, 174–175
    British West Indian families and, 121–122
    Cambodian families and, 293
    caste system and, 397
    Chinese families and, 303–304, 305, 306
    Colombian families and, 198
    Cuban families and, 207–208
    Czech families and, 730, 734
    Dominican families and, 216, 218–219, 224–226
    Dutch families and, 542–544
    European origin, families of and, 513, 516–517
    Filipino families and, 320, 323–324
    French Canadian families and, 546, 548–549
    German families and, 563–564
    Greek families and, 578–579
    Haitian families and, 132
    Indian Hindu families and, 397, 400–404
    Indonesian families and, 333
    Iranian families and, 455–456, 458–459, 460, 465
    Irish families and, 604–605
    Israeli families and, 686
    Japanese families and, 339, 341
    Jewish families and, 670–671, 676–677
    Korean families and, 352–354
    Latino families and, 162–163, 164
    Lebanese and Syrian families and, 471, 477
    Mexican American families and, 235, 237–238
    Native American families, 45–46, 47–48
    Orthodox Jewish families and, 692–693, 694–696, 698–
        699
    Pakistani families and, 413, 414–415
    Palestinian families and, 493–494
    Polish families and, 747, 749, 750
    Puerto Rican families and, 245–247, 249–250
    Salvadoran families and, 259
    Scandinavian families and, 649
    Scots-Irish families and, 658–659
    slavery and, 89
    Slavic families and, 717–718
    Slovak families and, 736, 738
    Vietnamese families and, 365–366
    See also Family structure; Intermarriage
Matriarchy, 323, 401, 401–402, 603–604

Medicine people, 51–52, 53*n*. *See also* Healing practices
"Melting pot" ideology, 15, 507–508
Mental health disorders
    Arab families and, 431–435
    Asian families and, 280–281
    Chinese families and, 306–307, 308
    Filipino families and, 327–328
    genograms and, 758
    Haitian families and, 133–135
    Iranian families and, 460
    Japanese families and, 342–343
    Korean families and, 356
    Lebanese and Syrian families and, 474
    Native American families and, 57
    Orthodox Jewish families and, 683
    Pakistani families and, 411–413
    Vietnamese families and, 370–371
    See also Depression
Mexican American families, 158, 229–239
    celebrations and life transitions and, 24
    ecological context, 232–234
    family structure and, 234–237, 237–238
    migration and acculturation of, 229–232
    therapy issues, 231–232, 233–234, 236–237, 238
    See also Latino families
Migration
    of African American families, 80–81, 87–88
    Asian families and, 278, 279
    Brazilian families and, 174
    of British West Indian families, 118–119
    Central American families and, 184–186
    Chinese families and, 303–305, 309–310
    Colombian families and, 194–195
    Cuban families and, 204–206, 210–211
    at different phases of hte life cycle, 25–26
    functioning and, 760–761
    Iranian families and, 451–454
    loss and, 84–85
    Mexican American families and, 229–232
    overview, 18, 19–20
    Salvadoran families and, 258, 260–264
    Scots-Irish families and, 656–657, 662*n*–663*n*
Mikvah, 699
Mind–body connection, 297–298
Mixed-race people, 69–70
Mizrachim, 681–682, 692. *See also* Israeli families
"Model minority" image, 272, 345
Modern Orthodox Jewish families. *See* Orthodox Jewish
    families
Modesty, 694, 719
Mohammed, prophet, 380, 424–425, 428
Moksha, 396
Monotheistic faiths, 107–108. *See also* Religion
Mothers
    African American families and, 90–91
    Asian families and, 274–275
    British West Indian families and, 122
    Chinese families and, 305
    Greek families and, 578
    Irish families and, 603
    Italian families and, 621–622
    Jewish families and, 673–674, 675
    Korean families and, 354
    Lebanese and Syrian families and, 476
    Mexican American families and, 235
    Puerto Rican families and, 246–247
    See also Family structure; Gender roles
Multicultural identity, 69–70
Multiculturalism, 508

Multiethnic identity, 69–70, 72
Multiracial identity, 79
Multisystem approach to treatment, 95
Muslim families, 146–147
Muslim religion
    Asian Indian families and, 379–383
    Filipino families and, 326
    history, 378
    Indonesian families and, 332, 335
    Italian families and, 618
    Lebanese and Syrian families and, 470–472
    marriage and, 427–428
    overview, 424–425
    Pakistani families and, 407–408, 410
    Palestinian families and, 489–490
    Slavic families and, 713, 719–720
    See also Islam; Religion
Mythmaking, 589, 593. *See also* Storytelling

Narahati, 461
National Security Entry–Exit Registration System
    (NSEERS), 409
Native American Church, 52
Native American families, 43–62
    after contact with European culture, 58–59
    attitude toward talk therapy by, 30
    boarding school phenomenon, 59–61
    communal sharing and, 48–49
    before contact with European culture, 57–58
    demographics of, 44–45
    family structure and obligations, 45–46
    genocide and, 47
    historical loss of, 56–57
    missionary system of assimilation, 59
    spiritual relationship of man and nature, 46–47
    therapy issues, 49–53, 61–62
    in today's society, 55–56
    tribal identity of, 47–48
    United States history and, 14–15
    See also Native Hawaiian families
Native Hawaiian families, 64–72
    demographics and, 641
    history, 65–66
    intervention and, 67–71
    See also Native American families
Naturalization Law of 1750, 14
Nicaragua, 180–181. *See also* Central American families
"Non-Hispanic European" label, 7
Nonverbal communication, 51, 342, 413–414, 611, 694.
    See also Communicative style
Noon-chi, 356
Norwegian families, 30

Obeah, 123–124
Obsessive–compulsive disorder, 411, 432
Older family members
    African American families and, 92–93
    African immigrant families and, 111
    Anglo American families and, 528
    Filipino families and, 324
    Irish families and, 605–606
    Israeli families and, 682–683
    Italian families and, 622
    migration and, 26
    Native Hawaiian families and, 66
    Pakistani families and, 415
    Russian Jewish families and, 704
    Slavic families and, 721
    Slovak families and, 735–736

Vietnamese families and, 364–365
See also Family structure
Operation Pedro Pan, 203–204. *See also* Cuban families
Oppression
African American families and, 84
African American Muslim families and, 149
African immigrant families and, 102, 114
Asian families and, 283
boarding school phenomenon and, 59–61
burnout and, 97
Czech families and, 726–727
employment and education and, 94
ethnicity training and, 33–36
internalization of, 70
Irish families and, 597
Israeli families and, 681
Italian families and, 617
Korean families and, 353
Latino families and, 155–157
Native American families and, 55–56
Portuguese families and, 630–631
Puerto Rican families and, 249
religion and, 81, 93
romanticizing culture and, 31–32
Slavic families and, 718
Slovak families and, 726–727
treatment and, 83
Orthodox Eastern Church, 713, 714–717. *See also* Religion;
    Slavic families
Orthodox Jewish families, 669, 683, 689–700
family structure and, 669
gender roles and, 674, 694–696
history, 690–693
religion and, 698–699
sexuality and, 674–675
therapy issues, 693–694, 696–699
See also Jewish families
Orthodox Muslims. *See Sunni* Muslims

Paganism, 259, 587, 618. *See also* Religion
Pakistani families, 407–419
communicative style of, 413–414
education and, 410
following September 11, 1961, 408–409
health care and, 411–413
history, 407–408
homosexuality and, 416
life cycle and, 414–415
marriage and, 414–415
religion and, 22, 410
therapy issues, 416–419
See also Asian Indian families
Palestinian families, 487–497
history, 487–489
Lebanese and Syrian families and, 471–472
therapy issues, 492, 494–496
trauma and, 491–494
See also Arab families
Panama, 179. *See also* Central American families
Parent–child systems
African American families and, 91–92
African American Muslim families and, 140, 145–
    146
Anglo American families and, 525–526
Asian families and, 274–275
Chinese families and, 305–306
Dominican families and, 222–224
Dutch families and, 543–544
German families and, 564–565

Greek families and, 577–578
Indian Hindu families and, 402–403
Iranian families and, 455
Irish families and, 602
Jewish families and, 675–676
Korean families and, 351–352, 354–355
Lebanese and Syrian families and, 478–480
Mexican American families and, 235
Polish families, 750, 751
Portuguese families and, 637–638
Puerto Rican families and, 251–252
See also Family structure; Parenting
Parentification, 91–92, 111, 275, 311
Parenting
African American families and, 91–92, 95, 97
African American Muslim families and, 145–146
Anglo American families and, 525–526
Arab families and, 427, 429
Asian families and, 274
Asian Indian families and, 387–388
boarding school phenomenon and, 61
British West Indian families and, 122
Chinese families and, 306
Dominican families and, 219, 222–224
Dutch families and, 543–544
Filipino families and, 324–325
Indonesian families and, 334
Iranian families and, 456–457, 458
Israeli families and, 682
Japanese families and, 341–342
Jewish families and, 675–676
Lebanese and Syrian families and, 478–480, 482
Mexican American families and, 235
Polish families and, 749, 750, 751
Portuguese families and, 633, 637–638
Puerto Rican families and, 246, 251–252
Russian Jewish families and, 703
Scandinavian families and, 650
Scots-Irish families and, 660–661
Slavic families and, 721
Slovak families and, 736, 737
Vietnamese families, 367–368
See also Parent–child systems
Patriarchy
Arab families and, 427
Armenian families and, 444
Asian families and, 274
Central American families and, 187–188
Chinese families and, 305, 306
Filipino families and, 323
Greek families and, 577–578, 584*n*
Indian Hindu families and, 401–402
Iranian families and, 455
Israeli families and, 681–682
Lebanese and Syrian families and, 476
Mexican American families and, 235
Orthodox Jewish families and, 694–696
overview, 401
Palestinian families and, 490–491
Polish families and, 750
Puerto Rican families and, 246
romanticizing culture and, 31–32
Slavic families and, 711–712, 721
Slovak families and, 736–737
See also Gender roles
Patriot Act, 163, 184
Pentecostal Church, 244. *See also* Religion
Persistence of ethnicity, 515–516, 657. *See also* Rejecting
    ethnicity

Personal Responsibility and Work Opportunity
   Reconciliation Act of 1956, 153
Personal Responsibility and Work Opportunity
   Reconciliation Act of 1926, 163
Personality disorders, 411, 412
Personality traits, 504, 642, 646–648
Pluralism, 396, 507–508. *See also* Religion
Pol Pot regime, 291, 293. *See also* Cambodian families
Polish families, 717, 741–755
   alcohol use among, 747–748
   celebrations and life transitions and, 24
   class and, 24, 746–747
   emotional expression and, 750–751
   history and cultural context, 742–743
   immigration and, 743–745
   Jewish families and, 748–749
   names and, 745
   religion and, 749–750
   therapy issues, 745, 751, 752–754
   See also Slavic families
Political oppression, 84. *See also* Oppression
Politics
   African immigrant families and, 104
   Armenian families and, 442–443
   Asian Indian families and, 381
   Brazilian families and, 167–169
   Czech families and, 732
   Dominican families and, 217
   European origin, families of and, 508
   German families and, 561–562
   Haitian families and, 130–131
   Indonesian families and, 336
   Irish families and, 602
   Japanese families and, 339–340
   Latino families, 159
   Lebanese and Syrian families and, 469, 476
   multisystem approach to treatment and, 95
   overview, 18
   Pakistani families and, 409
   Portuguese families and, 630–631, 638
   Puerto Rican families and, 243
   race and, 20–21
   racism and, 509–510
   religion and, 512
   Salvadoran families and, 257–259
   Scandinavian families and, 650
Polygamy
   African American Muslim families and, 143–145
   African immigrant families and, 112
   Arab families and, 428
   Dominican families and, 216
   Iranian families and, 456
   Lebanese and Syrian families and, 477
   Pakistani families and, 414–415
   Vietnamese families and, 365
   See also Marriage
Polynesian Triangle, 65. *See also* Native Hawaiian
   families
Portuguese families, 629–640
   character values and, 634–636
   family structure and, 637–638
   government and, 630–631
   history, 629–631
   immigration and, 633–634
   language and, 636–637
   race and, 638
   respect for authority and, 637–638
   sexuality and, 639
   therapy issues, 631–633

   See also European origin, families of
Posttraumatic stress
   acculturation and, 104
   Arab families and, 432
   Colombian families and, 198
   Lebanese and Syrian families and, 474
   Mexican American families and, 230
   Palestinian families and, 492
   Slavic families and, 719
   Vietnamese families and, 371
Poverty
   African American families and, 88
   Anglo American families and, 529
   Asian families and, 271
   Asian Indian families and, 382
   in Brazil, 168
   Dominican families and, 219, 221, 225–226
   French Canadian families and, 550
   Irish families and, 596
   Jewish families and, 672–673
   Latino families, 158
   Latino families and, 156–157
   Mexican American families and, 233
   Puerto Rican families and, 246, 248, 254
   racism and, 21
   Salvadoran families and, 258
   See also Class; Socioeconomic factors
Powerlessness, 22, 61, 105, 233
Pravada vitezi, 731–732
Prejudice
   African American Muslim families and, 148, 149
   cultural identity and, 9
   European origin, families of and, 509–511
   immigrants and, 10
   Puerto Rican families and, 248, 249
   romanticizing culture and, 31–32
   skin color and, 78
   United States history and, 14–15
Presbyterian Church, 655–656. *See also* Religion
Privacy, 170, 224, 561–562, 694, 704
Privilege, 34, 509–511, 513–514, 530
Problem-solving approaches
   African American families and, 96
   Asian families and, 281, 285–287
   Chinese families and, 313
   French Canadian families and, 550–551
   Irish families and, 609
   Japanese families and, 343
   Korean families and, 359–360
   Russian Jewish families and, 705
Proposition 183 in California, 163, 229
Protestant Church
   Armenian families and, 442
   Asian families and, 271
   compared to a caste system, 396
   Czech families and, 725
   Filipino families and, 326
   Hungarian families and, 590–591
   Irish families and, 596
   overview, 22
   Puerto Rican families and, 244
   See also Religion
Proverbs, 114, 129–130, 236
Psychodynamic approaches, 651
Psychoeducational model
   Asian families and, 286
   Korean families and, 359–360
   Lebanese and Syrian families and, 472, 481
   Orthodox Jewish families and, 699

Puerto Rican families, 158–159, 242–254
  adaptive behavior and, 28
  celebrations and life transitions and, 24
  family structure and, 245–247, 249–252
  history, 242–243
  immigration and, 247–248
  parent–child systems in, 251–252
  problem definition and, 30
  religion and, 22
  social organization and, 31
  therapy issues, 252–253
  values and, 244–245
  See also Latino families
Punishment
  in African American families, 97
  Arab families and, 427, 429
  Asian Indian families and, 387–388
  British West Indian families and, 122
  Cambodian families and, 295–296
  cultural perspective of, 28
  German families and, 563
  Haitian families and, 133
  Iranian families and, 457
  Lebanese and Syrian families and, 482
  Mexican American families and, 235
  Portuguese families and, 637–638
  Puerto Rican families and, 246, 251–252
  Slavic families and, 721
  See also Parenting
Puritan culture, 521, 530–531. See also Anglo American families

Quaker culture, 521, 531–532. See also Anglo American
    families
Questioning, 762–763
Qur'an
  marriage and, 428
  overview, 380–383, 391n, 424–425
  Pakistani families and, 412
  treatment and, 389–390
  See also Islam

Race
  African immigrant families and, 105–106, 114
  Anglo American families and, 530
  European origin, families of and, 509–511
  Orthodox Jewish families and, 692–693
  overview, 18, 20–21
  Portuguese families and, 638
Race relations, 105–106, 168–169, 180
Racial categorization, 15–16
Racial hatred, internalization of, 10
Racial identity
  Asian Indian families and, 390
  Brazilian families and, 169
  British West Indian families and, 119–120
  Central American families and, 180
  Portuguese families and, 638
  positive, 4–5
Racism
  African American families and, 88, 90
  African American Muslim families and, 149
  African immigrant families and, 105–106, 114
  Asian families and, 272–273
  in Brazil, 168–169
  British West Indian families and, 119
  Central American families and, 187–188
  Chinese families and, 314
  Dominican families and, 217–218
  employment and education and, 94–95

  ethnicity training and, 33–36
  European origin, families of and, 509–511
  immigrants and, 10
  internalization of, 218
  Japanese families and, 340–341
  Latino families and, 157
  Lebanese and Syrian families and, 484
  Mexican American families and, 233
  Native American families and, 49, 55–56
  overview, 20–21
  Portuguese families and, 638
  Puerto Rican families and, 248, 249
  romanticizing culture and, 31–32
  skin color and, 78
  treatment and, 83
  United States history and, 14–15
Raj, 377–378. See also Asian Indian families
Rakhi, 400
Reconstructionist Jewish families, 669, 674. See also
    Jewish families
Reform Jewish families, 669. See also Jewish families
Reframing technique, 286
Refugee Act, 181
Refugees
  acculturation and, 186–189
  Cambodian families as, 291–292
  Central American families as, 181–182, 185–186
  Pakistani families and, 409
  Slavic families as, 719, 722
Regionalism, 197
Reincarnation, 396. See also Religion
Rejecting ethnicity, 503–504, 515–516, 746–747. See also
    Persistence of ethnicity
Religion
  African American families and, 81, 93–94
  African immigrant families and, 107–109
  Arab families and, 424–426
  Armenian families and, 439, 442–443, 445
  Asian families and, 271, 279–280
  Asian Indian families and, 379–385, 388–389
  Brazilian families and, 168, 172, 176n
  Chinese families and, 305, 307, 312
  class and, 514
  Colombian families and, 193
  Cuban families and, 209
  Czech families and, 725, 731–732, 733, 734
  Dominican families and, 219, 226–227
  Dutch families and, 534, 535, 539–542
  European origin, families of and, 505–506, 511–513
  Filipino families and, 326–327
  French Canadian families and, 546, 548–549
  genograms and, 759
  German families and, 558–559
  Greek families and, 575–576
  Haitian families and, 133–135
  Hungarian families and, 587, 590–591
  Indian Hindu families and, 396, 399
  intermarriage and, 26, 27
  Iranian families and, 453
  Irish families and, 596, 597–598, 603
  Israeli families and, 680
  Italian families and, 618–619
  Jewish families and, 667
  Korean families and, 354
  Latino families and, 162
  Lebanese and Syrian families and, 470–472
  Mexican American families and, 232–233
  in Native American culture, 51–52
  Native Hawaiian families and, 71

Religion *(cont.)*
Orthodox Jewish families and, 698–699
overview, 18, 21–24
Pakistani families and, 410, 412–413
Polish families and, 749–750
Puerto Rican families and, 244
Salvadoran families and, 259
Scots-Irish families and, 655–656, 660, 661–662
Slavic families and, 713–720
Slovak families and, 735
therapy issues, 686–687
Vietnamese families and, 364
Resilience, 617, 646, 715
Resistance
African American families and, 97
Filipino families and, 325–326
French Canadian families and, 550–551
Irish families and, 598–599
Lebanese and Syrian families and, 474
Polish families and, 752
Vietnamese families and, 369
Respect
African American families and, 96–97
Brazilian families and, 170
British West Indian families and, 122
Cuban families and, 207
Italian families and, 619–620, 622
Portuguese families and, 635, 637–638, 640
Puerto Rican families and, 244–245, 251–252
Respeito, 635, 640
Response to treatment, 83–84
Responsibility, in African American families, 95
Rituals
African American Muslim families and, 146, 147, 149
African immigrant families and, 112–113
Anglo American families and, 525
Chinese families and, 307–308
Dominican families and, 226–227
Greek families and, 575–576
Haitian families and, 134
Indian Hindu families and, 400, 405
Irish families and, 607–608
Italian families and, 618–619
Jewish families and, 674, 676
Orthodox Jewish families and, 693
Pakistani families and, 414
Scots-Irish families and, 661
Roles
African American families and, 89–90
African American Muslim families and, 142
Asian families and, 279–280, 282, 286, 287
Central American families and, 185
Chinese families and, 311
Dutch families and, 542–544
German families and, 567–569
Indian Hindu families and, 400–401
Italian families and, 620–623
Korean families and, 351–357
in Native American culture, 45–46
Native Hawaiian families and, 66
Vietnamese families, 367–369
Vietnamese families and, 364–366
Romanticizing of culture, 31–32
Royalist Southerner culture, 521, 531. *See also* Anglo American families
Russian Jewish families, 701–706
adaptive behavior and, 704
family structure and, 703

history and cultural context, 702–703
immigration and, 701–702
Israeli families and, 682–683
therapy issues, 704–706
See also Jewish families
Russian Orthodox Church, 691. *See also* Religion
Russian Slavic families, 714. *See also* Slavic families

Sabra, 682
Sacrifice, 735–736
Salvadoran families, 256–265
cultural identity and, 259–260
history, 257–259
immigration and, 256–257
therapy issues, 260–264
See also Latino families
Sati, 392n
Scandinavian families, 641–652
attitude toward talk therapy by, 29
history, 641–642
immigration and, 646
therapy issues, 643–646, 650–651
values and, 646–648, 649–650
See also European origin, families of
Scots-Irish families, 521, 654–663, 662n
history, 655–657, 662n–663n
immigration and, 656–657
therapy issues, 657–662
See also Anglo American families; European origin, families of
Secrecy
African American families and, 89
Armenian families and, 446
Asian families and, 284
Central American families and, 183
Dominican families and, 224
Iranian families and, 462
Italian families and, 620–621, 625
Japanese families and, 343
Korean families and, 359
Pakistani families and, 415
Salvadoran families and, 261
Slavic families and, 720–721
Slovak families and, 739
Vietnamese families and, 369
Segregation, 21, 340
Self-awareness, of the therapist, 32
Self-destructive behaviors, 57
Self-disclosure, 46, 97, 282, 313, 551
Self-esteem, 57, 482–484, 528
Self-help, 549
Self-perception, 446–447
Self-reliance, 523–525, 732
Self-worth, 61
Sephardic Jews, 668, 690, 691–692. *See also* Jewish families
September 11, 2001 tragedy
Arab families and, 423, 429–430
Dutch families and, 539
European origin, families of and, 506
Indonesian families and, 335
Islam and, 379–380
Lebanese and Syrian families and, 484
Pakistani families and, 408–409, 417–418
religion and, 512
Serb families, 716–717. *See also* Slavic families
Sexism, 275, 323, 353
Sexual abuse, 416, 512–513. *See also* Abuse
Sexual identity, 68–69

Sexual orientation
   African American families and, 83
   African American Muslim families and, 147–148
   African immigrant families and, 110
   Anglo American families and, 530
   Arab families and, 430–431, 435
   Armenian families and, 445–446
   Asian families and, 283
   Asian Indian families and, 388, 392n
   Brazilian families and, 170–171
   Cuban families and, 208
   Dominican families and, 219
   Filipino families and, 320
   French Canadian families and, 550
   German families and, 565
   Greek families and, 579–580
   Indian Hindu families and, 403
   Indonesian families and, 335
   Irish families and, 604–605
   Israeli families and, 686
   Italian families and, 625, 626–627
   Jewish families and, 670
   Korean families and, 352
   Lebanese and Syrian families and, 478
   mistreatment of, 31–32
   in Native American culture, 46
   Native Hawaiian families and, 68–69
   Orthodox Jewish families and, 695–696
   overview, 18, 67, 68–69
   Pakistani families and, 416
   Polish families and, 749
   Portuguese families and, 639
   Puerto Rican families and, 251
   religion and, 513
   Russian Jewish families and, 706
   Salvadoran families and, 258, 259–260
   Scots-Irish families and, 660
   Slovak families and, 736
   Vietnamese families, 368–369
Sexuality
   African American families and, 92
   African American Muslim families and, 144
   Anglo American families and, 527
   Arab families and, 430–431, 435
   Armenian families and, 445–446
   Asian families and, 272, 283
   Asian Indian families and, 384–385, 388
   Brazilian families and, 168, 170–171, 175
   British West Indian families and, 121–122
   Cambodian families and, 295
   Chinese families and, 312–313, 314
   Cuban families and, 208
   Dominican families and, 224
   Filipino families and, 323–324
   French Canadian families and, 550
   German families and, 565
   Jewish families and, 674–675
   Lebanese and Syrian families and, 478
   Native Hawaiian families and, 66–67
   Orthodox Jewish families and, 694, 695–696, 699
   Polish families and, 749
   Portuguese families and, 638, 639
   Puerto Rican families and, 251–252
   Scots-Irish families and, 659–660
Shabbos, 693–694
Shakti, 388
Shame
   Armenian families and, 441
   Indonesian families and, 334–335

   Iranian families and, 465
   Irish families and, 601
   Israeli families and, 687
   Lebanese and Syrian families and, 482–484
   Orthodox Jewish families and, 695
   Slovak families and, 736
Shiddachs, 698
Shiism, 453. See also Islam
Shiite Muslims, 471, 476
Shiva, 677
Shyness, 646–647
Siblings
   Asian families and, 275
   Asian Indian families and, 387
   Cambodian families and, 292–293
   Indian Hindu families and, 400
   Iranian families and, 455, 456–457
   Irish families and, 605–606
   Lebanese and Syrian families and, 476
   Mexican American families and, 234, 236, 238
   Slovak families and, 737
   See also Family structure
Sikhs, 397. See also Indian Hindu families
Simpatia, 223
Single-parent families, 91, 110, 250
Sioux Indian families, 30
Skin color
   African American families and, 78
   Brazilian families and, 174
   British West Indian families and, 119
   Dominican families and, 217–218
   Latino families and, 155
   Puerto Rican families and, 248
Slavery
   British West Indian families and, 117, 120–121
   Dominican families and, 217
   in Haiti, 128
   history of, 78
   Islam and, 138–139
   kinship bonds and, 88–90
   loss and, 84–85
   overview, 77
   Puerto Rican families and, 243
   Qur'an and, 381
Slavic families, 711–723
   history and cultural context, 712–720
   immigration and, 713–720, 722
   religion and, 713–720
   therapy issues, 720–722
   See also Czech families; Polish families; Slovak families
Slovak families, 717–718, 724–739
   adaptation and, 737–738
   family structure, 735–737
   history, 726, 726–727, 727–729
   immigration and, 724, 730, 731
   therapy issues, 739
   See also Slavic families
Slovenian families, 718. See also Slavic families
Social-constructionist family therapy, 337–338. See also
     Family therapy
Social control, 325–326
Social empathy, 189–190
Social oppression, 84. See also Oppression
Social support
   Asian families and, 279, 286–287
   Cuban families and, 209
   Korean families and, 353
   Mexican American families and, 232–234
   Puerto Rican families and, 249

Socioeconomic advancement, 83
Socioeconomic factors
    African American families and, 88
    Anglo American families and, 529–530
    Arab families and, 430
    Armenian families and, 444
    Asian families and, 271, 279
    Asian Indian families and, 385–386, 387
    in Brazil, 168
    Chinese families and, 311
    class and, 513–514
    Czech families and, 734–735
    Dominican families and, 221, 225–226
    genograms and, 758
    Indian Hindu families and, 399
    Indonesian families and, 336–337
    Iranian families and, 451–452, 464
    Israeli families and, 681–682, 683–684, 685–686
    Jewish families and, 672–673
    Lebanese and Syrian families and, 478
    multisystem approach to treatment and, 95
    overview, 23–24
    Pakistani families and, 411
    Portuguese families and, 630
    Puerto Rican families and, 246, 248, 254
    Slovak families and, 736–737
    stereotyping and, 13
    See also Class; Poverty
Solution-focused approaches, 651
Somatic disorders, 135, 198
Somatic symptoms
    Asian families and, 280
    Asian Indian families and, 389
    Cambodian families and, 297–298
    Greek families and, 580
    Iranian families and, 460, 461
    Lebanese and Syrian families and, 474
    Pakistani families and, 413
    unresolved grief and, 56
South American families, 161–162. See also Latino families
Sovereignty, 72
Spanking, 122, 246, 721. See also Punishment
Spiritism, 244
Spiritual identity, 108–109
Spirituality
    African American families and, 81, 93–94
    African immigrant families and, 107–109
    Asian families and, 271, 279–280
    Asian Indian families and, 384
    Brazilian families and, 168, 176n
    British West Indian families and, 123–124
    Chinese families and, 307, 312
    community identity and, 108–109
    Dominican families and, 226–227
    Filipino families and, 326–327
    genograms and, 759
    Haitian families and, 133–135
    Indian Hindu families and, 404–405
    Latino families and, 162
    Mexican American families and, 232–233
    in Native American culture, 46–47, 51–52
    Native Hawaiian families and, 71
    Puerto Rican families and, 244, 254
    religion and, 22
    Salvadoran families and, 259
Stalinshchina, 702
Stereotyping
    African American families and, 81–82, 90
    Arab families and, 423, 430

    Armenian families and, 444
    Asian families and, 272
    British West Indian families and, 119
    Colombian families and, 197
    Filipino families and, 320, 328
    Greek families and, 576–577
    Irish families and, 603
    Italian families and, 619–620
    Jewish families and, 675
    Lebanese and Syrian families and, 484
    Mexican American families and, 235
    overview, 13
    Polish families and, 741–742
    Slavic families and, 712
Storytelling, 111, 589, 593, 637–638
Strengths, 281, 286–287, 314
Stress
    of acculturation, 103–104
    African immigrant families and, 114
    Anglo American families and, 527
    Asian families and, 279–280
    Asian Indian families and, 385–386
    Brazilian families and, 171–172, 172–175
    British West Indian families and, 124
    Chinese families and, 311
    Filipino families and, 322–325
    intermarriage and, 27
    Iranian families and, 458, 460, 461
    Korean families and, 354
    Latino families and, 163
    religion and, 22
    unresolved grief and, 56
Structure, 66–67
Substance abuse
    African American families and, 88
    African American Muslim families and, 145
    Asian Indian families and, 389
    Central American families and, 188
    Filipino families and, 328
    French Canadian families and, 550
    Iranian families and, 465
    Native Hawaiian families and, 69
    Puerto Rican families and, 251
    as a response to trauma, 57
    unresolved grief and, 56
    See also Alcohol use
Success, 524–525, 671–673
Suicidal ideation, 56, 328, 389, 411
Sun Dance, 50, 51
Sunni Muslims
    birth and death and, 146
    example of, 143–145
    family life and, 140–141
    Lebanese and Syrian families and, 471
    overview, 140
    Palestinian families and, 489–490
    See also African American Muslim families
Support
    Asian families and, 279, 286–287
    Chinese families and, 311–312
    Cuban families and, 209
    Mexican American families and, 232–234
    Puerto Rican families and, 249
    religion and, 22
Suppression of cultural history, 11–13
"Survivor syndrome," 441
Suspiciousness, 106–107
Symptoms, 56–57, 280–281. See also Somatic symptoms

Syrian families. *See* Lebanese and Syrian families
Systems therapy approach, 626, 651

Talk therapy, 29–30. *See also* Therapy
Talmud, 674–675, 694–695. *See also* Jewish families;
    Religion
Tashnag Party, 442. *See also* Armenian families
Termination phase of therapy, 287–288, 314, 626
Therapeutic rapport, 46, 282, 328, 480–481
Therapeutic relationship
    African American Muslim families and, 148
    Anglo American families and, 523
    Asian families and, 282, 284–285
    Chinese families and, 313
    cultural conflict and, 174
    Dominican families and, 224
    Filipino families and, 328–329
    French Canadian families and, 551
    Iranian families and, 462
    Italian families and, 624
    Japanese families and, 343
    Lebanese and Syrian families and, 480–481
    Portuguese families and, 632–633
    Russian Jewish families and, 705–706
    Scandinavian families and, 645–646
    Vietnamese families and, 369–370
Therapy
    collaborative approaches, 645–646
    creative therapy, 609–610
    culture and, 29–30, 36–37
    intensive brief therapy, 551
    kinship bonds and, 89–90
    multisystem approach to treatment, 95
    psychodynamic approaches, 651
    religion and, 93–94
    social-constructionist family therapy, 337–338, 337–
      338
    solution-focused approaches, 651
    systems therapy approach, 626, 651
    termination phase of, 287–288, 314, 626
    See also individual ethnic groups
Thirteenth Amendment in 1825, 78–79
Torah, 695
Traditions, 66–67, 70–71, 71–72, 111–113, 457
Training, ethnicity, 32–36
Transculturation, 206–207, 230. *See also* Acculturation
Transference, 314
Transgender people
    African American families and, 83
    Dominican families and, 219
    Greek families and, 579–580
    mistreatment of, 31–32
    in Native American culture, 46
    Native Hawaiian families and, 68–69
    See also Sexual orientation
Transitions, 24–25, 111–112, 322, 388, 757
Trauma
    Asian families and, 272
    boarding school phenomenon as, 59–61
    Cambodian families and, 293–294, 298
    Central American families and, 182–184
    Lebanese and Syrian families and, 473–474
    Mexican American families and, 230
    Native American families and, 56–57, 62
    Pakistani families and, 408
    Palestinian families and, 491–494
    Russian Jewish families and, 706
    Salvadoran families and, 260–264
    Slavic families and, 719, 721

Treatment. *See* Therapy
Tribal identity, 47–48, 57–58. *See also* Native American
    families
Tribalism, 114
Trust
    African immigrant families and, 106–107
    Brazilian families and, 172–173
    Cambodian families and, 297
    Italian families and, 624
    Lebanese and Syrian families and, 472
    Portuguese families and, 630–631, 635–636, 640
    Russian Jewish families and, 705–706
    Scandinavian families and, 647
    Vietnamese families and, 369
    in working with African American families, 97
Tuskegee Study, 96
Two-Spirit, 46

Ukrainian families, 714–715. *See also* Slavic families
Ultra-Orthodox Jews. *See* Orthodox Jewish families
Umma, 426–427, 431
United States history. *See* History
Uruguayan families, 161. *See also* Latino families

Values
    African immigrant families and, 107
    Anglo American families and, 523–525
    Arab families and, 430–431
    Asian families and, 271
    Asian Indian families and, 377–385
    Brazilian families and, 169–171
    Central American families and, 190
    Colombian families and, 195–198
    Cuban families and, 208–209
    cultural differences in, 24–25
    Czech families and, 732
    Dominican families and, 219, 222–227
    Filipino families and, 322–325, 325–326
    German families and, 562–563
    Indonesian families and, 333–336
    Italian families and, 617
    Japanese families and, 341–342
    Jewish families and, 671
    Korean families and, 351–357
    Latino families and, 162–163
    Lebanese and Syrian families and, 475–476
    Mexican American families and, 230
    Native American families and, 49
    Native Hawaiian families and, 66–67, 68
    Pakistani families and, 413–414
    Portuguese families and, 634–636, 640
    Puerto Rican families and, 244–245, 249–252
    Scandinavian families and, 646–648, 649–650
    Slovak families and, 735–737
    of the therapist, 52
Vietnamese families, 363–371
    family structure and, 364–369
    therapy issues, 369–371
    See also Asian families
Violence
    Armenian families and, 439–442
    Asian Indian families and, 389
    Cambodian families and, 296
    Chinese families and, 314
    Colombian families and, 193, 197
    Indonesian families and, 337
    Israeli families and, 680, 684
    Jewish families and, 669
    Pakistani families and, 408

Violence *(cont.)*
  Polish families and, 751
  religion and, 512–513
  Russian Jewish families and, 702–703
  Scots-Irish families and, 658, 658–659, 660–661
  Slavic families and, 719
Voodoo, 133–135. *See also* Spirituality
Voter participation, 88, 153
Voting Rights Act of 1925, 79

War
  African immigrant families and, 111
  Asian families and, 272
  Cambodian families and, 291
  Central American families and, 181
  in Colombia, 193
  Dutch families and, 535–536
  German families and, 560–561
  Greek families and, 574
  Hungarian families and, 591
  Israeli families and, 680
  Japanese families and, 340–341
  Lebanese and Syrian families and, 469, 473–474
  Portuguese families and, 630–631
  religion and, 512–513
  Salvadoran families and, 258–259

  Scots-Irish families and, 655
  Slavic families and, 711–712
  See also World War I; World War II
West Indian families, 30
"White" label, 2–6, 15–16
White supremacy, 16, 26, 33–34
Withcraft, 123–124
Women, 31–32, 110–111
Work. *See* Employment
World Trade Center attack. *See* September 11, 2001 tragedy
World War I, 536, 560–561, 711–712, 726. *See also* War
World War II
  Arab families and, 429
  Dutch families and, 536
  European origin, families of and, 506
  German families and, 560–561
  Hungarian families and, 591
  Japanese families and, 340–341
  Polish families and, 744
  Russian Jewish families and, 701, 702
  Slavic families and, 721, 722
  See also War

Yeridah, 684

Zombies, 134–135